Seeing Depression through a Cultural Lens

Seeing Depression through a Cultural Lens

Barry S. Fogel, MD
Xiaoling Jiang, PhD

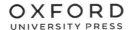

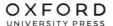

Oxford University Press is a department of the University of Oxford. It furthers
the University's objective of excellence in research, scholarship, and education
by publishing worldwide. Oxford is a registered trade mark of Oxford University
Press in the UK and certain other countries.

Published in the United States of America by Oxford University Press
198 Madison Avenue, New York, NY 10016, United States of America.

© Oxford University Press 2025

All rights reserved. No part of this publication may be reproduced, stored in
a retrieval system, or transmitted, in any form or by any means, without the
prior permission in writing of Oxford University Press, or as expressly permitted
by law, by license, or under terms agreed with the appropriate reproduction
rights organization. Inquiries concerning reproduction outside the scope of the
above should be sent to the Rights Department, Oxford University Press, at the
address above.

You must not circulate this work in any other form
and you must impose this same condition on any acquirer.

Library of Congress Cataloging-in-Publication Data
Names: Fogel, Barry S., author. | Jiang, Xiaoling, author.
Title: Seeing depression through a cultural lens / Barry S. Fogel, Xiaoling Jiang.
Description: New York, NY : Oxford University Press, [2025] |
Includes bibliographical references and index.
Identifiers: LCCN 2023023460 (print) | LCCN 2023023461 (ebook) |
ISBN 9780190850074 (hardback) | ISBN 9780190850098 (epub) |
ISBN 9780190850104 (online)
Subjects: MESH: Depression | Depressive Disorder | Cultural Characteristics |
Cross-Cultural Comparison
Classification: LCC RC537 (print) | LCC RC537 (ebook) | NLM WM 171.5 |
DDC 616.85/27—dc23/eng/20230901
LC record available at https://lccn.loc.gov/2023023460
LC ebook record available at https://lccn.loc.gov/2023023461

This material is not intended to be, and should not be considered, a substitute for medical
or other professional advice. Treatment for the conditions described in this material is
highly dependent on the individual circumstances. And, while this material is designed
to offer accurate information with respect to the subject matter covered and to be current
as of the time it was written, research and knowledge about medical and health issues is
constantly evolving and dose schedules for medications are being revised continually,
with new side effects recognized and accounted for regularly. Readers must therefore
always check the product information and clinical procedures with the most up-to-date
published product information and data sheets provided by the manufacturers and
the most recent codes of conduct and safety regulation. The publisher and the authors
make no representations or warranties to readers, express or implied, as to the accuracy
or completeness of this material. Without limiting the foregoing, the publisher and the
authors make no representations or warranties as to the accuracy or efficacy of the drug
dosages mentioned in the material. The authors and the publisher do not accept, and
expressly disclaim, any responsibility for any liability, loss, or risk that may be claimed
or incurred as a consequence of the use and/ or application of any of the contents of this
material.

DOI: 10.1093/med/9780190850074.001.0001

Printed by Integrated Books International, United States of America

The manufacturer's authorised representative in the EU for product safety is Oxford University Press España S.A. of El Parque Empresarial San Fernando de Henares, Avenida de Castilla, 2 - 28830 Madrid (www.oup.es/en or product.safety@oup.com). OUP España S.A. also acts as importer into Spain of products made by the manufacturer.

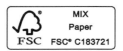

Barry Fogel dedicates this work to our children – Susanna, Juliana, and William.
Xiaoling Jiang dedicates this work to Professor Keizo Yamada and to the memory of Professor Patrick Hanan.

Contents

Preface *xv*

List of Abbreviations and Acronyms *xxiii*

Part I Constructing the Cultural Lens

1 Picturing Depression: Faces, Backgrounds, and Foregrounds *3*
  From *Obasute* to *Kodokushi* *4*
  Twenty-Four Filial Exemplars—Ancient and Modern *9*
  States of Mind: Depression and American Regional Cultures *11*
  A Low-Context Primary Care Physician Encounters a High-Context Patient *17*
  Conclusion *21*

2 Faces of Clinical Depression *23*
  Culture-Related Issues with the Diagnosis of MDD *25*
  Alternative Diagnostic Criteria for Clinical Depression: A Prompt for Dialogue *32*
  Suggested Criteria for Clinical Depression (All Must Apply for the Diagnosis to Be Made) *33*
  The Middle Zones of Depression and Bipolar Illness *36*
  Depression Screening Questionnaires *38*

3 Beyond Shades of Gray: Depression and the Bipolar Spectrum *48*
  Defining a Bipolar Spectrum *50*
  Screening Questionnaires for Bipolarity *52*
  Biomarkers of Bipolarity *57*

4 Dimensions and Implications of Cultural Identity *60*
  Dimensional Characterization of Cultures *62*
  Trust *72*
  Social Capital *74*
  Communication Culture and Talking About Depression *79*
  Inference from Metaphor and Word Choice *81*
  Religious Identity and Its Implications *83*

5 Cultural Identity and Personal Biography *88*
  Acculturation: Not Just for Immigrants *93*
  Normalization of Trauma *95*

6 Unnatural Deaths *99*
  Cultural Dimensions of an Interpersonal-Neuropsychiatric Model of Suicide *101*
    Thwarted Belongingness (TB) and Perceived Burdensomeness (PB) *101*
    Acquired Capacity for Suicide (ACS) *102*
    Behavioral Activation *104*
    Behavioral Inhibition *105*
    Experience of Pain *106*
    Experience of Pleasure *107*
    Hope *108*
    Reason to Live *108*
  Availability of Highly Lethal Means of Self-Harm *109*
  Suicidality Through a Cultural Lens *110*

7 Depression and Social Class: A Four-Dimensional View *113*
  Depression Risks of Middle-Class and Upper-Middle-Class Jobs *120*
  When Determinants of Socioeconomic Class Conflict *121*
  Class and Mood Disorder Phenomenology *124*
  Class and Mood Disorder Epidemiology *126*
  The Importance of Subjective Social Status *130*
  Troubles of the Upper Class *133*

8 Cultural Correlates and Clinical Consequences *140*
  Culture, Diet, and Depression *140*
  Culture, Sleep, and Depression *142*
  Culture, Environmental Hazards, and Depression *143*
  Culture, Psychoactive Substance Use, and Depression *145*
  Culture and the Phenomenology of Depression *146*
  The Perspective of Traditional Medical Systems *147*
  Biomarkers of Depression and Cross-Cultural Dialogue *149*
  Stigma of Depression Is Universal; Its Details Are Culture-Dependent *151*
  Culture and the Choice of Treatment for Depression *155*
  "Patient" as Cultural Identity *157*
  Cultural Mnemonics: Comparisons, Themes, Narratives, Unexpected Facts *159*

9 Ancient Wisdom Meets Modern Science: Depression in Traditional Medicine *161*
  From Hippocrates to Galen: Classical Greco-Roman Medicine *163*

From the Yellow Emperor to the King of Medicines: TCM *167*

From Rhazes to Maimonides: TAIM *175*

Illness or Demonic Possession? A Brief History of Stigma *180*

The Contemporary Relationship of Mainstream and Traditional Medical Approaches to Depression *182*

Tradition, Diet, and Depression *189*

The Past Recaptured: Integrative Medicine and Depression *194*

Part II Depression and the Cultures of Places

10 China: Confucian Harmony and Dissonance *201*

Loved and Abused: The Success and Suicide of Nikita Guo *203*

Masked Depression: The Sadness of Linka Liu *206*

Achievement, Bipolarity, and Christianity in an ABC Student: The Death of Luke Tang *208*

No Time to Get Well: Luchang Wang's Leap to Her Death *210*

When Olivia Kong Screamed for Help, She Was Serious *212*

The Imperial Examination *216*

Trauma of the "Lost Decade" and the Restoration of the National Examination *219*

Filial Piety, Bonds of Love, and Unspoken Rules *222*

Face (*Miànzi*; 面子), Upward Comparison (*Pānbǐ*; 攀比), and Climbing the Ivy (*Páténg*; 爬藤) *225*

Report the Good News, Conceal the Bad (*Bào xǐ bù bào yōu*; 报喜不报忧) *228*

Issues of Chinese International Students *229*

Intergenerational Cultural Conflicts of ABCs and "Generation 1.5" *232*

Encounters with Student Health and Counseling Services *238*

Potential for Social Media Analysis *243*

Expression of Negative Emotions in the Chinese Language *246*

Depression with Near-Tragic Consequences in a Left-Behind Rural Wife *249*

Depression and Suicide in Older Chinese Americans *262*

Expression of Depression Among Chinese Americans *264*

Culturally-Aware Depression Screening and Rating *266*

The Chinese PHQ-9 *268*

Cultural Customization of the PHQ-9? *271*

The Chinese CES-D and the Varied Faces of Depression among Chinese People *274*

Acculturation, Stigma, and Therapeutic Strategy *281*

Trust and Adherence to Antidepressant Medication *285*

Postscript: Universities' Responses to International Student Mental Health Issues *291*

11 Japan: Invisible Double-Edged Swords *293*
   Syncretism and the Yamato Spirit *298*
   Wabi-Sabi, *Mujō* (Impermanence), and *Mono no Aware* (the Pathos of Things) in Daily Life: Japanese Aesthetics and Depression *301*
   Modern Consequences of Samurai Culture *304*
   Mental Health and Self-Construal *307*
   "Reading the Air" (ba no kuuki wo yomu; 場の空気を読む) and Ambiguity (aimai; 曖昧)— The Communication Code *309*
   Japan's Alternative to Psychiatry—*Shinyrōnaika* (心療内科) *313*
   Self-indulgent (*Wagamama*), Spoiled (*Amae*), or Modern Type Depression? *314*
   Heart (*Kokoro*; 心), Chest (*Mune*; 胸), Belly (*Hara*; 腹): Metaphors for Emotional States *319*
   Normalization of Bullying (Ijime; 虐め) *321*
   Shame (Haji; 恥) and Suicide *323*
   Japan's Varied Faces of Depression *327*
   A "Culture-Bound Syndrome" Goes Global: The Story of *Hikikomori* *327*
   Kodokushi (Lonely Death)—*Hikikomori*'s Elderly Relative? *331*
   Problems in Recognition of Bipolarity *333*
   Depression in Japanese Americans *334*
   Cultural Concerns in Antidepressant Treatment *338*

12 South Korea: *Han* and Passionate Intensity *342*
   The Historical Context of Modern Korean Culture *345*
   Han (한) and *Jeong* (정): Korea's "National Emotions" *346*
   Depression-Related Syndromes Reflecting Korean Culture *347*
   Confucianism in Korea *354*
   Korean Drinking Culture and Its Relationship to Depression and Suicide *358*
   Cosmetic Surgery and the Culture of "Face" *360*
   A Young Woman Who Did Not Want Cosmetic Surgery *363*
   Sexual Harassment in the Workplace and Bullying at School *365*
   Suicide in Korea *366*
   Rating and Screening for Depression in Koreans: Culture and Psychometrics *370*
   Korean Americans—Family Acculturative Stress *373*
   Stigma of Depression and Cultural Barriers to Treatment *376*

13 Depression and Suicide in the "World's Happiest Countries" *380*
   Taking the Measure of Happiness and Depression *384*

Values and Cultural Dimensions in the Nordic Countries and Switzerland *385*

Social, Economic, and Demographic Issues *388*

Diet and Depression at the National Level *393*

Sisu, Historical Trauma, and Binge Drinking: Finland *397*

Sisu: True Grit, Finnish Style *402*

Lagom, Sexual Harassment, and Cultural Conflict in an Industrial Champion: Sweden *404*

Hygge Culture, Indulgence, and Its Consequences: Denmark *411*

Gender Equality, Male Ambivalence, and Collective Action: Norway *414*

Subarctic Warmth: Iceland *420*

Picturesque but Sad Countryside: Switzerland *423*

14 American Regional Cultures and Geography of Mood *430*

Salient Categories of Immigrants to the U.S. *433*

Describing Regional Cultures *435*

Culture of the Deep South *437*

Culture of the American Southwest *438*

Regions with Hybrid Cultures: The Midwest, the Mountain States, and the Pacific Northwest *440*

Region, Personality, and Mental Health *443*

Regional Variations in Mental Health *444*

Lessons from Cultural Comparison of Eight Pairs of States *447*

Regional Variation in Social Capital *455*

Regional Personality *459*

Religion, Depression, and Suicide *465*

Differences in Education and Their Impact *467*

Income Inequality, Poverty, and the Context of Depression and Its Treatment *472*

Behavioral and Environmental Risk Factors *480*

Regional Differences in Lifestyle Risk Factors for Depression *487*

Interstate Differences in Firearm Culture *490*

Environmental Influences on Depression Risk *493*

Linking Regional Culture with the Epidemiology of MDD, Bipolar Disorder, and Suicide *499*

Culture and Variability in Suicide Rates *505*

Depression During the COVID-19 Pandemic *512*

Concluding Comment *518*

Part III Depression and the Cultures of Occupations

15 The Dark Side of Creative Talent *521*
Productive, Eminent, and "Touched by Fire" *522*
A Spectrum of Misconception *526*
The Culture of the Creative Professions *529*
Suicide and Premature Death *533*
Why Depressed and Bipolar Creative Professionals Often Avoid Treatment *539*
Lessons from Tragic Lives: Mishima, Hemingway, Kawabata *540*
Creative Productivity and Its Relationship to Illness *543*
Working Conditions of Creative Professionals *546*
"Stairway to Hell": The Toxicity of Pop Music Stardom *547*
Lonely at the Top *553*
Parasocial Relationships and the Culture of Fandom *554*
Issues of Specific Musical Genres *555*
Comedians' Lives: Not So Funny *560*
The Role of Undiagnosed Medical Problems *562*
Bipolar Illness and the Creative Biography *563*
The Promise of Personalized Treatment *566*

16 Physicians in Pain: Depression in the Medical Profession *571*
Physicians' Complex Cultural Identities *577*
Physicians' Motives and Career Anchors *578*
Gender-Related Challenges *581*
Cultural Conflict, Working Conditions, and the Commodification of Healthcare *584*
Trials of Physicians in Training *588*
Professional Burnout *591*
Biomarkers of Burnout *597*
Treatment of Physician Burnout *598*
A Toxic Tetrad of Job Stress: Demand–Control Imbalance, Effort–Reward Imbalance, Organizational Injustice, and Illegitimate Tasks *600*
Questions for Characterizing Physicians' Job Stress *603*
Moral Injury on the Clinical Battlefield *607*
Physicians and Financial Stress *609*
Stigma and Its Consequences *611*
Stigmatizing Policies of Medical Licensing Boards and PHPs *614*
Substance Abuse *618*
Clinical Care of Physicians with Depression or Bipolar Disorder *619*

Pharmacologic Treatment *623*
Assessment and Management of Suicidal Physicians *624*
A Psychiatrist Is the Clinician of Choice for a Depressed Physician *625*

17 Flying High, Feeling Low: Depression in Airline Pilots *627*
Regulations and Institutional Stigma *630*
Depressed Pilots Often Conceal Their Illness *632*
Financial and Psychological Impact of Pilots' Health Conditions *635*
Stigma and Choice of Treatment *636*
Suicide in Active and Retired Pilots *637*
The Culture of Airline Pilots *638*
Special Issues of Female Pilots *639*
Financial Aspects of Pilots' Careers *640*
Health Hazards—Generic and Specific *643*
Working Around Stigma and Denial *646*

18 Truck-Driving Blues *652*
The Work of Long-Haul Truck Drivers *657*
Health Consequences of the Truck-Driving Lifestyle *660*
Additional Health Risks: Vibration, Noise, and Poor Air Quality *662*
Loneliness of the Long-Distance Trucker *666*
Masculine Occupational Culture and "Male Depression" *668*
Drivers' Relationships with Their Jobs *671*
Truck-Driving Women *672*
Institutional and Personal Stigma *676*
Prevention and Treatment *678*
Clinical Evaluation of Truckers with Suspected Depression *679*
Personalized Treatment *682*

Afterword *685*
Acknowledgments *687*
References *689*
Index *799*

Preface

Each year, the *World Happiness Report* is published by the Sustainable Development Solutions Network, based primarily on analysis of survey data obtained by the Gallup World Poll. The five Nordic nations—Denmark, Finland, Iceland, Norway, and Sweden—have consistently ranked in the top ten, with one of them, currently Finland, in first place (Helliwell et al., 2023). Yet, all but Norway had per capita antidepressant drug consumption above the Organisation for Economic Co-operation and Development's (OECD's) median in 2020, and in 2021, Iceland had the world's highest rate—161.1 standard daily doses per 1000 inhabitants per day (OECD, 2023). The 2021 suicide mortality rates for Finland and Sweden are significantly higher than the benchmark rate for Western Europe overall (Institute for Health Metrics and Evaluation [IHME], 2024).

In the United States, a physician dies by suicide almost every day (300–400 per year), and suicide is the leading cause of death of medical students (Andrew, 2018). *Burnout*, an occupational syndrome of emotional exhaustion, depersonalization, and a reduced sense of personal accomplishment—accompanied often by depression and sometimes by suicidal ideation—was widespread in the medical profession before the COVID-19 pandemic began and increased further as the pandemic progressed (Bailey et al., 2023; Duarte et al., 2023; Harvey et al., 2021; Kumar, 2016; Laboe et al., 2021; Shanafelt et al., 2015). An online survey of 9175 American physicians conducted in the summer of 2022 found that 53% were burned out, and 23% were depressed (Kane, 2023).

In April 2018, Swedish recording star Avicii (1989–2018) died after cutting himself with a shard of glass (Ibrahim, 2021). In June 2018, iconic fashion designer Kate Spade (1962–2018) hanged herself (Katersky & Hutchinson, 2018). In the same month, chef, writer, documentarian, and culture critic Anthony Bourdain (1956–2018) died by suicide in the same way (Margaritoff, 2023). In October 2019, K-pop superstar, model, actress, and activist Sulli (1994–2019) died of a suicidal drug overdose (Fortin, 2019). In December 2021, acclaimed Japanese singer and voice actress Sayaka Kanda (1986–2021) fell to her death from a hotel room window in an apparent suicide (Wang, 2021). In April 2022, country music legend Naomi Judd (1946–2022) died by a self-inflicted gunshot wound one day prior to her induction into the Country Music Hall of Fame (Hulpuch, 2022). On July 5, 2023, Coco Lee (1975–2023), an international superstar Chinese singer-songwriter, died of complications of a suicide attempt. She had been receiving treatment for depression but had not attained a stable remission (Broadway, 2023). On October 28, 2023, actor Matthew Perry (1969–2023), famous for his role on the TV series *Friends*, was found dead in his hot tub with significant levels of ketamine and buprenorphine in his blood. At the time of his death, he was under treatment for depression, anxiety, and a substance use disorder (Radcliffe, 2023). All were in their creative prime. All suffered from depression. They are exemplary of the unnatural deaths of thousands of writers, artists, and performers.

In the past several years, many Chinese students at elite American universities have died by suicide. Most were extraordinarily accomplished, ambitious young adults who suddenly took their own lives with no public hint of their despair. A frequently-cited survey of Chinese international students at Yale University revealed a 45% prevalence of depressive symptoms (Han et al., 2013). In a broader sample of Chinese international students at American universities surveyed in the summer of 2020, 24.5% were clinically depressed, as indicated by a score of 10 or greater on the nine-item Patient Health Questionnaire (PHQ-9) (Lin et al., 2022).

Living in a "happy country" does not prevent depression. Neither wealth, fame, elite education, creativity, nor professional success prevents depression or suicide.

Globalization has been a double-edged sword. It has enriched the world but has inevitably entailed emotional stress, practical challenges, and interpersonal conflicts, not only for migrants but also for natives of host countries confronting changes in their economy and cultural landscape. These side effects of globalization are common antecedents of depression.

Depression and bipolar disorders are medical conditions. Melancholia and mania—and their well-established physiological and biochemical accompaniments—are recognized similarly around the world. However, the epidemiology, phenomenology, idioms of distress, and illness narratives of depression and the bipolar spectrum vary greatly among cultural groups. Variability in the expression of depression is especially evident in cases falling in the "middle zone" between flagrant mental illness and quotidian, non-pathological human suffering.

Medical care in the United States—and in most high-income nations—is a multicultural activity. Cultural differences between clinicians and patients can cause miscommunication or mistrust that interferes with accurate diagnosis and effective treatment. Critical points can be lost in translation.

In 2019, approximately 300 million people worldwide experienced major depression or dysthymia, and another 40 million had bipolar disorder. Depression was the primary reason for more than 5% of all years lived with disability. Approximately 759,000 deaths were known to be suicidal, and if the count were to include a modest proportion of deaths due to drowning, poisoning, drug overdose, or falls under ambiguous circumstances, the global number of suicides in a single year would greatly exceed one million (IHME, 2023). Worldwide, suicide is the fourth leading cause of death among adolescents and young adults (World Health Organization [WHO], 2023a). In the United States it is the second leading cause—accounting for more deaths than cancer or heart disease among people aged 15–29 (National Institute of Mental Health, 2021). Most people who die by suicide are depressed at the time of their fatal decision.

In 2020, the mental health consequences of the global COVID-19 pandemic included over 50 million additional cases of major depressive disorder (MDD), with females and younger people disproportionately afflicted (COVID-19 Mental Disorders Collaborators, 2021). As depressing as these statistics might be, they underestimate the magnitude of the "second pandemic" of mental illness. Millions of cases of depression serious enough to impair function, diminish quality of life, and/or involve suicidal risk do not fully meet diagnostic criteria for MDD. Furthermore, the survey methodologies typically used to detect depression usually do not adequately adjust for cultural differences in the psychometrics of screening tests and questionnaires. For example, when WHO mental health survey data from Nigeria were reanalyzed with such adjustment, the prevalence of depression jumped from 3% to over 21% (Scorza et al., 2018).

Even in high-income countries, most cases of depression remain untreated or are treated ineffectively. In low- and middle-income countries, more than 75% of people with depression receive no treatment (WHO, 2023). Timely diagnosis and effective treatment of depression would save many lives and would prevent disability, suffering, and grief.

The scope of the depression epidemic, the gaps in care, and the evident value of cultural awareness in addressing the problem provoked the authors to write this book. One author is an American academic physician with a low-context, direct communication style; the other is a humanities scholar educated in China, Japan, and the United States, with a high-context, indirect communication style. The authors' aim is to construct a *cultural lens*—a syncretic methodology for better understanding depression, the bipolar spectrum, and suicide in transpersonal context.

The authors' cultural lens is constructed by combining concepts, findings, and narratives from social sciences, literature, epidemiology, and biological psychiatry that seldom are integrated. It accounts for cultures defined by features other than race, ethnicity, or nationality—including occupation, socioeconomic class, religion, immigration and acculturation status, age, gender, and generation—and, importantly, it sees each person's cultural identity as intersectional.

Normalized or rationalized traumatic experiences and their consequences are recognized as prevalent and powerful in a range of cultures. Biologically relevant correlates of cultural identity including diets, sleeping habits, and environmental exposures are considered. Persistent shared historical memories, foundational texts, and ancient traditions are related to depression in contemporary times. Dimensions are preferred over categories and, figuratively, movies over snapshots.

In addition to literature found by searching the PubMed and PsycINFO databases, the authors used several other sources of material for constructing the cultural lens. Social scientists interested in depression and culture were interviewed, as were clinicians from North and South America, Europe, and Asia who see patients with depression. Primary sources—historical texts and literary narratives—were closely read in their original languages, including classical Chinese and classical Japanese, English, and Spanish. Epidemiologic databases were analyzed to test hypotheses about the cultural and structural determinants of depression and suicide.

Assessments of cultural–clinical relationships sometimes lump when they should split and split when they should lump. Neighboring countries, like China and Japan, that have related languages and cultural roots can differ sharply on dimensions especially relevant to the causation and expression of depression. Countries on different continents, like Finland and South Korea, can share historical themes, types of normalized trauma, and customary patterns of alcohol use that contribute to their high rates of suicide or intimate partner violence. This book takes a strategic approach to lumping and splitting not only for cultures of place but also for those of occupation and of social class.

When writing descriptions of cultures and their relationship to mental health, one immediately encounters a paradox. Efforts to raise cultural sensitivity by presenting generalizations about cultural groups risk the unwanted consequence of stereotyping; avoiding it was one of our greatest challenges in writing this book. Cultural identity is always intersectional, and the cultural identity most relevant to a person's sense of self and their mental health might not be their racial/ethnic identity—it might be their occupation, socioeconomic class, age/generation, gender, immigration status, or any combination of such identities. People can be multicultural, expressing different cultural identities in different contexts. Structural factors, personal history, and present circumstances can be far more important in individual cases than cultural identity. For all these reasons, generalizations about cultural groups should be seen as sources of hypotheses rather than a source of oversimplified assumptions, so the cultural lens can enhance perception and inform empathy.

Trenchant concepts, salient statistics, and engaging stories are useful mnemonics that can prompt productive questions. We will have achieved our purpose if our readers—clinicians, social scientists, public health professionals, and people with a personal or intellectual interest in depression—find that the cultural lens described in this book meaningfully and usefully broadens and sharpens their views of depression, the bipolar spectrum, and suicide, in individuals and in populations.

Barry S. Fogel is a psychiatrist and neurologist, a founder of the American Neuropsychiatric Association and the International Neuropsychiatric Association, a professor of psychiatry at Harvard Medical School, and a staff physician at the Brigham and Women's Hospital and the Dana-Farber Cancer Institute in Boston. He is a graduate of the University of California, San Francisco School of Medicine and of the MIT/Sloan School of Management. Xiaoling Jiang is a humanities scholar, with an M.A. in Japanese literature from Beijing Normal University; a Ph.D. in Structure of Culture from Kobe University, Japan; and postdoctoral studies in comparative literature at Harvard. She has served on the editorial board of *Culture Studies*, China's leading journal of comparative culture.

References

Andrew, L. B. (2018, August 1). Physician suicide. *Medscape*. Article 806779. https://emedicine.medscape.com/article/806779-overview

Bailey, J. G., Wong, M., Bailey, K., Banfield, J. C., Barry, G., Munro, A., Kirkland, S., & Leiter, M. (2023). Pandemic-related factors predicting physician burnout beyond established organizational factors: Cross-sectional results from the COPING survey. *Psychology, Health & Medicine*, 28(8), 2353–2367. https://doi.org/10.1080/13548506.2021.1990366

Broadway, D. (2023, July 6). Coco Lee, Hong Kong-born singer-songwriter, dies at 48 after suicide attempt. *Reuters*. https://www.reuters.com/world/china/coco-lee-hong-kong-born-singer-songwriter-dies-48-after-suicide-attempt-2023-07-05/

Congressional-Executive Commission on China (2023). *Criminal law of the People's Republic of China*. https://www.cecc.gov/resources/legal-provisions/criminal-law-of-the-peoples-republic-of-china

COVID-19 Mental Disorders Collaborators (2021). Global prevalence and burden of depressive and anxiety disorders in 204 countries and territories in 2020 due to the COVID-19 pandemic. *Lancet*, 398(10312), 1700–1712. https://doi.org/10.1016/S0140-6736(21)02143-7

Duarte, D., El-Hagrassy, M. M., Couto, T., Gurgel, W., Minuzzi, L., Saperson, K., & Corrêa, H. (2023). Challenges and potential solutions for physician suicide risk factors in the COVID-19 era: Psychiatric comorbidities, judicialization of medicine, and burnout. *Trends in Psychiatry and Psychotherapy*, 45, 1–9. https://doi.org/10.47626/2237-6089-2021-0293

Fortin, J. (2019, October 14; updated November 25). Sulli, South Korean K-Pop star and actress, is found dead. *The New York Times*. https://www.nytimes.com/2019/10/14/arts/music/sulli-dead.html?searchResultPosition=1

Han, X., Han, X., Luo, Q., Jacobs, S., & Jean-Baptiste, M. (2013). Report of a mental health survey among Chinese international students at Yale University. *Journal of American College Health*, *61*, 1–8.

Harvey, S. B., Epstein, R. M., Glozier, N., Petrie, K., Strudwick, J., Gayed, A., Dean, K., & Henderson, M. (2021). Mental illness and suicide among physicians. *Lancet*, *398*(10303), 920–930. https://doi.org/10.1016/S0140-6736(21)01596-8

Helliwell, J. F., Layard, R., Sachs, J. D., De Neve, J.-E., Aknin, L. B., & Wan, S. (eds.) (2023). *World Happiness Report 2023 (11th ed.)*. Sustainable Development Solutions Network.

Hulpuch, A. (2022, May 12). Naomi Judd died of a self-inflicted gunshot wound, her daughter says. *New York Times*. https://www.nytimes.com/2022/05/12/arts/music/naomi-judd-death-mental-illness.html

Ibrahim, S. (2021). Avicii's final words before suicide revealed in a new book. *New York Post, December 29*. https://nypost.com/2021/12/29/aviciis-final-words-before-suicide-revealed-in-new-book.

IHME (2024). *Global Burden of Disease 2021*. http://ghdx.healthdata.org/gbd-results-tool

Kane, L. (2023). "I cry but no one cares": Physician burnout & depression report 2023. *Medscape*. https://www.medscape.com/slideshow/2023-lifestyle-burnout-6016058

Katersky, A., & Hutchinson, B. (2018). Fashion designer Kate Spade found dead in apparent suicide: Police sources. *ABC News, June 5*. https://abcnews.go.com/US/fashion-designer-kate-spade-found-dead-apparent-suicide/story?id=55664239

Kumar, S. (2016). Burnout and doctors: Prevalence, prevention and intervention. *Healthcare*, *4*, Article 37. https://doi.org/10.3390/healthcare4030037

Laboe, C. W., Jain, A., Bodicherla, K. P., & Pathak, M. (2021). Physician suicide in the era of the COVID-19 pandemic. *Cureus*, *13*(11), Article e19313. https://doi.org/10.7759/cureus.19313

Lin, C., Tong, Y., Bai, Y., Zhao, Z., Quan, W., Liu, Z., Wang, J., Song, Y., Tian, J., & Dong, W. (2022). Prevalence and correlates of depression and anxiety among Chinese international students in US colleges during the COVID-19 pandemic: A cross-sectional study. *PLOS One*, *17*(4), Article e0267081. https://doi.org/10.1371/journal.pone.0267081

Margaritoff, M. (2023). How did Anthony Bourdain die? Inside the beloved chef's troubled final days. *All That's Interesting, March 25*. https://allthatsinteresting.com/anthony-bourdain-death.

National Institute of Mental Health (2021). *Mental health information: Suicide*. Retrieved December 20, 2021, from https://www.nimh.nih.gov/health/statistics/suicide

OECD (2023). *Pharmaceutical consumption—Antidepressants*. Retrieved March 26, 2023, from https://data-explorer.oecd.org

Radcliffe, S. (2023). Matthew Perry's cause of death raises concerns about the effects of ketamine. *Healthline, December 19*. https://www.healthline.com/health-news/matthew-perry-cause-of-death-acute-effects-of-ketamine

Scorza, P., Masyn, K., Salomon, J. A., & Betancourt, T. S. (2018). The impact of measurement differences on cross-country depression prevalence estimates: A latent transition analysis. *PLoS One*, *13*(6), Article e0198429.

Shanafelt, T. D., Hasan, O., Dyrbye, L. N., Sinsky, C., Satele, D., Sloan, J., & West, C. P. (2015). Changes in burnout and satisfaction with work–life balance in physicians and the general US working population between 2011 and 2014. *Mayo Clinic Proceedings, 90*(12), 1600–1613. https://doi.org/10.1016/j.mayocp.2015.08.023

Wang, J. (2021). Sayaka Kanda, Japanese actress and singer, dies at 35. *Entertainment Weekly, December 21*. https://ew.com/movies/sayaka-kanda-dead-35/

WHO (2023a). *Suicide* [Fact sheet]. Retrieved August 28, 2023, from https://www.who.int/news-room/fact-sheets/detail/suicide

WHO (2023b). *Depressive disorder (depression)* [Fact sheet]. Retrieved March 31, 2023, from https://www.who.int/news-room/fact-sheets/detail/depression

List of Abbreviations and Acronyms

BD	Bipolar disorder	IHME	Institute for Health Metrics and Evaluation
BDI	Beck Depression Inventory		
BD-I	Bipolar I disorder	MDD	Major depressive disorder
BD-II	Bipolar II disorder	MDE	Major depressive episode
BD-III	Bipolar III disorder	MDQ	Mood Disorder Questionnaire
CES-D	Center for Epidemiologic Studies Depression Scale	ODQ	Oxford Depression Questionnaire
DCI	Demand-Control Imbalance	OECD	Organisation for Economic Co-operation and Development
DSM	Diagnostic and Statistical Manual of Mental Disorders	PHQ	Patient Health Questionnaire
DSM-4	DSM, Fourth Edition	PHQ-2	Patient Health Questionnaire, two questions
DSM-5	DSM, Fifth Edition		
DSM-5-TR	DSM, Fifth Edition, Text Revision	PHQ-8	Patient Health Questionnaire, eight questions
ERI	Effort-Reward Imbalance	PHQ-9	Patient Health Questionnaire, nine questions
GBD	Global Burden of Disease	SES	Socioeconomic Status
HADS	Hospital Anxiety and Depression Scale	SNRI	Serotonin and Norepinephrine Reuptake Inhibitor
HCL-32	Hypomania Checklist	SSRI	Selective Serotonin Reuptake Inhibitor
ICD	International Classification of Diseases		
		US or U.S.	United States
ICD-10-CM	International Classification of Diseases, Tenth Edition, Clinical Modification	WHO	World Health Organization

Part I

Constructing the Cultural Lens

Chapter 1

Picturing Depression: Faces, Backgrounds, and Foregrounds

Like a photographic portrait, a picture of a person's depression shows a face, connected to a body, framed by a background, and set within a foreground. As a person might have a prominent forehead, a dimple in the chin, or a few missing teeth, an individual's syndrome of clinical depression strongly expresses some characteristic symptoms and expresses others weakly or not at all. In the background are many transpersonal features that influence mood and its somatic and behavioral expressions, including cultural norms and social determinants of health. In the foreground are individual circumstances that caused or contributed to the person's illness and that currently offer hope or worsen despair. Depending on the photographer and when the photo was taken, background and foreground are complex or minimal, blurred or in focus. Lighting might accentuate or attenuate specific facial features—as diagnostic criteria for major depressive disorder count some symptoms of clinical depression and exclude others. The entire body might be visible or just the head—as general health issues, nutritional state, and biomarkers are variably included in a case history.

An expert photographer has multiple lenses for their camera. They might take many photos of the same subject, varying the lenses, lighting, and viewpoints. Ultimately, subject and photographer choose a picture that best represents the subject, and that photo is enlarged. A clinician's ticking through a list of standard diagnostic criteria and making a binary judgment about a patient's illness is like a photographer taking one standard picture of each subject, always with the same lens and lighting, and then sorting the prints into piles with little or no input from the subject.

Metaphorically, a cultural lens offers wide-angle and telephoto views and foci from infinity to a few centimeters away. The authors encourage clinical photographers to take diverse images of each of their subjects and to engage their subjects in collaboratively choosing the ones that best capture the essence of their illness.

From *Obasute* to *Kodokushi*

Orin, a 69-year-old widow, lived with her 45-year-old, recently widowed son Tatsuhei and her grandchildren in a remote, impoverished mountain village in the Shinshū area of Nagano Prefecture, during the Edo period (1603–1868). Food was scarce. A strictly enforced rule of the village required that when people reached age 70 their children take them up the slope of Narayama, a nearby mountain, and leave them to wait alone in the wilderness until they died from starvation or exposure, thus leaving more food for other members of the family. Orin was a strong and energetic woman, well respected in the village, who accepted her fate and acted with great determination to prepare for her day of *Narayama mairi* (楢山参り; going to Narayama). In her eagerness, she was very different from her neighbor Mata, a man already 70 who had refused to go to the mountain.

Orin's story is told in *Narayama Bushikō* (楢山節考), a novella by Shichirō Fukazawa (1914–1987) that was first published in *Chūōkōron* (中央公論), Japan's leading literary magazine, in 1956. It won that publication's award for the year's best literary debut—reviewed and praised by the eminent writers Yukio Mishima (1925–1970), Sei Itō (1905–1969), and Taijun Takeda (1912–1976). Itō praised the novel as describing the essence of Japanese life as it has been for "thousands of years." Takeda attributed the novel's success to the character of Orin, who eagerly volunteered to go to the mountain (Mishima et al., 1956).

Narayama Bushikō clearly moved many Japanese hearts. When the story was republished as a book the following year, it immediately became a bestseller (Fukazawa, 1956). It was adapted for the screen in 1958 and 1983 as *The Ballad of Narayama* (Kinoshita, 1958; Imamura, 1983). Director Shōhei Imamura's version won the Palme d'Or at the Cannes Film Festival.

After Tatsuhei had found a new wife, a widow from a neighboring village, Orin immediately began preparing to go to the mountain. She welcomed her son's new wife and showed her a secret place to catch fish. She found a local woman with whom her younger son—mentally slow, odd, and often bullied—could have his first sexual experience. She cooked, worked in the fields, cared for her younger grandchildren, and attended to a sick neighbor. Orin was ashamed of her intact teeth, a rarity in the starving village, which her grandson ridiculed. She secretly knocked out her front teeth with a stone and then danced among the villagers with a toothless, bloody mouth.

Orin wanted to go to the mountain before the birth of her expected first great-grandchild. Tatsuhei was pained about his mother's impending death and was reluctant to take her up the mountain earlier than her 70th birthday. Orin fathomed her son's feelings but nonetheless pushed him to go. Three days before the

New Year, in the dark of night, Tatsuhei carried her up the slope of Narayama on his back. Nearing the mountaintop, mother and son saw piles of skeletons, and vultures circling in the sky. Tatsuhei left Orin and had started down the mountain when it began to snow, a good omen and a sign that Orin would die quickly of cold rather than slowly of starvation. He returned to his mother, crying out "Mom, snow is falling." She calmly waved him away.

On the way home, he witnessed a struggling, screaming Mata being thrown over a cliff to his death by his son. Orin died with dignity, in accordance with the village's *okite* (掟; a rule or law people are obliged to follow) but on her own terms.

Orin was healthy and vigorous and had proved she still could contribute much to the family and to the community—but Orin accepted the injustice and sacrificed herself, even going to die earlier than required, once she had accomplished what she felt was most important. At times, she seemed euphoric as she prepared for her death. By contrast, Mata, who fought his fate, was sad and angry. The characters of Orin and Mata suggest hypomanic versus depressed reactions to an inescapable situation.

The story ends with Orin sitting on the mountaintop, snow falling, awaiting her death. Back home, Tatsuhei returned to his usual family life. The family accepted the village's merciless *okite* with no sense of injustice or tragedy. In the context of the story, Orin's behavior was heroic and Mata's was shameful. Orin's death was noble; Mata's was humiliating. The story normalizes the abandonment and solitary death of a healthy older person.

The story illustrates the legendary Japanese practice of *obasute* (姨捨て; "throwing away the aunt"). It is sometimes called *ubasute* (姥捨て; "throwing away the old woman") or *oyasute* (親捨て; "throwing away the parents"). *Obasute* was first described in two 10th-century anthologies, *Kokin Wakashū* (古今和歌集; 905; Saeki, 1981; McCullough, 1985) and *Yamato Monogatari* (大和物語; 951; Amagai & Okayama, 2006; Tahara, 1980). Of 173 tales in the latter collection, the one about *obasute* was selected for the high school textbook of classic Japanese readings (Iwasaki et al., 2023). It concerns an orphaned man who was brought up by his aunt. After he married, his wife, who loathed his old aunt, insisted that he take her to the mountain to die. The man complied with his wife's request. The night he returned from the mountain he gazed at the moon and was overcome by regret:

> Waga kokoro nagusamekanetsu sarashina ya obasuteyama ni teru tsuki o mite
> 我が心なぐさめかねつさらしなや姨捨山にてる月を見て

> My heart cannot be tranquilized,
> Here in Sarashina,
> As I gaze at the moon above Mount Obasute. (authors' translation)

The next morning, he returned to the mountain and retrieved his aunt.

Matsuo Bashō (松尾 芭蕉; 1644–1694), Japan's master of haiku, visited Sarashina in 1688 and wrote,

> Omokage ya oba hitori naku tsuki no tomo
> 俤や姨ひとり泣く月の友. (Ueno, 2008)
>
> The look on her face—
> An old woman is weeping—
> The moon is her only company. (authors' translation)

The theme of *obasute* appears in many other Japanese literary works. Fukazawa's novella is especially poignant because there was no last-minute reprieve for the old woman destined to die and because Orin accepted her fate with enthusiasm. Mount Obasute, in the city of Chikuma, Nagano Prefecture, is a popular tourist destination, known for beautiful views of moonlight over its terraced rice paddies. It is served by trains stopping at Obasute Station. Whether *obasute* was a historical fact is outside the scope of this book, but Japan's literature and popular culture show that its people have long been fascinated by tales of *obasute*. For over a thousand years, Japanese have tolerated and normalized the idea of abandoning older people, though some classic stories of *obasute* do have endings in which the older person's life is spared.

On January 30, 2010, NHK (Japan Broadcasting Corporation) aired a shocking documentary characterizing Japan as a *muen shakai* (無縁社会; "disconnected society"). The film noted that 32,000 Japanese people annually died alone, with no one claiming their bodies (Nippon Hōsō Kyōkai, 2010). Such deaths are known as *muenshi* (無縁死; "disconnected deaths"). The cause of death usually is a chronic medical illness, though some die by a sudden acute illness, an accident, or suicide. In most cases of *muenshi* the deceased is identified, but either no living relatives can be located, or the relatives who can be found reject involvement. The corpses are cremated, and their ashes are buried in a *muenbo* (無縁墓; "unrelated people's cemetery") established by a local government.

Related to *muenshi* are *kodokushi* (孤独死; "lonely deaths"), in which people die alone at their homes and are not initially discovered for days to weeks afterward. Corpses are identified, and efforts are made by local authorities to contact living relatives. In most, but by no means all, cases, there are relatives who acknowledge a connection with the deceased. While some take responsibility for a funeral and might express regret about their long-term disconnection from the one who died, others do not want the trouble and expense of arranging a funeral (Taylor, 2012).

While the Japanese government maintains no national statistics on lonely deaths specifically—remarkably, given its meticulous maintenance of statistics on suicides—*Yomiuri Shinbun*, one of Japan's newspapers of record, published an investigative report on lonely deaths based on data from prefectural police in 19 of Japan's prefectures and from the Tokyo medical examiner's office. There were 17,433 such deaths in areas comprising 38% of Japan's population, implying about 46,000 lonely deaths per year if the sample is representative (Suzuki, 2018).

Most lonely deaths involve middle-aged or older men or older women, who are single, widowed, or divorced and either have no children or have children with whom they seldom have contact or communication. Most deaths are from chronic diseases, combined with malnutrition and dehydration. They involve the older person's intention to remain alone and await death rather than seek medical help or a personal connection. Some reject assistance that is offered. People who have living adult children and are considering a lonely death do not want to *meiwaku* (迷惑; burden) them and would prefer to die alone. Adult children's attachment to their older parents may be weak and contact infrequent. In extreme cases, the parent and child have not communicated in decades. Weeks can pass before the child knows that a parent has died.

In the Edo period of Japanese history, filial piety was promoted by the ruling Tokugawa shogunate, and abuse of older family members was a crime. There are specific historical records of older people's adult children being punished for neglecting or abusing them (Takagi, 2016). Official endorsement of respect and care for elders has been weaker in modern times. Though many Japanese adults maintain close relationships with their parents and display filial piety, contemporary Japanese culture does appear to normalize weak connections of middle-aged children with their older parents. This leads to cases of neglect that end in lonely deaths. Lonely death reflects the social isolation of millions of Japanese, an increasing problem as the population ages (more than one in four Japanese are over 65), fewer Japanese marry, and the country's fertility rate continues to fall (Siripala, 2018).

An important concept in Japanese culture is *en* (縁), which is not precisely translatable by a single word but conveys the sense of a personal connection, bonds of relationship, shared destiny, and linked fates. It is applied to ties a person might have with family (*chi-en*; 血縁), with community (*chi-en*; 地縁), or with an organization (*sha-en*; 社縁). The person with a lonely death has lost all three types of *en*. For men in their late 50s through early 70s, the group with the highest rate of lonely deaths, family connections might have been broken by the loss of a wife through divorce or her death and by children moving away. Community connections might have been maintained by the wife who is no longer present. Organizational connections might have been lost when the man lost his job or was required to retire once he had reached a mandatory retirement age.

Lonely deaths rarely are classified as suicides. Most people with lonely deaths do not receive a diagnosis of depression (*utsubyō*; 鬱病). However, it is likely that most are depressed before they die. Either they first become depressed and then choose a lonely death or, like Mata in *Narayama Bushikō*, they struggle with their fate, feeling sad, irritable, or angry. They might plan a lonely death with a positive sense of self-determination and autonomy, like Orin, but nonetheless become depressed as mortality approaches. Social isolation, poverty, untreated medical problems often associated with pain or discomfort, and lack of nutrition, sunlight, and exercise all are powerful antecedents of depression. Older Japanese who are suffering alone and lack positive reasons to live may choose to disconnect from everyone and practice radical self-neglect until they die weeks or months later of malnutrition or an untreated medical problem—a peaceful and gradual suicide (*odayaka na jisatsu*; 穏やかな自殺). Along the way such people would clearly meet diagnostic criteria for some form of clinical depression. A systematic lack of recognition of the role of depression and of suicidal intent in lonely deaths is symptomatic of Japanese society's denial of the scope of these problems.

Japan—both its government and its medical profession—have made modestly successful efforts to increase the rate of treatment of depression and to decrease the suicide rate. Its overall age-standardized suicide rate (both sexes) fell from a peak of 19.3 per 100,000 in 2005 to 14.2 per 100,000 in 2019, a decrease of 26% (Institute for Health Metrics and Evaluation [IHME], 2023). The demographic challenges faced by Japan require larger changes in Japan's policies regarding compulsory retirement and public financing of care for its "oldest old"—the growing population of citizens over age 80, who in 2019 had suicide rates of 42.0 for men and 17.8 for women. Though in Japan over 400,000 people await beds in nursing homes, there are insufficient staff for the facilities that already exist; and in 2015, the Japanese government cut reimbursement of nursing home care, making it even harder for long-term care facilities to attract nurses and aides (Matsuyama, 2015).

In contemporary Japan there is no need to bring old people to a mountainside wilderness. They can be left to die alone and unsupported in an urban apartment or of neglect in a dismal and poorly staffed nursing home. Though Japan has the greatest longevity of high-income countries, many of its older citizens live in poverty and squalor. Devaluation, neglect, and abandonment of older people by families, and by the broader society, are deeply rooted in the nation's culture, from 10th-century Mount Obasute to 21st-century Tokyo.

Twenty-Four Filial Exemplars—Ancient and Modern

The Chinese Confucian classic *The Twenty-Four Filial Exemplars* (*Èrshísì Xiào*; 二十四孝), written by Guo Jujing (郭居敬; ca. 1289–1354) during the Yuan Dynasty (1271–1368), includes the story "He Buried His Son to Serve His Mother" ("Mái Ér Fèng Mǔ"; "埋儿奉母") (Yu & Yu, 2012). Guo Ju (郭巨), a very poor man, lived with his wife, his 3-year-old son, and his mother. Lacking enough food for four, he and his wife decided to bury their young son alive so that there would be more food for his mother, reasoning that they could have another child but his mother could not be replaced. As Guo Ju dug a grave for his son, he uncovered a pile of gold, Heaven's reward for his outstanding filial piety (Jordan, 2016).

Filial piety (*xiào*; 孝) is the preeminent Confucian virtue—the foundation of the Chinese moral code for over two millennia. In the often-quoted words of the famous Qing Dynasty scholar Wang Yongbin (王永彬; 1792–1869), *Bǎi shàn xiào wéi xiān* (百善孝为先; "Among all the virtues filial piety comes first"; Wang, 1854/2008). The Chinese character for *xiao*, 孝, has two components, one representing "elder" placed on top and one representing "child," underneath. Children are supposed to obey and submit (*shùn cóng*; 顺从) to their parents earlier in their lives and to do their filial duty as adults by respecting and supporting them (*jìn xiào*; 尽孝) later in their lives. In China, filial piety is more important than loyalty to any organization or individual outside the family, and children's success or failure brings glory or shame to their families. The trust level in society overall is low, reliance on family is essential, and commitment to family is required.

In contemporary China, a land of filial piety, obedience to, and submissiveness toward parents are expected from a child's earliest years. In some Chinese families, children are treated as their parents' property rather than as autonomous individuals. China has a popular proverb: "Under the rod a child learns filial piety" (棍棒底下出孝子; *Gùnbàng dǐxià chū xiàozǐ*). If a parent beats a child in public, bystanders rarely intervene because parents harshly punishing their children is normalized, and it is not seen as other people's business. Article 260 of the Chinese Criminal Code prescribes shockingly mild penalties for domestic violence including the injury of a child at their parents' hands; even when a child dies from parental abuse, the maximum prison term is seven years (Congressional-Executive Commission on China, 2023).

Many parents have unrealistic expectations of their children, setting goals for them that are not compatible with their abilities and interests. Such parents often compel their children, from a very early age, to engage in incessant study that interferes with sleep, play, and relaxation, and punish them—verbally, physically, and by withholding their affection—for less-than-perfect academic performance or for disobedience with actions that would be classified as abuse in most Western countries. Many parents are relatively unconcerned with their children's happiness and seldom communicate with their children about their feelings or their emotional well-being. Even when parents realize that a child suffers from depression or is considering suicide, they tell the child to keep the problem a secret (to avoid a loss of face), and they do not seek professional help. Often, children internalize their parents' harsh discipline and become self-abusive perfectionists.

Trauma to children at the hands of their parents is normalized, but its normalization does not reduce its harmful effects on children's developing brains and minds. It increases their lifetime risk of depression, bipolar illness, and suicide. Additional adverse effects of extreme authoritarian parenting include diminished self-esteem, performance anxiety, loss of creativity, and a lack of psychological resilience.

Chinese children may normalize harsh treatment by their parents—an experience shared by many of their peers—as an expression of parental love and good intentions. This perspective does not necessarily continue into adult life, especially if they come to study or work overseas in a place where abusive authoritarian parenting is neither common nor acceptable. Young adults who are already vulnerable to depression because of adverse childhood experiences can develop clinical depression or become suicidal when they first realize they have been abused and recall their traumatic experiences.

In China, adult children are obligated by law to contribute to the support of their elderly parents if they are able and the parents are in need. The All-China Women's Federation—an agency of the Chinese government—in 2012 published a set of recommendations for how adults should treat their aged parents, entitled *The New Twenty-Four Filial Exemplars* (Jacobs & Century, 2012; National Committee on Aging et al., 2012). It instructs the younger generation to keep track of their parents' health and living situations, to make sure their parents have health insurance and get regular medical checkups, to call them at least weekly, to spend weekends and holidays with them, to see them often, to celebrate their birthdays, to join them in visiting old friends, to tell their parents they love them, etc.

Cultural memory is persistent and powerful. Tales of *obasute* can be linked to Japan's current epidemic of lonely and disconnected deaths and to the normalization of poverty, neglect, and social isolation of Japan's elders, with their consequences of depression and suicide. The literature on filial piety and obedience can be linked to the present reality that in China lonely or disconnected deaths of older people are relatively rare. On the other hand, severe depression culminating in death by suicide of talented and promising Chinese university students is tragically commonplace.

With these contrasting narratives in mind, one would not conflate Japanese and Chinese cultures as "East Asian" when considering issues of depression and suicide in their cultural context. In this book we will expand further on the history and ethos of China, Japan, and Korea and how they connect with salient differences in the occurrence and phenomenology of depression, bipolar illness, and suicide in their citizens, in their international students, and in immigrants from those countries to the United States (U.S.).

States of Mind: Depression and American Regional Cultures

While there are many distinctively American manners, cultural differences between regions, states, and localities within the U.S. are profound in ways that affect the occurrence, phenomenology, and narratives of depression, bipolar illness, and suicide. Subjective and narrative perspectives on interstate differences are complemented by, and often corroborated by, the numbers—social, economic, and demographic metrics aligned with epidemiologic measures, such as depression prevalence and suicide mortality rate.

Among the states, Utah has one of the highest suicide rates—in 2019 its age-standardized, both sexes rate was 18.84 per 100,000 population—58% higher than the national rate of 11.93. Connecticut's rate of 9.63 is one of the lowest in the nation. Table 1.1 shows selected 2019 data on major depression, substance use, and suicide from the Global Burden of Disease (GBD) 2019 database (IHME, 2023), along with data from the United Health Foundation (2023) on self-rated mental health status and suicidal ideation. Values of statistics that are significantly higher than the national benchmark are displayed in bold face, and those significantly lower are displayed in italics. Table 1.2, formatted similarly, provides demographic, socioeconomic, and environmental context helpful to understanding the differences displayed in Table 1.1.

Comparing the rates for Utah with those for Connecticut, Utah's male suicide rate is 2.29 times higher, but its female suicide rate is 3.50 times higher! The ratios of suicide rates between the two states are much larger than the ratios of their rates of major depression and bipolar disorder (BD), for both genders. It is more likely in Utah than in Connecticut that a depressed person will die by suicide. While a purely physical difference between Utah and Connecticut—Utah's

Table 1.1 Selected Epidemiologic Statistics for Connecticut, Utah, and the United States

2019 Prevalence data (%) and mortality data (per 100,000) from IHME (2023). Other data sources are cited the first time they are used.	Connecticut	Utah	United States
Major depression—Male	*2.0%*	**3.6%**	2.6%
Major depression—Female	*3.5%*	**6.4%**	4.6%
Major depression Male aged 15–49	*2.7%*	**5.0%**	3.6%
Major depression Female aged 15–49	*4.8%*	**9.1%**	6.3%
Drug use disorders—Male	**4.7%**	3.9%	4.0%
Drug use disorders—Female	3.1%	**3.4%**	3.0%
Drug use disorders Male aged 15–49	**8.8%**	6.7%	7.2%
Drug use disorders Female aged 15–49	5.8%	5.7%	5.4%
Alcohol use disorders—Male	3.2%	*2.7%*	3.4%
Alcohol use disorders—Female	1.9%	1.7%	1.9%
Alcohol use disorders Male aged 15–49	4.5%	*3.8%*	4.7%
Alcohol use disorders Female aged 15–49	2.8%	2.5%	2.7%
Suicide—Male	*15.5*	**29.6**	21.6
Suicide by firearm—Male	6.3	**17.5**	6.3
Suicide—Female	*4.6*	10.4	12.5
Suicide by firearm—Female	*0.6*	**2.7**	2.0
Percentage of suicides by firearm—Male	**41%**	**59%**	29%
Percentage of suicides by firearm—Female	14%	**26%**	16%
Suicide—Male aged 15–49	*14.0*	**35.0**	22.7
Suicide—Female aged 15–49	*5.1*	**12.7**	7.3
Suicide—Male aged 50–69	*23.5*	**46.1**	30.2
Suicide—Female aged 50–69	*6.8*	**17.6**	9.5
Suicide—Male aged 70+	*23.8*	**48.2**	35.7
Suicide—Female aged 70+	*3.9*	**8.7**	4.9
Youths aged 12-17 with severe major depression in past year (Mental Health America, 2020)	*10.2%*	**16.4%**	11.5%
Serious thoughts of suicide in past year, adults of both sexes (Mental Health America, 2023).	*4.4%*	**7.6%**	4.8%
Residents fully vaccinated for COVID-19 as of 5/10/2023 (USA Facts, 2023)	**83%**	*67%*	70%

Note. State values significantly and meaningfully lower than the national value are highlighted in italics. Values significantly and meaningfully higher than the national value are highlighted in bold face.

Table 1.2 Demographic, Socioeconomic, and Environmental Statistics for Connecticut, Utah, and the United States

Demographic, socioeconomic, or environmental feature	Connecticut	Utah	United States	Data source if not Kaiser Family Foundation (2021)
Population under 18 (2020)	22%	**31%**	23%	
Population over 65 (2020)	**20%**	12%	17%	
Adults who live with children under 18 (2019)	32%	**41%**	33%	
Percentage non-Hispanic White (2019)	**66%**	78%	60%	
Percentage Hispanic (2019)	17%	14%	19%	
Percentage Black (2019)	10%	1%	12%	
Percentage Asian (2019)	5%	2%	6%	
Median household income (2019)	**$78,833**	$75,780	$65,712	
Gini coefficient (higher → more inequality) (2020)	**0.496**	0.427	0.481	US Census Bureau (2023b)
Income equality rank (out of 50)	49	1	–	US Census Bureau (2023a)
Adults 19–64 in poverty (2022)	10%	9%	11%	US Census Bureau (2024)
Children under 18 in poverty (2022)	13%	8%	15%	US Census Bureau (2024)
Older adults (over 65) in poverty (2022)	9%	8%	10%	US Census Bureau (2024)
Gender Equity Score: Rank on Women, Peace and Security Index	**.696** **(2nd of 51)**	.400 (36th of 51)	.486	Berman-Vaporis et al., (2020)
Paid family and sick leave	Yes	No	15 states + DC	

(continued)

Table 1.2 Continued

Demographic, socioeconomic, or environmental feature	Connecticut	Utah	United States	Data source if not Kaiser Family Foundation (2021)
Men over 25 with a college degree (2019)	**39%**	**37%**	32%	US Census Bureau (2024)
Women over 25 with a college degree (2019)	**41%**	33%	34%	US Census Bureau (2024)
Men over 25 with a graduate degree (2019)	**17%**	**14%**	12%	US Census Bureau (2024)
Women over 25 with a graduate degree (2019)	**18%**	9%	13%	US Census Bureau (2024)
Two most prevalent religious affiliations of adults and percentage unaffiliated	**Catholic (33%),** Mainline Protestant (17%), Unaffiliated (23%)	**Latter-day Saints (55%),** *Evangelical Protestant (7%),* Unaffiliated (22%)	Evangelical Protestant (25%), Catholic. (8%), Unaffiliated (22.8%)	Pew Research Center (2018)
Adults for whom religion is "very important" in their lives	*42%*	**58%**	53%	Pew Research Center (2018)
Adults who attend church at least once a week	*28%*	**53%**	37%	Pew Research Center (2018)
Adults living in a household with a firearm.	*19%*	**47%**	40%	Schell et al. (2020)
Births per year per 1000, women aged 15–44 (2019)	*51.1*	**66.7**	58.3	
Abortions per 1000 women aged 15–44 (2019)	13.7	4.2		

Table 1.2 Continued

Demographic, socioeconomic, or environmental feature	Connecticut	Utah	United States	Data source if not Kaiser Family Foundation (2021)
Median age at first marriage—women (2017)	**29.7**	*24.8* (lowest in US)	28.6	Payne (2019)
Women aged 15-49 with no health insurance (2019)	*7%*	12%	12%	
Adults with mental illness reporting unmet need	27%	**34%**	28%	Reinert et al. (2022)
State mental health budget per capita	**$216.76**	*$70.86*	$119.62	
Psychiatrists per 100,000 people	**24.8**	*7.5*	12.4	HRSA (2024)
Average elevation	*500 feet*	**6100 feet**	2500 feet	Wikipedia (2023a)

Note. State values significantly and meaningfully lower than the national value are highlighted in italics. Values significantly and meaningfully higher than the national value are highlighted in bold face.

higher altitude—is associated with a higher prevalence of depression and a higher suicide rate, several cultural differences are salient in understanding why so many Utahns die by suicide.

First, an adult in Utah is more than twice as likely as one in Connecticut to live in a household with a firearm. Suicide attempts made with firearms usually are fatal. In Utah, firearms are used in more than half of all suicides by men and in more than a quarter of those by women. In Connecticut, only 8% of women's suicides use a firearm, and only 36% of male suicides (Schell et al., 2020). Second, timely access to mental health services is much more difficult in Utah than Connecticut; Utah's public mental health services are poorly funded, and there is a shortage of psychiatrists. Young women—the highest risk group for depression—often lack health insurance. 9% of all Utah adults in 2019, before the COVID-19 pandemic, reported an unmet need for mental health treatment, and half of those gave cost as the main reason. By contrast, only 5% of Connecticut adults reported an unmet need for mental health treatment, and only a quarter of them cited cost as the main reason. The large differences in mental health care are not attributable to state-level economics; both states have median household incomes well above the national benchmark. The differences can be associated with Utah's culture—one that is averse to an important role for government in addressing social and health issues, that accepts significant gender inequality, and that stigmatizes mental illness and its treatment by psychiatrists. In mainstream Utah culture, adults are expected to seldom need psychological help, and they are expected to turn to family or to the church if they do. The state's resistance to public solutions to health problems comports with its below-average COVID-19 vaccination rates during the pandemic, despite the state's having a higher COVID incidence and mortality rate than the national average.

The differences between Utah and Connecticut in women's mental health are especially marked, in keeping with Connecticut being one of the most gender-equal states (in second place among the 50 states plus the District of Columbia) and Utah well below average (in 36th place) (Berman-Vaporis et al., 2020). Compared with Connecticut's women, Utah's women marry younger and have more children, have less higher education, and are more likely to lack health insurance. Unlike Connecticut, Utah has no state requirement for paid family and sick leave. Utah is a highly religious state, with most of its residents attending church at least weekly and the dominant faith being the Church of Jesus Christ of Latter-Day Saints (also known as the LDS or Mormon Church), one with high gender inequality, authoritarian norms, and perfectionistic expectations for the performance of women as wives and mothers (Peer & McGraw, 2017).

More pregnancies imply more occasions for postpartum depression; a culture strongly opposed to abortion implies that more unwanted pregnancies come to term. Women who work outside the home and have young children are especially likely to experience stress balancing work and family obligations.

While Connecticut has lower rates of depression and suicide than Utah, it has a significantly higher rate of substance use disorders. While it has relatively low gender inequality, its income inequality is the second highest in the U.S.; Utah's is the second lowest. In Connecticut, an "unnatural death" due to a drug overdose is much more likely than an explicit suicide. In a narrative of depression, it is more likely in Connecticut than in Utah that social class will play a role. Details might include a rise or fall in class, distress over comparing oneself to wealthier neighbors or co-workers, a diet loaded with depressing foods, or problematic use of alcohol or drugs. Socioeconomic status and its structural correlates help explain which demographic groups in Connecticut have the highest prevalence of depression, comorbidity of depression with substance use disorders and general medical conditions, and the role of drug overdoses in suicides and other unnatural deaths in that state.

It should also be noted that Utah's elevated rates of depression and suicide are not expressions of a generally high prevalence of mental disorders. Its prevalence rates of schizophrenia, of anxiety disorders, and of alcohol use disorders do not differ significantly from national benchmarks; and its prevalence of drug use disorders in men is significantly below the national rate (IHME, 2023).

Utah is a mountainous state with an average elevation over 6100 feet above sea level; Connecticut is a coastal state with an average elevation of 500 feet. Living at higher elevation has been linked to a higher prevalence of depression and a suicide rate disproportionately higher than the rate of depression, even after controlling for many known correlates of depression and suicide, such as poverty and rates of gun ownership. In some studies, the correlation of suicide rate with altitude is significantly greater than its correlation with other recognized risk factors. The phenomenon has been related to the effect of hypoxia on serotonin metabolism and brain bioenergetics (Kious et al., 2018). The U.S. states through which the Rocky Mountains pass all have high average elevation, high gun ownership, and high suicide rates.

The environmental correlates of cultural identity deserve consideration in understanding rates of depression, the distribution of depression among demographically-defined subsets of a cultural group, and the relationship of depression to suicide. These issues will be explored in detail later in this book.

Cultural differences between Utah and Connecticut reflected in quantitative data suggest explanations for the strikingly different epidemiology of depression and suicide in the two states. They are representative of the differences between regions of the U.S., which on many parameters can exceed the differences between neighboring nations. In a chapter devoted to regional differences within the U.S., a qualitative segmentation of the country by regional culture will be related to quantitative data on the demographics, economy, environment, and health service landscape of the region, as well as to the epidemiology of depression, including relative rates of depression and suicide among age groups and between men and women.

A Low-Context Primary Care Physician Encounters a High-Context Patient

Sophie, age 41, a decorous Frenchwoman, the only child of a wealthy and highly educated Parisian family, presented for an urgent visit with Dr. T., an internist covering for her usual primary care physician (PCP) at a Boston teaching hospital. Sophie was married; she met her husband Mike, age 40, when he was an undergraduate at Stanford spending his junior year in France, and she was an undergraduate at Sorbonne University. After college, Mike earned an MBA from an elite business school and joined a well-known Boston venture capital firm, where he eventually became a managing partner. The couple had two sons, aged 12 and 9. They lived in Weston, Massachusetts, one of Boston's most affluent suburbs. Sophie was an introvert, who focused her life on home and family. She was active in her sons' education, committed to bringing them up to be fully bilingual.

Several months before the primary care visit, when Sophie was organizing Mike's luggage after a business trip, she was shocked to find that Mike was involved in an ongoing affair with a business school classmate; several of his "business trips" were actually romantic trysts. Sophie was heartbroken; the man she had deeply loved and fully trusted had betrayed her. Though furious at Mike, Sophie was not ready to confront him. She had mixed feelings about divorce because of its potential effect on her sons, and she feared that opening up the issue of Mike's infidelity might lead to the end of the marriage.

Sophie felt trapped and hopeless, anxious, and sad. Though a light drinker before she discovered her husband's infidelity, she started drinking two full glasses of wine to calm herself before bedtime and often took 3 mg of over-the-counter (OTC) melatonin as well. She usually awoke at dawn, feeling physically and emotionally miserable. Lumbar spine pain, dating from a skiing accident in her 20s, flared up and became intolerable.

Sophie started sleeping in a separate room from Mike, telling him she did not want her nighttime wakefulness to interfere with his sleep. Mike did not suspect the underlying reason for his wife's behavior.

Sophie had planned to take her sons to see their grandparents in Paris on their summer vacation. Two days before their scheduled departure, she abruptly canceled the trip, feeling she was too miserable to enjoy it, fearing that a long flight would make her back pain worse, and worried that her parents would sense that she had a problem with Mike. They loved Mike and accepted Sophie's living far from them because they thought she had a near-perfect life.

She called her PCP's office for an urgent appointment. Her PCP was on vacation, and Dr. T. was covering. Dr. T. fit Sophie into his busy schedule, seeing her at five in the afternoon, at the end of a long clinical day.

During the visit, Sophie *smiled with a doleful and faraway look* in her blue eyes. She told Dr. T. she hoped for some relief from insomnia and back pain— *she hadn't had a good night's sleep in weeks.* She told Dr. T she'd had lower back pain on and off for years. She had managed it with yoga and exercises; but recently *she couldn't concentrate* on yoga, and her usual exercises made her pain worse. She had developed insomnia; the pain made it hard to fall asleep or to get back to sleep if she awoke during the night. Sophie told Dr. T. that she'd just had to call off her planned trip to Paris with her sons and that *she felt guilty* about disappointing them and her parents.

She said she had tried different OTC medications for pain and for sleep, but they didn't help. She wanted prescriptions for medicines that could give her sufficient pain relief and decent sleep. Dr. T. reviewed her medical record. Apart from an old lumbar spine injury, there was nothing remarkable; there was no history of insomnia and no mention of anxiety or depression. She had never sought opioid analgesics or sleeping pills, there was nothing in the record to suggest a problem with substance use, and the Massachusetts controlled substance monitoring website showed she hadn't had any prior opioid prescriptions. When he asked her about drinking, she said she drank socially and sometimes *drank a glass of wine to relax at night if something worried her.* He asked if having a drink helped, and Sophie nodded. Dr. T. didn't ask further about her drinking; Sophie didn't fit his idea of a woman with a drinking problem. He pointed out that if he prescribed any medication for her, she would have to abstain from alcohol while she was on it. Sophie nodded again.

On physical examination, Dr. T. found tenderness over the fourth and fifth lumbar vertebrae and bilateral lumbar muscle spasms. Based on her medical history and her complaints of insomnia and pain in her back, he ordered lumbar spine imaging and a physical therapy evaluation. He gave her one-week non-refillable prescriptions for a low dose of hydrocodone, a moderate-potency opioid analgesic, and eszopiclone, a prescription hypnotic. He emphasized that he would consider refilling the prescriptions at most once and then only if she followed through on the imaging study and the physical therapy evaluation. He arranged a follow-up with Sophie's usual PCP in two weeks but expressed the hope she'd feel better enough to take her sons to Paris before they had to go back to school: "Let's see if we can give you enough relief so you can make that trip." He said he had a nine-year-old son himself and could relate to how hard it could be for a parent to disappoint a child expecting to go see their grandparents and to visit an exciting city. Dr. T's comment, intended to show empathy, made Sophie despondent.

In Dr. T.'s note of the office visit, he mentioned the possibility that Sophie might be mildly depressed; this would prompt Sophie's regular PCP to follow up on the point. He didn't have the time that day to get into a detailed mental status examination, and he would not want to prescribe an unnecessary antidepressant medication. As evidenced by his care with the opioid and hypnotic prescriptions, he was cautious and conservative in his practice.

In the evening after her primary care visit, Sophie tried the sleeping pill. She got to sleep easily but awoke three hours later in severe pain. She took the hydrocodone and got another three hours of sleep. On awakening in the morning, she felt hungover, miserable, and hopeless and saw no way out of her situation. She resolved to die by suicide. That day, she wrote letters to her sons, to her parents, and to Mike. She told her sons and her parents that she loved them very much and was sorry that she had to leave them. She told Mike she had loved him deeply, but he had broken her heart and that she could not live with his betrayal.

That evening, after her sons were asleep, she drank a pint of brandy and took all the remaining eszopiclone and hydrocodone. Mike, who had a business meeting, came home unexpectedly early and found Sophie unresponsive but still alive. Mike called an ambulance, and Sophie survived.

In Sophie's case, the covering PCP did not identify that Sophie was desperate and at risk for suicide, although there were hints to her state of mind throughout the clinical encounter, which are indicated by the italicized phrases above. The thought crossed his mind that there could be an emotional issue contributing to her pain, but to him she had looked self-possessed and in control, uncomfortable but not miserable, and not like someone ill with major depression and at risk of suicide. The problem faced by Dr. T. is a common one: 64% of people who attempt suicide visit a physician during the month before their attempt, and 38% do so in the week before (Ahmedani et al., 2015). When depression is mild, PCPs make the diagnosis in only one third of cases; when it is moderate or severe, they still miss it more than 40% of the time (Mitchell et al., 2011). Furthermore, the relationship of suicidality to the number, severity, and frequency of other symptoms of depression is weak. A person with mild major depression or subsyndromal depression (clinical depression meeting fewer than five of the criteria for major depressive disorder) can have strong suicidal ideation or even a specific plan for suicide (Wakefield & Schmitz, 2017).

An important reason that Dr. T. missed Sophie's communication of her depression and despair is the incompatibility of their communication styles. Dr. T. employed the usual "low-context" communication style of Americans and of primary care medicine everywhere—direct, explicit, and not greatly dependent on attention to paralinguistic communication, prior shared knowledge, hints, and allusions. Sophie's communication was "high context," conveying critical information about her mental state in an understated and indirect way, by her facial expressions and by combining observations of what she said and what she did not say. As an example of the latter, she made no mention of her husband despite her being highly family oriented. Her despair "leaked out" in various ways, without her intending to talk about it explicitly, or perhaps not even fully appreciating it herself. And Dr. T., meeting Sophie for the first time, had no historical context or knowledge of Sophie's emotional baseline.

Sophie had several cultural identities contributing to her high-context communication style. She was from France, a nation with higher-context communication than the Nordic, Germanic, or English-speaking countries. She was from Paris, which, like many capital cities, has higher-context communication than the country in general. She was from an educated, upper-class background in which people of the same social circle share distinctive knowledge and attitudes that need not be mentioned explicitly when they talk with one another. Finally, as the wife of a powerful and socially prominent man, she would be inclined to tact and understatement.

There are many other reasons PCPs fail to diagnose—or misdiagnose—clinical depression and bipolar illness or fail to appreciate suicidality. Insufficient time is a common one, as is the physician's awkwardness about bringing up the subject of depression—let alone suicide—with a patient who presents with a somatic symptom or general medical problem and no explicit emotional concern. When a patient presents an explicit concern about depression, a PCP typically will address it like any other potentially serious illness. When the presentation is sufficiently indirect, however, it is easy to avoid the subject. Utilizing a modified approach to communication that accounts for cultural differences can remove one barrier to accurate diagnosis and help build empathy and trust with a patient that can make treatment more successful. When a patient has a high-context communication style, it is important to recognize it promptly. Doing so increases the clinician's attention to indirect, understated, and non-linguistic forms of communication. Knowing that a patient has several cultural identities associated with high-context communication makes it reasonable to start with the assumption that they will communicate in that style. If the patient turns out to communicate directly and explicitly, nothing is lost; but if not, the clinician has been tuned in from the outset to hints, clues, understatements, inconsistencies, facial expressions, and other details essential to apprehending the patient's full story. In the chapters that follow we will present a multidimensional framework for understanding cultures' communication styles, including further explanation of the useful and widely accepted concept of high-context versus low-context communication.

Conclusion

This chapter has illustrated several aspects of a cultural lens through which depression can be seen more clearly and understood more accurately, aiding clinicians in empathic connection with patients and with personalization of their care. Cultures have folklore and literature that illustrate their values and morals. Cultures' rules—often unwritten—can lead to stresses, losses, traumatic events, and disruptions of social bonds that can precipitate depression. The quantitative data on demographic, social, economic, and environmental dimensions of cultures can confirm or contradict hypotheses based on theory or clinical experience. The sometimes-profound differences in communication style across cultures can be a barrier to clinical understanding—though simply recognizing the issue starts one down the path to resolving it—because high-context, indirect communication usually makes up in redundancy what it lacks in explicitness.

A cultural lens does not apply ethnic stereotypes. Intersecting cultural identities are the rule, and ethnic identity is just one of them. However, in a case like that of Sophie and Dr. T., a patient's combination of cultural identities together with the clinical presentation can support a confident judgment about communication style that can make a clinical encounter more meaningful and a diagnosis more accurate, even lifesaving.

A major idea of this book is that items of cultural knowledge that are easily recalled can prime the mind to recognize cultural aspects of depression—depression-related, culture-specific "themes and memes"—in an individual or in a population. Salient differences between groups often lumped together, statistics of shocking magnitude, clinical narratives of avoidable error, and dramatic stories, like *The Ballad of Narayama* and "He Buried His Son to Serve His Mother," are hard to forget.

Chapter 2
Faces of Clinical Depression

Objects to be seen through a cultural lens are clinical depression, episodes of bipolar disorder (BD) with predominantly or entirely depressive symptoms, depression with mixed features (i.e., including some hypomanic symptoms), and suicide and "unnatural deaths" related to these conditions. Dealing effectively with depression as a clinical problem or population health issue requires attention not only to conditions that would meet criteria for major depressive disorder (MDD). MDD is defined in the *Diagnostic and Statistical Manual* of the American Psychiatric Association, *Fifth Edition, Text Revision* (DSM, Fifth Edition, Text Revision [DSM-5-TR] or simply Diagnostic and Statistical Manual of Mental Disorders [DSM]; American Psychiatric Association, 2022), and the *International Classification of Diseases, Tenth Revision, Clinical Modification* (ICD-10-CM or simply *International Classification of Diseases* [ICD]; National Center for Health Statistics, 2023). It is the form of depression most often cited in reports of prevalence and most often studied in clinical trials of antidepressant therapies. Although the DSM and the ICD are the standard references for psychiatric nosology worldwide, their criteria for MDD do not capture depressive illness equally well across cultures. Their highly specific criteria for MDD can exclude many people with depressive conditions that are "major" concerns in the common sense of the word—conditions that cause painful distress, impair social, occupational, and/or instrumental functioning, and sometimes threaten life. Though the criteria for MDD explicitly exclude people whose depressive symptoms represent self-limited and normal emotional reactions to major losses and other stressful events, people with situational depression frequently will be misdiagnosed if a checklist approach is taken to diagnostic assessment (Frances, 2013).

Fortunately, the DSM-5-TR and the ICD-10-CM offer alternative diagnostic labels that can be accurately applied to people who have clinically significant depressive syndromes that do not fit MDD criteria. They provide clinicians with a way to record, code, and legitimate a depressed patient's illness that allows room for individual differences in the expression of depression, including those related to transpersonal identity. However, in our experience these alternatives are relatively seldom used. Three useful alternatives are *other specified depressive disorder* (ICD-10-CM code F32.89), *unspecified depressive disorder* (ICD-10-CM code F32.A), and *unspecified mood disorder* (ICD-10-CM Code F39) (American Psychiatric Association, 2022).

Other specified depressive disorder applies to presentations of depression that cause "clinically significant distress or impairment in social, occupational, or other important areas of functioning," do not meet full criteria for MDD, dysthymia, or other disorders in the depressive disorders diagnostic class, and do not meet criteria for an adjustment disorder with depressed mood or with mixed anxiety and depressed mood. To make the diagnosis, the clinician must record specifically the reason why the patient does not meet criteria for a specific depressive disorder. For example, an episode might last less than two weeks, or there might be an insufficient number of discrete symptoms to meet criteria for MDD.

Unspecified depressive disorder applies to presentations of depression that do not meet full criteria for a more specific depressive disorder, where the clinician either has insufficient information to make a definitive diagnosis or chooses not to specify the reason that full criteria for MDD or another specific depressive disorder are not met.

Unspecified mood disorder applies to presentations of a mood disorder with possible bipolar features (see Chapter 6) that do not meet full criteria for either a more specific depressive disorder or a bipolar disorder. As with unspecified depressive disorder, the clinician might lack complete information, or might have information they do not choose to utilize and/or disclose at the time of the initial diagnosis.

The "unspecified" diagnoses can be particularly useful when a clinician is in the process of evaluating a patient from a culture they do not know well, where there is a significant risk of miscommunication and of false positive or false negative assessments of the presence or severity of symptoms. Using one of them, a clinician can determine and document that their patient is ill with a form of depression and provide a predicate for treatment, without making premature conclusions about the scope, severity, and specifics of the illness.

Referring to a non-usual and clinically important state of mood, thought, perception, and/or behavior as a *disorder* can have negative implications. For example, *disorderly conduct* is a crime. *Disease* or *condition* perhaps inspires more sympathy and a less judgmental and critical view. *Disorder* and *condition* are used in this book to describe syndromes (i.e., groupings of symptoms and signs). *Disease* is reserved for describing syndromes associated with demonstrable biochemical or physiological abnormalities. The term *illness* is primarily used to describe syndromes in connection with personal experiences and narratives. *Mental illness* is consistently used to refer to mental disorders that include behavior consistently viewed within its cultural context as outside of normal limits.

Clinical depression is used here to encompass conditions that deserve clinical attention because they cause significant distress and/or significantly affect function and are persistent or expected to persist without treatment. It excludes self-limited emotional reactions to external events, such as uncomplicated grief after the loss of a loved one.

MDD requires five out of nine specified symptoms, for a duration of at least two weeks. There clearly are people with syndromes with fewer than five of the specified symptoms or a duration shorter than 14 days who deserve the label of *clinical depression*. If a person has been ill for 10 days with a recurrent depressive syndrome and they are getting gradually worse, it would be necessary to wait four days before the criteria for MDD were met, but clinical depression can be diagnosed immediately.

In this book, episodes of depression related to bipolar disorder are included in the scope of clinical depression, including episodes in which symptoms both of depression and of hypomania are present but the former predominate. As will be discussed in detail below, people with bipolar illness often present for care with symptoms of depression, and their bipolarity is not initially appreciated.

More severe forms of depression, including melancholia, psychotic depression, and the depressed phase of bipolar I disorder (BD-I) (manic-depressive illness with a manic phase having psychotic features or requiring hospitalization), are recognized as *mental illness* worldwide, and their phenomenology is similar across cultures. This book's main concern is people with clinical depression who do not have one of these severe conditions, a group that includes people with mild to moderate non-psychotic MDD or bipolar II disorder (BD-II); dysthymia, subsyndromal MDD, or clinically significant depressive reactions to grief, trauma, or extraordinary stress. The phenomenology and narratives of these conditions show more cross-cultural differences, and these conditions are more likely than melancholia or psychotic disorders to go unrecognized, undiagnosed, misdiagnosed, untreated, or ineffectively treated. Even though it is less symptomatically extreme than melancholia or psychotic depression, depression in the "middle zone" between normality and mental illness can cause disability, death by suicide, and changes in comorbid general medical conditions that affect life expectancy and quality of life. *Middle zone depression* is encompassed by the definition we propose below for *clinical depression* as it might present to a clinician with cultural awareness.

Culture-Related Issues with the Diagnosis of MDD

Making a diagnosis of MDD according to DSM or ICD criteria is an act of converting several dimensional assessments into a single binary judgment. A categorical diagnosis of this kind might be necessary for epidemiologic studies or for selecting subjects for clinical trials. However, it is not ideal when the purpose is greater understanding of depression within a cultural group, attributing the causes of suicides, or engaging clinically with a person on the boundary between normal life experience and depressive illness. Clinical depression—depression that is a medical condition worthy of study and clinical care—is not necessarily depression that would be classified as *major* in terms of a count of specified symptoms. A person with only four of the nine defining symptoms of major depression should meet valid criteria for *clinical* depression if, in addition to severe hopelessness, they have a specific and imminent plan for suicide or are occupationally disabled because of fatigue and cognitive slowing.

In considering the limitations of the diagnosis of MDD, and the other depressive syndromes described in the DSM, it is relevant to consider the process whereby DSM criteria are periodically revised and established as a standard. A proposed set of criteria is written by a subcommittee of the American Psychiatric Association, which is then circulated, reviewed, and critiqued by a wider circle of its members (with input from non-psychiatrist consultants), before being revised and presented for endorsement by a larger committee with responsibility for approving the DSM as a whole. The criteria thus represent a consensus of Western-trained medical specialists who are members of an American professional association. The clinical experience of most committee members with depressed people will be especially rich in encounters with people who become psychiatric patients in the American mental health system. Continuity with the criteria of the previous edition of the DSM is an important consideration, given the use of DSM diagnoses in epidemiologic research, clinical trials, US Food and Drug Administration evaluations of antidepressants, payers' coverage criteria and utilization reviews, diagnostic coding, and clinician payment. Thus, the process for adopting criteria for MDD and other depressive syndromes is culturally biased from the outset, and there is great resistance to modifying criteria. Recognizing that DSM criteria can sometimes be a barrier to valuable research and clinical observations, the National Institute of Mental Health (2021), beginning in 2010, developed a parallel set of diagnostic criteria called the Research Domain Criteria (RDC), which take a multidimensional rather than a categorical approach to psychopathology harmonious with contemporary thinking about the brain dysfunctions that correlate with the different symptoms and syndromes of mental disorders. Because they are multidimensional, the RDC necessarily accommodate cultural differences better than the DSM criteria. However, they are not used in clinical practice, regulation, or payment, nor are most clinicians familiar with them.

The DSM definition of MDD requires that a person have five or more symptoms out of a list of nine present during the same two-week period, representing a change from the person's baseline and not "clearly attributable" to another medical condition or the physiological effects of an exogenous substance. The symptoms must cause "clinically significant" distress or impairment in social, occupational, or other "important areas of functioning." One of the symptoms must be either depressed mood or a loss of interest or pleasure in activities (*anhedonia*), and that symptom must be present for most of the day, almost every day. If a person has a depressed mood or anhedonia but has fewer than four of the other symptoms on the list, the diagnosis cannot be *major* depression. Unfortunately, *not major* can carry the connotation of *less serious*, an implication that often is not valid.

The authors' view is that the DSM definition of MDD is culture-bound and that to see depression through a cultural lens, the criteria for diagnosing clinical depression must be different. The nine criterial symptoms of MDD are now reviewed with comments on how they might be adapted to account for cultural differences while still capturing the essence of what makes depression an illness distinct from a period of ordinary, quotidian sadness or unhappiness. The analysis is followed by an informal set of criteria for clinical depression that defines the scope of this book's exploration of depression. The criteria might be useful to clinicians having dialogues with depressed people about their symptoms. We designed the alternative criteria to allow for consideration of cultural differences in determining whether a person's depression is of clinical severity and to address the relative insensitivity of the DSM criteria for MDD to patients with depression in the middle zone.

For each of the MDD criteria below we note a cultural issue that could lead to a false-positive or false-negative determination that the criterion applied. When issues related to ethnicity are mentioned, they are not meant to be stereotypes or always-present correlates of ethnic identity. Many potential combinations of individual differences, non-conformity, intersecting identities, and acculturation can make them irrelevant or even misleading. However, they apply often enough that they expose a weakness of the DSM criteria when applied to individuals of that ethnic origin. In many of the examples offered in the comments, the issue associated with cultural identity has a large structural component, in which objective circumstances correlated with membership in a cultural group are more consequential than culture per se.

The nine symptoms of MDD in the DSM, Fifth Edition (DSM-5) are as follows:

1.. Depressed mood most of the day, nearly every day, as indicated by either subjective report (e.g., feels sad, empty, hopeless) or observation made by others (e.g., appears tearful). (Note: In children and adolescents, can be irritable mood.)

    Comment: People with depression can experience anger or resentment, as they do in the Korean syndrome of *hwa-byung* (화병), rather than a feeling they would describe as sadness. They might feel desperate but not hopeless, as they could be if they came from a religious community where the hope of divine intervention was never lost. Irritability as the primary symptom is not limited to children and adolescents, as cultures differ in the age at which young adults are expected to transition from adolescence to adulthood, and people with depression in later life may be more concerned about irritability than about sadness. The DSM acknowledges that depression with mixed (i.e., bipolar) features often presents with prominent irritability. In conceptualizing clinical depression in a world where most people with depression don't seek treatment and would not be pre-assorted into unipolar and bipolar categories, people with mixed features should be captured by criteria that will be applied in non-psychiatric contexts to decide who requires further assessment and possible treatment.

In a culture that requires suppression of emotion at work or even forced smiling regardless of one's inner state—as does the majority culture of Japan and occupational cultures of the hospitality industry—people might not characterize their negative moods as felt "most of the day." In a culture where sadness or emptiness is a common "background" emotion, the relevant change with depression might not be feeling sad or empty but feeling *more sad than usual* or finding one's usual sadness to be *unusually unbearable*.

2. Markedly diminished interest or pleasure in all, or almost all, activities most of the day, nearly every day (as indicated by either subjective account or observation).

Comment: For people who must spend most of their time on goal-directed activities they don't like—such as "model minority" students striving to get top grades in classes they enrolled in only because of parental pressure or working poor people taking two full-time minimum-wage jobs to support their families—interest and pleasure might be experienced as occasional luxuries. A depression-related loss of engagement in work or study or loss of incidental daily pleasures would be determined by observation of changes in a person's engagement with work or study and their expressed affect when involved in usual activities. There might be no one in the person's life willing or able to make the observations to establish this criterion. In the future, analysis of data from widely available wearable devices, or smartphone-based ecological momentary assessment (EMA), might enable the reliable, quantitative assessment of changes in engagement, interest, and incidental pleasure (Shiffman et al., 2008). When EMA is employed to assess depressive symptoms, cultural differences should be considered in the interpretation of the assessments.

3. Significant weight loss when not dieting or weight gain (e.g., a change of more than 5% of body weight in a month or a decrease or increase in appetite nearly every day). (Note: In children, consider failure to make expected weight gain.)

    Comment: For people living in poverty, with food insecurity, or with only poor-quality food available, either weight gain or weight loss can reflect external conditions more than mental state. Such people might also have clinical depression provoked by their difficult circumstances or associated with nutritional deficiencies, but the weight change per se would not be attributable to depression.

4. Insomnia or hypersomnia nearly every day.

    Comment: Insomnia can be a consequence of excessive work and/or study time or of chronobiological disruption by shift work, fluctuating work schedules, or frequent travel across time zones. Chronobiologically unhealthy schedules are normalized by some occupational cultures, such as those of long-haul airline pilots, truck drivers, and emergency medical personnel. They might be adopted because of parental expectations of extreme study such as those seen for high school students from traditional Chinese families in which academic achievement is a filial obligation and a determinant of status for both oneself and one's family. They can be a consequence of poverty or discrimination in employment related to a person's ethnic identity or immigrant status, leading them to accept work with unusually demanding and unhealthy schedules. The latter include jobs involving long commutes and work with "on-call" assignments and/or last-minute changes in hours of work. In such circumstances attribution of insomnia to depression is difficult, while at the same time the culturally-associated chronobiological disruption could contribute to the development of depressive illness in which sleep disturbance was a symptom.

5. Psychomotor agitation or retardation nearly every day (observable by others, not merely subjective feelings of restlessness or being slowed down).

    Comment: These symptoms are relatively culture-independent. However, in some personal contexts partially determined by culture, there might be no one to notice them, for example, if the person with depression were socially isolated or if the culture normalized depression and minimized the significance of its symptoms. Millions of retired older adults in Japan would have no one to regularly observe their behavior because they are relatively disconnected from their families and have lost their workplace-based social connections. The same lack of "others" to observe behavioral changes might be the case for a recently widowed or recently divorced introvert with limited non-familial social connections and no family members living nearby. A clinical encounter with a socially isolated person would provide a small sample of daily behavior that might not capture symptoms that vary throughout the day. A standardized determination of psychomotor agitation or retardation via analysis of actigraphy data collected by smartphones or wearable devices might in the future be adopted as a more reliable and consistently obtainable measure of agitation or retardation. Should that occur, the normal range applicable to the interpretation of actigraphy data might differ by demographic or other dimensions of cultural identity.

6. Fatigue or loss of energy nearly every day.

   Comment: The symptom of fatigue is a generic presentation of illnesses of many kinds in many cultures. In some occupational cultures, for example those of laborers, agricultural workers, and long-haul truck drivers, fatigue is endemic. Non-specific or occupational fatigue can be mistaken for a symptom of depression, or depression-related fatigue can be misattributed. Fatigue often is the presenting complaint when depressed people seek primary medical care in cultures where depression is heavily stigmatized.

7. Feelings of worthlessness or excessive or inappropriate guilt (which may be delusional) nearly every day (not merely self-reproach or guilt about being sick).

   Comment: In collectivist cultures, self-shaming or anticipated shame, rather than guilt, can be the self-conscious feeling that arises or is intensified during an episode of depression. In some cultures, individuals of minority ethnicity and lower social class are stereotyped as worthless, and the feeling of worthlessness sometimes is internalized by those who are stereotyped. This can be a contributing cause of depression rather than a symptom of it.

8. Diminished ability to think or concentrate, or indecisiveness, nearly every day (either by subjective account or as observed by others).

   Comment: While cognitive dysfunction can be assessed objectively, *change* in cognition requires knowledge of a person's baseline that might not be available for cultural reasons. The affected person might have poor insight into current function or have an inaccurate recollection of prior function. If the person is socially isolated, there might be no one available to comment on baseline function. This might be the case in older, widowed immigrants who are not proficient in the language of the host country and who do not have adult children they see frequently. Cognition might fluctuate with the ingestion of substances commonly used in a person's cultural group or with the course of medical conditions not diagnosed because of poor access to healthcare. Attribution of cognitive problems, rather than identification of them, is the usual diagnostic problem.

People who are illiterate or have little formal education can have low scores on standardized cognitive screening tests although they have no cognitive impairment. People with higher education and cognitively intense occupations can suffer a clinically significant loss of cognitive function and still score perfectly on standard screening tests for cognitive impairment. At both the high and the low ends of expected cognitive performance, screening for depression-related impairment may require adaptation.

A reliable history that a task a person does regularly is now done more slowly, with mistakes, only with assistance, or not at all for cognitive rather than physical reasons is useful in establishing the cognitive criterion for depression. Useful tasks to ask about are ones intrinsic to a person's role given their age, gender, and occupation and within their context of race/ethnicity, location of residence, and socioeconomic class.

9. Recurrent thoughts of death (not just fear of dying), recurrent suicidal ideation without a specific plan, or a suicide attempt or a specific plan for committing suicide.

Comment: The criterion is valid, but in many cultures, including those with low trust and high-context, indirect communication, many people would be unlikely to explicitly disclose suicidal feelings on a survey, questionnaire, or first clinical encounter—and disclosure to a clinician might vary according to the clinician's identity. For example, a Chinese patient might be less likely to disclose suicidality to a Chinese clinician than a White clinician (Albert Yeung, personal communication, 2016). Ascertaining whether suicidality is present might require multiple interviews or clinical encounters, information from third parties, or analysis of non-clinical data, like social media posts. Furthermore, engaging in high-risk behavior entailing a substantial risk of serious injury or even death is not a suicide attempt, but it might be an indicator of depression. In "male depression," a syndrome seen in national, regional, and occupational cultures with high gender role differentiation, engaging in dangerous behavior is a primary symptom (Oliffe et al., 2019; Rice, Oliffe et al., 2018). People with bipolar depression, especially those with mixed symptoms, may display behavior when ill that involves a high risk of death or serious injury but not conscious suicidal intent.

Onset or increase in distressing somatic symptoms is a major symptom of depression missing from the list of nine criteria. The syndrome of clinical depression often includes symptoms like somatic pain, shortness of breath, or indigestion that either are unexplained by another medical condition, are worse in parallel with other depressive symptoms, or have recently become unbearable. Worsening or new intolerability of pain or other somatic symptoms—usually accompanied by insomnia and/or fatigue—is a common presenting symptom of depression in cultures where people with depression usually see traditional practitioners first or where seeing a psychiatrist or other mental health professional is highly stigmatized and seeing a primary care provider or traditional medicine practitioner is not.

The requirement that the symptoms are associated with distress or dysfunction should be seen in cultural context. For adults working in perfectionistic occupational cultures or for students in cultures where perfect test scores are expected by parents, even a minor change in function can be distressing. Distress and self-reproach associated with not meeting perfectionistic expectations might be perceived by the depressed person as natural, even when the person's performance is objectively satisfactory. Subtle changes in function can be difficult to bear in occupational cultures where people are continually operating at the limits of their abilities and expect this of themselves. This can be seen in elite creative and performing artists, athletes, scientists, and entrepreneurs. Functional changes a person from such a culture might find unbearable might be difficult for others to appreciate. Occupationally outstanding, perfectionistic depressed people who think their best work is forever behind them might be at risk for suicide. Suicides by writers and visual artists will be discussed in detail later in this book. Often the co-occurrence of bipolar depression with an unsuccessful creative project is the trigger for suicidal behavior.

Alternative Diagnostic Criteria for Clinical Depression: A Prompt for Dialogue

Alternative, culturally adaptable criteria for clinical depression should accommodate cultural variations by design. They should recognize clinically serious cases that might be subsyndromal by DSM criteria, while not mischaracterizing people with intense but normal sad moods as being clinically depressed. Dr. Allen Frances, leader of the group that developed the DSM, Fourth Edition (DSM-4), eloquently pointed out in his book *Saving Normal* (2013) the clinical and societal downside of over-diagnosing clinical depression in people with strong emotional reactions to loss or disappointment. We here propose a model of culturally aware criteria for clinical depression. It is intended not to replace the DSM criteria for MDD but to prompt dialogue between clinicians and their patients and stimulate productive conversations about depression by people concerned with depression as a problem of populations.

The criteria are both more inclusive and more rigorous: They are more inclusive because culturally related variations in the core symptoms of depression are accepted. They are more rigorous because to be diagnosed as clinically depressed a person must meet *all* of the proposed criteria, not merely a subset of them.

In the proposed alternate criteria for clinical depression, suicidal thoughts, plans, and actions are not listed as core symptoms of depression. While most people with severe depression do have suicidal thoughts, cultural differences in the disclosure of suicidal thoughts and plans are so great that including them in the core symptoms can decrease the reliability of the criteria, and it is inconsistent with a design concept that requires a depressed person to meet all listed criteria. Of course, any clinical assessment of a person with depression would include assessment of suicidality. Supporting this approach is research comparing the PHQ-9 and PHQ-8 (Patient Health Questionnaire for depression, either with all nine original items or dropping the item inquiring about "thoughts that you would be better off dead or of hurting yourself" during the past two weeks). In a meta-analysis of 54 studies from five continents that tested both versions against an MDD diagnosis using a semi-structured diagnostic interview and the same cutoff score for both tests, the PHQ-8 was 2% less sensitive and 1% more specific for MDD, and the correlation between PHQ-8 and PHQ-9 scores in the total study population of 16,742 participants was .996 (Wu et al., 2019). The results of the meta-analysis leave one thinking that the ninth item on the PHQ-9 would perhaps be better off dead.

Suggested Criteria for Clinical Depression (All Must Apply for the Diagnosis to Be Made)

1. *There is a persistent change—or one expected to persist—from one's usual state of health*, affecting the experience of one's life, and one's behavior, in ways that are distressing or unpleasant or make it more difficult or more effortful to conduct daily activities or effectively pursue personal goals. At least three of the symptoms characterizing the change must be present every day. Functional performance is assessed relative to the person's reasonable expectations and past performance.
2. *The change is unlikely to be entirely due to another illness or the effects of a drug or substance*, although another illness or a substance might contribute to it.
3. *Negative thoughts and/or feelings are more frequent, more intense, and/or less tolerable.* Negative thoughts include pessimism, hopelessness, self-criticism, regrets, suspicions, doubts, and sad or painful memories. Negative feelings

include sadness, disappointment, discouragement, fear, irritation, anger, hatred, guilt, shame, envy, and jealousy. (To meet the criterion, at least one type of negative thought or feeling must be more frequent, more intense, or less bearable than before.)

4. *Positive thoughts and/or feelings are less frequent, weaker, and/or less gratifying than before.* Positive thoughts include hopes, optimistic ideas and expectations of future success, confidence in one's abilities, appreciation of others, thoughts of having helped or pleased others or of being appreciated by them, and memories of happy times or of satisfying accomplishments. Positive feelings include happiness, joy, pleasure, interest, satisfaction, love, and affection. (To meet the criterion, at least one type of positive thought or feeling must be less frequent, weaker, or less gratifying than before.)

5. *Less energy is available for useful activity.* The experience might be one of apathy, tiredness, fatigability, slowing down, or being restless or agitated in a way that makes it harder to carry out intended actions or makes purposeful activity less efficient.

6. *Cognition is slower, less accurate, less efficient, and/or less confident.* Executive cognitive functions (e.g., abstract reasoning, organization, and planning) and working memory (maintenance of memories and intentions despite distraction) might be the only functions to change.

7. *Sleep is worse in some way.* Sleep trouble might be difficulty falling asleep, waking up during the night, waking up too early in the morning, sleeping fewer hours, waking up feeling unrested, feeling tired or sleepy during the day, and/or sleeping excessively. One or more sleep symptoms must be new, worse, less tolerable, or more functionally impactful than before.

8. *There is at least one new, worsened, and/or less tolerable physical symptom such as fatigue or weakness, somatic pain or headache, dizziness, shortness of breath, constipation, or indigestion.* The symptom might be preexisting and might be due to a chronic illness or past injury.

9. *The illness is associated with a known or expected, measurable change or abnormality in one or more biomarkers with an established relationship to depression.* Biomarkers of depression currently studied include those related to endocrine function, systemic inflammation, autonomic function, resting state brain activity as measured by functional imaging or quantitative electroencephalography, sleep architecture, circadian rhythm, metabolomics, the lipidome, and the gut microbiome (Deif & Salama, 2021; D. Lee et al., 2021; Lombardo et al., 2021; Lucidi et al., 2021; Mosiołek et al., 2021; Saadat et al., 2020; Tarasov et al., 2021).

Measurement of biomarkers is not currently the standard of practice for assessment and treatment of depression, and biomarkers are unlikely to be measured in epidemiologic surveys of non-clinical populations. However, if a person met all other criteria but either they or another interested party were reluctant to accept the diagnosis, establishing the presence of an abnormal biomarker to corroborate the presence of an illness might be useful. Also, if there were uncertainty about the person's meeting one or two of the symptomatic criteria, an abnormal biomarker would reduce diagnostic uncertainty; and finding no abnormality on a comprehensive panel of biomarkers would help rule out the diagnosis. An emerging option for assessment of a diagnostically significant biomarker is determination of sleep architecture with a relatively inexpensive wearable device in the form of a ring or wristband. Such devices can identify sleep-related biomarkers of depression such as increased sleep latency and time awake after sleep onset, decreased REM sleep latency, and decreased slow wave sleep (Antonijevic, 2008; Assche et al., 2021; Bernert, Luckenbaugh et al., 2017; Bertrand et al., 2021; Chee et al., 2021; Hutka et al., 2021; Lüdtke et al., 2021; Zhang et al., 2021).

Clinical depression is a serious diagnosis that can have profound effects on a person's life, altering the life course for years after the acute illness, even if there is a full remission. While its impact as a global epidemic is recognized by the World Health Organization, it is not consistently recognized, diagnosed, and treated. The lack of consensus in the non-academic community that depression is a serious medical condition is a large part of the problem. Investment in obtaining and using biomarkers might help change perceptions of the nature of depression in the medical profession and among policymakers and others whose decisions affect the availability of effective care.

In addition, biomarkers might be helpful in individualizing treatment so that from the outset a depressed patient would receive treatment that is highly likely to be effective. For example, depressed patients with predominant somatic symptoms including pain and fatigue and abnormally high levels of inflammatory mediators are more likely to attain a full remission of their depressive symptoms on an antidepressant regimen that includes an anti-inflammatory drug or nutraceutical (Bhattacharya & Drevets, 2017; Chi & Lee, 2021; Corrigan et al., 2023; Guo & Jiang, 2017; Sarno et al., 2021). If sleep architecture is consistently measured with a wearable device and there are consistent abnormalities, correction of those abnormalities can be made one of the targets of the patient's treatment. If antidepressant treatment personalized using biomarkers showed >80% efficacy rather than the more typical 60% efficacy seen in antidepressant clinical trials and if most patients treated for depression had full remissions rather than partial ones, there might be wider appreciation of depression as a "real disease" and its treatment as offering more than mere relief of its most unpleasant symptoms. This is highly relevant to treatment persistence and adherence, particularly among cultural groups very cautious about medications and fearful of becoming dependent upon them. As will be discussed in Part II of this book, many Asians and Asian Americans fear that if they or a loved one take an antidepressant drug, they will become addicted to it. They would be unlikely to have a similar fear of a diabetic becoming addicted to insulin because insulin would be viewed as treating an illness and not merely masking its symptoms.

Membership in cultural groups defined by race, ethnicity, or other attributes might be associated with differences in normal ranges for the values of potential biomarkers of depression. These should be considered when biomarkers are used to confirm a depression diagnosis, subtype clinical depression, or personalize treatment. Culturally correlated variation in biomarkers does not make them less useful if the variation is sufficiently understood to enable valid interpretation of the biomarkers.

Examining the DSM criteria for MDD demonstrates the culture dependence of its criteria and the non-equivalence of MDD to clinical depression. Two additional issues emerge when the criteria are examined critically. The first is the importance of bipolar phenomena in subdividing the phenotypes of depression to better interpret illness narratives, engage patients, and plan treatment. Bipolarity is often missed by clinicians from high-income Western nations, even when they and most of their patients have similar cultural backgrounds; when clinicians and patients have cultural differences, the rate of missed diagnoses must be even higher. Recognizing bipolar phenomena less dramatic than hypomania is clinically consequential. Doing so with cultural awareness requires the concept of a bipolar spectrum that includes cyclothymia, subsyndromal bipolar disorder, and depression with mixed features, as well as the variable expression of the bipolar spectrum across cultures. For both unipolar and bipolar depression, screening tests and rating scales are essential to defining the epidemiology of the disorders, identifying people in need of care, individualizing treatment, assessing new treatments, and evaluating clinical outcomes. Subsequent chapters in this section will address culturally aware assessment of bipolarity and cultural issues with the most frequently used questionnaires and rating scales for mood disorders.

The Middle Zones of Depression and Bipolar Illness

The domains of depression and bipolar illness in which cultural considerations matter the most to accuracy of diagnosis, and in which cultural awareness in research and practice might be especially helpful, lie between normality and conditions like mania and melancholia that are universally recognized as "mental illness." In this book these domains are called *middle zones*. People with illness in a middle zone know their condition is not usual for them and find it problematic, but they would not necessarily see themselves as ill, let alone "mentally ill." Middle zone depression does not refer to negative feelings and thoughts that normally accompany a situation of loss or trauma or the heightened emotionality and exploration of the "dark side" often seen in normal adolescent development. The criteria for labeling a difficult time as an episode of clinical depression require *persistence, distress,* and *adverse effect on function.*

Of those who regard themselves as ill, those with relevant experience from prior episodes of illness, or applicable knowledge gained from study, online interactions, or from talking with people they know well often can accurately label their condition as depression or bipolar illness. Others who see themselves as ill will focus on a physical symptom or on the worsening or lesser tolerability of a preexisting general medical condition, perhaps defining their problem as insomnia, fatigue, or worsening of chronic pain. In this case, most of the cognitive, emotional, and behavioral symptoms of depression can be elicited, although people often are reticent about symptoms related to sexuality, suicidality, and occupational performance. Furthermore, the non-somatic symptoms of depression will not necessarily be disclosed on a questionnaire or on a first interview. Either more than one encounter will be needed, or a clinician may need to rely on empathy, cultural awareness, and hypothesis-testing dialogue to determine if they are present. This is often the case when the depressed person comes from—and communicates in the typical manner of—a culture with a high-context, indirect, and/or understated communication style.

Part of the middle zone of depression is occupied by *psychosomatic* or *somatoform* cases—illnesses that present with physical symptoms but include cognitive, emotional, and/or behavioral components that are denied, minimized, or explained away by circumstances. Psychosomatic syndromes of this kind are recognized as illnesses in traditional medical systems and are not classified by them in the same category as psychoses, mania, or melancholia. If a culture stigmatizes them, the stigma is less severe than that of psychotic disorders. In many cultures, cases in the middle zone of depression that are not psychosomatic are not distinguished from normality—they are judged to be unusually strong reactions to life events, perhaps reflecting personal weakness or a sensitive personality. In these cultures, people with middle zone depression that is not psychosomatic might know they are ill but their conditions don't fit into a culturally acceptable category of illness.

Another part of the middle zone of depression comprises cases in which people—usually, but not always, men—express their depression as "externalizing behavior" with such symptoms as problematic substance use, irritability or anger with arguments and altercations, and impulsive behavior, such as high-risk sex or reckless driving. A syndrome of "male depression" was first described in Sweden and subsequently validated in several other countries (Barrigon & Cegla-Schvartzman, 2020; Oliffe et al., 2019; Rice et al., 2020). It will be elaborated in Chapter 13.

The middle zone of depression also comprises cases of occupational *burnout*—a combination of emotional exhaustion, depersonalization, and cynicism related to a person's work. The negative thoughts and feelings of a burned-out person center on their work and might be absent when they are away from work, but they are sufficiently persistent and troublesome that they affect occupational function and cause distress. Mild cases of burnout usually would not meet the criteria for MDD, but most cases of even mild burnout would fit the proposed criteria for clinical depression.

The concept of the middle zone of depression can be helpful in thinking across cultures about depression as a public health, public policy, or educational issue. A campaign to destigmatize mental illness in general can make matters worse for people with middle zone depression, if its effect is to encourage the lumping of middle zone depression—a condition that might be regarded with sympathy and at most mild stigma—with conditions universally stigmatized as mental illness. The problem of stigma and the sometimes-paradoxical effects of anti-stigma messaging will be addressed later in Part I.

Depression Screening Questionnaires

Population screening for depression—including screening of patients in primary care practices and on medical specialty services—usually is done with self-rated questionnaires. Three often used for the purpose in the general population and in primary care are the nine-item Patient Health Questionnaire (PHQ-9; Kroenke et al., 2001), the Beck Depression Inventory (BDI-II; Beck et al., 1996), and the Center for Epidemiologic Studies Depression Scale (CES-D [revised]; Eaton et al., 2004; Radloff, 1977). Similar questionnaires have been tailored for special populations like hospital inpatients (the Hospital Anxiety and Depression Scale (HADS; Zigmond & Snaith, 1983), postpartum women (the Edinburgh Postnatal Depression Scale; Cox et al., 1987), and people with epilepsy (the Neurological Depressive Disorders Inventory for Epilepsy; Gilliam et al., 2006). When a person scores at or higher than a threshold ("cutoff score") on the questionnaire, a clinical interview is performed to confirm the diagnosis of a depressive disorder. In epidemiologic contexts, the interview will be structured with branching logic, based on DSM/ICD criteria. In clinical contexts the interview is less standardized, but the interviewer usually aims to confirm a diagnosis of MDD, another depressive disorder, or a bipolar disorder.

The PHQ-9 has nine questions, one item for each of the nine DSM criteria for MDD. (There are two commonly used variations: The PHQ-8, which omits the item about suicidal ideation, and the Patient Health Questionnaire, two questions (PHQ-2), which includes only the items about mood and anhedonia.) The lookback period is two weeks, in line with those criteria. The respondent (subject or patient) is asked to rate each of the symptoms on a scale of zero to 3, according to the number of days per week on which they were "bothered by any of the following problems." The choices are not at all, several days, more than half the days, and nearly every day. Note that the severity of the symptoms is not considered, only whether the respondent was "bothered" by them. A person from a culture with a stoic outlook might have significant symptoms but not endorse being "bothered" by them, while a person from an emotionally expressive culture might say they were bothered every day by relatively minor symptoms. If a person has a high threshold for acknowledging being bothered, they might have symptoms every day but only count the days when the symptoms were at their worst—leading to underrated symptoms and perhaps a missed diagnosis.

The PHQ-9 does not ask respondents to distinguish symptoms in the last two weeks from their usual condition. A person who had long-standing issues with self-esteem because of low status in their cultural group might answer the question about "feeling bad about yourself" with "nearly every day" or "not at all"—depending on whether they normalized the experience of feeling inferior. In patients from disadvantaged populations, social determinants of health might provide a better explanation of symptoms like weight loss or sleep disturbance than the medical problem of clinical depression.

If the PHQ-9, a test known to be internally consistent, had uniform sensitivity to depressive symptoms across their range of severity and the prevalence of severe depression is lower than the prevalence of moderate depression, one would expect for each item to see more zeros than 1s, more 1s than 2s or 3s, and more 2s than 3s. However, 3s would not be rare because a substantial minority of cases of clinical depression are severe—and in unusual external circumstances there might be slightly more 3s than 2s on some PHQ-9 items. Cultural factors can change the distribution of PHQ item scores, and consequently change the test's psychometric properties if the same cutoff score is used in every context.

If a culture normalizes, minimizes, or rationalizes a symptom unless it is both severe and continual, there will be fewer nonzero scores, but relatively more of the nonzero scores will be 3s. Many cases of middle zone depression will be undetected. If a culture or subculture has a norm of understatement of emotion, the PHQ will be less sensitive for clinical depression in that group if its cutoff score is not adjusted downward. If young men within a culture commonly deal with distressing feelings by using psychoactive substances or by seeking pleasure or adventure, they might rarely report feeling bothered by symptoms "nearly every day" because their symptoms were relieved, masked, or disregarded every weekend. In that situation, a scale more sensitive to externalizing behavior than the PHQ-9 would miss fewer cases of clinical depression and would be less likely to underrate a depression's severity.

The PHQ-9 has an item concerning suicidal thoughts, described as "thoughts you would be better off dead, or of hurting yourself." In a culture where having such thoughts would be highly stigmatized, a person probably would deny them, especially if the questionnaire were not anonymous. Because the item does not measure severity or seriousness of the thoughts, it would give a higher score to someone who had idle thoughts about meaninglessness of life every day than to someone who had an active suicidal plan one day but chose not to act on it.

When treating or studying any specific cultural group, a clinician or epidemiologist would examine PHQ-9 data from a few hundred patients/subjects to see how individual item scores and the summary score were distributed. Application of item response theory (IRT), factor analysis, and a sensitivity/specificity analysis of the PHQ-9 with an interview-based "gold standard" has been done for a range of populations defined by nationality, age, gender, occupation, and other determinants of cultural identity. If in the study population most relevant to the current purpose, an item on the PHQ-9 almost always was rated "not at all" or the item's score did not correlate well with the sum of the other eight items, it would be unsuitable for screening patients for MDD or measuring antidepressant treatment response in that population. Using the sum of the other eight items as the score and adjusting the cutoff score for clinical depression downward would make the scale a more effective and valid screen for depression. An example of this strategy is the use of the PHQ-8 to screen for depression in cultural contexts where respondents are unlikely to disclose or acknowledge death wishes and thoughts of self-harm.

The CES-D is a 20-item questionnaire that provides a list of ways a respondent "might have felt or behaved" during the past week. Like the PHQ-9, it is scored by frequency, measured by day. The responses are "rarely or none of the time (less than one day in the past week)," "some or a little of the time (1–2 days)," "occasionally or a moderate amount of time (3–4 days)," and "most or all of the time (5–7 days)." A typical cutoff score is 16. Four items, which are reverse-scored, relate to positive feelings of being hopeful, enjoying life, being happy, and feeling "just as good as other people." The remaining 16 items cover the core symptoms of major depression but also cover territory not found either in

MDD criteria or in the PHQ-9. There are items about problems in interpersonal relationships, such as feeling that "people disliked me" or that "people were unfriendly." Other items mention feeling lonely and feeling fearful. The CES-D does not have any item related to suicide, self-harm, or death wishes.

Questions tapping into the loss of positive thoughts and feelings and questions about fear, reticence, and negative interpersonal experiences make the CES-D sensitive to a broader range of depression phenotypes than the PHQ-9. A person who would be reluctant to say they were sad, depressed, or having crying spells—for example, a man in a "masculine" culture in which "boys don't cry"—might be willing to acknowledge a lack of joy and happiness or feeling that people seemed unfriendly to him.

However, the same items that make the CES-D more sensitive to depression in people who deny a sad or depressed mood make it possible for a person to score at or higher than the clinical cutoff score for the CES-D because of social problems related to their ethnic/cultural identity. Consider the case of a male Central American immigrant to the United States whose family did not accompany him. Every day he might feel lonely and fearful and that people disliked him and were unfriendly to him. He would talk less than usual. All these feelings would reflect the realities of his experience as an immigrant from a negatively stereotyped minority. It is unlikely that he would be happy and enjoy life five to seven days per week. Based on the items just mentioned, he could score above the cut point for probable clinical depression even if he had no mental disorder whatever.

The BDI comprises 21 sets of one-sentence statements about symptoms of depression. For each group of sentences, the respondent picks the one that "best describes the way you have been feeling during the past two weeks, including today." The sentence scored 0 always refers to the absence of the symptom. The other three sentences increase by number in some combination of frequency, severity, tolerability, and functional impact. For the item on sadness, "I do not feel sad" scores zero, "I feel sad much of the time" scores 1, "I am sad all of the time" scores 2, and "I am so sad or unhappy that I can't stand it" scores 3. The four sentences on sadness do not cover the full spectrum of possibilities; if a person felt extreme, unbearable sadness only on the day of the test, their situation would not fit with any of the options. The scope of items on the BDI goes well beyond DSM criteria for major depression, covering eight discrete negative sentiments that can be increased in depression, including pessimism, a sense of past failure, guilt, self-dislike, feelings of being punished or expecting punishment, self-blame/self-criticism, and worthlessness. The sole item about mood refers to sadness, not depression, the "blues," or unhappiness. There are separate items on irritability and agitation and on tiredness/fatigue and loss of energy.

The BDI is the only one of the three that explicitly mentions sexual interest, referring only to a *change* in sexual interest. Unlike the CES-D, it does not have content on interpersonal aspects of depression like loneliness or feeling disliked. While it has items concerning trouble concentrating and indecisiveness, there is no item that captures psychomotor slowing.

On the BDI with its most commonly used cutoff scores, mild depression begins with a score of 14, moderate depression with 20, and severe depression with 29. It is possible to screen in for moderate depression on the BDI without any physical symptoms and without sadness or depressed mood. At the same time, a person with a somatic or externalized expression of depression might not screen in for depression at all or might score as mildly depressed when they had profoundly disruptive symptoms. Somatic emphasis in the experience and expression of depression is typical of cultures with a traditional mind–body perspective on depression and of those that heavily stigmatize purely "mental" illness. Highly "masculine" and self-enhancing cultures encourage men to express depression with behavior that distracts them from their emotional pain or expresses it interpersonally—rather than with articulating negative sentiments like feelings of guilt, regret, or inadequacy.

The non-trivial differences between the three scales explain why they are imperfectly correlated. They have approximately the same power to predict a diagnosis of MDD, but their false positives and false negatives are different; and analysis of population-specific data would be needed to determine which of the three would be most accurate for use in a specific population. The PHQ-9 is an efficient way to screen for MDD as defined by the DSM. It can miss other phenotypes of clinical depression than MDD, so it should not be relied on for comprehensive screening for clinical depression, especially in cultural groups where non-MDD presentations of depression are common.

The CES-D is especially sensitive to interpersonal aspects of depression. It may be especially useful in collectivistic cultures in which a person's self-concept is closely linked to what they think about their relations with others in the collective. For a person in a collectivistic culture, feeling lonely and disliked and that others are unfriendly is a particularly painful part of depression and one that can lead to suicidality. When the CES-D is used, the occurrence of interpersonal symptoms of depression without other symptoms does not imply clinical depression (let alone MDD). However, a very high level of interpersonal symptoms raises an issue of suicide risk even in the absence of a diagnosis of a depressive disorder. Inquiry about suicidality in the clinical interview is important if a person screens in for depression on the CES-D with prominent interpersonal symptoms since the questionnaire has no item specifically dealing with suicidality or death wishes.

Cutoff scores for triggering an interview for diagnosing MDD can be adjusted to emphasize sensitivity or specificity. If the goal were to capture 90% of cases of MDD, then a false-positive rate of 50% would not be unusual. *Sensitivity* is the percentage of people with depression on clinical examination who would be above the cutoff score on the questionnaire. *Specificity* is the percentage of people without depression on clinical examination who would be below the cutoff score on the questionnaire. *Positive predictive value* is the percentage of people with scores above the cutoff who would be diagnosed with depression on clinical examination. If the prevalence of clinical depression is low in a population, a screening test can have high specificity but low positive predictive value. If the prevalence of clinical depression is high in a population, a screening test with relatively low specificity might have an acceptably high positive predictive value.

Several issues are not visible in a simple analysis of sensitivity and specificity of a screening questionnaire for the diagnosis of MDD. People might have clinical depression without meeting the criteria for MDD, and "non-major" depression can have consequences as severe as long-term disability, loss of employment, divorce, or suicide. Even when clinical depression is equated with MDD, the expected trade-off of sensitivity and specificity is based on sometimes-tacit assumptions that the relationship between screening test scores and the presence and severity of depression is consistent across cultures. However, some cultural groups so stigmatize depression and/or value stoicism that people will not acknowledge depressive symptoms unless they are severe enough to be obvious to all. Even then, many people of the culture will understate them both on a screening questionnaire and in a clinical interview. In such a situation, a test like the PHQ-9 with a standard cutoff score wouldn't identify milder cases of MDD at all, and a small decrease in the cut point for the scale could dramatically increase sensitivity without much loss of specificity or positive predictive value.

Numerous studies of the three rating scales show that the optimal cut points for identification of MDD differ by culture, gender, and clinical context—a few representative ones will be cited in this chapter, and others will be cited in chapters on the cultures of place (Adams et al., 2020; Barbosa-Leiker et al., 2021; Benuto et al., 2021; Blodgett et al., 2021; Getting It Right Collaborative Group, 2019; Kato, 2021; Kiely & Butterworth, 2015; Lopez et al., 2021; Saadat et al., 2020; Suchy-Dicey et al., 2020). A consistent finding is the interaction of gender with other dimensions of identity in determining the psychometrics of depression questionnaires. For example, in a study of secondary school students in Chile, the optimal cut point for the BDI for identifying MDD was 20 for girls and 14 for boys. The study's authors point out that if the usual BDI cut point of 16 were used, the test would identify 89.7% of the girls with MDD but only 55.7% of the boys (Araya et al., 2013).

The findings of psychometric studies of depression rating scales sometimes run counter to one's first impressions of a culture, and when they do, they call attention to how the commonly used questionnaires differ and the importance of the study's context. When the PHQ-9 was studied in a Japanese outpatient psychiatric clinic, the optimal cut point for diagnosing a current major depressive episode was 14, rather than the cut point of 10 typically used to identify moderate depression in primary care (Inoue et al., 2012). How could a *higher* cut point for diagnosing MDD make sense when Japan is a country known for an understated communication style and a literature that normalizes sadness and often condones suicide? Without the data in hand, one can't be sure; but two explanations are plausible: First, the patients with scores of 10–13 were almost certainly clinically depressed even if they didn't meet the criteria for MDD, and many Japanese people clinically depressed by this chapter's criteria wouldn't meet MDD criteria. Second, in a country where most depressed people don't seek treatment, those who sought treatment in the clinic probably had their symptoms more than half of days or almost every day, implying that each item of the PHQ they endorsed would have contributed 2 or 3 points to the total score.

When the CES-D was used as a screen for MDD in low-income women in primary care clinics in Louisiana, a cut point of 34—more than double the conventional cut point of 16—was necessary to reach a positive predictive value of 50% (Thomas et al., 2001). When the CES-D was evaluated as a screener for MDD in low-income Alabama adults on parole or probation, the optimal cut point for women was 23, while for men it was 15. The optimal cut point for White subjects was 3 points higher than for non-White subjects (Henry et al., 2018). Findings like these suggest that people facing multiple adversities might score many points on the CES-D for reasons unrelated to MDD and that gender and race/ethnicity interact with socioeconomic class in the expression of depressive symptoms. So, clinicians working with culturally-distinctive populations should not expect standard depression questionnaires with generic cut points to efficiently find patients needing treatment for clinical depression while not missing many people urgently in need of help for suicidality or depression-related functional impairment.

As noted above, the CES-D has the benefit of broader coverage of depressive symptoms than offered by the PHQ-9, including symptoms relevant to clinical depression that are not included in the criteria for MDD. Such symptoms may be the most distressing ones for an individual patient, and thus an especially important target of treatment. If the goal of screening with a questionnaire is limited to finding cases of MDD, the presence of non-MDD depressive symptoms on the CES-D will lead to false positives for MDD that are not false positives for clinical depression. A systematic review of the CES-D as a screen for MDD in the general population and primary care settings, English-speaking or Spanish-speaking, concluded that a cut point of 20 offered a better trade-off of sensitivity and specificity than a cut point of 16 (Vilagut et al., 2016). From the perspective of this chapter, this is further evidence that people can have clinically significant depression-related distress, suicidality, and impairment of occupational function or family relationships without meeting the diagnostic criteria for MDD. Most of the patients with CES-D scores of 16–19 in the meta-analysis would fit that description.

The PHQ-9, CES-D, and BDI were developed in English, the international language of business and medicine. Commonly used structured interviews for clinician confirmation of diagnoses of major depression and other mood disorders are the Structured Clinical Interview for DSM, Fifth Edition (DSM-5) (First et al., 2015), which was developed in the United States, and the Mini International Neuropsychiatric Interview (MINI; Sheehan, 2015), which was developed by a group of clinical researchers from the United States and Western Europe. The MINI is based on ICD-10 criteria, which are very similar (though not identical) to DSM-4 criteria. Thus, the standard interview-based instruments for confirming categorical diagnoses of depression are based on the DSM concept of major depression and the language used in the DSM to describe its symptoms. To the extent that clinical depression doesn't look like MDD phenotypically, or its symptoms are described with different language from what is typical in high-income Western nations, the self-rated scales and the interview-based standards of diagnosis are subject to similar culture-related limitations and considerations for their valid interpretation.

The three rating scales and the two diagnostic interviews have been translated into many languages, but the psychometric properties of the rating scales—their reliability, internal consistency, and ability to predict the findings of structured clinical interviews—are similar in English and in most published translations. While the patterns and correlates of individual item responses can vary between cultures, total scores on the scales are less sensitive to intercultural differences.

However, the psychometric findings only establish that the questionnaire-based rating scale/screening test accurately predicts the result of a diagnostic interview based on the same underlying diagnostic criteria. That is, if in a specific cultural context, people with clinical depression usually would meet the MDD criteria of the DSM, then a questionnaire like the PHQ-9, BDI, or CES-D with a standard cutoff score usually would find them. If clinical depression in a culture often takes a form that does not fit MDD criteria, both DSM-based clinical interviews and the three standard screening questionnaires would be likely to miss it. In other words, accurate translation of DSM criteria, structured diagnostic interviews, and depression screening tests *between languages* does not ensure equivalence of the phenotypes of clinical depression and optimal screening procedures *between cultures*.

If, in a culture with high-context communication, a rating scale and a structured clinical interview are conducted in the same context, the rating scale score might accurately predict the diagnosis resulting from a structured interview. But if the rating scale were conducted in one context and the structured interview in a different one, prediction might be less valid. In a low-trust culture, people might conceal or minimize symptoms on a non-anonymous questionnaire or in a face-to-face interview with a clinician with whom trust has not been established. If people begin with low trust, depression can increase their suspiciousness because it tends to increase all negative thoughts and emotions. An anonymous online questionnaire or a clinical interview with a trusted primary care physician might yield different answers to the same questions.

The difference made by anonymity is exemplified by the case of airline pilots, an occupation discussed in detail in Chapter 17. Pilots have a high prevalence of depressive symptoms, as assessed by anonymous web-based questionnaires, but a very low rate of diagnosed depression because a diagnosis of depression can cost an airline pilot the medical certification that is required to fly professionally. Within a clinical relationship, answers to some questions may change as treatment continues even when there has been no change in the patient's symptoms. In another scenario, improvement in the patient's depression might initially be offset by the patient's greater candor in acknowledging symptoms as they develop trust in the clinician. If so, a rating scale score might not change even though the patient has improved.

The correlation coefficients between the three most commonly used general-purpose depression questionnaires are in the range of .7 to .8, implying that between one third and one half of the variance in one scale is not explained by variance in another. The scales are not measuring the same construct. If for cultural/linguistic reasons a patient scores over the threshold for clinical depression on the CES-D but not on the BDI, either the CES-D is giving a false positive or the BDI is giving a false negative. The overall predictive power of the three tests might be the same, but one of the three might be better for assessing the presence and severity of a specific phenotype of depression within a specific culture. In the future, computerized adaptive testing will permit depression screening to flexibly adapt to a person's culture, language, and personality.

The most often used depression rating scales have been studied exhaustively using IRT to identify differential item functioning (DIF). (Hagquist and

Andrich [2017] describe application of IRT to the CES-D; see De Ayala [2008] for a comprehensive reference on IRT.) DIF characterizes specific rating scale items that do not correlate with the construct of interest within a given population. For example, the BDI item on sexual interest might have no correlation with depression when the test is administered to women in a traditional masculine culture where the norm is for women not to openly acknowledge sexual interest. The PHQ-9 item on suicidality might be of little value in a cultural group that so heavily stigmatizes suicide that a depressed person already fearful of stigma would be especially unlikely to disclose suicidal thoughts. Because the PHQ-9, the BDI, and the CES-D have very high internal consistency, any individual item can be dropped without greatly affecting the test's psychometric properties as a scale of depression severity or as a predictor of a clinician's diagnosis of MDD on a subsequent interview. However, to the extent that the symptoms behind individual items are a focus of interest for clinical care or population health, a user of a scale would want to know what the literature on DIF has shown for the scale in the cultural group of interest. If DIF hasn't been studied for a given test in a clinical population of current interest, the possible presence of non-functioning or atypically functioning test items should be recognized as an open question.

The relevance of culture to the choice and interpretation of depression questionnaires will be revisited in several chapters of this book. It has often been considered in connection with validation of translations of depression questionnaires from English to another language. Accuracy of translation as determined by back-translation, revision, and review by bilingual expert clinicians does not imply that items will perform equally well as indicators of depression, that factor analyses will yield the same number of factors, or that optimal cutoff scores will be the same. In fact, cross-cultural differences in the psychometrics of common depression questionnaires are so common that studying them proves to be a valuable source of insight into cultural differences in the phenomenology and narratives of depression.

Chapter 3

Beyond Shades of Gray: Depression and the Bipolar Spectrum

Once a person is identified as having clinical depression, it is important to determine if they have a condition in the bipolar spectrum. Compared with those who have only depression (e.g., MDD or dysthymia), those with bipolarity have more episodes of major depression in their lifetimes, and their depressive episodes are more likely to have atypical features such as concurrent hypomanic symptoms. They are more likely to be disabled by their illness, to have suicidal ideation at the same level of depression severity, to make suicide attempts, and to die by suicide (Kamali et al., 2019). More than half of patients with recurrent major depressive episodes (MDEs) and a poor response to medications may have bipolar I disorder (BD-I) or bipolar II disorder (BD-II) (Francesca et al., 2014).

People with bipolar disorders have a high rate of comorbid substance use disorders, especially alcohol use disorders. They have a relatively high rate of comorbid neurological diseases such as migraine, epilepsy, and multiple sclerosis (MS) and a significantly higher rate of hypothyroidism (Sinha et al., 2018). The increased risk of substance use disorders is greater in men than women, and the increased risks of migraine and MS are greater in women than men (R. S. Patel et al. 2018). Despite the high medical comorbidity of bipolar disorder (BD), psychiatrists treating bipolar disorder frequently fail to promptly identify and address medical comorbidities; and neurologists treating migraine, MS, or epilepsy often fail to promptly identify and address comorbid bipolar disorder. Despite the high comorbidity of substance use disorders and bipolar disorder, substance abuse treatment programs often focus narrowly on the substance use issue and do not provide timely diagnosis or adequate treatment of the bipolar condition. This worsens the prognosis for both conditions.

The lack of coordination of psychiatric and general medical care is found throughout the American healthcare system, but the problem is especially acute among patients disadvantaged by race/ethnicity, poverty, and/or limited English proficiency. Routinely providing clinicians with estimates of the probability of comorbidities may be helpful in overcoming clinicians' natural inclination to keep things simple, "stay on their own turf," and use time efficiently. Knowing that the prevalence of hypothyroidism in patients with bipolar disorder exceeds 8% is likely to prompt a mental health provider to order or recommend a thyroid function test if their bipolar patient has not recently had one. Knowing that approximately one third of depressed MS patients will have bipolar disorder is likely to prompt a neurologist or primary care physician (PCP) caring for an MS patient with depression to screen the patient carefully for bipolarity or to refer them to a mental health professional who is likely to do it.

People with bipolar depression respond less well to antidepressant drugs than patients with unipolar depression, and many if treated with an antidepressant alone will get worse, develop a mixed bipolar state ("driven dysphoria"), have new or worsening suicidal ideation, or begin rapidly cycling between depression and hypomania (Rolin et al., 2020; Yalin & Young, 2020). They are more likely to recover from depression and remain euthymic if treated with some combination of pharmacologic therapy and lifestyle modification with involvement of significant others, treatment of general medical comorbidities, and non-pharmacologic therapies including psychotherapy and chronotherapy or light therapy to aid in normalizing sleep and circadian rhythm (Dallaspezia & Benedetti, 2020; Esaki et al., 2021; Geoffroy & Palagini, 2021; Gottlieb et al., 2019, 2021; Hirakawa et al., 2020; McIntyre et al., 2020).

The often-complex treatment needed to attain full remission and prevent relapse in bipolar depression ideally would be managed by a psychiatrist, as few non-psychiatric physicians will have the necessary knowledge, skills, and time; and non-medical mental health professionals will not be able to directly make the multiple medication adjustments often needed to find a regimen that is effective, acceptable to the patient, and compatible with the patient's general medical comorbidities and their treatments. However, in many contexts, direct treatment of bipolar depression by a psychiatrist is infeasible because of a shortage of psychiatrists or because a patient who would accept treatment from a PCP or a non-medical counselor would be unwilling to see a psychiatrist because of stigma or fear.

Because bipolar depression is common and requires different treatment from unipolar depression, it is surprising that standard depression screening questionnaires do not have questions about past hypomanic symptoms. PCPs who prescribe antidepressants to outpatients newly identified as clinically depressed often neglect the issue of possible bipolarity. Screening depressed patients more consistently for bipolar symptoms is an opportunity to improve practice, but it requires even more cultural awareness than diagnosing the syndrome of current clinical depression.

Defining a Bipolar Spectrum

The syndrome of major depression can present for a discrete period —a major depressive episode (MDE)—within a long term course comprising one or more MDEs and no episodes of hypomanic or mixed bipolar symptoms. In this case the Diagnostic and Statistical Manual of Mental Disorders (DSM) and International Classification of Diseases (ICD) classify it as MDD. In practice, an MDE without a history of hypomania or mania is presumed to be MDD, and articles about the psychometrics of screening tests usually relate rating scale scores to an MDD diagnosis, rather than to the diagnosis of an MDE with an open question about bipolarity. If it is an episode within a course of illness with one or more episodes of mania or hypomania, it is properly labeled as *bipolar depression*; and the long-term illness is called *bipolar disorder*, either BD-I if there is at least one episode of mania or BD-II if there are hypomanic episodes only. An implication of this scheme is that when a patient presents with a first MDE, the diagnosis of unipolar MDD is necessarily provisional because if the person has an episode of hypomania in the future, the original illness would be better described not as MDD but as bipolar disorder presenting with an MDE. Other recognized diagnoses in the bipolar spectrum include cyclothymia, depression with mixed features, hypomania with mixed features, and subsyndromal combinations of depressive and hypomanic symptoms. Clinicians treating patients with depression and a suspicion of bipolarity without meeting the criteria for bipolar disorder or cyclothymia might find the diagnoses of "other specified bipolar disorder" and "other specified depressive disorder" useful if a formal diagnosis is required during a protracted process of diagnosis and therapeutic engagement.

To receive a DSM or ICD diagnosis of hypomania a person must have elevated/euphoric mood or irritability plus several associated symptoms such as decreased need for sleep, rapid speech/racing thoughts, or hypersexuality. Three additional symptoms are required if the mood is elevated/euphoric and four if it is irritable but not elevated. If a person has a persistently elevated, euphoric, or irritable mood without the minimum number of associated symptoms, they can be described as having *subsyndromal hypomania*. If they have three or more of the associated symptoms but do not have an elevated, euphoric, or irritable mood, they can be described as having *bipolar features, bipolarity*, or a *bipolar specifier*. If the associated symptoms occur together with a depressed mood, they have *depression with mixed features*. Non-psychiatrist physicians typically don't know the latest formal subdivision of the bipolar spectrum and might lose patience with diagnostic hair-splitting. The frequent and unfortunate result is that the most critical distinction is not made, between depressed people with hypomanic symptoms indicative of a condition in the bipolar spectrum and those without them. Medical students usually see manic and/or hypomanic patients during their psychiatry rotations, so most physicians would recognize overt hypomania in one of their patients. Missed diagnoses usually involve patients on the milder end of the bipolar spectrum—exactly where culture can have the most effect on the expression of illness, whether its symptoms are normalized, and how much the diagnosis is stigmatized.

Among patients with MDEs, disorders in the bipolar spectrum are especially prevalent among those with recurrent, treatment-resistant depressive episodes. The spectrum includes BD-I and BD-II and conditions in which MDEs occur along with episodes of depression with mixed symptoms, subsyndromal hypomania, and/or hypomania seen only when the patient is taking antidepressant drugs. The last of these conditions is sometimes referred to as bipolar III disorder (BD-III).

Optimal treatment for bipolar depression includes not only pharmacologic therapy with medication with established efficacy for that condition but also treatment of substance use disorders and general medical comorbidities if present (as they often are), lifestyle modification focusing on risk factors like inadequate sleep, and psychotherapy. Light therapy—the administration of precisely timed periods of bright artificial light to regulate circadian rhythm and promote normal chronobiology—can facilitate the recovery of some patients with BD (Cuomo et al., 2023; Fregna et al., 2023; Wirz-Justice & Terman, 2022).

First-line medications for bipolar depression comprise lithium, the antiepileptic drugs lamotrigine and valproate, and the second-generation antipsychotic drugs lurasidone, quetiapine, olanzapine, cariprazine, and lumateperone (Kadakia et al., 2021; Kishi et al., 2020; McIntyre et al., 2013, 2020, 2022). Lamotrigine and lithium are as efficacious as antipsychotic drugs for treating bipolar depression, and neither of them carries the stigma of an "antipsychotic" medication or the risk of a drug-induced movement disorder or metabolic syndrome (Yatham et al., 2018).

Unless there is a well-established history of a durable remission on an antidepressant drug alone, antidepressant drugs should not be used initially in the treatment of bipolar depression. They are best reserved for the treatment of residual depressive symptoms that remain after the patient is established on an optimal dose of a well-tolerated mood stabilizer or atypical antipsychotic drug and appropriate nonpharmacologic therapies are under way.

Although a minority of patients with bipolar depression will do well on an antidepressant alone, if an antidepressant is given without a mood stabilizer or antipsychotic drug to a patient with known bipolar depression, the patient must be monitored very closely for signs of hypomania, worsening mental status, risky behavior, or increased suicidal ideation. When a PCP diagnoses an MDE but doesn't appreciate bipolarity and prescribes a selective serotonin reuptake inhibitor (SSRI) antidepressant with a follow-up appointment a month later, there is a significant risk of a poor clinical outcome. The problem of bipolar depression misdiagnosed as (unipolar) MDD is seen worldwide, even in places with easily accessible mental health care and psychiatrically informed PCPs (Hashimoto, 2018; McIntyre & Calabrese, 2019; Shen et al., 2018; Stiles et al., 2018).

Culture-related issues contribute significantly to the problem of misdiagnosis, and greater cultural awareness by physicians might help solve it. Culture-related issues in the diagnosis of bipolar spectrum disorders are most salient at the milder end of the bipolar spectrum, where there is an overlap between adaptive (or at least tolerable) behavioral variations and symptoms of a mental disorder. Emerging biomarkers that distinguish bipolar depression from MDD might be part of the solution, but they are unlikely to substitute for cultural awareness in identifying patients with middle zone depression and bipolar conditions milder than BD-II.

In non-psychiatric settings, depressed patients with bipolar features rarely give histories of mania that would support a diagnosis of BD-I. In a high-income country with wide availability of mental health services, people with frank manic episodes will be seen early in their illness by psychiatrists, or they will be hospitalized and subsequently receive care from mental health professionals. (By DSM criteria, a diagnosis of mania requires hospitalization or evidence of psychosis.) In locales with adequate mental health systems, a patient with a bipolar spectrum disorder who presents to a PCP with depression usually has either had a hypomanic or subsyndromal hypomanic episode for which they were not seen by a psychiatrist, has had an episode of depression with mixed symptoms, or has cyclothymia. They might report or acknowledge periods of decreased sleep, increased activity, risk-taking behavior, expansiveness, or hypersexuality. However, such symptoms might have credible explanations unrelated to hypomania. Sometimes, symptoms truly due to bipolarity are regarded by both the clinician and the patient as normal for a person of the patient's culture with the same age, gender, social class, and occupation.

Screening Questionnaires for Bipolarity

Two screening questionnaires composed of yes–no items are commonly used worldwide to detect bipolar spectrum disorders, much as the PHQ-9 is used globally to detect clinical depression: the 32-item Hypomania Checklist (HCL-32; Angst et al., 2005) and the 13-item Mood Disorder Questionnaire (MDQ; Hirschfeld et al., 2000). Both introduce the idea that everyone has high and low moods and ask respondents to check off behaviors and subjective experiences that characterize their high periods. Both have additional questions concerning the impact of the items checked "yes." The MDQ appears to be slightly more accurate than the HCL-32 in predicting a diagnosis of BD-I or BD-II on a subsequent psychiatric interview, while the latter, with its broader scope, is more sensitive to the milder end of the bipolar spectrum (Camacho et al., 2018; Y. Y. Wang, Xu et al., 2019). Because diagnoses at the milder end of the spectrum are most affected by cultural considerations, the HCL-32 will be discussed further here.

Factor analysis of items on the HCL-32 consistently yields two factors that account for much of the variance in total scores. One comprises items related to elevated mood and increased energy and activity—things that often are positive. The other comprises items related to irritability, distractibility, and risk-taking behavior (Gamma et al., 2013). These two factors have emerged consistently from analyses of HCL-32 scores when the instrument has been used with people of different nationalities and cultural groups. Studies in patients and non-clinical subjects from different contexts and different ethnic groups sometimes yield a third or fourth factor which isn't consistently associated with either of the two principal factors. In an Iranian sample, there were four factors—two positive ones (*physically and mentally active* and *positive social interactions*) and two negative ones (*risky behavior and substance abuse* and *difficulties in social interaction and impatience*) (Haghighi et al., 2011). In a Korean sample, *elated mood* and *increased energy* accounted for most of the variance, but *increased sexual activity* was a third, independent factor (An et al., 2011). In a relatively small American sample, three factors best fit the data: *activity/increased energy*, *risk-taking/irritability*, and *novelty-seeking* (Glaus et al., 2018). The separability of substance use and increased sexual activity from other signs of hypomania according to culture makes sense because there is much intercultural difference in prohibitions against sexual behaviors and variability in permissiveness according to gender, social class, and other intersecting identities.

The items of the HCL-32 associated with each of the two main factors are listed in Table 3.1. The items of Factor 2 more consistently distinguish illness in the bipolar spectrum from adaptive hyperthymia.

In a 12-country study of the HCL-32, men with or without bipolar spectrum disorders score slightly higher on the HCL-32 than women because of higher scores on the second (negative) factor. The positive factor was highest in northern and eastern Europe (Belgium, Germany, the Netherlands, Sweden, Croatia, and Russia) and lowest in Brazil. Some items worked differently according to location and/or gender. For example, in Chinese patients, there was a weaker association of Factor 1 with "higher mood"; and at the same level of hypomania, Chinese women were less likely to smoke than those from the other countries studied. In northern Europe, women were much more likely than men to express hypomania in dressing more colorfully or extravagantly (Angst et al., 2005). These observations can be related to different behavioral

Table 3.1 Two Factors of the 32-Item Hypomania Checklist (Angst et al., 2005)

Factor 1: Potentially positive (elevated mood; increased energy)	Factor 2: Often negative (irritability/distractibility; risk-taking)
Mood is higher, more optimistic	Is more impatient and irritable
Is more self-confident	Is more easily distracted
Needs less sleep	Thoughts jump from topic to topic
Has more energy	Tends to bug other people
Is more physically active	Gets into more quarrels
Has more ideas, is more creative	Takes more risks in daily life
Does things more quickly/easily	Spends more/too much money
Thinks faster	Drives faster, takes more risks when driving
Talks more	Drinks more coffee
Makes more plans	Smokes more cigarettes
Is less shy or inhibited	Drinks more alcohol
Is more sociable, goes out more	Takes more drugs or medicines
Meets more people	Gambles more
Travels more	
Engages in lots of new things	
Enjoys work more	
Makes more jokes or puns	
Dresses more colorfully or extravagantly	
Flirts more, has more sex	

norms: The more unusual or discouraged a behavior is in a given culture, the more hypomanic one would have to be to display it.

In an international study of MDEs (both MDD and bipolar depression) in outpatient psychiatric practices, factor analyses and differential item response analyses were conducted on HCL-32 responses from 5635 patients from Iberia, western Europe (Germany and the Netherlands), eastern Europe (Armenia, Bulgaria, Georgia, Macedonia, Slovakia, and Ukraine), North Africa/the Near East (Bosnia, Egypt, Iran, Morocco, and Pakistan), and the Far East (China, Korea, and Vietnam) (Gamma et al., 2013). Eleven of the 32 potential expressions of hypomania measured by the HCL-32 varied by age and gender in one or more regions, as reflected by different average item scores at the same total score on the scale.

Hypomanic women were more likely than hypomanic men to dress more colorfully or extravagantly. Flirtatiousness and increased sexuality were more frequent in men than women, with a larger gender difference in more "masculine" cultures. In the Far East, increased sexuality decreased with age. Excessive drinking by women was most often seen in western Europe. Excessive drinking by men decreased with age in East Asia but increased with age in North Africa. Risky driving by women was less common in eastern Europe and Iberia than in the other regions.

Average scores for the entire patient population (including outpatients with both unipolar MDD and bipolar depression) were highest in Iberia and North Africa/the Near East and lowest in the Far East, with most of the difference in Factor 1. The difference can be associated with the greater extraversion of Iberian, North African and Middle Eastern cultures than those of the Far East. In studies comparing HCL-32 scores with psychiatric diagnoses, optimal cutoff scores on the HCL-32 for distinguishing bipolar depression (including BD-II) from unipolar MDD have varied by cultural group—for example, 17 for Portuguese (Camacho et al., 2018), 15 for Koreans (Yoon et al., 2017) and Italians (Sasdelli et al., 2013), 14 for Russians (Mosolov et al., 2014), and 12 for Chinese (Yang et al., 2012). The Portuguese study's authors noted that measuring Factor 2 only and using a cutoff score of 2 was more accurate in predicting bipolar depression than using the entire HCL-32. However, given the stigma associated with several of the items in Factor 2 in restrained cultures, using negative items only to diagnose past hypomania would be unlikely to work well with Asian patients. In fact, questionnaires with only positive items proved effective at identifying bipolar depression in Chinese patients.

Zimmerman et al. (2014) developed the Clinically Useful Depression Outcome Scale supplemented with questions for DSM, Fifth Edition (DSM-5) mixed features (CUDOS-M), a questionnaire-based measure for MDD. Patients rate each item on a 5-point scale to indicate the frequency of the symptom during the past week (0 [*not at all true*], 1 [*rarely true*], 2 [*sometimes true*], 3 [*often true*], 4 [*almost always true*]). The 13 items used to screen for hypomanic features are listed in Table 3.2. Note that the emphasis is on elevated mood and increased energy, rather than on irritability, distractibility, risk-taking, and impulsiveness. In the initial validation of the CUDOS-M on a population of 1170 depressed patients from Rhode Island Hospital, some with MDD and some with bipolar disorder, the 13-item hypomania symptom scale showed high internal consistency. The final three items of the scale had correlations of .56, .43, and .46 with the total score. The sample studied was 88.5% White.

The final three items of the 13, those mentioning "wild, impulsive things," spending money, and thinking about sex, did not correlate with the other 10

Table 3.2 Hypomania Items of the CUDOS-M (Zimmerman et al., 2014)

1. I felt so happy and cheerful it was like a high.
2. I had many brilliant, creative ideas.
3. I felt extremely self-confident.
4. I slept only a few hours but woke full of energy.
5. My energy seemed endless.
6. I was much more talkative than usual.
7. I spoke faster than usual.
8. My thoughts were racing through my mind.
9. I took on many new projects because I felt I could do everything.
10. I was much more social and outgoing than usual.
11. I did wild, impulsive things.
12. I spent money more freely than usual.
13. I had many more thoughts and fantasies about sex.

Note. CUDOS-M = Clinically Useful Depression Outcome Scale supplemented with questions about mixed features as described in DSM-5 (Zimmerman et al., 2014).

items when a Chinese translation of the scale was used in a study of 300 depressed inpatients and outpatients from hospitals in eastern China. In that study, factor analysis of the CUDOS-M yielded two discrete factors, one comprising the first 10 items and the other the final three. Even though the items were phrased to avoid mentioning sexual *behavior*, or *excessive* spending, they were associated with "wild, impulsive things" (Du et al., 2021). Further study of the CUDOS-M in diverse cultural groups would be welcome. Social class is particularly relevant to judgments about hypomanic symptoms. If a person has sufficiently high status, their optimism and extraversion might be rationalized, their talkativeness and irritability tolerated, their problematic substance use kept secret with the aid of servants or subordinates, and their gambling and shopping sprees affordable even if later regretted. The same symptoms in a person of the middle class might cause the loss of a job, criticism by family and rejection by friends, and/or financial distress. People of the lower class who are already the targets of stereotyping, prejudice, and disdain from middle class people might suffer no additional loss of reputation and status.

The potentially positive and usually negative groups of hypomanic symptoms are universal. Like depression, hypomania is a medical illness with characteristic biology and not merely a culturally determined phenomenon. However, the cultures of nations and regions, occupations, and religions take different views on the acceptability, tolerability, and potential normality of specific behaviors associated with hypomania. In a nation, region, or ethnic group with a collectivistic and restrained culture, a combination of talkativeness, extraversion, and excessive optimism, coupled with one or more usually negative symptoms like risk-taking or substance use, might evoke a judgment of moral deficiency, poor upbringing, or a mental health problem. In a cultural group with an individualistic, indulgent culture, the same behavior might not evoke either a moral or a clinical judgment unless the consequences of the behavior were clearly negative. This difference might explain why, in the above-cited multinational study, the accuracy of the HCL-32 in predicting psychiatric diagnoses of bipolar spectrum disorders was weakest in Germany and the Netherlands, the nations in the sample that have the most individualistic and indulgent cultures (Gamma et al., 2013).

According to culture, aspects of hypomanic behavior in an adolescent or young adult might or might not fall within the scope of non-pathological follies and adventures of youth. In this respect, young men generally have more latitude than young women. In highly masculine, traditional cultures, behavior that often would be tolerated in a young man typically would provoke a moral or clinical judgment if displayed by a young woman. Feminist subcultures in countries and regions with high gender equality and cultural "looseness" might tolerate in young women hypomanic-like behavior that traditional cultures would allow only for young men. As will be discussed in detail in the chapters on depression and occupational cultures, the culture of the creative professions often accepts hypomanic symptoms as normal or as an admittedly pathological but nonetheless acceptable accompaniment of talent and creative productivity.

Because Factor 1 items are sometimes positive and often acceptable within a culture if not too extreme or discordant with a person's age, gender, class, and occupation, the items of Factor 2 more consistently distinguish people with bipolar spectrum disorders from those without them. Factor 2 has recognized biological correlates. For example, people who score higher on the irritable/risk-taking factor of the HCL-32 have greater variability in sleep–wake times and a preference for a later bedtime even when their moods are normal. They also have more seasonal variation in mood (Bae et al., 2104).

Biomarkers of Bipolarity

There is a clinical need for rapid and reliable identification of bipolar spectrum conditions when people present for assessment and treatment of clinical depression. Optimal methodology would be quick and affordable, would not involve unusual expertise, and would be applicable across a wide range of settings, cultures, and demographic groups. Fulfilling the need will require combining traditional clinical methods with a panel of biochemical, physiological, and digital biomarkers that are either culture-independent or culturally adaptable.

Digital biomarkers that help distinguish unipolar MDD from a depressive episode in a bipolar spectrum disorder already appear feasible. For example, data from any consumer wearable device that accurately records sleep and activity can identify the consistently diminished activity and early morning awakening of a patient with melancholic MDD and distinguish the pattern of late and variable bedtimes, decreased sleep duration, and intermittent hyperactivity shown by patients with a bipolar spectrum disorder or depression with mixed features. Data collected from a wearable device showing distinctive changes in patterns of sleep and activity would have the same physiological meaning regardless of the patient's cultural identity. On the other hand, baseline patterns of sleep and activity are highly dependent on culture and its associated structural factors (e.g., work schedules).

The potential has been demonstrated for using biochemical markers to distinguish bipolar from unipolar depression and to subdivide unipolar depression into phenotypes that are more or less likely to respond to specific antidepressant treatments. For example, bipolar depression and unipolar depression with prominent somatic symptoms have been associated with increased levels of the cytokine IL-6 (interleukin 6; Y. R. Lu et al., 2019; Sarno et al., 2021). A diagnostic algorithm based on patterns of blood levels of specific pro-inflammatory and regulatory cytokines—the "immune-inflammatory signature"—distinguished bipolar depression from unipolar MDD with >90% accuracy in a recent Italian study (Poletti et al., 2021). In a sample of 115 Chinese psychiatric inpatients, elevation of the IL-4 level was most useful in separating those with MDD from those with BD (Lu et al., 2023). A 2023 meta-analysis of cytokines in major psychiatric disorders reached the conclusion that elevated IL-10 distinguished BD, while elevated IL-1β (interleukin 1 beta) was characteristic of MDD. (Zhang et al., 2023). Establishing a standard biochemically based approach to the differential diagnosis of clinical depression will require studies in diverse cultures that would either demonstrate the invariance of a diagnostic algorithm's validity across demographic/cultural groups or validate an algorithm that included one or more demographic/cultural descriptors as independent variables. In addition, the cost of measuring the biochemical parameters and implementing the algorithm would have to be acceptable within diverse systems of care. However, given the high likelihood of an expensive adverse outcome if bipolar depression is misdiagnosed as unipolar and treated with an antidepressant drug alone, highly accurate biomarker-based diagnosis of mood disorders is likely to be cost-effective.

Clinical researchers are beginning to apply machine learning to large sets of physiologic, biochemical, and imaging data of depressed patients from diverse cultural and demographic groups, hoping to create useful diagnostic and prognostic algorithms and to support personalized antidepressant and/ or mood-stabilizing therapy. If diagnostic algorithms focus solely on existing DSM/ICD diagnoses of MDD, BD-I, and BD-II, they will have little to offer patients whose syndromes of clinical depression lie outside of their limits. On the other hand, if biomarkers are used to better understand the full spectrum of depression phenotypes and to personalize treatments, their use will significantly improve the care of people with clinical depression in the middle zone. Broad acceptance of diagnostic biomarkers of depression by the general medical community might help destigmatize depression, by spreading the news that clinical depression is a genuine disease.

Artificial intelligence (AI) for identifying, distinguishing, and phenotyping mood disorders might also be applied to records of smartphone activity, including the number, length, timing, and diversity of phone calls and text messages; spelling errors in texts; the use of emojis; and people's locations when making calls and sending texts. The data to which AI would be applied would include demographic and cultural context. One challenge in developing such technology will be obtaining consent from people to share their medical histories and allow their linkage with details of their smartphone use. This is likely only within high-trust cultures.

Until utilization of biomarkers becomes the standard of practice, there is great clinical value in establishing the presence or absence of bipolar features ("bipolarity") in depressed patients who don't warrant a diagnosis of BD-I or BD-II. Since identifying and noting bipolarity or "mixed features" does not necessitate the recording of a stigmatizing diagnosis, questionnaires like the HCL-32 can be used to enhance depression care if clinicians consider cultural identities in interpreting patients' responses. For tracking the course and treatment response of a person with a bipolar spectrum disorder in clinical practice, a suitable depression rating scale can be combined with a personalized, ad hoc hypomania scale that includes only the items on the HCL-32 that the patient indicates are typically present in their discrete periods of elevated or irritable mood.

Chapter 4

Dimensions and Implications of Cultural Identity

The *Oxford English Dictionary*, third edition, offers three related definitions of *culture* relevant to the cultural lens, viz. definitions 7a, 7b, and 7c of culture as a noun (Oxford University Press, n.d.). Simplified, and with examples for each, they are as follows:

a. *The distinctive ideas, customs, social behavior, products, or way of life of a nation, society, people, or period.* Examples: Japanese culture, Mexican American culture, Afro-Caribbean culture, the culture of the antebellum Deep South.
b. *A way of life or social environment characterized by or associated with a specified quality or thing.* Examples: upper-class culture, millennial culture, gun culture.
c. *The philosophy, practices and attitudes of an institution, business, or other organization.* Examples: the culture of Hollywood, the culture of elite universities, military culture, the culture of truck drivers.

A complementary and elegant definition was given by Professor Geert Hofstede (1928–2020), a social psychologist who devoted his career to studying (and ultimately to influencing) culture's impact on organizations. He described culture as "software of the mind," a "form of collective programming that distinguishes groups from one another, influencing their behavior, reflected in the meanings they give to various aspects of life, and embodied in the groups' organizations and institutions" (Hofstede et al., 2010).

People belong simultaneously to several cultural groups; cultural identity goes beyond nationality or ethnicity. Cultural identities can combine or "intersect"; for example, the intersection of nationality, ethnicity, socioeconomic class, occupation, gender, and life stage can describe a cultural identity associated with characteristic narratives of depression. One of a person's cultural identities might give insight into the precipitating cause of a depressive episode or the trigger of a suicide attempt, another might best explain the symptom profile, a third might account best for the person's self-stigmatization, and a fourth might aid in choosing a treatment acceptable, feasible, and likely to be effective.

People's self-perceived cultural identities can differ greatly from the ones assigned to them by others. For example, physicians from negatively stereotyped ethnic minorities might identify themselves with their profession rather than with their ethnicity, but some of their patients might discriminate against them because of ethnic stereotypes that they apply without regard to the physicians' qualifications, skills, or conduct as clinicians. Gender or age often triggers stereotyping, as when a young female physician is assumed by patients to be a nurse. At a world-renowned Boston teaching hospital, physicians' ID badges now display the word *DOCTOR* in large, bold, capital letters so that patients won't do this.

In constructing the cultural lens, three facets of cultural identity are considered:

- *Cultural background*: To which cultures and subcultures does a person belong, as defined by nationality and ethnicity, socioeconomic status, education, occupation, religion, gender, age, relationship status, and, if applicable, identity as a first-, second-, or third-generation immigrant or refugee? Is the person's cultural identity best characterized by an intersection of cultural group memberships? Is the person in the process of acculturation? If acculturating, is the person best described as bicultural, assimilated, isolated, or alienated? Is the person a non-conformist or outlier within an ethnic or other cultural group? (The issue of non-conformity is especially salient for people with non-conforming gender identities and/or a homosexual or bisexual orientation. Ethnic and occupational cultures differ greatly in their acceptance of non-conformity related to gender or to sexual orientation, and the group culture of similarly non-conforming individuals differs according to their other intersecting identities.)

- *Self-definition*: Which cultural identities are most important to the person's concept of self and presentation of self? Are there cultural identities that the person minimizes, denies, disavows, or does not recognize? Does the person feel pride or shame about a cultural identity? Does the person feel different in an important way from others of the same culture? Is the person in a process of changing cultural identity, related to entering a new occupation, to acculturation following immigration or inter-regional migration, or to an event like marriage, divorce, childbirth or adoption, retirement, development of a new chronic disease or disability, a major change in wealth or income, or "coming out" as gay, lesbian, or bisexual?

- *Others' perceptions*: With what cultural groups does the person have regular contact? How is the person seen and treated by members of those groups? Does the person experience stereotyping, prejudice, discrimination, hostility, or microaggressions based on one or more of their cultural identities?

If a member of a community defined by ethnicity or by occupation, how is the person treated by other members of that community? Is the person seen as a loyal group member or as a non-conformist or rebel? Does the person receive support or experience ostracism or indifference?

Dimensional Characterization of Cultures

Cultures have been characterized dimensionally by social scientists interested in the functioning of organizations around the world. The same dimensions of culture used to explain variations in organizational function are relevant to depression, via their influence on the experiences, values, and relationships of individuals. They relate to the circumstances that trigger depressive episodes; to self-disclosure; to help-seeking; to normalization, rationalization, and/or justification of trauma; to social capital that buffers stress and protects against depression; and to the stigma of depression. They affect the probability of suicide through their relationship to individuals' meaning and purpose in life, their hopefulness or hopelessness, and their social resources in adversity. In constructing the cultural lens, three valuable characterizations of culture are Geert Hofstede's (2011) six dimensions, the dimension of trust explored in detail in the work of Francis Fukuyama (1995), and the trust-related dimension of social capital. The latter concept, first introduced early in the 20th century, has been elaborated and specified by many contemporary social scientists, of whom Robert Putnam (2000) and Pierre Bourdieu (1997) are often-cited examples.

Geert Hofstede (1928-2020), a Dutch sociologist, originally identified four characteristics ("dimensions") that distinguish national or ethnic cultures; two more were added later in collaboration with his colleagues Michael Bond and Michael Minkov (Hofstede et al., 2010). These dimensions are general tendencies; there are many exceptions even in the majority population, and there may be even more exceptions among ethnic minorities or regional subcultures within a national culture. For each of the six dimensions there are countries with majority cultures that are close to one pole of the dimension. Such cultures have most (but usually not all) of the features that Hofstede and his colleagues describe for a cultural dimension. Following are descriptions of the dimensions, with examples of countries high, intermediate, and low on them. Contrasts between nations with obvious commonalities are pointed out. Inferences are drawn concerning the relevance of the dimensions to depression and the bipolar spectrum. Nations' relative scores on Hofstede's dimensions cited here are taken from a reference website established and maintained by Hofstede and his colleagues and successors (Hofstede-Insights, n.d.). The following paragraphs describe Hofstede's dimensions. They are accompanied by tables with salient examples of differences between countries on the dimensions. Hofstede-Insights scores cultural dimensions on a scale of 1 to 100. In the tables, countries are grouped into quintiles by their scores. The tables include the English-speaking countries, the Nordic nations, and selected nations of Asia, the Middle East, western Europe, and Latin America. The text includes some comments on nations not shown in the tables.

1. *Individualism/collectivism* (Table 4.1): In an individualistic culture, people are expected to take care only of themselves and their immediate families, personal expressions of opinion are expected and valued, other people are judged as individuals, and a right to privacy is recognized. Guilt is the principal self-conscious emotion felt when a person transgresses a norm. In a collectivistic culture, people identify with clans or extended families that offer protection in exchange for loyalty, maintenance of harmony is more important than everyone having a say, other people are judged according to group membership, and privacy is less important than belonging. Transgressions lead to shame—both external shaming and self-shaming.

   The United States, the United Kingdom, and Australia have the highest individualism scores overall, with Ireland and New Zealand close behind, though individualism is lower in specific regional and ethnic subcultures. For example, in the American state of New Mexico, a more collectivistic Mexican American subculture is expressed by a plurality of residents. The major nations of Asia are high on collectivism, except for India, which is intermediate. Taiwan is more collectivistic than mainland China, perhaps reflecting greater adherence to tradition, as in its continuing to use traditional Chinese writing. The Nordic nations are all moderately individualistic (Iceland scores 60, just below the breakpoint between quintiles), as is Switzerland. Thus, moderate individualism is a feature shared by the "world's happiest countries." The Central and South American nations are collectivist except for Argentina, which is intermediate. Central America, poorer and

Table 4.1 Individualism/Collectivism

Individualistic	Australia, United Kingdom, United States
Moderately individualistic	Canada, Denmark, Finland, France, Germany, Ireland, Italy, the Netherlands, New Zealand, Norway, Sweden, Switzerland
Intermediate	Argentina, Iceland, India, Israel, Japan, Spain
Moderately collectivistic	Brazil, Chile, China, Hong Kong, Mexico, Portugal, Saudi Arabia, Turkey
Collectivistic	Costa Rica, Guatemala, South Korea, Taiwan

more unequal than South America, is more collectivistic. In both the Nordic nations and Latin America, indigenous minorities are more collectivistic. Apart from Spain and Portugal, the nations of western Europe tend toward individualism. Moving eastward, Poland, Austria, the Czech Republic, and Hungary are significantly more collectivistic than the nations of western Europe, though still intermediate by world standards. The African countries are collectivistic, except for South Africa, which falls within the range of European countries. Within the nations of sub-Saharan Africa, there are tribal differences in the extent of collectivism.

Like other cultural dimensions, collectivism cuts both ways with respect to its effect on depression, bipolar illness, and suicide. People with harmonious relationships with their collectives—extended families or organizations—can access social support and assistance in adversity that helps them deal with stress and protect them against depression. However, if people are rejected by their collectives for non-conformity with their explicit or implicit rules or because of an illness stigmatized by their collectives, they suffer a major loss that can cause or exacerbate depression or bipolar illness. At worst, such rejection contributes to suicidal intentions and actions. A discrete episode of depression or hypomania can cause a change in a person's status within the collective that persists long after the mood disorder has remitted.

Those respected and supported by a collective (e.g., an extended family) might feel lonely and vulnerable after migration alone or with their nuclear families to a country or region with an individualistic culture. On the other hand, those experiencing ostracism in their native country or region for non-conformity with the collective's rules and expectations might find greater tolerance or even support after their move. These losses and gains affect the risk of emotional distress or clinical depression in response to stresses in their new home, which include those related to acculturation, separation from loved ones, and being the target of stereotyping or discrimination.

2. *Power distance* (Table 4.2): When a culture has high power distance, authority is a fundamental aspect of culture; authorities are to be respected whether they are right or wrong. Children are to be obedient, and elders are to be respected. Government is authoritarian, and corruption is expected and tolerated. Regimes change through coups and revolutions rather than through legitimate elections with widely accepted results. There usually is high inequality of wealth and income, though Japan is an outlier in this respect.

In a culture with low power distance, authority is contingent, with leaders held to moral standards. Adults treat children more as equals and do not

Table 4.2 Power Distance

High	Guatemala, Mexico, Saudi Arabia
Moderately high	Brazil, Chile, China, France, Hong Kong, India, Portugal, Turkey
Intermediate	Argentina, Italy, Japan, South Korea, Spain, Taiwan
Moderately low	Australia, Canada, Costa Rica, Finland, Germany, Iceland, Ireland, Norway, Sweden, Switzerland, United Kingdom, United States
Low	Denmark, Israel, New Zealand

accord elders special respect or deference. Government is democratic; corruption is relatively rare, and it is not accepted as normal. There usually is relatively low inequality of wealth and/or income—but the United States is a salient exception.

In Asia, power distance is moderately high in mainland China, Hong Kong, and India and intermediate in Japan, South Korea, and Taiwan. Taiwan's lesser power distance than mainland China might be related to its longer relationship with the West, its being a high-income country, and its decades of democratic government. Power distance is moderately high or high in most of Latin America but intermediate in Argentina and moderately low in Costa Rica. The latter two countries have distinctive ethnic compositions and political histories that help explain their lower power distance. The English-speaking countries and the Nordic nations have moderately low or low power distance.

Among countries with low power distance overall, those with high wealth and/or income inequality have relatively greater power distance. Regional or ethnic subcultures can differ in power distance from the majority culture of a nation or region. For example, there is more power distance in the Deep South or greater Appalachia than in New England or the Pacific Northwest. Religious subcultures like those of Hindus, Muslims, and LDS Christians have high power distance; and those of liberal Protestant sects and reform Judaism have low power distance.

While countries with high power distance virtually all have large inequality of wealth and/or income, the converse is not true. In the past half-century, wealth and income inequality have increased dramatically in the United States. However, the power distance has not increased in parallel because high power distance is contrary to American tradition.

In cultures with high power distance, mild hypomania might be tolerated in a person with power and authority but have dire social consequences in a person with low status in the hierarchy. Cultures with high power distance tend to have relatively low upward mobility. An ambitious and talented person who is low in the hierarchy of power might find their path to success blocked and become depressed as a result.

3. *Uncertainty avoidance* (Table 4.3): *Uncertainty avoidance* is difficulty accepting change and ambiguity. In cultures with high uncertainty avoidance, people rely on rules that rarely change; authorities are relied upon to teach and enforce rules; people believe in ultimate truths that do not change with context or new evidence; people with deviant or non-conforming opinions or behavior may suffer bullying or social ostracism; and people rarely change jobs, even if they are dissatisfied with their working conditions. In cultures with low uncertainty avoidance, ambiguity is expected, rigid rules are disliked, and authorities don't have all the answers. Doubt and skepticism are common. Strongly held opinions are subject to change if scientific experiments or factual observations show them to be wrong. People change jobs relatively easily. Non-conformity is acceptable.

In western Europe, the United Kingdom and Ireland have moderately low uncertainty avoidance, as do Denmark and Sweden. Finland, Iceland, and Norway have intermediate uncertainty avoidance, as do the Netherlands and Switzerland. The larger nations of western Europe are high or moderately high on that dimension. In Asia, Hong Kong, Singapore, and Malaysia have low uncertainty avoidance; Japan, Pakistan, and Taiwan have high uncertainty avoidance; and mainland China, India, Indonesia, the Philippines, and Thailand all are intermediate. The United States has intermediate uncertainty avoidance that varies significantly by region. Jamaica has remarkably low uncertainty avoidance, second only to Singapore and even lower than Denmark or Sweden.

Living in a culture with high uncertainty avoidance can be difficult for people with non-conforming opinions; they may suffer loneliness

Table 4.3 Uncertainty Avoidance

High	Costa Rica, France, Guatemala, Japan, Israel, Mexico, South Korea, Turkey
Moderately high	Germany, Italy, Saudi Arabia, Taiwan
Intermediate	Australia, Canada, Finland, Iceland, Netherlands, New Zealand, Norway, Switzerland, United States
Moderately low	China, Denmark, Hong Kong, India, Ireland, Sweden, United Kingdom
Low	Jamaica, Singapore

or emotional trauma from social ostracism. Difficulty in changing jobs without damaging one's career or reputation implies that a person may feel compelled to stay in a job with noxious, dangerous, or otherwise depressing physical conditions; adverse social conditions (e.g., bullying); or high work demands without commensurate control (e.g., continually changing shifts, excessive overtime, schedule changes on short notice). Uncertainty avoidance is associated with greater stigmatization of depression and especially of bipolar illness.

4. *Masculinity/femininity (high gender role differentiation)* (Table 4.4): The dimension of culture labeled *masculinity/femininity* by Hofstede refers to the extent of gender role differentiation—how much men and women are expected to conform to traditional stereotypes of male and female behavior. We prefer to designate this dimension as *gender role differentiation*. In cultures with high gender role differentiation, men are expected to be assertive and ambitious, to privilege work over family, to fight back if challenged, and not to cry or display weakness. Strong men are admired. Sexual activity, especially for men, is primarily a form of performance rather than an expression of intimacy (dopamine vs. oxytocin, metaphorically speaking). In cultures with lesser gender role differentiation, both men and women are expected to be modest and caring, both men and women seek work–family balance, men may cry without a loss of dignity or status, and fighting is discouraged. There is sympathy for the weak. Sexual activity is primarily a way of relating.

Japan is high on the dimension of gender role differentiation, as are Austria, Hungary, Italy, and Switzerland. China, Germany, the United Kingdom, the United States, and Australia have similar moderately high ratings. Among the Spanish- and Portuguese-speaking countries, Venezuela and Mexico have high scores on this dimension, while Chile, Costa Rica, and Portugal have relatively low scores. The Nordic countries are known

Table 4.4 Masculinity/Femininity (Gender Role Differentiation)

High	Japan
Moderately high	Australia, China, Germany, Ireland, Italy, Mexico, Switzerland, United States, United Kingdom
Intermediate	Argentina, Brazil, Canada, France, India, Hong Kong, Israel, New Zealand, Saudi Arabia, Taiwan, Turkey
Moderately low	Chile, Finland, Guatemala, South Korea
Low	Costa Rica, Denmark, Iceland, Norway, Sweden

for low gender role differentiation and low gender inequality in the workplace and the political sphere. Among them, Finland has the lowest gender role differentiation with a score of 26 out of 100—though, as will be detailed in Chapter 13, it might normalize intimate partner violence that usually involves a male perpetrator and a female victim. On the same scale, the United States scores 62, and China scores 66. In the United States, there is substantial regional and ethnic variation in the dimension of gender role differentiation, with its more politically conservative and religiously observant regions scoring higher. Immigrants to the United States from Latin America and from Islamic nations have higher gender role differentiation, consistent with the cultures of their native countries.

Greater gender role differentiation is associated with more gender inequality; but the concepts are different, and there are nations relatively high on gender role differentiation but relatively low on gender inequality, such as Ireland (ranked ninth out of 156 for "gender parity") and Switzerland (ranked 10th). In this comparison, gender role differentiation is measured by questionnaire-based surveys using Hofstede's criteria, and gender inequality statistics come from the World Economic Forum's *Global Gender Gap Report* (2023), which measures and ranks countries on women's political empowerment, health and survival, educational attainment, and economic participation and opportunity.

With respect to depression, non-conformity with the expected gender role for one's culture can have negative social consequences, including conflicts with one's family and disapproval or emotional distance from peers and colleagues. In cultures with high gender role differentiation, men who openly express sadness or seek professional help for depression may be viewed negatively as weak and unmanly, with the consequence of shaming, self-shaming, or loss of social status or occupational opportunity. Hyperthymic or mildly hypomanic behavior may be more tolerated in men and less tolerated in women in cultures with more gender role inequality. Finally, given the importance of assertive behavior, physical strength and aggressiveness, and sexual performance in the definition of masculinity, a man in such a culture is likely to suffer a significant loss of status and self-esteem if he has a physical illness or injury that makes him physically weaker or less mobile, or causes sexual dysfunction. Men who have such illnesses or injuries have a high depression risk. Depression, if it occurs, is likely to affect physical and/or sexual function, implying further negative impact on their self-esteem and social status.

5. *Short-term orientation/long-term orientation* (Table 4.5): In cultures with a *short-term orientation*, the past and the present are more important than the

Table 4.5 Short-Term Orientation/Long-Term Orientation

Short-term orientation	Argentina
Moderately short-term orientation	Australia, Canada, Chile, Denmark, Finland, Iceland, Ireland, Israel, Mexico, New Zealand, Norway, Saudi Arabia, United States
Intermediate	Brazil, India, Sweden, Turkey, United Kingdom
Moderately long-term orientation	France, Hong Kong, Italy, Switzerland
Long-term orientation	China, Germany, Japan, South Korea, Taiwan

future, good and evil are absolutes, service to others is an important goal, people consume freely, and students attribute success or failure mainly to luck. In those with a *long-term orientation*, the future is more important than the present or the past, good and evil are contingent on circumstances, thrift and perseverance are valued over altruism and savings over consumption, and students attribute success to effort and failure to lack of effort.

China (including Taiwan and Hong Kong), Japan, and South Korea have a long-term orientation. The United States, the United Kingdom, Australia, New Zealand, and Norway have short-term orientations. Among nations in the Western Hemisphere, Brazil has the most long-term orientation, though it is not as high on this dimension as China, Japan, and South Korea. The Philippines has the most short-term orientation of the major Asian nations.

In cultures with a long-term orientation, excuses for failure at school or work are not accepted, and there is relatively little sympathy for people who are unemployed or financially distressed, even when the cause is external and beyond the individual's control. Financial problems, job loss, or other practical problems due to depression or bipolar illness would more likely lead to disapproval rather than to offers of assistance. People from cultures with a long-term orientation live frugally relative to their incomes, save money, and prepare for adversity—and thus might avoid some of the personal catastrophes that trigger episodes of depression. During the COVID-19 pandemic, the financial hardship of people with moderate incomes pre-pandemic has been worse for those with a short-term orientation as they typically had accumulated less wealth before the economic disruptions of the pandemic began. A higher rate of financial distress (e.g., food or housing insecurity) has been associated with a higher prevalence of depression. In Chapter 14 we present analyses of survey data that show how financial hardship, cultural identity, and region of residence interacted as determinants of depression among Americans during the pandemic.

Life-threatening illness, natural disasters, and global economic crises can be overwhelming even to those with substantial savings and a cautious outlook. A case of metastatic cancer can exhaust a family's savings, from a combination of lost income and healthcare costs not covered by insurance. Major earthquakes, hurricanes, and floods can destroy houses beyond repair; and even when losses are insured, life and work can be disrupted for months. In the Great Recession of 2007–2009 many thrifty people lost their jobs, their homes, and/or their small businesses. In the COVID-19 pandemic, many previously successful small businesses failed because of a loss of business related to lockdowns and other restrictions. However, even when bankruptcy or business failure is attributable to extraordinary circumstances, it might nonetheless be stigmatized in cultures with a long-term orientation, raising the risk of depression for a person facing financial adversity.

People from cultures with a short-term orientation are more likely to be sympathetic and forgiving toward people who suffer financial reversals, even when their troubles were made worse by their emotional reactions to them. Mildly hypomanic behavior is less likely to be stigmatized in cultures with a short-term orientation.

6. *Indulgence/restraint* (Table 4.6): In an indulgent culture, leisure, having fun, sports, free speech, and enjoyment of food, sexual activity, and sensual pleasures are valued. People are more likely to remember positive experiences and emotions. In a restrained one, immediate gratification is valued less, and people are expected to control their appetites and their self-expression. People are more likely to remember the negative feelings and experiences in their lives.

North America, Latin America, and western Europe have relatively indulgent cultures. Most Asian countries and Islamic countries have restrained cultures. Japan is the most indulgent of the major Asian nations. Although

Table 4.6 Indulgence/Restraint

Indulgent	Mexico
Moderately indulgent	Argentina, Australia, Canada, Chile, Denmark, Iceland, Ireland, New Zealand, Sweden, Switzerland, United States, United Kingdom
Intermediate	Brazil, Finland, France, Japan, Norway, Taiwan, Turkey, Saudi Arabia
Moderately restrained	China, Germany, India, Italy, South Korea
Restrained	Hong Kong

its culture is more restrained overall than the cultures of western Europe or the United States, Japan has a long tradition of hedonism, celebrated in the *ukiyo* (浮世; "floating world") of the Edo period (1603–1868)—a sensual, materialistic, and erotic lifestyle of Japan's urban merchant class documented in the art and literature of the period (Fiorillo, n.d.). A nation known for geishas, karaoke bars, *washoku* (和食; traditional Japanese cuisine), and the association of corporate work with extensive after-hours drinking and entertainment cannot be characterized simply as a restrained culture. Japan's paradoxical culture of hard work and pleasure-seeking will be explored further in Chapter 11.

People from restrained cultures are more likely to have depressive symptoms because of their focus on the negative, but they are not necessarily more likely to develop clinical depression. Their behavioral conservatism makes them less likely to engage in risky behaviors with potentially depressing consequences. They tend to be stoic, and thus may be able to tolerate mild clinical depression better than people from indulgent cultures. In such cultures, mildly hypomanic behavior is unacceptable except for people from specific subcultures, like those of successful creative professionals and of male university students from upper-class families. (Even then, intersecting identities such as religious affiliation might still make hypomanic behavior unacceptable.) In more indulgent cultures, hyperthymia or even mild hypomania might be more acceptable, though not among people in occupations requiring highly controlled behavior, punctuality, and reliability. The populations of more indulgent countries tend to have lower average levels of depressed mood than those in more restrained ones because they find more enjoyment in daily life. Their greater pleasure in daily life makes them happier, but it does not protect them from clinical depression. If they become clinically depressed, they may be less able to bear it than someone from a restrained culture who was enculturated to be stoic and has had more practice in self-denial and in bearing frustration and disappointment.

The six dimensions of culture described by Hofstede and related to nationality are subject to interaction with or preemption by other identities. In all nations, the culture of the armed services is collectivistic, with high power distance, high uncertainty avoidance, and high gender role differentiation. In collectivistic nations with high power distance, the upper class might be more individualistic and indulgent than other socioeconomic classes. Women in individualistic cultures might be more collectivist than men. Rural areas often have more collectivistic, long term–oriented, uncertainty-avoidant, and restrained cultures than urban areas of the same countries.

Trust

Trust is a dimension of national or regional culture largely independent of the six described by Hofstede, though it is lower in cultures with high power distance and often is low with respect to "out-groups" in collectivistic cultures. It is a component of social capital. *Trust* at the individual level is a person's willingness to rely on another's actions, attributing to the other honesty, fairness, benevolence, and competence. At the cultural level, *trust* is the widespread acceptance of norms of behavior and the rule of law and confidence in the predictability of others' behavior. In a high-trust culture, people are willing to rely upon other people they don't know personally. Contracts are honored, and loans are repaid. Signatures are trusted to be valid without a fingerprint or notary's stamp. Employees can be relied upon to do their jobs without continuous supervision and checking up. Corruption in government is a scandal with consequences and not something accepted as inevitable. Physicians and lawyers can be counted on to respect confidentiality.

High trust in a culture is associated with higher economic productivity (Fukuyama, 1995) and with lower crime rates and less fear of crime. One way it is assessed in surveys is by asking people whether they think most people in their society are trustworthy. Variations among nations in the answer are remarkable, but the question is inadequate by itself. In a place with high power distance, a middle-class or working-class person might feel that "ordinary people" in their country are trustworthy but that people with power and high status cannot be trusted by people of lower status. In addition, the citizens of a country might hold opinions about the trustworthiness of people from specific ethnic minorities or occupations that differ from their general view of the trustworthiness of their neighbors. In the Social Capital Project of the U.S. Senate, to be discussed in detail in Chapter 14, the measure of trust includes answers to questions about trust in corporations, the media, and the public schools to "do the right thing" (Joint Economic Committee, 2018a).

Even in low-trust cultures, physicians or clergy might be trusted. In high-trust cultures, physicians usually are trusted. Clinicians of other types, such as traditional healers, might be trusted to be honest but not necessarily to consistently be competent or effective. On the other hand, in lower-trust cultures, trust in physicians often is conditional, varying according to the setting of care, the nature of the problem, the ethnic background of the physician, and the physician's qualifications and reputation.

In the United States many people rely on online reviews to select physicians. Phony reviews or false credentials are not a major worry for most people. In China there is widespread suspicion of the validity of online reviews. While there are fraudulent reviews in the United States and valid ones in China, the difference in general attitudes distinguishes one culture as high-trust and the other as low-trust. In China the usual choice for a person of means who is seriously ill is to consult a physician who is famous or has a leadership position in a hospital or clinic, often using personal connections to arrange a timely appointment (X. Zou et al., 2018). To ensure the physician gives the patient the very best care, the patient might discreetly present the physician with a gift—a cash gratuity in a *hong bao* (红包; "red envelope")—at the time of the first visit (Zhu et al., 2018).

Trust can affect the validity of depression screening procedures, including both questionnaires and face-to-face interviews. People who do not presume that strangers are trustworthy may be reluctant to disclose personal information relevant to depression to someone they have just met. Questions about suicidal ideation, substance use, and sexual interest can be especially problematic. First encounters with physicians may entail the same issues: Many clinicians we have interviewed observed that their patients' accounts of their depressive illness and answers to questions about specific symptoms changed between the first appointment and the second or third. Irrespective of a person's culture, a clinician can build trust with a new patient by showing respect, interest, empathy, patience, and cultural awareness. Tacit communication by the clinician that immediate, complete self-disclosure is not expected can aid in the process. A patient's response to a question about whether they or a family member have had a negative experience with healthcare can both alert the clinician to a potential trust issue and help begin a process of trust-building.

Depression itself can affect patients' level of trust. While suspiciousness is not part of the core syndrome of depression, the bias of depressed people toward negative thought content can intensify mistrust and doubt that are already present. Culturally based pessimism, doubt, and/or negative stereotyping can be part of the thought content that is amplified when a person is depressed.

A specific trust issue relates to medications. Cultures can have common beliefs about medications that influence people's willingness to try medications or to continue with them if there are side effects or no immediate benefit or if symptoms remit and continued medication is for prevention of recurrence. Chinese culture is an example: Virtually every Chinese person has heard the saying *shì yào sān fēn dú* (是药三分毒), which is literally translatable as "every medicine is 30% toxic" but is understood as "every medicine has its side effects or toxicity." Its implication is that because negative effects can be expected, medications should be started—or continued—only if essential for preserving health, function, and life expectancy. People of Chinese ethnicity tend to be particularly cautious about conventional Western medications, especially if the condition they treat is, correctly or not, thought of as self-limited, bearable without treatment, and not disabling or life-threatening. Clinicians considering prescribing or recommending drug treatments for depression can make better decisions and communicate them more effectively if they know when their patients have culturally based suspicions and attitudes that discourage their use. When patients begin with a bias against medications, they tend to take medications to relieve symptoms only if they are unbearable and to take medications long-term only if they are prescribed for a serious medical condition that would be uncomfortably symptomatic, immediately disabling, or life-threatening if not treated, like heart failure or cancer. Perhaps surprisingly, patients with cultural biases against long-term use of medications can be non-adherent to treatments for significant chronic diseases like Type 2 diabetes or atherosclerotic vascular disease with a history of myocardial infarction or stroke.

Social Capital

Social capital comprises characteristics of people and populations related to interpersonal relationships that, like economic capital, enable productivity and problem resolution. Like trust, the concept has gained increasing prominence among social scientists as one that helps explain large differences in well-being and economic success between regions and cultural groups with apparently similar material resources. Aspects of social capital include the size, stability, and function of social networks; norms of trust and reciprocity; and people's trust in institutions. In a region or culture with high social capital, people would socialize informally with others outside their families, do favors for one another, and call on one another for assistance. They would be likely to participate in community organizations like clubs, sports leagues, religious congregations, charities, or political groups. They would start with an assumption that most people—including strangers—can be trusted, and they would assume that institutions like schools and government agencies, and their leadership, could be trusted to be honest and non-corrupt. They would see dishonesty, deception, and corruption as exceptional rather than usual.

The dimensions of social capital are structural, relational, instrumental, and cognitive. *Structural* social capital refers to organizations that bring people together and coordinate their efforts, including clubs, teams, religious congregations, charities, and political groups. *Relational* social capital refers to relationships between people outside their immediate families. Its three subtypes are *bonding* (relationships between people with similar cultural identity), *bridging* (relationships between people with different cultural identities) and *linking* (relationships between people at different levels in the social hierarchy). *Instrumental* social capital refers to people offering support and assistance to one another. *Cognitive* social capital refers to trust in individuals and institutions, norms of generosity and reciprocity, and satisfaction with the relational and instrumental social capital.

Measurement of social capital usually is based on population surveys using questionnaires or in-person interviews. In some studies, these are supplemented by analysis of statistics such as numbers of non-profit organizations, rates of voting participation, attendance at religious services, rates of charitable donation, or crime rates. Further assessment of social capital has been done with behavioral experiments, such as giving a person a "lost wallet" with a request to contact its owner and observing what the person will do with it (Cohn et al., 2019). In Cohn and colleagues' study of people from 40 countries with varying levels of social capital, most people from high-trust countries contacted the owner of the lost wallet, while most people from low-trust countries did not. For example, fewer than 10% of Chinese people attempted to return a lost wallet that contained business cards, a shopping list, and a key but no cash, while 75% of Swiss did so.

Social capital can be measured at the individual level and at the level of a region, nation, or cultural group. In relating social capital to mental health, an important distinction should be made between the level of measurement for the two variables. An individual's personal assessment of their social capital—relational, instrumental, and cognitive—can fluctuate with their current mood. The relationship of social capital and depression is circular. Loneliness and a lack of trust reduce mental well-being and increase the risk of clinical depression. A person's depression can increase their suspicion of others, and social connections can be weakened or lost because of the person's depression-related apathy, withdrawal, irritability, and/or disagreeableness. Aggregated assessments of social capital at the neighborhood level or higher will be more stable over time than individuals' assessments, though they will vary with the prevalence of depressive symptoms in the population. Populations with higher social capital tend to have lower levels of depressive symptoms and a lower prevalence of clinical depression.

Cognitive social capital—especially individuals' level of trust and norms of reciprocity—appears more relevant to depression risk than structural social capital. The relative importance of relational versus cognitive social capital, and of different forms of relational social capital, vary across cultures (Son & Feng, 2019). In the analyses of depression in the United States during the COVID-19 pandemic presented in Chapter 14, measures of state-level cognitive social capital are shown to correlate negatively with depression prevalence after controlling for many other variables.

In Cali, Colombia, a city with high crime and violence, the rate of subjective mental illness (feeling mental distress at least 14 days out of the past month) dropped as people scored higher on a survey item rating "interpersonal trust in unknown people" on a scale of zero to 10, and the effect was greater in men. The effect persisted after controlling for economic status, family structure, and number of close friends (Martinez et al., 2019).

Among over 20,000 residents of Chinese cities, neighborhood-level social capital was associated with lower average levels of depressive symptoms as measured with the Center for Epidemiologic Studies Depression Scale (CES-D) (R. Wang et al., 2019). Among urban Chinese adults aged 18–45, both bonding and bridging social capital were protective against depression, but the effect of bonding social capital was stronger (Chen et al., 2018). The effect of different types of social capital on depression in China varies according to the age and urban–rural status of the population: Older and rural Chinese experience antidepressant effects of bonding but not bridging social capital. Younger, urban Chinese benefit from both types of social capital, though the effect of bonding social capital is larger (Jiang & Kang, 2019).

In South Korea, trust as assessed by the question "Do you think most people are reliable?" was more protective against incident depression than reciprocity as assessed by the question "Are you willing to help your neighbor who urgently needs your help (e.g., blood donation)?" (Kim et al., 2012). Another study from South Korea assessed how the balance of negative versus positive social support affected depression risk in people with low incomes. Negative social support was evaluated by asking subjects to answer true or false to six statements with the stem "There is a person who." The end of the sentence is one of the following phrases: "who objects to or meddles with what I do," "who blames me for all the problems I have," "who forgets or ignores me," "who gives me unwanted help and makes me uncomfortable," "who is indifferent to me and my affairs," or "who turns me down most of the time when I ask for help." As might be expected, negative social support increased the risk of depression even when the subject received positive social support (Lee et al., 2019). Negative stereotyping, discrimination, and microaggressions against a stigmatized minority by the majority cultural group can be conceptualized as a lack of cognitive and relational bridging social capital, sometimes including negative social support.

In the metropolitan area of Vancouver, Canada, residents with a higher "sense of community belonging" had a lower prevalence of major depressive disorder

(MDD) and lower levels of self-reported "negative mental health" and "psychological distress." A neighborhood having more greenspace (parks, trees, etc.) and "blue space" (water views) was associated with more people having a high sense of community belonging (Rugel et al., 2019). There appears to be a bidirectional relationship between environmental quality and neighborhood social capital. One of the several ways in which improving a community's environmental quality can be expected to reduce its prevalence of depression is an indirect effect through enhancement of social capital.

A study of older adults in 702 Japanese communities (123,760 individual subjects) assessed the relationship between community-level social capital and the community's prevalence of depression (scores of 5 or higher on the 15-item Geriatric Depression Scale). Of the three components of social capital—participation in organized groups, reciprocal assistance, and social cohesion (trust in neighbors, norms of reciprocity, and attachment to the community)—group participation had the strongest negative correlation with depression prevalence. In the highly homogenous society of Japan, trust and reciprocity bring burdens as well as benefits (Saito et al., 2017). Group participation translates into enjoyable activity and less loneliness, apparently a less mixed blessing than a norm of reciprocal obligation.

In the Czech Republic, Russia, and Poland, lower levels of self-reported social cohesion were associated with a higher prevalence of clinical depression three years later, with a stronger effect in men (Bertossi Urzua et al., 2019). This supports a causal connection, not simply a correlation, between low social capital and more depressive symptoms at the individual level. In the Netherlands, relational and cognitive types of social cohesion at the municipal level were associated with a lower prevalence of depression, severe headache, and medically unexplained physical symptoms. Once age, gender, socioeconomic status, household income, and social cohesion were included in a multivariate predictive model of depression, air pollution was the only physical environmental variable tested that remained significant (Zock et al., 2018).

A study of migrant Filipina domestic workers in Macau, China, demonstrated the subtlety of the relationship between social capital and depression in people under stress from ethnic discrimination. As expected, experiencing discrimination was associated with a lower level of cognitive social capital (e.g., trust) and a higher level of depression. Overall, the women with more cognitive social capital had fewer symptoms of depression and anxiety; but among those who experienced the highest level of discrimination, those with moderate or high cognitive social capital had worse mental health. Apparently, trusting others may not be protective against depression in an objectively hostile environment (Hall et al., 2019).

An Australian study of depression following a natural disaster (wildfires in southeastern Australia in 2009) showed a non-monotonic effect of individuals' post-disaster community involvement on depression 3–5 years later. Both non-participation and high participation in community organizations following the disaster were associated with a future higher risk of MDD or post-traumatic stress disorder (PTSD) than moderate participation. At the community level, widespread moderate community involvement was associated with a lower prevalence of PTSD and MDD than a mix of highly involved and uninvolved residents (Gallagher et al., 2019).

The importance of social capital in protecting against depression can vary according to an individual's personality. In an African American population, people who were more neurotic, more introverted, and less conscientious showed a stronger correlation between high social capital and lower depression rate than people who were less neurotic, more extraverted, and more conscientious (Clark et al., 2018). The lesser sensitivity of the latter to their community social environment appears to reflect a combination of their lesser disposition to depressive symptoms and their greater resourcefulness and resilience. They are perhaps more able to find the emotional and instrumental support they need even when community-level social capital is low.

Social capital may have a critical role in the well-established relationship between income inequality and depression. Since the late 1980s income inequality has dramatically increased in many countries, as has the rate of depression. Income inequality is associated with depression at national, neighborhood, and individual levels. At the neighborhood level, excessive income inequality is associated with lower social capital, through the perception of unfairness leading to lower trust and through the contradiction between society's valuation of acquiring wealth and the lower class's lack of access to opportunities to acquire it. Lack of opportunities can be exacerbated by discrimination on account of ethnicity, age, and/or gender. At the individual level, upward comparison and/or lack of class mobility can make individuals feel stressed and/or defeated. The impact of income inequality is greatest among women and people with low incomes, but it is present in both men and women across the entire spectrum of socioeconomic class. It is more salient in high-income and middle-income countries than in low-income countries where poverty is a more immediate social determinant of mental health than inequality (V. Patel et al., 2018).

Communication Culture and Talking About Depression

A third set of dimensions used to describe cultures, useful in understanding and deconstructing depression narratives, characterizes cultures' typical communication styles. As with other cultural characteristics, group measures of communication styles are central tendencies, with respect to which there will always be many individual differences. Of a person's several intersecting identities, one or two may predominate and interact with social context in determining a person's communication style.

The best-known dimension of cultural communication style is the high-context/low-context distinction first described by the sociologist Edward Hall (1976). High-context communication, typical of collectivistic cultures, relies on the physical and social contexts of the communication, the preexisting knowledge of the people communicating, and appreciation of gestures, facial expressions, and paralinguistic features of speech (i.e., prosody, pitch, rhythm, and "paralinguistic respiration" such as sighing or saying "Hmm"). High-context communications are, in the extreme, merely cues or references to an implicit message that remains unspoken. At times, the explicit spoken message is opposite to the intended message. Low-context communication is typical of individualistic cultures. It is explicit and interpretable without much attention to the contemporaneous physical and social environment, reference to unspoken assumptions, or precise decoding of paralinguistic features.

Japan has the highest-context communication style of any major high-income nation; Japanese are enculturated to "read the air" (*ba no kuki wo yomu*; 場の空気を読む) to understand others' messages. Japanese communication style is at the extreme end of three other dimensions of cultural communication style: It is also indirect, self-effacing, and understated. Chinese and Korean communication styles are also high-context, though less so than Japan's. (The three countries' cultures and the impact of their communication styles on depression will be discussed in detail in the chapters devoted to each one.) The United States' majority culture has a low-context communication style, but some members of ethnic minorities retain the high-context communication styles of their countries of origin or ancestry. France and Italy have communication styles intermediate between high-context and low-context.

Three other dimensions of cultural communication style, described by other social scientists, were recently summarized in a review by Liu (2016):

1. *Direct versus indirect.* In direct communication, people say what they mean and mean what they say. Indirect communication conceals the true opinion, preference, or intention of the speaker, though it may offer a subtle hint of it.

Japanese communication is indirect, German communication is direct, and the communication style of India is intermediate.

2. *Self-enhancing versus self-effacing.* In self-enhancing speech, people "talk big" about themselves, emphasizing their strengths and minimizing their weaknesses, faults, and doubts. Self-effacing speech is modest and self-critical. Japanese communication is self-effacing, Australian communication is self-enhancing, and Swedish communication is intermediate.

3. *Elaborate versus understated.* In elaborate speech there are many words and abundant details, with liberal use of adjectives and adverbs. In understated speech less is said, and more is implied. High-context communication typically is understated. Sentences are shorter, and there may be pauses and periods of silence. Understatement is preferred to emphatic statements. Japanese communication is understated, French communication is elaborate, and Greek communication is intermediate.

Dimensions of communication style should be considered in assessing people for depression, bipolar symptoms, or suicidal intent. More care must be taken to confirm the accuracy of the message received when the sender is a high-context or indirect communicator, especially when the clinician is not from the same culture. Without consideration of cultural communication style, self-enhancing speakers might be judged to be less depressed or more hypomanic than they are, and with self-effacing speakers, the opposite might be the case. Similar considerations apply to elaborate versus understated communication. An important risk management issue is accurate assessment of suicidality in high-context, indirectly-communicating people. There is no shortcut to doing this, though suggestions will be offered throughout this book. The solution begins with recognizing the problem.

Acculturating or bicultural individuals often combine or mix communication styles or change their communication style in response to circumstances. For example, a second-generation Japanese American (*Nisei*) might use a high-context, understated communication style with family and with Japanese friends but be less indirect and self-effacing than a Japanese native when interacting with Americans of the majority culture. Such a person, if interviewed about symptoms of depression, might express feelings of despair and hopelessness in the understated terms they might use with family and friends, or make self-effacing statements. If understood out of context and with no clarification, the person's understatement could lead to underestimation of depression severity and suicide risk, or self-effacing statements about their role and accomplishments could be misinterpreted as a lack of self-esteem related to depression. Critical information can be lost in *cultural* translation even when dialogue is between two native speakers of the same language, as it is when a clinician from a country's majority culture interviews a patient who is a second-generation immigrant.

An essential part of the cultural lens is *the use of qualitative aspects of people's illness narratives to (provisionally) infer their communication style.* The inferred communication style can then be used as a frame of reference for interpreting statements about the symptoms of depression and answers to questions about them. Periodically, and when the inference is about a critical issue, like suicidal ideation, a clinician interpreting indirect communication should tactfully validate their inferences with the patient. This need not be disruptive when the clinician and the patient have already acknowledged that there are cultural differences between them.

Inference from Metaphor and Word Choice

In every language there are metaphors—often involving body parts—that convey emotional states, from "heartbroken" to "a pain in the neck." Metaphors relating to the heart are especially numerous, as will be illustrated in this book's chapters on China, Japan, and Korea (Chapters 10–12, respectively). Languages also have alternative terms for negative moods that capture both their flavor and their intensity; consider in English the differences between 20 synonyms for depressed: *dejected, desolate, despairing, despondent, disconsolate, dispirited, doleful, down, forlorn, gloomy, glum, grief-stricken, inconsolable, melancholy, miserable, morose, sad, sorrowful, unhappy, wretched*. A person who felt desolate and despondent two days in the past week probably would be at greater risk for suicide than someone who felt dispirited and glum every day. The items on typical depression screening instruments use generic words to describe thoughts, emotions, and behavior, and people are asked to assign a frequency or severity level to them. This is not the same as judging the seriousness of a person's depression through the connotations and meanings of the words they choose to describe it.

The Montgomery-Åsberg depression rating scale (MADRS; Montgomery & Åsberg, 1979), a clinician-rated scale that is frequently used in clinical trials of antidepressants, is a notable exception to the linguistic blandness of most psychiatric rating scales and questionnaires. The point scores assigned to symptoms and signs describe them in ways that combine the dimensions of persistence and severity, using well-chosen synonyms to convey qualitative differences that map onto ordinal scores. For the sign of *apparent sadness*, a patient scores 2 points for "Looks dispirited but does brighten up without difficulty," 4 points for "Appears sad and unhappy most of the time," and 6 points for "Looks miserable all the time. Extremely despondent." While the item does refer to persistence and variability of the sign, the comparison of *dispirited, unhappy,* and *miserable/despondent* prompts the rater to listen to the details of the patient's account of their feelings. A similarly colorful contrast is found in the item on *inner tension*, which offers descriptions including "occasional feelings of edginess and ill-defined discomfort," "continuous feelings of inner tension," and "unrelenting dread or anguish." Edginess or ill-defined discomfort, even felt every waking minute, is not the same thing as unrelenting dread or anguish.

In any language and culture there are words and metaphors that express emotional pain outside the realm of everyday experience or capture emotional experience of deep significance. A 60-year-old Japanese man saying he has lost his *ikigai* (生き甲斐; reason to live) is cause for great concern even if he has not had any thoughts of suicide or death in the past two weeks. The word *tsurai* (辛い; literally translatable as "hot, spicy, or harsh") is not used by Japanese to talk about everyday unhappiness or disappointment. When the word is used to describe feelings, it connotes major emotional suffering. For example, *tsurai* might be used in the sentence *Ikiru koto ga shinu koto yori haruka ni tsurai* (生きることが死ぬことよりはるかに辛い; translatable as "Sometimes, it is much harder to live than to die"). *Zetsubou* (絶望; despair, hopelessness) is another word most often used to describe the hopelessness of depression and one that carries a suggestion of increased suicide risk.

The German word *lebesmüde*, literally "life-tired" or "weary of life," describes a state that could lead to suicide or to doing something risky that could have fatal consequences. It clearly is not a synonym for ordinary sadness. If someone were *lebesmüde*, they would be facing either an existential crisis, clinical depression, or most likely both. German has alternate words for being suicidal: *Selbstmordgefährdet* is a compound of "self-murder" and "endangered," and *selbstmörderisch* is "self-murder-ish." Both words are translated into English as "suicidal," but the former word connotes more immediate risk of self-harm. In Spanish *deprimido* means very sad, while *depresivo* means depressive (i.e., inclined to be depressed). A person who is *depresivo* has a persistent tendency to feel sad and blue, as would someone with a depressive personality or dysthymia. *Abatido* means dejected, despondent, or dispirited in response to a specific situation.

While it is unrealistic to expect all clinicians to be multilingual, it is feasible for clinicians to learn from the languages (including dialects) that their patients speak a handful of words and phrases that strongly suggest clinical depression or suicide risk. They can ask their patients what words—in any language—would most precisely describe how they feel and ask them to explain how those words have a meanings different from generic words like *sad* and *unhappy*.

The feasibility of automated analysis of text messages, email, and social media posts to identify depression or suicidality has been established (Coppersmith et al. 2016; O'Dea et al. 2017; Seabrook et al., 2018; Settanni & Marengo, 2015). In many cultural groups such analysis might prove to be superior for depression screening than a questionnaire. Even more promising is the combination of a questionnaire or a clinician-rated scale with depression or suicide risk scores derived by artificial intelligence or machine learning from social media posts or text communications submitted by patients for clinical analysis (with rigorous privacy protection). Before such technology matures, undergoes rigorous validation, and becomes broadly available, recognizing language- or culture-specific key words and metaphors can help clinicians interpret borderline scores on depression rating scales and screening tests and can improve the sensitivity and specificity of screening for suicide risk.

Religious Identity and Its Implications

Religion is another intersecting identity associated with circumstances that can cause stress and with attributes that can make stress more bearable. Religion and cultural groups defined by religion often are associated with norms and expectations for males and females at specific points in the life course. The personal choices of an individual make them a conformist or a non-conformist relative to the religion's life script, and this can have both psychological and social consequences.

Religious identity has many aspects that are not necessarily correlated. To fully understand a person's unique intersection of cultural identities and its significance for depression, their religious identity must be characterized and not just labeled. While labeling a person with the name of a religious denomination will convey some insight, a depressed person's relationship with their religious identity may be more important than the label when assessing the relationship of religion to the cause of a depression and how best to treat it. Following is a sequence of related questions to guide exploration of a person's religious identity and their relationship with it.

Does the person identify with a religion? Do other people identify the person with a religion? If a person is identified with a religion, what are the social consequences of that identification? Is the person stereotyped positively or negatively or targeted for discrimination?

If a person identifies with a religion, are they affiliated with a congregation or religious organization or with an informal religious community? Does the person live in an area with many people of the same religion? Do they have personal connections with others of the same religion? Do people of the same religion account for most of their personal connections? Are religious ritual and compliance with religious rules important parts of their life? Is it important for members of their family or community to conform with the religion's rules regardless of their personal beliefs? How much time does the person spend in religious activities? How much of that time is spent alone and how much in the company of others, as in a prayer or study group? Is the person involved in charitable or service activities related to religion?

Does the person have faith in God or an equivalent higher power? Do they personally believe in the doctrine and moral code of the religion? Do they pray or engage in meditation or another spiritual practice?

Has the person given up a religion or adopted a new one? Is the person's religious identity today the same as it was in their childhood? If it is different, when and how did it change? Has their religion become more important or less important recently?

If a person identifies with a religion, do they conform to the norms of the religion? Is the person a conspicuous non-conformist? If they are a non-conformist, how do people of the same religion in their social network react to the non-conformity?

Has the person ever turned to religion when feeling distressed? Did they use prayer or meditation, counseling by clergy, or support by peers of the same religion? Did they rely on faith as a reason to live? Was any sort of religion-related activity helpful to them in tolerating their distress, relieving it, or changing their personal situation for the better?

Are there important negative aspects of their religious experience? Did they, or do they now, experience guilt or shame related to their religion? Is there a history of trauma at the hands of religious people, or harsh punishment given in the name of religion?

Does the person wish they had a sincere religious belief but not yet found one? Are they actively searching for faith?

Religious people regularly use religious beliefs and practices to cope with stressful life events and physical or emotional pain. Religious coping can have positive or negative effects on mental health and behavior. The Brief Religious Coping Scale (Brief RCOPE) is a 14-item, psychometrically validated questionnaire for assessing people's relative use of positive and negative religious coping strategies (Pargament et al., 2011). The items of the scale are presented in Table 4.7. Each is rated by the subject on a 4-point Likert scale ranging from *not at all* to *a great deal.*

The Brief RCOPE has been validated in a broad range of cultural groups, ranging from Black American women with a history of intimate partner

Table 4.7 The Brief RCOPE: Positive and Negative Subscale Items

Positive religious coping subscale items
1. Looked for a stronger connection with God.
2. Sought God's love and care.
3. Sought help from God in letting go of my anger.
4. Tried to put my plans in action together with God.
5. Tried to see how God might be trying to strengthen me in this situation.
6. Asked forgiveness for my sins.
7. Focused on religion to stop worrying about my problems.

Negative religious coping subscale items
8. Wondered whether God had abandoned me.
9. Felt punished by God for my lack of devotion.
10. Wondered what I did for God to punish me.
11. Questioned God's love for me.
12. Wondered whether my church had abandoned me.
13. Decided the devil made this happen.
14. Questioned the power of God.

Note. The brief RCOPE (Pargament et al., 2011) is an abridged version of the RCOPE Religious Coping Scale (Pargament et al., 2000).

violence to Pakistani Muslim university students. Both the positive and negative religious coping scales have high internal consistency—a median alpha statistic of .92 for the positive scale and a median alpha of .81 for the negative scale. Negative religious coping has been significantly correlated with depression in various studies; the evidence that positive religious coping protects against depression is weaker (Pargament et al., 2011). In a study of first-episode clinically depressed patients treated at a medical center in Chandigarh, India, patients who had attempted suicide in the past 14 days had significantly higher negative religious coping scores than those who had only thought about suicide (Dua et al., 2021). In a study of Italian, Dutch, and American psychiatric outpatients with a first episode of MDD, positive religious coping was strongly and inversely correlated with scores on the Hamilton Depression Rating Scale (HAM-D). Controlling for HAM-D scores, negative religious coping was associated with greater suicidal ideation and positive religious coping with less (De Berardis et al., 2020). A similar association of negative religious coping and suicidal behavior—present after controlling for depressive symptoms—was found in a sample of recently returned U.S. war veterans (Kopacz et al., 2017).

Positive religious coping was protective against depression, and negative religious coping was a risk factor for depression in a sample of 200 Malaysian healthcare workers (mainly physicians) working on the front lines at an academic medical center specializing in the treatment of COVID-19 patients. In a multivariate model that included age, gender, ethnicity, marital status, occupation, monthly income, site of work, and work schedule, only positive and negative religious coping had significant effects on depressive symptoms, with a greater (adverse) effect of negative religious coping (Chow et al., 2021).

In a primarily Black, Christian sample of low-income residents of Houston, Texas, aged 50 and over, scores on the PHQ-8 were strongly associated with negative religious coping, but simultaneous positive religious coping moderated the effect (O'Brien et al., 2019).

Other studies of religious coping and its relationship to depression, encompassing diverse cultural groups and intersectional identities, confirm a highly significant association of negative religious coping with depression, with a weaker though often meaningful beneficial effect of positive religious coping. Groups recently studied include Somali college students in Minnesota (Areba et al., 2018).

Though most published studies on religious coping and depression have been cross-sectional, a longitudinal study of a national sample of 937 community-dwelling Black Americans showed that negative religious coping at baseline predicted increased CES-D depression scores 2.5 years later, even after controlling for age, gender, education, general health status, and depressive symptoms at baseline (C. L. Park et al., 2018). In a study of adults aged over 60 treated for MDD at an academic medical center, positive religious coping at baseline predicted lower ratings on the MADRS 6 months later. (In a multivariate model, negative religious coping was correlated with higher depression scores at baseline, but it did not significantly affect the 6-month outcome [Bosworth et al., 2003].)

If a clinician knows that a patient is a typical adherent of a religion or that the patient belongs to a specific sect or congregation, they might make assumptions about the person's behavioral norms, moral principles, and social capital. Because such assumptions might be wrong in ways critical to the patient's current illness, it is best to treat them as hypotheses. Membership in a religious community (with associated belief) offers, at its best, much to reduce the risk of depression and enable a person to bear adversity without becoming depressed. Potential benefits include a reason to live, hope, social capital that relieves loneliness and offers practical support in hard times, empathy and counsel, rituals to relieve emotional distress, and group solidarity when facing external discrimination or prejudice. At its worst it can cause or exacerbate depression. Potential adverse effects of religious affiliation and belief include childhood trauma or intimate partner violence normalized or even encouraged by a religious community, shaming or stigmatization if one transgresses a norm, social ostracism if one is a non-conformist, receiving religious counsel instead of medical treatment when the medical approach is more likely to be effective, and being a target for prejudice, discrimination, or social exclusion because one's religious group is a negatively-stereotyped minority in the broader community.

Given the complexity of the issue, it is tempting for a clinician to simply "not go there" when assessing a depressed patient. However, if religion is central to a patient's identity, a diagnosis of depression and a recommendation for its treatment may not be accepted unless the issue of religion is considered and addressed. For example, it will be observed in Chapter 9 that Islam has unique perspectives on both depression and suicide. If a patient is a devout Muslim, a clinician will be more helpful to the patient if they give advice that is compatible with the patient's religious beliefs.

The same information informs a decision about whether to suggest that a depressed patient seek religious or spiritual counsel or social support in their religious community. When the depressed person remains positive about their religious identity and retains their belief or sense of affiliation with a community of faith, consideration of religious resources is appropriate. When religious disillusionment contributes to a patient's hopelessness, the clinician would be wiser to focus on secular sources of support and counsel. A clinician with many religious patients can benefit from identifying local pastoral counselors with mental health literacy, cultural awareness, and compatible beliefs about the role of mainstream medical treatments of depression.

Chapter 5

Cultural Identity and Personal Biography

The onset of clinical depression is salient event within a life course and often one that is a sequel of other events involving trauma, loss, pain, stress, and/or disappointment. A person's cultural identity, including the structural accompaniments of that identity (e.g., the experience of discrimination, food insecurity, or living in a polluted environment), affects the likelihood and nature of negative life events. A culture might prescribe a pattern of gender relations that normalizes intimate partner violence (IPV) or a strict form of parenting that easily turns abusive. It might entail modes of dress, social behavior, and communication that target individuals for stereotyping and discrimination when they are in the minority in a nation or region. Conversely, life events can lead to a fundamental alteration of a person's identity. Immigration with subsequent acculturation is an obvious example, but becoming an officer in the U.S. Marines, a neurosurgeon, a priest, or a nun involves a transformation no less consequential. More prosaic but equally powerful changes in identity take place when a person marries, when a woman bears her first child, or when a person retires after a long career or loses a job held for many years.

Ethnic groups have characteristic attitudes toward people based on their age, gender, and location on the "family organizational chart." Employing a cultural lens includes considering the intersection of age and gender with national or ethnic identity. Japanese salarymen offer a good example. A salaryman in his 50s who has accumulated seniority at a lifetime job at a large corporation enjoys respect, authority over more junior employees, a relatively high salary, frequent pleasurable work-related social events, and (at least) ritualized affection from his wife at the beginning and end of the workday. A recently retired salaryman in his 60s, forced to retire at a fixed retirement age, has no authority, no subordinates, reduced income, and no work-related social events to enjoy. His relationship with his wife, after decades of his putting work ahead of family, might be distant or awkward. In the worst case, his wife is overtly condescending or humiliating to him, seeing him as worthless if he no longer earns money. (A Japanese slang expression, *sodai gomi* (粗大ごみ; "oversized trash"), is attributed to disgruntled wives of recently retired Japanese salarymen describing their husbands who now passively sit around the house.) Even when there is goodwill between husband and wife, the relationship often is not emotionally intimate. Given his nationality and occupation, his age has a profound effect on his social role, his sources of stress, and his social and material resources for buffering stress and dealing with adversity.

A person's age is inseparable from their generational cohort—an American in their 60s also has a cultural identity as a member of the baby boom generation – they are a Boomer. Boomers are the first generation in America to see their seventh decade as late middle age rather than as old age and to not have a normative expectation of retirement in their early 60s. Being involuntarily unemployed and in a financially precarious position in one's late 60s might precipitate depression, and millions of Americans experience this situation. The unhappiness of such a person might relate to a loss of status and purpose as well as to financial hardship. A French or Swedish person of the same age would not be expected to work; their retirement would not entail a loss of status, and they would be much less likely than an American of the same age and social class to face poverty or financial precarity.

National cultures, ethnic minority cultures, and many occupational cultures have expectations and norms for life stages that entail specific stresses that are potential triggers for episodes of depression. People with life trajectories, desires, or aspirations that conflict with cultural norms for life stages can feel oppressed or thwarted, leading to depression.

In a country or an occupation with a mandatory retirement age or a normative retirement age, with few exceptions, a person who loves their work and wants to continue it will, when obliged to retire, lose a major source of meaning and satisfaction in their life. If there has been no change in work performance that would appropriately warrant retirement, they are likely to find the situation unfair. If they are conscious of declining job performance prior to retirement, there may be a loss of self-esteem. Other losses following an unwanted retirement include a loss of status, a loss of income, and a loss or weakening of their social network of fellow employees or colleagues. If the person's work–family balance has been tilted toward work, relationships with family members will change, sometimes for the worse, as in the above example of Japanese salarymen.

In ethnic groups in which there are ages by which women or men are expected to be married, a person who reaches the usual age limit for a first marriage and is still single might feel disappointment or a sense of failure or inadequacy. If the single person's desires regarding marriage are discrepant from those of their parents, conflict or discomfort in family relations might increase. This issue often arises when the parents are first-generation immigrants and differ from their second-generation children in their expectations regarding age of marriage, the role of parents as matchmakers, and/or the ethnicity or religion of the spouse. People who are gay, lesbian, bisexual, or otherwise queer, especially if they have not "come out" to their parents, can experience stress or conflicts related to expectations of (conventional) marriage when they reach the age by which marriage is expected in their cultural group.

Cultural expectations that married women will have children are another source of depression. Married women whose cultural identity implies a strong expectation of motherhood are especially vulnerable to depression if they wish to have children but encounter a fertility problem. The latter might be blamed on the woman even if the man is the infertile member of the couple. Those who do not want to have children might experience their families' disapproval or might become more distant from women friends who are mothers of young children. In South Korea, where not having children is the norm for women with serious careers, a college-educated businesswoman who chooses to have a child probably will find herself excluded from after-work social activities essential for advancement in her occupation.

The postpartum period is one of known vulnerability to depression. Many ethnic groups have detailed rules for how women are to conduct themselves postpartum. In some cases, the woman's following cultural rules for postpartum behavior can make postpartum depression worse. In others, difficulty in following the rules because of current circumstances, such as those related to immigration or distance from family, is a source of emotional distress. Dissenting from a culture's rules for postpartum behavior can precipitate family conflicts, with attendant loss of emotional or practical support from the older generation—circumstances that make depression more likely and make it worse if it has already occurred. Conflict between a new mother and her parents or her husband's parents over postpartum conduct is especially common when the new mother is an immigrant or child of immigrants who, unlike the older generation, is assimilated and has expectations for postpartum life based on the norms of her new home country. Similar issues can arise when the new mother is a rural-to-urban migrant, living in a city where historical postpartum traditions frequently are not followed.

Menopause or andropause can be associated with changes in people's sexuality—in the direction of greater or lesser interest in sex or sexual dysfunction including erectile dysfunction in men and dyspareunia in women. The interpersonal consequences of changes in sexuality will depend on the relationship status of the person going through the change. How a man or woman judges the quality of a marriage or other intimate relationship can change as well. A person not in an intimate relationship and wanting one, who newly experiences sexual dysfunction or a loss of sexual interest, might conclude that their prospect of finding love has become much worse. Cultural expectations regarding sexuality in later life partly determine the role of sexuality in a man's or woman's self-esteem, in their actual or perceived status in the eyes of others, and in the likelihood that a single person without sexual interest or with diminished sexual performance will be able to find a mate. Sexual dysfunction or loss of sexual interest can cause emotional distress or worsen clinical depression in a person from a culture in which older people often are devalued and in which diminished sexuality is a cardinal sign of transition to old age. A widow's lack of sexual interest might contribute to feelings of hopelessness if in her cultural group widows are expected to remarry and an older woman would be expected to sexually satisfy her husband.

In cultures in which older people are expected to be asexual, a person with little sexual interest would not be troubled by it and might even be relieved that they no longer have sexual needs or performance expectations to fulfill. Such a person would be unlikely to report diminished sexual interest as a symptom when evaluated for depression as it would not be a cause for complaint. In such a culture, a person with an active sexual interest might have cause for emotional distress, either if they had no partner or if their spouse or partner were uninterested in having sexual relations or unable to enjoy sex for medical reasons.

Worldwide, old age is a time of vulnerability to depressive symptoms, though the latter are not necessarily expressed as a typical syndrome of major depressive disorder (MDD). Prevalence statistics for MDD show peak rates in young adulthood. Our view is that the high level of general medical comorbidity seen in old age and age-related cognitive impairments can make it difficult to attribute depressed people's physical and cognitive major symptoms, so that accurately diagnosing MDD often is problematic. A persistent and personally consequential increase in negative thoughts and feelings and decrease in positive ones, together with physiologic dysfunction, sleep problems, and either distress or impaired function—the core of clinical depression as defined here—is a highly prevalent syndrome in old age. As in other life stages, culture affects the details and shapes illness narratives.

In the COVID-19 pandemic, the prevalence of clinical depression in the United States, as estimated via scores on the PHQ-2 in national surveys, increased dramatically. However, the increase was far greater for younger adults than older ones, with the percentage of people aged 18–29 with PHQ-2 scores in the clinical range during the pandemic approximately three times higher than that of people aged 70–79 (US Census Bureau, 2022).

The definition of old age and the boundary between the *young-old* and the *oldest old* are culturally determined, with geography (including region) and socioeconomic class having a critical role. In the U.S., the current difference in life expectancy at age 40 between the top and the bottom 1% of the income distribution is 15 years for men and 10 years for women. People in the bottom 1% have life expectancies like those of people from Sudan or Pakistan. Differences in expected age at death between the top and bottom quartiles of income, adjusting for race and ethnicity, exceed 7 years in several states (Chetty et al., 2016). For a man of the working poor or lower class, age 70 is old. A lower-class man of that age would probably be either disabled or retired, and if he worked, it would probably be driven by financial necessity and not by finding meaning or pleasure in his work. An upper-class or upper-middle-class man of age 70 would be young-old. If he liked his work, he probably would still be working at least part-time even if he were financially secure. The situation for women regarding biological and social age is like that of men, but it is different with respect to work because the current cohort of women over 70, born in the early 1950s or before, did not have the same educational and employment opportunities as today's young women. Relatively fewer rose to high positions in business, government, academia, and the professions. As a result, high-income women over 70 are less likely than men over 70 to be working currently even though they might remain biologically young-old into their 80s.

In the U.S., people over 50 who have a college education and hold technical or managerial jobs are vulnerable to age discrimination if they seek a new job. Even if their résumés show excellent education and work for well-respected employers at progressively increasing pay, they often lose to younger workers in competition for attractive positions. Employers might inappropriately assume that an older candidate for a job is less current with developments in their field, less technically adept, or less energetic. A younger worker qualified for the same position might accept a lower salary. Productive older workers might lose their jobs because of layoffs, geographical moves, or restructurings of the firms that employ them. In some egregious cases, employers outsource work to firms that hire low-wage foreign workers, require loyal long-term employees to train their replacements, and then terminate their employment. An employee over 50 in such a situation might find it very difficult to find work that did not involve a large cut in salary.

Similar issues arise with skilled blue-collar industrial workers who are laid off in midlife. They might have worked for the same company for 20 years or more at gradually increasing wages. Following a layoff, they might be unable to find similar work without a geographical move, and the jobs available to them in their field without their moving might have much lower wages. New employers in their area of residence might prefer to hire younger people. Middle-aged women seeking new jobs frequently encounter discrimination related to gaps in their résumés or periods of part-time work related to their care of young children or dependent elders.

Being the target of discrimination adds to stress from loss of income, uncertainty about the future, and disruption of employment-based social connections. These circumstances can lead to disillusionment, loss of trust, and loss of hope, implying an increased risk of depression.

Acculturation: Not Just for Immigrants

Three references offer three different definitions of acculturation:

Oxford English Dictionary: "Adoption of or adaptation to a different culture, especially that of a colonizing, conquering, or majority group" (Oxford University Press, n.d.).

Merriam-Webster: "Cultural modification of an individual, group, or people by adapting to or borrowing traits from another culture; also, a merging of cultures as a result of prolonged contact" (Merriam-Webster, 2019).

Wikipedia: "A process of social, psychological, and cultural change that stems from the balancing of two cultures while adapting to the prevailing culture of the society" ("Acculturation," 2019).

Between the above definitions, which reflect 19th-, 20th-, and 21st-century concepts of acculturation, the meaning moves from the imposition of a majority culture on a minority to borrowing and adaptation of traits to blending between cultures accompanied by psychological changes as well as changes in social behavior. The third definition fits well with the acculturation taking place as majority cultures mutate in the face of globalization and increasing demographic diversity. Cultural groups that were once a solid majority but now have lost that position or are losing it, such as Protestant Christian non-Hispanic Whites in many parts of the U.S., are challenged to adjust to their new status within contemporary American culture.

Acculturation implies *acculturative stress*, an issue most often discussed with respect to immigrants but with relevance to many other groups, as will be elaborated below. Acculturating immigrants often need to learn or become more proficient at a new language and communication style, and even if they begin with fluency in the language of the host country, they must adopt new social behaviors typical of the host country but not of their native country. Adolescent and young adult children of immigrants—whether born in the host country or having arrived in early childhood—are likely to differ from their parents in their level of acculturation, including differences in communication style and in values. They often are not fully enculturated in the language, heritage, values, and everyday behavior of the family's country of origin. The usual consequence is *acculturative family distancing*, a phenomenon that comprises four dimensions—verbal communication difficulties, non-verbal communication difficulties, general cultural values incongruency, and family values incongruency (Fujimoto & Hwang, 2014). Acculturative family distancing is associated with an increased risk of depression and other mental health problems in both parents and children. Similar phenomena have been described in studies of families of Chinese and Latinx immigrants to the U.S. (Carrera & Wei, 2014; Hwang, 2006; Hwang & Wood, 2009; Hwang et al., 2010). Bicultural competence of the younger generation partially mitigates the problem.

Acculturation can take the form of assimilation to the host culture, isolation in an ethnically homogeneous community, or the development of a bicultural (and often bilingual) identity, with meaningful social connections in both the immigrant and the host communities. The last of these forms of acculturation is associated with the best health outcomes, including the lowest prevalence of depression. Not adapting to the host culture reduces economic opportunity and increases the likelihood of being a target of discrimination. Attempting full assimilation and not maintaining meaningful ties with the immigrant community can make a person more vulnerable to depression. When a person with preserved ties to the immigrant community encounters discrimination or social rejection from people of the host culture, they usually can draw on connections in the immigrant community to help with both practical and emotional issues. An immigrant who has pursued full assimilation for years might no longer have relationships with members of the immigrant community that are strong enough to provide meaningful support in a highly stressful situation.

Possibly excepting a few isolated ethnic/religious communities, each successive generation following immigration becomes more assimilated to the host culture. Yet, even fully assimilated people from racial minorities—including those of mixed race—might not be accepted socially by members of the majority and might face stereotyping, prejudice, and discrimination. For example, third- or fourth-generation Chinese Americans talk about the discomfort they feel when people compliment them on their excellent English. At the same time, they face disapproval when they visit China and do not speak fluent Chinese. People in this situation can have painful identity issues, feeling rootless or "culturally homeless."

In the U.S., a person of mixed race, White on one side and Black, Asian, or Latinx on the other, might look like their racial minority parent but identify with their White parent and with the majority (White) American culture. At worst, they feel unwelcome among White people and uncomfortable among those of the same race/ethnicity as the minority parent. Non-White adopted children of White parents often face similar issues. Conversely, a person of mixed race who "passes for White" might be regarded with suspicion by members of the minority race, feel like an impostor, or meet with disapproval from the minority parent for denying their heritage.

Acculturative stress or "cultural homelessness" can precipitate depression. Depression can make acculturation more difficult and effortful via its effects on energy, cognition, and self-presentation. In applying a cultural lens to a person with symptoms of depression, it is always relevant to consider whether they are acculturating and whether acculturative stress or acculturative family distancing might be contributors to their current emotional distress.

A person need not be an immigrant to encounter a need to adapt to a challenging new culture. Acculturative stress can accompany the adaptation of a person from a lower-class background to sudden wealth, as might occur with extraordinary success in business, sports, or the performing arts or with marriage to a much wealthier person. It is a common issue for young adults who are the first in their families to ever attend college. In J. D. Vance's memoir *Hillbilly Elegy*, he poignantly describes his experience starting at Yale Law School following a poor and chaotic childhood in Appalachia, service in the U.S. Marines, and undergraduate education at Ohio State University. He had no academic difficulty at Yale but felt out of place, not knowing the unwritten rules for conversation with highly educated, upper-class professionals (Vance, 2016).

Normalization of Trauma

Traumatic experiences are common in the life courses of people with depression for several reasons. A traumatic event can precipitate a depressive episode in someone already vulnerable to it for genetic, epigenetic, developmental, or environmental reasons. People with depression and with bipolar spectrum conditions are at increased risk for having traumatic experiences. Repeated physical and/or emotional trauma in childhood—including neglect or vicarious trauma such as witnessing IPV between parents—can create a lifetime increase in the risk of depression, bipolar illness, and suicide, as well as an increased risk of general medical disorders associated with comorbid depression (Chang et al., 2019; LeMoult et al., 2020; Nelson et al., 2020; Sahle et al., 2021).

Childhood traumatic events with adverse effects on adult mental health include trauma from harsh discipline or family violence, verbal and emotional abuse, neglect, sexual abuse or exploitation, and disruption of parent–child attachment by a parent's illness, injury, incarceration, divorce, or desertion. Such occurrences are collectively referred to as *adverse childhood events* (ACEs).

Growing up in an unsafe neighborhood, witnessing violent encounters and trauma to others, experiencing discrimination, experiencing bullying, or having lived in foster care—collectively known as expanded ACEs—can have effects on lifetime emotional vulnerability like those of personally experienced ACEs (Cronholm et al., 2015). The persistent effects of ACEs on mental health are greater if there is a family history of depression or bipolar illness. Trauma to parents, especially to mothers but to fathers as well, can increase the risk of mood disorders in their children via epigenetic mechanisms. Clinicians' knowing the traumatic events that patients and their parents have experienced improves diagnoses and risk assessments and can make treatment of depression or bipolar illness more effective. Clinicians' awareness of their patients' traumatic experiences enhances their empathy, with the benefits for diagnostic accuracy and for treatment process and outcome that come with greater empathy. On a population basis, knowledge of highly prevalent traumatic events and adverse childhood experiences can be used to target primary and secondary prevention (Wade et al., 2016).

The likelihood of specific ACEs is strongly associated with cultural identity. Harsh physical discipline of children is common in some ethnic groups but is exceptional in others. The likelihood that a child will witness physical, verbal, or emotional abuse of their mother by her husband or partner varies greatly by ethnicity. Bullying in school is common within certain ethnic groups, and in those groups most children will at some time in their childhood be bullied, will bully another child, or will suffer emotional distress from witnessing the bullying of another child. When ethnic minorities are targeted for discrimination by the majority population, their children often are victims of bullying. The prevalence of expanded ACEs is significantly higher among people with low incomes who live in neighborhoods with high poverty rates (Wade et al., 2016).

Statistics on the prevalence of harsh discipline, IPV, bullying, and other ACEs are available for many ethnic groups and for the intersections of ethnicity with socioeconomic class, place of residence, and immigrant status. These provide useful background for culturally aware assessments of people with depression. Statistical estimates of the risk of various traumatic events provide a more valid basis than ethnic stereotypes for focusing a clinician's efforts to elicit a comprehensive life narrative of a depressed patient. A PubMed search on the intersection of ACEs and descriptors of a patient's identity is an efficient way to find if relevant risk estimates are available.

Adult traumatic events similarly vary by culture—with occupational cultures being important. Culturally related traumatic events include IPV, bullying at work, sexual harassment, trauma from dangerous employment (e.g., military service or work as a police officer or firefighter), and repeated witnessing of violence in one's neighborhood. Ethnic groups may have shared traumatic experiences such as those related to war, displacement, difficulties related to immigration or rural-to-urban migration, or a major natural disaster. Bullying at work is common in organizations with an authoritarian, hierarchical structure with high power distance. These include units of the armed services in which humiliating treatment of new recruits is a valid stereotype. Sexual harassment is common in the media and entertainment industries and can be especially egregious in countries with highly "masculine" cultures.

When a form of trauma is common in a cultural group—typically an ethnic group, an occupational group, or a group defined by the intersection of ethnicity and occupation with age, gender, and class—it often is normalized. Normalization can take several forms, all of which can have adverse effects on the health of the traumatized person.

In one form of normalization, the trauma is acknowledged within the cultural group. The traumatic events are regarded as undesirable but as common and not necessarily avoidable—in other words, normal in a statistical sense but not a moral one. There may be an unspoken rule that the high incidence of such trauma should not be complained about or talked about with others outside the group. In a related form of normalization, the trauma is acknowledged as undesirable and painful to undergo but nonetheless a potential positive that can eventually make the victim stronger for having endured it. A victim who responds to the normalized trauma by becoming depressed might be shamed for a lack of expected resilience.

In an especially malignant form of normalization, the cultural group sees the trauma as beneficial for the victim and for the group. The group directly or indirectly encourages the infliction of the trauma. Victims are told, or are expected to think, that the trauma is for their own good. Traumatic experiences "for one's own good" can be especially pernicious psychologically because unhappy victims might criticize themselves for weakness or feel ashamed or guilty about feeling anger or resentment toward the perpetrator of the trauma.

When a group of people share the same traumatic experience, they might offer one another practical and emotional support. This can reduce the adverse psychological effects of trauma but usually does not eliminate them. When, because of migration, acculturation, education, or changes in family relationships, people newly enter a social context in which the trauma they have suffered is not normalized, they might experience new distress over past events. If people are already depressed when their previously normalized trauma is denormalized, the depression can worsen since depression can intensify unhappy memories. Longer term, however, denormalization of their trauma in a new and supportive context might help with emotional healing and might help prevent intergenerational transmission of the trauma.

Hints to a history of culturally normalized trauma often occur in people's depression narratives, especially when they go beyond a history of recent symptoms and touch on their childhoods and on milestones in their personal development, including their education and their work experiences. Traumatic events are more likely to be recognized if they are suspected by a clinician or other interviewer who is aware of the types of trauma normalized by the culture. Awareness of cultural groups' normalized traumas is a critical piece of a cultural lens.

Chapter 6

Unnatural Deaths

Suicide is the most dramatic expression of depression's impact on life expectancy and the most common way for a single, acute episode of clinical depression to end in death. Chronic or recurrent depression can cause death not only by suicide but also via exacerbation of comorbid general medical conditions. Either acute or chronic depression—possibly accompanied by bipolarity and its associated risk-taking—can play a role in "unnatural deaths" not conclusively deemed to be suicides. These include deaths during high-risk recreational activities, falls and drownings under ambiguous circumstances, drug overdoses not known to be intentional, motor vehicle crashes, and violent altercations that might have been avoided.

In the United States (U.S.), psychological autopsies are rarely done after deaths known to be suicides and are done even less frequently after unnatural deaths of people with no history of depression or a suicide attempt. When carried out, they often are inconclusive. Some "unnatural deaths" would be classified as suicides if all the facts were known. Others would best be classified as mortality due to intentional acts undertaken with knowledge of significant mortality risk but without an explicit expectation of death. Such acts are the complement of "suicide attempts" in which a person commits a deliberate act of self-harm from which death could result but is not the most likely outcome, as when an adolescent girl living with her parents communicates distress by taking an overdose of sleeping pills or slashing her wrists at home, at a time when the most likely outcome is discovery and rescue. Deaths from self-neglect, a common form of depression-related mortality, are more frequent than suicides in some demographics. As mentioned in Chapter 1, lonely deaths (*kodokushi*) are epidemic among poor, widowed Japanese elders. A less dramatic form of "giving up on life" is encountered among depressed and lonely older Americans who die of cardiopulmonary disease because, indifferent to life or death, they don't get immunizations, eat poorly, and don't adhere to treatment for their chronic disease. They may succumb to influenza, pneumonia, sepsis, or decompensation of heart failure, having "natural deaths" that would have been prevented had the person not been depressed, passive, and fatalistic. During the COVID-19 pandemic, many people without a positive desire to live expressed their fatalistic mental state by intentionally disregarding recommendations on social distancing, mask-wearing, and handwashing, and declined to receive vaccinations even when they were free and easily accessed.

If a person died in a motor vehicle crash while driving at twice the speed limit on a narrow, poorly lit road while intoxicated with alcohol and cannabis, their death would not be classified as a suicide, though it would not have occurred without a decision to engage in obviously dangerous behavior. If the decision was the result of the "driven dysphoria" of bipolar depression with mixed features, the death would in fact be depression-associated mortality, but it is unlikely that it would be recorded as such in vital statistics. If a depressed person with an opioid use history, currently abstinent, injected a dose of fentanyl purchased on the street, with no one around to administer naloxone if it were needed, they would know that death from overdose was a significant risk. But death from overdose under such circumstances would not be deemed a suicide if the proximate reason for the injection was craving for an opioid rather than an expressed wish to die.

Suicide is not always due to a mental disorder, and people who die by suicide might never have qualified for a psychiatric diagnosis. It can be a thoughtful, deliberate act by a person who prefers to choose the time, place, and manner of their death. This view of suicide was articulated by Stoic philosophers two millennia ago (Seidler, 1983). In many societies people die by suicide to conform to a cultural norm. In Japan and, to a lesser extent, in China and South Korea—all nations with cultures rooted in Confucianism—a high government official or business leader caught in a major scandal might choose suicide not only to escape humiliation but also to salvage his family's honor. In the historical Hindu tradition of *sati*, the widow of an upper-caste man would throw herself on her husband's funeral pyre so that she could burn to death and join him in the afterlife. When *sati* was first practiced, a widow's suicide would be voluntary and would be respected as evidence of her devotion to her husband and her strength of character, rather than as implying that she would be desperately unhappy and suicidal without him. In 21st-century India, the self-immolation of young women has been associated with dowry disputes, in which a woman's in-laws, disappointed with gifts and remittances from her family of origin, compel her to burn herself to death (Kumar, 2003).

The joint suicide of lovers whose marriage is impossible within their society is a popular theme in literature. It is now rare in high-income, Western nations. Joint suicides of ill-fated couples continue to occur in Asian and African countries that have high power distance, gender inequality, and violent sectarian or tribal conflicts. For example, interfaith Hindu–Muslim couples in India have carried out joint suicides when forbidden to marry by their parents (Brennan, 2018). In societies with arranged marriages, women might choose to die by suicide rather than marry at an early age a man they do not love and might even actively detest (Arango, 2012).

While suicide does not necessarily entail a mental *disorder*, it almost always involves mental *distress*, with a judgment that suicide would relieve it. Modern theories of suicide have focused on individuals' mental distress considered in an interpersonal context. A prevalent theory of suicidal behavior with cross-cultural empirical support is Joiner's interpersonal-psychological theory of suicide (IPTS; Chu et al., 2017; Smith & Cukrowicz, 2010; Van Orden et al., 2010). According to the IPTS, a person who dies by suicide has experienced thwarted belongingness (TB) and perceived burdensomeness (PB) and has an acquired capacity for suicide (ACS). People experiencing TB want to feel connected to specific others but think it is not possible. People experiencing PB feel they are a burden to their families, to other significant people, or to society—that people they care about would be better off with them dead than alive. ACS is the lack of a fear of pain and/or death that would deter suicidal action.

In relating culture and depression to suicide risk, the authors find it useful to complement the three elements of the IPTS with a second set of seven related elements—four elements related to brain functions, two to higher-level cognitions, and one to environment—to constitute an interpersonal-neuropsychiatric (IPNP) model of suicide. Several of the additional elements proposed are mentioned in full descriptions of the IPTS such as those referenced in the cited review by Chu and colleagues, but they are not called out explicitly as separate factors. The model is summarized in Table 6.1. The interactive effects of culture and of depression (including bipolar depression) on suicide can be understood in terms of their effects on each of the 10 elements. Application of the model suggests ideas for suicide prevention at the individual and population levels.

Cultural Dimensions of an Interpersonal-Neuropsychiatric Model of Suicide

Thwarted Belongingness (TB) and Perceived Burdensomeness (PB)

A fundamental cultural element of the relationship between depression, TB, and PB concerns the acceptability versus stigmatization of depression. A person with public stigma may experience TB if they desire connection with those who stigmatize them. Anticipated public stigma can have the same effect as actual stigma on a person's sense of TB. A person with intense self-stigma may feel that their presence, or even their existence, burdens those they care about and that they deserve rejection and ostracism. If a culture conspicuously stigmatizes depression, it is likely that a depressed person will internalize the stigma so that public stigma, anticipated public stigma, and self-stigma combine to intensify TB and PB.

Table 6.1 An Interpersonal-Neuropsychiatric Model of Suicide

Category	Element	Description
Interpersonal/ psychological	Thwarted belongingness	Frustrated wish for interpersonal connection
	Perceived burdensomeness	Feeling like a burden on others or society—"worth more dead than alive"
	Acquired capacity for suicide	Loss of fear of death and/or the pain of dying
Brain function	Behavioral activation	Initiating and persisting in intentional behavior (vs. apathy)
	Behavioral inhibition	Inhibiting actions cued by immediate circumstances but inconsistent with plans or learned prohibitions (vs. impulsiveness)
	Experience of pain	Physical and/or emotional pain that is aversive and difficult to bear
	Experience of pleasure	Feeling pleasure or reward from a sensation or activity
Higher-level cognitions	Hope	Belief that the future will be better—for oneself or for loved ones
	Reason to live (aka *ikigai* or raison d'être)	Life's meaning and purpose (long-term *ikigai*) and daily joys (short-term *ikigai*)
Environment	Availability of highly lethal means of self-harm	Highly lethal means of suicide available quickly and without planning or extraordinary effort or expense

Depression can operate to either increase or decrease ACS. It can increase the capacity if the potentially suicidal person feels they have nothing to lose by dying. It can decrease ACS if it increases their fear of death and/or the pain of the contemplated suicidal act. Depression with mixed features can include feelings of fearlessness. This phenomenon helps explain why the rate of death by suicide is higher in bipolar depression than in unipolar major depressive disorder (Grande et al., 2016; McIntyre & Calabrese, 2019).

Acquired Capacity for Suicide (ACS)

Cultural attitudes toward suicide have a powerful effect on Acquired Capacity for Suicide (ACS). Singapore is a city-state with a multiethnic population and centralized recording of suicide attempts requiring hospital care. This permits analysis of ethnicity-specific suicide attempt incidence and interethnic comparison of the details of attempts. The frequency and potential lethality of attempts are greatest for Chinese, intermediate for Indians, and lowest for Malays.

Differences are attributed to the religiosity of Malays and the effectiveness of their religious and familial injunctions against suicide (Choo et al., 2017). Islam strongly discourages suicide, and the effectiveness of its prohibitions is reflected by the low suicide rates of predominantly Muslim countries.

Among Christian sects, Catholicism might discourage suicide more effectively than most Protestant denominations. The point was made by Emile Durkheim (1897/1951) when he noted higher suicide rates in majority-Protestant countries than majority-Catholic countries. Spoerri et al. (2010) examined the relationship of the religious affiliation of Swiss people aged 35 to 94 as reported on the 2000 census to suicides over the next five years. The study classified people by religious affiliation without regard to their participation in services or membership in a specific church. They found that compared with Protestants, Catholics had lower suicide rates and those with no religious affiliation had higher suicide rates, after adjusting for age, marital status, education, and type of household (single person, multi-person, or institutional). The benefit of Catholic identity was greater in men than in women, and the harm of non-affiliation was greater in women than in men. All effects increased with age in both men and women. For men under age 55, the harm of non-affiliation was not statistically significant. For women under age 64, the benefit of Catholic identification was not statistically significant. Viewing the results from a generational perspective, religion is a less important determinant of suicide for Swiss Boomers than for those of the Silent Generation.

In a longitudinal study of 89,708 female nurses in the U.S., those who attended religious services weekly or more had a five-fold lower suicide rate over the next 14 years. After adjusting for covariates, the hazard ratio was 0.05 (95% confidence limits [0.006, 0.48]) for Catholics and 0.34 (95% confidence limits [0.10, 1.10]) for Protestants (VanderWeele et al., 2016).

With respect to religion and suicide, "the devil is in the details." In a comprehensive review of 10 years of articles on religion and suicide, Lawrence and colleagues (2016) provided evidence that religion has little effect on suicidal ideation and that its effects on suicide attempts (and thus on suicide mortality) are different for people who adhere to a minority religion within their area or have a diagnosis or other identity that is stigmatized within their religion. For example, adolescent Protestant students attending Catholic schools in Scotland had a significantly higher risk of suicide attempts or self-harm than their Catholic classmates (Young et al., 2011). In rural China, where religious people are a minority, suicides in adults aged 15–34 were more frequent among those with a religious affiliation than those without one (Jia & Zhang, 2012). In young adults serving in the U.S. Air Force, suicide attempts and serious suicidal ideation were more common in those with a non-Christian religious affiliation (Snarr et al., 2010).

The impact of religion on an individual also differs according to the specific doctrines they accept. A person who expects to go to heaven when they die does not necessarily believe that death by suicide will disqualify them if their life was extremely painful. If so, the religion having a general prohibition against suicide might not protect them from attempting it.

A Hungarian case–control study based on interviews with family members of people who had died by suicide offers a provocative perspective on how intersecting identities modify the effect of religion on suicidal behavior. In Hungary, 85% of Protestants belong to Calvinist sects, the doctrine of which bases a person's fate on God's mercy or its absence, with little effect of the person's deeds during life—a fundamentally gloomier outlook than that of Catholicism, which offers believers absolution from sin via confession. Among the Christians studied, Protestant affiliation associated with higher suicide risk. However, the effect of religious identity for an individual was influenced by their education and their level of participation in religious activity. For Protestants, there was a higher risk of suicide in people who had less than a high school education or who were college graduates who attended religious services weekly or more frequently. For Catholics, more frequent service attendance was associated with lower suicide risk for people regardless of their level of education, and both college graduates and people without high school diplomas had lower risk than those other levels. The authors' inference was that, at least in the Hungarian context, religious culture rather than religion-based social integration was a more relevant contributor to suicide (Moksony & Hegedűs, 2019).

In assessing the ACS of a patient with suicidal ideation or death wishes, religious affiliation is less important than the specifics of the patient's use of religion to cope with stress, the frequency and intensity of their involvement with religious activities, the place of their religion within the relevant local community, and the intersection of the patient's other cultural identities with their religious affiliation. Knowing that a patient with suicidal ideation or death wishes sees religious affiliation as important to their personal identity should prompt a more detailed exploration of the role of religion in the person's life and the specific beliefs the patient has adopted from the religion with which they identify.

Behavioral Activation

Suicidal acts require behavioral activation; a person too apathetic to get out of bed may not be able to plan and execute a suicidal act. The weeks immediately after starting an antidepressant drug can be a time of increased suicide risk because apathy can improve more rapidly than dysphoric mood, anhedonia, and suicidal ideation. When depression is associated with substance abuse and the depressed person gives up alcohol, an opiate, or other addictive substance, they may experience a combination of behavioral activation and increased dysphoria, both due to drug withdrawal. People with bipolar depression or depression with mixed features can experience *driven dysphoria*—a combination of emotional pain and negative thoughts with increased energy and motivation to act. Increased behavioral activation at miserable times is one of the reasons for the high risk of suicide in people who are depressed with mixed features.

Because behavioral activation is needed to initiate a suicidal act, the three situations just described are times of increased suicide risk. Culture affects the likelihood that they may occur and the likelihood that suicide will be prevented even when a depressed person is willing to seek treatment. If family, friends, or influential community members question the diagnosis or minimize the problem of a depressed person who has sought treatment, they may discourage the person from returning for a follow-up visit to the clinician. If the person has little disposable income, practical necessities, family pressures, or cultural values may not allow money to be spent on mental health care or medications for treating their depression. In cultures where husbands control family money and wives may spend only with their husband's consent, a depressed woman might be denied the resources to pay for follow-up care, to make a co-payment on a prescription, or to spend money for transportation to a clinician's office. She might also be discouraged from taking time off work for mental health care if it would imply a loss of wage income for the family. If substance use is heavily stigmatized within a culture, it is likely that medication-assisted treatment for substance use disorders will be unacceptable and that depression will be dismissed as an accompaniment of substance use that requires no treatment other than quitting the use of the substance. The person might be pressured to withdraw from a drug or alcohol and experience behavioral activation from substance withdrawal while miserable from an untreated depression.

Behavioral Inhibition

Motivation to harm oneself or to risk death does not translate into self-injurious or dangerous behavior if it is inhibited by executive control. Normal brains have neural pathways that enable rational considerations (e.g., judgment of danger and learned rules of appropriate behavior) to inhibit self-injurious or risky behavior that would otherwise occur in response to strong emotions or environmental cues. Just as behavioral activation is necessary for planning and preparing to take a suicidal action, behavioral inhibition can stop a person from carrying it out. Behavioral inhibition is reduced by alcohol, benzodiazepines, phencyclidine, and several other abusable substances. It is impaired by sleep deprivation. A person's capacity for behavioral inhibition normally develops throughout childhood and adolescence into young adulthood; for this reason wrongdoers in their childhood or early teens usually are tried in a separate juvenile court system because they are seen by the law as being less fully responsible than adults for their criminal acts. The brain's behavioral inhibition system can be impaired for life by severe trauma or multiple adverse childhood experiences (ACEs), by neurodevelopmental disorders, by malnutrition, by traumatic brain injury, or by acute or chronic exposure to neurotoxins. Cultural identity and its structural accompaniments are associated with the prevalence of causes of both long-term and acute impairments of behavioral inhibition. There are cultures that expect long hours of work or study at the expense of adequate sleep. Others condone intimate partner violence and harsh discipline of children, common sources of adult trauma and of ACEs. Poverty and/or discrimination can lead to chronic toxic exposures, as when neighborhoods or entire cities are exposed to lead from contaminated public water supplies or when agricultural workers living on or next to farms are chronically exposed to the neurotoxicity of organophosphate pesticides. Poverty also can place a family in an unsafe neighborhood or a food desert where healthy groceries are hard to find or are unaffordable.

Experience of Pain

When people feel persistent, severe physical and/or emotional pain, they will do what they can to relieve it, including engaging in life-threatening behavior like taking large quantities of opioids. Depression can increase suicidal behavior by increasing the experienced intensity of pain and/or making it less tolerable. Depression is a very common comorbidity of chronically painful medical conditions. Treating comorbid depression is a central principle of chronic pain treatment.

Culture will determine the social acceptability of complaints of pain for people according to their life circumstances, health issues, and status in the group. It might condone or prohibit specific approaches to pain relief and might offer traditional alternatives for treating it. If complaints of pain are contrary to his culture's masculine ideal, a man in pain might not seek treatment for it. If the diagnosis and treatment of depression are stigmatized, he might avoid treatment of comorbid depression. He might use opioid analgesics, alcohol, cannabis, or other potentially abusable substances without medical supervision, entailing mortality risks related to overdose or dangerous driving.

On the other hand, if a person comes from an ethnic group with a well-developed system of traditional medicine, seeking traditional treatment as a complement or alternative to mainstream medical care might be appealing. If traditional practitioners are available in the community, the person might seek help from one of them. Traditional treatment for their painful condition would probably be holistic and would include elements directed at improving the patient's mental state and at making their lifestyle healthier. This option could decrease suicide risk by reducing pain or making it more bearable, without worsening TB and PB via stigmatization.

Experience of Pleasure

Anhedonia, the inability to experience pleasure, is a major symptom of depression and one that depressed people find most unbearable in the long term. Anhedonia is associated with greater suicidal ideation after controlling for psychiatric diagnosis and the overall level of depressive symptoms (Ducasse et al., 2018). It is increasingly appreciated as a dimension of the depression phenotype important for understanding pathophysiology and personalizing treatment. Its measurement, like the measurement of mood, requires measures sensitive to culture as well as to the condition of the depressed person. The standard measure has been the Snaith-Hamilton Pleasure Scale (SHAPS; Snaith et al., 1995). A respondent to the SHAPS questionnaire is asked to agree or disagree with each of 14 statements, all of which begin with "I would enjoy," "I would be able to enjoy," or "I would find pleasure." If the person disagrees with three or more items, they are deemed to have a clinically significant degree of anhedonia. Items include such activities as having a favorite meal or a cup of coffee or tea, taking a warm bath, reading, seeing a beautiful view, helping others, and being praised; they touch on sensual, intellectual, aesthetic, and social pleasures. In a sample of British psychiatric inpatients under treatment for depression, anhedonia measured with the scale was significantly correlated with suicidal ideation as well as with the anhedonia item on the Montgomery-Åsberg Depression Rating Scale (MADRS). The questions on the SHAPS are relatively bland and culture-independent, though specific items might not be useful in some cultures: For example, a strictly observant Mormon would not drink caffeinated beverages. A more significant concern about the SHAPS is that does not cover the loss of pleasure in areas that are intensely important to many people, such as the pleasure of meaningful work and the pleasure of intimacy. Another shortcoming is that it does not deal with the anticipation of pleasure or with the pursuit of pleasure. These dimensions of anhedonia can contribute to suicide risk. Measures of these other aspects of anhedonia are more likely to require cultural adaptation (Rizvi et al., 2016).

People willingly make exhausting efforts at work, in avocational activities, and in family-related contexts, looking forward to experiencing pleasure and/or satisfaction if their efforts succeed. With no prospect of feeling pleasure, satisfaction, or happiness, a person can rapidly lose their will to live. A person with severe depressive anhedonia cannot be "cheered up" by pleasant experiences.

One with moderate depressive anhedonia might lose their motivation to pursue pleasant experiences, and thus have very few of them even if the capacity to feel pleasure is not completely lost. A person with mild to moderate depression with a retained ability to experience pleasure is less likely to become suicidal if they frequently have pleasant experiences. This is part of the rationale for *behavioral activation therapy*, a treatment for depression that encourages patients to systematically pursue activities they will enjoy (Knittle et al., 2019). The prevailing culture and the person's role in it affect whether their everyday life frequently offers opportunities for daily pleasures without requiring special effort to pursue them.

Hope

Hope for the future cues the brain's behavioral inhibition system (BIS) to prevent self-harm and its behavioral activation system (BAS) to promote actions that might improve a person's situation. While hopefulness is an individual trait, cultures and subcultures are well known to have characteristic average levels of hope and optimism. Pessimism can coexist with hopefulness: A person might think that their life on earth will continue to be miserable, but they look forward to some form of life after death (heaven or reincarnation into a better situation) or to a better life for their children and grandchildren. In religions including Catholicism, Islam, and certain Buddhist sects, there is a belief in an afterlife or next life (reincarnation) that will reward the faithful—but only if they die naturally rather than by suicide. This belief is a source of hope, as well as a cue to the BIS to prevent suicidal acts.

Hope that one's children will have a better life is the rule in first-generation immigrants. It is one of the reasons first-generation immigrants to most high-income countries have lower rates of suicide than subsequent generations of the same immigrant group (Bauwelinck et al., 2017; Di Thiene et al., 2015; Ide et al., 2012; Nasseri & Moulton, 2011; Peña et al., 2008; Puzo et al., 2018).

Reason to Live

A strong reason for living, including a sense of meaning and purpose in life, can offset factors that favor suicide, especially if the BAS is sufficiently intact for a person's purpose in life to translate into positive, life-affirming actions and if the BIS is sufficiently intact for self-destructive impulses to be inhibited. As elaborated in Chapter 11, the Japanese concept of *ikigai* (reason to live) has a quotidian and a long-term/life-course dimension. Everyday meaning of life comprises, among other things, the enjoyment of food and drink, nature, music or art, productive work, novelty and learning, sports or hobbies, positive relationships, generosity, affection, and sexuality. Long-term meaning of life can come from an occupation or profession one experiences as a vocation or life purpose; a marriage or other long-term intimate relationship; the care and education of children or grandchildren; creating, maintaining, or growing a business; religious practice; philanthropy; military service; or political action. During a young person's growing into maturity, having primary and secondary education, and being enculturated, they will develop personal reasons for living. These will evolve over the life course, influenced by education, life experiences, and relationships. Enculturation can endow a person with a strong reason to live, as religious education and practice can do when they are positive and nontraumatic. In other circumstances, the culture imposes a purpose in life on a young person that is incompatible with their authentic self. Entering adulthood, they may feel empty, rootless, or like an impostor, with no real purpose in living. If depression makes the person unable to enjoy mundane pleasures, they might experience neither long-term nor everyday meaning of life and feel no positive reason to live that would deter a suicidal act.

For example, growing up in a family that is part of a highly religious community can place a late adolescent or young adult in a difficult situation if they do not share the family's faith or find that their religion rejects or stigmatizes the life choices they would want to make. Many religions reject homosexuality or non-binary sexual identity. Some religious communities will not accept a young woman wanting to pursue higher education and an independent career while rejecting marriage and/or having children. A person in such a situation might find that establishing an authentic purpose in life will come at the cost of family conflict, loss of friendships, disruption of social support, and loss of practical assistance from others. Until the person comes to believe in another way of life, whether a secular philosophy or a different religion, there will be greater vulnerability to suicidality if they become depressed. Religions with tight communities of faith and detailed specifications for the life course (e.g., Hasidic Judaism, Latter-Day Saints Christianity, traditional Islam) can at their best supply young people with a reason to live in both the mundane and the long-term senses. Social support from a community of faith can protect against depression, and a powerful, explicit reason to live can reduce the risk of suicide. However, the benefits of the religious community are unlikely to be shared by non-conforming and/or skeptical members of faithful families.

Availability of Highly Lethal Means of Self-Harm

Firearms, highly toxic pesticides, and high bridges or towers easily accessible and suitable for jumping offer suicide methods that are highly lethal and difficult to reverse once initiated. By comparison, some types of drug overdoses can be reversed (e.g., opioid overdoses can be reduced by timely administration of naloxone) or managed by giving supportive treatment while the drug is eliminated from the body. A person who begins a suicide by hanging, drowning, or slashing a wrist sometimes can be rescued. Making the most lethal and irreversible means of suicide less accessible (e.g., by banning the sale of paraquat, having waiting periods and other restrictions for handgun sales, blocking pedestrian access to the rooftops of prominent towers, or placing nets below bridges popular for jumping) have reduced total suicide rates in places that have implemented them. When highly lethal means of self-harm are restricted, people do not necessarily find alternative means, so overall suicide rates decrease (Jin et al., 2016). Even modest delays and inconveniences in undertaking a suicidal act can be lifesaving. It is quick and convenient to use a gun that is kept loaded and unlocked in one's bedroom or to swallow a pesticide already stored in a lethal quantity in a shed in one's backyard. The need to unlock a gun safe and to load a gun with ammunition stored separately, or to specifically purchase enough of a pesticide to be irreversibly toxic, can put a lifesaving interval between a suicidal impulse and a highly lethal act. A person's cultural identity, including the place they live, is associated with the availability of highly lethal means. For example, in the U.S. there are regions in which most adult men own guns and many of them store their guns unsafely, and regions where the rate of gun ownership is low and few gun owners fail to lock their guns and securely store their ammunition. In all of America, gun ownership is lower among women and members of racial/ethnic minorities than it is among non-Hispanic White men.

Suicidality Through a Cultural Lens

At the individual level, cultural identity affects suicide risk through its effects on the 10 elements of the IPNP model. It also is related to the willingness of a suicidal person to seek help and to disclose to another person their suicidal ideas, plans, and contributors to suicide risk.

A cultural group at a given time and place has shared perspectives on life and its prospects and shared experiences of the suicides of group members. If the rate of suicide is sufficiently high in a group, virtually every individual will have experienced the suicide of someone with whom they have a connection. The connection might be familial, via a network of friends and acquaintances, via relationships with organizations like employers or educational institutions, or via social media. Or the connection might be a parasocial relationship, with the person being a fan, follower, or admirer of one who recently died by suicide. (Parasocial relationships will be discussed in detail in Chapter 15.) After a suicide, survivors often talk about the death as tragic, exceptional, and unnecessary. Even so, a high incidence of suicide in a cultural group tends to normalize suicide within that group, and multiple deaths by suicide among a person's connections in many cases increase their ACS. Within a culture there can thus be a positive feedback loop with negative consequences. A high suicide rate creates conditions that might increase the rate further if neither deliberate action nor changes in circumstances oppose the trend.

Beyond individual risk factors, there appears to be an influence of the physical and social environment on suicide rates. Known risk factors in the physical environment are the length of the day (season), amount of sunlight, and average temperature. News of a celebrity suicide predicts an increase in the suicide rate over the subsequent month, controlling for many other known population-level factors. Other relevant aspects of the prevalent social environment can be estimated by analysis of a large volume of social media posts. A South Korean study used data from the country's most popular blogging platform to determine whether words frequently used in social media posts, when combined with known predictors like day of the week, season of the year, and recent celebrity suicides, would predict future suicide rates (K. S. Lee et al., 2018). The authors modeled suicide rates for 730 days, using independent variables from the 5 years ending 1 week before the day predicted. On 82.9% of the days covered by their models, the actual suicide rate was within the 85% confidence limits of the model's prediction.

Not surprisingly, high counts of posts mentioning depression—either psychological or economic—predicted higher suicide rates, and high counts of posts that included at least one positive word predicted lower rates. Less expected was the finding that frequent posts containing certain words with no apparent emotional content were predictive of higher suicide rates. For example, the count of posts containing the Korean word *siljejeokg*, implying "practical," "matter-of-fact," or "businesslike," was a more powerful contributor to the estimated rate of suicide than the count of posts mentioning "depressive disorder."

The study of Lee and colleagues suggests that spikes in a nation's suicide rate often can be predicted, and if so, public health interventions to prevent suicide could be focused on periods where expected suicide rates are high. In many places, anti-suicide messaging and offers of telephone crisis counseling are now triggered by celebrity suicides. More can be done to focus suicide prevention efforts, and utilizing social media analysis to do so offers the additional benefit of uncovering themes worth exploring when counseling a suicidal person within a specific cultural and social context.

At the individual level, there are copycat suicides following the suicide of a celebrity, suicide pacts of people who meet online, and joint suicides of people who encourage one another to act on their shared suicidal ideation (Durkee et al., 2011; S. Y. Lee & Kwon, 2018; Ozawa-de Silva, 2008). From the standpoint of the IPTS, these situations involve an increase in ACS. Suicides of respected or admired people can increase hopelessness or reduce reason to live: A suicidal person feels that if someone they admire and respect finds life hopeless or meaningless, how could they have hope or find meaning?

Social media have a potential positive role to play in reducing suicide. Analysis of posts at the population level can help estimate the environmental contribution to suicide risk in people already known to have suicidal ideation and can help public health organizations to target and time educational messages about depression and suicide and links for information, support, and clinical services. Analysis of posts at the individual level can potentially complement clinical assessment and enhance its completeness and accuracy.

Clinical suicide risk analysis should be applied to people who disclose suicidal ideas or plans, who have made suicide attempts, who have mood disorders or other psychiatric conditions associated with suicide, or who have a pattern of recent healthcare use that raises a suspicion of suicidality. When the technology has sufficiently matured, confidential automated analysis of social media posts and mobile device data at the individual level will be helpful in identifying when a person known to have chronic suicide risk should be urgently reassessed.

In a review of studies from 2000 to 2017 of contacts with primary care prior to suicide, an average of 80% of suicidal people contacted a primary care provider within 1 year of a suicide, and an average of 44% did so within 1 month of their deaths (Stene-Larsen & Reneflot, 2019). Women and people over age 50 were more likely to seek primary care in the month before their suicide. The typical reason for primary care visits of people in the month before suicide usually is not depressed mood. The example of "Sophie" in Chapter 1 illustrates a typical presentation of a suicidal person to a primary care physician. She came to her physician seeking prescriptions for an opioid and a hypnotic, with a chief complaint of insomnia related to somatic pain. Such a patient might be seeking the means of suicide by drug overdose—or might have increased risk of suicide but not yet be thinking of it.

A presentation like Sophie's should prompt a physician to screen for depression and for suicide risk before considering the prescription of medications that could be combined with alcohol in a fatal overdose. In her case, there was severe physical and emotional pain, her pain and interpersonal conflict increased behavioral activation, insomnia and alcohol reduced inhibition, and marital problems decreased her reason to live. An overdose of opioids and hypnotics together with alcohol would be a painless means of suicide she would not find frightening, and if she received the prescriptions that she was requesting, she would have lethal means at hand.

Chapter 7

Depression and Social Class: A Four-Dimensional View

Social class or socioeconomic status (SES)—as determined within a person's nation and region by the four dimensions of wealth/income, education, occupation, and heritage—is essential to the definition of cultural identity. It is significant in determining an individual's risk of depression, the typical illness narratives of depression, treatments available, engagement with treatment, and treatment outcomes. In any locality, people living in poverty have higher rates of depressive symptoms, of clinical depression including MDD, and of general medical illness than those with secure food and housing and access to affordable healthcare. However, rates of depression and suicide do not consistently correlate with income or education *across* nations and regions. And, once basic needs are met, the relationship between social class and depression becomes more complicated. This chapter will focus on exceptions to the association of higher status with less depression, the modifying effect of intersecting identities on depression in lower classes, and the implications of social class for timely recognition, accurate diagnosis, and effective treatment of depression and bipolar illness.

Reference to four dimensions brings in the concept of time. A person's social class identity and its implications for depression are determined not only by where a person currently lives and their current wealth and income but also by a person's past and future residence and financial circumstances, by the path that the person and their fortunes take over time, by intergenerational differences, and by acculturation. For example, during the COVID-19 pandemic and its aftermath, many people's economic status changed. Many small businesses closed, with significant losses to their owners. At the same time, income increased for many providers of essential services.

In the literature of the social sciences, populations are divided into a hierarchy of socioeconomic classes, based on combinations of income, education, occupation, and parental status. Two commonly encountered stratifications are based entirely on household income, presuming that the dimensions that determine social class are sufficiently correlated for an income-based approach to be valid. Since dimensions are not perfectly correlated, understanding class effects at an individual level requires modification of the income-based approach. If people initially are sorted into classes based on their income, their class assignments should be modified so that higher education, higher-class background, a more prestigious occupation, and membership in a non-stigmatized ethnic group or subculture will raise a person's status; and opposite attributes will lower it.

The simplest income-based stratification is upper class, middle class, lower class: For example, people in the top 20% of household incomes are upper class, the next 40% are middle class, and the lowest 40% are lower class. The characterization of people in the top quintile of income as "upper class" undoubtedly would seem ironic to a couple with two young children in San Francisco or a similarly high-cost city with an income at the national 80th percentile. Such a family would have trouble finding affordable housing close to work, and the cost of childcare and obligations to repay college student loans might make their financial situation precarious.

A more nuanced and interesting stratification by household income divides the American population into seven groups: upper-upper class (>99th percentile of income—"the 1%"), lower-upper class (96th–99th percentile), upper-middle class (82nd–96th percentile), middle class (58th–82nd percentile), working class (28th–58th percentile), working poor (15th–28th percentile), and underclass (<15th percentile). The seven-level model makes culturally relevant distinctions between people with annual household incomes in the millions and those with household incomes around $100,000, between the working poor and the underclass, and between the working class (often with blue-collar occupations) and the middle class (typically white-collar workers, highly skilled tradespeople, or proprietors of small businesses). The working poor support themselves by working at poorly paid jobs in service industries or by doing minimally skilled manual labor. Members of the underclass are unemployed, disabled, or inconsistently employed, relying all or part of the year on some form of public assistance or charity. Part of the underclass comprises people with severe and chronic mental illness. Most of the working poor have low educational attainment, often lacking a high school diploma or equivalent. The same is true of non-disabled members of the underclass.

In 2013 the British Broadcasting Corporation conducted the Great British Class Survey, a survey of 161,000 people intended to provide a basis for updating the conception of social class in the United Kingdom. The survey aimed to identify the three types of 'capital' identified by French sociologist Pierre Bourdieu as differentiating social classes: economic (wealth and income), cultural (educational credentials and cultural tastes), and social (especially relational social capital that can be utilized for practical purposes). A team led by Mike Savage of the London School of Economics analyzed the data and using latent class analysis identified seven groups with characteristic combinations of capital (Savage et al., 2013):

1. The elite: Wealth, high income, social connections, degrees from prestigious universities, and highbrow tastes. Examples: People with substantial inherited wealth, successful lawyers and medical specialists, top executives.
2. The established middle class: Relatively high income, significant wealth but less than the elite, a broad range of social contacts, and engagement with a mixture of highbrow and "emerging" culture. Examples: Upper management, career government officials.
3. The technical middle class: Relatively high income, high savings, and expensive housing but with limited social networks and limited cultural engagement. Examples: Engineers and airline pilots.
4. New affluent workers: Moderate on economic and social capital with above average income but not much savings and engaged with emerging culture. Mostly young; in skilled occupations, either white- or blue-collar; usually without elite education.
5. Traditional working class: Modest income but usually own their own homes. Limited social contacts, limited engagement with culture. Examples: Truck drivers, plumbers.
6. Emergent service workers: Modest income, little savings, probably rent rather than own their residences. Engaged with emerging culture, many social connections. Many have degrees in arts or humanities and/or are pursuing creative careers.
7. Precariat: Low income, little or no savings, rent their residences, low social capital, little cultural engagement. Examples: Unemployed, house cleaner.

Similar distinctions can be made in all high-income countries and upper-middle-income countries. Divisions between classes defined solely by annual household incomes will be different across nations. This reflects not only differences in the purchasing power of different nations' currencies but also the extent to which public services or income transfers mitigate the effects of unequal gross household incomes. Within a single nation, there can be major differences between regions in the most valid definition of class in relation to income. In Memphis, Tennessee or Albuquerque, New Mexico, a 2020 family income of $310,000 would have put a family in the top 1%, with corresponding social status. In the San Francisco metropolitan area, the same income would not even be in the top 10% (DQYDJ.com, n.d.).

Basing social class on income alone also disregards the important effect of wealth in providing economic security and resources to deal with random shocks like the loss of a job, the need for major repairs on one's house, or a serious illness in one's family. Two people with the same household income can have dramatically different net worth—one might be loaded with debt, and the other might have savings to support their household for one year or more. Major life stresses, even ones that are not directly involved with financial losses, often are associated with unbudgeted costs such as medical or legal bills, costs of travel, or loss of income due to disruption of work. The likelihood of depression in the face of a stressful life event will be higher for people with negative net worth and lower for those with substantial savings. In this connection, racial/ethnic identity, age, and gender are strongly associated with median household wealth and with wealth inequality; and the differences among racial/ethnic groups in median household wealth are disproportionate to the differences in their median household income. Black Americans are especially likely to have low or negative household net worth, in part because of historical barriers to homeownership. Age effects are large as well. Younger people are more likely to have outstanding educational debt, and older ones are more likely to own real estate and have savings for retirement. Table 7.1 displays the contrast between median household net worth by race/ethnicity and by age band (Table 7.1).

Within a racial group in the United States (U.S.) there are subgroups of people who would describe themselves as "American" preceded by an ethnic adjective. Comparison among these groups reveals striking intergroup differences

Table 7.1 2020 Household Net Worth by Race/Ethnicity and by Age (US Census, 2022)

Racial/Ethnic Group	Median Net Worth in 2020
Non-Hispanic White	$217,500
Black	$18,430
Asian	$64,800
Hispanic	$39,800
Age of Head of Household	
Less than 35 Years	$22,000
35-44 Years	$97,740
45-54 Years	$166,600
55-64 Years	$230,900
65 Years and Over	$300,000

in median household income within the same broader racial/ethnic group (Table 7.2). While Blacks overall have a much lower median household income than Whites, Appalachian Whites (typically of remote British ancestry) have a much lower median household income than Blacks of Nigerian or West

Table 7.2 Median Household Income by Race and Ethnicity: Illustrative Examples (Wikipedia, 2023b)

Race/Ethnicity	2021 Median Household Income
Non-Hispanic White	$74,932
Appalachian	$49,747
Armenian	$83,756
British	$87,288
French	$75,783
Irish	$78,949
German	$78,960
Italian	$84,416
Russian	$90,296
Swedish	$82,731
Black	$46,774
Ethiopian	$58,507
Haitian	$60,169
Jamaican	$65,789
Nigerian	$71,465
Asian	$100,572
Bangladeshi	$67,187
Chinese	$93,007
Filipino	$101,157
Indian	$141,906
Japanese	$87,789
Korean	$82,946
Pakistani	$100,730
Taiwanese	$119,022
Vietnamese	$77,884
Hispanic	$57,981

Indian origin. Among ethnic minorities, some subgroups have median household incomes markedly higher than the median for non-Hispanic Whites overall, while others have median household incomes well below the median for their broader group. The relevance of the intergroup income differences to depression relates both to the likelihood of financial distress (e.g., food insecurity, homelessness) and to what is normal for one's group. If a 35-year-old Indian American had a household income of $80,000, they would probably be a disappointment to their parents and would have relatively low status in their local ethnic community. An African American with the same household income living in a lower-income region of the U.S. would probably be seen as successful by their peers in the local Black community.

There are clinically significant economic differences between nationalities that might initially be lumped by a clinician of a different race. For example, the median household income of families of Taiwanese background is significantly higher than those of families from mainland China, and the differences between Indians, Pakistanis, and Bangladeshis are even larger. The median household income of Russian Americans is almost twice that of those who describe their heritage as Appalachian. Awareness of subgroup norms is especially important for clinicians treating patients from racial/ethnic minority populations they do not know well. Awareness of the large differences between subgroups prompts appropriate skepticism and follow-up questions when reading research findings that group patients by broad racial categories.

During the COVID-19 pandemic, many Americans had large drops in their incomes related to job loss or disruption of their business or professional work. Analysis of data from Wave 13 of the U.S. Census Bureau's Household Pulse Survey, conducted nine months into the pandemic (December 9 to December 21, 2020) shows that, even after controlling for 2019 household income, groups definable by gender, age/generation, racial/ethnic identity, educational level, and region of residence differed greatly in their level of difficulty paying bills and/or concerns about food or housing security (US Census Bureau, 2023d). Some examples: Americans aged 65 or older were less likely than those of other ages to have difficulty paying usual household expenses. Black and Hispanic Americans were more likely to have insufficient food sometimes or often. In Utah and in the District of Columbia, only 25% of households had difficulty paying their usual household expenses, while in several states of the South and Southwest, more than 40% of households faced such insecurity.

When people loaded with debt develop clinical depression, they often feel they cannot afford treatment and therefore delay seeking help until their depression is more severe and difficult to treat or until they come to medical attention because they are suicidal. In the U.S., income-based federal health insurance subsidies, tax deductions for medical expenses, and fee adjustments by healthcare providers would not be sufficient to help patients with middle-class household incomes but little or no net worth and significant debt service obligations. Functional impairments due to depression can reduce a person's work performance and put their income at risk. Negative net worth heightens anxiety about income loss and makes its personal consequences much worse. In the U.S. Federal Reserve November 2020 Survey of Household Economics and Decisionmaking, 16% of respondents were unable to pay some of their current bills, and 13% stated that a $400 emergency expense would make them unable to do so. More than half reported an unexpected major medical expense of $1000 or more during the past 12 months. 20% stated they went without a needed doctor visit or mental health care because they couldn't afford it (US Federal Reserve, 2021). For an individual with negative net worth and little cash, a $20 co-payment for an antidepressant drug would be reason to not fill a prescription. Timely and consistent treatment for depressed people in financially precarious circumstances requires insurance that covers antidepressant drugs, physician visits, and psychotherapy without substantial and often unaffordable co-payments, or adjustment of prices and fees by suppliers of medications and clinical services.

Higher education—especially if connected with a respected profession like medicine or law—can raise a person's social status beyond where it would be based on household income alone. The relationship of higher education to depression risk is dependent on economic and cultural context. For example, in the U.S. low education is associated with MDE, in Europe it is not, and in Japan it is associated with *lower* risk of major depression (Kessler & Bromet, 2013).

The relationship between dropping out of college and subsequent vulnerability to depression persists after controlling for income and wealth. There are several potential mediators of the relationship. Though there are highly publicized cases of college dropouts who became billionaire entrepreneurs, failure to complete college usually implies lesser occupational opportunity and lower lifetime income. If a person has borrowed money to pay college tuition and living expenses, the impact is even greater. The reason for dropping out of college might be a traumatic event in the person's life which by itself would increase their subsequent vulnerability to depression. A woman might have had an unplanned pregnancy that exposed her to the risk of postpartum depression and would make her life more stressful for years after her child was born. Adverse childhood experiences (ACEs) and neurodevelopmental issues can cause both lifetime vulnerability to depression and difficulty completing college.

Depression Risks of Middle-Class and Upper-Middle-Class Jobs

Employment typically associated with middle-class or upper-middle-class status can entail depression risk related to *job strain*—a potential consequence of an employee's role within the organization that employs them. Job strain is associated with positions that have high demands but little control over working conditions and positions where the great effort required for the job is disproportionate to its modest financial, social, and organizational rewards. Job strain due to either demand–control imbalance (DCI) or effort–reward imbalance (ERI) is associated with elevated levels of inflammatory biomarkers and with high scores on depression rating scales (Almroth et al., 2021; Arango et al., 2021; Duchaine et al., 2021; Matthews et al., 2021; Niedhammer et al., 2021a).

Examples of DCI can be offered from the healthcare and the retail sectors of the economy. A licensed practical nurse (LPN) working in a hospital caring for acutely ill patients will be held accountable for the outcomes of their patients' care but will be less able than a registered nurse to question or challenge physicians' orders (Rajbhandary & Basu, 2010). Especially when there are staffing shortages, as there were during the COVID-19 pandemic, they might be called upon to work additional shifts on short notice, entailing disruption of family life as well as fatigue and sleep disturbance. LPNs working on the front lines during the pandemic were continually exposed to infection and early, in the pandemic, might have been required to do so without vaccination or adequate personal protective equipment. A middle manager in a "big box" store might be responsible for the performance of employees who lack skill, motivation, or reliability, without the authority to deviate from company policies even when they think that changes in employees' hours, training, or procedures would lead to better results.

Long-haul truck drivers offer an example of ERI. As will be detailed in Chapter 18, the work is physically demanding, entails substantial risks of work-related injury or illness, and often adds stress to significant relationships. During the COVID-19 pandemic, most truck drivers were subjected to repeated, involuntary exposures to the virus, whether when picking up and delivering goods or visiting truck stops with numerous unmasked customers (Crizzle, 2022). In part because of occupational hazards, truck drivers have an increased prevalence of major chronic diseases and a relatively short life expectancy (Apostolopoulos et al., 2010). Notwithstanding, the median pay for truck drivers in the U.S. is below the national median for all occupations. The job does not have high social status, nor do years of reliable driving typically lead to a pay raise or promotion.

Apparently secure, well-paid, and even prestigious employment does not exclude an occupational contribution to a patient's depression. Examples abound in the medical profession. In high-income countries, physicians have secure employment, typically with pay in the top quintile nationally. But, depending on their specialty and work setting, they can face various combinations of harmful or risky occupational exposures, overwork, and/or chronobiological stress, work–family conflict, and job strain from DCI and/or ERI. In institutions with an unhealthy organizational culture, physicians who are junior, are female, or have minority identities can be subjected to bullying, harassment, discrimination, and/or microaggressions. Physicians on the front lines during the COVID-19 pandemic faced the additional challenge of *moral injury*—circumstances in which a person engages in, fails to prevent, or witnesses an act that conflicts with deeply held values or beliefs. If a hospital lacked sufficient resources (e.g., intensive care unit beds or ventilators) to give lifesaving treatment to all patients with respiratory failure, a physician might have had to deny optimal treatment to some patients while providing it to others—an occasion for moral injury if they felt all patients deserve equally intensive care. In some countries, physicians faced humiliating and sometimes violent stigmatization by people seeing them as vectors of COVID transmission, an excruciating situation for healthcare providers risking their lives to treat people afflicted by the illness.

When Determinants of Socioeconomic Class Conflict

Income-based stratification works best to explain class-related culture and vulnerability to depression when wealth, income, education, and occupation all cluster together in a typical way. When the four determinants of class do not correspond for an individual, the discrepancy can be relevant to the cause or the narrative of depression. When a person with a graduate degree is struggling financially, they may be more self-critical than one who has only a high school diploma and lives among others with modest education and a working-class identity.

When a person's financial situation differs greatly from that of their parents, the parents' socioeconomic class can be important in determining the person's place in society. The young adult offspring of wealthy parents pursuing careers in the arts, teaching, or social services might have relatively low and/or unstable incomes and personal wealth but probably can turn to their parents for assistance in case of financial need and probably will have social relationships with people of significantly higher income. They will not have a working-poor, working-class, or middle-class identity. When considering class and depression, identifying a person as *working poor* by income alone is analogous to identifying a person as *Asian* or *Hispanic*—there is risk of lumping cultural attributes that should be considered separately to construct an accurate cultural perspective on a person's depression.

Cultural differences between "old money" and "new money" and between the merely rich (top 1%) and the super-rich (0.1%) can be highly relevant to the circumstances and narratives of depression, especially in places or in ethnic subcultures that have a large upper-class population. People at the lower end of the upper class might be rejected socially by those of extreme wealth or from "old money," and they might feel discouraged and unsuccessful when they compare themselves with people in their social network who are far more fortunate. When they become depressed, issues of social exclusion and upward comparison can worsen or become less bearable.

Parents' socioeconomic class has significant impact on their children's vulnerability to depression. In the U.S. and in other high-income nations without a "safety net" of the sort found in the Nordic countries, many children of parents of the working poor or the underclass are periodically exposed to food and/or housing insecurity (Gundersen & Ziliak, 2015). After controlling for income, age, and gender, food insecurity is associated with significantly higher odds of clinical depression (Leung et al., 2015). ACEs related to family poverty make a person more vulnerable to losses and other stressful events later in their lives, and the effect is worse if the person has had other ACEs—and most do. Middle-class and upper-class adults who experienced poverty in childhood have a higher risk of depression as adults than those who did not.

Though most of the working poor lack a high school education, a person can join the working poor despite a high school education or even some college education. Circumstances that move people from the middle class to the working poor include living in an economically depressed area, working for a failing business or in an industry in decline, physical or mental health problems including substance use disorders, facing discrimination based on race or ethnicity, or having a family obligation such as caring for a seriously ill spouse or child.

The working poor often are subject to adverse living and working conditions and to overwork. They might be exposed in their jobs to the risk of occupational illness or injury (e.g., from exposure to toxic chemicals or frequent heavy lifting). Those paid minimum or near-minimum wages might regularly need to work overtime, have continually changing work schedules, or have more than one job, to pay their bills. If they are in the "gig economy," they might have low wages and lack the benefits of regular employment, feeling pressure to take every job they are offered even if they are tired and the hours of work conflict with personal or family needs. Overwork is associated with poor sleep, which directly increases the risk of depression. It also increases the risk of chronic medical conditions and the risk of occupational injury that leads to depression via job loss, disability, and/or chronic pain. Many low-wage jobs involve work schedules that can change on short notice, further disrupting sleep and creating practical problems with transportation and childcare. Because of low family incomes, they may live in areas with environmental risk factors for depression, including air and/or water pollution, excessive noise, violent crime in the neighborhood, and difficulty accessing healthy food. The prevalence of clinical depression is high among the working poor, and treating their depression poses specific challenges that will be detailed further below.

The prevalence of severe mental illness, including severe MDD and bipolar disorder (BD), is highest in the underclass, with a bidirectional relationship between SES and mental health. People with severe and chronic mental or physical illnesses who do not have family support or substantial wealth tend to fall in SES. Many people with chronic mental disorders who are born into the middle or working class will descend into the underclass over the course of their lives. Substance abuse and behavioral addictions also can lead to a fall in SES/social class, as can a period of incarceration for crime. A working-class adolescent might be arrested for an offense like illicit drug use, vandalism, or petty larceny; might be tried as an adult and sentenced to a prison term; and, when released from prison, may find it virtually impossible to find stable and adequately paid employment, even when with greater maturity their risk of reoffending has decreased.

Those in the underclass are subject to adverse social and environmental determinants of health—including poor-quality diets; polluted, noisy, or unsafe environments; homelessness; and lack of social support. These greatly increase the risk of depression and interact with other vulnerabilities including those due to genetics, ACEs, and trauma. Successfully treating depression and bipolar illness in underclass patients, including maintenance of remissions, usually requires attention to social determinants of health. Sometimes clinical depression will remit with improvement in the depressed person's economic, social, and environmental circumstances alone, with no need for antidepressant drugs or psychotherapy.

It is not surprising that the working poor and the underclass have the highest risk of depression of all social classes, but there are several factors that can offset the increased risk: favorable genetics, social capital (e.g., positive ethnic or religious identity, neighborhood social support), personal resilience, and a realistic hope that one's life will improve and/or that one's children's lives will be significantly better. The antidepressant value of these attributes persists in the face of material adversity. It contributes to the "immigrant paradox" of better mental health in first-generation immigrants than in natives of the same socioeconomic class or in second-generation immigrants of the same class and ethnicity (Hausmann-Stabile & Guarnaccia, 2015; Perreira et al., 2019; Salas-Wright et al., 2014, 2018).

"Cultural antidepressants" for low-income people vary greatly according to their intersecting cultural identities, including those related to ethnicity and its interaction with locality. For example, the prevalence of depression in low-income rural African Americans in the Deep South is reportedly lower than that of non-Hispanic Whites and of urban Blacks at the same level of household income, though there is some controversy about the details of measurement and interpretation of findings (Keyes et al., 2015; Weaver, Himle, et al., 2015; Weaver, Taylor, & Himle, 2015). If low-income rural Blacks do have a decreased risk of depression, it might be related to *bonding social capital*, to personal and material assistance to people under stress by members of their extended families, to positive religious coping, and to a culture of John Henryism—high-effort coping with stress and disadvantage. The latter is associated with better mental health but worse long-term physical health (Brody et al., 2013; Gaydosh et al., 2018). Religion can operate through faith or through social or material support by clergy or members of the same congregation. Religious belief alone without a social network of co-religionists is less protective against depression (Moreno & Cardemil, 2018).

Class and Mood Disorder Phenomenology

Variations in the presentation of depression sometimes associated with social class identity include externalizing behaviors (anger/irritability/violence, high-risk behavior, alcohol and/or drug misuse), a disproportionate expression of the somatic symptoms of depression, and normalization of depression. Normalization can take the form either of denial that depression is an illness at all or viewing depression as a condition that is inevitable and must be accepted and tolerated. Mild hypomania might be normalized, attributing it to personality or to exciting life events rather than to an illness.

The expression of depression in men through externalizing behavior occurs among all social classes, but it is relatively more common in men with less-than-college education. Wealth and income don't protect against externalization, though they can influence how depression is externalized. Men with more money can engage in more expensive high-risk behavior—metaphorically, binge-drinking cognac rather than beer, or recklessly driving a new Lamborghini rather than a Toyota Corolla with high mileage. In those with the wealth or income to have trusted assistants or subordinates at work, depression-related impairment of job performance might be less evident. In that situation, a person's depression (or hypomania) might be expressed through problems in their relationships with employees.

People with a somatic emphasis in their expression of depression are found in all social classes. While a mainly psychological expression of depression can be seen in any social class, emotional complaints may be more acceptable among people with higher education and/or an upper-middle or upper-class identity. University students, academics, and people in the artistic professions might be middle class by income but be part of an academic or occupational culture that accepts and sympathizes with verbal expressions of emotional distress. Members of the upper-middle and upper classes, including academics and successful creative professionals, usually can afford to see psychotherapists or counselors and are more likely than members of the middle class, working class, or working poor to have employment that allows them to take time for therapy or counseling during the workweek.

Melancholy moods have been less stigmatized among those of higher social class for hundreds of years, in many countries. The stigma of emotional complaints for people of lower classes might be related to their need to work without interruption and their socialization to work in circumstances of low control and autonomy. Melancholy may not be as fashionable now as it was in the 19th century, but people of means might more readily acknowledge and express ennui and Weltschmerz than those needing to work two jobs to keep their families afloat. For the latter, complaints about fatigue, aches and pains, hard work, and tough bosses would be more common than talk about feeling depressed or sad.

People with high-level professional positions often can accommodate temporary depression-related diminution of productivity and/or temporarily alter their work schedules without losing their jobs. People of independent means and proprietors of well-established family businesses need not suffer a loss of income or status if they suffer transient functional impairment from depression. People with lower-paid, lower-status jobs are at risk of losing them if depression makes them inefficient, unreliable, or occasionally absent from work. Depressed people might be less able to work overtime or hold a second job because of fatigue or decreased energy. People—usually women—with service jobs that require them to engage pleasantly with customers or clients can find the social aspect of their work very difficult when they are depressed. Presenting a somatic reason for impairment in work sometimes can help a depressed person keep their job, and if there is a decrease in income, the worker's family might be more accepting if the reason is somatic than if it is explicitly emotional. " In many localities it is easier for a depressed worker to get temporary disability or workers' compensation income if the ostensible reason is a painful condition apparently related to the job, such as low back pain in a warehouse worker or in a nursing assistant responsible for turning, repositioning, and transferring bedfast patients.

Expressions of hyperthymia, hypomania, and non-psychotic mania are influenced by social class and its underlying elements of education, wealth, income, occupation, and family background. A wealthy person can undertake more grandiose and ambitious projects and spend or lose more money before experiencing financial distress or imposing financially-related strain upon their family. A person with modest income and negative net worth can create a personal and family crisis by a single error in financial judgment.

Class and Mood Disorder Epidemiology

People in the first (lowest) quintile of income have more frequent mental distress, higher average levels of depressive symptoms, and a higher prevalence of MDD than people in the third or fourth quintile of income (Gresenz et al., 2001). Depending on the country, the mental health of people in the second quintile of income will be more like that of people in the lowest quintile, or more like that of those in the middle quintile.

Income is roughly correlated with education, but in lower-income countries with a high prevalence of poverty, income usually predominates as a determinant of depression risk. In middle-income countries, income and education have significant and partially independent correlations with depression and general mental health. Which effect is larger varies by country (Araya et al., 2013; Maselko et al., 2017). A recent meta-analysis of 60 studies with data on social class and depressive symptoms in U.S. residents showed a nonlinear effect of education on depression in non-Hispanic Whites only: People with the least education and those with the most education had more depressive symptoms than those in the middle (Korous et al., 2023). Such findings support an important effect of intersecting cultural identities on the risk of depression.

Higher education is the most important route from the lower classes to the upper ones. Educational inequality in the U.S. is the main reason for its lower upward mobility than Canada or the countries of western Europe. Elementary and secondary education in low-income neighborhoods is inferior, making it difficult for children of the lower classes to be admitted to highly ranked colleges and universities. Because college tuition and fees are so high in the U.S., even those who are admitted might not attend for financial reasons or might be unable to complete their college degrees.

Adult immigrants from poorer countries to richer ones typically have incomes lower than the median for their new country of residence but higher than their incomes in their country of origin. After controlling for major issues like exposure to trauma, such immigrants tend to have less mental distress, lower average depressive symptoms, and a lower rate of MDD than people with the same levels of education and income who have always lived in the richer country. For example, the 12-month prevalence rate for MDD in people who had immigrated from China to the U.S. as adults was significantly lower than that for second-generation Chinese Americans. Even after controlling for age, education, income, marital status, BMI, and income-to-needs ratio, China-to-US immigrant women had a lower lifetime prevalence of MDD than US-born Chinese Americans (Tan, 2014).

Notwithsanding, in the U.S., immigrant women (but not men) whose occupational prestige is lower or higher after immigration than it was in the host country have a higher rate of depression, suggesting that mobility in either direction can be stressful (Ro, 2014). Those who are exploited in their jobs or who face chronic discrimination have higher rates of depression regardless of their incomes (Clark et al., 2015; Muntaner et al., 2015).

Children of immigrants born in the receiving country (the second generation) or brought to it as young children ("generation 1.5") do not have a lower prevalence of depression than natives of the new country from the same socioeconomic class. They often are worse off than their peers from non-immigrant families, especially if they are targets of prejudice and discrimination or if they or their parents were victims of trauma.

Lower-middle-class people who in high-income countries tend to have high school educations and vocational skills acquired from training and/or experience, if physically healthy and employed, do not have an increased prevalence rate of depression. This is true whether rates are measured by average depressive symptoms or by prevalence of MDD. Many will live in working-class neighborhoods where they have accumulated social capital by assisting friends and neighbors and being assisted by them. Childcare, emergency transportation, and household repairs are occasions for members of a working-class or middle-class community to help one another; in upper-middle-class and upper-class neighborhoods it would be more common for people to hire the help they needed. Exchanges of favors are a basis for establishing bonding social capital, which can help people get through emotionally stressful times without developing depression. When working-class people live in disadvantaged neighborhoods, they are less likely to develop social capital. The contrast is exemplified by a neighborhood in which most working-class people have steady jobs with high wages and benefits versus one in which most have precarious and/or poorly paid employment. Qualitative interviews with working-class men living in the two types of neighborhoods in an industrial English city illustrate differences in neighborhood social capital that underlie their differences in physical and mental health (Dolan, 2007).

If a working-class man or woman becomes unemployed, develops a major illness, or is seriously injured, ensuing events can overwhelm their personal coping capacity, even with the benefits of a supportive social network. The household might lack savings or have negative net worth. In this case bankruptcy, housing instability, food insecurity, and neglect of medical conditions are significant risks if income from employment is lost.

If the worker and family must move to a poorer neighborhood, or in the worst case become homeless, neighborhood-based bonding social capital is less useful because it is more distant. The worker's spouse or partner may need to work more hours outside the home, creating or increasing work–family conflicts that can increase tension in the household. Finally, if the worker's job is important to personal identity and illness or unemployment might continue for a long time, life might have less meaning and purpose. This combination of stressors can precipitate clinical depression and/or suicidal thoughts and behavior. In times of economic recession there have been localized epidemics of depression and clusters of suicides in economically disadvantaged municipalities (Alarcão et al., 2019; Fontanella et al., 2018). Women of the working class with children have two gender-specific issues. Working-class women are more likely than working-class men to be single parents with children at home. In this situation, they often have no reliable financial support for the children other than their own earnings, as their children's fathers may be unable or unwilling to pay child support. When such women lose jobs or suffer impaired occupational function because of illness or injury, there will be impact on the children's health and well-being, a major source of emotional pain for any mother. In addition, childcare needs can limit mothers' options for a new or different job.

Members of the middle class—typically people with some post-secondary education and stable employment—have class-related influences on vulnerability to depression that are shaped by their other cultural identities. If they have significant savings and positive net worth, they can manage the consequences of a national or local economic downturn, such as unemployment, decreased income from a small family business, or the profound disruptions of the COVID-19 pandemic, without the risk of bankruptcy, losing their home, food insecurity, or inability to pay for needed healthcare. A middle-class person with negative net worth and minimal savings can be tipped into a financial crisis not only by an economic event but also by a large, unexpected expense related to their house, car, or healthcare. Living in a region with a weak economy heightens economic insecurity, while living in a region with a booming economy and a high cost of living can have the same effect if the person's income does not rise as the local economy grows. If a person's social capital is local and related to their neighborhood, moving to find employment—or to find a better job—implies a loss of social capital that can combine with the stress of the move to precipitate depression.

The upper-middle class defined by income alone comprises people with household incomes well above the median but below the threshold for the upper class, the specific cut points depending on the country and the region. Most members of the upper-middle class are college graduates. Typically, at least one adult in the household has a professional or managerial occupation or is an owner of a successful small business. As with the middle class, an upper-middle-class household income can be associated with a wide range of net worth, with the range extending from negative to several million dollars. Members of the upper-middle class usually pay for services like childcare and household repairs and rarely rely on their neighbors for practical assistance. As a result, neighborhood social networks tend to be weaker, and there is less bonding social capital. This is a source of vulnerability to depression among the upper-middle class. It is offset partially by the ability of most upper-middle-class families to access and pay for treatment if a member of the family develops depression.

Much of the American upper-middle class lives in suburban single-family houses spaced far enough apart that significant social interaction with neighbors is optional. New social connections are made at workplaces and via membership in organizations, including clubs, religious congregations, professional and trade associations, groups related to children's schools and activities (e.g., PTA, scouting), charitable organizations, and political groups. Despite opportunities for forming social connections, many upper-middle-class people have relatively small social networks. Some are introverted, while others are too busy with work and family obligations to participate in organizations outside of work or to do much socializing outside the family. The proprietor of a small business or a professional in solo or small-group practice might have few opportunities for social connections with peers during the workday. While people who live with a spouse or a partner or have children at home may not be lonely in the strict sense, there are many *lonely families*, for which the couple or family has little or no social or practical support nearby to rely upon for assistance if it is needed and few or no close local friends with whom to share the joys and disappointments of daily life. Members of lonely families are at increased risk of depression. This type of loneliness might be more frequent in more prosperous regions than in poorer ones. In less affluent regions, there tend to be more social relationships across class lines (bridging social capital), and local organizations like churches play a stronger role.

When a person has a small social network outside their immediate family, the risk of loneliness and depression is high if there is a loss—or change in closeness—of an important relationship. In addition to divorce or separation or the death of a close friend, relative, or beloved pet, even positive events can contribute to loneliness. An adult child's educational or occupational success can lead to their moving away. A promotion at work or a move to a different worksite can lead to the loss of close relationships with co-workers. A friend's occupational or financial success may make them more physically or emotionally distant.

Sociologist Philip Slater wrote a classic book, *The Pursuit of Loneliness* (Slater, 1970/1990), about Americans becoming lonelier as they rise in status, distanced from their neighbors by competitiveness, individualism, and "wealth addiction." He anticipated America's decline in social capital. While poverty is associated with loneliness, higher income beyond a certain point does not bring further protection against it. Chapter 15 describes the potential adverse effects of celebrity on social relationships—the lonely at the top phenomenon. The point made by Slater, Putnam, and other writers on social capital is that one need not be anywhere near the very top of the socioeconomic ladder for success to bring loss or impairment of social connections.

The Importance of Subjective Social Status

An accumulating body of research supports the idea that subjective social status (SSS)—where people place themselves on a 10-rung ladder of social position—has an independent effect on physical and mental health outcomes beyond its association with objective SES as determined by income, occupation, and education (Hoebel et al., 2017). If there is an extreme discrepancy between SSS and SES, depression or hypomania might be suspected. If there is a meaningful but plausible discrepancy between SSS and SES in a person—or a population—not suffering from a mood disorder, higher SSS reduces the risk of depression, and lower SSS increases it. SSS has similar effects on general well-being and on stress-related general medical illness.

A striking example of SSS eclipsing SES as a social determinant of health is offered by a study of social determinants of long COVID—persistent symptoms including fatigue, headache, dyspnea, cognitive and mood complaints—following the resolution of acute COVID-19 (Thomason et al., 2021). The investigators surveyed 1584 patients who had been treated for COVID-19 in the New York University Langone health system, obtaining data on persistent symptoms and on social determinants of health. In their sample, 19.4% of the subjects reported persistent mood symptoms, and 25% reported persistent cognitive or memory problems. A subject's objective SES was based on their educational level and household income. Perceived social status combined four elements: the subject's self-assessed position on a socioeconomic ladder between the best-off and the worst-off people in the U.S. based on wealth, education, and occupational prestige; their frequency of worry about financial matters; their level of satisfaction with their financial status; and whether they generally know how much money they will have to live on from one month to the next. Persistent cognitive complaints were significantly associated with subjective status and not with objective status.

Several mechanisms can make SSS differ from objective SES. A depressive or hyperthymic temperament can alter one's self-assessment and assessment of one's status and reputation. Upward or downward comparison can decrease or increase SSS: If a person lives among people with greater wealth and income, higher education, and/or more prestigious employment, they might place themselves lower on the ladder of status. If a person has more wealth or income, education, or occupational prestige than their neighbors, the opposite may occur. However, both upward and downward comparison can be offset by the quality of neighborhood resources (Roy et al., 2016). If a lower-middle-class person moves to an upper-middle-class neighborhood, the sense of status they get from enjoying well-maintained and safe public parks, having great service from the police and fire department, using a well-appointed public library, and sending children to excellent public schools might outweigh negative feelings related to upward comparison. In addition, they might develop positive relationships with higher-class people who can be of practical help to them or to family members. If a middle-class person moves to a poorer neighborhood, perhaps so that a larger home will be affordable, a lack of greenspace, less safe streets, and lower-quality public schools might outweigh any positive feelings related to downward comparison. Growing up in a low SES family can increase depression risk even when SSS increases in adulthood. In a study of SSS and its correlates in college students, those with low family SES and higher current SSS had greater positive affect, but their risk of depressive symptoms was greater than for those with a higher family SES (Niu, Hoyt et al., 2023). For a retired person, a high income and high occupational status when they were employed can support higher SSS than their situation in retirement might suggest.

Unexpectedly low or decreasing SSS leading to depression is a risk encountered by Americans of the upper-middle class, especially those residing in prosperous regions of the country. Even when members of the upper-middle class have household incomes in the top 5% (but not in the top 1%), they can feel relatively unsuccessful or economically vulnerable because of some combination of upward comparison, low or negative net worth, a high local cost of living, or downward mobility within their families. Any of these can impact self-esteem and self-confidence with downstream effects on social connections.

For many upper-middle-class people in countries with a competitive ethos and a high level of income inequality such as the United States and China, the effect on SSS of living among the upper class is negative. In countries or subcultures with lesser income inequality and traditions of community solidarity, the benefits of linking social capital would be greater than the negative effects of upward comparison.

In prosperous regions of the U.S., there are many people in the upper-middle class by income who have low or even negative net worth despite well-compensated employment and high educational attainment. Examples include young professionals with substantial college debt, people who have recently had an expensive divorce, and couples in midlife who have recently paid for their children's higher education and might also be providing aid to older and functionally dependent parents. The last group might have anxiety about saving enough money for their retirement.

Young professionals may be aware of living less prosperous or comfortable lives than their parents, despite having studied for years to acquire their professional credentials and currently working long hours to establish their careers. Consider the exemplary case of an early-career female primary care physician with two young children and a husband in a less well-paid occupation, living in a high-cost metropolitan area of the Northeastern United States or California. With a salary of $150,000 and a household income of $250,000, she and her husband might just be covering the cost of childcare, a mortgage, and general living expenses. If her father were an established primary care physician in a small Midwestern city whose wife did not work outside the home, he might be a member of the local elite, owning his house without a mortgage, having substantial savings, and having a prominent role in several local organizations. She might experience an uncomfortable feeling of downward mobility and be vulnerable to depression even though by personal and household income she and her father would have the same SES.

Upper-middle-class people, even those with respected occupations, can have cultural identities that make them targets of prejudice, discrimination, negative stereotyping and/or microaggressions. In one common scenario, a person's higher education and success at business or in a profession leads them to move out of a working-class or middle-class neighborhood in which many of the residents are of the same cultural group, into an upper-middle-class suburb or urban neighborhood in which their cultural group is a small minority. In the new neighborhood there may be more social distance from neighbors, no close friends may live nearby, and the person might have frequent experiences of minor discrimination or microaggressions. Continual reminders that one's economic success has not brought full social acceptance can lead to a depressed mood.

A final depression risk of the upper-middle class applies to families with adolescent children. Upper-middle-class parents often have anxieties about their children's ability to retain or improve their SES as they usually do not have the financial and social resources to practically ensure that their children will have the same or higher status than they. In affluent communities, there is a significant risk of adolescents becoming involved with alcohol, illegal drugs, and/or risky sexual behavior—these risks are not limited to lower-income youths (Racz et al., 2011). At the same time, high school students in affluent neighborhoods are competing for admission to the most prestigious colleges. Parents with anxiety about their children's success might pressure their children to achieve—for some parents, their child's receiving anything less than an "A" grade in a class is equivalent to failure. Parents may be overinvolved and controlling or emotionally distant. In either case the adolescent may feel unsupported, angry, and vulnerable. Achievement pressure can lead to unhealthy lifestyles with too little sleep, too much time online, and/or inadequate relaxation. Some pressured adolescents will express their distress through substance use or risk-taking behavior. These external expressions of adolescent distress can make parents anxious even when they were previously insensitive to their children's unhappiness. Either the pressured adolescent or the anxious parent—or both—might develop clinical depression.

Troubles of the Upper Class

The upper class can be defined by income, wealth, education, occupation, and family background. Defining the upper class by household income might start with the "top 1%." In the U.S. in 2020 the 99th percentile for annual household income ranged from $300,774 in New Mexico to $913,312 in Washington, DC (DQYDJ.com, n.d.). The difference between the average income of the top 1% and the bottom 99% is so great that in many U.S. cities the upper class truly lives in a different world from those who are less fortunate. An extreme example is Jackson, Wyoming, where the average household income of the top 1% in 2015 was $16,161,955, while the average income of the bottom 99% was $122,447—a top-to-bottom ratio of 132. In the same year, the top-to-bottom ratio was 39.4 in New York City, 33.5 in Los Angeles, and 27.8 in Chicago (Sommeiller & Price, 2018).

If factors other than income are considered, a person with a graduate degree and a sufficiently prestigious profession (e.g., lawyer at a major firm, successful medical specialist, or senior executive at a respected company) might qualify for the upper class with household income below the top 1%, as might the offspring of a locally well-known wealthy family. There are depression-relevant distinctions within the upper class. At the lower end of the upper class, individuals can afford luxuries, usually could have a comfortable (though not necessarily luxurious) life if they chose not to work or were unable to work, and can provide their children with elite higher education and help launch them in their adult lives (e.g., by providing them with money to start a business or make a down payment for a house). In the middle of the upper class, individuals can, if they choose, enjoy a luxurious standard of living without working. They also can provide their children with a similar life situation in which life can be luxurious and paid employment is optional. At the high end of the upper class, people have vast sums of money to spend, if they choose, on extravagant living (e.g., owning multiple large houses or apartments in prime locations, owning a yacht or private jet, collecting museum-quality art), highly visible philanthropy (e.g., donating and naming a hospital or a college), and/or building even more wealth by large-scale investment.

At the lower end of the upper class as determined by household income, people might feel negative emotions like envy, disappointment, or self-criticism when making comparisons with people richer than themselves—their SSS is not upper class. They often describe themselves as "middle class" or "upper-middle class." The San Francisco Bay Area and metropolitan Boston, New York City, Washington, DC, and Los Angeles are full of "upper-middle-class" multi-millionaires. They might worry about their children's ability to maintain their status as they grow into adulthood. Their children are exposed to the perils of affluent adolescence (drugs, alcohol, reckless driving, etc.), while feeling competitive pressure and their parents' insecurity.

Some people at the lower end of the upper class will commit a large part of their income and a great deal of time spending money in a conspicuous, status-building way (e.g., by custom building, remodeling, and/or elaborately decorating their homes; dressing stylishly; building collections of luxury items; taking expensive vacations at exclusive resorts). Doing so might require them to earn more money, and they might work more hours or take more risks to do so. People focused on pursuing status in this way might lack self-awareness and resilience, and they might have trust issues related to their intense competitiveness. These attributes make them vulnerable to depression if they experience losses—financial or relational—or other traumatic events. Competition and status-seeking do not have the stress-buffering effect of positive and mutual human relationships, exercise, spiritual or religious activities, or altruistic behavior. Further, the children of such nouveau riche status seekers sometimes suffer emotional neglect from their parents, who are absorbed in their work and their conspicuous consumption.

Membership in the lowest stratum of the upper class can be precarious if it relies on ownership of, or an executive position in, a business subject to major fluctuations in performance and value. Losing upper-class status can be emotionally devastating to people—usually men—for whom a high income and identification with a successful enterprise are central to their personal identities. Major professionals (e.g., physicians and lawyers) are in general less likely to suffer a sudden work-related loss in status. However, there are situations emotionally equivalent to the decline or failure of a business for an owner or executive. These include a costly and publicized malpractice case against a physician or a major legal or ethical issue involving a lawyer, accountant, money manager, or management consultant.

Adolescent and young adult children of the upper class are in general less likely to have had multiple and severe ACEs than those of the lower classes. However, there are common exceptions to the rule. There are cultural groups defined by nationality and/or religion that condone authoritarian parenting and harsh discipline, and high-income families in such a group might follow its norms. Couples with high incomes sometimes entrust their children's care to nannies or other domestic employees, who might neglect or abuse their charges. When parents rose to the upper class from poor circumstances and had many ACEs themselves, they might express their traumatic history through domestic violence.

An adolescent or young adult with a privileged and non-traumatic childhood might have increased vulnerability to depression if they had lacked opportunities to build resilience and self-reliance, and some may lack the empathy, generosity, and interpersonal skills needed to build their social capital. The need to build resilience and self-reliance may underlie the tradition of hereditary upper-class families to send their children to boarding schools and to summer camps where they will be appropriately and safely challenged—cognitively, physically, and interpersonally. Their parents do not want to "spoil" their children. Some old-money upper-class parents see spoiled children as a problem primarily of *nouveau riche* families, which they try to avoid.

When a person enters the upper class through a dramatic personal achievement like writing a bestselling novel or being a co-founder of a successful startup, they might experience a period of ennui, feeling a lack of purpose or questioning the value of their work apart from money. Other people following sudden wealth or celebrity develop marital or family conflicts or become involved in problematic substance use, inappropriate relationships, or risky behavior. Especially when the person has bipolar traits, as do many entrepreneurs and creative professionals, these events can lead to depression with mixed features.

Upper-class status can contribute to loneliness. Upper-class people who grew up poor, working class, or middle class might not be fully accepted socially by those born into the upper class. At the same time, their upward mobility often weakens their ties with people of the same background who were not as successful. If newly rich people belong to an ethnic minority that is a target of discrimination and they live outside a large metropolitan area, they might have difficulty finding a suitable place to live. If they live in an upper-class neighborhood, they might be socially isolated, and they and/or their children might experience stereotyping and microaggressions. If they continue to live among less affluent members of their own ethnic group, frequent reminders of status differences can lead to social distance.

Adult children of upper-class families sometimes are significantly less successful than their parents. While it is unlikely that they will drop below the upper-middle class, their remaining in an upper-class neighborhood or social milieu may be uncomfortable. Upward comparisons will lower their SSS, and their circumstances might continually remind them that they did not meet their own or their parents' expectations. If they move to a middle-class neighborhood, they may feel out of place or not fully accepted by their neighbors.

A person in the "lower-upper" class might have enough household income to have an upper-class lifestyle and live in an upper-class neighborhood but lack commensurate wealth. They are at risk of dropping out of the upper class if there is a personal or family misfortune. Social connections made with other upper-class people might not survive the drop in their status. They might be reluctant to reveal their anxiety about their financial circumstances for fear of reputational damage. If clinical depression develops in this context, it can intensify feelings of social and economic insecurity at the same time as illness-related cognitive and functional impairments increase the risk that something else will go wrong with their health, business, or family.

When people in the "new money" upper class become depressed and have no prior experience with the condition, they might doubt themselves—how could they be depressed when they are so fortunate? Such feelings might delay their seeking professional help for their depression. People from "old money" might not have such feelings as they grew up with wealth and would be very likely to know people in their social circle who suffered depression. However, beliefs and attitudes about depression related to other, intersecting identities might deter them from seeking treatment.

Another reason depressed people with new money might not seek treatment is fear of stigma. If they are already sensitive to rejection by people with old money and high social status in their community, they might fear that being known as depressed or bipolar and needing treatment might make them even less acceptable. In the U.S., concern about stigmatization is greater in smaller communities in more traditional/conservative locales. In such places, a relatively small number of wealthy families might function as "nobility." Mere financial success would not suffice to make one "noble" if they were deviant in some way. Publicly known treatment for a mental illness could be a disqualification, as could minority ethnicity or religious non-conformity. Further, the relatively small number of healthcare and mental health care providers in a small community might make it hard for a person to keep their treatment secret. The rapid growth in telepsychiatry during the COVID-19 pandemic is beginning to change the landscape as it is now much easier for a prominent person in a small community to get psychiatric care remotely and completely confidentially.

When very wealthy people become hypomanic, they can afford to display their mood expansively and expensively, for example, by purchasing luxury goods or "trophies," throwing extravagant parties, making large gifts to people or charities, gambling, or impulsively making large and risky investments. When people can afford such expenditures, it may not be obvious at first that their spending is abnormal and a sign of illness. A diagnosis of hypomania would be supported by such symptoms as decreased need for sleep, disorganized thoughts and speech, grandiosity, unusual anger and/or irritability, inappropriate sexual behavior, or dysphoric excitement. Such symptoms would not be normalized by a person's wealth.

Normalization of non-psychotic hypomania can also occur with eminent writers and artists, a topic that is covered at length in Chapter 15. If the writer or artist also is wealthy—either from sale of creative work or otherwise—a diagnosis of hypomania is even more likely to be missed. When a highly successful entrepreneur or eminent creative person presents with depression, a very careful and wide-ranging review of the person's history for signs of hypomania or depression with mixed features is essential because such a patient has a relatively high probability of having a condition in the bipolar spectrum based on their social class and occupation.

When upper-class people with depression or bipolar spectrum illness acknowledge they are ill and seek treatment, they can afford the best care available. However, for reasons related to their social class background, they sometimes don't get the care they need. The risks of class-related problems with treatment are greatest when the status of the patient is widely known, either because they are a celebrity, have had a conspicuous business success, come from an eminent family, or hold a high position in a prominent organization.

Many clinicians, including non-psychiatric physicians and non-medical mental health professionals as well as psychiatrists, find it difficult to take the emotional suffering of a very privileged person seriously and to respond with appropriate empathy. Training in psychodynamic psychotherapy addresses this issue along with other types of countertransference, but most physicians don't get such training. Schadenfreude, or excessive scrupulousness as a reaction to it, can be unconscious on the clinician's part but nonetheless be sensed by the patient as a lack of empathy.

People from upper-class subcultures might have an attitude of low trust toward people outside a relatively small "in-group" of people of similar status and a few people of lower status who have loyally served them for years. It may be based on fear of financial exploitation or a more generic in-group/out-group dynamic. Some upper-class people who are accustomed to being treated with deference—as VIPs—are embarrassed to reveal weakness and vulnerability to anyone, even to a psychiatrist or other qualified clinician.

A final impediment to clinical care with some upper-class depressed people is frequent travel related to their occupations or usual social life. This can impede regular in-person meetings for psychothreapy or close monitoring of their response to psychiatric medication.

Clinicians might be so accustomed to controlling costs of care and to justifying care to health plan utilization reviewers that they don't recommend intensive, expensive, or personalized treatment even when such a treatment would be best for the individual patient and the patient is willing and able to pay for it. For example, a depressed patient with many years' history of recurrent severe MDD, incomplete responses to several different antidepressants, and two past suicide attempts might have the best chance of a full remission, and the lowest risk of self-harm, with several weeks of inpatient treatment at a mood disorders specialty unit. However, health insurance plans frequently have policies that require continual reauthorizations for inpatient psychiatric treatment and won't cover inpatient treatment for patients who are not dangerous to themselves or others, nor seriously disabled by their current symptoms. A clinician who regularly works within the framework of typical health insurance plans might not even include a multi-week hospitalization on their list of therapeutic options to consider and discuss with the patient in a shared decision-making process.

On the other hand, a clinician might specialize in an expensive treatment for depression often not covered by insurance such as intensive psychoanalytic psychotherapy, transcranial magnetic stimulation, intravenous ketamine infusions, or psychedelic treatment. They might almost always propose, recommend, prescribe, or insist upon such a treatment for a depressed upper-class patient, even when a less costly treatment might work as well or better and be equally well tolerated.

Regardless of the preconceptions of the patient, the attitudes of payers, or the subspecialty of the clinician, the patient (and, if appropriate, a family member or significant other of the patient) must have the information necessary to make an informed, collaborative choice among a range of evidence-based treatments. A patient's ability to pay for treatments not covered by insurance broadens the range of options to be considered.

In high-income countries outside the U.S. that have national health systems rather than commercial health insurance, payment mechanisms and the organization of care are different, but the issue is essentially the same. Depressed upper-class patients have a broader range of treatment options because they can pay out of pocket if necessary. A clinician treating upper-class patients should be familiar with the full range of options both inside and outside the restricted set preferred by the national health system or the most prevalent health insurance plans.

Chapter 8

Cultural Correlates and Clinical Consequences

Cultural identity is associated with lifestyle including diet, sleeping habits, and psychoactive substance use, and with exposure to physical and environmental hazards. Unhealthy lifestyles and risk exposures associated with culture sometimes are intrinsic to the culture, but often they are not, especially in the case of migrants. They can be consequences of socioeconomic disadvantage or discrimination, side effects of acculturation, or results of intersecting identities. Applying a cultural lens to a person or a population with depression includes identifying lifestyle and environmental issues contributing to the problem. Addressing them often is necessary for a full, stable remission of depression in an individual, or for reducing the depression prevalence and suicide mortality in a population. Identifying and dealing with lifestyle and environmental issues with a depressed patient helps establish a therapeutic relationship, can reduce self-stigma, and sometimes brings improvement in mood without other treatment.

Culture, Diet, and Depression

Eating habits are associated with culture, either directly or indirectly through socioeconomic class and differential access to healthy food based on affordability and location of residence. Traditional diets of ethnic groups tend to be healthy ones for people with genetics, environments, and lifestyles typical for the group. Studies focusing on diet and depression specifically have shown that the traditional Mediterranean diet (Davis et al., 2015), the Tuscan diet (Vermeulen et al., 2016), the Nordic diet (Mannikko et al., 2015), and the traditional Japanese (*Washoku*) diet (Miki et al., 2018; Sanada et al., 2021) are associated with lower rates of depressive symptoms. On the other hand, diets associated with increased systemic inflammation, such as ones with high consumption of sweet soft drinks (either sugar-sweetened or artificially sweetened), processed grains, added sugar (especially high-fructose corn syrup), margarine, and red meat, and/or low in green leafy vegetables, yellow vegetables, coffee, and wine, increase the risk of depression (Lucas et al., 2014; Kashino et al., 2021). South

Asian diets that heavily use anti-inflammatory spices such as turmeric and saffron might have associated antidepressant benefits (Ng, Koh, et al., 2017). A prospective study of diet and depression in Australian women differentiated "traditional" diets that emphasized vegetables, fruit, meat, fish, and whole grains from "Western" ones emphasizing processed or fried foods, refined grains, sugary products, and beer. After controlling for many potential confounders including age, education, socioeconomic status, calorie intake, exercise, body mass index, smoking, and alcohol consumption, the incidence of MDD or dysthymia was 2.3 times higher in women who consumed Western diets as compared with those who consumed traditional ones (Jacka et al., 2010).

Because obesity is directly and indirectly connected with depression, dietary patterns associated with obesity increase depression risk. Departure from traditional, healthy diets can of course increase the risk of major diseases other than depression, notably certain cancers, Type 2 diabetes, and cardiovascular disease. For example, Japanese women who eat Western diets are more likely to develop breast cancer than those who eat traditional Japanese diets (Shin et al., 2016).

When people migrate, their traditional foods might become unavailable or unaffordable, while less healthy foods might be ubiquitous. When people's diets shift toward higher consumption of refined carbohydrates, processed foods with high added sugar, and sugary drinks, they are more likely to develop obesity, glucose intolerance, and chronic systemic inflammation, all risk factors for depression. Employment involving much overtime or frequent travel can lead to excessive consumption of fast food, which often leads to obesity and systemic inflammation. Poor food quality can entail vitamin or mineral insufficiencies. A calorie-dense but nutrient-poor diet can lead to insufficiency of folate, vitamin D, magnesium, or zinc, any of which can contribute to the onset of clinical depression or to the severity of depressive symptoms.

When assessing depression in a person from an ethnic minority with a distinctive traditional diet, the dietary impact of assimilation should be considered. Also, cultural groups can, for reasons of discrimination or economic disadvantage, be concentrated in *food deserts*, where healthy food is unavailable or prohibitively expensive, making it difficult for people to adhere to traditional diets even if doing so was their preference. When people for cultural reasons might prefer to eat healthier and more traditional diets, there is opportunity to reduce their depression risk by helping them find practicable and affordable ways to get their traditional foods. When immigrants or ethnic minorities express their assimilation to mainstream Western culture by adopting unhealthy diets, targeted education on diet and health sometimes helps. While most educated people in high-income countries know about dietary risks for diabetes and cardiovascular disease, they often are not aware of dietary risks for depression.

The issue of diet and depression is discussed in detail in Chapter 9, in connection with the role of diet in the treatment of depression in traditional medical systems. That chapter provides referenced tables listing antidepressant foods and foods that increase depression risk.

Culture, Sleep, and Depression

Adequate sleep is essential to maintaining good health. Insufficient or poor-quality sleep is associated with depression, as well as with obesity, diabetes, the metabolic syndrome, hypertension, cerebrovascular disease, and sexual dysfunction (Covassin & Singh, 2016; Grandner, 2017; Nowakowski et al., 2016; Sluggett et al., 2019; Worley, 2018). Chronically inadequate sleep causes impairment in cognition, memory, and judgment that can impair academic or occupational performance (Chen & Chen, 2019; Judd, 2017; Wernette & Emory, 2017). It can increase the stress reactivity of the hypothalamic–pituitary–adrenal axis and thus increase the likelihood of stress-related psychopathology (van Dalfsen & Markus, 2018). It is a risk factor for motor vehicle crashes, occupational injury, and sports-related injuries (Owens & Weiss, 2017; Worley, 2018). Poor sleep is associated with an increase in suicidal ideation and self-harm (Chakravorty et al., 2014; Kohyama, 2011; Sarchiapone et al., 2014). Sleep variability assessed with actigraphy has been shown to be a warning sign of acute suicidal ideation in young adults at high risk for suicide (Bernert, Hom, et al., 2017).

Persistently inadequate sleep in a person's childhood alters brain development in ways that make them more vulnerable to depression as adolescents and adults (Young et al., 2019). Inadequate sleep in a person's midlife increases the likelihood of their cognitive decline with aging (Virta et al., 2013). Inadequate sleep exacerbates age-related cognitive deficits in older people. The cognitive impairments, obesity, and vascular disease associated with chronically poor sleep increase the risk of late-onset depression.

Cultural factors associated with poor sleep are thus indirectly associated with depression. An anonymous questionnaire-based study of over 5000 professional and administrative staff at 10 hospitals in Japan showed that 13% of men and 19% of women reported insomnia and that insomnia was a significant risk factor for depression. Nurses and workers over age 50 were most likely to suffer from insomnia (Koyama et al., 2017).

Immigrants and ethnic minorities might, because of discrimination or limited proficiency in the host country's language, be limited to jobs with relatively low wages and might need to work overtime, accept frequently changing work hours, or work several jobs to support themselves and their families. If their homes and work are far apart—often the case when jobs are in cities with high housing costs—commuting time can be an additional impediment to adequate sleep. If jobs require working evening or night shifts or if working hours or shift assignments frequently change, sleep can be inadequate even though total working hours are not excessive.

Several culture-related issues can interfere with the sleep of children and adolescents. When children are pressed to study incessantly in pursuit of perfect test scores and organized after-school activities are the norm, time allowed for sleep often is below guidelines for optimal health. (The consensus of the American Academy of Sleep Medicine is that preschool children aged 3–5 should sleep 10–13 hours per day [including naps], children aged 6–12 years should sleep 9–12 hours per day, and teens aged 13–18 should sleep 8–10 hours per day [Paruthi et al., 2016]). In low-income families, older children may be expected to work to help support the family or to help provide care for younger children or elders who need assistance so that their parents are free to work outside the home. Time for these activities combined with time for school and homework can interfere with adequate sleep. When living conditions are unstable, unsafe, or excessively noisy, as might be the case for low-income children and especially for those from ethnic minorities that are targets of discrimination, children's sleep is likely to suffer. Parents often do not appreciate the harm that insufficient sleep can cause their children's developing brains and its relationship to behavioral problems, academic performance, and the future risk of depression.

Specific occupational groups are susceptible to depression or bipolar illness precipitated or exacerbated by frequent chronobiologic disruption by flights across multiple time zones. These include long-haul airline pilots, people involved in global business operations, journalists/foreign correspondents, and performing artists with multinational audiences.

Culture, Environmental Hazards, and Depression

Whether lower socioeconomic status is viewed as a cultural identity, a correlate of certain ethnic identities, or a personal characteristic that intersects with ethnic identity, assessing the indirect impact of lower-class status on depression via environmental exposures is part of the cultural lens. People with lower incomes, and/or from minority groups subject to discrimination in housing, are more likely to live in neighborhoods with high noise levels, polluted air and/or water, and/or a higher prevalence of violent crime, all of which raise depression risk.

Effects of environmental noise on mental health include increases in depressive symptoms, anxiety symptoms, and suicidal behavior (Leijssen et al., 2019; Ma et al., 2018). Air pollution has been related to increased rates of depression and of suicide attempts (Fan et al., 2019; Generaal et al., 2019; Gu et al., 2019; Lu, 2019). Fluctuations in air quality have been correlated with fluctuations in suicide rates in urban areas where air quality often is poor (Gładka et al., 2018). Frequent exposure to violent crime in one's neighborhood has adverse health effects even on people who are not personally victimized (Ma et al., 2018; Mueller et al., 2019). These environmental influences operate without respect to individuals' incomes. When middle-class people must live in unhealthy neighborhoods because discrimination excludes them from healthier ones, their higher incomes and education do not protect them from the depressing effect of noise, air pollution, and neighborhood street crime.

Chemical exposures via air, water, or food, can have profound effects on brain health, including effects that cause depression or make preexisting depression worse. Beyond gross examples like the lead poisoning of an entire community in Flint, Michigan, there are more subtle examples like exposure to endocrine-disrupting or neurotoxic chemicals from living near a chemical plant or in an agricultural area with high pesticide use.

In the United States, much of the agricultural work is done by immigrants. When farms utilize neurotoxic pesticides like chlorpyrifos, entire families are exposed to them sufficiently to affect their brains. Children's brains—from infancy through adolescence—are especially vulnerable to damage from neurotoxic pesticides that impair their cognitive performance, attention, and self-control (Eadeh et al., 2021; Ismail et al., 2010; Marsillach et al., 2016; Rohlman et al., 2016; van Wendel de Joode et al., 2016). Living near farms that use neurotoxic pesticides has been associated with lower IQs in 7-year-old children (Gunier et al., 2017). Problems with attention and cognition make school more challenging and less rewarding, and impaired self-control can lead to emotional trauma from either harsh discipline, humiliation by adults, or bullying by peers. In contexts in which adolescents of specific cultural backgrounds are differentially employed doing farm work including application of pesticides, the issue of neurotoxic brain injury becomes a structural correlate of cultural identity.

Depression in the parents can be an indirect effect of the child's exposure to toxins. If toxins damage a child's developing nervous system, the parents may experience a loss of hope for their child's future, the pain of empathy with their child's suffering, and the costs in time, energy, and worry of addressing their child's medical, academic, and possibly legal issues. These losses and stresses can precipitate or worsen depression in the child's parents.

Culture, Psychoactive Substance Use, and Depression

Cultures and subcultures have psychoactive drugs ("substances") of choice, be they medical or recreational, legal or illegal. They are used either to enhance positive experiences or to reduce negative experiences, or both. Cultures have different criteria for judging that a pattern of substance use is pathological. Substance use that is condoned or normalized by a culture can be harmful to some individuals as people's vulnerability to harm from substances is based on their genetics, preexisting medical conditions, consumption of medications, and concurrent use of other non-prescribed psychoactive substances. A depressed person might start or increase substance use with the intention of easing their symptoms, using substances that are available legally and might be used without stigma in the person's culture. Potential consequences of self-medication with non-prescribed psychoactive substances include direct exacerbation of depression by the substance or withdrawal from the substance after habitual use, and worsening of depression via the substance's effects on general health, occupational performance, or behavior in important relationships.

When substance use is the primary problem, depression can develop as a side effect of the substance used or can emerge when the person stops using it. Effective treatment of the depression requires addressing the substance use problem. When a person with a substance use disorder has comorbid depression, long-term abstinence is much more likely if the depression is effectively treated. The expectation that abstinence alone usually will resolve the depression of a person with a "dual diagnosis" is commonly encountered but not supported by evidence.

Some cultures normalize or even expect harmful or risky patterns of substance use. For example, both Finland and South Korea have cultures in which drinking to intoxication in a group is commonplace (Mäkelä et al., 2015; Ryu et al., 2013). In these cultures, many men consume eight or more alcoholic drinks on one occasion, thus attaining blood alcohol levels well above the threshold for intoxication. Binge-drinking cultures are associated with high rates of suicide. In countries with binge-drinking cultures, the demographic groups with the most binge drinking (typically men of working age) show suicide mortality rates disproportionate to their rates of MDD. Finland and South Korea are two examples (Institute for Health Metrics and Evaluation [IHME], 2023). Cultural normalization of binge drinking can persist through immigration and acculturation. For example, surveys of Asian Americans from 2002 to 2008 showed a 24.8% 1-month prevalence of binge drinking in Korean American adults, compared with 8.1% for Chinese Americans. Uniquely among Asian American ethnic groups, Korean Americans showed a frequency of binge drinking that was not significantly different between women and men. Among all other Asian American ethnic groups, men are significantly more likely than women to binge-drink (Lee et al., 2013).

In the U.S., teenagers and young adults have high rates of past-year alcohol and drug use. These are significantly higher in youths from affluent communities. For example, in a 2010 survey of high school seniors from two New England suburbs with median home prices over $1 million, 69.8% of boys and 71.5% of girls had drunk to intoxication in the past year, compared with 46.8% and 40.8%, respectively, for the same age cohort for the U.S. overall. For past-year use of marijuana, the rates were 58.2% and 39.0% for boys and girls in the affluent communities versus 38.3% and 30.7% in national samples. One year later, all rates were higher, but the differential between the affluent youths and the national sample persisted (Luthar et al., 2018). Risks associated with problem drinking and with drug use include a decline in academic performance, injuries from high-risk activities including driving or playing sports while intoxicated, and arrest for unlawful drug use. Any of these can be a major disruption of life plans that triggers an episode of depression.

Culture and the Phenomenology of Depression

Clinical depression is an illness that always includes both physical symptoms and changes in mood, thinking, and behavior. It is intrinsically a mind/body problem—*somatopsychic* or *psychosomatic*. In this respect it is like chronic pain. It virtually always includes a measurable disturbance in the body's physiology or chemistry that could be found if looked for specifically—that is why the presence of such a disturbance is part of this book's suggested criteria for the illness. However, no biological marker of depression is 100% sensitive and specific for depression. Further, some cases of depression are accompanied by significant state-related changes in a physiological or biochemical measure that nonetheless remains within the normal range for the population.

When people have a combination of physical and psychological symptoms they make causal attributions: Either the psychological symptoms are thought to be a reaction to the physical ones, the physical symptoms are thought to be an expression and/or consequence of the psychological ones, or both are regarded as an expression of a common inner disturbance (e.g., imbalance of *yin* and *yang*), as an effect of a common external factor (e.g., trauma or "stress") or as symptoms of a multisystem disease that affects the brain. Regardless of the attribution, people experiencing clinical depression for the first time often consult a primary care physician first, with insomnia, fatigue, or pain/discomfort as a chief complaint.

In our proposed criteria for clinical depression, any unpleasant physical sensation, or the worsening or lesser tolerability of a preexisting one, can substitute for the problems with sleep, changes in appetite, and fatigue/lack of energy that are part of standard DSM, Fifth Edition (DSM-5), diagnostic criteria for MDD. Depression's effects on the nervous, endocrine, and immune systems imply that depression can produce somatic pain, worsen existing somatic pain, and/or make somatic pain less bearable. It can, similarly, cause, worsen, or make less bearable other distressing symptoms like dyspnea or dyspepsia. Exacerbation of distressing physical symptoms can be mediated by systemic inflammation, autonomic changes, or lack of sleep. Increased intolerability of physical symptoms is a direct result of depression's effects on brain function.

An individual person with depression will have a characteristic physical face of the illness (e.g., insomnia and fatigue or neck pain and upset stomach). Culture is a determinant of what somatic symptoms are typical for depressed people; they often are ones that are prevalent in the population for other reasons. Back and neck pain are widespread among people who do physical labor, and depressed patients from cultures with many people who do physically strenuous work frequently present to clinicians with such pain. Mothers of infants and toddlers often have disrupted sleep. Poorly tolerated insomnia and distressing fatigue are typical presenting physical symptoms of depression in mothers of young children.

In highly masculine cultures, men with sad or depressed mood are unlikely to present to physicians with mood complaints. Often, they don't even acknowledge sadness or unhappiness if asked about it directly. Anhedonia is more frequently mentioned or acknowledged. Anger or irritability might be substituted. Impulsive or risky behavior, or substance use, can be the behavioral expression of the inner disturbance (i.e., negative affect is externalized; Sigurdsson et al., 2015). The consequences of substance use or risky behavior might bring the person to see a physician. Presenting symptoms might be physical complaints related to recent unhealthy behavior, injury or illness related to risk-taking, occupational injury, and/or a chronic painful condition like low back pain.

Cultural identity can be associated with specific unpleasant physical symptoms or negative emotions. For example, in Korean culture, a depressed person might acknowledge feelings of anger and vengefulness and complain of physical sensations of heat and chest discomfort. This culturally characteristic face of depression known in Korean as *hwa-byung* is explored in detail in Chapter 12.

The Perspective of Traditional Medical Systems

Depression without melancholia or psychosis that presents with prominent physical symptoms is a condition recognized by traditional medical systems worldwide. The patient's illness might be explained in spiritual terms. This form of depression is treated with some combination of physical treatments such as acupuncture or massage, herbs (taken orally, applied to the skin, or burned and inhaled), recommended changes in diet or daily routine, and/or participation in ceremonies that target the spiritual dimension of the disease.

Though no complementary or alternative treatment of depression taken from a traditional medical system currently meets the standard for the highest level of evidence of efficacy, several traditional treatments of depression have scientific support, and research on them continues (Cutler et al., 2023, Liu et al., 2015; K. S. Yeung et al., 2018). Acupuncture has shown positive results in small controlled clinical trials in patients with major depression, but the quality of evidence is low compared with the evidence supporting the efficacy of approved antidepressants (Li et al., 2020). It has been shown to improve sleep quality in depressed patients (Sun & Wu, 2023) In recent meta-analyses, acupuncture was shown to be as effective as antidepressant drugs in relieving cancer-related depression (F. Wang et al., 2022) and post-stroke depression (Lam Ching et al., 2023), and depression associated with chronic pain (Yan et al. 2020). Furthermore, acupuncture can significantly augment the effects of an SSRI in the treatment of depression (Y. Wang et al., 2022).

There is substantial evidence that herbal remedies for depression, or their active ingredients, have effects on neurotransmitters, inflammation, and/or endocrine regulation much like those of approved prescription antidepressants (Martins & Brijeshjsuku, 2018). For example, *yueju* (越橘), an herbal preparation used in traditional Chinese medicine (TCM) to treat depression accompanied by gastrointestinal distress, has effects on glutamate transmission and brain-derived neurotrophic factor (BDNF) levels like those of ketamine. Like ketamine, it shows rapid effects in several animal models of depression (Ren & Chen, 2017). Other examples are provided in Chapter 9, which deals with depression in three traditional medical systems.

In many ethnic cultures, people with symptoms of depression prefer to consult a traditional practitioner first, rather than a conventional physician or nonmedical mental health professional. This is especially true when traditional practitioners are covered by health insurance, as is the case with practitioners of Korean Oriental medicine in South Korea, or when they are more accessible or affordable than conventional physicians, as is the case with practitioners of *curanderismo* in parts of the American Southwest. *Curanderos/as* treat immigrants from Mexico and Central America using a system of traditional medicine that, like TCM and traditional Arabic and Islamic medicine (TAIM), has a religious/spiritual dimension. Among their clients are people suffering from depression, anxiety disorders, and post-traumatic stress disorder (Hoogasian & Lijtmaer, 2010; Hoskins & Padrón, 2018; Tafur et al., 2009). Consulting a traditional practitioner is less stigmatized than consulting a psychiatrist, and using traditional herbal treatments is less stigmatized than taking prescription psychotropic drugs.

The perspectives of traditional medical systems on depression and the bipolar spectrum are similar across cultures. TCM and its Japanese and Korean variants, Ayurvedic medicine, TAIM, *curanderismo*, and the medical traditions of ancient Greece and Rome share a holistic and comprehensive view of mood disorders. Common and distinctive themes in three traditional medical systems will be explored in depth in the next chapter.

A main objective of this book is to elicit changes in how clinicians interact with depressed patients and in how policymakers act to improve population mental health. As America's diversity has increased, medical and mental health–related organizations have encouraged clinicians to approach depressed patients with "cultural sensitivity" or "cultural competency." Clinicians are urged to learn about culture-specific *idioms of distress*—the language and behavior in which patients of specific cultures communicate the details of their condition—and about culture-specific beliefs about the causes and meaning of mental disorders. As a practical matter, it is equally important for clinicians to know about culture-associated aspects of lifestyle and/or environment that might contribute to a patient's depression—knowledge known as *structural competency*. This book uses the term *cultural awareness* to encompass structural competency, cultural sensitivity, and *cultural humility*—the latter entailing the clinician's respecting cultural differences, acknowledging the limits of their own knowledge of the patient's culture and circumstances, avoiding stereotyping, and understanding the large effects of economic and environmental circumstances on people's mental health. For policymakers and others concerned with the high prevalence of depression and high suicide mortality in disadvantaged minorities—an important aspect of health inequity in the U.S. and other ethnically diverse high-income nations—cultural awareness would include an understanding that addressing issues like food and housing security and quality, the safety of neighborhoods and workplaces, adequate greenspace, and unpolluted water and air is likely to have greater antidepressant benefits at the population level than mental health services narrowly defined.

Biomarkers of Depression and Cross-Cultural Dialogue

Depending on the presentation of clinical depression in the middle zone— initially somatic or initially psychological—cultures that do not accept depression as a bona fide and distinctive disease typically characterize it either as a primarily physical condition or as an extreme variation of normality. If the latter, the culture's expectation usually is that depressed people deal with their troubles alone—with stoic strength—or with the support of family, friends, and/or religion. Demonstrating that people with middle zone depression have abnormal biomarkers—including laboratory tests and brain images—can help bring cases into the realm of "real" illness both for the person with depression and for important people in the person's life. On the other hand, abnormal biomarkers would in some cultures increase stigma. The abnormal test findings would be misinterpreted as meaning the person was abnormal in a way that would warrant stigmatization. This might happen in a culture or subculture that stigmatizes diabetes, as some still do. Like many other strategies for reducing stigma, presenting depression "biologically" also cuts both ways.

Demonstration of abnormal biomarkers might help people with primarily somatic presentations of clinical depression to be more respected by conventional physicians. Many non-psychiatric physicians dislike treating patients who "somatize" (Pridmore et al., 2004). It may also help engage families who felt disappointment or perhaps embarrassment when their adolescent or young adult child showed undeniable signs of depression. If they can see their child as ill rather than as weak, spoiled, or lacking in character, resolve, or appropriate filial piety, they might be more supportive of their child's psychiatric treatment.

Targeting an abnormal biomarker as an indicator of progress in treatment can be helpful in encouraging patients to remain on treatment if they come from a culture in which there is a widespread fear of dependency on medications or a culturally embedded view that side effects frequently outweigh medications' benefits. When engaging with people from cultures averse to the long-term use of medications, a physician might successfully argue for a patient's staying on a medication until a laboratory test becomes and remains normal. Targeting a biomarker might also help in "selling" the idea that antidepressant treatment is disease-modifying and not merely symptomatic. Most optimistically, analysis of biomarkers combined with more refined phenotyping of depression probably will enable more precise matching of patients with treatments early in their course of illness. If it were widely known (and true) that depressed people had an 80% probability of remission with the first treatment they received, patients with depression would be more willing to accept the diagnosis and adhere to treatment, and middle zone depression would be perceived in more cultures as an ordinary illness rather than one deserving of special stigma or skepticism.

Examples of biological markers for depression, all based on multiply replicated studies, include altered sleep architecture (more rapid onset of REM sleep), impaired regulation of cortisol secretion (lack of normal diurnal variation and/or failure to suppress afternoon hypercortisolemia with dexamethasone), decreased levels of BDNF and other neurotrophic factors, decreased low-frequency heart rate variability, changes in electroencephalographic measures (e.g., increased loudness dependence of auditory evoked response), increased pro-inflammatory peptides (e.g., C-reactive protein, interleukins 6 and 1β, and tumor necrosis factor-α), altered levels of microRNAs, and decreased frontal cortical metabolism on functional brain imaging (Gadad et al., 2018; Hacimusalar & Eşel, 2018; Kidwell & Ellenbroek, 2018; J. S. Kim et al., 2016; Kraus et al., 2019; Levy et al., 2018; Strawbridge et al., 2017). In people with middle zone depression, blood tests might reveal nutritional insufficiencies relatively common in apparently well-nourished people, such as vitamin D insufficiency and borderline low magnesium or folate, that can contribute to the development of depression or make it harder to treat successfully with antidepressants. Finding and addressing a mild nutritional insufficiency is an easy and sometimes helpful way for a clinician to engage a patient in the medical treatment of depression. Sometimes simply correcting nutritional insufficiencies improves the patient's mood, and taking supplements often is more acceptable to people from low-trust, suspicious, cultures than treatment with antidepressant drugs.

Stigma of Depression Is Universal; Its Details Are Culture-Dependent

Public stigma, self-stigma, and anticipated stigma are critical aspects of the experience of depression, which, like the somatic symptoms of depression, are universally encountered but are variable across cultures. When seeing depression through a cultural lens, one begins with a hypothesis that stigma in some form may be an issue. Clinicians should listen for experienced stigma, anticipated stigma, and self-stigma in their depressed patients' narratives. The interpretation of a clinical encounter should include consideration of how anticipated stigma and self-stigma might have altered the patient's narrative and responses to the clinician's questions.

Mental illnesses—especially psychotic conditions—are stigmatized in virtually all cultures. Even in cultures that have sympathy for the mentally ill, most people would not want a mentally ill person as a neighbor, friend, or employee; most would not want their son or daughter to marry one; and very few would want one to take care of their children or grandchildren. By contrast, non-pathological negative mood states, like normal bereavement, are responded to with sympathy in almost all cultures. The status of patients with clinical depression in the middle zone is more complex, with more variation among individuals with the same principal cultural identity.

Reasons for stigma and discrimination against people with clinical depression in the middle zone range from fear that they will become psychotic and therefore dangerous to others (as unfair as the latter association might be) to a disapproving judgment that they have not been strong enough and have not tried hard enough to deal with life's vicissitudes. In some cases, they are suspected of malingering or exaggerating symptoms to escape responsibilities. Another source of stigma is the belief that antidepressants are addictive, a view widely held by Asian Americans from a range of national origins. (Jung et al., 2019). Stigma associated with antidepressant medication is shared by people of other ethnicities, for example, Mexican American women and Central American women with less than a high school education (Lopez et al., 2018).

In Japan, there is an entity of "new type" or "modern type" depression, *shingata utsu byo* (新型うつ病), most often seen in younger male salaried employees, who complain of physical and psychological symptoms of depression while at work but feel and appear much better outside of work. When employees with "new type depression" seek sick leave or disability benefits, their supervisors frequently doubt their sincerity and the validity of their illness. This is especially the case for employees who are witnessed enjoying themselves or who post images or accounts on social media of happy activities outside of work. A similar phenomenon can occur with depressed college students, who offer depression as an excuse or explanation for worse-than-expected academic performance but appear to occasionally have fun and sometimes share their enjoyment on social media. There are plausible reasons why a person with clinical depression might occasionally enjoy activities. For example, their depressive anhedonia might be incomplete or intermittent, and enjoying life when possible eases their emotional pain. Or, their depression might have mixed (bipolar) features. The suspicion of depressed people in situations like these is a form of stigmatization since people with other chronic diseases like diabetes, arthritis, or cancer who occasionally forget about their illness and enjoy life are not suspected of dishonesty in the same way.

People with depression often stigmatize themselves, blaming themselves for not performing better. This is particularly a problem when physical and/or cognitive performance is diminished because of depressive slowness, fatigue, or the consequences of insomnia. Depressed people might accept a diagnosis of depression but not embrace the idea that depression is a disorder that affects physical and cognitive performance and can impair a person's ability to do their best at work or school. If they accept the diagnosis of depression, they might think they should be able to overcome functional consequences through application of a strong will and extra effort, or they might blame themselves for getting depressed in the first place.

Perceived stigma of mental illness worsens self-stigma and usually decreases willingness to seek treatment for mental health problems (Jennings et al., 2015). When people experience discrimination based on gender, age, ethnicity, or another personal attribute, a common response is for them to identify more strongly with that attribute and draw strength from a sense of connection with other people who share it. A professional woman who has experienced discrimination based on her gender might respond by thinking of herself as a *woman* first—and a *strong* woman like her sister professionals. A Chinese immigrant who experiences discrimination based on their nationality might feel more connected with other Chinese people, feel proud of their heritage, and not be discouraged. A person who repeatedly encounters discrimination based on being depressed—if not assisted in dealing with it—might come to think of "depressed person" as their most salient identity. Such an identification usually is not helpful in building resilience. In fact, someone who self-identifies as a depressed person might pick up additional negative thoughts, feelings, and expectations from other depressed people they meet and with whom they identify (Cruwys & Gunaseelan, 2016). A clinician treating a depressed patient should be aware of whether the patient has experienced discrimination because of their depression, specific expressions of it, the diagnosis, or its treatment. Talking with the patient about the issue of discrimination or other public stigma—and how to deal with it—helps prevent the patient leaving treatment because they hope to avoid stigma by transforming themselves from a *patient diagnosed with a mental illness* to merely a *depressed person*—like lots of other depressed people. While disconnecting from formal treatment might have some short-term benefits, the patient might adopt an identity that is more hopeless and miserable even if less explicitly stigmatized.

People with depression often anticipate that they will be stigmatized if they reveal their diagnosis or others find out about it. Anticipated stigma is a major impediment to people seeking help for depressive symptoms. In many cultural and occupational contexts, the anticipation of stigma is realistic. Patients can be caught in a bind that leads to hopelessness and sometimes to suicide: Untreated, their depressive symptoms are unbearable, while if diagnosed and treated, they may be stigmatized in a way that affects their livelihood, their chances for happiness, or even their reasons for living.

The situation is especially poignant when the stigma of depression is institutionalized, as it is for airline pilots. In the U.S., an air transport pilot who discloses a diagnosis of depression or reveals its treatment with medication will at least temporarily lose the first-class medical certificate required to pilot scheduled airline flights. If a diagnosis is of any form of bipolar disorder (BD), the certificate is lost permanently. On many treatments for depression well supported by evidence and not often associated with cognitive or motor side effects, a pilot would never be permitted to fly professionally, even though the treatment was effective, the depression was in a stable remission, and there were no adverse effects of the treatment on flying performance (Federal Aviation Administration, 2023/2018). Consider the situation of a man for whom flying was a raison d'être in addition to a job, who took on substantial debt for pilot's training, and felt he could not marry his beloved fiancée without stable, well-paid employment. He might think the loss of his first-class medical certification would be personally catastrophic. He would keep his depression secret, go untreated, and perhaps eventually die by suicide. Similar, realistic anticipation of life-altering institutional stigma can affect the course of depression in physicians. In many U.S. states, a physician must report a diagnosis of depression to the state medical licensing board and may be subject to loss of privacy and to intrusive and expensive monitoring, even if the depression and its treatment have no adverse effect on their performance as a clinician.

In many ethnic groups, a history of formally diagnosed depression would diminish a person's hopes of making a favorable marriage, of marrying the person they love, or of marrying at all. In countries where young adult men significantly outnumber young women, as is the case in several Asian nations, becoming undesirable as a potential husband is a major loss. In cultural groups defined by nationality, ethnicity, or religion in which a woman's status, opportunities, and quality of life depend greatly on the man she marries, stigmatization as a potential wife because of a depression diagnosis has a similarly painful significance. In both cases the major, lifetime consequences of depression-related stigma can increase the risk of suicide.

Cross-cultural study of the stigma of depression suggests that stigma is least when the depression is attributed to a tough life situation and worst when it is viewed as endogenous and genetically determined (Zimmermann & Papa, 2019). Across cultures, people are inclined to sympathize with those who have suffered major losses and life troubles for which they are not personally responsible. Even though a person has no control over their genome, depression related to genetic risk factors may be, incorrectly, seen as impossible to fix and as making a person less trustworthy and less desirable as a friend, employee, or spouse.

The stigma of depression among Asian Americans has been studied systematically. In this group, depression often is seen as a sign of personal weakness and a reason for shame and family disappointment. The belief that antidepressants are addictive is common. Greater stigma is associated with more recent immigration, less acculturation and/or English proficiency, less education, older age, and Asian Indian or Korean ethnicity. Among major Asian ethnic groups, depression is least stigmatized by the Chinese (Jung et al., 2020). A similar study in Singapore confirmed that the stigma of depression was greater among Asian Indians than among Chinese. Those who stigmatized depression commonly held the belief that depressed people are weak, not sick (Subramaniam et al., 2017).

In many cultures, men are more stigmatized for depression than women, and this contributes to their lesser likelihood of seeking treatment (Oliffe et al., 2016; Pedersen & Paves, 2014). Stigma is associated with conceiving of depression as a sign of weakness of character (Cook & Wang, 2011). Those who stigmatize others with mental health issues may be especially unwilling to seek help for their own problems (Schnyder et al., 2017).

The universal and sometimes punitive stigma faced by people with depression in some cultural contexts suggests there is clinical value in identifying and intervening with people at risk for depression before they cross the line of diagnostic criteria for MDD or bipolar depression. A person with poor sleep, fatigue, and intermittent low mood, with genetic, historical, or environmental risk factors for depression but not meeting diagnostic criteria might be engaged in a program to "improve sleep and build resilience," to "promote health through mindfulness," or to "learn a healthier lifestyle." The interventions used would have evidence for antidepressant efficacy when used in people with middle zone clinical depression and would have justification for use in non-depressed people based on published demonstration of benefits for general health, well-being, and/or disease prevention. For example, people with subsyndromal depression and chronic chronobiologic stress might be taught how to use bright light therapy.

Culture and the Choice of Treatment for Depression

An "evidence-based best practice" approach to treatment of depression with medication calls for the use of an adequate dose of an antidepressant taken for several months. The dosage of the medication is adjusted, and changes are made in the drug and the dose to bring the patient to a full remission of symptoms. Medication is continued for several months after the remission is reached to prevent relapse. Patients with a history of recurrence might remain on medication indefinitely. Patients with bipolar depression are treated with mood-stabilizing medication on a long-term basis.

This plan of treatment conflicts with cultures in which taking medication for a condition like depression that is not linked to an abnormal biopsy, image, or laboratory test is regarded as merely relieving symptoms rather than controlling or curing a disease. Such cultures might have fears of drug dependency that are disproportionate to the actual risk or concerns about side effects that are excessive in relation to the reported incidence and seriousness of known adverse effects of antidepressant and mood-stabilizing medicines. The durations of first antidepressant treatment episodes of depressed patients over age 65 were compared between the United States (Boston), the United Kingdom (national sample), Canada (Ontario and Quebec separately), and Taiwan (national sample). Focusing on patients who received just one drug rather than two or more different treatments, the mean duration of treatment in Taiwan was 104.7 days, much shorter than the mean treatment duration in the United States (225.7 days), the United Kingdom (192.8 days) or Canada (289.1 days in Ontario and 340.9 days in Quebec City; Tamblyn et al., 2019). The short treatment duration seen in Taiwan is incompatible with the practice standard of continuing treatment for at least 6 months after attainment of remission. In South Korea, premature discontinuation of antidepressants appears to be the rule rather than the exception. In an analysis of national health insurance claims data, 57% of patients treated pharmacologically for depression stopped treatment less than 4 weeks after it was started (N. Kim et al., 2019).

It might seem paradoxical that national cultures like the Chinese and the Koreans that have a long-term orientation often are averse to long-term antidepressant use. However, the phenomenon makes sense if depression treatment is seen as merely symptomatic and not disease-modifying.

Non-pharmacological treatment of depression (e.g., psychotherapy, counseling, or behavioral healthcare) is preferred to medications by many people. In addition to personal preferences, cost, coverage, and availability of services, culture is a determinant of attitudes toward such treatment. Psychotherapy is less stigmatized than taking medication, everywhere. However, in low-trust cultures in which healthcare professionals are not excluded from a general suspicion of people not in their own extended family, depressed people might be reluctant to trust a therapist to be competent, to be honest, or to maintain confidentiality. In cultures (including intersections of "masculine" culture and male gender) that highly value stoicism or self-reliance, people might feel that if their depression can improve solely with psychotherapy, they should be able to manage it on their own.

Choosing a culturally compatible or culturally adapted treatment for depression is based on understanding the depressed person's conception of the disease and narrative of the illness and appreciation of the cultural issues that would make a treatment acceptable or unacceptable. There are many evidence-supported treatments for clinical depression other than prescription medications and conventional psychotherapy. Nutritional supplements, bright light therapy, non-invasive brain stimulation, and psychotherapeutic smartphone apps are four examples. Traditional medical practitioners offer additional options including herbs and acupuncture. While clinicians without a special interest in complementary and alternative medicine may not be familiar with many of the options, alternative therapies can be much more acceptable—and consequently more effective—than antidepressant drugs that a person doesn't take consistently or psychotherapy that is soon abandoned.

In considering the potential effectiveness of an alternative treatment for a patient's depression, weaker (but still substantial) evidence for efficacy of a treatment might be outweighed by the patient's greater acceptance of, adherence to, and persistence with it. When the depressed patient of a clinician practicing mainstream Western medicine prefers alternative treatment that is not within the clinician's scope of practice, the clinician can meaningfully assist the patient in several ways. They can discourage the patient from pursuing an alternative treatment that has no scientific support and/or that entails significant risks to someone with the patient's clinical profile. If the alternative does have an evidence base and is not unacceptably risky, the clinician can offer to see the patient regularly to monitor their response to the alternative treatment, with attention to the adequacy of improvement and to potential adverse effects or interactions with treatments for the patient's other medical conditions. If the clinician is familiar with providers of alternative treatments such as specific practitioners of traditional medicine or reliable sources of herbal antidepressants, they might share the information. Along the way, the patient would be reminded of viable mainstream treatments that might be effective if the alternative treatment does not yield a remission.

"Patient" as Cultural Identity

Physicians have written eloquently about the experience of being a patient with an illness of their own, describing the change in their self-identity and the challenge of accepting their vulnerability, loss of control, and sometimes a loss of the respect they have come to expect from others (Jones, 2005; Klitzman, 2008; Mandell & Spiro, 1987). People of other occupations who have high status in the broader culture from occupational prestige, wealth, and/or family connections can face a similar challenge.

The communication style of conventional Western medicine is low-context and direct, and physicians prefer patients who are both trusting and trustworthy. Patients with chronic illnesses will have more satisfactory clinical relationships if they can collaborate with their physicians and have unambiguous, uncomplicated communication with them. However, people from cultures with low trust and high-context, indirect communication might not be able to immediately adapt to the mainstream physician's ideal style of relationship and communication. An acculturation process is required, which sometimes involves acculturative stress. A patient might need to make changes in their lifestyle, conception of self, and communication style to best cope with a chronic illness.

The physician–patient relationship typical of a person's culture (taking both ethnicity and class into account) might not be optimal when the patient's chronic condition is depression or bipolar illness. In a hierarchical culture, a patient might be clearly above the physician or clearly below the physician in social status or authority. Even so, either a controlling or a submissive position of the patient with respect to the physician is likely to produce a poor outcome. If they become members of a "classless" patient culture, patients will aim for mutually respectful, collaborative relationships with their physicians with a norm of shared decision-making for major treatment decisions. They will listen to physicians' advice with open minds, and they will be willing to consider in-person or online connections with other people suffering from the same illness. They will explicitly share responsibility with their physicians for outcomes of care. People who fully identify with "patient culture" are likely to adhere to treatment and to promptly report problems with treatment because they have participated in the treatment decision and "own it."

For depression and bipolar illness, the process of acculturating to the patient role usually begins when a person has a relapse of symptoms after several months of responding well to treatment, has a second episode of depression after being well for months or years, or has a first episode of hypomania following one or more episodes of depression, thus unequivocally establishing the diagnosis of bipolar illness. These experiences establish that the person is dealing with a chronic illness and not a once-in-a-lifetime episode of clinical depression. Awareness of "patient" culture and the challenge of acculturation to it is another function of the cultural lens. It is especially helpful to clinicians when they work with patients who begin with low trust or with being accustomed to a position of authority.

Cultural Mnemonics: Comparisons, Themes, Narratives, Unexpected Facts

The essence of cultural awareness in the clinical context is primed perception and informed empathy. *Primed perception* is hearing themes in patients' narratives and making observations in clinical encounters that are especially pertinent to understanding depression in people with patient's cultural identity. Prior exposure to *facts, theory, and illness narratives* related to the patient's culture primes the clinician to note important details when they emerge: Priming makes what is *relevant, salient. Informed empathy* entails that the clinician metaphorically puts themselves in the patient's shoes, after carefully examining different styles and sizes of shoes to find the ones that fit best and appeal most to the patient's taste. When the clinician knows enough about the special issues of depression in people of the patient's cultural identity, they will not just feel the patient's pain but know where it hurts the most. Patients can sense the difference between informed empathy and a sincere but more generic variety of empathy. A well-timed, perspicacious comment or question by the clinician about a culture-related dimension of the patient's illness often can establish for the patient that the clinician understands, cares, can be trusted, and probably will help. Several principles are relevant to the cultivation of cultural awareness and the practice of primed perception and informed empathy:

People's cultural identities are suggested by their illness narratives and presentations of themselves.

A suspected cultural identity links to a set of testable hypotheses about the dimensions of the culture, its communication style, and trust or distrust in clinicians and their practices. Cultural features relevant to primed perception and informed empathy are more memorable when they are part of comparisons between obviously related or superficially similar cultural groups that nonetheless differ in ways especially important to depression, bipolar illness, or suicide.

Each national or ethnic culture has historical memories, adages, cautionary tales, and basic rules of conduct that almost every child from that culture learns and almost every adult from the culture keeps in mind.

Culturally typical stories—narratives from literature, from film, and from clinical encounters—evoke a reader's, viewer's, or clinician's emotions and tend to be more memorable than the theories of social science or the data analyses of medical research. Effective and efficient preparation for beginning clinical work with a new and different cultural group might include seeing a movie or reading a novel exemplifying depression in that group and hearing from colleagues about a few of their most memorable patients from that culture.

Single words, metaphors, or idioms of a language or cultural group can convey precious information about a person's mood state, level of emotional pain and hopelessness, and suicide risk. Patients can, one by one, teach the clinicians who treat them such words, metaphors, and idioms and their connotations and implicit meanings.

Chapter 9

Ancient Wisdom Meets Modern Science: Depression in Traditional Medicine

Whether mood disorders are treated as genuine illnesses and whether they are stigmatized depend upon the meanings ascribed to their symptoms. The meaning of an illness is shaped by a culture's prevailing system of medicine and the philosophy and worldview behind it. Religion, popular culture, and politics can influence it as well. This chapter describes the surprisingly congruent conceptions of depression and bipolar disorder (BD) in three antique medical systems—those of classical Greece and Rome, of imperial China, and of the medieval Islamic world. These conceptions are comprehensive, holistic, and dimensional. Some ancient viewpoints are surprisingly compatible with current concepts of mood disorders in mainstream Western medicine. In the case of traditional Chinese medicine (TCM), ongoing research by academic TCM specialists on the mechanisms of action of its antidepressant treatments is congruent with other contemporary explorations of mechanisms that address inflammation and disorders of the microbiome and metabolome as well as alterations in neurotransmission.

In approaching the comparison of ancient and modern perspectives, it is helpful to recall the broader definition of clinical depression that extends beyond major depressive disorder (MDD) and the concept of a bipolar spectrum that includes bipolar disorder I (BD-I) and bipolar disorder II (BD-II) but also mixed mood states and dysfunctional cyclothymia. As noted throughout Part I, narrow categorical definitions may be useful for reliable classification for epidemiological purposes, but they do not capture the observed variability of distressing and functionally significant depressive and bipolar syndromes in the general population.

In TCM and in several other historical systems of medicine, depression is subdivided into discrete phenotypes that respond best to different treatments. Prevention, treatment, and rehabilitation go beyond pharmacology and psychotherapy to include physical treatments and modifications of diet, activity, and environment. All the senses are involved; aromatherapy and music therapy are found in the major traditional medical systems. Specific therapies with ancient origins are being reassessed using rigorous scientific methodology, and those with evidentiary support are slowly being integrated into conventional Western medicine. Worldwide, more people with depression consult practitioners of traditional medicine than seek treatment from mental health professionals. In most cases people with depression regard traditional medicine as an alternative to standard mental health care. Sometimes it is a complement, as when a person sees a non-medical counselor to talk about emotional and interpersonal issues while getting treatment for somatic symptoms from a traditional medicine practitioner. True integration of traditional and mainstream Western medicine is found at academic medical centers in both high-income countries and middle-income countries, but it is not widespread.

The holistic and dimensional views of mood disorders in traditional medical systems have historically coexisted with a narrower categorical view of people as either healthy or "mentally ill," accompanied by reductionistic explanations of mental illness. The views of mood disorders described in the literature of traditional medical systems minimize stigma and entail empathy and compassionate care for people who suffer from them. By contrast, the categorization of people as "mentally ill" usually has entailed stigmatizing attitudes, blame, irrational fear, and superstition.

This chapter describes mood disorders as seen in three traditional medical systems: classical Greco-Roman medicine, TCM, and traditional Arabic and Islamic medicine (TAIM). These medical systems share a holistic, comprehensive approach and multidimensional view of the nature and treatment of depression and the bipolar spectrum. Other similar systems include Kampo, the Japanese adaptation of TCM; traditional Korean medicine (TKM), a synthesis of TCM with local elements; and Indian Ayurvedic medicine. The practice of complementary, alternative, and integrative medicine (CAIM) in Western academic medical centers draws specific concepts and therapeutic modalities from these and other traditional medical systems while not adopting their underlying philosophies and explanations of illness. Systematic reviews by leading academic psychiatrists have summarized best practices and supporting evidence for applying CAIM to mood disorders and other psychiatric illness (Gerbarg et al., 2017).

Traditional medical systems explain non-psychotic forms of depression, BD-II, and cyclothymia in terms of quantitative rather than qualitative deviations from normal function, such as an imbalance of yin (阴) and yang (阳) or an excess of black bile. Nothing supernatural is involved. They do less well with affective psychoses, which before the modern era often were attributed to supernatural influences.

From Hippocrates to Galen: Classical Greco-Roman Medicine

Ancient Greek medicine, which was adopted and further developed by the Romans, was built on the idea that health was a balance of four humors (liquids), with analogies drawn between the four humors, the stages of a person's life, and the seasons of the year. They were yellow bile (youth, spring), blood (maturity, summer), black bile (old age, autumn), and phlegm (senility, winter). Illness reflected an imbalance of the four humors (Jouanna & Allies, 2012; National Library of Medicine, 2019).

Hippocrates (ca. 460-370 BCE) described symptoms fitting the profile of major depression, mentioning aversion to food, despondency, sleeplessness, irritability, and restlessness. He emphasized that *persistence* of emotional symptoms was essential to the diagnosis: "Fear or sadness that *lasts a long time* means melancholia" (emphasis added). At any specific time, a person not ill with melancholia might have intense feelings of sadness, despair, or fear. *Abnormal duration* of these feelings was the sign of disease. Hippocrates attributed depression to an excess of cold black bile in the spleen. Humoral imbalances were not endogenous; they reflected a combination of factors including a person's diet, lifestyle, living conditions, and atmospheric conditions (Horwitz et al., 2016). A minimum duration of symptoms is a major criterion for the diagnosis of mood disorders in the American Psychiatric Association's *Diagnostic and Statistical Manual*, fifth edition (DSM, Fifth Edition [DSM-5]; American Psychiatric Association, 2013) and in the *International Classification of Diseases*, 10th revision (ICD-10; World Health Organization, 1992). Hippocrates appreciated that depression can only be diagnosed with a proper history. In the words of Dr. Allen Frances, an eminent American psychiatrist and critic of "disease mongering" in psychiatry, a diagnosis requires "a movie rather than just a snapshot" (Frances, 2013).

Hippocrates appreciated the role of the brain in producing mental and behavioral symptoms:

> It is the brain which makes us mad or delirious, inspires us with dread and fear, whether by night or by day, brings sleeplessness, inopportune mistakes, aimless anxieties, absentmindedness, and acts that are contrary to habit. These things that we suffer all come from the brain when it is not healthy, but becomes abnormally hot, cold, moist, or dry. (Hippocrates, 2023, p. 175)

The function of the brain would, of course, be influenced by the imbalance of humors in the body. For Hippocrates, depression was a condition with a physical cause and a combination of physical, cognitive, and emotional symptoms. In addition to herbal medication, Hippocrates recommended baths, exercise, a special diet, and bloodletting. (At the time of Hippocrates and for another two millennia, bloodletting was a standard medical therapy throughout the world—one now thought worthless for all but a handful of conditions.) One of the herbal treatments for depression used by the school of Hippocrates probably was *Hypericum perforatum* (St. John's wort), which has been shown by several credible clinical trials (but not in all published clinical trials) to be more efficacious than placebo for treatment of mild to moderate depression (Linde et al., 2008; Ng et al., 2017).

Hippocrates noted a relationship between depression (melancholia) and epilepsy (Hoppe, 2018). In fact, depression is the most common psychiatric comorbidity of epilepsy, and suicide is a major cause of death in people with epilepsy (Christensen et al., 2007; Hesdorfer et al., 2012). In correctly noting the connection, Hippocrates identified both depression and epilepsy, chronic conditions with invisible causes, as ordinary natural phenomena. Both have been stigmatized since ancient times, and at times epilepsy has been given a supernatural explanation. The development of electroencephalography in the 20th century definitively established the physical origins of epilepsy, with a consequent reduction (though not elimination) of its stigma. The connection between mood disorders and epilepsy is made in other traditional medical systems, notably TCM, as will be addressed further later in this chapter.

Hippocrates and other Greeks, notably Aristotle, emphasized that people who suffered serious losses like the death of loved ones, romantic disappointments, or reversals of fortune should not be labeled as ill merely because they experience sadness or even despair. Symptoms disproportionate to life events, or accompanied by major physical symptoms or functional impairment, would be the reason to diagnose disease (Horwitz et al., 2016).

Aristotle (384-322 BCE) recognized that eminent, successful creative people—whether in the arts, sciences, or political life—often had conditions in the bipolar spectrum (Doerr-Zegers, 2003). He applied the term *melancholy* (black bile) to describe both phases of their illness. Cold black bile was associated with depression and hot black bile with hypomania. His description of bipolar symptomatology parallels that of TCM, where yin takes the place of cold black bile and yang the place of hot black bile.

Aristotle described the need of people with bipolar spectrum disorders for ongoing mood-stabilizing treatment—rather than only treatment as needed for current distressing symptoms.

> Melancholics are in perpetual need of medicine because their mixture of bodily fluids keeps their bodies in a constant state of irritation and their passions are continually active. Depending on coincidence, they can become the victim of either an extreme exuberance or a deep sorrow. And through medical therapy these extremes become less pronounced. (Aristotle, 2023)

Aristotle, anticipating by more than two millenia the distinction between Axis I and Axis II of the Diagnostic and Statistical Manual of Mental Disorders (DSM), distinguished self-indulgence from a lack of self-control, the former a personality trait or a voluntary behavior, and the latter a potential sign of a medical problem.

In chapter 30 of his *Problemata*, Aristotle described depressive and hypomanic symptomatology as two faces of a single pathologic process. However, he did not explicitly describe BD as a cyclical condition. He also distinguished hypomania from mania ("frenzy"; Pies, 2007).

> Now black bile ... if it is in excessive quantity in the body, produces apoplexy or torpor, or despondency or fear; but if it becomes overheated, it produces cheerfulness with song, and madness. ... Those in whom the bile is considerable and cold become sluggish and stupid, while those with whom it is excessive and hot become mad, clever or amorous and easily moved to passion and desire, and some become more talkative. ... Many, because this heat is near to the seat of the mind, are affected by the diseases of madness or frenzy (Aristotle, 1965, pp. 155–169).

Aristotle's personal authorship of the just-cited description has been questioned by classical scholars. However, even if Aristotle was not the author, the quote is representative of more advanced thinking of Greeks during the classical period.

Aretaeus of Cappadocia (81–138 CE) described a cyclical condition like BD-I, noting that depression often was the state experienced first. He described euphoric patients who would "laugh, play, dance night and day, and sometimes go openly to the market crowned, as if victors in some contest of skill," only later to appear "torpid, dull and sorrowful." (Aretaeus, 1972, p. 302). Earlier writers had described syndromes of mania and depression, but Aretaeus was the first Western writer to explicitly identify a single illness that cycled between depressive and manic phases (Angst & Marneros, 2001; Fornaro et al., 2009).

Greco-Roman classical medicine was summarized in the first century CE by the Roman encyclopedist Aulus Cornelius Celsus (ca. 25 BCE–ca. 50 CE). In his work *De Medicina*, Celsus described "insanity" as one of the "affections of the body ... which cannot be ascribed to any definite part," an idea consonant with modern conceptions of depression being related to non-localized pathophysiology like systemic inflammation, endocrine disturbance, or alteration of the microbiome (Cui et al., 2024; Dabboussi et al., 2024; Kopera et al., 2024; Kouba et al., 2024). One type of "insanity" described by Celsus was *tristitia* (sadness), which "seems caused by black bile." The recommended treatment began with laxatives and emetics to detoxify the body. The patient was to have massages twice a day and to exercise frequently if they were strong enough. Causes of fright were to be excluded, and good hope was to be put forward and entertainment provided by storytelling and games, especially those the patient enjoyed when sane. If the patient had produced tangible work products (e.g., writings or crafts), they were to be set before the patient and praised. "His sadness should be gently reproved as being without cause, he should have it pointed out to him now and again how in the very things which trouble him there may be a cause of rejoicing rather than of solicitude" (Celsus, 1935/1971, book III, chapter 18).

Celsus appears to have proposed a combination of physical therapy, occupational therapy, and cognitive-behavioral psychotherapy. In addition, he recommended that any comorbid general medical conditions be identified and treated: "When there is fever besides, it is to be treated like other fevers" (Celsus, 1935/1971).

Celsus went on, however, to describe another type of insanity, in which the patient is "duped" by the mind or by "phantoms." If the patient "duped by phantoms" were sad, a laxative would be given; if the patient were "hilarious," the treatment was a drug to induce vomiting. If, unfortunately, the "madman" was deceived by their own mind, Celsus recommended "certain tortures." He described flogging, putting patients in chains, and starving them, all to draw the attention of the patient "duped by his mind" away from their preoccupations, delusions, and wrong thoughts—or to associate insane thoughts with frightening and unpleasant experiences, thus making them less likely to recur.

Regrettably, Celsus' prescription for highly aversive behavior therapy became part of historical basis and rationale for the torture and mistreatment of the mentally ill during the Dark Ages. His prescription for torture is followed by advice that insane people—even those duped by their own minds—should not be left alone, among strangers, or with people they despise or don't respect. He called for patients to be treated with kindness following the administration of harsh treatment (Celsus, 1935/1971). Celsus was not concerned with demonic possession, and the recommended treatment for mood disorders was not exorcism. He did not state or imply that insane people were evil or were being punished for past sins of their own or their ancestors.

Galen (129–216 CE) elaborated on Hippocrates' theory of the four humors by describing temperaments that reflect humoral excesses: melancholic, sanguine, phlegmatic, and choleric. A melancholic temperament would naturally be a risk factor for the illness of melancholia, but temperament and illness were not the same. Galen also saw hypomania and depression as related conditions; anger and fear were emotions common to both. He described how a depressed or manic person could have a single delusion without otherwise having a psychotic thought process—thus distinguishing a form of psychotic mood disorder from schizophrenia, a condition in which there is more pervasive abnormality of thought process and reality testing (Dols & Immisch, 1992).

The Greek and Roman physicians described conditions much like major depression, BD-I, and BD-II and treated them with multiple complementary modalities. They appreciated the relevance of life circumstances and life events to mood disorders but did not label intense emotional reactions as illness if they were not overly prolonged or disproportionate to their context. Their approach did not worsen stigma. They recommended a long-term therapeutic relationship for the best outcome in BD. Their descriptions and observations seem fresh and modern. Treatment of mood disorders in classical times included herbal medicaments, dietary changes, exercises, massage, music therapy, and aromatherapy. The emotional brain was accessed through all five senses.

The classical Greco-Roman approach to mood disorders did not survive in western Europe after the fall of Rome. However, it was carried forward by Arabs and Persians in the golden age of Islam. There it was developed further as it absorbed ideas and new treatments from Chinese, Indian, and central Asian traditional medicine. By contrast, TCM, a system of similar antiquity, has persisted continuously since its origin.

From the Yellow Emperor to the King of Medicines: TCM

The documentary history of TCM (*Zhōngyī*; 中医) can be said to begin with the *Huángdì Nèijīng* (黄帝内经; *The Yellow Emperor's Inner Canon*). The work, assembled by several eminent scholars of the time, originated during the Warring States period (475–221 BCE), which was followed by the establishment of imperial China. The *Huángdi Nèijīng* takes the form of a dialogue between the mythical emperor and his physician, whom the emperor asks about many issues concerning health and illness.

The book has its roots in Daoist philosophy. The Dao, literally the "way" or the "road," offers a path through human existence that is effortless and harmonious. Living in accordance with the Dao requires a proper balance of yin and yang, the two fundamental principles of the natural world. Yin and yang correspond to shadow and light, moon and sun, female and male, inside and outside, cold and hot, downward and upward. Yin and yang are two aspects of qi (气; vital energy/life force), which circulates through the body through channels called *meridian*s (*jīngluò*; 经络). Health is affected by the influence of the five elements (*wǔ xíng*; 五行), of which all matter is composed, each of which is associated with two internal organs. Wood (*mù*; 木) is associated with the liver and gallbladder, fire (*huǒ*; 火) with the heart and small intestine, earth (*tǔ*; 土) with the spleen and the stomach, metal (*jīn*; 金) with the lung and the large intestine, and water (*shuǐ*; 水) with the kidneys and bladder. The organs are nourished by the blood (*xuè*; 血). Symptoms of illnesses are produced by an imbalance of yin and yang, an excess or deficiency of qi or blockage of the flow of qi or *xue*.

Illness is characterized by two aspects, *bìng* (病) and *zhèng* (症), the first being the disease and the second the profile of symptoms, as determined by the TCM diagnostic process. Contemporary research has related *zheng* to subtypes of Western medicine's diseases that differ in their prognoses or responses to treatment. *Zheng* can be the basis of groupings of patients created by machine learning or artificial intelligence and validated by proving their association with different patterns of biomarkers or responses to different treatments (Quan et al., 2014; Y.-N. Song et al., 2013; P. Wang & Chen, 2013). Nonetheless, the explanatory framework of TCM is metaphorical: Most of its specific explanations are incompatible with modern science if taken literally. The five elements do not correspond to actual anatomical structures; the flow of *qi* along the meridians is not measurable with any known apparatus. However, conduction of low-voltage direct current through the subcutaneous tissue along meridians can be measured. Variations in current correspond to variations in resistance, which depend upon dermal autonomic activity along the meridian (Tsai et al., 2017).

Electroacupuncture has empirical support as an adjunct to selective serotonin reuptake inhibitors (SSRIs) or serotonin and norepinephrine reuptake inhibitors (SNRIs) in the treatment of MDD. A 2021 meta-analysis of relevant studies shows that the combination of electroacupuncture with an SSRI or SNRI is more efficacious than the medication alone (Zhichao et al., 2021).

The diagnostic process in TCM entails four parts: *wàng* (望), *wén* (闻), *wèn* (问), and *qiè* (切)—inspection, auscultation/olfaction, inquiry, and palpation. Inspection comprises systematic observation of the patient's appearance, movement, and behavior, with meticulous examination of the tongue. Auscultation attends to the sound of the patient's voice and breathing; olfaction comprises assessment of body and breath odors. Inquiry is taking a medical history and performing a review of symptoms of organ dysfunction. The history, as in modern medicine, includes the narrative of the present illness as well as the patient's life history, family history, and past medical history. Palpation is an advanced form of pulse-taking in which three locations on the radial artery of each arm are touched, respectively, by the examiner's index, middle, and ring fingers. In addition to rate, rhythm, strength, and volume, other qualitative aspects of the pulse are noted. Palpation also includes tactile examination of the abdomen and of specific acupuncture points. TCM in contemporary practice in China does not necessarily fully implement this ideal. However, the inspection and palpation aspects of TCM diagnosis might help a conventional, allopathic physician find signs of general medical or neurological conditions that can present with depression, such as thyroid disease or early Parkinson's disease. And its broad-ranging inquiry might uncover social and environmental aspects of mental health that deserve attention.

When CAIM programs in Western countries adapt methods of TCM to the diagnosis and treatment of mood disorders, the focus is not on diagnosing unbalanced yin and yang or on blockage, constraint, or excess or deficiency of qi but on doing a more comprehensive and holistic patient assessment and on making use of traditional treatments including herbal formulas, acupuncture, and *qìgōng* (气功; practice to cultivate qi). Qigong combines meditation with structured exercises and conscious breathing (Abbott et al., 2017). These treatments usually are accompanied by recommendations on diet and activity.

The *Huangdi Nejing* has two volumes, the *Sùwèn* (素问; *Basic Questions*) and the less frequently cited *Língshū* (灵枢; *Spiritual Pivot*). The *Suwen* lays out the basic theory and practice of TCM. The *Lingshu* concentrates on methods of acupuncture and bloodletting (a procedure that involves only a few drops of blood and is intended to enable *qi* to escape through the hole made by the acupuncture needle). Both the *Suwen* and the *Lingshu* have chapters referring to mood disorders. Chapter 22 of the *Lingshu* gives a clear picture of how the founders of TCM saw two mood disorders. One was *diān* (癫), a term used in modern Chinese to denote epilepsy but that in the *Lingshu* seems to refer to a form of depression as well. The other was *kuáng* (狂), a condition strongly resembling BD. According to the *Lingshu*, *dian* is due to excessive yin and *kuang* is due to excessive yang. *Dian kuang* began with sadness and evolved into euphoria and grandiosity. That is, mania preceded by depression. In modern usage, *kuang* simply means "crazy," "mad," or psychotic or, when used metaphorically, aggressive, wildly arrogant, and conceited. No specific psychiatric diagnosis is implied. *Dian* is now used exclusively to denote epilepsy. The modern term for clinical depression is *yōuyù* (忧郁; anxiety and depression). Major depression is *zhòngdù yōuyù zhèng* (重度忧郁症; literally "severe depression disease"). BD is *zào yù zhèng* (躁郁症; manic depressive illness).

> *Dian* begins with an unhappy feeling and a headache. When the patient looks up the eyes are red. They are irritable.
>
> To treat a patient with *dian*, the healer should live with the patient and observe their behavior throughout the day.
>
> In the prodrome of *kuang* the patient feels sad, forgetful, easily angered and often frightened ... then, *kuang* begins. The patient seldom lies down. They rarely feel hungry. The patient becomes euphoric, grandiose, feeling noble, smart, and eloquent, and disparaging others. They are sleepless day and night. (*Lingshu*, chapter 22)

Dian kuang as described in the *Lingshu* presents with a clinical syndrome resembling BD. It is a physical illness that reflects an imbalance of *qi*, involving neither a moral defect nor a supernatural influence. The treatment prescribed for *dian kuang* in the *Huángdì Nèijīng* emphasizes bloodletting at specified points. Thus, an accurate and non-stigmatizing description of a form of BD is combined in *Lingshu* with a theory of etiology that is more mystical than scientific and a method of treatment with no physiologic rationale.

Zhāng Zhòngjǐng (张仲景; 150–219 CE), was the leading physician of the late Han Dynasty (206–220 CE). Before his death he published *Treatise on Cold Damage Disorders* (*Shānghán Zábìng Lùn*; 伤寒杂病论), a medical textbook of broad scope. The original edition was lost, but the content was collected and republished hundreds of years later, with one of two parts of the work appearing under the title *Essential Prescriptions from the Golden Cabinet* (*Jīn Guì Yào Lüè*; 金匮要略) (Z. Zhang, 2012).

In the *Treatise on Cold Damage Disorders*, Zhang distinguishes two presentations of depression: liver qi stagnation and heart/spleen qi deficiency (Z. Zhang, 1999). Together the two presentations account for 31% of the patients with MDD described in a 2015 review of randomized controlled trials of TCM treatment (W.-F. Yeung et al., 2015). The other two TCM syndromes frequently described in the clinical trials reviewed were liver qi depression/spleen qi deficiency and liver qi depression. In *Essential Prescriptions*, he describes an illness understandable from a modern perspective as atypical depression with prominent somatic symptoms. *Bǎihé bìng* (百合病; usually translated as "lily disease" but also translatable as "a hundred illnesses combined") is remarkable because of its consistently demonstrated response to a simple decoction of lily bulbs and the root of *Rehmannia glutinosa*. Modern research has shown that the two phenotypes of liver qi stagnation and heart/spleen qi deficiency are correlated with abnormal metabolomes. In liver qi deficiency these include abnormal serum levels of catecholamine and amino acid neurotransmitter metabolites (L.-Y. Liu et al., 2018). One of the chemical components in the decoction of lily bulbs inhibits monoamine oxidase, potentially correcting the decreased levels of catecholamines found in liver qi deficiency. TCM depression phenotypes also have distinctive brain functional connectivity maps (Xu et al., 2018).

A comparison of four depressive syndromes (*zheng*) gives a sense of how TCM distinguishes conditions that might be lumped together by Western medicine as clinical depression, and specifically as MDD if a person had at least five of the nine essential symptoms for at least two weeks, accompanied by distress and impairment. The process of subdividing Western disease (*bing*) into discrete phenotypes (*zheng* in TCM) is an essential feature of integrative medicine that combines TCM and mainstream Western medicine. The process is called *biànzhèng lùnzhì* (辨证论治; pattern recognition and treatment determination). Applying *bianzheng lunzhi* to the management of diseases defined by Western medicine has been a focus of TCM medical centers in China (Karchmer, 2010). As shown in Table 9.1, TCM matches each of four *zheng* for clinical depression with herbal treatments specific to the symptom profile rather than with generic

Table 9.1 Four TCM Phenotypes of Clinical Depression

Lily disease	Mental symptoms	Anxious, restless, ill at ease; expects bad reactions to medications
	Physical symptoms	Insomnia, feeling hot or cold; nausea; appetite fluctuates; trouble getting moving; faint and rapid pulse; concentrated urine; looking well while feeling ill
	TCM herbal treatment	Decoction of lily bulb and *Rehmannia* root
	Western diagnosis	Anxious depression
Spleen *qì* deficiency	Mental symptoms	Apathetic, loss of interest and pleasure
	Physical symptoms	Headache, chronic or with exertion; weakness; dizziness; fatigue. Gastrointestinal: poor appetite, indigestion, bloating, gas, loose stools, abdominal discomfort worse with pressure
	TCM herbal treatment	*Xiaoyao* decoction
	Western diagnosis	Apathetic depression with prominent somatic symptoms, especially gastrointestinal
Heart *qì* deficiency	Mental symptoms	Mood swings, anxious, restless
	Physical symptoms	Sweating, palpitations
	TCM herbal treatment	*Ningcao* decoction
	Western diagnosis	Depression with mixed features (bipolarity) and anxiety
Liver *qì* stagnation	Mental symptoms	Depressed, irritable, angry, easily frustrated; a premenopausal woman may have premenstrual tension and irritability
	Physical symptoms	Sighing, hiccups, poor appetite, stomachache, epigastric pain worse with anger and better with massage, constipation. If a premenopausal woman may have irregular or painful periods. Pulse "wiry."
	TCM herbal treatment	*Chaihu Shugan* decoction, saffron, turmeric
	Western diagnosis	Depression with mixed features with prominent gastrointestinal symptoms and autonomic disturbance

treatments of depression. The efficacy of each matched treatment is supported by randomized controlled clinical trials, and one or more of the active ingredients of each herbal remedy has shown positive effects in an animal model of depression (W.-F. Yeung et al., 2015).

The most prescribed remedy for lily disease, first specified by the Chinese physician Zhang, is a decoction of the bulbs of *Lilium brownii* and the root of *Rehmannia glutinosa*. In a rat model of depression—cumulative unpredictable mild stress—the traditional remedy mitigates behavioral changes as well as biochemical abnormalities involving catecholamine and amino acid neurotransmitters, an increased level of cortisol, and a decreased level of brain-derived neurotrophic factor (Chi et al., 2019).

Enthusiasts for the integration of Western medicine and TCM foresee the convergence of *zheng* differentiation and the subdivision of Western disease categories using omics technologies (e.g., quantitative study of the genome, metabolome, proteome, and cerebral connectome; Y.-N. Song et al., 2013; P. Wang & Chen, 2013). The prospect is appealing, but research in the area is just beginning. It remains to be seen whether attempts to integrate the TCM *zheng* and Western omics perspectives will be productive.

The perspective of TCM on depression fits well with the methodology of the cultural lens. In this book we advocate using the term *clinical depression* to cover a range of disorders broader than the syndrome of MDD. We suspect that people who would meet our criteria for clinical depression would be found to be ill by a TCM physician—but could have any of a dozen or more *zheng*. The patient's cultural identity—as well as their genetics, developmental history, personality, comorbidities, and circumstances—would determine how depression would be expressed in an individual patient.

Most of the Chinese herbal remedies for forms of depression recognized in TCM have several plant-derived ingredients, and each has many specific chemical constituents with actions on the central nervous system, the immune system, and/or the endocrine system. The relative proportions of these constituents can differ between batches of an herbal remedy, even ones from the same supplier. It is extraordinarily difficult to anticipate the physiological consequences of consuming them, and there are additional concerns about how components interact with one another, the patient's genetically determined pattern of drug metabolism, and whatever other medications or supplements the patient might be taking. Some of the remedies were known by early TCM practitioners to be potentially toxic in high doses. Moreover, quality control of commercially available TCM remedies is variable; and contamination with heavy metals, prescription drugs, and undisclosed natural ingredients is common. This makes clear that, despite their regulatory classification in some countries, many TCM herbal remedies should be treated as drugs with potential adverse effects and interactions and not as presumptively safe nutritional supplements (Chan et al., 2010; Coghlan et al., 2015; García-Cortés et al., 2016; Parvez & Ricci, 2019).

Sūn Sīmiǎo (孙思邈; 581–682 CE) was a physician and scholar of legendary skill and erudition during the late Sui Dynasty (581–618 CE) and early Tang Dynasty (618–907 CE). He was a Daoist philosopher and one of the pioneers of medical ethics and often is referred to as China's "King of Medicines" (*Yàowáng*; 药王). His largest book, *Essential Prescriptions for Emergencies* (*Bèijí Qiānjīn Yàofāng*; 备急千金要方), includes over 5000 recipes for medications, many of which are utilized in contemporary TCM. Sūn attributed depression to abnormal qi and recommended treating it with acupuncture: Needling the correct meridians for the patient's *zheng* would allow the problematic qi to escape. A Cochrane review of controlled trials of acupuncture in depression found insufficient high-quality trial data to conclusively establish its therapeutic benefit (Smith et al., 2018). When patients have both depression and moderate to severe pain, the addition of acupuncture to antidepressant therapy can produce a significantly better outcome (Hopton et al., 2014). Controlled trials suggest that acupuncture might be specifically useful in perimenopausal depression (Zheng et al., 2023), post-stroke depression (Ching et al., 2023); Jiang et al., 2023; migraine-associated depression (Li et al., 2023); depression-related insomnia (Sun & Wu, 2023); late-life depression (Cai et al., 2023); and cancer-associated depression (Fangfang et al., 2023)

Sun's advice regarding physicians' proper conduct is classic and much like the advice of Hippocrates, Maimonides, and other legendary clinician-philosophers:

> A Great Physician should not pay attention to status, wealth or age; neither should he question whether the particular person is attractive or unattractive, whether he is an enemy or friend, whether he is a Chinese or a foreigner, or finally, whether he is uneducated or educated. He should meet everyone on equal grounds. He should always act as if he were thinking of his close relatives.
>
> Whenever eminent physicians treat an illness, they must quiet the spirit and settle the will, they must be free of wants and desires, and they must first develop a heart full of great compassion and empathy. They must pledge to devote themselves completely to relieving the suffering of all sentient beings. (Sun Simiao, 2019)

A contemporary physician who fully embraced the philosophy of Sun Simiao would stigmatize no one. It is hard to imagine such a physician condescendingly, dismissively, or abusively treating a patient with depression.

The Song Dynasty (960–1279 CE) was a glorious period in Chinese history, a time when China was extraordinarily productive in the arts, literature, and technology. The royal family during the Song was genetically predisposed to BD, and many emperors suffered from symptoms of depression, BD-I, or BD-II during their reigns. The treatment of people with mood disorders during the period reflected the simultaneous existence of a medical model and a supernatural model of illness. People with non-psychotic depression or mild bipolar spectrum conditions without grossly abnormal behavior might be treated by TCM physicians for "illness," especially if they had prominent physical symptoms. Those with psychosis or more severe behavioral disturbances were judged to be afflicted by spirits and were treated by shamans. Shamanic healing procedures could be dramatic, for example, torturing or burning an effigy of a patient to drive out evil spirits. Patients themselves were not tortured or injured, as they were at times in medieval Europe. Shamans varied in their skill and ethics; some sexually exploited their clients or financially exploited their families. Overall, however, stigma was not severe because people with mood disorders were not blamed as the sole cause of their afflictions. Genetic vulnerability, traumatic life events, shock, loss, grief, and the misconduct of ancestors could all have a role in causing a person's illness.

When a person with a mood disorder had abnormal behavior, it was expected that they would be kept at home by their family. Women especially were kept out of sight if they had unusual behavior. People with mood disorders were kept at home to avoid the family's losing face and the person being bullied, and in some cases to prevent the person from harming themselves or others. Mentally ill people without family protection might be homeless, living in the streets. If a person of high rank, like a court official, developed depression or bipolar illness, they might lose their position, leading to a loss of income as well as a loss of face. They would not, however, be persecuted (Yang, 2003).

For most of the two millennia of imperial China, the conception and treatment of people with depression and bipolar spectrum disorders lay on a continuum between TCM and shamanism, with severity of symptoms, urban versus rural location, and the social status of the ill person influencing where on the continuum they would fall. The systematic mistreatment of people as "mentally ill," heavily stigmatized and officially abused, did not occur until the 20th century, when China was influenced by the categorical and reductionistic perspective of the Western psychiatry of the time.

The legacy of TCM to contemporary integrative medicine includes its richness of clinical observation, its wide range of herbal remedies and therapeutic modalities, the methodology of *bianzheng lunzhi*, and its holistic mind–body perspective. Its conception of depression as reflecting an "imbalance" rather than a defect can make a diagnosis and treatment of depression more acceptable to people who stigmatize "mental illness." In a study of 3157 low-income Chinese Americans in metropolitan Chicago, 8.2% had moderate to severe depression on the nine-item Patient Health Questionnaire. Of those, 74% had used a TCM treatment in the prior year, and 60% had used a TCM herbal remedy. Herbal treatments were the only TCM treatment used by the majority of those with moderate to severe depression. People who were less acculturated, less educated, and more recently arrived in the United States (U.S.) were more likely to use TCM; but the use of traditional treatment was widespread even among well-educated and highly acculturated subjects (Chao et al., 2020).

Along with the non-stigmatizing language, holistic approach, and attention to discrete phenotypes of clinical depression, TCM brings treatments for depression that have such biochemical complexity that their risks are not fully understood, a lightly regulated herbal pharmacology industry that at times distributes dangerous or mislabeled substances, and a theoretical basis incompatible with modern science. TCM's most used treatments for depression have neurophysiologic rationales and some support from animal models, but their clinical evidence base would not be adequate to support their regular use in mainstream Western medicine, let alone incorporation into evidence-based practice guidelines.

The integrated mind–body treatment of mood disorders in TCM—and its Japanese and Korean offshoots—is appreciated by people worldwide, including many non-Asian people. People with depression or bipolar illness who would initially be unwilling to consult a mainstream Western physician or mental health professional for their symptoms might be open to seeing a practitioner of traditional medicine, who could earn their trust and eventually introduce them to a mental health professional if their symptoms were persistent and troublesome. A clinician who learns that a patient with depression has a positive view of TCM (or Kampo or TKM) might ask how the patient would present their account of the current illness to a traditional practitioner. The clinician could then frame the diagnosis in terms compatible with the patient's narrative. Deciding that a dimensional symptom like sleep quality or anhedonia has crossed the line and become an item on the checklist for a DSM/ICD disorder is a clinical judgment. A patient accepting of traditional medicine might appreciate the clinician's talking about a relationship between life circumstances and a physiologic "imbalance." The need for treatment would reflect the distress and dysfunction associated with the imbalance. A combination of medication and psychotherapy or lifestyle changes could be understood as addressing the imbalance while giving the patient strategies for better coping with, tolerating, or reducing the stressful circumstances that caused the imbalance.

From Rhazes to Maimonides: TAIM

From the seventh through the 15th centuries Islamic civilization was remarkable for its scientific sophistication and innovation. While Europe was in the grip of intellectual stagnation and religious reductionism, Islamic civilization carried forward and built upon the knowledge and wisdom of classical scholars. The perspective of TAIM on depression is expressed in the works of four of its most historically significant physicians: Rhazes, Ibn Imran, Avicenna, and Maimonides.

Rhazes (Abi Bakr Muhammad ibn Zakariyya al-Razi; 865–925 CE) was both a clinician and a scientist; he was one of the first physicians in history to describe the concept of controlled clinical trials for testing treatments (Ghaffari et al., 2017). He asserted that mind–body dualism was misguided: Mental health was relevant to physical well-being, and general medical problems produced psychological symptoms. He attributed depression (melancholia) to abnormal blood flow in the brain. This was not a bad guess; focally decreased cerebral blood flow is a known correlate of severe depression (Song et al., 2018; Toma et al., 2018).

Rhazes was the director of a hospital in Baghdad, where he introduced the idea of specialized wards in general hospitals (*bimaristans*) for treating patients with mental disorders. Treatment of depression included diet, medication (herbs and spices), aromatherapy, baths, and music therapy. It also included an encouraging and empathic personal relationship between physician and patient. Patients leaving the hospital after successful treatment of depression were discharged with a sum of money to aid in their return to society. Care was compassionate and holistic. Patients were hospitalized not to confine them and isolate them from society but to protect them and provide them with a greater intensity of treatment than would be feasible otherwise (Kasim Mohamad & Younis, 2018).

Ishaq Ibn Imran (died c. 905 CE), an Iraqi physician living in Tunisia, published his *Treatise on Melancholy* in 900 CE. It was the first book ever published that was solely devoted to the medical issues of depression and BD (Omrani et al., 2012). He defined melancholy as a condition that "affects the soul through fear and sadness—the worst thing that can befall it. Sadness is defined by the loss of what one loves; fear is the expectation of misfortune." He added that people with melancholia might also have pathological doubts and suspicions. Melancholia was caused by an imbalance of the four humors (yellow bile, blood, black bile, and phlegm). Differing from Hippocrates and Galen, Ibn Imran thought that an excess of black bile was not the only possible cause. The cause of the humoral imbalance could be hereditary, environmental, or a combination; his model of disease was biopsychosocial. He described mania as an inconsistent consequence of depression rather than part of a cyclic illness, and thus did not have a modern conception of BD. He noted that mania could be particularly hard to treat because people affected by it did not see themselves as being ill. Ibn Imran thought that the diagnosing of mania or melancholia required understanding the longitudinal course of illness and that deviation of the patient's symptoms from their premorbid temperament was a necessary condition for diagnosing depression as an illness. He described variations on mania that correspond to modern concepts of hypomania and subsyndromal hypomania. Ibn Imran's recommended treatments were combinations of plant-based medicaments, regular exercise, and a healthy diet (Omrani et al., 2012).

Avicenna (Abu Ali Hussein Ibn Sina; 980–1037 CE), in his *Canon of Medicine* (1025), described melancholia as a condition that could originate either in the brain or in the body but ultimately involved the whole body and affected the function of the brain. He noted that women, older people, malnourished people, and people recovering from acute illnesses were especially vulnerable to the condition. These observations are compatible with modern psychiatric epidemiology. Early symptoms of melancholia could include suspiciousness, irrational fear, quick anger, involuntary muscle movements, dizziness, and tinnitus. Later symptoms could include moaning, sadness, restlessness, fear of catastrophe, and fear of being deceived. Delusions of grandeur, involuntary laughter, and "affection for death" (suicidal ideation) are mentioned. The description encompasses several different syndromes that might now be classified as MDD with prominent somatic symptoms, MDD with mixed features, delusional depression, and the depressed phase of BD. All are concurrent mind–body disturbances (Araj-Khodaei et al., 2017).

Avicenna advised treating melancholia in its early stages because chronic melancholia could become refractory to treatment—another concept congruent with current research. Like Rhazes he described a range of treatments, including aromatherapy, music therapy, and increasing the patient's pleasant experiences. The idea of systematically increasing a person's pleasant experiences to treat a clinical depression is embodied in the modern concept of behavioral activation therapy, a treatment of empirically established efficacy for mild to moderate MDD. Avicenna opined that in some cases patients would do better if they moved to a different residence or even to a different country with a different climate. He suggested regular physical exercise and advised patients to be sexually active if it were feasible for them. Physical treatments comprised massage, phlebotomy, and cupping. Dietary supplements were suggested, including saffron, ginger, cinnamon, and turmeric. These were characterized by Avicenna as having "exhilarating effects." Modern research has shown these foods to have anti-inflammatory, antioxidant, and antidepressant effects. For example, a meta-analysis of 11 randomized trials showed that saffron is superior to placebo for treatment of mild to moderate depression and not inferior to several SSRIs (Tóth et al., 2019).

Like practitioners of TCM, the founders of TAIM considered individual differences in symptom profiles, underlying temperaments, lifestyle, and environment in prescribing treatment for patients with conditions that conventional Western medicine would regard as a single disease. In this way they anticipated today's personalized/precision medicine, and those who hope to integrate TAIM and Western medicine express the hope that omics technologies will corroborate distinctions made by traditional practitioners (Moeini et al., 2017).

Maimonides (Moses ben Maimon; 1135–1204 CE), was a Jewish philosopher and physician who lived and practiced medicine in the Islamic nations of Spain, Morocco, and Egypt; his 10 medical books were written in Arabic and widely used as references by Arabic-speaking physicians. Maimonides had an integrated mind–body perspective, regarding physical health and mental health as essential to each other. For example, he advised that following a non-injurious suicide attempt, a person see a physician because a general medical problem might be what provoked the attempt (Gesundheit et al., 2008). Maimonides made recommendations regarding psychological treatment of depression that anticipate modern concepts of guided imagery and cognitive-behavioral psychotherapy (Pies, 1997).

A non-Muslim physician who treated many adherents to Islam, Maimonides was "culturally sensitive" in his practice. He wrote a now-famous letter of advice to an Egyptian nobleman with bipolar depression, whom he thought would recover more rapidly with the aid of wine and song. He knew that these were forbidden to Muslims.

> A physician is bound, inasmuch as he is a physician, to present [the patient] with a beneficial regimen, whether it is forbidden or permitted; the patient is endowed with the freedom to choose whether to follow or not. If [the physician] fails to mention everything that may be helpful, be it forbidden or permitted, he is guilty of acting dishonestly, for he did not offer trustworthy advice

It is well known that religious law commands what is beneficial and prohibits what is harmful with respect to the world-to-come. The physician, on the other hand, instructs what will benefit the body and warns about what will harm it in this world (Gesundheit et al., 2008).While the classics of TAIM convey a thoughtful, non-mystical, and non-stigmatizing view of mood disorders, this coexisted with more superstitious views. As in China, when symptoms were worse and affected people had lower status and lived in rural areas, religious or mystical explanations for mental disorders were common, for example, possession by spirits (*jinns*; Islam & Campbell, 2014). Islamic and shamanic healing rituals probably were more common among the masses than herbal pharmacology and music therapy.

A salient feature of Islam relevant to depression is the religion's vigorous prohibition of suicide. The Quran specifies that people should reject suicide because Allah has been merciful to them. Other Islamic texts are more colorful, telling people that those who commit suicide will be punished in the next world by endless repetition of the suicidal act—if one stabbed oneself, one would do it again and again while burning in hell (Baasher, 2001; Sabry & Vohra, 2013). While a psychotic person would be forgiven for attempting suicide while insane, the suicide of a non-psychotic person for reasons of disappointment, humiliation, or existential despair would be a great sin. In fact, the rate of death by suicide in majority-Islamic nations is markedly lower than the average for nations with the same sociodemographic index (a composite of per capita income, average educational attainment, and fertility rate). This remains the case even if deaths by drowning and poisoning (e.g., by pesticides) are included in suicide mortality rates (Institute for Health Metrics and Evaluation [IHME], 2023).

The perspectives of TAIM and TCM on depression and the bipolar spectrum are compatible. Chinese herbal remedies, along with some of the theory underlying their use, were imported into the Islamic world by traders who visited China (Heyadri et al., 2015). During the Renaissance, the wisdom of TAIM was passed back to European physicians, who read the works of Rhazes, Avicenna, and Maimonides in translation. When European powers took control of Islamic nations, Western medicine partially displaced TAIM, with similar results as in China: There came to be more categorical thinking about mental disorders, more stigma of mental illness, and less respect for traditional medicine. In recent decades TAIM has functioned in Islamic nations as an accessible, less expensive alternative to conventional Western medicine.

The idea that integrating TAIM with Western medicine could improve care outcomes is relatively recent. A depressed person in an Islamic country might consult a TAIM practitioner because of cost, accessibility, and lesser stigma and fear. They would not necessarily view TAIM as more valid than Western medicine.

As with Chinese immigrants who have not fully assimilated mainstream American culture, clinicians treating depressed immigrants from majority-Islamic countries to the U.S. should inquire about their patients' use of TAIM. A patient who has experience with TAIM might be asked how they would describe the present illness to a practitioner of traditional medicine. Discussion of a diagnosis of clinical depression and prescription of treatment might make use of the words and concepts in the patient's illness narrative. Parallels between the current recommended treatment of depression and historical/traditional approaches might be pointed out.

Illness or Demonic Possession? A Brief History of Stigma

As discussed at length in Chapter 6, people with depression and bipolar disorders face several types of stigma: self-stigma, public stigma, anticipated public stigma, and institutional stigma. Stigma of all four types is related both to the affected person's behavior and to the diagnostic label and explanation of illness applied to them. The three traditional medical systems above—classical Greco-Roman medicine, TCM, and TAIM—explained illness, including depression and bipolar illness, in terms of imbalances of metaphorical substances. Their etiologic concepts taken literally have no evidentiary support. Yet, traditional medicine incorporates perspectives, clinical wisdom, and specific treatments that should be preserved as they can enhance patient engagement and can suggest viable alternative treatments when conventional therapy is unavailable, unaffordable, not tolerated, ineffective, or incompatible with a patient's beliefs and preferences. Seeing depression and bipolar illness through the lens of traditional medicine can reduce its stigma within a community that utilizes traditional medicine and respects its practitioners. Even when people with depression or bipolar illness come from a community without its own traditional medical system, they may be more comfortable with "alternative medicine" than with mainstream psychiatry.

A holistic and comprehensive perspective on mental disorders—such as that taken by traditional medical systems—has been shown to be associated with less stigma. The words chosen to name mental disorders are significantly associated with their level of stigmatization. Simply calling a person "ill" rather than "mentally ill" reduces stigma. For example, a study of high school students in Macao showed that calling a person with schizophrenia "ill" rather than "mentally ill" reduced the students' fear and desire for social distance. In Japan, the national health authorities in 2002 renamed schizophrenia to reduce its stigma-associated barrier to people's seeking treatment. The official name was changed from *seishin-bunretsu-byo* (精神分裂病; mind-split disease) to the new name of *togo-shitcho-sho* (統合失調症; integration disorder [literally, "comprehensive imbalance disorder"]). Following the change there was a large increase in the proportion of patients with schizophrenia who were informed about their diagnosis by their physicians. Patients and families became more optimistic, and surveys confirmed that public stigma was reduced (Sartorius et al., 2014). This issue will be discussed further in Chapter 11.

The history of stigma associated with depression and bipolar illness is one of loss and recovery. In classical Greece and Rome and in the Islamic world during its golden age, most people with non-psychotic mood disorders were regarded as "ill"—not "mentally ill"—and were treated by the same physicians who treated other kinds of illness. This enlightened perspective was lost in western Europe after the fall of Rome and replaced by powerful, religion-based negative judgments of depressed people. Augustine of Hippo (354–430 CE) saw depression as manifesting the sin of sloth and its suffering as punishment for sin. Thomas Aquinas (1225–1274 CE) believed in a rigid mind–body dualism, allowing for no influence of the general health on a person's mood and behavior. Suggestions that depressed people deserved punishment are found in the writings of many medieval clergy (Walker, 2008, pp. 33–34). The reduction of stigma during the Renaissance was partly due to the weakening of the intellectual hegemony of the Catholic Church. In medieval Europe, the abuse of mentally ill people, especially those with depression or BD-I, was sometimes extreme, including prolonged incarceration, beatings, starvation, ice water baths, and physical restraints including chains.

Trephination (surgically opening a hole in the skull) was performed on many people with melancholia or mania, with the expectation that the noxious material causing the person's mania or melancholy would escape to the outside. Physicians at the time thought their procedure was therapeutic and not punitive, though from a modern perspective it seems like harsh treatment. Use of the procedure as a treatment for melancholia and mania was described in 12th-century Italy and in subsequent European medical texts including one by the renowned neuroanatomist Thomas Willis. Ironically, Willis saw trephination and St. John's wort as treatment alternatives (Gross, 1999). From a modern perspective the former treatment would be criminal malpractice, while the latter is a viable alternative to prescription antidepressants for people with mild to moderate MDD who reject the latter and do not have medical contraindications to its use (Haller et al., 2019).

In Europe, an empathic, non-stigmatizing perspective on non-psychotic melancholia returned during the Renaissance among people with education and status, though probably not among the masses. Depression as a condition that could afflict a decent and civilized person was memorably described by Robert Burton (1577–1640) in his magnum opus *Anatomy of Melancholy* (Burton, 1620/2001). Burton distinguished melancholy moods, a universal human experience, from the illness that would now be called melancholic MDD or melancholia, a "serious ailment"—a "habit" that will "hardly be removed." He presented depressive illness as a complex phenomenon involving mind, body, and spirit, with both supernatural and purely biological aspects, the latter including genetics. Burton related the onset of depression to the experience of loss, whether of a loved one, of status, or of one's personal health. He cited Galen and Avicenna and appreciated the bidirectional relationship of mind and body in causing melancholia (Brink, 1979; Claman, 2012).

From the 17th through the 19th centuries, the upper class of western Europe accepted people of their social stratum suffering from non-psychotic depression or BD-II, possibly romanticizing their suffering and appreciating their creativity when it was displayed. On the other hand, for a person without means or status, being functionally impaired by symptoms of a mood disorder might end in poverty, homelessness, and social isolation.

In the late 19th and early 20th centuries the progress of general medicine in Europe and the U.S. included major advances in neurology and psychiatry, which ultimately changed the status of depression and bipolar illness, transforming their more severe forms into brain diseases and their milder forms into conditions primarily understood with a psychosocial model.

The Contemporary Relationship of Mainstream and Traditional Medical Approaches to Depression

In the second half of the 20th century the prevailing model of depression adopted by mainstream American medicine was biopsychosocial. With the waning of the influence of psychoanalysis and major advances in neuroscience, severe depression came to be seen in mainly biological terms, while individual psychology and social circumstances continued to be recognized as important in mild to moderate cases. BD came to be seen by most physicians in almost entirely biological terms—with many clinicians apparently neglecting the importance of personal beliefs, experiences, and lifestyle in determining the course of the illness. Social, environmental, and cultural dimensions of mood disorders—and their structural accompaniments—were of interest to academicians and specialists but not central to the wider society's view of mood disorders. Treatment became more evidence-based, with an initial implication that it was less personalized. Preferred pharmacologic treatments were those supported primarily by large industry-sponsored clinical trials that tested non-personalized treatments on subjects not representative of the general population. Non-pharmacologic treatments of depression were evaluated on smaller samples, and for many non-pharmacologic treatments, defining a suitable control group was problematic.

In the 21st century, mass migration and globalization have made cultural diversity impossible for the medical profession to avoid. Advances in technology are making it more feasible to personalize care while utilizing an empirical evidence base and monitoring patient outcomes objectively and rigorously. In the authors' opinion, the emergence of personalized medicine and increasing cultural awareness within the medical profession have led to mainstream psychiatry becoming more flexible in its approach to mood disorders. As this happens, there appears to be a lessening of the stigma of depression and greater compatibility of traditional and mainstream medical perspectives on depression.

In the late 19th century, China began a process of modernization that accelerated after the end of the Qing Dynasty in 1912. Part of China's modernization was the progressive replacement of TCM by conventional Western medicine. This included the importation of Western psychiatry, changing the characterization of depression and bipolar illness from the holistic and dimensional approach of TCM to the Western approach of categorical diagnosis focused on the individual and their mental and behavioral symptoms. In the Western model, treatment of depression—when given at all—was mainly biological. Moderately severe cases might be treated with medications on an outpatient basis, while hospitalization and sometimes electroconvulsive therapy were employed for severe cases. In the early 20th-century Chinese adaptation of Western psychiatry, a person was either "mentally ill"—and thus stigmatized—or not ill at all.

In TCM, patients with persistent and troublesome symptoms of non-psychotic depression would be diagnosed with one of several syndromes, such as liver *qi* deficiency or lily disease. However, in Republican China (1912–1949), TCM was under attack as one of the obsolescent legacies preventing China from becoming a modern nation. Prominent political leaders and public intellectuals such as Yan Fu (1854–1921), Sun Yat-sen (1866–1925), Liang Qichao (1873–1929), Lu Xun (1881–1936), and Hu Shi (1891–1962) called for abandonment of TCM, which they saw as folk belief or even witchcraft rather than legitimate medical practice (Gross, 2018). However, especially in the psychiatric domain, there was no real alternative to TCM for most of China. In the 1950s there were approximately 500,000 practitioners of TCM and no more than 20,000 physicians practicing Western medicine (Hsu, 2008).

After the establishment of the People's Republic in 1949, China began training more of its physicians in Western medicine, and Western medicine was added to the curriculum at colleges of TCM. Mental disorder diagnosis and treatment moved toward the Western model, especially for people who were more severely ill. There were few psychiatrists in China; they usually worked in hospitals and focused primarily on psychotic or otherwise severely ill patients (Hu et al., 2017). This associated psychiatrists and psychiatric care with psychosis, and thus with fear and stigma. People with depression would be classified either as "mentally ill," treated by psychiatrists and severely stigmatized or as "not mentally ill" not treated by psychiatrists, and stigmatized for their behavior (if socially deviant) rather than for a diagnosis. In this context, people with depression and prominent somatic symptoms were given—and were willing to accept—a diagnosis of "neurasthenia," which enabled them to assume a sick role without the stigma associated with "mental illness." Other people with depression, and those with a bipolar spectrum disorder such as BD-II or cyclothymia, might turn to TCM practitioners for symptomatic treatment.

Psychiatric diagnosis and treatment were heavily stigmatized in China after the Revolution, and the stigma became much worse during and after the Cultural Revolution. During the Cultural Revolution, political opponents of the regime with no mental disorder might be labeled as "mentally ill" and incarcerated in mental hospitals or prisons, where they would be severely abused and humiliated. People who were unable to work because of severe depressive symptoms would be criticized as enemies of the revolution unless they could find a credible physical explanation for their disability. This strongly reinforced a somatic presentation of clinical depression.

It has taken China more than a generation to deal with the massive historical trauma of the Cultural Revolution, and the nation's recovery is not yet complete. A residual effect has been the continued severe stigmatization of diagnosed major psychiatric illness and its treatment by psychiatrists. While most Chinese people with clinical depression do not get treatment at all, most who do seek treatment turn to TCM physicians, most of whom now also have training in Western medicine. TCM physicians have extensive training in mind–body syndromes that cover much of the territory of clinical depression, while students of Western medicine in China might receive as little as two weeks of training in psychiatry. Thus, a typical TCM physician in China would be more familiar with assessment and treatment of depression than a typical non-psychiatrist practitioner of Western medicine. Usual treatment of MDD in China combines Western medications like SSRIs with TCM treatments, and treatment of BD-I utilizes mood stabilizers and antipsychotic drugs, as it does in the West. A very small segment of educated urban society might consult a psychologist for psychotherapeutic treatment of clinically significant depression or anxiety. Psychiatrists in China continue to have lower status and lower pay than other medical specialists ("China Wakes Up to Its Mental Health Problems," 2017; Jiang et al., 2018; Yao et al., 2021).

From the late 19th century through the publication of DSM-3 in 1980, Western psychiatrists made use of the diagnosis of *neurasthenia* to describe a non-psychotic psychosomatic condition involving mental and behavioral symptoms but not tainted by the stigma of "insanity." The concept of neurasthenia was embraced by physicians in East Asia, first in Japan and then in China. The Japanese term *shinkei suijaku* (神経衰弱) and the Chinese term *shénjīng shuāiruò* (神经衰弱) both literally translatable as "nerve weakness," are written with almost the same characters. The diagnosis was applied to young and middle-aged people who presented as weak and sickly with no obvious systemic disease to explain their symptoms (Daido, 2013; Karchmer, 2013; Wu, 2016).

Several prominent early 20th-century Chinese physicians related the role of the nervous system in Western medicine to the role of the liver in TCM. Current TCM practitioners do not advocate mapping the organs of the traditional system onto standard Western anatomy. However, they do use medicines to treat depression that are recommended in TCM texts for treating disorders of the liver (Karchmer, 2013). The concept of depression currently prevalent in China is the Western one rather than that of TCM, reflecting the predominance of physicians practicing Western medicine and the concurrent training of TCM students in Western medicine.

In the medieval Islamic world, the thoughtful, holistic, and comprehensive approach to depression and the bipolar spectrum exemplified by the writings of its great physicians coexisted with magical and religious explanations of mental disorders. The thorough documentation of psychiatric thinking during the golden age of Islam makes it clear that a person with depression or a BD could get thoughtful, medically sophisticated, and non-superstitious care from the best hospitals and physicians of the time. Sophisticated psychosomatic thinking coexisted with folk beliefs that depression or mania was the consequence of a person's being possessed by a *jinn*—a spirit with the power to affect one's mind and body, sometimes with malign intent. *Jinn* possession is not a person's fault, though life events, heredity, and adverse circumstances can make a person more vulnerable to it. An interview study of women with postpartum depression in an Arabian Gulf nation suggests that belief in *jinn* possession persists into the 21st century in some Islamic communities (Hanely & Brown, 2014). Ridding a patient of *jinn* possession might require spiritual assistance.

In the context of European imperialism, a Western model of medicine, including psychiatry, was disseminated in the Islamic world in the late 19th and early 20th centuries. This weakened the authority and status of TAIM, and thus reduced the power that TAIM might have to counter the superstitious stigmatization of people with psychotic illness and the moralistic dismissal of non-psychotic depression as not a real disease. The concept of "mental" illness as a disembodied and individual spiritual problem—or brain disease (in either case unconnected with both general physical health and social/environmental issues)—persists in majority-Islamic nations to the present day, where it underlies personal and family stigma of mental illness. Such stigma can affect socialization, business relationships, and marriage proposals, all major issues in the highly collectivist cultures of such nations. Many contemporary Muslims believe that a psychotic illness like mania or schizophrenia might be due to demonic possession and that the cause of non-psychotic depression or anxiety might be insufficient prayer or a lack of faith (Attum & Shamoon, 2019). For religious Muslims, the direct support of their imam for psychiatric treatment reduces self-stigma and increases the likelihood that they will pursue treatment for depression. Psychiatrists working with Muslim communities have published suggestions that patients and families be reminded that superstitious beliefs about *jinns* are not based in the Quran and that the greatest Islamic physicians in history saw depression as a mind–body problem with no supernatural element (Lim et al., 2018). Alternatively, family members of depressed or manic patient who attribute the illness to *jinn* possession should be encouraged to "hedge their bets" by also pursuing conventional medical treatment. Clinicians should warn patients and their families with traditional beliefs about *jinn* possession about the potential for their exploitation by exorcists (Sheikh, 2005).

When assessing a religious Muslim patient with symptoms of depression, a culturally aware clinician might ask the patient whether they attribute a religious/spiritual meaning to their symptoms and, if so, whether they have sought help from a religious/spiritual source. Personal use of TAIM or knowledge of its use by friends or family would be another topic to explore, especially if the clinician senses a reluctance of the patient to accept a diagnosis of depression or a related condition.

Academic psychotherapists have observed that if religion and psychotherapy are presented as mutually exclusive alternatives for dealing with depression, people with strong faith will reject psychotherapy. Manuals for cognitive-behavioral therapy (CBT) of depression are available that integrate religious concepts and behavior into their content. Trials of CBT with integrated religious content have shown positive results with depressed patients professing Buddhism, Christianity, Hinduism, Islam, and Judaism (Pearce et al., 2015). Especially when dealing with immigrants to a Western country from majority-Islamic countries of the Middle East and Southeast Asia, allowing for a mixture of mainstream and religion-based treatment might help with patient engagement and ultimately improve outcomes (Kizilhan, 2014). It might also be necessary for the mental health professionals working in Muslim immigrant communities to engage local Muslim clerics in an educational dialogue since clergy often are turned to first by people seeking help for symptoms of depression or a bipolar spectrum disorder. In the absence of such dialogue, patients' relationships with clergy might undermine their acceptance of the clinician's diagnosis and their adherence to treatment. For example, when Muslim clergy in Sydney, Australia, were interviewed about the causes and treatment of mental illness, many did not give a role to biology. Even when they thought medications might be helpful, they were concerned about side effects (Youssef & Deane, 2013).

A survey of young, affluent college students in the United Arab Emirates indicated an open-minded view of depression as a problem that could happen to anyone, concurrent with the knowledge that disclosing one's depression or seeking psychiatric or "mental health" treatment would bring stigma and shame both to oneself and to one's family. Subjects in the survey also distinguished benign and situational psychological problems from "mental" problems, which were frightening and stigmatized conditions due to brain disease. A minority of students attributed mental illness to a religious/spiritual cause. Most would be willing to seek help if they needed it, with a strong preference for counseling/psychotherapy over either medication or a religious intervention. This preference related their widely shared belief that (non-psychotic) depression is most often explained by excessive stress in one's life (Al-Darmaki et al., 2016).

Since fluoxetine, the first approved SSRI antidepressant, was introduced in 1987, the Western concept of clinical depression has evolved into a condition that always involves altered brain function, often involves disturbances in the function of the endocrine system and the immune system, and usually includes abnormalities of sleep and/or chronobiology. These alterations in physiology represent the interaction of genetics, development (including the impact of trauma and loss), general medical status (including adequacy of nutrition and the presence or absence of pain or inflammation), the patient's beliefs and habits (cognition and behavior), and personal circumstances (social and environmental determinants of health). Once again, after many centuries, depression is an affliction of mind, brain, and body, rather than a disembodied "psychological," "emotional," or "spiritual" condition. The complexity and heterogeneity of depression are recognized, and physicians consider how patients' depression should be subtyped in ways that would support more personalized and more effective treatment.

As mentioned in Chapter 2, this more nuanced view of depression is implicit in the National Institute of Mental Health's (2019) Research Domain Criteria (RDoC), which are built around dimensions of dysfunction rather than on categorical diagnoses(NIMH, 2021). To quote the RDoC,

> These domains reflect contemporary knowledge about major systems of emotion, cognition, motivation, and social behavior. Within each domain are behavioral elements, processes, mechanisms, and responses, called *constructs*, that comprise different aspects of the overall range of functions. Constructs are studied along a span

of functioning from normal to abnormal, with the understanding that each is situated in, and affected by, environmental and neurodevelopmental contexts. Measurement of constructs can occur using several different methods termed *units of analysis*. Units of analysis can include molecular, genetic, neurocircuit, behavioral, and self-report assessments.

Domains comprise negative valence systems, positive valence systems, cognitive systems, systems for social processes, arousal/regulatory systems, and sensorimotor systems. In the framework of the RDoC, a major depressive episode following the death of a loved one might begin with dysfunction of the negative valence systems that deal with loss. The depressed person's anhedonia would reflect dysfunction of positive valence systems. The illness overall would be combination of dimensional dysfunctions.

In the past two decades, as China has become more prosperous, urban, and educated, its long-standing stigma around mental illness, and mood disorders specifically, has begun to be publicly discussed and questioned. Chinese young adults, who have had the opportunity to learn about depression in college or from educational or patient support websites, know that depression is widespread and that those who suffer from it are not crazy, evil, or dangerous. However, pursuing psychiatric treatment still can endanger a person's reputation, with potential impact on employment or marriage prospects, and can cause the family to lose face. Thus, even if the self-stigma of a depressed person is reduced by the person's better understanding of the illness, public stigma and anticipated public stigma will still attach to the diagnosis. In a collectivist, family-oriented culture, the family's loss of face would induce shame or guilt in the depressed person, increasing their self-stigma even if they have come to adopt a modern view of the causes, meaning, and consequences of the illness.

Depression is less stigmatized in the mainstream culture of the U.S. and other high-income English-speaking countries than it is in China. Chinese immigrants and expatriates commonly arrive in Western countries with views of mental illness typical of their home country. Mental illness, including non-psychotic depression if formally diagnosed, is stigmatized. There is a common fear that a history of psychiatric treatment will cause permanent harm to one's reputation and life prospects as well as a loss of face for one's family. There usually is less respect for psychiatrists than for other medical specialists.

Dealing with symptoms of depression or BD within the framework of TCM offers Chinese people—including immigrants from China to the West who are early in the process of acculturation—an opportunity to get some care for their conditions without accepting a stigmatizing diagnosis. When a clinician in a Western country sees a Chinese immigrant or expatriate for assessment of depression—especially one who is not highly acculturated—they should, if feasible, assess the patient's relationship with TCM since in China, TCM is widely seen as a useful, integrative complement to the Western medicine that is the country's mainstream model of healthcare. In 2020, visits to TCM hospitals constituted 15.6% of all clinical visits to Chinese hospitals. When a national sample of hospital outpatients was surveyed, 76.3% of respondents said they would use TCM for disease prevention, 34% said they would use it to treat a chronic disease like hypertension or diabetes, 26.3% said they would use it to treat a sleep disorder, and 11.1% said they would use it to treat a condition like chronic pain or a mental disorder. Attributes associated with greater willingness to use TCM were an age over 35, female gender, not having a low income, and having a college education (Zhao et al., 2023).

While there is a significant likelihood that a Chinese patient presenting to a clinician with symptoms of depression has consulted a TCM practitioner, the consultation might not have been specifically about depression or the prescribed treatment specifically addressing depression. The problem presented to the TCM practitioner might be pain, insomnia, or general medical condition for which depression is a common comorbidity. A patient who denies a history of depression might have been treated for a syndrome described by TCM syndrome that overlaps with clinical depression.

In some cases, collaborative care involving a mental health professional and a TCM practitioner will be more acceptable to a patient than mainstream clinical care. Strategy for collaboration is discussed further later in this chapter.

Tradition, Diet, and Depression

Traditional medical systems' approach to the treatment and prevention of diseases of all kinds, including depression and the bipolar spectrum, includes dietary recommendations. Components of foods affect moods, cognition, and the somatic symptoms of depression. Deliberate action by people to change what they eat activates them behaviorally and helps instill hope of recovery. Action by a depressed person's family members to help the person make a change in diet can involve them constructively in the recovery process and may reduce intra-family stigma and self-stigma by reinforcing the idea that there is a biological component to the person's illness. Dietary advice can be given to any depressed patient, based on common principles of antidepressant diets. If a patient comes from a culture with a traditional diet that is antidepressant, the advice might be to eat more traditionally. If a patient comes from a culture that does not have an antidepressant diet, their dietary preferences can be explored—including enjoyment of foods of other nations—to identify antidepressant foods the patient would enjoy eating. When feasible, a patient is encouraged to do more of something they might enjoy—or at least not mind—that might help them recover fully from depression sooner and with less risk of relapse. Some unhealthy foods might need to be cut down or given up, but the clinician's priority should be to find locally available and affordable antidepressant foods that the patient will like and therefore will be inclined to continue.

Specific traditional diets known to have antidepressant benefits include the traditional Japanese diet ((*washoku*), the Mediterranean diet, and the Nordic diet (Opie et al., 2016; Quirk et al., 2013; Suzuki et al., 2013). People of various nationalities who eat Western-style diets heavy on meat, saturated fat, sugar, salt, and processed foods and low on fiber, fish, whole grains, and fresh fruit and vegetables tend to show more depressive symptoms and have more cases of clinical depression. In addition to the benefits or harms of individual foods, consuming a "whole foods" diet with fresh fruit and vegetables is associated with less depression than consuming a "processed foods diet" heavy on sweets, refined grains, fried foods, and processed meats (Akbaraly et al., 2009). Most nations' traditional cuisines are closer to a "whole foods" diet than a "processed foods diet."

A clinician working regularly with a specific nationality or cultural group can learn the patterns of healthy and unhealthy eating that are typical of that group in its current environment. Dietary advice can be tailored to take advantage of healthy foods that are readily available and fit with the person's lifestyle and budget.

The following tables list foods for which consumption has been correlated in population studies either with depressive symptoms or with an increased risk of MDD. *Antidepressant foods* are those for which one or more studies have shown a negative correlation with depressive symptoms or MDD (Table 9.2). *Depressing foods* are those for which one or more studies have shown a positive correlation with depressive symptoms or MDD (Table 9.3).

Dietary advice should include counsel on avoiding food additives and contaminants that can have adverse effects on brain function. In addition to refined sugar, single dietary elements known to add depression risk are cured meats containing sodium nitrate and foods from cans lined with bisphenol-A (BPA)–containing plastic. Nitrate exposure is associated with an increased risk of hypomania and with an increased likelihood of suicide attempts in people with psychiatric illness and a history of hospitalization (Dickerson et al., 2019; Khambadkone et al., 2020). BPA, a plasticizer used in formulating the plastic linings used in commercially canned foods, disrupts the metabolism of sex hormones, with downstream effects on neurotransmitter systems related to depression (Kajta & Wójtowicz, 2013). Cured meats and canned foods commonly are consumed by people in personal situations and/or social and environmental

Table 9.2 Antidepressant Foods

Food	References
Whole grains	Gibson-Smith et al., 2020; Huang et al., 2018; Jacka et al., 2010; Lai et al., 2014; Y. Li et al., 2017; Z. M. Liu et al., 2016; C. J. Wang et al., 2018
Legumes	Grases et al., 2019; Sanhueza et al., 2013
Fish and seafood (especially fatty fish and mollusks), fish oil	Eltgeest et al., 2019; Huang et al., 2018; Jacka et al., 2010; Khanna et al., 2019; Lai et al., 2014; Y. Li et al., 2017; Parletta et al., 2017; Sanhueza et al., 2013; Skarupski et al., 2013
Soybeans and soy products: tofu, miso, natto (fermented soybeans)	Messina, 2016; Messina & Gleason, 2016; Miki et al., 2018; Miyake et al., 2018; Nanri et al., 2010; Yu et al., 2015
Mushrooms: several species, including honey mushrooms, lion's mane, maitake, and oyster mushrooms	Lazur et al., 2023; Miki et al., 2018; Nanri et al., 2010
Seaweed	Allaert et al., 2018; Miki et al., 2018; Miyaki et al., 2014
Green leafy vegetables and cruciferous vegetables (e.g., broccoli, cauliflower)	Cheng et al., 2019; Jacka et al., 2010; Khanna et al., 2019; Lai et al., 2014; Y. Li et al., 2017; Z. M. Liu et al., 2016; Sanhueza et al., 2013; Skarupski et al., 2013; C. J. Wang et al., 2018
Fruit, especially citrus and berries	Cheng et al., 2019; Jacka et al., 2010; Khanna et al., 2019; Lai et al., 2014; Y. Li et al., 2017; Z. M. Liu et al., 2016; Miki et al., 2018; Sanhueza et al., 2013
Fermented foods, including pickled vegetables, full-fat yogurt, and kimchi	Selhub et al., 2014; Winter et al., 2018
Olive oil	Khanna et al., 2019; Y. Li et al., 2017; Pagliai et al., 2018; Sanhueza et al., 2013
Tree nuts	Arab et al., 2019; Frésan et al., 2019; Khanna et al., 2019; Sanhueza et al., 2013; Su et al., 2016.
Tea	Dong, Yang et al., 2015; Hidese et al., 2017; Kim & Kim, 2018; F. D. Li et al., 2016; Miki et al., 2018
Orange juice	Park et al., 2020
High-polyphenol foods: apples; berries; grapes; plums; cabbage; eggplant; onions; peppers; plant-derived beverages including coffee, tea, and fruit juices; seeds; nuts; dark chocolate; red wine (in moderation)	Kontogianni et al., 2020
Carotenoids—beta-carotene, lycopene, lutein, and zeaxanthin. Foods include brightly colored fruits and vegetables: spinach, kale, broccoli, corn, tomatoes, carrots, watermelon, pink grapefruit.	Rasmus & Kozlowska, 2023
Saffron	Ali et al., 2022; Shafiee et al., 2024; Esmaealzadeh et al., 2023.

Table 9.3 Depressing Foods

Food	References
Refined sugar, high-fructose corn syrup, and sweets made from them	Eltgeest et al., 2019; Grases et al., 2019; Huang et al., 2018; Khanna et al., 2019; Z. M. Liu et al., 2016; Lustig, 2013
Sugar-sweetened beverages	Grases et al., 2019; Huang et al., 2018; Khanna et al., 2019; Y. Li et al., 2017; Sanchez-Villegas et al., 2018
Processed/cured meats	Khanna et al., 2019; Y. Li et al., 2017
Fried foods	Jacka et al., 2010; Khanna et al., 2019; Z. M. Liu et al., 2016; Yoshikawa et al., 2016
Refined grains	Jacka et al., 2010; Z. M. Liu et al., 2016
Trans-fatty acids	B. Liu et al., 2019
"Ultra-processed" foods	Arshad et al., 2023

circumstances that already contribute to an increased risk of depression, bipolar spectrum disorders, and suicide. An example of the former would be a depressed, lonely widower who eats unhealthy processed foods because he lacks the energy or skill to prepare alternatives. An example of the latter would be a person living in a low-income urban neighborhood with exposure to excessive noise, particulate air pollution, and street crime that also is a "food desert," with poor availability and/or affordability of healthy foods.

Healthy diets help prevent depression in people facing stress, whether from work, chronobiological challenges, family or other relationship issues, or general medical conditions. They also help prevent relapses in people who have recovered from depression. Cultural groups with specific risk factors for depression sometimes have traditional diets that address them. For example, people in the Nordic nations have limited exposure to winter sunlight, putting them at risk for vitamin D insufficiency. Even without frank vitamin D *deficiency* (serum 25-hydroxyvitamin D <20 ng/mL), vitamin D *insufficiency* (20 ng/mL ≤ serum 25-hydroxyvitamin D ≤ 30 ng/mL) is associated with increased rates of prevalent and incident depression (Briggs et al., 2019; Parker et al., 2017). The Nordic diet (admittedly not consistently followed by many residents of Nordic nations) includes the regular consumption of fatty fish such as salmon and herring, one of the best natural sources of vitamin D (14; Bendik et al., 2014; Biltoft-Jensen et al., 2015). Short winter days can provoke depression on a chronobiological basis, but the omega-3 fatty acids abundant in fish have antidepressant and mood-stabilizing effects that partially mitigate the depressant effects of darkness. (Outdoor winter activities with associated sunlight exposure—a Nordic tradition—also help mitigate the depressing potential of vitamin D insufficiency and short winter days.)

Controlled clinical trials of dietary change as a primary treatment of clinical depression suggest that a consistent change in diet can have an effect size equivalent to that of an SSRI antidepressant (Francis et al., 2019; Jacka et al., 2017). It is not known whether the same patients would respond to SSRIs as would respond to dietary changes. It can be anticipated that biomarkers will eventually identify a subset of patients with depression especially likely to respond to dietary change alone or a subset unlikely to respond to an SSRI unless there were a change in diet.

Migrants (whether between nations or within a large country) often make clinically significant changes in their diets when they move away from an area where their ethnic group is in the majority. In places where there are few others of their ethnicity, their traditional foods might be harder to find and might be more expensive. If they assimilate into the dominant culture of their new home, they will adopt its diet at least partially, and that diet may be less healthy for them than their traditional one. Similar phenomena can occur without migration due to demographic or economic changes in an area (Satia, 2010). The "immigrant paradox"—better mental health in the first generation than the second generation—might be due in part to differences in diet between the parents and the children. Opposing unhealthy dietary acculturation might require an immigrant community's collective action to ensure its access to healthy food.

A nation's or ethnic group's cuisine and eating habits are essential aspects of its culture, often the ones that come to mind first when one thinks about nations famous for their wonderful food. However, individuals' cultural identities are intersections of their nationality and ethnicity with attributes related to religion, education, social class, gender, occupation, age, and generational cohort. For example, people living in poverty in urban "food deserts" may be unable to consistently purchase fresh fruit and vegetables even though they are an important part of the cuisine of their ethnic group. Long-haul truck drivers can for days at a time be limited to eating what they can purchase at truck stops. Hospital interns working long hours might eat on irregular schedules because they must give priority to their patients' care. An aged widow or widower living alone might not want to invest energy in preparing the foods that constituted their usual diet for decades of family life. If a clinician identifies a barrier to a depressed patient's eating a healthy diet, they—or a dietitian working in the same clinical context—might be able to help the patient find a feasible workaround for the practical barriers to their maintaining a healthier diet.

Globalization has had both positive and negative effects with respect to diet and depression. It has increased the variety of foods easily available, especially in cities, offering people a better chance of finding antidepressant foods they like to eat. At the same time, unhealthy fast food, processed foods, and foods high in sugar, saturated fat, and salt are ubiquitous and tirelessly promoted by commercial interests. Young Japanese people may prefer a hamburger, French fries, and a high-sugar soft drink to *washoku* and green tea.

The Past Recaptured: Integrative Medicine and Depression

Traditional medicine and CAIM exemplify a comprehensive, holistic, and dimensional approach to mood disorders. They encourage patients to pursue positive health, with full remission of their troublesome symptoms and lifestyle changes to help prevent recurrence. They put changes in diet and activity on the table for discussion between clinicians and patients and teach mindfulness-promoting practices like meditation, yoga, and *qigong* that can reduce depressive symptoms and promote mental health. They recognize subtypes of clinical depression that require different treatments for optimal outcomes. They bring attention to herbal preparations and nutritional supplements that can augment the effects of prescription psychotropics and can in some cases be a preferable alternative to them.

Traditional systems' conception of depression and the bipolar spectrum—one of "illness" rather than "mental illness"—is virtually incompatible with severe stigma. It does not support people with MDD or BD-I being demonized, blamed, or harshly treated. Even where traditional thinking predominates, however, there will nonetheless be stigma. If people show social behavior that is far out of the bounds of appropriateness for the culture and the person's role within it, they might evoke fear, anger, disgust, mistrust, or other negative feelings and a desire for social distance. Individuals might stigmatize themselves for failing to meet their own expectations or those of their families. In addition, many cultural groups attach mild stigma to chronic illness of any kind.

People seeking treatment for depression or BD might initially feel more comfortable consulting a practitioner of traditional medicine or CAIM rather than a psychiatrist, a primary care physician (PCP), or a non-medical mental health professional. In many parts of the world, beginning with traditional medicine is the norm. In addition to raising less fear of stigma, traditional practitioners might be more accessible and less expensive. If a conventional physician is consulted, it is much more likely that it will be a PCP rather than a psychiatrist.

The integration of conventional Western medicine with traditional medicine or complementary or alternative medicine offers meaningful opportunities for improving clinical outcomes. A depressed patient with a partial response to an initial dose of an SSRI who cannot tolerate a dosage increase might attain a remission without unacceptable side effects by adding a daily dose of saffron or turmeric or using aromatherapy with lavender oil. A depressed patient with chronic anxiety might find relief from anxiety by taking up daily meditation. A depressed patient with chronic low back pain might find that acupuncture treatment combined with an antidepressant drug gives far better relief of both pain and depression than either treatment alone (Gerbarg et al., 2017).

Practitioners of traditional medicine might lack adequate knowledge of general medical and neurological disorders that can present as depression or bipolar symptoms, especially if they have not trained in a program that included several years of instruction in Western medicine. They might have limited knowledge of conventional evidence-based psychotherapy, medications, and non-pharmacologic somatic therapies like electroconvulsive therapy (ECT), transcranial magnetic stimulation (TMS), and light therapy. To deliver optimal care for the many depressed and bipolar patients who will consult them rather than a conventional physician, they need to have an ongoing referral relationship with a psychiatrist. Ideally, the relationship is bidirectional, with the psychiatrist referring appropriate patients to the traditional practitioner for complementary treatment.

PCPs usually know the basics of categorical DSM/ICD diagnosis of mood disorders and guidelines for their first-line treatments with medications like SSRIs. They usually will know psychotherapists to whom they can refer patients who desire talk therapy as an alternative or complement to medication and a psychiatrist or mental health clinic to whom they would refer a patient with BD-I or severe depression. Knowledge of alternative therapies and practitioners—including practitioners of traditional medicine—is less common among PCPs. Patients of minority ethnicity or nonconformist outlook who reject prescription drugs or cognitive-behavioral psychotherapy might be open to seeing a traditional medicine practitioner; to prescriptions for diet, exercise, meditation, herbs, and/or supplements; and/or to faith-based or spiritual counseling or support. There is thus great value in PCPs—and psychiatrists—being familiar with a broad range of alternative and complementary treatments for depression, focusing on those that are available in their community and likely to be used by patients in their area. This would include knowing which locally available traditional treatments are scientifically supported and which ones have known risks for significant adverse effects and/or adverse interactions with prescription drugs. Even better, they, or someone in their practice group, would know the traditional practitioners in their area and their areas of competence. They could then be resources for providing complementary and alternative treatments. For safe and effective integration of conventional and traditional psychopharmacology, the conventional physician should be familiar with interactions between commonly used herbal preparations and prescription psychotropics, with special attention to treatments that are popular with local ethnic communities and their traditional medicine providers. Peer-reviewed articles in the mainstream medical literature periodically review herbal treatments for common psychiatric disorders and offer conventional practitioners a useful perspective on which treatments have substantial scientific support (L. Liu, C. Liu, et al., 2015; Zhuang et al., 2023; Dang et al., 2024; Ding et al., 2024).

The addition of traditional medical care as a complement to conventional therapy of depression or bipolar illness can enhance the patient's acceptance of a diagnosis, engagement in their care, and adherence to long-term treatment. It can also decrease self-stigma, by offering a patient a holistic framework for understanding the illness and an additional supportive, empathic relationship with a trusted clinician.

Use of traditional medicine or other forms of alternative medicine alone, rather than as a complement to conventional medical care, for depression or bipolar illness entails significant risks. It can lead to delays in the correct diagnosis of significant medical comorbidities. Numerous patients treated with ineffective traditional treatments have required psychiatric hospitalization, become disabled by their illnesses, or died by suicide. Hospitalizations, disabilities, and deaths might have been prevented if the patients involved had received timely evidence-based conventional treatment. If a mental health professional sees a depressed patient who wants traditional treatment but not conventional treatment, they might suggest a division of responsibilities. They would ensure (typically via advocacy or liaison with medical specialists) that the patient was properly screened for general medical conditions that can cause or exacerbate depression and that the patient's known chronic medical conditions were optimally treated. They would propose seeing the patient periodically to reassess the patient's depression, to confirm that the patient was improving with traditional treatments, and to screen the patient for their potential side effects.

Many people utilize herbs and supplements to self-treat depression without the oversight of a clinician skilled in their use. By doing so they avoid the expense and inconvenience of clinical care. And a person who is subject to institutional stigma, such as an airline pilot or a physician, can in this way treat a depression without having the diagnosis on their medical record or having a legal obligation to disclose such treatment. There are specific risks of this kind of self-treatment. As noted above, herbal remedies and nutritional supplements vary in potency and purity, some have toxic ingredients, and many have clinically significant interactions with common prescription drugs. For people with undiagnosed bipolar spectrum disorders, taking an effective herbal or nutritional antidepressant can trigger hypomania or rapid cycling. This problem might not be recognized if there is no clinician involved, especially if the person lives alone or among people with limited mental health literacy or belongs to a subculture (e.g., the subculture of popular musicians) that normalizes mild hypomania or cyclothymia. Mainstream physicians, including both PCPs and psychiatrists, can mitigate these risks by letting their patients know they are interested in herbs and supplements and that if their patients are using them, they'd like to help with monitoring and advice to make that self-treatment safer and more effective. Physicians can advise their patients on reliable sources for herbs and supplements and inform them of personally relevant interaction risks.

A PCP or psychiatrist caring for a patient planning to take an herbal remedy or nutritional supplement for depression can set up a schedule for follow-up contacts and provide questionnaires for monitoring symptoms and screening for adverse effects. The patient can be reminded that conventional pharmacologic treatment is available if they are not satisfied with the outcome of self-treatment with herbs and supplements and that immediate help and support are available if the depression gets worse and the patient feels hopeless or suicidal. In this way the physician continues to take responsibility for the patient's medical care while showing respect for the patient's perspective (which may have significant roots in their cultural background). This creates a stronger foundation for more conventional treatment if the patient chooses it in the future.

The more comprehensive menu of treatments provided by CAIM makes it more likely in an integrated care model that a treatment can be found that a depressed patient will accept, tolerate, ultimately find effective, and consider continuing to prevent a relapse. Because its range of treatments goes far beyond medications and talk therapy, CAIM can enable a clinician to circumvent culturally related suspicion of medications or a patient's culturally based reluctance to disclose personal matters to someone outside of their family.

Part II

Depression and the Cultures of Places

Chapter 10

China: Confucian Harmony and Dissonance

In this chapter a cultural lens on depression in Chinese people is illustrated by focusing intensively on the problem of depression and suicide in two exemplary groups of people: Chinese and Chinese American students at universities in the United States and "left-behind women" in rural China. The narratives and analyses presented are intended to stimulate cultural awareness and clinical hypothesis generation. The cases are not put forward as stereotypes. For any person with depression, transpersonal features provide context for a unique personal illness narrative, and national origin is just one of several characteristics that intersect to form an individual's cultural identity.

China, the world's second most populous nation, is the largest source of international students at the world's universities, and students of Chinese descent constitute a plurality of ethnic minority students at highly ranked universities in the United States and the United Kingdom. Approximately 5.4 million ethnically Chinese people, immigrants and U.S.-born, live in the United States (Budiman, 2021a). In academic year 2019–2020 there were 372,000 Chinese international students at American universities, constituting 35% of the total international student population (McGregor, 2021).

Chinese students at American universities, whether international students, first-generation immigrants, or American-born Chinese (ABCs, or second-generation immigrants) are at increased risk for clinical depression—higher than that of Chinese university students in their home country and higher than that of American university students overall (J. A. Chen, Liu, et al., 2015). In a 2017 survey of Chinese international students, of whom 84.7% were graduate students, 77.9% reported being depressed at some time during the past year, and 58% reported experiencing depression in the past 30 days (Lian & Wallace, 2020). In a 2007 study using the Center for Epidemiologic Studies Depression Scale (CES-D), 32.2% of a 189-student sample had scores of 16 or higher (above the cutoff score for probable major depression), and most of those scoring below 16 had symptoms of potential clinical significance. Clinically relevant symptoms of depression were detected by the PHQ-9 in 45% of a sample of 130 Chinese international students at Yale in 2009. In that study, 27% of respondents were unaware that mental health services were available on campus. Using different depression rating scales, depression prevalence rates of 47.5% and 32%

had previously been found in Chinese students at two other U.S. universities (Han et al., 2013). More recent studies of Chinese international students from other universities in U.S., Canada, and Australia have shown prevalence rates of clinical depression ranging from 25% to over 50% (Bi et al., 2023; Ke et al., 2023; Lian & Wallace, 2020; Lin et al., 2022; Yu et al., 2023).

ABCs (second-generation immigrants) have 2.64 times the lifetime risk of major depression or dysthymia compared with first-generation immigrants (J. Zhang et al., 2013). The overall 12-month prevalence of depression in a sample of ABC adults of all ages was 21.5% (Jackson et al., 2011). An even higher prevalence rate would be expected for university students in their 20s.

There is no published study of bipolar disorder (BD) prevalence in Chinese international or Chinese American students at U.S. universities. However, in a 2001–2002 national survey of American college students that diagnosed subjects using face-to-face structured interviews, college students of all ethnicities aged 18–24 showed a 7.0% prevalence of MDD and a 3.2% prevalence of BD (Blanco et al., 2008). If the Chinese student population shows a similar ratio of BD to MDD, it would imply there are many currently undiagnosed cases of bipolar spectrum disorders.

College students overall have a high lifetime prevalence of suicidal ideation— 22% in a 2018 meta-analysis (Mortier et al., 2018). Chinese Americans—ABCs and Generation 1.5—are more likely than Caucasian students to have suicidal ideation; in one 2011 study, they had 60% higher risk after controlling for other demographic factors (Wong et al., 2012). The epidemic of depression among university students of Chinese origin, with its associated suicide mortality, warrants a vigorous response from America's universities.

College students of all nationalities and ethnicities are vulnerable to depression related to stresses common to their life stage: academic pressures, financial issues, general health concerns, and problems with important relationships, including those with their families of origin, their romantic partners, their peers (friends and classmates), and authorities (teachers, advisors, and employers) (Karyotaki et al., 2020). Illness narratives of depression in Chinese American and Chinese international university students usually include mention of one or more of these generic stresses, often with details and emphasis that reflect students' Chinese cultural identity. Chinese students' patterns of disclosure of symptoms, help-seeking, and engagement in treatment often have important cultural dimensions. Seeing depression in this at-risk population through a cultural lens reveals potential opportunities for primary and secondary prevention of clinical depression, timelier and more effective treatment, and prevention of suicide. Five cases of depression in Chinese or Chinese American students that ended in death by suicide are now described in detail, to set the stage for a culturally aware view of the problem. The reports are based on published news about the cases and social media posts by and about the students that were freely available on the internet when we researched them. They are not based on review of medical records.

Loved and Abused: The Success and Suicide of Nikita Guo

In the fall of 2012, Heng "Nikita" Guo, a second-year MBA student at the MIT/Sloan School of Management, hanged herself in her apartment in Cambridge, Massachusetts. She was 28.

Nikita was the only child of a working-class couple in a small town in northwestern China. Her mother, a strong-willed woman whose opportunities had been limited by her lack of secondary education, was determined that her daughter would have an elite higher education and a much richer life than hers. When Nikita was only two years old, her mother began teaching her to read and write. Play and sleep time were sacrificed. Her parents set the goal that Nikita would have a perfect score on every examination, in every subject. In the fourth grade, Nikita took the elementary school examination a year early, earned the top score in the county, and was admitted directly to the county's "number one" middle school. Her parents' objective for middle school was that she be first in her grade in every subject and one of the top three students in the region in every subject. Continuing with intensive and rigorous study vigorously monitored by her mother, she won competitive examinations in physics, chemistry, mathematics, English, and essay writing. She received press and television coverage as a child prodigy (*shéntóng*; 神童). Her parents gained face and enjoyed their local celebrity.

Nikita deeply resented being characterized and admired as a prodigy. She attributed her outstanding test performance not to talent or intelligence but to countless hours of study and practice, compelled by her parents and enforced with harsh discipline. Since age five, she went to bed at midnight or later and was up at 6 a.m. to begin studying. Her sleeping hours were always far shorter than the nine-hour minimum recommended by pediatricians and sleep specialists (Paruthi et al., 2016). When she got a less-than-perfect score on a test or when she was disobedient, she would be physically punished, for example, by being forced to kneel on a washboard with bare legs. In her own words, she felt she was "beaten like a boy," although she was a "vulnerable girl." For several days before major examinations, she became extremely anxious and lost her appetite. No matter how well she performed, her parents never praised her in her presence. She only recalled their reprimands and their dissatisfaction.

Nikita's parents' fortunes improved; her father started a successful business in Shenzhen, and Nikita and her mother joined him there when she was 14. Newly affluent, her parents were able to send her at age 17 to a summer chemistry program for high school students at Harvard. She finished the program second in her class, but she noticed with disappointment that her American classmates of the same age were more mature and experienced than she. After her summer course, she took the advice of a Chinese mentor, Yanding Gao, and enrolled as an undergraduate electrical engineering major at Texas A&M University. She had hoped to transfer to Stanford and to study biochemistry through a doctorate, but her mentor argued that it would be better to be first in her class at Texas A&M than to be in the middle of her class at Stanford, and better to study a discipline that would lead to a well-paid and prestigious position immediately after her graduation from college. Her mentor was a professional consultant to students in China seeking to study in the United States. In 2005, he published a bestselling book on educational strategy and career planning. In the book, he included a full account of how Nikita had succeeded with the aid of his advice. The title can be translated as *Life Design in Childhood, a Harvard Dad Has Something to Say* (人生设计在童年—哈佛爸爸有话说), (Gao, 2005.). In 2015, three years after Nikita's death, Gao published another book elaborating a similar approach to "Life Design" (Gao, 2015).

Nikita graduated at the top of her class and moved to New York City to work as a financial analyst for Citibank. After five years working in finance, she moved to Cambridge and began the MBA program at MIT/Sloan School of Management. Her parents in China arranged a marriage for her, to a Chinese-born New York cardiac surgeon five years her senior. Getting married at age 26, she could plan on having a baby at age 28 while in business school—perfect timing.

The wedding, arranged by her parents and taking place in China on her 26th birthday, was picture-perfect, but Nikita's marriage was not happy. Her husband complained that he wanted a wife and not a "perfect learning machine" and soon sought a divorce. Nikita blogged that she was lonely and miserable but consoled herself: By leaving the husband picked by her mother she was now breaking free of her mother's control and could pursue her own happiness, like a butterfly emerging from a cocoon.

Nikita could not stop competing despite her many successes. In her first year at MIT, she was disillusioned to find that her midterm test scores placed her in the middle of her class. And it seemed to her that her classmates were not only smart but also worldly and sophisticated, and some were accomplished in the arts or in sports in addition to academics and business. Comparing herself with them, she felt her only distinction was her fluency in Mandarin. Wanting to be more competitive, she began a plan of "devilish training," resolving to study four hours a day beyond the time needed to complete her homework. Thinking that it would help for her to be physically stronger, she also began intensive physical training that included a daily 3-km run, 100 pushups, and other exercises.

On her breaks she traveled extensively, visiting 33 countries in addition to returning to China to visit her parents. While presenting a lively personality and smiling face to the world, her writings reveal that inside her apartment, behind her social mask, she felt pessimistic, discouraged, self-critical, and hopeless. She felt mediocre when she compared herself to classmates who seemed both happier and more accomplished. In the autumn of her second year at MIT she wrote a suicide note stating that she had no purpose or place in the world since her classmates were far more successful than she. Competition and winning were her purpose in life, and at that she had failed.

Nikita's short life was entirely scripted by her parents, with assistance from a consultant. From earliest childhood, she was subjected to corporal punishment, sleep deprivation, and withholding of parental affection. She internalized and normalized her parents' harsh treatment, accepting that it was "for her good" rather than mainly a function of her parents' ambition and unhealthy traditions. After celebrating her "breaking free" from her mother, she continued to mistreat herself as her parents had mistreated her. The story of her childhood experience and subsequent emotional life evoke the themes of psychoanalyst Alice Miller's classic book *The Drama of the Gifted Child: The Search for the True Self* (Miller, 2008). Miller pointed out that a sensitive child yearning for their parents' love often conforms to their expectations with compunction rather than developing a true autonomous self. When the child confronts the stresses of an independent adulthood, inner coping resources may be inadequate. Kaiwen Xu, a psychologist at the Beijing University Student Mental Health Education and Counseling Center, describes seeing many students with "hollow disease." His patients, who presented with depressed mood and suicidality, had childhoods full of utilitarian, exam-focused education and a sense of living for others, with no space for the cultivation of an authentic personality (Xu, 2019).

Nikita's mother had lost her opportunity for higher education and wanted her daughter to have the education and status she had missed. The mother's dream became the daughter's obligation. The focus of Nikita's education was attaining perfect scores on tests—winning in competition. The aims of her higher education, conceived with the suggestions of her Chinese mentor, were entirely utilitarian and instrumental. The harsh treatment she had received beginning in preschool increased her lifetime risk of mental health problems including depression, BD, and suicide.

Had Nikita sought treatment for her mood symptoms, a clinician might have considered a diagnosis of a bipolar spectrum disorder in view of her driven, hyperactive behavior, her façade of positivity, and her chronically short hours of sleep. However, it might have been hard for the clinician to distinguish Nikita's behavior pattern from that of many students of Chinese origin with no mental illness who are similarly obsessed with winning in academic competition and willing to sacrifice sleep for study and work. While a certain diagnosis of a bipolar spectrum disorder cannot be made in retrospect, some of her behavior (extreme travel and intense physical workouts) had no obvious link to academic or occupational success, and thus suggests hypomania. Adverse childhood experiences of the type Nikita had are known to hasten the onset of adult BD in adolescents with subclinical bipolar symptoms (Aas et al., 2016).

Masked Depression: The Sadness of Linka Liu

> When people read this note I will probably already be gone from this world. Of course, I hope I am already gone at that point. I will no longer be as if in a vegetative state, in coma but still breathing. It took me a long time to make this decision. I had wished I had accomplished everything I planned on. The world is beautiful, but I am a coward. The heaviness of life is unbearable to me, so I have chosen to quit and escape. This is totally my own decision. It's not caused by anyone else. ... If someone wants to die, it's not determined by external events—it's based on how a person feels.

Weiwei "Linka" Liu, a Chinese international student at the University of California at Santa Barbara (UCSB), a sophomore majoring in German and psychology, died by suicide in February 2017. She was 20. Her suicide followed many months of pondering the meaning of existence and whether she "deserved to live." Her suicide shocked her family and her friends, several of whom described on social media her beautiful smile and cheerful disposition.

Linka grew up in Foshan, a city of 7.2 million population in Guangdong Province. She was an intelligent girl with special aptitude for learning languages; in addition to Mandarin, she spoke the local Cantonese dialect and was proficient in English, Japanese, and German. Without extraordinary effort she was first or second in her class throughout middle school and high school.

Linka was different in many ways from Nikita. She was not an only child, she was not treated harshly by her mother, and she did not have Nikita's hyperactivity. Her personality was sensitive and moody, and throughout her adolescence she mused about the meaning of life.

Linka probably would have scored high enough on the *gāokǎo* (高考; National College Entrance Examination) to gain admission to a top university in China. But, like many outstanding Chinese high school students, she opted to pursue an American college degree and full fluency in English. The cost of education at UCSB, over $60,000 per year, was a financial burden that her parents willingly accepted.

Linka was not adventurous by nature, and she was anxious about her new circumstances, 11,530 km from home. Despite her timid nature she resolved to be brave and to deal resolutely with the challenges of life in America. She was well liked and made many friends. She began posting regularly on social media sites in both English and Chinese. Her posts describe joyful experiences, and the associated photos always show her with a sweet smile.

In the fall of her sophomore year, she fell into a depressed mood that got progressively worse. Her ruminations about the meaning of life and whether she deserved to live became more intrusive. Around the New Year, her parents and younger sister came to visit for a month. She did not tell them about her severe depression.

She floated the idea of her transferring to the University of Southern California (USC), an institution with almost 5000 students from China and a reputation as one of the best universities in America for Chinese international students. She thought she might be less lonely and homesick there, but her parents did not favor a transfer, saying they were worried about USC's location in a potentially dangerous urban neighborhood. Her parents apparently could not conceive of something as intangible as depression being more dangerous than street crime near an inner-city college campus.

While Linka's parents were visiting shortly before her death, she posted notes on social media describing her loving and supportive parents and how happy she was to be together with her family. After her family returned to China, Linka felt hopeless, miserable, and desperate. She struggled every day with thoughts of suicide. She consulted a psychiatrist, describing her mood and mentioning a recent romantic breakup. She did not find the psychiatric visit to be helpful. She recounted that the psychiatrist had said she had had a loss and naturally she felt sad. She should give herself time and space to experience her sadness. Apparently, the psychiatrist did not assess Linka as clinically depressed or as at imminent risk for suicide. It is possible that the assessment would have been different if the cultural context had been appreciated. Considering prevalent Chinese attitudes toward psychiatry, Linka's seeking treatment at all made it probable she had a serious problem. Given her personal issue of loneliness, the time immediately following her family's return to China would be one of especially high risk for suicide.

Did Linka successfully mask her depression during her family's visit? Did she minimize her distress and suicidality with the psychiatrist? Did her family and/or her psychiatrist interpret her academic success and apparent coping with the life of an international student as evidence that her mental health issues could not be of life-threatening magnitude? All of these are reasonable hypotheses, based on the cultural context.

Achievement, Bipolarity, and Christianity in an ABC Student: The Death of Luke Tang

ABC students at elite universities do not have many of the generic stresses of Chinese international students. They are less often lonely. They are not so far from their families, and they usually have hometown friends with whom they stay connected. They do not have issues with English proficiency or with visa status. Even so, ABC students have higher rates of depression than White students. And, like Chinese international students, they often conceal their depression from their parents.

In September 2015, Luke Tang, a Chinese American Harvard sophomore, was found dead by suicide in his dormitory room. He was 19. His classmates, professors, and parents were shocked by his death. Two years later, a documentary about his story, *Looking for Luke*, was selectively exhibited throughout the United States.

Luke's parents immigrated from China to the United States in 1990. Both parents had graduate degrees. Luke, the younger of two sons, was born in Hawaii. After several moves, his family settled in New Orleans when he was 11. Luke attended a charter high school for gifted students, where he displayed extraordinary talent and industriousness. An outstanding young violinist, he was concertmaster of the New Orleans Youth Orchestra. He was honored as a Presidential Scholar, receiving an award from the U.S. Department of Education that is given to only 121 students per year. He was a practicing Christian, active in the New Orleans Chinese Baptist Church. He graduated second in his high school class, had near-perfect Scholastic Aptitude Test (SAT) scores, and was admitted to Harvard College.

An autobiographical sketch Luke wrote in high school offers insight into his mental state. He describes gratitude to his parents for their "daring move from China in 1990 and their judicious parenting." He describes his "relationship with God as the most important aspect of my life." He explains that he was driven to teach and offers examples: teaching Bible study and offering counseling to fifth and sixth graders at his church, teaching violin at an elementary school, teaching competitive mathematics to his peers on the math team, and tutoring another high school student in physics. His autobiography is remarkable for its many expressions of expansiveness, enthusiasm, and euphoria. In intellectually gifted adolescents, self-documented exuberance often represents healthy and adaptive hyperthymia. However, if a hyperthymic person repeatedly becomes depressed, bipolarity should be considered seriously.

Arriving at Harvard, Luke decided to major in physics and took a demanding course load. He immediately became involved in a student Christian group, participating in religious services several times a week and often leading them. On April 11, 2015, he made a suicide attempt in his Harvard dormitory. Eleven days later, on April 22, because of continuing suicidal ideation, he was referred by student health services to McLean Hospital for inpatient psychiatric care. He remained at McLean for one week, during which he had several psychiatric evaluations and underwent psychological testing. While his records from McLean are not public, they were quoted in a legal complaint against Harvard—ultimately unsuccessful—that was subsequently made by Luke's parents. He was described by a McLean psychiatrist as "immature, a contrarian, stubborn and lacking full insight." Another clinician wrote about his "nonchalant and suboptimal appreciation for the gravity of his suicide attempt."

The day of Luke's discharge from McLean he met with a counselor at Harvard who reported that Luke "demonstrates little insight into the nature or feelings of depression." Despite his signing a written agreement stating that treatment was a requirement for his returning to Harvard in the fall, Luke did not follow through with treatment over the summer or check in with a therapist when he returned to Harvard in the fall after a visit to China. Two weeks into the fall term he died by suicide (Middlesex Superior Court, 2018; Ricciuti, 2019).

Luke's story is one of a boy with a strong internal drive to achieve rather than one of a child submitting to his controlling parents. In retrospect, Luke's story suggests a bipolar spectrum condition, but at the time his bipolarity might have been invisible. To his parents he was a gifted, energetic, high-achieving, and loving son. To others, he might have been another Chinese American "model minority" student with a stereotypically impressive list of accomplishments. It is unknown whether a bipolar spectrum disorder was in the differential diagnosis at McLean, but it is unlikely that Luke received a formal diagnosis of BD given that the recommended follow-up was weekly counseling, rather than medical treatment by a psychiatrist that included mood-stabilizing medication. The healthcare system's response to his suicide attempt suggests that it was not interpreted as a presenting sign of a serious mental illness.

Luke's impressive drive, his excellent academic and musical performance, and his passion for Christianity all could have looked normal for an ABC. However, his suicide attempt and persistent suicidal ideation after the attempt, his expansiveness and high goal-directed activity, and his profound lack of insight suggest that he had a bipolar spectrum condition. People who consistently achieve despite significant negative emotions have found ways to cope. These can be positive, like mindfulness or altruistic behavior, or problematic, like denial or deliberate concealment of distress even when help is at hand. In Luke's case, denial was conspicuous to several clinicians, and he did not make use of counseling that was offered to him. It is known that bipolar spectrum disorders are common among intellectually and artistically gifted people, and the diagnosis of a bipolar spectrum disorder should be considered seriously whenever a creative professional has a major depressive episode or a makes a suicide attempt. (The relationship of exceptional talent and the bipolar spectrum is explored further in Chapter 15.)

Was Luke perceived by those around him as one more gifted Chinese student intensely—but normally—driven to excel in every discipline he touched? Did anyone consider the possibility of bipolarity? Was Luke's tendency to "minimize and under-report" his emotional and behavioral symptoms interpreted as a sign of possible BD, as an indication of emotional immaturity, or as a reflection of Chinese culture?

No Time to Get Well: Luchang Wang's Leap to Her Death

> Dear Yale:
> I loved being here. I only wish I could've had some time. I needed time to work things out and to wait for new medication to kick in, but I couldn't do it in school, and I couldn't bear the thought of having to leave for a full year, or of leaving and never being readmitted.
> Love, Luchang

Luchang Wang, an ABC sophomore mathematics major, was last seen at Yale on January 25, 2015. Soon afterward, she bought a one-way ticket to San Francisco. On January 27, she posted the above note on her Facebook page and leaped to her death from the Golden Gate Bridge. She was 20.

Luchang was born in California to Chinese parents and grew up near Des Moines, Iowa, where she attended public school and excelled in math and science, winning national competitions in both. She also was a varsity distance runner. She succeeded academically and athletically despite suffering from dysthymia (chronic non-major depression). She was discreet about her psychiatric issues, which did not interfere with her having many friends and many achievements. In her freshman year at Yale, she was active in political and charitable activities and declared a life goal of "making the world more beautiful."

That year, she had a major depressive episode for which she ultimately took a leave of absence for treatment. According to Yale's policy at the time, taking leave more than 10 days into a semester required her to fully withdraw from the university, remain away for an additional semester, and formally apply for readmission. There was no guarantee that a student could return after leaving, and, if a student withdrew in this way for a second time, it was very likely that they would not be readmitted. Luchang recovered from her depression and was readmitted to Yale. In the fall of her sophomore year at Yale, the depression recurred. She had poor sleep and was unable to concentrate on her classwork. She sought treatment from Yale's student health service and was started on an antidepressant drug. After a few weeks on the medication, Luchang had not yet recovered sufficiently to keep up with her studies. Taking leave would require withdrawal from Yale with a poor chance of readmission, while not taking leave would have involved a risk of failing one or more classes. Luchang felt that if she were permanently rejected by Yale, she would have no reason to live—it would be too humiliating to her and to her family.

Being forced to withdraw from the college of one's choice because of a health problem would be disappointing to anyone. Luchang's Chinese identity might have aggravated her emotional distress and made suicide more likely. An elite education has been of central importance to Chinese people for centuries, mental illness has always been stigmatized in China, and either academic failure or mental illness would imply a painful loss of face for one's family as well as oneself. In terms of the interpersonal theory of suicide, Luchang's rejection by Yale would constitute thwarted belongingness, and her bringing shame to her family through her illness and its consequences would imply perceived burdensomeness. There have been many well-publicized suicides of Chinese and Chinese American university students in the United States. In their obituaries it is typical for their wonderful qualities and accomplishments to be recalled. For some students, the prospect of death by suicide with a laudatory obituary might be more appealing than that of a personal and familial loss of face followed by a lifetime of stigma. Acquired capacity for suicide is assisted by role models.

At the time of Luchang's death, Yale's policy for health-related leaves of absence—still the rule at many universities—was poorly suited for adolescents and young adults facing the specific challenges of depression and bipolar spectrum disorders. In students with these conditions, transient periods of serious functional impairment can punctuate a usually consistent pattern of high motivation and high achievement. Once a student with a major mood disorder and very high baseline functioning attains a full, stable remission, they can rapidly make up for missed classes or assignments. There would rarely be a need for a prolonged period of rehabilitation away from the university. In fact, return to academic work, positive social interactions, and an active, structured daily routine can accelerate recovery and help a person maintain a remission of illness.

It is bitterly ironic that Yale's leave of absence policy, with literally fatal consequences for Luchang Wang, was implemented at a university with one of the world's best departments of psychiatry. There was plenty of knowledge about depression available on campus, but neither that knowledge nor the anti-stigma messaging of Yale's psychiatry faculty informed the university's policies regarding leave for treatment of mental illness. The interaction of those policies with Luchang's cultural context was fatally toxic. Should it cause irreversible damage to a student's lifetime educational and occupational prospects; her social life, status, and reputation; and, for a Chinese student, the face of her family, if an episode of major depression remits in 5 weeks instead of 3 weeks or if its onset is in the middle of a term rather than during a summer or winter break?

When Olivia Kong Screamed for Help, She Was Serious

On April 11, 2016, Ao "Olivia" Kong, a junior at the University of Pennsylvania Wharton School of Business, lay down on the tracks of a nearby commuter train. The train could not stop in time, and she was killed. She was 21 (*Xianguo Kong v. Trustees of the University of Pennsylvania*, 2018; Malfitano, 2022).

Olivia and her parents had immigrated to the United States from China when she was nine years old and had settled in Philadelphia. Olivia had an outstanding academic record, played the violin, was a member of her high school's varsity tennis team, and placed first in a national mathematics competition. She was admitted by early decision to the Wharton School of Business, the nation's top-ranked undergraduate business school. She received a scholarship covering most of the school's annual tuition and fees, which were over $53,000 the year Olivia died.

Her first two years at Wharton were psychiatrically uneventful. In March of her junior year, she developed an episode of clinical depression, with severe insomnia, anxiety, impaired concentration, and thoughts of suicide. Because of her poor concentration, she was having difficulty with one of her six classes. She was worried she would fail the class, causing her to lose her scholarship and her upcoming paid summer internship at the Bank of America. She tried to withdraw from the problematic class but was told that her request was too far into the term to be honored.

On a visit to the student health service in late March for an upper respiratory infection, she completed a PHQ-9, indicating symptoms of clinical depression and endorsing suicidal ideation. The primary care physician attributed her depression to her physical illness and told her to get a good night's sleep—apparently not considering that one of the main symptoms of Olivia's depression was insomnia. Over the next two weeks she mentioned her suicidal ideation to a Counseling and Psychological Services (CPS) psychiatrist twice, to a CPS social worker three times, and to her academic adviser once. The final time that she confided her suicidal ideation, she described academic difficulties as her specific reason to die, a plan to overdose on sleeping pills and a date for carrying out her plan. She urgently telephoned the on-call psychiatrist and asked about psychiatric hospitalization. The psychiatrist suggested it was a "last resort" if nothing else worked. He said she might go to the emergency room (ER) "if she felt desperate." When she expressed worry about the cost of the ER visit, he "offered that the cost of an ER visit is likely less than the cost of funeral arrangements." His note included a comment that Olivia had "said she had actually planned to return to campus Sunday and kill self."

That same weekend she visited her parents. They could see she was not happy, but she did not talk with them about her depression or her thoughts of suicide. The night before her death, her parents stopped by the campus to check on her, meeting her outside her dormitory. Her mother felt her daughter's forehead for fever and gave her some homemade dumplings.

Unlike many Chinese and Chinese American college students, Olivia had no difficulty seeking help for her depression. She cried for help repeatedly and was very explicit about her suicidality. One possible reason for the lack of alacrity of the CPS response is that the clinicians did not appreciate that it is extremely unlikely that a successful Chinese Ivy League student with no prior psychiatric history would repeatedly say she was suicidal unless she were truly ill and at high risk for self-harm. At the time Olivia called for help she was already desperate. Her expressed worry about the cost of an ER visit can be understood as a further expression of her depression and its context. She was explicitly worried about money, including potential risk to her scholarship and her summer job. Unless and until some combination of mental health education, anti-stigma efforts, and healthy acculturation changes Chinese college students' reluctance to seek mental health care and disclose mental health problems, it will be safer for a clinician to take the forthright disclosure of a suicidal plan by a Chinese student very seriously.

Table 10.1 briefly describes 13 additional Chinese and Chinese American students at major American universities who died by suicide between 2012 and 2019. The cases are included here because information about them is available from public records. All 13 used highly lethal means of suicide, with virtually no chance of rescue. All had demanding majors—all but two were in science, technology, engineering, and math (STEM) fields. Three were openly depressed; the remainder gave no clue of their distress to others. Only two mention seeking or receiving treatment.

Depression, either unipolar or bipolar, usually not diagnosed or treated, was the apparent underlying cause of suicide in the 18 cases described in the case histories and in Table 10.1. Most of the students did not seek help. Their external presentation usually was positive. Their misery was hidden by high levels

Table 10.1 Additional Representative Suicides of Chinese and Chinese American Students

Student, age, and gender	International student, immigrant, or Chinese American	Month of death	University, year, major	Brief background	Mode of suicide
Wendy Chang, 22, F	Chinese American	April 2012	Harvard senior, English	From Irvine, CA; memorable laugh	Hanging
Andrew Sun, 20, M	Immigrated as teenager	April 2014	Harvard sophomore, economics	Practicing Christian; no disclosure of depression	Jumping from a building
Yangkai Li, 20, M	International student from Guangzhou	October 2014	Johns Hopkins University sophomore, physics	Diagnosed depression	Jumping from a building
Xiao Lu, 28, M	International student	January 2016	University of Chicago MBA student	Mood normal on video chat with mother three days before death	Jumping into a frozen lake
Shuqin Zhang, 22, F	International student from Beijing	January 2016	UC Berkeley statistics graduate student	Perfectionistic; developed acute depression after failing a course	Jumping from a cliff
Kaifeng Liu, 24, M	International student from Tianjin	December 2016	Ohio State physics graduate student	Came to United States for college and remained	Firearm
Xin Rong, 27, M	International student	March 2017	University of Michigan PhD candidate in information technology	Married; interned at Microsoft and Google; blogged in late 2016 about depression in graduate students	Jumping out of a rented airplane (was a licensed pilot)
Xiaolin Tang, 32, F	International student	October 2017	University of Utah PhD candidate in astrophysics	BS from Beijing University; introvert; seventh year in graduate school with no hope of finishing dissertation	Jumping from a bridge

Table 10.1 Continued

Student, age, and gender	International student, immigrant, or Chinese American	Month of death	University, year, major	Brief background	Mode of suicide
Miaoxiu Tian, 21, F	International student from Chengdu	December-2017	Cornell University senior, materials science and engineering	Early achiever; near perfect score on TOEFL; sentimental personality; got psychological counseling	Unknown
Annie Wang, 20, F	Chinese American	Mary 2018	UCSB sophomore, psychological and brain science with minor in art	Grew up in San Diego; happy, cheerful extravert	Jumping from a bridge or cliff
Andrea Liu, 26, F	Chinese American	May 2018	New York University senior medical student	Grew up in suburban New Jersey; mathematics undergraduate; died one month before graduation; blogged that medical school was stressful	Hanging
Shengyu Jin, 20, M	International student from Harbin	June 2018	UCSB sophomore, physics	Well respected by classmates	Died in a car; probable carbon monoxide toxicity
Ziwen Wang, 26, M	International student	February 2019	Stanford fifth-year PhD candidate in materials science	Undergraduate physics degree from a Chinese university	Hanging (in the laboratory)

Note. TOEFL = Test of English as a Foreign Language; UCSB = University of California, Santa Barbara.

of productive activity. Their sadness often was masked by social smiles. Their suicides were shocking to everyone around them.

The narratives of these suicides, and of the depressions that preceded them, reflect an interaction of three factors: the personal and family history of the student, their life circumstances and life events, and the effect of Chinese culture on the meaning of their life situation and on the expression of their psychiatric condition including help-seeking. Sometimes culture is relevant to the cause of a depression but has little effect on its symptomatic expression. Sometimes a depression has a largely endogenous/biological/genetic cause, but culture strongly affects how it is (or isn't) displayed in the depressed person's daily behavior.

All international students face challenges beyond academic ones. Depending on the student's national origin and personal background, these might include some combination of limited proficiency in colloquial English, acculturative stress, the great expense of higher education, distance from loved ones, and experiencing prejudice and discrimination, stereotyping, and/or microaggressions. Even when there is no gross prejudice or discrimination, minority students can face subtle forms of social exclusion. Second-generation immigrants might have identity issues, feelings of deracination, and conflicts with parents or distance from them because of differences in acculturation. In addition to these, Chinese and Chinese American students often have concerns relatable to the special role of education in Chinese history and culture. The relationships of Chinese parents and children are shaped by a collectivistic, family-oriented Confucian ethos that has persisted through modernization, globalization, and political upheavals. Ancient traditions and Confucian principles can lead many well-meaning Chinese parents to adopt childrearing practices that can traumatize their children and catalyze the development of mental illness many years later. (The usual caveat about stereotypes applies. There are, of course, many Chinese families without problematic behaviors, beliefs, and dynamics relatable to Confucian ideology. Our aim is to raise cultural awareness and facilitate "informed empathy.")

The Imperial Examination

"Give up sleep, forget about food" (*fèiqǐn wàngshí*; 废寝忘食).
"Tie your hair to the roofbeam, jab your thigh with an awl" (*xuánliáng cìgǔ*; 悬梁刺股).
"Get your name on the golden scoreboard" (*jīn bǎng tí míng*; 金榜题名).

In the Sui Dynasty (581–618 CE), China began using a standardized examination to identify talent for administrative posts. The examination was an aid to the unification of separate states into a single empire, and it helped reduce corruption and nepotism in the selection of civil servants. In the early

Tang Dynasty (618–907 CE) the examination took its enduring form as the *Imperial Examination* (*kējǔ*; 科举), which China used to select its civil servants through the end of the Qing Dynasty in 1905. The examination lasted around 1300 years, with only one interruption, from 1279 to 1315, under Mongolian rule. Examinees—candidates for public office—were tested on their verbatim recall of Confucian texts, as assessed by fill-in-the-blank questions; on their ability to write essays in a highly structured format on topics related to Confucian teachings; and on their skill at writing poetry in classical style on specified themes. Additional content varied over the centuries, but the rote recall of Confucian texts and writing in formal classical style was central.

The procedure was extremely rigorous. For three days, examinees were locked in small rooms with wooden benches and chamber pots. They brought food, water, pens, and ink and were expected to remain in their cells from the beginning to the end of the examination. If an examinee needed to leave his cell, for example, to deal with gastrointestinal distress, he was escorted to an outhouse; but the episode was recorded on his examination paper and might be held against him in scoring it. The examination area was policed to discourage cheating, which was severely punished if it occurred. After examinations were completed, test papers were copied by scribes before passing them on to the readers so that the readers would not be able to identify examinees by their handwriting. The fixed content of the examination, the standard testing environment, and the anonymity in grading tended to limit corrupt influences on scoring of the test.

The *keju* was given at four successive levels: local, provincial, national, and imperial. Local (county-level) examinations were annual, and the others were triennial. The national- and imperial-level examinations were given in the capital, with the imperial-level examination personally overseen by the emperor. There were strict quotas for how many examinees could pass each test; local, provincial, and ethnic quotas were set to ensure that civil servants were sufficiently representative of the empire's different constituencies. A consequence of the quotas was that passing the examination was more difficult for men from the wealthier and more populous provinces of China. The overall pass rate was less than 1%. Passing each examination gave the successful examinee a title that brought honor and privileges to him and his family. Two such titles survive today—*xiùcái* (秀才) historically denoted a man who had passed the county-level examination, and *zhuàngyuán* (状元) denoted a man who was the top scorer at the imperial level. In modern times, *xiucai* sometimes is used to denote intellectuals, either straightforwardly or sarcastically. *Zhuangyuan* is used, always without sarcasm, to denote a person with the highest score on some part of the *gaokao*. In the era of the *keju*, the names of those who passed at the imperial level were posted on a list written in calligraphy on a background of gold leaf. In colloquial Chinese, to get one's name on the golden list (*jin bang ti ming*) means to pass an examination with high honors.

Historically, success on the *keju* at the county level—becoming a *xiucai*—would immediately give a man social status, exemption from military service, and lighter punishment if he committed a misdemeanor. It would improve a single man's prospects for a favorable marriage. Success at the provincial level would guarantee a man lifetime employment in the civil service. A man who passed the keju was set in life. By passing the examination at the provincial or national level a man could move from the middle class to the nobility, attaining status beyond what he might have from wealth alone. Passing the test at the imperial level made a man famous in his time. In over 1300 years of the *keju* there were only 596 *zhuangyuan* (Xiao, 1992).

Because passing the *keju* truly had extraordinary value, men spared no expense to hire tutors and protect their time for study. Women were not eligible to take the examination, but a literate mother or wife might help a man prepare for it. Chinese literature is full of stories of the *keju*, its overwhelming importance in examinees' lives, and the extremes men went to in the hopes of passing it. The obsession with study is captured by numerous ancient Chinese idioms and sayings which survive and are widely used today to encourage diligence. Following are three of them:

Wànbān jiē xiàpǐn, wéi yǒu dúshū gāo (万般皆下品，唯有读书高; "Being a scholar is exalted above all other occupations"). Historically, the implication of the adage was that learning—meaning study to pass examinations—is the purpose of life, rather than the means to any other end or an expression of personal interest.

Xuanliang cigu (悬梁刺股; "To tie one's hair to the house beam and jab one's thigh with an awl"). The idiom combines two historical references. Su Qin (380–284 BCE) was a very poor man who became a diplomat through years of diligent study followed by self-promotion. He had a crucial role in uniting six kingdoms in an alliance against the more powerful state of Qin during China's Warring States period (475–221 BCE). He eventually became the prime minister of the six kingdoms. During his years of intensive study, he would stab himself in the thigh with an awl to keep himself awake. In the later years of the eastern Han Dynasty (225 CE–220 CE), a man named Sun Jing was a widely renowned scholar. In his youth he would study through the night, keeping himself awake by tying one end of a rope to his hair and the other to a roofbeam to keep his head erect. While gross physical self-abuse seldom happens among contemporary Chinese students, sleep deprivation is widespread, and idioms like *xuanliang cigu* encourage it. Sleep deprivation, usually related to late-night homework and study, is associated with both depression and externalizing behavior problems in contemporary Chinese adolescents (Y. Wang et al., 2017).

Feiqin wangshi ("Stay up all night, forget about food"). This idiom was initially used in *The Family Instructions of Master Yan*, a book of personal philosophy and practical advice by Yan Zhitui (531 CE – 591 CE), a talented man from a noble family who served in official positions in several Chinese states. Yan was also a painter, calligrapher, and musician. Yan wrote the idiom to encourage his descendants to study. In modern times it refers both to intense study and to diligent work. Students might use it to describe cramming before an examination. Interestingly, in Yan's book he advises his progeny to study music and arts but not to become excessively proficient at them, lest they be called upon to provide entertainment for men of higher rank. This idea is carried forward by those contemporary Chinese parents who provide their children with extracurricular instruction in music and art but would discourage their child if they wished to pursue a career in the visual or performing arts.

The obsession of generations of Chinese with the *keju* was captured and ridiculed in a collection of satirical stories, *Rúlín Wàishǐ* (儒林外史; *The Scholars*) by Wu Jingzi (吴敬梓, 1701–1754), which was published in 1750 (Wu, 2008). *Rulin Waishi* rapidly became a classic in China. Stories described men going to absurd lengths to pass the examination. In one tale, a studious protagonist passes the test at the provincial level in his 50s after years of attempts, only to babble incoherently after hearing he had passed. Before passing, he was treated with scorn and abuse by everyone including family members; immediately afterward, he was treated with respect and deference. Those who had scoffed now humbled themselves before the noble scholar.

Wu ridiculed the idea of choosing civil servants by their knowledge of Confucianism, pointing out the hypocrisy of the system. He told stories about men with excellent formal knowledge of Confucian ethics whose actual behavior was immoral, corrupt, and sometimes cruel and exploitative. He conveyed both genuine respect for the Confucian moral code and contempt for how it was vainly cited by despicable characters.

Trauma of the "Lost Decade" and the Restoration of the National Examination

The *keju* ended with the fall of the Qing Dynasty in 1905. A national examination for college entrance was instituted by the People's Republic of China in 1952, but it did not assume its current form until 1977, a year after the end of the Cultural Revolution of 1966–1976. During the "lost decade" of the Cultural Revolution there were official persecution of intellectuals, attacks on educational institutions, disparagement of ideas and culture associated with the West, and humiliation of people thought to be too "bourgeois" in their background or outlook. Merely being well educated or from a prosperous family could make a person a target even if they personally were apolitical. University professors, urban medical specialists, performing artists, successful businesspeople, and people with relatives living in Western countries would be sent to internal exile in rural areas, where they were required to do manual work, were treated disrespectfully, and often were physically and verbally abused. Critics of the regime might be imprisoned, tortured, or executed. Capital punishment was given for purely ideological offenses, sometimes targeting public intellectuals whose opinions were influential with the masses. Millions were forced to undergo sessions of "self-criticism" in which compulsory confession of their "reactionary bourgeois thinking" would be followed by public humiliation.

Some critics of the Cultural Revolution were labeled as *jīngshénbìng* (精神病; "mentally ill") and incarcerated and abused in mental hospitals or in prisons. This added to the already great stigma of inpatient psychiatric treatment. Depression and post-traumatic distress disorder (PTSD) were frequent consequences of the abuse of well-educated people. Many eminent academics, professionals, and writers died by suicide.

Between 1970 and 1976, admission to China's universities was determined solely by political considerations, with workers, peasants, and soldiers (*gōngnóng bīng dàxuéshēng*; 工农兵大学生) receiving preference without regard for their academic performance. This subsequently lowered the perceived value of university degrees received in China during the 1970s.

China's intellectual class, its universities, and its social capital were rehabilitated starting in 1977 under the leadership of Deng Xiaoping (1904–1997), who later initiated a process of "reform and opening up" (gǎi gé kāi fàng; 改革开放). Since 1977, China has had the *gaokao*, the modern equivalent of the the *keju*, as the sole criterion for admission to the universities of mainland China. Of course, the *gaokao*, is only a college entrance examination and it does not ensure lifetime status and security as the *keju* once did. The content of the *gaokao* now includes Chinese, mathematics, a foreign language (most often English), and three elective subjects drawn from the sciences and humanities. Recalling the *keju*, the Chinese portion of the *gaokao* includes content on ancient poetry and "ancient cultural knowledge," including precise memory of classical quotations (Chinese Ministry of Education, 2018).

When the *gaokao* was instituted in 1977 there was a huge backlog of qualified applicants for higher education, from teenagers to adults in their late 30s, whose academic aspirations had been thwarted for 10 years. Competition was extreme: 5.7 million people took the examination, but only about 4% were admitted to China's universities that year (Gu & Magaziner, 2016; Y. Wang, 2017).

Much irreversible damage had been done. It was impossible for many talented and ambitious people to resume their education or to return to professional work at the same level as before the Cultural Revolution. People who were in their late teens at the beginning of the "lost decade" were now in their late 20s, and most of those who would have qualified for admission to a university before the Cultural Revolution were not able to attend one in the period after it. The faculties of Chinese universities had been decimated, and it took many years for the quality of their education to be fully restored.

Many people who emigrated from China to Western countries in the wake of the Cultural Revolution came with personal histories of trauma, loss, and/or depression related to that catastrophic period. When immigrant parents' educational or occupational aspirations had been thwarted, they usually expected their children to fulfill their dreams. In a culture of filial piety, parental wishes easily become children's obligations. In addition to culturally-based expectations, children's natural sympathy for their parents' suffering would add to their motivation to achieve for their parents' sake as well as their own.

While the *keju* ended in 1905, its spirit still pervades the Chinese educational system. Chinese education is focused on examinations. While there are critics of test-centered schooling among educated Chinese and some contemporary urban Chinese schools place non-traditional emphasis on teamwork, creativity, and problem-solving, the predominant culture of Chinese schools remains test-centric. Both parents and schools often "teach to the test"—an approach to education described by the metaphor of force-feeding a duck to create foie gras (*Tiányā shì jiàoxué*; 填鸭式教学; literally "duck-filling teaching").

Worldwide, many Chinese people regard receiving top scores on standardized examinations like the SAT, the Test of English as a Foreign Language (TOEFL), or the Graduate Record Examination and subsequently entering Harvard (or another similarly iconic university) as equivalent to passing the *keju* in imperial China. Such an accomplishment would imply a lifetime of status and security for the successful examinee and would bring honor to the student's parents and ancestors.

While college entrance examinations like the SAT and the *gaokao* are most important, stereotypical Chinese parents have strong feelings about their child's performance on every test. Children are expected to get perfect scores on tests in primary and secondary school. If they are not native English speakers and plan to study in the U.S., they are expected to ace the TOEFL. Test scores, rather than the underlying learning, are the explicit goal; and a child's getting anything less than a perfect score on any test can be an occasion for criticism, the withholding of affection, or even punishment, as described in the case history of Nikita Guo. If a child has neither interest in nor aptitude for a subject, that is simply a reason for them to study it longer and harder, still aiming for a perfect score on every test.

Many Chinese parents worry that their child will "lose at the starting line"— that they will already be behind their peers at the start of the first grade. In a famous case, a 2-year old boy began to lose his hair (develop alopecia areata) from the stress of taking five courses: English, mathematics, piano, painting, and how to emcee a show. The boy's parents sought to enroll him in a prestigious preschool at age 3, and the courses were intended to prepare him to compete for admission. When he was "too naughty to sit still" for the five classes, his mother would urge him to try harder. He frequently would awaken at night with anxiety attacks (LaiTimes, 2022). A Hong Kong television series, *No Starting Line*, depicted parents' extreme behavior related to their children's education. In one episode, a mother reads to her unborn child in English so that her baby could "win in the womb." Some of her friends aimed to "win before conception" by planning for their child to be born in January, the birth month associated with the highest rate of acceptance at some sought-after preschools (Daydaynews, 2019).

Filial Piety, Bonds of Love, and Unspoken Rules

The ethical basis of Chinese society has been, and continues to be, Confucianism, a collectivist ethos that creates a harmonious society through a structure of hierarchical, authoritarian relationships: rulers over subjects, parents over children, and men over women. While the superior parties hold power over the inferior ones, they are expected to develop their own morality so that they do not abuse their authority.

Of the three hierarchical relationships, that of parents and children is given greatest emphasis in Confucian thought. As discussed in the first part of this book in connection with the care of older adults in China, *filial piety and obedience (xiàoshùn;* 孝顺) is an organizing principle of Chinese society that touches everyone, irrespective of their personal religious/spiritual/philosophical beliefs or their familiarity with the Confucian classics. Confucian principles are the basis of the national ethos of Japan and South Korea, which deliberately imported Chinese philosophy and customs hundreds of years ago. However, filial piety, though important in Japanese and Korean cultures, does not predominate in them as it does in the culture of China.

Filial piety is the subject of the book *Xiàojīng* (孝經; usually translated as *The Classic of Filial Piety*; Zeng, 2008), one of the 13 Confucian texts that would be memorized by a candidate for the Imperial Examination. *Xiaojing* is attributed to Confucius' disciple Zeng Shen (aka Zengzi; 曾子; 505–435 BCE), the teacher of Confucius' grandson, who subsequently taught Mencius (aka Meng Zi; 孟子; 372–289 BCE). To quote some of its main ideas:

身体发肤，受之父母，不敢毁伤，孝之始也.
"The body, hair and skin, all have been received from the parents, and so one doesn't dare damage them—that is the beginning of *xiao*." (chapter 1)

立身行道, 扬名于后世, 以显父母, 孝之终也.
"Establishing oneself, practicing The Way, spreading the fame of one's name to posterity, so that one's parents become renowned—that is the end of *xiao*." (chapter 2)

用天之道，分地之利，谨身节用，以养父母，此庶人之孝也.
"Using Heaven's Way, sharing in Earth's bounties, being prudent with their persons and thrifty in their expenditure, in order to support their parents—this is the *xiao* of the common people." (chapter 6)

孝莫大于严父.
"In *xiao* nothing is greater than revering the father." (chapter 9)

子曰：孝子之丧亲也，哭不偯，礼无容,言不文, 服美不安, 闻乐不乐, 食旨不甘, 此哀戚之情也.
"The Teacher said, 'When a *xiao* son loses his parent, he cries without trying to stop himself, his politeness is without pleasantry, his words are without adornment, when he dresses in fine clothes, he feels uncomfortable, when he hears music, he does not feel joy, and when he eats delicious food it is not tasty. This is sadness and grief.'" (chapter 18)

Many Chinese parents feel that their children are their possessions, making it natural that they would dominate them, "design their lives," and be both controlling and protective. According to the Confucian ethos, a child's goal is to enhance their parents' and ancestors' status through accomplishments—and not to pursue their own dreams and ambitions. Thrift is a great virtue, and support of parents is the highest priority. When parents sacrifice materially to support their children's education, the children should feel guilty and ashamed if they fail to meet high expectations for their performance. As suggested by the adjective *yán* (translatable as "strict," "severe") in the adage about revering the father, harsh discipline is permitted if done with the goal of reinforcing filial piety.

Severe and persistent anhedonia—as distinguished from sadness and heartache from missing the deceased person—would be a sign of depression from a modern psychiatric perspective, but it is praised here if the bereaved person has lost a parent. Ideal filial piety requires symptoms of depression after loss of a parent, not just ordinary grief.

Of all Confucian principles, filial piety has shown the most universality and the greatest persistence. The ideas of material support and unconditional respect for parents are endorsed by adults in China regardless of their generation, region of the country, urban or rural status, gender, level of education, knowledge of a foreign language, and employment status (Y. Hu & Scott, 2016).

Filial piety provides Chinese children with goals and direction—their aim is to obey, please, and bring honor to their parents. When the children's best efforts to obey their parents and meet their expectations are not adequate in their parents' eyes, under Confucian ethics the parents are authorized to utilize whatever means seem necessary to enforce compliance—including harsh discipline or the withholding of affection. More than half of Chinese parents acknowledge using corporal punishment, and more than 75% use various forms of psychological aggression with their children (M. Wang & Liu, 2014). Occasions for harsh discipline include a child's speaking disrespectfully to parents, being disobedient, engaging in risky behavior, and performing academically below expectations.

Traditional Chinese parents' discipline of their children can be arbitrary and capricious, and sometimes it is the consequence of a parent's problem with substance use, PTSD, depression, or BD. When children's punishments are related more to their parents' issues and less to their behavior, adverse effects of harsh discipline on children's mental health are greater. The long-term consequences of parental physical abuse also are greater when the abuse is combined with a lack of parental warmth and affection (Carroll et al., 2013). It is not unusual for Chinese parents to withhold their affection from their children when they are disappointed in their behavior or academic performance. Well-intentioned traditional parents may view their discipline as being for the good of the child's moral development and success in life, even when it causes their children emotional distress and might contribute to future mental health problems. The laws of modern China reflect a conception of children as virtually the property of their parents. If a child in China is severely injured by a parent's physical abuse and the injuries lead to death, the responsible parent will be imprisoned for between 2 and 7 years—a remarkably light punishment by Western standards (Criminal Law of the People's Republic of China, Article 260, English translation by International Labour Organization, 2023). When parents in China beat their children in public, bystanders rarely comment, and police rarely pay attention.

While filial piety has its dark side, expressed as an excess of harsh discipline in Chinese childrearing, it has a positive aspect related to the development of children's self-discipline and goal-directedness. When children know they can both please and honor their parents by hard work and academic success, they have a positive motivation to study that ideally becomes internalized and persistent. Under this scenario the child transitions "from learning for love to love of learning" (Ekstein & Motto, 1969). However, this genuinely positive phenomenon—one that contributes to the widely appreciated accomplishments of Chinese students—can turn into a negative if the goal of obeying, pleasing, and honoring parents interferes with the child's normal development of autonomy, age-appropriate independence, self-confidence, and the sense of an authentic identity.

Face (*Miànzi*; 面子), Upward Comparison (*Pānbǐ*; 攀比), and Climbing the Ivy (*Páténg*; 爬藤)

Confucian culture is one in which self-construal is interdependent; there is no self without a context of relationships to others. In such a culture the way one is seen by others is not just a *reaction* to who one is—it is essential to *determining* who one is. Among the self-conscious emotions, shame is more powerful than guilt. A person's external face—how they are seen by others—is essential to their self-concept, so a loss of face can be felt very deeply. A gain or loss of face by a child always implies a gain or loss of face by the parents. One would virtually never hear Chinese parents say, as some Western parents do, that they would take neither credit for their children's accomplishments nor blame for their faults.

In Chinese culture there are two aspects of face: *mianzi* and *liǎn* (脸). *Mianzi* is the aspect related to physical appearance, social status, credentials, connections, accomplishments, material circumstances, and social behavior. Loss of *mianzi* (*diūmiànzi*; 丢面子) is a loss of status that can be embarrassing or humiliating but is not deeply shameful. *Lian* connotes a loss of face related to personal failure, misconduct, or, at worst, immoral behavior. Loss of *lian* (*diūliǎn*; 丢脸) is always associated with shame (*xiūchǐ*; 羞耻). A parent could gain *mianzi* from a child's acceptance by Harvard or MIT and could lose *mianzi* from a child's performing poorly on the SAT. The parent would lose *lian* if the child were caught cheating on a test or plagiarizing an essay. Loss of face of either kind can cause emotional distress for everyone in the family. Fear of losing face can block Chinese people from considering ways out of personal distress that would otherwise be attractive—such as a student's seeking treatment for clinical depression or returning to China to complete college if their initial experience as an international student were unbearably lonely.

Conspicuous display of wealth does not necessarily bring people or their families a good face, though it may evoke envy or admiration in others that the wealthy person might appreciate. The term used to describe hedonistic and ostentatious offspring of newly rich Chinese, *fùèrdài* (富二代; "rich second generation"), has a pejorative connotation. Young adults seen as merely rich are widely disliked and disrespected in mainland China. The pursuit of *mianzi* motivates many rich young Chinese to pursue elite education in the West so that they will not be regarded with contempt as merely wealthy and not worthy. *Fuerdai* ccount for a meaningful slice of Chinese international students. Some *fuerdai* are conspicuously wealthy yet naïve because of overprotected childhoods. If such students develop impaired judgment due to depression, substance use, or extreme loneliness, they can become targets for personal victimization and financial exploitation.

A Chinese person pursuing *mianzi* will be continually conscious of the face of other Chinese people (whether in China or in a Chinese immigrant community). They will take notice of others with more accomplishments, higher status, or greater wealth. Because a child's education is a family project and a child's accomplishments directly affect a parent's face, a parent will be highly aware of the accomplishments of other Chinese parents' children. They will take little comfort in knowing of others who are worse off or whose children have accomplished less. The eyes of comparison are always directed upward. *Pānbǐ* (攀比; the two ideograms signify "climbing comparison") is a usual practice for many Chinese parents, both in their dialogues with one another and in their conversations with their children. If another family's child has outperformed their own on a test or in a competition, a parent will be critical of their child and very likely anxious and/or self-critical. Parents might shame their children, telling them to look at another family's child who has outperformed them, perhaps saying that their child lacks ability and must do more to make up for it or that their child is smarter or more talented than the competitor and ought to do much better. The child is blamed for causing the parent to lose face. In the process of *panbi* it is not important whether the parents' expectation for their child is realistic. There often is an underlying belief that nothing is impossible if one works hard enough at it.

There is, of course, nothing uniquely Chinese about basing one's subjective social status on comparison with others deemed to be sufficiently like oneself. What distinguishes the process of upward comparison engaged in by many Chinese people is a combination of three elements: especially great importance of subjective social status to one's self-concept, extreme valuation of academic accomplishment among potential bases for subjective social status, and comparison with other Chinese families even when there are many relevant differences apart from nationality.

Panbi can produce symptomatic anxiety in the parents that drives them to be more extreme in the pressure they put on their children and to be deeply distressed if their children do not meet their expectations for academic performance. Competition of parents with one another can lead a parent to make choices that go against their intuition about what would be best for their own child. Competition between parents might underlie the publicized cases of urban Chinese parents enrolling their children in intensive preschool programs that are grossly developmentally inappropriate. *Panbi* might also be at work when middle-class Chinese parents—either in China or in Western countries—sacrifice financially to move to expensive neighborhoods with outstanding public schools and then engage in upward comparisons with their wealthier neighbors that lower their own subjective status. Parents, painfully feeling their loss of subjective status, might then pressure their child by reminding them how much they have sacrificed to move for the sake of the child's education.

The idea of moving to a different neighborhood for a child's education, though seemingly contemporary, has ancient roots in Chinese culture. The Chinese idiom *Mèng mǔ sān qiān* (孟母三迁; "Mencius' mother moved three times") refers to the widowed mother of the Mencius moving from one neighborhood to another when he was a child, until she found one near a school of Confucianism. In that neighborhood her son observed and emulated the courteous and studious behavior of the scholars around him, rather than the irreverent and crass behavior that he had observed and copied when he and his mother had lived close to a cemetery and close to a marketplace.

Competition between parents related to their children's academic success can have adverse effects on parents' mental health. It can diminish bonding social capital that helps people tolerate stress without becoming depressed. If the parents become depressed, there is a greater likelihood that they will unreasonably criticize, harshly discipline, or withhold affection from their children, with traumatic effects that raise their children's lifetime risk of depression.

A child's admission to an Ivy League university, Harvard above all, is a consuming goal for many Chinese families. This goal is described by the word *pateng*—literally, "climbing the vine," but in this context, "climbing the ivy." Getting into the Ivy League is like climbing a vine. A child's Ivy League education raises the status of the family. China has had several bestselling books on how to get one's child into Harvard, for example, *Harvard Girl Liu Yiting* (W. Liu & X. Zhang, 2000).

Pateng is more about face and upward comparison than it is about what would necessarily be best for a child's education, let alone the child's mental health. But if climbing the ivy is the parents' passion, a filial child will make it their own and might feel great disappointment if they do not reach the top of the vine. If a student has successfully climbed the ivy and then fails academically or must take leave because of depression, concern over loss of face and its potential impact on parents can make it much harder for the student to find a way forward. A gifted college student with depression or a bipolar spectrum condition might be able to complete undergraduate and graduate degrees at a different highly ranked university on a more flexible schedule compatible with the course of their illness. But from the psychologically myopic viewpoint of depression, they might only see failure—falling off the vine and crashing to earth.

Report the Good News, Conceal the Bad (*Bào xǐ bù bào yōu,* 报喜不报忧)

Unlike many American parents who encourage their children to express their feelings, many Chinese parents pay little attention to children's complaints unless they suggest physical illness or an urgent need. Similarly, Chinese parents tend to be less physically demonstrative with hugs and kisses and affectionate words than American parents of non-Asian ethnicities. A secondary school student living at home typically would not be encouraged to tell their parents about feeling low, and if they did express sadness or discouragement, the parental response might be "you'll get over it." In several of the cases at the start of this chapter, students not only did not disclose their distressed mental state to their parents but even had positive conversations with their parents a few days before their deaths. They concealed their negative moods and reported only good news.

A culturally based pattern of concealment of negative emotion is one reason that Chinese and Chinese American students usually do not seek help (including consultation with a psychiatrist or psychologist) when ill with depression. Another is stigmatization of psychiatric diagnoses and treatments, with inpatient treatment stigmatized most of all. Most depressed Chinese adolescents and young adults would be reluctant to tell their parents about depression, to avoid causing them worry and concern. Filial piety and concern about face will make a depressed student even more likely to conceal their problem.

Many of those Chinese parents who would take their child's complaint of depression seriously would be concerned about not only their child's health but also the potential adverse effects on the child's academic performance and the potential for a loss of face from either diminished performance or the stigma of a psychiatric diagnosis. On the other hand, they might see the child's complaining, rather than their depressive symptoms, as the problem. Such parents might think that their child will get over whatever is bothering them and see mental health care as a negative, risking stigma and costing money better spent directly on their child's education. They might be worried that a diagnosis of depression

would "go on their record" at the university and damage their child's prospects. Frequently encountered beliefs include the following:
- Depression if mild is to be borne without complaint.
- Depression if more severe might be acknowledged to family but should be hidden from outsiders if feasible.
- Treatment should be pursued with great caution because it will be stigmatizing, expensive, probably unnecessary, and possibly dangerous if it involves medications.
- Even if one is miserable with depression, study or work should continue.

Students whose parents have these beliefs are likely to behave in conformity with them because a child who properly respected their parents would not challenge them over such opinions.

Issues of Chinese International Students

In addition to the generic stresses of college and graduate/professional school, and the further stress of studying outside one's native country, Chinese international students at universities in Western countries may have issues associated with Chinese culture and its differences from the culture of high-income Western countries. One set of issues concerns adaptation to Western (and especially American) academic culture. Students with secondary education in China are skilled at listening attentively, carefully reading texts, and extracting the main ideas and details; but some have difficulty writing essays with original perspectives on what they have learned. Students who do extremely well on standardized tests may be less adept at expressing their opinions or personal perspectives, especially in real time during classroom discussion. Some, whose lives before going to college were narrowly focused on academics, lack life experiences that inform the viewpoints of most classmates who had grown up in the West. International students in the U.S. who are unfamiliar with American history and culture might lack knowledge of people and events often referenced in essays and dialogues by Americans—potentially putting them at a disadvantage when making written and oral presentations of their opinions.

American academic culture contrasts with the authoritarian culture of education in China and in many other non-Western countries. Though in China's largest cities there are some schools with more liberal educational practices, in most Chinese schools, teachers are authorities not to be questioned, and teaching is focused on preparing students for examinations that emphasize rote recall of facts and concepts. When essays are required, the structure, style, and content are highly specified. Students are largely passive consumers of content delivered by or assigned by the teachers.

The acculturative stress for Chinese international students will be greater in courses that require more creative output and/or impromptu classroom dialogue from students. Even students with high scores on written examinations of English proficiency might not initially have the verbal skills to perform well in spontaneous interchanges.

The authoritarian, examination-oriented model of secondary education entails intense competition among students for top test scores, with relatively few collaborative activities. International students initially educated in that model might lack the skills and experience needed for effective teamwork. When they first participate in academic team projects, they might be oversensitive to their peers' constructive criticism and suggestions, have trouble contributing to others' work, or compare themselves unfavorably with their American teammates, as Nikita Guo did when she did her first team project at MIT.

Another difference between American and Chinese academic culture concerns the basis of grading in undergraduate courses. The norm in China is for grades to be based on a final examination, or perhaps a final and a midterm. In America, course grades often give significant weight to class participation, homework assignments, and/or quizzes. When this is the case, the traditional Chinese approach of cramming for the big examination will not work, and it is possible that a student with a history of top test performance in China will not do as well in the American system.

Most Chinese international students will successfully respond to the academic acculturative challenge by learning—and sometimes perfecting—new skills (Heng, 2018). They will find faculty and/or peers willing to help them acquire new speaking and writing skills. For some Chinese students, this is a main attraction of study in the U.S. (Z. Li et al., 2017). However, students with fragile self-esteem, cognitive inflexibility, and a catastrophic approach to disappointment and criticism might be unable to deal with an acculturative challenge of several months a period of less-than-perfect grades and occasionally below-average performance.

For most undergraduates and for all graduate students, mentorship and advice from faculty are important aspects of education. The most productive mentoring relationships require mutual trust, good communication, and a measure of self-disclosure by the student. Chinese students often have little experience with Western-style student–faculty relationships and might not be forthcoming about their concerns or be willing to disagree with a professor. Even when a faculty member understands the acculturative challenge for a Chinese student, the student might be reluctant to reveal a need for help in adapting to Western academic culture.

For Chinese international students from middle-class families, the cost of higher education in English-speaking countries can be formidable. The average annual cost of a year of college in America can be five to ten times the annual income of a Chinese family. This places enormous pressure on the student to excel in college and to succeed occupationally afterward. However, starting salaries in China for people with American undergraduate degrees are not much higher than those for people with degrees from first-rank Chinese universities. If the student has majored in STEM, economics, business administration, or another in-demand field, they might be able to have a high starting salary in the U.S., but getting a visa permitting long-term employment beginning immediately after graduation can be problematic. Anxiety about money and post-graduation plans can add to students' stress, with students especially vulnerable to mental health concerns if their future plans are not settled as graduation approaches.

If an international graduate student is accustomed only to hierarchical relationships with authoritarian professors, they may be vulnerable to exploitation by a thesis advisor. For example, an unscrupulous faculty member might withhold approval of a Chinese student's doctoral thesis to take advantage of the student's low-paid labor as a teaching or research assistant. Such a situation can lead to depression or even suicidal despair. Other students might have difficulty making the transition from working under a professor's direct supervision to fully independent research and scholarship.

Chinese international students' concerns about face have complex effects. In a survey of Chinese international students at American universities, respondents endorsing more face concerns (e.g., "I do not want to make mistakes in front of other people," "I hesitate to ask for help because I think my request will be an inconvenience to others,") had more symptoms of depression and anxiety than those who didn't; but they were more likely to endorse a statement that they would seek professional help if they had a mental health problem, perhaps hoping that such help would prevent them from losing face by visibly displaying signs of the problem. However, they were also more likely to experience self-stigma, endorsing statements like "It would make me feel inferior to ask a therapist for help," and "Seeking psychological help would make me feel less intelligent." Students with lower proficiency in English had more face concerns (Ma et al., 2021).

Because face concerns have complex effects, a clinician beginning work with a depressed Chinese international student should be aware of how important face is to the student and whether in their case self-stigma or a wish to prevent loss of face is a larger issue. In the former case, anti-stigma education might be especially relevant, where in the latter case reassurance about privacy and advice on how to prevent disruption of the student's studies might be a higher priority. When a clinician evaluates a depressed Chinese international student with limited English proficiency, the student's potential face concerns should be assessed when considering a referral to a Chinese-speaking psychotherapist. For most such students, easier communication about emotional issues will be most important; but for some, a concern about loss of face with a member of the Chinese-speaking community will have a greater negative effect on the potential for a therapeutic relationship.

Chinese international students are less likely to pursue treatment for diagnosed mental health conditions than students who are U.S. residents. In addition to stigma, the cost of care, and finding time for therapy in a packed schedule, students can have realistic concerns about the disruption of their education by unwanted medical leave and the impact of such leave on their student visa status. And, since sharing of sensitive clinical information with university authorities is required to receive medical leave, they can have concerns about confidentiality and the potential for downstream effects on their academic and occupational prospects. Universities vary in how effectively they address such concerns. Because China is a low-trust country, many students would start with the assumption that unknown others would find out about one's mental health problems, with probable negative consequences.

Intergenerational Cultural Conflicts of ABCs and "Generation 1.5"

American students with Chinese immigrant parents, whether they were born in America (ABCs, or second-generation immigrants) or in China and arrived in America as children or early adolescents ("Generation 1.5"), have different culturally-related depression risk factors from those of Chinese international students. They are proficient in colloquial as well as formal English and are familiar with American history and American campus culture. (Even so, those who arrived in adolescence probably will speak English with a foreign accent, which will increase their risk of being stereotyped.) They will have extensive contact with mainstream American culture through school, relationships with peers, and the media. They will be acculturated by the time they enter college; and, depending on how they are educated, how they are parented, and their personal interest in their heritage culture, they will be largely assimilated or largely bicultural. Even if they enter college as largely assimilated, they might choose while in college or post-graduation to explore their Chinese identity and perhaps embrace it, becoming better speakers of Chinese, spending more time with Chinese people, and engaging more with Chinese culture. Whether they are assimilated or bicultural, they almost always will be more acculturated than their parents—setting the stage for family conflict (S. Y. Kim et al., 2013).

Two major sources of intergenerational cultural conflict are communication problems and discrepant values. Cultural conflict can be expressed explicitly or indirectly by emotional distancing (*acculturative family distancing* [AFD]) (Hwang, 2006). Because the Chinese culture of filial respect and parental authority is not conducive to parent–child argument or to collaborative problem-solving in which a child's views are given equal weight, emotional distancing probably is more common than explicit conflict. At worst, adolescent and young adult ABCs and Generation 1.5 Chinese Americans will both feel distant from their parents and unaccepted by their American peers. Youths of Generation 1.5 might be more prone to acculturation-related family conflict than ABCs because their parents usually have spent less time in the U.S. than the parents of ABCs, and thus tend to be less acculturated (Ying et al., 2001). AFD is associated with depressive symptoms and an increased risk of clinical depression in both parents and children (Hwang & Wood, 2009; Hwang et al., 2010). Even if a Chinese American adolescent or young adult is depressed for reasons unrelated to family issues, AFD can reduce the emotional support they might get from their parents.

Communication issues are of two types: those related to direct spoken communication and those related to indirect communication. Problems in direct communication typically occur when parents are not proficient in English and children are not proficient in Chinese. Problems in indirect communication usually reflect parents' customarily using traditional Chinese high-context communication and children's customarily using mainstream American low-context communication.

Even when neither parents nor children are fully bilingual there seldom are problems with mundane communication about practical matters. However, details and nuances of important life events and feelings about them can be lost. Mainstream American culture allows for frank expression of strong feelings, including negative ones, with an expectation that family members will frequently speak of their affection for one another and that parental instructions and injunctions will be explicit. Traditional Chinese parents are sparing in their explicit expressions of affection for their children no matter how much they love them; their nurturing, protection, and care of their children are sufficient evidence of their love. (Parents see this as especially obvious if they have made extraordinary efforts or sacrifices to immigrate or to provide their children with an excellent education.) They expect their children to be restrained in their expression of negative emotions and disagreement and to know their parents' expectations for their behavior—requiring only occasional and subtle reminders of them. If children are highly acculturated, they may find their less acculturated parents to be cold and unsupportive and miss some of their parents' messages about what behavior is acceptable and what is not. At the same time, their parents may find them lacking in filial respect, self-control, and/or age-appropriate manners.

A clinician assessing the contribution of intergenerational cultural conflict to depression in a patient of either generation might explore the dimensions of communication differences and value differences in a way that recognizes that the two dimensions are themselves multifaceted. For both communication and value issues, the two generations can have discrepant views of the same issue—for example, a parent finding a child's communication disrespectful, while the child sees nothing wrong with it. Positive and negative aspects of communication are not necessarily correlated; a person of the younger generation might share very little with their parents but not say they feel a communication barrier. Understanding the details of a depressed patient's intergenerational cultural conflicts can help a clinician determine how much cultural conflict should be addressed in the treatment and whether it is realistic and desirable to directly include the other generation in the patient's treatment.

A psychometric analysis of AFD questionnaire responses by Chinese American high school students and their immigrant parents provides a useful framework for a clinician to explore the topic with a patient (Fujimoto & Hwang, 2014). The outcome of a factor analysis suggests the following content for an interview with a patient of the younger generation (each theme is illustrated by sample questions):

- Positive communication to parents: "Can you communicate how you feel to your parents?" "Do you talk about your problems with your parents?"
- Positive communication by parents: "Are your parents able to communicate how they feel to you?" "Do your parents share personal things with you?"
- Communication problems from the student's perspective: "Do you find you can get your basic point across with your parents, but it's hard for you to talk about things with them in greater depth?" "Do you feel like there is a communication barrier between you and your parents?"
- Communication problems from the parent(s)' perspective: "Do your parents feel like there is a communication barrier between them and you?" "Can your parents communicate basic or concrete needs to you but have a hard time communicating feelings and emotional needs?"
- Non-verbal communication problems from the student's perspective: "Do you sometimes misunderstand your parents' non-verbal communication?" "Do you sometimes have a hard time understanding the implied meanings behind your parents' verbal and non-verbal communication?"

- Non-verbal communication problems from the parents' perspective: "Do your parents sometimes misunderstand your non-verbal communication?" "Do your parents sometimes have a hard time understanding the implied meanings behind your verbal and non-verbal communication?"
- Understanding physical expressions of emotion (in both directions): "If your parents communicated emotional distress through physical symptoms, would you understand what the physical symptoms meant?" "If you communicated emotional distress through physical symptoms, would your parents understand what the physical symptoms meant?"
- Agreement on general values: "Do your parents and you share the same values?" "Do your parents and you agree on the relative importance of academics and social life? On when a person should begin dating? On the definition of success in life?"
- Disagreement on general values: "Do you and your parents disagree on what is important in life? On the roles that men and women should have? On how parents should treat children? On the importance of a social life? On the qualities that are important in a romantic partner?"
- Agreement on family values: "Are you and your parents equally concerned about how you appear before others? About how older people should be treated? About how much time family members should spend together? About the importance of family harmony? About putting family needs before individual needs?"
- Disagreement on family values: "Do you and your parents disagree on the importance of family?"

If there is insufficient time in a clinical interview to assess intergenerational cultural conflict, a clinician can ask a patient to complete a questionnaire dealing with the issue. Two such questionnaires that have been specifically validated with Chinese Americans are the Asian American Family Conflict Scale (FCS; R. M. Lee et al., 2000; S. Wu et al., 2017) and the Intercultural Conflict Inventory (ICI; Chung, 2001).

The FCS asks respondents how likely each of ten types of conflict is in their family—ranging from *almost never* (1) to *almost always* (5). For example, "Your parents tell you what to do with your life, but you want to make your own decisions." "Your parents want you to sacrifice personal interests for the sake of the family, but you feel this is unfair." "You have done well in school, but your parents' academic expectations always exceed your performance."

The ICI asks respondents how much each of 24 issues causes conflict in their family, with issues related to each of three domains. *Family Expectations* includes issues related to the young person's desire for greater independence and autonomy, with specific items including following cultural traditions, learning one's Asian language, expectations related to gender and birth order, closeness versus distance in various family relationships, and how much time to spend with the family, helping around the house, and helping in the family business (if applicable). *Education and Career* includes how much time to spend on studying, practicing music, and sports; the importance of academic achievement, materialism, and success; being compared to others; what college to attend, what to major in, and what career to choose. *Dating and Marriage* includes when to begin dating, whom to date, and whom to marry.

When engaging a depressed person from either the older or the younger generation in treatment and intergenerational cultural conflict is a relevant factor, it can be useful to identify the cultural conflicts explicitly and to reframe intergenerational conflict as acculturation-related rather than a reflection of personal faults or hurtful intentions on either side. Exploration of intergenerational cultural conflict that might contribute to an adolescent's or young adult's depression can be helpful in combatting the stigma of seeking psychotherapy or counseling: Such conflict can be legitimately normalized as a typical phenomenon in immigrant families where children acculturate more rapidly than their parents. Counseling to help an adolescent or young adult deal with acculturation-related conflict does not imply that anyone is "weak" or "mentally ill," and it might even be framed in terms of enabling the young person to be a better son or daughter to their immigrant parents.

When feasible, a clinician should encourage parents and children to develop bicultural competence, with the aim that adult immigrants better understand the values and communication style of mainstream American culture and that children of immigrants better understand those of traditional Chinese culture (Hwang, 2006). A therapeutic intervention with a family might help a child and their parents express positive feelings of attachment and commitment to the family while allowing for different levels of acculturation. The young person would be encouraged to show respect for their parents, to communicate with them frequently about important matters, to spend time together frequently, and to offer help when their parents need it. The parents would be encouraged to acknowledge that a devoted, loving, and respectful child might make some choices that break with tradition and that attachment, loyalty, and commitment to the family, time together, and honest communication can be preserved even when there are generational differences in other values and tastes.

In mainstream American culture, issues of autonomy and separation from parents usually are dealt with during a young person's adolescence. This often is followed by a stable and positive relationship between the young adult and the parents. By contrast, many young Chinese Americans do not address autonomy issues and challenge parental control until they are already young adults, shifting the task of negotiating a separate identity to a time when they are less able to rely on their parents for support.

Many Chinese parents have strong opinions—accompanied by expectations of their child's compliance—concerning which colleges are preferable, what they should study in college, what occupations would be acceptable, and whom they should and should not date or marry. If a student's parents made great personal sacrifices to immigrate for their children's sake, students might feel deeply indebted to their parents and be reluctant to disagree with them about important life choices. A student can face a painful choice between being true to themselves and deeply disappointing their parents.

AFD is a lesser problem, but still a relevant one, for those ABCs whose parents are highly educated, highly proficient in English, and relatively assimilated. Even in families of educated, successful, and highly-acculturated immigrants, parents' and children's values and priorities may differ, and communication about disagreements and negative emotions might be avoided or delayed.

Parenting style is relevant to the potential for conflict and the likelihood of depression both in children and in parents. Authoritarian parenting utilizes physical coercion, verbal hostility, and punitive practices to compel compliance with the parents' agenda. Authoritative parenting uses education, reasoning, and positive reinforcement of desirable behavior to enable children to become appropriately autonomous. Traditional, unassimilated Chinese parents typically tend toward authoritarian parenting, while those with a more bicultural or integrated identity typically have a less authoritarian, more authoritative style. Authoritative rather than authoritarian parenting by mothers is associated with less depression in mothers as well as in their children (Yu et al., 2016).

The association of intergenerational cultural conflict with depressive symptoms in second-generation adolescents and young adults has been shown not only for Chinese Americans but also for Asian Americans of several nationalities and for American Latino/as. Though specific values and their relative importance vary among nationalities, a common feature among immigrant families from non-Western cultures is that the native national culture is more collectivistic, is more gendered, and has more authoritarian parent–child relationships than mainstream American culture (Juang et al., 2007; S. Y. Kim et al., 2009; Lim et al., 2008).

ABCs and early childhood immigrants who are fully acculturated (either bicultural or assimilated) are likely to want social acceptance from classmates of other ethnicities. However, they may encounter stereotyping, social exclusion, and/or microaggressions; general anti-immigrant sentiment; and, in the U.S. since the COVID-19 pandemic began, overt or even violent expressions of anti-Asian hatred. When an assimilated student with weak ties to Chinese culture, who feels distant from their parents and other native Chinese people, encounters discrimination from Whites and from students of other ethnicities, they can feel alienated. If the student is not fluent in Chinese, they might experience social rejection from Chinese international students, adding to a feeling of cultural homelessness. Many ABCs experience the "perpetual foreigner" stereotype in America (e.g., "Your English is so good"), while also encountering disapproval or ridicule on a trip to China when they reveal they are not proficient in Chinese. Being stereotyped as a foreigner is associated with depressive symptoms in ABCs, as it is in second-generation immigrants of other Asian nationalities (Armenta et al., 2013). Chinese American adolescents from Generation 1.5 with low English proficiency often are treated as foreigners, experiencing either chronic daily discrimination or discriminatory victimization, both of which are associated with depressive symptoms (S. Y. Kim et al., 2011).

For even the most talented and privileged Chinese American adolescents, issues of acculturative stress, intergenerational cultural conflicts, and the aftereffects of authoritarian parenting can set the stage for depression. In less exceptional and advantaged Chinese American adolescents, an intersection of social determinants and culture-related issues underlies many cases of clinical depression. Factors predisposing to depression in Chinese American adolescents and young adults include intergenerational cultural conflict, harsh parenting, being a victim of discrimination or bullying, and being exposed to neighborhood violence, poverty, or economic precarity. Those born outside the U.S. will face additional stresses related to acculturation, and their English might be less than perfect. Chinese American adolescents, whether ABCs or of Generation 1.5, are more vulnerable to depression in their late teens than earlier (Zou et al., 2021).

Encounters with Student Health and Counseling Services

Whenever a suicide is reported in a university newspaper, it is accompanied by information for students about where to call for "help" or "counseling" if they feel desperate or suicidal. (The situation is seldom framed as a medical issue to be addressed by physicians, let alone psychiatrists.) In their orientation of new students, universities inform them about student health services, including psychological services. It would seem reasonable to assume that all students are aware of the existence of services for those with depression or suicidal ideas, but at least for Chinese international students this has not been the case. In the study of Yale students cited above (Han et al., 2013), 27% responded that they did not know about mental health and counseling services on campus.

Relatively few Chinese and Chinese American university students make use of counseling or psychological services when they are depressed or even suicidal (Tummala-Narra et al., 2021; Zheng & West-Olatunji, 2016). Depression of moderate or greater severity is itself associated with a diminished likelihood of seeking help (J. E. Kim et al., 2015). Worries about stigma or cost, hopelessness about treatment effectiveness, and impatience with delays in connecting with a counselor all will be greater when a person's depression amplifies negative thoughts and feelings. Even when services are used, they might be ineffective. Many Chinese students who died by suicide did talk to clinicians from their university's student health or counseling service in the days or weeks before their deaths. A culturally-aware perspective suggests some reasons why Chinese and Chinese American students might avoid student health services and why the outcomes of counseling migt be disappointing.

The public stigma of depression is greater in China than in the United States. Chinese immigrant parents commonly stigmatize depression and may be reluctant to acknowledge it in their children. The combination of a tradition of filial piety, parental stigmatization of depression, and concerns about loss of face can make a Chinese student relatively immune to anti-stigma messaging from the university or mental health advocacy organizations. Depression itself is associated with decreased stigma tolerance, and intolerance of perceived stigma is a major reason depressed students do not seek help (Ting & Hwang, 2009). Both perceived stigma and self-stigma prevent help-seeking (Pedersen & Paves, 2014), and self-stigma alone can prevent help-seeking even when the depressed person is in a supportive and non-stigmatizing environment. This argues for designing student mental health services to detect and intervene quickly with mild depression, taking advantage of a time when a student perceives a need but does not fear stigma so much that they will not seek help.

Often, a Chinese American or Chinese international student who suffers from depression in college has had an episode of clinical depression—or ongoing symptoms and signs of depression—that began when they were in secondary school. Parents of such students have directly seen the signs of their children's illness. If a teenager is evidently depressed and their parents express no concern and take no action, they convey a powerful message to their child that they should accept and cope with the situation—and perhaps that their parents would be disappointed if they needed mental health care.

Students not worried about parental stigmatization might still be worried about stigmatization or distancing by Chinese or Chinese American peers. It is striking how often the friends and classmates of a Chinese student who died by suicide say that the person said nothing to them about their emotional distress. This was true for many of the students in the case histories. Classmates' postmortem recollections usually describe smiles, warmth, and good feelings rather than expressions of distress that might warn of a potential suicide.

Some depressed students will not contact student health services for fear of being forced to leave the university if they are open about their depression and/or suicidal ideation. Even occasional cases of Chinese students not being readmitted after taking leave for treatment of depression or students being forced to withdraw after disclosing suicidal ideation will become widely known and influential in the Chinese student community. While any student of any ethnicity might feel distressed about being forced out of a college because of depression or suicidality, Chinese students can bear an additional burden of shame or guilt relating to loss of face and/or to distressing awareness that their extended families had made financial sacrifices to help support their education. This can make their forced withdrawal from classes even harder to bear. The combination of thwarted belongingness and perceived burdensomeness can set the stage for suicide, as it did in the case of Luchang Wang.

The tradition of confidentiality and patient autonomy in healthcare is less established in China than in the United States. Chinese international students might be especially concerned about a getting a formal record of "mental illness" that could have negative implications for advanced study opportunities, employment, or immigration. The parents of an ABC or Generation 1.5 Chinese student might have similar concerns and pass them on to their child.

If these concerns are not limiting, students can be deterred by a long wait to be seen by a clinician or counselor. A person suffering acute emotional distress can find waiting for a week or more to see a counselor to be unbearable. They might deal with the pain in a less adaptive way, through some form of self-destructive behavior. Even students expressing explicit suicidal plans to university staff or on-call clinicians might have to wait several days for an appointment with a counselor. At many universities' student health services, it is difficult for a depressed student who needs one to find a bilingual counselor or one familiar with their culture. Another limiting concern is the capacity of most college counseling services to provide continuing care. Several months of weekly or twice-weekly psychotherapy might be clinically optimal for a student with moderate to severe depression accompanied by family and acculturation-related issues, but a college counseling service would rarely have the resources to provide it.

Referring students to hospital emergency services, psychiatric clinics, and other outside resources might reduce waiting time; but outside services usually would involve substantial out-of-pocket cost for the student or family. A depressed student from a family of modest means might feel that they cannot afford such care, are undeserving of care, or should be ashamed of spending the family's money on it. Although globalization has begun to have an impact on attitudes toward mental health issues, mainstream Chinese culture does not at present support the expenditure of large sums of money on something as intangible as psychotherapy.

Students with milder forms of depression might get substantial benefit from education in stress management and interpersonal conflict resolution, assistance in building their local social capital, and coaching on academic strategy. These will be insufficient, however, for a student with a severe major depressive episode, a bipolar spectrum disorder, or depression comorbid with another problem like chronic anxiety, problematic substance use, an eating disorder, PTSD, or a significant general medical illness. The likelihood of one of these more serious problems being present in someone seeking student mental health services is greater in Chinese and Chinese American students because presenting for care at all often requires their overcoming significant reluctance. When a Chinese international student or an unassimilated Chinese American student actively pursues mental health care, they should initially be presumed to have a serious problem, even if they appear to be to coping well with academic demands. Academic performance usually is the last thing to be lost as a Chinese student sinks into a severe depression.

The attitude of many traditional Chinese or Chinese American parents toward their child's getting psychotherapy can be contrasted with that of many Americans of Ashkenazic Jewish background. Often the latter would conceive of a child's getting psychotherapy as a positive action that might increase their chances of a happy life, and they would expect the therapist to be helpful. The child's acceptance of psychotherapy might be a viewed as a sign of maturity. While this is admittedly a comparison of stereotypes, empirical studies support group-level ethnic differences in attitudes toward psychotherapy (Midlarsky et al., 2012).

Effective management of depression, preventing functional impairment, and reducing suicide risk require rapid and accurate diagnosis. This almost always requires the involvement of a psychiatrist or an internist/psychologist team in carefully screening the student for the bipolar spectrum and for common psychiatric and general medical comorbidities of depression. An indiscriminate prescription of "counseling"—usually by a non-medical clinician, possibly with a prescription for a SSRI from a peripherally involved primary care provider—is not an acceptable substitute. Unfortunately, full psychiatric evaluations sometimes take place only after a student's academic performance has suffered greatly or there has been a suicide attempt.

Traditional Chinese culture includes caution about medications. To Chinese students and their parents, potential side effects can loom larger than potential benefits. Education about psychopharmacology and the biology of clinical depression can help build collaboration between patients and prescribers. Especially close follow-up might be needed to ensure adherence to a prescription for an antidepressant or mood stabilizer. Practical strategies for close follow-up can be based on frequent secure electronic communication. Options include daily global self-ratings of mood, distress, function, and side effect concerns; weekly questionnaire-based self-ratings of depressive symptoms; and tracking sleep and activity with a wearable device. The objectivity of the last of these might especially appeal to students in STEM fields.

Many Chinese and Chinese American students with mild depression, without comorbidities, functional impairment, suicidal ideation, or bipolarity, can benefit from services in a non-psychiatric model that involves the promotion of positive mental health and resilience, teaching techniques of stress management such as mindfulness meditation and exercise, and education in healthy sleeping and eating habits. Services of this kind should not require a student's seeking formal mental health services at all.

Education in skills to build positive mental health and resilience can be offered by a university at no additional cost to all students of all ethnic and cultural backgrounds, with no need for them to indicate they have any problem, difficulty, or diagnosis. However, even that option will be rejected by some students if getting such education is associated with being "weak," "soft," or unable to "take care of oneself without help." The time involved for mental health education would be time taken away from studying for examinations. To avoid culturally-based resistance to seeking help and to fully destigmatize education in self-care, prevention, and positive mental health, a university might make a for-credit, graded course in mental health an academic requirement for entering students. To get an "A" in the course, a student would have to learn to take care of themselves and prove on an examination that they knew about depression, substance use disorders, eating disorders, non-suicidal self-injury, social media addiction, and other mental health problems common in college students. The course might include skill training in mindfulness, sleep hygiene, relaxation, time management, and effective conflict resolution. It would teach the relationship of diet, exercise, and sleep habits to mental health and optimal function and would describe practical strategies for maintaining a physically and mentally healthy lifestyle. Making mental health literacy a universal requirement associated with grades and credits would be a far more powerful message than anti-stigma platitudes and phone numbers to call if feeling desperate.

While there are few controlled studies of educational interventions for the primary prevention of suicide (Zalsman et al., 2016), a study conducted on secondary school students in ten Europen Union countries showed a significant reduction in suicide attempts one year after students received a structured, manual-based educational intervention that included three hours of role-play sessions, distribution of a 32-page booklet, educational posters in participating classrooms, and lectures about mental health. The program's aim was to raise awareness of risk and protective factors associated with suicide, knowledge of depression and anxiety, and skills for dealing with adverse life events and stress. The intervention reduced suicide attempts and severe suicidal ideation by approximately 50% with respect to controls who received no mental health education. By contrast, screening and referral programs had no significant effect on either suicide attempts or severe suicidal ideation (Wasserman et al., 2015).

In the study, students were not examined on the content of the educational program. If knowledge were the active ingredient in the group receiving mental health education, one might expect even greater effects if the content were part of the formal curriculum.

Another educational approach to primary prevention of suicide that does not require self-disclosure or entail stigma is the use of mobile applications that provide self-guided education and training in the management of suicidal thoughts and behaviors. The value of such applications in reducing suicidal ideation is supported by controlled trials, though sample sizes have been too small to assess their impact on suicide attempts (Torok et al., 2020).

Academicians in China concerned about depression and suicide in students have put forward a similar idea about making positive mental health part of the academic curriculum. In China, physicians get undergraduate medical degrees. Medical students are a particularly stressed group; in China their prevalence of clinical depression is 30%, and their prevalence of suicidal ideation is 10% (Pan et al., 2016). However, most medical schools have no curricular content related to physician wellness or mental health. Medical school faculty knowledgeable about psychiatry have observed that building content into the curriculum ensures that all students will be exposed to it, without having to declare themselves as having trouble or being in need of counseling (Sobowale et al., 2014). The "second pandemic" of mental health problems that accompanied the COVID-19 pandemic offers an additional rationale for requiring mental health education for college students.

Potential for Social Media Analysis

Given the popularity of social media among all students, it is surprising that analysis of social media posts is not more often employed as a tool by student health services. As the case histories at the start of this chapter illustrate, many students post details of their emotional states and mental health online that they do not share in face-to-face conversations with clinicians or even with personal friends. Even when messages on social media do not relate explicitly to mental health, automated analysis of the qualitative and quantitative attributes of messages, including words preferred and words avoided, frequency and length of messages, and qualitative features of attached images, yields information about a person's state of mind. Identification of suicidal ideation and suicide risk would be especially valuable because many people who die by suicide make social media posts less than a week before their death.

Automated analysis of social media posts for mental health content is a rapidly growing and promising area of research, though its technological and clinical aspects have not yet been fully integrated (Chancellor & De Choudhury, 2020; J. Kim et al., 2021; Rassy et al., 2021; Resnik et al., 2021). False-positive identification of people needing professional help is a major problem.

While use of social media analysis to screen populations for suicide risk and intervention is fraught with ethical issues and problems of false positives, analysis of posts by people already in treatment for depression is less complicated, both ethically and psychometrically. Ethical practice requires informed consent with an explicit, shared understanding between patients and clinicians of its purposes and limitations (Marks, 2019).

Used under appropriate conditions, automated social media analysis offers the promise of efficiently capturing impending mood changes in people with BD and periods of elevated risk for suicide attempts in people under treatment for depression. Valid algorithms for clinical interpretation of social media posts would include independent variables correlated with cultural identity. If algorithms were developed for use in student populations, characteristics of cultural identity could be submitted at the same time as the student offered (appropriately circumscribed) consent for analysis of their posts.

The mood states associated with specific words and phrases used in social media posts vary by culture. For example, in Chinese young adults, frequent references in social media posts to achievement (e.g., "good at," "master") are associated with a higher level of depression, while references to work (e.g., "salary," "factory") are associated with a lower level of depression (Cheng et al., 2017). Such relationships have not been reported for non-Hispanic White Americans.

Chinese expatriate students and Chinese American students who are not fully assimilated might be reluctant to trust mental health professionals whom they experience as ignorant of Chinese culture. Chinese students who have used campus counseling services have complained about counselors' lack of cultural awareness. This is an addressable problem: Groups of Chinese and Chinese American students could help define a curriculum for introducing student health counselors to Chinese culture. On the other hand, if a student is part of a close-knit local Chinese community and a counselor is part of the same community, the benefit of the counselor's cultural competence might be outweighed by a student's concerns about confidentiality and loss of face.

Depression and suicide are epidemic at American universities. Prevalence and mortality statistics are worse for international students and for some ethnic minorities, but the problem affects all students. Seriously addressing depression, suicidal behavior, and related mental health issues of Chinese and Chinese American students—and other international and ethnic minority students—will require universities to invest new resources. Elite universities with multibillion-dollar endowments have an extraordinary opportunity to address depression in their undergraduates, including international students and ethnic minority students, to reduce suicide rates, to prevent disruption of students' education, and to reduce the stigma of depression. A comprehensive response to the epidemic of depression among their students would include universities' funding work of their own faculty in mental health–related curriculum development, treatment outcome research, application of artificial intelligence to case identification and risk assessment, and development and optimization of mobile applications to support psychological wellness and mental health care. Projects would include the creation and maintenance of a required undergraduate course in mental health and wellness and rigorous evaluation of the outcomes of the university's mental health and suicide prevention programs as a basis for their continual improvement. Goals would include a suicide rate of zero and a significant reduction in depressive symptoms among the student body. When students had a recurrent major depression or a bipolar spectrum disorder, they would be engaged in effective treatment with the expectation that such students rarely would withdraw from the university or fail to earn a degree as expected. An important aim would be for outcomes to be as favorable for international students and minority students as for non-Hispanic White students. The global effects of several highly ranked, world-famous universities making a well-funded, multidisciplinary, and persistent *academic* effort in student mental health and wellness could be profound. Part of the work might be funded by philanthropists as it would further the universities' mission. It could permanently reduce the stigma of depression and its treatment.

Universities' policies about withdrawing from classes for health reasons should be revisited. Ejecting students from college because of a diagnosis of depression or a single suicide attempt has no legitimate justification, and it affects not just the student asked to leave but many other students who need help and would have sought it if not for fear of dire consequences for their education, future work opportunities, or visa status. Policies should aim to assist patients with major depression or BD in getting the treatment they need while completing their degrees on time or with minimal delay. They should be based on the best evidence about the time needed to attain remission of symptoms and recovery of function in patients whose mood disorders are associated with transient impairment in academic performance.

Universities should be prepared to fund co-payments for students who require outside mental health services and for whom co-payments would be a hardship. Outside services might be needed because of the limited capacity of student health services, because students might have legitimate concerns about confidentiality, because some international students would do better with a therapist fluent in their native language, and/or because students have clinical issues that need subspecialist involvement for the best outcome. Examples of the latter include depression with significant general medical comorbidity (e.g., epilepsy, chronic migraine, inflammatory bowel disease), treatment-refractory depression, and BD not currently in remission.

Expression of Negative Emotions in the Chinese Language

China's being a "low-trust" society (Fukuyama, 1995), its people tend to be reluctant to share negative emotions with people outside of a small circle of trusted family and friends. Even with a family member or close friend, there will be concern about burdening the other person with an unhappy situation they cannot do much about. Notwithstanding, the Chinese language has many metaphors that enable its people to precisely communicate negative emotions in a few words. Regardless of their level of education, most Chinese people will use them when they do acknowledge negative emotions or confide about them to those they trust. In Chinese tradition the heart is the locus of emotion, and metaphors concerning feelings usually involve the heart rather than the brain or the mind. The historical Chinese view of health, as expressed in traditional Chinese medicine (TCM), is essentially psychosomatic or somatopsychic, as discussed in Chapter 9. There is thus an overlap between expressions used to describe emotional states often accompanied by physical sensations and those used to describe symptoms of general medical illness.

Chinese "heart" metaphors distinguish between everyday moods and extraordinary ones of the sort associated with major losses, personal tragedies, or clinical depression. A clinician assessing depression in a Chinese speaker can make use of this fact even if they do not speak Chinese, by asking what Chinese expressions the person might use to describe the current state of their heart. They could then be asked to explain the meaning of the expression. Understanding the patient's choice of words can sometimes give a more accurate assessment of the severity and character of a depressed mood than asking the patient to give their depressive symptoms numerical ratings as on the BDI or state how often in the past two weeks they have had them as on the PHQ-9. Table 10.2 lists a few of the many "heart" metaphors used for describing negative emotions.

Table 10.2 Chinese "Heart" Metaphors for Negative Emotions

Chinese metaphor	Pinyin	Literal translation	Connotation
心病	xīn bìng	Heart disease	Secret sorrow or trouble (e.g., older unmarried daughter or unemployed son)
无心	wú xīn	No heart to do things	Not in the mood, no energy, apathy
多心	duō xīn	Much heart	Overthinking, suspiciousness
伤心	shāng xīn	Injured heart	Grieving, brokenhearted
痛心	tòng xīn	Pain heart	Heartbroken, sad
心难受	xīn nán shòu	Heart receives with difficulty	Afflicted, sad if related to a situation; can be empathic; can be physical
心疼	xīn téng	Heart ache	Feel bad for a loved one's suffering; sympathy or concern
揪心	jiū xīn	Pulling on the heart	Extreme, agonizing worry or anxiety (event-related)
心闷	xīn mèn	Heart blocked or suppressed	Emotional distress; also used to describe physical chest pressure
心紧	xīn jǐn	Heart (is) tight	Extremely anxious or uptight; also used to describe physical chest tightness
心情不好	xīn qíng bù hǎo	Heart's condition is no good	Bad mood, having a bad day; does not imply illness
心烦	xīn fán	Heart (is) bothered	Weary, fretful, and impatient; "leave me alone"
心乱	xīn luàn	Heart (is) disorderly	Disturbed, emotionally disorganized, overwhelmed
心事重重	xīn shì chóng chóng	Things on the heart, layer by layer	Preoccupied, may be concerned about something (usually used to describe another person)
忧心重重	yōu xīn chóng chóng	Worried heart, layer by layer	Full of anxiety, loaded down with worries (usually used to describe another person)
担心	dān xīn	Lifted heart	Worried (usually related to a mild everyday concern)
心慌	xīn huāng	Heart (is) nervous or fluttering	Panicky feeling—restless, may be with palpitations (can be physical)
心焦	xīn jiāo	Heart (is) scorched	Uneasy, anxious
灰心	huī xīn	Gray heart	Discouraged, disappointed, disheartened
心寒	xīn hán	Heart (is) chilly	Bitterly disappointed by another person (e.g., by betrayal or lack of gratitude)

(continued)

Table 10.2 Continued

Chinese metaphor	Pinyin	Literal translation	Connotation
心碎	xīn suì	Heart (is) shattered	Devastated, heartbroken, extreme sadness or grief (always event-related)
心酸	xīn suān	Heart (is) sour	Sadness or grief, usually tearful; can be used to express pity or sympathy
心悸	xīn jì	Heart (is) throbbing	Extremely stressed; scared, possibly with strong physical sensations; can be used to describe palpitations with anxiety
万箭穿心	wàn jiàn chuān xīn	Ten thousand arrows pierce the heart	Great pain with sorrow or grief (severe and event-related)
撕心裂肺	sī xīn liè fèi	Torn heart, cracked lung	Intense grief or emotional pain (severe and event-related)
提心吊胆	tí xīn diào dǎn	Hanging the heart, lifting the gallbladder	Being on tenterhooks, haunted with fear
心如刀绞	xīn rú dāo jiǎo	A knife twisted in the heart	Intense emotional pain (event-related)
绞心	jiǎo xīn	Twisted heart	Great emotional pain (or physical pain in the region of the heart)
心虚	xīn xū	Heart (is) weak	Afraid that one's misdeed will be revealed
心死	xīn sǐ	Heart (is) dead	Hopeless, completely given up
负心	fù xīn	Lack of heart	Betrayal of or disloyalty to a spouse or partner; also can refer to a lack of gratitude
恶心	ě xīn	Nausea (literally "evil heart")	Disgusted, nauseated (can be physical)
堵心	dǔ xīn	(Something) stuck (in the) heart	Having a disturbing feeling
不开心	bù kāi xīn	Closed heart	Unhappy (applies to everyday moods)
疑心	yí xīn	Suspicious heart	Suspicious
亏心	kuī xīn	Deficient heart	Feeling guilty or ashamed because of wrongdoing (e.g., because of dishonesty)
心力交瘁	xīn lì jiāo cuì	Heart and energy (are) weary and distressed	Mentally and physically exhausted

Table 10.2 Continued

Chinese metaphor	Pinyin	Literal translation	Connotation
心神不定	xīn shén bù dìng	Heart (and) spirit (are) not stable	Agitated, distracted, no peace of mind
心如死灰	xīn rú sǐ huī	Heart (is) like dead ashes	Utterly dispirited, extremely downhearted
心烦意乱	xīn fán yì luàn	Heart (is) bothered and distracted	Upset, distracted, thoughts disordered, can't think clearly
心灰意冷	xīn huī yì lěng	Heart (is) gray, mind (is) cold	Downhearted, disspirited, despairing, hopeless
伤心欲绝	shāng xīn yù jué	Injured heart, want to die	Extremely grieved, inconsolable, lost will to live (event-related)
心疚	xīn jiù	Heart (is) remorseful	Full of regret for mistake or wrongdoing (self-conscious emotion, may be event-related)
心不在焉	xīn bù zài yān	Heart is not here	Absent mind

Depression with Near-Tragic Consequences in a Left-Behind Rural Wife

Xiaojuan Wang, a native of Jiangsu Province, was a 35-year-old married woman who lived with her nine-year-old daughter and her parents-in-law in her husband's home village on the outskirts of Chengdu in Sichuan Province. One afternoon, after an angry scene with her mother-in-law, she decided to kill herself and her daughter. She found a bottle of organophosphate insecticide in the shed behind their cottage; she mixed it with apple juice, served some to her daughter, and drank the remainder herself. Minutes later she and her daughter began to cough and gasp for air. Her mother-in-law heard what was happening and called for an ambulance. Mother and child were fighting for their lives when the ambulance arrived.

Xiaojuan met her husband, Gong, when both were migrant workers in Shenzhen. Xiaojuan worked in an electronics factory, and Gong worked in construction. They married, and their first child was born a year later. They lived in Shenzhen when their daughter was young. As their daughter reached school age, they had a painful choice: They did not have a Shenzhen *hukou* (户口; resident registration), so it would be hard to ensure their daughter's access to public education. Even though Shenzhen has a relatively liberal policy about public education for the children of rural migrants, there are practical obstacles for families who wish to take advantage of it (S. Zhou & Cheung, 2017). So, when their daughter reached school age, Xiaojuan moved to her husband's hometown in Chengdu. There she and her daughter lived with her husband's aging parents, supported by remittances from her husband, who continued to work in Shenzhen. Chengdu is 19 hours from Shenzhen by regular train; a flight or high-speed train is quicker but more expensive. Between the time and the money required, Gong could afford to visit his family only twice year. Xiaojuan provided physical assistance to Gong's father, who had trouble walking because of a past injury to his legs. She raised chickens and tended the vegetable garden. Gong's mother was an extremely disagreeable, irascible woman who continually complained that she and her husband had to care for a granddaughter but had no grandson to carry on the family name (Gong was their only child and his daughter their only grandchild). She often treated Xiaojuan disrespectfully. Gong's father had only a primary education, and his mother was illiterate.

Xiaojuan as a young woman had been bright and beautiful, extraverted, and sociable. Her family was more affluent than Gong's. Now she was "left behind"— effectively a widow, though her husband was still alive. She felt she was aging rapidly. Her husband gradually had become emotionally distant, telephoning her less frequently and seeming impatient with her when she called him. She began losing sleep. She would look around her house, perceiving the interior as dark, unhappily noticing dirt everywhere, and noticing chores undone. She felt trapped and hopeless. She blamed herself for making bad life decisions. She considered divorce but felt she could not leave her daughter without a father or leave her father-in-law without a caregiver. She kept her distress secret from her own parents, whom she would seldom see as they lived in a village outside of Nanjing, 20 hours from Chengdu by train. She avoided people outside the family; she didn't want to reveal her misery to anyone else and didn't want people to gossip about her as they surely would if she socialized with a man outside her family. She had women friends in her hometown who also had been left behind. One had been raped one evening when she was out by herself. Another was poor and alone, having been abandoned by both her husband and her lover following an extramarital affair.

Xiaojuan developed back pain and joint pain, for which she took over-the-counter medication in steadily increasing amounts. At night in bed, she felt a stone on her chest; she secretly cried under her quilt; she began to lose weight. Time passed very slowly. She lost interest in her favorite television shows. Grooming herself became so effortful that she became disheveled. Her parents-in-law seemed not to notice or not to care. Xiaojuan did not recognize that she was ill with depression and did not think of asking anyone for help with her low mood, her physical symptoms, and her impairment of function.

Gong returned home for a summer holiday with many gifts for Xiaojuan and their daughter, but she was unmoved. She smiled for him halfheartedly; he did not seem to notice how miserable she was. Xiaojuan had little interest in sex with her husband, and, surprisingly to her, Gong didn't seem to mind. The day before her husband left for Shenzhen, Xiaojuan found his mobile phone; and by scrolling through his text messages on WeChat, she discovered that he was having an affair with another woman. She felt total despair. She had sacrificed her youth, beauty, and health for a man who had exploited and betrayed her. Perhaps she would kill herself after her husband returned to Shenzhen. If she did, she would kill her daughter as well. She thought her daughter would be lonely and vulnerable without her, and she couldn't bear the thought of her girl having her husband's lover as her stepmother. She hadn't resolved to act on her suicidal thoughts until the afternoon she quarreled with her husband's mother. She then remembered seeing a bottle of insecticide on the shelf in a closet.

When notified that his wife and daughter were hospitalized after nearly dying, Gong, guilty and ashamed, immediately flew to Chengdu. He gave up his life in Shenzhen, found a job near Chengdu, and permanently rejoined his wife and daughter.

Xiaojuan was seen by a psychiatrist while in the hospital following her poisoning. He diagnosed major depression and prescribed an SSRI. Xiaojuan took the medication for 2 months. Feeling better and reconciled with Gong, she discontinued it and remained well.

Since the end of the Cultural Revolution China has experienced unprecedented economic growth, transforming from a low-income, mainly agricultural nation to a global power with the world's second largest economy. The benefits of China's growth have been unevenly distributed, with its urban areas, especially those of eastern China, having much greater wealth, higher incomes, better educational institutions, and more developed social welfare systems than the rural areas of China's interior. A consequence has been a massive migration of Chinese people from rural areas to the metropolitan areas of eastern China, seeking more highly paid work and a better life in a more modern environment. In 2018 there were 288 million migrant workers in China's cities, approximately one third of the nation's entire workforce ("China's Migrant Workers and Their Children," 2019).

China has a system of household registration—the *hùkǒu* (户口) system—which links each citizen and their children to a specific region and to urban or rural status. Effectively, it is an internal passport. Even if a child is born in a city, they will have a rural *hukou* if their parents did (Y. Hu, 2017). A Chinese person's *hukou* is the basis for their receipt of public benefits including pensions, healthcare, housing, and children's access to public schools. All such benefits are far less in rural areas than in cities. Thus, a rural-to-urban migrant works and pays taxes in a city but does not have commensurate benefits. While migrant workers' children can by national law attend public school in the city where they work, there are in practice many practical barriers to enrolling a child; and rural children in urban schools often face prejudice, discrimination, and bullying (S. Zhou & Cheung, 2017).

The original aim of the *hukou* system was to ensure that there was adequate agricultural labor—the government was concerned that too many farmers would move to the cities. As China industrialized and agriculture became more mechanized, the need for labor was increasingly in the cities; but the *hukou* system did not change. Of China's 297.4 million migrant workers in 2023, long-distance migrants working outside their home province comprised 67.51 million, more than the population of France. About two thirds of China's migrant workers are employed in either manufacturing, construction, sales, or transport. Only 15.8% have any post-secondary education (Statista, 2024).

The working conditions of migrants are poor. Their average monthly income in 2023 was approximately 4,780 RMB ($614 USD). Most employment is precarious, with no contractual protections. Only about a quarter of migrant workers have health insurance or insurance for work-related injuries. Their typical workday is 11 hours. However, as tough as life is for long-distance migrant workers, their wages are significantly higher than they would have been had they remained in their home provinces. ("China's Migrant Workers and Their Children," 2019; Statista, 2024). Among parents who leave children behind in the country, most will return home no more than twice a year; and some do not see their children for more than a year at a time (Su et al., 2013).

A migrant from a Chinese rural village to a metropolis like Shenzhen would essentially be treated like an immigrant from another country and might face discriminatory treatment from the city's permanent residents. Migrants are paid less than permanent residents for similar work and usually live in poorer, more polluted, and higher-crime neighborhoods. Because their wages are relatively low, housing costs are high, and their children have difficulty accessing public education, they often cannot keep their children with them once they reach school age. Because older adults living in rural areas would not be entitled to urban pensions or healthcare benefits if they migrated to a city, they do not have a realistic option of going to the city to live with or near an adult child who migrated. The effect of these contingencies is that older adults, school-age children, and wives often are "left behind" in the country when rural men migrate to the cities for work. A rural woman might migrate to the city for work, enjoy urban life, and prefer to remain; but if she marries and has a child, she might choose to return to the country when her child reaches school age.

If the child is left behind in a rural area without one or both parents—a situation characterizing over 40 million rural Chinese children—their life prospects and mental health can be permanently harmed by circumstances related to left-behind status (X. Li et al., 2020; X. Li et al., 2021; X. Li et al., 2022; Mao et al., 2020; H. Wu et al., 2021; H. Zhang et al., 2021). Left-behind children attend inferior schools, and they are at increased risk for neglect or abuse by caregivers, malnutrition, inadequate healthcare, injury in accidents, and victimization by peers (bullying) and by predatory adults (M. Chen & Chan, 2016; H. Zhang, Chi, et al., 2019; H. Zhang et al., 2019, 2021).

These problems contribute to a high risk of anxiety, depression, and externalizing behaviors in left-behind children (Lei et al., 2021; X. Sun et al., 2021; Y.-Y. Wang, Xu et al., 2019). Left-behind children often do not complete high school. If they do complete high school and take the *gaokao* for college entrance, their inferior education puts them at a disadvantage. Left-behind children who attend college are more than twice as likely to have mental health problems as students who were not left behind, after controlling for other common risk factors (H. Liu et al., 2020). Left-behind children under the care of poorly-educated grandparents cannot benefit from family members' help in studying for examinations. In many cases, the grandparents speak only a regional dialect rather than standard Mandarin. This is a great disadvantage for a child, who will have limited educational and employment opportunities if they are not highly proficient in China's official national language.

When left-behind children with emotional problems are reunited with their parents, their symptoms usually will improve (H. Hu et al., 2014). However, if a child has been neglected or abused while the parents were away, they will continue to have an increased lifetime risk of mental health problems.

If a child's mother is present with her child in the country, she can supervise and supplement her child's education, ensure that they are well nourished, and help keep them safe. However, the mother left behind is likely to be less educated than the father who migrates. A male migrant typically will send remittances to left-behind family members in his hometown that might exceed what he would earn there if he had stayed and still leave himself enough money for his expenses as a single man. However, he will be separated from his family for all but a few days a year. He is likely to be lonely, and he might begin an extramarital relationship with a woman in the city in which he works.

Depression is a common problem of left-behind people of three generations—children, wives, and parents. In a culture where adult children have traditionally been responsible for their aging parents, community resources for support and care of left-behind older adults often are inadequate. Left-behind older adults, who constitute 37% of all rural elders, have an extremely high rate of clinical depression. In a study in Hunan Province, left-behind women over age 65 had a 45% rate of clinically significant depressive symptoms, as did 33% of left-behind older men. Only 2% of those with depression received any mental health services (He et al., 2016). Social capital, in the form of relationships with friends and neighbors, participation in group activities, and a higher level of trust in friends, neighbors, and extended family, has protective effects against depression in older adults left behind by their children (Ke et al., 2019).

Left-behind married women face challenges related to living in a traditional Confucian culture in which women have inferior status, a husband's parents have authority over his wife, and an adult woman without a husband present is vulnerable and unprotected. A left-behind wife may be responsible for childcare, eldercare, housework, agricultural labor if the family has a small farm, and perhaps working outside the home if the family needs the money. Left-behind women who work outside the home are vulnerable to exploitation and sexual harassment by employers. In families without domineering in-laws, the woman's hard work might be associated with autonomy and a sense of agency. In the worst cases, however, she works even harder than she might if she were living in the city with her husband, while at the same time having little say in the household.

Left-behind women live in locales where mental health services usually are unavailable except for people with severe mental illness and where mental health care is highly stigmatized. Half of the counties in China have no psychiatrist at all (Liang et al., 2018). Psychiatrists who do work in rural areas almost all work in hospitals and concentrate on the care of patients with severe mental illness. Clinical psychologists and other non-medical psychotherapists are even rarer than psychiatrists. The association of psychiatric care with psychosis and hospitalization enhances its stigma. Even when mental health services are available and a person can overcome the barrier of stigma to seek help, ongoing care usually is unaffordable for China's rural residents. The out-of-pocket cost of a single outpatient psychiatric visit could be more than a quarter of a rural resident's monthly disposable income.

Historically, middle-income countries have reported lower rates of major depression than high-income countries, and in almost all countries the suicide mortality rate for men has been much higher than that for women. In most countries there is a lower prevalence of depression and a lower rate of death by suicide for women who are married than for those who are single. Rural China is an exception to the rule. In the Chinese countryside there is a high prevalence of depression in both men and women, and suicide rates in women are as high as those in men and in some areas higher. For women in rural China, marriage is associated with worse mental health, regardless of whether their husbands live with them or leave them behind (Phillips et al., 2002; J. Zhang, 2010). Marriage has no protective effect against suicide in young women in rural China, and cohabitation without marriage has been associated with a markedly increased risk of suicide by young rural Chinese women. Jie Zhang and his colleagues (2011) have framed a central issue for many suicidal young women as "conflicting social values between communist gender equalitarianism and Confucian gender discrimination."

Zhang and Lv (2016) analyzed data on depression and its risk factors from interviews of 1618 relatives and friends of rural Chinese people who had died by suicide. In addition to the usual demographic items, subjects were asked about their religious identity, their "relative deprivation," and their "social value conflict." Depression was measured with the CES-D. The question about "relative deprivation" asked subjects whether they saw their family's economic status as very good, good, so-so, poor, or very poor in comparison with people around them in the same community or village. Five questions about value strain asked subjects how difficult it would be for them to make decisions concerning working outside the home, having a son rather than a daughter (e.g., by terminating a pregnancy if the fetus were female), choosing a spouse based on love rather than family directives, obeying a husband or father, or having more education.

Multivariate models showed that older age was associated with more depressive symptoms, but that women were not more depressed than men, and that marriage did not have a protective effect. Value strain, relative deprivation, and religion were significant depression risks in both sexes; the effects of all were stronger in women than in men. Education was strongly antidepressant in men but had an insignificant effect in women.

The study by Zhang and Lv clearly demonstrates the powerful effect of gender on the determinants of depression in rural China. Widespread economic hardship affects everyone's mental health, and older adults have fewer options for escaping from it, for example by migrating to an urban area for higher-paid employment. Women experience more distress than men related to conflicts between mainstream modern values and traditional Confucian concepts of women's roles and status, and having secondary or higher education is less empowering for rural Chinese women than for rural Chinese men. While the study of Zhang and Lv was based on data collected in 2005–2008, the World Economic Forum's *Gender Gap Report 2023* suggests that little has changed since then with respect to women's relative status. For example, in China there are 89 girls born for every 100 boys. China's statistics on the differential mortality of female fetuses put it in 145th place of among the 146 nations rated by the organization (World Economic Forum, 2023, page 143).

In rural China, single women tend to have better social support than married ones because they can turn to their own parents and siblings as well as to their peers. After marriage, a rural woman's personal connections are mainly with her husband and his family, and her time may be taken up with caregiving. If a woman is left behind, she might experience a progressive deterioration in her health-related quality of life. If a left-behind woman loses function or stamina because of depression, she will be less able to cope actively with stress and effectively assert herself within the family. Her status within the family might decline further, contributing to feelings of worthlessness and/or hopelessness.

Suicide is facilitated by the ready availability of means for impulsive self-harm that are usually lethal. In America, Switzerland, and other countries with gun cultures, firearms are the usual means for impulsive suicides. In rural China, highly concentrated and highly toxic organophosphate and carbamate pesticides are the preferred means. While hanging, jumping from a height or in front of a train, and drowning are equally highly lethal, they usually require planning; and fear of pain can deter people from attempting them. In agricultural areas of China, pesticides are ubiquitous. A lethal dose can readily be located and swallowed on impulse, and people do not appear to fear swallowing pesticides as much as they fear hanging or jumping from a height. Pesticides are used in approximately one half of rural suicides in China, and the proportion is higher in women and in people with no diagnosed mental disorder. They are used more in unplanned, impulsive suicide attempts than in planned ones (L. Sun & Zhang, 2016; B. Wang et al., 2020). Marital and family conflicts are typical precipitants of pesticide ingestion in younger rural Chinese women (Kong & Zhang, 2010).

When rural women and children live on or near farms, they can be passively exposed to toxic levels of organophosphate pesticides. Chronic exposure to such pesticides at levels too low to cause acute intoxication can increase the likelihood of clinical depression and can cause subtle impairments in executive cognitive function that impede adaptive problem solving and thus reduce resilience. Chronic low-level organophosphate pesticide exposure causes an increase in impulsiveness and an associated increase in the incidence of suicide attempts (Lyu et al., 2018).

Migrant workers in China's urban factories have long work hours, and factory environments can be noisy, polluted, and/or dangerous; but many rural women prefer to migrate to the cities and work in factories rather than remain in the country, marry in their early 20s, and be in a position with no power, control, or independence. In the city a young working woman will have some money of her own and more autonomy than she would have in a traditional rural Chinese household.

The prevalence of depression in rural women in China in 2012 was estimated in a representative sample of 1898 women from Sichuan Province (Qiu et al., 2016). The investigators used the Chinese version of the CES-D to identify depressive symptoms and the Mini International Neuropsychiatric Interview to establish a categorical psychiatric diagnosis: 12.4% of women had CES-D scores of 16 or higher, suggesting clinical depression, and half of those met current Diagnostic and Statistical Manual of Mental Disorders (DSM) International Classification of Diseases (ICD) criteria for a MDE; 62% of the women with probable clinical depression (7.7% of the sample) had CES-D scores of 21 or higher, indicating moderate or severe depression. Those without MDE criteria would have met this book's criteria for clinical depression. Item-level data that would have enabled characterization of women with high depressive symptoms and no MDE diagnosis were not published. Some would be expected to have somatoform presentations. Others might have had an anger-predominant pattern like that of *hwa-byung*, a syndrome that will be discussed in detail in Chapter 12.

Yue et al. (2018) studied the qualitative aspect of depression in an interview-based study of rural Chinese women responsible for the care of children under age three. Women related their depression to the burden of caregiving, which often included the care of an older or disabled adult in addition to the young child; a lack of control and agency within the household; conflict within the family; and poverty coupled with the perception of wealth as a measure of self-worth. There were several reasons the depressed women did not find it useful to talk with family members about their troubles. In some cases, the women worried that they would be burdening the person with whom they shared their distress. In others, they felt that the other person would not understand, would dismiss their concerns as unimportant, or would give token reassurance that would leave them feeling worse than if they had kept silent about their depression.

A case–control study of a representative sample of 519 Chinese who died by suicide and 523 who died of unintentional injuries found eight risk factors that distinguished the two groups and had significant coefficients in models that controlled for age, gender, and region of the country: having a high level of depressive symptoms, a previous suicide attempt, acute stress at the time of death, severe interpersonal conflict in the two days before the death, low quality of life, high chronic stress, a blood relative with previous suicidal behavior, and a friend or associate with previous suicidal behavior (Phillips et al., 2002). Xiaojuan, the woman in the case vignette, had five of the eight risk factors: clinical depression, chronic stress from her caregiving roles, acute stress from learning of her husband's infidelity, interpersonal conflict with her mother-in-law, and a low quality of life. In China, the rural suicide rate is twice as high as the urban suicide rate (Sha et al., 2018). For Chinese adults aged 65 and over, the rural suicide rate is more than three times the urban rate (M. Li & Katikireddi, 2019).

Rates of pesticide-related suicide are similar in men and women in China. The difference in overall suicide rates between genders in rural areas is due to a higher rate of male suicide by other highly lethal means, especially hanging. People involved in agriculture—even part-time—are significantly more likely to use pesticides in suicide attempts, as are people with less education (Page et al., 2017). Women like Xiaojuan of the case vignette usually will not substitute other means if pesticides are hard to access at their time of most intense suicidal thinking (Reifels et al., 2019).

Zhang and colleagues in 2001–2003 conducted a remarkable series of psychological autopsies of suicides in the northeastern Chinese subprovince of Dalian (J. Zhang et al., 2004; J. Zhang & Zhou, 2009). For each of 66 people who had died by suicide, their research team did extensive face-to-face interviews of two family members or close friends of the deceased. They found that 68% of the suicides met DSM-3-R criteria for a mental disorder, and the remainder did not. However, the mean estimated Hamilton Depression Rating Scale (HAM-D) score among the suicides without a mental disorder diagnosis was 10.9 ± 6.7, indicating that more than half had depressive symptoms of potential clinical relevance. Suicides in people with no mental disorder were more likely to use pesticides and to be unplanned. The most common proximate causes of impulsive suicide by pesticides were fights with family members, a loss of face, and criticism or punishment by a parent, a teacher, or a superior at work. The study's authors suggested that improving access to mental health services might address suicide risk among those with diagnosable mental disorders but would be unlikely to affect rates of impulsive suicide among those without them. Their prescription for the latter group was a combination of tighter control of pesticides and "improving social support networks."

In the past two decades China's overall suicide mortality rate has declined significantly, but much of the change can be attributed to the nation's urbanization and greater prosperity rather than to public health measures. The trend is

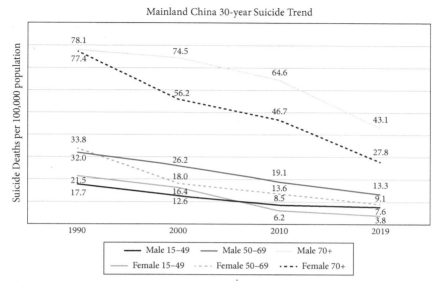

Figure 10.1 Mainland China Suicide Mortality Trend 1990–2019
Data from IHME (2023).

likely to reverse as China's population ages since suicide rates in both rural and urban China rise progressively with age. Also, China's economic growth and its rural-to-urban migration have slowed. Figure 10.1 shows the 30-year trend in China's suicide mortality, subdivided by gender and age bands.

While the downward trend in China's suicide mortality is real, its reported rates of suicide in people aged 70 and over are almost certainly underestimates as it has high rates of "unintentional" drownings and poisonings in its older population, and a significant proportion of them are likely to reflect death wishes or explicit suicidal plans. While officially recognized suicides of Mainland Chinese women 70 and over decreased by 64% between 1990 and 2019 and those of men decreased by 45%, deaths by drowning in the same groups decreased only slightly, and deaths by poisoning *increased*. Over the same three decades, unnatural deaths in Taiwan and Singapore took a different course. In Taiwan, deaths of older people by drowning and poisoning decreased dramatically, but rates of suicide did not. In Singapore, suicide rates dropped by more than half, and rates of death by drowning or poisoning, already low in 1990, fell even further. Mainland China, Taiwan, and Singapore all are places where Chinese culture is dominant (Singapore is 75% ethnically Chinese); but they differ in ways especially relevant to older adults' risk of suicide or possibly suicidal unnatural death. The persistence of deaths by drowning and poisoning of older people in mainland China can be attributed to a large rural population

Table 10.3 Unnatural Deaths of Older People in Mainland China, Taiwan, and Singapore: 1990–2019 (Rates per 100,000 People)

Cause of death	Men 70 and over				Women 70 and over			
	Mainland China							
Year	1990	2000	2010	2019	1990	2000	2010	2019
Suicide	78.0	74.5	64.6	43.1	77.4	56.1	46.7	27.8
Drowning	15.1	14.2	14.8	13.2	16.0	14.0	14.2	11.7
Poisoning	7.2	6.7	10.3	8.5	4.1	4.3	8.1	6.5
Total	100.4	95.5	89.7	64.8	97.5	74.5	69.0	46.0
	Taiwan							
Year	1990	2000	2010	2019	1990	2000	2010	2019
Suicide	50.6	59.6	53.9	52.9	35.0	36.1	28.8	26.2
Drowning	17.9	10.9	7.7	7.0	10.5	6.7	3.2	2.8
Poisoning	11.1	3.7	1.2	1.1	9.5	3.3	0.9	0.8
Total	79.6	74.2	62.7	61.0	55.1	46.1	32.9	29.8
	Singapore							
Year	1990	2000	2010	2019	1990	2000	2010	2019
Suicide	75.5	57.3	42.3	34.4	45.0	28.1	20.1	16.1
Drowning	3.2	2.1	1.6	1.2	1.0	0.8	0.6	0.4
Poisoning	0.5	0.3	0.2	0.1	0.3	0.2	0.2	0.2
Total	79.2	59.7	44.1	35.7	46.3	29.2	21.0	16.7

Note: Data from IHME (2023).

of older people living in absolute or relative poverty, with little access to mental health care. The decreasing rates of drowning and poisoning in Taiwan can be related to its prosperity and urbanization. The initially low and decreasing rates of drowning and poisoning in Singapore, and its consistently decreasing rates of suicide, reflect its status as a high-income city-state with an intense focus on public health and safety and general availability of healthcare including mental health services. Statistics on unnatural deaths of people aged 70 and over are presented in Table 10.3.

Statistics on unnatural deaths in people under age 70 during the same three decades are shown in Table 10.4. Among young and middle-aged Taiwanese, rates of suicide did not fall over three decades in which suicide mortality fell sharply both in mainland China and in Singapore. Suicide mortality rates for Taiwanese males aged 15–49 were twice as high in 2019 as they were in 1990.

Table 10.4 Suicides of Young and Middle-Aged Adults in Mainland China, Taiwan, and Singapore: 1990–2019 (Rates per 100K People)

Age range	Male suicide mortality				Female suicide mortality			
	Mainland China							
	1990	2000	2010	2019	1990	2000	2010	2019
Age 15–49	17.7	12.6	8.5	7.6	21.5	16.4	6.2	3.8
Age 50–69	32.0	19.1	26.2	13.3	33.8	18.0	13.6	9.1
	Taiwan							
Age 15–49	11.1	19.3	25.3	22.5	7.3	9.8	12.1	10.4
Age 50–69	23.4	36.8	35.8	32.2	13.2	16.6	15.3	13.7
	Singapore							
Age 15–49	19.8	15.2	10.3	8.9	11.9	8.8	5.7	4.7
Age 50–69	30.0	17.7	23.0	13.9	15.8	12.1	9.6	7.4

Note: Data from IHME (2023).

The difference between Taiwan and mainland China and Singapore might lie at the intersection of culture and economics. While both Singapore and mainland China continue to have rapidly growing economies broadly offering opportunities to younger adults, Taiwan's growth has slowed, implying that more young and middle-aged adults will be "losers." In addition, its culture has become more globalized and "connected," increasing the likelihood that people will frequently and unhappily compare their situation with that of others more successful than they.

In China of the 1970s and 1980s the female suicide rate was higher than the male rate (Ji et al., 2001). By 1990 the age-standardized suicide rate for females, while still higher than that for males, was not statistically significantly different. A difference in age-standardized rates indicating significantly more suicides in males did not emerge until 2001. Over 30 years, a steep age gradient in suicide was observed, with rates much higher in older adults (age 70 and up). The ratio of female to male suicides remains much higher in China than it is in most high-income and upper-middle-income countries, where the male rate is typically three times the female rate below age 70 and greater than three times the female rate for age 70 and above. In China in 2019 the male rate was twice as high as the female rate below age 50 and approximately 1.5 times higher for age 50 and above.

Striking gender inequity might partially account for China's relatively high female-to-male suicide rate ratio. While prospects for women have improved in absolute terms as the country has developed, China has had a large and persistent gap in women's economic opportunities, educational attainment, health and survival, and political empowerment, in 107th place among the 156 countries ranked by the World Economic Forum on these dimensions of gender equity (World Economic Forum, 2023, pp. 143–144). The issue appears to be more cultural than economic: Taiwan, an autonomous province of China with a much higher per capita income, also has a relatively high female-to-male suicide rate ratio and shares with mainland China a greater rise in suicide rate with age for women than for men (IHME, 2023).

Taiwan's gender-specific suicide rates for people under age 70 far exceed those of mainland China, and those for people over age 70 are similar. The two places share female suicide rates far above world benchmarks for high-income or upper-middle-income countries. Compared with mainland China, Taiwan has a smaller gender gap politically and economically—it has a female head of state, women are well represented in the national legislature, and the gender pay gap is small for Asia. However, women have inferior status within families, and older women are more likely than older men to be neglected and poor, as they are more likely to be widowed; and when they were of working age there was lower female workforce participation and a greater gender pay gap than there is today.

Depression and Suicide in Older Chinese Americans

In today's America, older Chinese adults are more likely than younger ones to be first-generation immigrants, to have limited English proficiency, to have a high school education or less, and to have low incomes (Budiman, 2021a). 80% of Chinese American older adults were born outside the U.S., and 30% came to the U.S. after age 60. Because of their age and social determinants of health, they are as a group at higher risk for clinical depression and for suicide. Most will be unacculturated or partially acculturated, and for that reason they will be likely to express their depression in traditional Chinese idioms of distress, experiencing and describing their illness as a mind–body problem rather than "psychologizing" it (Dong, Bergren, & Chang, 2015). Stressors that often precipitate depression in older adults (e.g., financial hardship, chronic medical conditions, bereavement, loneliness, caring for a sick or disabled spouse, or suffering maltreatment such as physical abuse, emotional abuse, financial exploitation, or neglect) apply to older Chinese Americans but can have distinctive features related to Chinese culture as well as to their status as immigrants. In a study of Chinese immigrants aged 60 and over in metropolitan Chicago, 15.8% of women and 14.3% of men had experienced one or more forms of maltreatment. In the sample, 6.5% of women and 2.6% of men had had suicidal ideation in the past 12 months, and of those, more than 40% had experienced maltreatment. Maltreatment was a particularly potent risk factor for suicidal ideation in older women. Even after controlling for age, medical comorbidity, education, income, and social support, women experiencing maltreatment were 2.46 times more likely to have considered suicide in the past year. Maltreatment did not have the same impact on men after controlling for social support (Dong, Chen, et al., 2015).

Estimated rates of clinical depression in older Chinese Americans are high (A. Yeung, R. Chan, et al., 2004). While Chinese Americans overall have lower suicide rates than non-Hispanic White Americans, Chinese American women have suicide rates significantly higher than those of White American women. White women's suicide rates fall with increasing age, while Chinese American women's rates increase. There are both structural and cultural reasons. Because most Chinese American women—and their husbands if they were married—immigrated after age 60, they are not eligible for Social Security or Medicare. Because they have no public "safety net," many rely on their adult children for financial and/or practical assistance; and if their children are unable or unwilling to provide the help they need, they will experience poverty and lack timely and adequate healthcare. If they become depressed and/or suicidal, they are unlikely to seek help or treatment, whether from a mental health professional, a primary care physician, or a friend. Most do not have religious or philosophical beliefs that oppose suicide.

With respect to poverty and loneliness, an older Chinese American immigrant typically has a culturally-based expectation of support from the younger generation. If an older Chinese immigrant has an adult child in the U.S. who does not offer expected financial, practical, and/or emotional support, they would be likely to feel deep disappointment and might also lose face (or fear losing face) in the local Chinese community (Dong et al., 2017). Social support from other Chinese people might relieve loneliness and be protective against depression, but a depressed older Chinese immigrant probably would be reluctant to socialize, let alone make new social connections. Social withdrawal can be a sign of depression in any culture. Among unacculturated Chinese immigrants, concerns about loss of face can contribute to it.

Among older Chinese Americans, caring for a sick or disabled spouse is especially burdensome for wives, from whom much is expected. In a study of distress in family caregivers of older adults with dementia, wives found their obligations more burdensome than husbands or adult children, even when their practical tasks were the same (J. Liu, 2021).

Asian Americans of all ages underutilize mental health services compared with non-Hispanic Whites. In a large-scale study of deidentified patient records from a large general hospital in Massachusetts in 2009, Asian Americans (Chinese being the most frequently-occurring nationality) had an 8.6% prevalence of *diagnosed* mental disorders versus 18.1% for non-Hispanic Whites. Remarkably, the rate of psychotropic medication use was higher than might be expected from the rate of mental disorder diagnoses (C. Wu et al., 2018). There are two likely reasons that Asian Americans' rates of mental disorder diagnoses and psychotropic medication use are insignificantly different. First, despite the caution and suspicion many Asian Americans have about medications, they usually are preferred to psychotherapy by people with self-stigma and concerns about acknowledging emotional or psychological problems to others. Second, psychotropic medications often are used as treatments for insomnia, fatigue, and physical pain—common somatic chief complaints for depressed Asian Americans who seek treatment from primary care physicians.

Expression of Depression Among Chinese Americans

Chinese American immigrants vary in their presentation of depression, but a consistent theme is their low utilization of mental health services when they are depressed. Acknowledgment of emotional issues or "stress" as playing a role in their illnesses and of affective or cognitive symptoms as part of the illness usually is not the main issue. Personal or anticipated stigma associated with seeing a psychiatrist or getting "mental health" care is relevant for many patients, but practical concerns probably are a bigger issue for older first-generation immigrants. For those still working, finding time for therapy appointments compatible with long working hours can be difficult; and in the U.S., many do not have health insurance or have insurance with poor coverage of mental health services. The latter comprises not only unaffordable copayments for psychotherapy visits but also high copayments for antidepressant drugs that might be best tolerated by patients, and cumbersome, discouraging processes of referral and prior authorization. Getting psychotherapy is especially difficult for patients with limited English proficiency.

For these reasons, it is not surprising that depressed first-generation Chinese Americans who seek formal treatment first consult a primary care physician. When they do, they usually will present a somatic chief complaint, either one associated with depression like fatigue or insomnia or one associated with a preexisting chronic illness. In China, the typical presentation of a depressed person to a health professional would be a visit to a primary care physician with some combination of fatigue, sleep problems, body aches, and other somatic symptoms. The depressed person's doing this would not reflect denial of depressed mood or negative thoughts, or the translation of emotional symptoms into physical ones, but rather a strategic emphasis on symptoms that would elicit treatment by a primary care physician and would enable the patient to be "sick without stigma" (Ahmad et al., 2018).

Whether somatic or psychological symptoms are emphasized by a depressed Chinese American can vary with how the information is obtained. When offering their chief complaints to a clinician or responding to questions on a structured clinical interview, somatic symptoms often predominate. When they complete standard depression questionnaires that include a full range of depressive symptoms, somatic symptoms usually are accompanied by mood symptoms. Less-educated Chinese immigrants might be reluctant to complete depression questionnaires in writing, and if so, they will give a fuller response if the questions are asked verbally by a Chinese-speaking member of the physician's or clinic's staff.

Younger, urban, more educated, and higher-status adults are more likely to accept the psychological concept of depression. They are likely to anticipate stigma in the Chinese community if they are open about a diagnosis of depression. Self-stigma is variable, with less among those who are better educated and of higher socioeconomic class. Among Chinese people, the status of depression lies on a spectrum, from an initially somatic presentation with minimal stigma to a combined psychological and somatic presentation with personal and anticipated public stigma, to a mainly psychological presentation with low personal stigma and anticipated public stigma dependent upon social circumstances.

The challenge for a Western, English-speaking clinician treating a depressed Chinese immigrant patient is engagement. Engagement is based on getting sufficient agreement with the patient on a conception of the illness, its cause, and the method and goals of treatment, so that the patient feels understood and respected. An engaged patient will collaborate with the clinician and be honest with them and will adhere to treatment prescribed through a process of shared decision-making.

Albert Yeung, a psychiatrist at the Massachusetts General Hospital who has published extensively on depression in Chinese Americans, described a culturally-adapted diagnostic interview to facilitate such engagement, the Engagement Interview Protocol (EIP; A. Yeung et al., 2011). Critical elements of the protocol include the following:

1. Eliciting the patient's personal illness narrative.
2. Eliciting the patient's explanation of their illness:
   a. What do you call your problem?
   b. What do you think has caused your problem?
   c. Why do you think it started when it did?

d. What does your sickness do to you? How does it work?
   e. How severe is it? Will it have a long or a short course?
   f. What do you fear most about your sickness?
   g. What are the chief problems the sickness has caused for you?
   h. What kind of treatment do you think you should receive? What are the most important results you hope to receive from the treatment?
3. Disclosure of the diagnosis in stages, with flexibility in the use of terminology, aiming to harmonize the diagnosis as communicated with the patient's illness beliefs and explanatory models.
4. Negotiating a treatment plan that considers the patient's understanding and preferences and addresses potential side effects and possible remedies for them.

Yeung and colleagues found the EIP to be feasible within a context of one-hour initial clinical visits. However, if the clinician must work through an interpreter, the patient has multiple comorbid conditions, and/or the patient is accompanied by family members with concerns of their own, even a full hour might be insufficient to carry out the EIP. If a clinician foresees one or more of these complications or if the clinic where they work does not schedule a full hour for an initial visit, a potential option is to divide the assessment and treatment planning process between two separate, closely-spaced visits. A diagnosis and treatment plan would not be offered until the second visit, which would begin with the patient (and possibly a family member) asking questions or offering information that occurred to them following the first visit. The two-visit structure exemplifies a process of personalizing care, thus addressing a common concern of Chinese people that Western allopathic medicine neglects individual differences, including those related to personal identity.

Culturally-Aware Depression Screening and Rating

Questionnaire-based screening tests and rating scales are emerging as a standard of practice in the diagnosis and treatment of depression as they enable earlier identification of depression needing treatment and permit more detailed and frequent assessment of depressed patients' symptoms without excessive demands on the patient's or the clinician's time. The three most popular questionnaires—the PHQ-9, the CES-D, and the BDI—have been translated into more than 80 languages, showing acceptable psychometric properties when their scores are used with a cutoff criterion to predict the binary outcome of a major depressive episode—or, less commonly, the outcome of any depressive disorder—as ascertained by a structured clinical interview. The three tests have been revised since their original development to accommodate changes in DSM/ICD criteria for MDD and to optimize their psychometric properties. The PHQ-9 and the CES-D are in the public domain. Chinese versions of depression questionnaires are validated by back-translation, modifying the Chinese translation successively until the back-translation into English is essentially identical to the original English version. However, attaining an equivalent back-translation does not imply that terms reciprocally translatable have the same connotations and significance within Western and Chinese culture. Evidence of a "lost in translation" phenomenon can be seen when factor analyses of the English and Chinese versions of the same questionnaire yield different structures.

A questionnaire's accurate prediction of diagnoses of major depression does not imply that it is optimal for identifying clinical depression as defined in this book, especially cases in the middle zone that can be associated with functional impairment, somatic distress, or suicide risk while not meeting DSM/ICD criteria for major depression. When depression symptom questionnaires are used in a primary care practice, non-psychiatric medical specialty practice, social services, or educational setting with people not diagnosed with depression or any other mental disorder, their most important function is the identification of non-obvious cases of clinical depression in people who don't complain of depression and are not actively seeking help or treatment for a mental health problem. In primary care and medical specialty practices, depressed people might present with somatic symptoms or cope conspicuously poorly with a general medical condition. In other contexts, people screened with questionnaires might have interpersonal problems or changes in academic or occupational function that they do not initially attribute to a mood disorder.

In psychiatric practice, questionnaire-based rating scales that measure the response of depressive symptoms to treatment must be able to identify residual symptoms indicating that the patient is not yet in full remission and thus is at risk for relapse if treatment is discontinued. That purpose also requires that a test be sensitive to relatively mild symptoms.

Another function of questionnaire-based depression scales in psychiatric practice is the qualitative characterization of a depressive illness—matching a case with a discrete phenotype such as melancholia, anxious depression, depression with prominent somatic features, or depression with predominant anhedonia and apathy. Patients with different depression phenotypes can respond differently to treatments. And, talking with patients about depression in terms of the symptoms that trouble them the most can aid in patient engagement—building a high-trust, empathic relationship that promotes adherence to prescribed treatment and maximizes non-specific benefits of treatment (aka placebo effects).

The psychometric properties of Chinese versions of the PHQ-9, CES-D, and BDI have been assessed in clinical and non-clinical populations in mainland China, Hong Kong, and Taiwan and in Chinese immigrants and international students in English-speaking countries. The three tests are internally consistent, reliable, and, in most Chinese populations, predictive of a diagnosis of MDD as ascertained by a structured clinical interview. However, the most appropriate cutoff score for predicting a diagnosis of depression (MDD or any DSM/ICD depressive disorder) varies dramatically by the population and context of use, and individual questionnaire items can work differently with Chinese people than with English-speaking people of European heritage. For example, among people identifying with traditional Chinese culture and its gender roles, a depressed man would be less likely than a depressed woman to report crying spells, and those of either gender would be less likely than depressed people of European origin to endorse crying spells on a questionnaire.

The Chinese PHQ-9

病人健康状况问卷-9
Patient Health Questionnaire – 9 (PHQ-9)

在过去两周您经常受到以下问题的困扰吗？ (请用 "√" 勾选您的答案) Over the past two weeks, how often have you been bothered by any of the following problems? (Use "√" to indicate your answer.)	从来没有 Not at all	有几天 Several days	刚超过一半天数 More than half the days	接近每天 Nearly every day
1. 做任何事都觉得沉闷或者根本不想做任何事 Having little interest or pleasure in doing things	0	1	2	3
2. 情绪低落，抑郁或绝望 Feeling down, depressed, or hopeless	0	1	2	3
3. 难以入睡；半夜会醒，或相反，睡觉时间过多 Having trouble falling or staying asleep, or sleeping too much	0	1	2	3
4. 觉得疲倦或没有活力 Feeling tired or having little energy	0	1	2	3
5. 胃口极差或饮食过量 Having a poor appetite or overeating	0	1	2	3
6. 不喜欢自己——觉得自己做的不好， 对自己失望或有负家人期望 Feeling bad about yourself – or that you are a failure and have let yourself or your family down	0	1	2	3
7. 难以集中精神做事，例如看报纸或看电视 Having trouble concentrating on things, such as reading the newspaper or watching television	0	1	2	3
8. 其他人反映你行动或说话迟缓；或者相反， 你比平常活动更多——坐立不安，停不下来 Moving or speaking so slowly that other people could have noticed? Or the opposite – being so fidgety or restless that you have been moving around a lot more than usual	0	1	2	3
9. 想到自己最好去死或自残 Having thoughts that you would be better off dead or of hurting yourself in some way	0	1	2	3

Among the three most common scales, the PHQ-9 offers the quickest administration and the tightest linkage to DSM/ICD criteria for major depression. The other two scales take longer to administer as they have more questions and, in the case of the BDI, response choices are not merely indications of the frequency of symptoms, so many more lines of text must be read carefully and considered by the respondent. PHQ-9 responses capture a single factor (depression) or at most two (somatic and cognitive/affective); the CES-D and BDI usually capture three or more aspects of depression and so can give more insight into a person's depressive phenotype. The CES-D and BDI capture symptoms of depression not included in the criteria for MDD, such as interpersonal problems and a lack of positive affect. Asking people about a broader range of depressive symptoms reduces the risk of a false-negative result if the condition to be predicted is clinical depression as described in this book. An additional limitation of the PHQ-9 is that among patients diagnosed with MDD and receiving treatment for it, the PHQ-9 can be relatively insensitive to improvement in symptoms with treatment. This issue has been specifically reported when the PHQ-9 was used to rate the responses of Chinese psychiatric inpatients to antidepressant treatment (Feng et al., 2016).

The Chinese PHQ-9 has been evaluated across a wide range of populations and contexts, as defined by age, education, place of residence (urban vs. rural, mainland vs. Hong Kong or Taiwan), and clinical status (non-patient vs. medical patient vs. psychiatric patient). In all published studies, the Chinese PHQ-9 was found to be internally consistent and to have a high area under the receiver operating characteristic curve for predicting MDD. However, the population and the context of administration had dramatic effects on the optimal cut point for an MDD diagnosis and on the factor analysis of the scale. The effects are large, supporting this book's premise that the intersection of other identities with nationality matters far more than nationality per se in determining the phenomenology of depression and how depressed people experience and describe their condition.

The optimal cut point for diagnosing major depression in Taiwanese high school students with the Chinese PHQ-9 was ≥15—much higher than the cutoff score of ≥10 most often used with the English PHQ-9 (Tsai et al., 2014). A plausible interpretation of the number is that, for Taiwanese high school students, occasional depressive symptoms are normal and that MDD should be suspected strongly only if symptoms are multiple, continual, and persistent. Among college students in Changsha, the optimal cutoff score was ≥11, again suggesting some normalization of intermittent depressive symptoms (Y. L. Zhang, Liang, et al., 2013). However, an optimal cutoff score of >10 for diagnosing MDD does not mean that lower scores—indicating less frequent or fewer depressive symptoms—are clinically irrelevant. Most adolescents and young adults who die by suicide would not have met the criteria for MDD at the time of their deaths. In a recent study of suicidality in 6836 students enrolled in 2016 at a public university in Shanghai, only 10.8% of the 992 students assessed as high suicide risk had scores ≥10 on the PHQ-9, and only 12 of the 66 students with a history of suicide attempts scored above that threshold (R. Wu et al., 2021).

When a sample of new fathers in Hong Kong consisting mostly of middle- and upper-middle-class men with secondary or tertiary education (average income approximately 57,000 USD) was screened for postnatal depression with the Chinese PHQ-9, the optimal cut point for diagnosing postnatal MDD was ≥4 (Lai et al., 2010). In a study population of typically happy and often sleep-deprived new fathers, having cognitive/affective symptoms of depression would be unusual unless one were ill, and somatic symptoms like fatigue probably would not "bother" the men, who would naturally attribute them to their current circumstances.

A study of the Chinese PHQ-9 in 1045 people from the general population of Shanghai showed an optimal cutoff score of ≥7, also well below the usual cutoff score for the English PHQ-9 (W. Wang et al., 2014). The relatively low cutoff might indicate a tendency of Shanghai residents to understate depressive symptoms or alternatively to normalize them and thus not be "bothered" by them.

In a non-clinical sample of rural people age 60 and above in Hunan Province, most of whom had low incomes and less than a high school education, the optimal PHQ-9 cutoff score for predicting MDD was ≥8. Somatic symptoms were similarly correlated with the total score, while cognitive symptoms like psychomotor slowing, trouble concentrating, and suicidal thoughts had correlations of <.5 with the total score (Z. W. Liu et al., 2016). The numbers suggest that, for most of the subjects, depression was a mind–body problem and that people were less likely to report cognitive problems or suicidality than more educated and/or urban Chinese.

In studies at Chinese primary care clinics, optimal Chinese PHQ-9 cutoff scores for predicting a diagnosis of MDD have been ≥10 or ≥9 (S. Chen et al., 2010, 2013). In Chinese medical specialty clinics, optimal cutoff scores have varied by patients' primary medical diagnoses, for example, ≥9 in a psoriasis clinic (Ye et al., 2020) and ≥7 in an epilepsy clinic (Xia et al., 2019) and in a diabetes clinic (Y. Zhang, Ting, et al., 2013). A person's identity and perspective as a primary care patient, or one with a specific chronic disease, are likely to be more significant than national origin as influences on the psychometrics of the PHQ-9.

Factor analyses of the Chinese PHQ-9 have yielded one of three patterns: one factor, two factors, and one factor with two or more secondary factors. In the first pattern, somatic, affective, and cognitive symptoms of depression all correlate with one another, describing depression as a mind–body illness. In the second, there are separable somatic and cognitive/affective factors, with some depressed people experiencing primarily psychological distress and other experiencing mainly somatic illness. In the third, a mind–body experience of depression is the norm, but a substantial minority of people with depressive symptoms will have disproportionate problems with a specific aspect of depression like low mood/anhedonia or disturbed sleep/fatigue.

While for most people in China depression remains a mind–body problem, a substantial proportion of the population can psychologize their suffering like Westerners and can describe intense emotional distress without equally severe somatic complaints. A separate cognitive/affective dimension of depression is more likely in more educated, urban populations, such as students at major universities (Y. Zhou et al., 2020). Optimal cutoff scores for student populations tend to be higher than those for the general population or for non-psychiatric patients. In China, students might have a greater "license to complain" than the general population, while patients with general medical conditions might normalize some of the somatic symptoms of depression as inevitable accompaniments of their physical problems.

Cultural Customization of the PHQ-9?

Clinicians diagnosing and treating depression in first-generation Chinese immigrants to the U.S. have noticed limitations of the PHQ-9 when used with less acculturated patients, especially when the purpose is identification of milder but clinically significant cases. A group of clinicians and researchers working with the Chinese community in San Francisco solicited the input of patients regarding potential modification of the PHQ-9 to focus more on their typical concerns, to avoid terms associated with stigma and shame, and to minimize effects of age, gender, or level of acculturation on item responses.

They then created a new nine-item questionnaire based on patients' suggestions, the Chinese American Depression Scale (CADS-9) (Wong et al., 2012). They showed that the scale was especially sensitive to mild clinical depression in less-acculturated Chinese immigrants.

美国华人移民心理健康问卷
Chinese American Depression Scale (CADS-9)

在过去两星期，你是否被以下事情所困扰？如果是，被困扰多少天？请阅读每题，并圈上最合适的答案。 Over the last two weeks, were you bothered by the following problems? If so, how many days? Please read each statement carefully and circle the most appropriate answer.	完全没有/ 没有一天 (0 天) Not at all/ No days	非常少/ 几天 (1-3 天) A little bit/ A few days	有时/大约 一半时间 (4-10 天) Quite a bit/ About half the days	经常是/差 不多每天 (11-14 天) Extremely/ Nearly every day
1. 很多事情让你感到很担心。 Many things make you very worried.	0	1	2	3
2. 你难以集中精神。 You are unable to concentrate well.	0	1	2	3
3. 你非常害怕自己健康有问题。例如：患癌症或心脏病。 You are very afraid that you have health problems. For example, you might have cancer or heart disease.	0	1	2	3
4. 你感到非常不开心。 You feel very unhappy.	0	1	2	3
5. 你很容易发脾气和发怒。 You have tantrums and get angry very easily.	0	1	2	3
6. 你隐瞒自己生活有困难。 You hide your life difficulties from other people.	0	1	2	3
7. 你感到很害怕。 You feel very afraid.	0	1	2	3
8. 你完全不想和别人接触，交往，或外出。 You don't want to have contact with people, socialize, or go out at all.	0	1	2	3
9. 你想过伤害自己。 You have thought about hurting yourself.	0	1	2	3

Note: This version of the CADS-9 was modified by the authors from the original version of Wong et al. It uses simplified rather than traditional Chinese characters, to facilitate its comparison with the official literal translation of the PHQ-9 into simplified Chinese.

Three items of the CADS-9 concern worry and fear—symptoms that are not part of the DSM/ICD definition of MDD but are highly correlated with non-melancholic depression and are relatively non-stigmatized emotions that do not carry a connotation of "mental illness" in Chinese culture. The CADS-9 also explicitly refers to concealing one's problems and to avoiding socialization—typical reactions to depression in a cultural environment where revealing emotional trouble might entail a loss of face. Like the PHQ-9, the CADS-9 asks patients how many days in the past two weeks they were bothered by a "problem." However, the questionnaire offers the respondent the alternative of giving a higher score to an item if a problem bothered them "quite a bit" or "extremely" even if the problem was not present seven days or more in the past two weeks.

When used for assessing Chinese-speaking immigrants for major depression in a medical or social service setting, optimal cutoff scores for diagnosing mild, moderate, and severe clinical depression were 10, 15, and 20 for women and 9, 14, and 19 for men, respectively. Using a lower cutoff score for men was supported by the study's data and attributed to expectations of traditional Chinese culture that men should not complain.

There would be no obvious advantage to an instrument like the CADS-9 when screening or rating depression in acculturated immigrants or in an adolescent or young adult student population in which disclosure of negative affect would not be stigmatized. In such populations, optimal cutoff scores for diagnosing clinical depression—or MDD specifically—might not differ between males and females.

As a practical point, the staff in a clinic serving Chinese immigrants and using the PHQ-9 as a depression screen might notice that many significantly depressed people were not being detected by it. They might then consider whether the PHQ-9 would work well with a lower cutoff score or whether the problem was that even quite depressed patients would not endorse specific items on the PHQ-9 because of cultural incompatibility or anticipated stigma or loss of face. If the latter, an instrument like the CADS-9 could be tried and evaluated as a substitute.

The choice of items and the precise wording of item translations on a depression symptom questionnaire can make a clinically meaningful difference when assessing patients from cultures different from the Anglo American one in which the PHQ-9, CES-D, BDI, and other commonly used depression questionnaires were developed. The psychometric and clinical impacts of imperfect translation are greater when scales are used with less-acculturated people, and when detecting milder forms of clinical depression is the main aim of using the questionnaire. Non-Chinese clinicians working with Chinese patients might find that adjustments in item choice, item wording, cut points, and scoring method can make depression questionnaires more useful both for screening patients for clinical depression in their practices and for providing points of departure for productive diagnostic interviews.

The Chinese CES-D and the Varied Faces of Depression among Chinese People

For establishing whether a person is likely to meet DSM/ICD criteria for major depression, the PHQ-9 is efficient, but it is relatively insensitive to clinically significant conditions that are "subthreshold" with respect to those criteria and might completely miss forms of clinical depression in which the loss of positive experience and the presence of new or worsened interpersonal problems are more salient than somatic symptoms or negative thoughts. By the criteria of this book—and in the experience of many clinicians—decreased positive thoughts and emotions and impairments in social function and relationship quality can be symptoms of depression more troubling to patients than negative thoughts and blue moods. Psychological autopsy studies of suicides and interviews with people who have attempted suicide suggest that new or increased problems with important relationships and feeling there is nothing positive to live for can lead to suicidality. People who are suicidal because of interpersonal problems and a loss of positive affect do not necessarily meet DSM/ICD criteria for MDD, and they don't necessarily reach cutoff scores on the PHQ-9 or a similar depression screening questionnaire. To gain more insight into a patient's depression phenotype, the CES-D and BDI are more informative than the PHQ-9 because they have more questions about symptoms of depression that are not explicit DSM/ICD criteria. Factor analyses of CES-D and BDI data in diverse populations have shown multiple factors even in cultural groups in which depression typically is experienced as a mind–body illness. In this chapter we focus on the CES-D as the scale is in the public domain.

A Chinese translation of the CES-D has been used to screen for and measure the severity of depression since the 1980s. There have been several Chinese translations of the CES-D since the scale was introduced; a representative one is shown.

流行病學研究中心抑鬱量表
The Center for Epidemiologic Studies Depression Scale (CES-D)

以下句子描述一些自我感覺或行為。請圈出最接近您**過去一週**的狀況。

Below is a list of some of the ways you may have felt or behaved. Please indicate how often you have felt this way during the **past week**. (circle **one** number on each line)

過去一週 During the past week...	很少或 完全沒有 Rarely or none of the time (少過1日) (Less than 1 day)	有幾天 Some or a little of the time (持續1-2日) (1-2 days)	間中或 一半時間 Occasional or moderate amount of time (持續3-4日) (3-4 days)	經常或 近乎每天 Most or all of the time (持續5-7日) (5-7 days)
1. 我被一些平時不會困擾我的事情困擾 I was bothered by things that usually don't bother me	0	1	2	3
2. 我不想吃東西,我的胃口很差 I did not feel like eating; my appetite was poor	0	1	2	3
3. 即使有家人和朋友的幫忙,我仍然覺得憂鬱 I felt that I could not shake off the blues even with help from my family	0	1	2	3
4. 我覺得我不比其他人差 I felt that I was just as good as other people	0	1	2	3
5. 我很難集中精神工作 I had trouble keeping my mind on what I was doing	0	1	2	3
6. 我覺得情緒低落 I felt depressed	0	1	2	3
7. 我覺得我做每件事情都很吃力 I felt that everything I did was an effort	0	1	2	3
8. 我對將來抱有希望 I felt hopeful about the future	0	1	2	3
9. 我覺得自己一生很失敗 I thought my life had been a failure	0	1	2	3
10. 我覺得恐懼 I felt fearful	0	1	2	3
11. 我睡眠不安寧 My sleep was restless	0	1	2	3
12. 我很開心 I was happy	0	1	2	3
13. 我比平時少說話 I talked less than usual	0	1	2	3
14. 我覺得孤獨 I felt lonely	0	1	2	3
15. 我覺得其他人不友善 People were unfriendly	0	1	2	3
16. 我很享受生活 I enjoyed life	0	1	2	3
17. 我會經常無故哭泣 I had crying spells	0	1	2	3
18. 我覺得不開心 I felt sad	0	1	2	3
19. 我覺得其他人不喜歡我 I felt that people disliked me	0	1	2	3
20. 我提不起勁 I could not get "going"	0	1	2	3

In the original conception of the CES-D, the 20 items on the questionnaire were designed to capture four aspects of depression: Seven items deal with depressed affect, seven with somatic symptoms, four with positive affect (scored inversely), and two with interpersonal problems.

Among rural Chinese people, depressed mood and somatic symptoms group together as a single factor, in keeping with the traditional Chinese mind–body concept of depressive illness (J. Zhang et al., 2012). Factors related to lack of positive affect and to interpersonal problems remain separate. Using the Chinese CES-D rather than the Chinese PHQ-9 to screen for depression would be an appealing choice in the rural Chinese population, where suicide rates are high, and suicide in a depressed person who wouldn't meet MDD criteria could be precipitated by interpersonal conflicts, especially when there were few positive experiences to counterbalance a person's distress.

In a 1999 study of three groups of college students—Chinese and White students at two American universities and students at a university in China, none of whom had sought mental health services—the Chinese students were significantly less likely to endorse somatic symptoms of depression than either group of American students, and they were less likely to endorse items related to positive mood—to see less hope for the future and to lack joy and happiness in the present. When the study was conducted in 1999, acknowledgment of mood symptoms by urban, educated young adults was already acceptable, and university students in China might have had realistic concerns about their careers and personal prospects in a country undergoing rapid socioeconomic change. Their objective situations rather than cultural differences might better explain their responses to the positive affect items on the CES-D (Yen et al., 2000).

Among adolescents in Hong Kong, responses to the CES-D were consistent with a three-factor model in which somatic, negative cognitive/affective, and interpersonal problems were separable dimensions of depression. The absence of positive affect was poorly correlated with the remainder of the symptoms of depression (S. W. Lee et al., 2008). Among mainland Chinese adolescents, depressed affect, somatic symptoms, and the lack of positive affect were independent aspects of depression. Interpersonal problems did not appear as a separate factor but simply accompanied depressed affect (M. Wang et al., 2013). A study of middle school students in urban China showed a similar three-factor structure in which somatic symptoms were distinct from depressed affect and interpersonal problems covaried with depressed affect (Zhu et al., 2021). In these studies, subjects' identities as adolescents appear more relevant than their Chinese nationality. Teenagers around the world will express negative moods without necessarily including somatic complaints, and it is typical of adolescence for interpersonal problems and low mood to have a reciprocal relationship.

A recent study compared the factor structure of the CES-D in university undergraduates in Changsha (the capital of Hunan Province, with a population of over 10 million) and outpatients in mental health clinics in the same city. A five-factor model best fit the data—with the same model working for the college students and the psychiatric outpatients. The model comprised the four original factors of depressed affect, somatic complaints, positive affect, and interpersonal problems and a fifth factor, *alienation*, which included items about loneliness, fear, and crying spells. Not unexpectedly, women scored higher on alienation and men on interpersonal problems ("people were unfriendly" and "I felt that people disliked me") and somatic complaints (Niu et al., 2021). Women were more likely to acknowledge internal emotional problems and men to make a somatic or external attribution of their distress—gender-related differences typical of a "masculine" culture like that of China.

Jiang, Wang, et al. (2019) took an alternative approach to deconstructing the CES-D with a population of students at Universities in Guangzhou. They found the test to have excellent psychometric properties in identifying clinical depression (including both MDD and "subthreshold depression") when six items were removed from the scale. The items eliminated were those related to crying spells, interpersonal problems, feeling that one's life had been a failure, talking less than usual, and feeling fearful. Crying spells were rarely endorsed by depressed males. The other dropped items appeared less consistently related to depression than the core 14 items. With a cutoff point of 16, the 14-item scale identified clinical depression in 31% of the sample. Neither gender, grade, nor college major had a significant relationship to the CES-D score. Three factors accounted for more than half of the total variance: somatic symptoms, depressed affect, and anhedonia.

Chinese psychiatric outpatients with depression as a primary diagnosis or as a comorbidity in contemporary China express their illness multidimensionally much as university students do. Among people in ongoing psychiatric treatment, the "patient" identity usually eclipses national origin as a determinant of how depression is experienced and described. If the patient and a treating mental health professional don't arrive at a common understanding of the illness being treated, the patient is likely to drop out of treatment, not adhere to prescribed therapies, or pursue treatment in a non-psychiatric context like that of primary care or TCM. Even if a depressed person presented with a somatic chief complaint, if they accepted a diagnosis of major depression, acknowledged their depressed mood to a clinician, and adhered to antidepressant medication and/or psychotherapy, somatic symptoms of the depression would become merely an aspect of the patient's depressive phenotype.

While historically somatization was thought to be more common in women, the somatic expression of depression, this may no longer be true where, as in today's Chinese cities, the cultural environment might allow the direct expression of negative feelings without unacceptable stigma. In a 2016–2017 study of medical outpatients at hospitals in five large Chinese cities, the prevalence of somatic symptom disorder (preoccupation with somatic symptoms without a medical explanation) was no greater in women than in men. In both men and women, higher levels of depressive symptoms were associated with a greater likelihood that the patient would meet diagnostic criteria for somatic symptom disorder (Cao et al., 2020). If in China's "masculine" culture men are discouraged from expressing negative affect, they would be more likely than women with the same level of depression to express their depressed mood somatically. A greater prevalence of clinical depression in women combined with a lower level of somatization would lead to an insignificant gender difference in preoccupation with somatic symptoms.

In the present century the psychometrics of the CES-D in Chinese people has been studied in diverse clinical and non-clinical populations, the latter usually comprising secondary school and university students. While the scale's reliability and internal consistency have been shown to be acceptable in most studies, factor analysis has revealed differences in the CES-D's function depending on attributes other than Chinese nationality. Over the two decades beginning in 2000, China became wealthier and, at least in urban areas, developed a more globalized culture. Its citizens became more "connected," with near-universal smartphone ownership and internet access. Coincident with these changes, "Western" expressions of depression appeared more often, especially in younger, urban, and more educated people. Recent Chinese immigrants to the U.S. typically express depression in the same way as people of the same age who remained in China. Those who immigrated from China to the U.S. in the 1980s and 1990s would show tighter linkage of the somatic and cognitive/affective dimensions of depression than those who immigrated after 2000. Inseparability of the somatic and cognitive/affective dimensions of depression was found in a factor analysis of CES-D data from telephone interviews of Chinese Americans in the late 1980s (Ying, 1988). More recent immigrants from China to the United States are more likely to be college-educated, to be of working age, and to have above-median incomes—all attributes associated with a more Western expression of depression in which somatic and cognitive/affective symptoms constitute separate factors.

Patients with major medical conditions are another group in which somatic and cognitive/affective dimensions of depression can be relatively independent in Chinese people whether in urban China, rural China, or an English-speaking country. A person with cancer or a recent stroke would be unlikely to be stigmatized for having negative emotions and thoughts, and the attribution of somatic symptoms to the medical condition or to depression often would be ambiguous. Furthermore, an inpatient at a general hospital who showed signs of severe depression could easily be seen by a psychiatrist, even in places with major shortages of mental health services. If a patient were seen in consultation by a psychiatrist who made a diagnosis of major depression, the patient's acceptance of the diagnosis would translate into their greater recognition of cognitive and affective symptoms and greater comfort in acknowledging them.

Chinese patients receiving primary care who are not highly educated are more likely than outpatients receiving medical specialty care to show close association of CES-D items for negative affect and items for somatic symptoms (Chin et al., 2015). In that population, items related to positive affect and interpersonal problems constitute independent factors. In establishing a therapeutic relationship and in choosing personalized therapy for a Chinese patient in whom depression has a prominent somatic face, it can be helpful to identify the loss of positive experience and the presence of new or worse interpersonal problems. The CES-D, or interview questions with similar content, can aid in the process.

Findings of these and other recent studies suggest that somatization of depression among Chinese people can be usefully understood as a phenomenon related to the intersection of Chinese ethnicity with age/generation, education, social class, and place of residence. The expression of the depressive experience will be influenced by context—clinical or non-clinical, and among clinical contexts whether the patient is a medical specialty patient with a serious illness, a primary care patient, or a psychiatric patient. Clinically depressed Chinese people, regardless of their cultural identity, are likely to have a combination of somatic and affective/cognitive symptoms. If somatic symptoms are clearly more prominent, targeting somatic symptoms with medication and addressing "stress" with a psychological intervention are suggested. If affective and cognitive symptoms predominate, targeting mood with medication and negative cognitions with counseling or psychotherapy (the latter potentially including a psychotherapeutic smartphone app) would be better initial treatment. The dimensions of loss of positive affect and new or increased interpersonal problems can be identified and addressed, further demonstrating the clinician's attention to the patient's personal narrative and the personalization of treatment.

In 1998 and 1999, Chinese-speaking first-generation immigrant patients in a Boston primary care clinic were screened for depression with the BDI, and those who screened positive were evaluated for MDD with a structured diagnostic interview. Of the 40 patients confirmed to have MDD, with a mean age of 46 ± 15 years and a mean length of stay in the U.S. of 6 ± 5 years, 29 were interviewed about their illness beliefs with the Explanatory Model Interview Catalogue, a structured exploration of illness beliefs including those related to etiology, stigma, and treatment (A. Yeung, D. Chang, et al., 2004): 76% of the patients had a somatic chief complaint, with fatigue, insomnia, and headache being the most common. None complained of a depressed mood, but 93% of the sample—all but two patients—endorsed a depressed mood on the BDI. When asked if they would agree with a diagnosis of MDD, 48% said they'd never heard of MDD, and only three patients thought they had any form of psychiatric condition. 90% of the patients thought they had an illness that affected their mind but was not intrinsically mental. 93% saw stress as causing or contributing to their illness; but only one patient had sought mental health services. Treatment by a general healthcare provider and support from family and friends were their preferred options for coping with their illness. Most of the patients attributed no stigma to their condition.

A decade later, between 2009 and 2012, an overlapping group of investigators screened Chinese primary care patients with the PHQ-9 and, among those with scores of 10 or higher, found 190 who had a diagnosis of MDD confirmed by a structured clinical interview and were willing to be interviewed about their illness beliefs (J. A. Chen, Hung, et al., 2015). Their sample had a mean age of 49.9±14.5 years—not significantly different from those of the earlier study—and 51.6% had less than a high school education. In marked contrast to the previous study, more than half of the patients (52.1%) had a chief complaint of depression (depressed mood, unhappiness, or "mood problems"). Of those who did not mention mood as a chief complaint, most mentioned common components/concomitants of major depression, including problems with sleep, loss of appetite, low energy, difficulty concentrating, ruminating, and/or agitation/irritability. Only 10% of the entire sample had a chief complaint of somatic pain or other physical symptoms not directly relatable to depression.

More than two thirds of the patients (68%) attributed their illness to psychological stress, of which problems marital problems, work or job problems, family relationship problems, or financial problems were identified most often. Another 17% attributed their illness to a psychological problem other than an external stress, such as their personality or their personal history. Remarkably, 75% saw self-help (e.g., reading or exercise) or assistance from friends and/or relatives as their most important resource for dealing with their illness. Only nine out of the 180 subjects (5%) viewed a general health professional as their most important resource; the same proportion thought a psychiatrist or psychotherapist would be their best source of help. Most of the patients showed signs of self-stigma: 40% would not tell another person about their illness.

Neither sample is fully representative of the Chinese American immigrant population, but the results strongly suggest a shift in Chinese American immigrants' typical views of depression since the late 1990s. By 2010 depression was now acknowledged as a medical problem—one acceptable to present to a physician as a chief complaint. Mood complaints often were presented in association with other symptoms of the major depressive syndrome. Somatic symptoms not relatable to depression were not mentioned. The patients studied saw depression as a mental disorder, one with a psychological rather than a biological cause. In that context, however, depression was more stigmatized, and clinicians of any kind were less likely to be sought as an important source of help. Apparently, for middle-aged and older Chinese American immigrants without higher education, the concept of depression as an integrated body–mind illness amenable to medical treatment had been replaced by a stigmatized mental condition with no biological cause, for which medical treatment would be irrelevant and perhaps useless.

The findings of Yeung, Chen, and colleagues suggest a complex effect of acculturation on Chinese American immigrants' views and narratives of depression. Similar complex effects can be seen in residents of mainland China who, in connection with higher education and living in a prosperous metropolitan area, have come to have a more "globalized" cultural identity.

Acculturation, Stigma, and Therapeutic Strategy

Unacculturated Chinese immigrants to the U.S. (or rural-to-urban migrants within China) with a traditional view of depression typically would experience depressive illness as a somatic problem and would seek treatment from a primary care physician if their symptoms were sufficiently distressing or disabling. They would acknowledge depressed mood or anhedonia if asked about it. They would be open to seeing stress as a cause or contributor to the illness. They probably would acknowledge to others that they were ill, though they might emphasize their main somatic problem (e.g., fatigue or insomnia) rather than name their illness as depression. They usually would not stigmatize themselves or anticipate being stigmatized by others. They would not initially think of consulting a mental health professional for their problem. If the primary care physician were to consider a referral for therapy or counseling, it would best be framed as help in coping better with stress, rather than as treatment for a "mental disorder" or "mental illness." The language of psychiatric diagnosis would, of course, be unavoidable if the patient had severe symptoms requiring hospitalization, antipsychotic medication, or electroconvulsive therapy (ECT) or the condition caused occupational or other disability for which the patient sought compensation or formal assistance.

Relatively unacculturated Chinese immigrants—and older people in China with traditional views and illness narratives of depression—can do well with collaborative care, in which treatment of depression is provided by a primary care physician who is assisted by a psychiatrist. The patient regularly sees both physicians; the primary care doctor prescribes antidepressants, treats comorbid medical problems and symptoms, and offers general support, while the psychiatrist makes a psychiatric diagnosis, recommends specific antidepressant treatment, monitors the response to treatment, and oversees psychoeducation and/or psychotherapy. The approach has proved effective in Boston and in Taiwan (H. C. Huang et al., 2018; Huang, Liu, et al., 2018; A. Yeung et al., 2016).

Partially-acculturated Chinese Americans typically would recognize depression as a syndrome characterized by low mood as the essential feature, accompanied by some associated physical symptoms like insomnia or fatigue and perhaps some irritability or agitation. They would blame it on a combination of external stress and personal weakness/vulnerability and would be reluctant to seek general medical care for it, to consult a mental health professional, or even to disclose it except possibly to highly trusted people. They would stigmatize themselves for being depressed and would anticipate being stigmatized by others if they knew of their problem. While they probably would not seek clinical treatment for their illness, if they did see a clinician, they would present with a chief complaint of a persistently low or depressed mood together with associated physical problems. They probably would be more open to taking medication targeting their physical symptoms (e.g., insomnia or low energy) than to seeing a psychotherapist or counselor. If the patient stigmatized themselves and anticipated public stigma for being depressed, internet-based psychotherapy might be more acceptable. Internet-delivered manual-based psychotherapies for depression, especially cognitive behavioral therapy (iCBT), have shown efficacy for both major depression (PHQ-9 scores of 10 or higher) and "subthreshold depression" (PHQ-9 scores of 5–9). Subthreshold depression is equally responsive to guided and unguided iCBT. While major depression has responded better to guided iCBT in clinical trials, its response to unguided iCBT has been clinically and statistically significant (Karyotaki et al., 2020). Recently, specialized iCBT programs were shown to significantly help Chinese people with depression following illness with COVID-19 (Z. Liu et al., 2021) and with insomnia and depression due to pandemic-related stress (Song et al., 2021). Patients with severe depression, regardless of their nationality, usually prefer face-to-face treatment (Choi et al., 2015).

A publicly available iCBT program, MoodGYM, was developed by the Center for Mental Health Research at the Australian National University (Christensen et al., 2004). In its Chinese translation it was tested and found effective for treating depression in Chinese Australians (Choi et al., 2012) and effective as an adjunct to standard outpatient care at a teaching hospital in Beijing (K. S. Yeung et al., 2018). People who know they are depressed and actively seek treatment will do better with unguided iCBT than those who seek clinical care for a somatic concern, are diagnosed with depression, and are prescribed online treatment. The latter will do better with iCBT that is supported by interaction with a therapist (Iakimova et al., 2017).

Fully-acculturated Chinese Americans would recognize depression as a "real illness" that was not entirely their fault, for which medical or psychological treatment of some kind might be helpful. They would still be more likely to consult a non-psychiatric physician than a psychiatrist or non-medical mental health professional. They probably would be open to considering either medication or counseling if suggested by a trusted physician. They might be embarrassed about their illness and reluctant to disclose it but would not blame themselves, stigmatize themselves severely, or think that others were justified in stigmatizing them. While fully-acculturated Chinese Americans would not be free from self-stigma or misinformation about depression, their beliefs and attitudes about depression would be associated more with their age and generation, educational level, and social class than with their race and national origin.

The idea that partial acculturation can be especially problematic is supported by analysis of data from a study of the health and healthcare of a panel of 3159 older Chinese Americans in Chicago. The subjects in the study, whose ages ranged from 60 to 109, with an average age of 76.3 years and an average of 20 years' residence in the U.S., were assessed for depression with the PHQ-9, for pain with ordinal self-ratings of severity and interference with daily life, and for acculturation with a standard scale based on language preferences, social relations with Chinese versus non-Chinese people, and engagement with Chinese versus non-Chinese media. The three variables of depression, pain, and acculturation were considered to be predictors of the number of visits to a doctor's office or clinic over a two-year period, controlling for age, education, income, years in the U.S., gender, health insurance coverage, number of chronic diseases, and the presence of disabilities affecting either physical or instrumental activities of daily living. Among people with low acculturation levels and high acculturation levels, pain and depression had independent, significant effects on the number of doctor visits; but among those with intermediate levels of acculturation, the effect of depression on the number of doctor visits was entirely mediated by somatic pain (Jiang, Sun, et al., 2019).

The impact of acculturation on the presentation and acknowledgment of depression in Chinese immigrants has also been observed in Australia, and, as in the U.S., its impact is a simple one of decreasing somatization and increasing willingness to seek treatment (Parker et al., 2005). Also, as in the U.S., acculturation effects are confounded with effects of age and education since, compared with younger Chinese Australians, older ones are more likely to be born in China, to have immigrated as adults, and not to have tertiary education.

Gordon Parker and his colleagues studied Chinese immigrants (first- and second-generation) in Sydney primary care practices, comparing those who chose to complete questionnaires in Chinese (less acculturated) and those who completed them in English (more acculturated), with each other and with non-Chinese patients from the same practices. Patients were presented with scenarios of fatigue, insomnia, and loss of appetite and were asked to choose a "somatic," "normalizing," or "psychologizing" explanation as most likely. For example, the options for fatigue were "There is a medical cause (e.g., anemia)," "I've been over-exerting myself or not exercising enough," and "I'm emotionally exhausted or discouraged." The patients were also given a screening questionnaire for current clinical depression, the ten-item Depression in the Medically Ill (DMI-10), which specifically excludes somatic symptoms, and were asked about their lifetime history of periods of two weeks or longer during which they felt worthless and hopeless, had decreased energy and motivation, and had decreased ability to cope. The authors found that, for fatigue and insomnia, the subjects who completed questionnaires in Chinese were significantly more likely than more acculturated Chinese or non-Chinese patients to offer somatic explanations and less likely to offer psychologizing ones for descriptions of other people's symptoms. However, the less-acculturated Chinese patients were more likely to have DMI scores in the range suggesting clinical depression, indicating their willingness to endorse mood-related symptoms when asked specifically about them.

When queried about a lifetime history of periods of altered mood, energy, and motivation, Chinese Australians were less likely to report them than non-Chinese. Among those who did, less-acculturated Chinese patients usually characterized their episodes as "normal blues," while more acculturated Chinese patients were more willing to characterize them as a "distinct disorder." Most of the non-Chinese patients with a history of such episodes had consulted their primary care physician or a psychiatrist when ill, while fewer than half of the Chinese patients did so, regardless of their level of acculturation. Of the Chinese patients who saw a mental health professional, most saw psychologists rather than psychiatrists, a preference not shown by the non-Chinese patients. In China, psychiatrists are associated with the treatment of severe—and highly stigmatized—mental illness. Less-acculturated Chinese patients who experienced an episode of probable clinical depression were more than four times more likely to consult friends or family about their problem, a significant difference from the more-acculturated Chinese patients that suggests lower anticipated stigma in the less acculturated patients.

The results of the study suggest that along the path of acculturation, Chinese immigrants to English-speaking countries come to accept the concept of depression as an illness, but as a stigmatized one for which they are reluctant to seek medical treatment or support from friends and family. At the same time, while less-acculturated Chinese are more inclined than non-Chinese to think of fatigue and insomnia as somatic problems unrelated to mood, they tend to have little difficulty acknowledging mood symptoms if asked about them.

A depressed, unacculturated Chinese American immigrant might present to a primary care physician with somatic symptoms of depression rather than with depressed mood, but would acknowledge a depressed mood or anhedonia if asked about it and would see a role for psychological stress in causing or contributing to the problem. They probably would be open to medical treatment by the primary care physician for their somatic symptoms of depression and might consider a referral for counseling to improve their coping with stress. Some might accept collaborative care involving a psychiatrist and their primary care physician, while others would prefer a non-medical counselor. Psychiatrists are associated with mental illness and thus with stigma, whereas a counselor helping them manage stress would not imply they were mentally ill. A primary care physician need not use the language of *mental illness* or *mental disorder* in dialogue with a depressed patient, unless the patient has symptoms requiring antipsychotic medication, ECT, or another treatment not given in mild to moderate cases.

Trust and Adherence to Antidepressant Medication

Patients' trust in their physicians is variable and a known correlate of better adherence to prescribed treatment and better ultimate treatment outcomes. Compared with patients in the U.S. and other high-income countries, those in mainland China have less trust in their physicians. Trust in physicians in China has been decreasing as the country has transitioned from a socialized medical system to a profit-driven system, as there is widespread suspicion by patients that doctors order unnecessary tests, procedures, and medications for personal financial gain (W. Wang et al., 2018; Zhao & Zhang, 2019; Zhao et al., 2018).

As trust in physicians and respect for the medical profession has decreased, a vicious circle has developed in which violence against physicians is common and sometimes normalized, fewer talented people are interested in becoming physicians, the standard of care declines, and patients find even less reason to trust and respect their doctors.

In contrast to current residents of mainland China, older Chinese Americans have relatively high trust in their physicians, especially with respect to their physicians' knowledge, skills, and judgment (Simon et al., 2013). Many emigrated from China at a time when public trust in physicians had not yet deteriorated. Some came to America with low trust in physicians but through acculturation and positive experiences developed greater trust. And, among wealthier and more educated Chinese immigrants, the U.S. has long been seen as the locus of the world's best medical care, if one can connect with the right physicians and institutions for one's specific case.

However, mistrust of physicians can be encountered in Chinese Americans of any age, and it is relevant not only to treatment of depression but also to the risk of depression. In a longitudinal study of a panel of 2713 older adult Chinese Americans in metropolitan Chicago, subjects' trust in their physicians was measured using the Trust in Physician Scale of Anderson and Detrick (1990). The scale has patients rate their level of agreement with each of 11 statements, such as "I doubt that my doctor really cares about me as a person," "My doctor is usually considerate of my needs and puts them first," and "I trust my doctor so much that I always try to follow his/her advice." Higher trust in physicians was correlated with a lower level of depressive symptoms at a baseline assessment and with a lower risk of developing depression over the next two years (Dong, Bergren, & Simon, 2017).

Chronic medical illness and/or the risk of serious acute medical illness is universal in later life. A person who trusts physicians is more likely to seek medical care promptly if a new symptom develops and to collaborate with their physician(s) in the treatment, prevention, or monitoring of disease. Such behavior reduces medically-related stress, improves subjective health, and sometimes prevents major acute medical problems that often entail secondary depression.

Chinese American immigrants who left China after the nation's trust in physicians had deteriorated might bring with them a high level of suspicion of physicians' knowledge, judgment, or motives. Or, perceiving obvious positive differences between the Chinese medical system and the American system, they might idealize American medical care and have unrealistic expectations of its quality and effectiveness. In the latter case, they might be disillusioned as well as disappointed if the care they receive does not meet their expectations.

Beyond issues of personal trust in physicians or in the healthcare system, people can begin their treatment with biases about the value and risk of medical treatments, both generally and specifically for depression. Traditional Chinese views of Western (allopathic) medications and of depression and its treatment entail a high risk that a Chinese patient prescribed an antidepressant drug will discontinue it too soon, either stopping it before its maximal effect on depressive symptoms or stopping it too soon after symptoms remit. Another way that patients might express their concern about the potential harms of medication or mistrust of physicians' motivation or expertise is taking antidepressants at a lower dosage and/or lower frequency than prescribed.

Patients might be non-adherent from the outset—not filling a prescription or starting prescribed medication with a different dosage and/or on a different schedule than prescribed—or might become non-adherent in response to symptoms they consider to be side effects of the medication. Often the prescriber is not involved in the patient's decision, and often they are not notified of it. Both patients in China and immigrants from China to Western countries have shown a relatively high rate of antidepressant non-adherence or premature discontinuation. In a study broadly representative of patients treated for major depression with antidepressants at mental health centers and general hospitals in China, the rate of spontaneous discontinuation of medication was 38% (Zhu et al., 2020). In a sample of older Chinese people treated with antidepressants, high adherence was reported by 37.8%, moderate adherence by 39.2%, and low adherence by 23%. Among antidepressant-treated patients at a Hong Kong outpatient psychiatric clinic, 46% discontinued their medication within six months of its start. Those who did had an 8.4 times greater risk of relapse or recurrence within the year following the start of treatment (Yau et al., 2014). In a study of prescription drug adherence in residents of urban British Columbia, Chinese patients were significantly less likely than patients of White, South Asian, or mixed ethnicity to fill prescriptions for antidepressants (Morgan et al., 2011).

In the study of Zhu and colleagues, the three main reasons offered by usually adherent patients for their deliberate discontinuation of antidepressant drugs were concern about long-term side effects (36%), no perceived need for taking medications long-term (34%), and believing themselves to be completely cured (30%). Many Chinese patients' mixed feelings about allopathic medications—and their high frequency of non-adherence to prescribed treatment—are not confined to psychotropics. For example, in a 2014 study of patients with stroke, diabetes, and rheumatoid arthritis at two urban Chinese hospitals, non-adherence to prescribed medication was seen in more than half of those with strokes and more than a quarter of those with diabetes. Approximately 90% of the patients appreciated the necessity of their medication. Their non-adherence usually was based on concern about side effects and often a belief that they were personally sensitive to the negative effects of the prescribed treatment (Wei et al., 2017). In the just-cited Canadian study, Chinese-Canadian women were significantly less likely than those of other ethnicities to fill prescriptions for antihypertensives, antibiotics, and respiratory drugs; and Chinese-Canadian men were significantly less likely to fill prescriptions for statins (Morgan et al., 2011).

A patient's adherence to prescribed medication is associated with a balance of necessity and concern. On one side are the patient's beliefs that they need medication to recover and maintain their health and that the medication is likely to be effective. On the other side are concerns that the medication might have distressing or dangerous side effects either in the short term or with longer-term treatment, that it will be ineffective or that its benefit will not persist, and/or that they will become dependent upon the medication and unable to live without it. The balance of necessity and concern applies to medications in general and to the medications prescribed for a specific illness. Traditional Chinese beliefs about medications emphasize that all medications have side effects, that side effects that are not present at first can emerge with long-term use, that most health problems can be resolved without medications, and that relying on a medication to feel well will make one dependent upon it in an unhealthy way.

These beliefs can be accompanied by views that Western medications are prescribed too readily, that the dosages prescribed often are excessive for Chinese people, and that Western physicians are relatively insensitive to medications' negative effects on their patients. If a Chinese patient has had experience with TCM, they will know that in TCM the precise combination of ingredients and dosages for treating a patient's illness will be individualized according to their pattern of symptoms, physical findings, and individual personal characteristics. The personalized, holistic TCM approach, which is seen as safe, benign, and often effective, contrasts with the Western approach of giving a single drug (rather than a personalized mixture) at a dosage that is similar for all patients—either the same for all patients or varied in a simple way, e.g., according to a person's weight or a blood test result (Cao & Brown, 2020).

Either a clinician's interview or a questionnaire—the Beliefs about Medicines Questionnaire (BMQ) (Horne et al., 1999)—can be used to elicit a patient's preexisting beliefs about medications before an antidepressant prescription is written. Questions deal with the patient's perception of their need for antidepressant medication; concerns about its risks, including specific side effects and the potential for drug dependency; and general sentiments about the harmfulness of medications and whether medications are overused. What are the patient's concepts of how long they must take an antidepressant before knowing it will or won't work and of how long they should remain on the drug if it is effective? Does the patient worry that the drug can have dangerous long-term effects even if there are no short-term problems? Does the patient think that most prescription drugs do more harm than good and that natural remedies are safer and more effective in the long run? Does the patient think it is a good idea to stop medications from time to time to see if they are still needed? In a study of university undergraduates in the U.K., students with a self-reported Asian background were more likely than those reporting a European background to see medications as being intrinsically harmful, addictive substances that should be avoided if possible (Horne et al., 2004). If a clinician thinks that an antidepressant drug is indicated for a patient who has culturally-based risk factors for non-adherence or non-persistence with treatment, they should consider a combination of strategies for "culturally-aware prescribing":

1. The patient should be educated on how the medication works, including the time needed for maximal symptom relief, when and how dosage will be adjusted, the value of its longer-term use in preventing a relapse and facilitating full recovery, and the evidence supporting the continuation of antidepressants for several months following remission of symptoms. The patient can be told that once symptoms have been relieved with medication, they will be more able to improve important relationships, to perform better at school or work, to cope better with non-psychiatric illness, to get more benefit from counseling or psychotherapy, and to make lifestyle changes like healthier eating and increased exercise. Changes in one's life made while feeling better can help prevent another episode of depression—and if the medication is stopped too soon, the patient might find it difficult to make the most helpful changes. Taking medication for several months does not imply lifetime dependency upon it.

2. The clinician should make it clear to the patient that their antidepressant regimen—the specific drug(s), dosage(s), and schedule—will be individualized. If there are several viable options, the patient should join the clinician in a shared decision-making process regarding the specific drug tried first (or next), whether the dosage should be built up gradually rather than starting with the usual full dose, and how dosages should be timed and coordinated with meals and other medications the patient might be taking. The patient should be asked what side effects they are most worried about, and the prescription might be modified if doing so will minimize the risk of those effects. There should be a specific plan for checking in frequently about side effects, perhaps by secure text or email. When it is indicated by the patient's experiences with other drugs, specific comorbidities, and/or

family history, pharmacogenomic testing and/or monitoring of medication blood levels should be considered.

3. The clinician should ask whether the patient has used or plans to use TCM or some other form of complementary or alternative treatment. If so, the patient should be asked about it in detail; and when feasible, the allopathic treatment should be described and explained, to make it and the alternative treatment truly complementary. If appropriate and acceptable to the patient, the clinician should communicate directly with the provider of the alternative treatment.

4. Since there will always be ways a patient can improve their lifestyle, exercise routine, sleep hygiene, diet, and/or management of comorbid general medical problems, the treatment prescription should include one or more of these in addition to antidepressant medication. In this way, the patient will not be relying on a drug alone to recover from their depression but will be using medication as part of a comprehensive and holistic plan of treatment.

5. If there is a significant other person with whom the patient talks about their health, the clinician should suggest including that person in the treatment. The other person can then be educated to support the prescribed treatment and to encourage the patient to report any negative effects or lack of expected benefit.

6. If the patient's limited English proficiency is a barrier to adequate patient education, shared decision-making, and communication about side effects and other concerns, the clinician should attempt to work around it. In a clinic setting, a bilingual health coach might be an option. In a private practice setting, that patient might be asked to identify a bilingual person who they would be comfortable including in the treatment process. (Note that neither a time-pressured professional interpreter nor a patient's child functioning as a "language broker" is equivalent.)

Typically, clinicians in high-income countries and especially in those with high-trust cultures assume that patients will trust them unless there is something in their history or their demeanor that would suggest otherwise. In approaching an unacculturated or partially-acculturated Chinese immigrant, a clinician should not assume the patient's trust. Instead, a few questions about past experiences with physicians or important vicarious experiences with physicians, both in China and in the U.S., can be included in the first or second visit. The clinician should not only listen for explicit comments about disappointment with prior treatment or fears about future treatment but also attend to paralinguistic communication suggesting mixed or negative feelings about the medical profession. If the clinician directly hears about negative experiences with physicians or clinics, or senses reluctance or negativity in the patient's responses to questions or recommendations, they can explore the patient's concerns in greater detail and develop a treatment plan that addresses them.

Postscript: Universities' Responses to International Student Mental Health Issues

Since the deaths by suicide described at the start of this chapter, the universities involved have responded in various ways to the events, publicity, group advocacy, and litigation that followed them. One dramatic, positive response was a change in academic regulations on "time away and return" made by Yale University in January 2023 (Yale College Programs of Study, 2023). The change is responsive to depressed students' fears of being forced out of the university if they acknowledge suicidality or need time for intensive psychiatric treatment. Under the new policy, a student facing a mental health crisis is permitted to take medical leave rather than withdraw, or to reduce their course load to as few as two classes per term. A student on leave can keep health insurance through Yale that would cover mental health care out of state. They can have access to the campus, use the library in person or online, consult their mentors and advisors, and work as student employees. When the student on leave is ready to return to Yale full time, they must submit a personal statement about why they left, the treatment they received, and why they feel ready to return, accompanied by a letter of support from a clinician. Formal reapplication for admission, with all its costs, burdens, and uncertainties, is not required (Wan, 2023).

However, under the new policy, involuntary medical leave still could be imposed on a student in a case of "significant risk to the student's health or safety, or to the health and safety of others." An advocacy group that was one of the plaintiffs in a lawsuit against Yale alleging discrimination against students with mental health disabilities acknowledged that the policy was a major improvement, but it gave Yale a grade of incomplete for its work on student mental health. It noted that Yale's policy required students to disclose extremely private information and that a student who revealed thoughts of suicide might face involuntary leave based on their risk of self-harm (Wan, 2023). Both concerns would be especially salient to an international student who was depressed, suicidal, and anxious about their academic and occupational prospects. On August 25, 2023, Yale reached a settlement in the case that entailed even greater support for students dealing with depression. It agreed to provide training to its mental health counselors on providing "culturally competent" mental health services, and to further liberalize its new medical leave policy. Medical leaves of absence will no longer require a minimum time away. Students who take medical leave within the first two weeks of a term will receive a 100% refund of tuition and fees, and those who take leave later in the term will receive a partial refund. Students will be permitted to drop all but two of their courses for mental health reasons at any point in the term while remaining in good academic standing. Students who did not have health insurance prior to requiring medical leave will have the option to purchase it, with a possible subsidy for students receiving financial aid (Svrluga & Wan, 2023).

Yale's new approach to students with serious mental health issues is now more progressive than those of many elite universities that attract international students. Most international university students with life-threatening depression still face realistic fears of involuntary leaves with inflexible terms, financial and/or visa-related problems, and trouble accessing or paying for effective mental health care. Moreover, Yale's exemplary new policy appears to be a response to tragic events, adverse publicity, and litigation, suggesting that the stigma of mental health problems persists and that a full solution to the problem of depression and suicide in international students will require persistent, fundamental, and visible changes in universities' institutional cultures. When an American clinician works with an international student—of which Chinese students constitute a plurality—they should identify the patient's fears and realistic concerns about issues related to confidentiality and stigma, disruption of studies, financial stress, and student visa status. A clinician's serving as the student's ally, advocate, and source of reliable information can strengthen a therapeutic relationship and improve the ultimate prognosis of the student's depression.

Chapter 11

Japan: Invisible Double-Edged Swords

One evening after work, Hideo Kimura, 50, rushed to catch a train to the Umeda neighborhood of downtown Osaka. He was looking forward to his weekly dinner and conversation with Midori, a 20-year-old women's college student he'd met online about a year earlier. They had built a close relationship that had relieved the painful loneliness both he and she had felt before they met through a social media site. Kimura felt distant from his wife Ayako, 46, and alienated from their two sons; and before he met Midori he had yearned for a sympathetic listener. Midori was an introverted only child whose parents had divorced when she was three years old; she barely knew her father. She had been bullied in middle school and had thought about suicide at the time. She had been depressed during her first year of college but had recovered with counseling and medication. She was doing well in her classes but had no close friends. Midori wanted a mature man to confide in without the complications of dating. Neither Kimura nor Midori wanted a physical relationship.

Kimura had looked online for female companionship at a point when he felt painfully lonely and vulnerable. He really needed a friend to talk to, and Ayako seemed particularly insensitive. When Kimura and Midori met, they felt an immediate connection despite their age difference, and their friendship had deepened over time.

Kimura was a section chief at a prestigious electronics company. He had worked for the same company since graduating from one of the top universities in Osaka. Kimura was hardworking and ambitious and saw a bright future with lifetime security and opportunity. He worked long hours, often taking the last train to his home in Nishinomiya, a small city between Osaka and Kobe. He sometimes fell asleep on the train and missed his stop. His long hours at his desk had led to back and neck pain, and the stress of the job contributed to his hypertension. He never complained to anyone about overwork.

After more than 25 years with the company, Kimura knew he was not a winner. Several of his college classmates who worked at other companies were now *buchō* (general managers; 部長) with hopes to become senior executives before they reached retirement age. He knew he had no chance of promotion after being passed over for so long. Over his career he had seen the system of lifetime employment with pay by seniority (*nenkō joretsu*; 年功序列) deteriorate as the nation's economic growth slowed. Years ago, his immediate supervisor was reassigned to a meaningless job, becoming one of the *madogiwa zoku* (窓際族; literally "the tribe sitting by the window," a term denoting managers no longer needed by a company, who were moved to desks by a window and given boring busywork to do until they chose to retire). More recently, another section chief got a "tap on the shoulder" (*katatataki*; 肩たたき) from his boss and got transferred to an *oidashibeya* (追い出し部屋; forcing-out room), where he was given tedious tasks to do without proper support and then humiliated when the work wasn't done on time. Eventually, his colleague got fed up with being bullied and quit. Kimura feared he would be the next one out the door. He had worked long hours for years and used less than half of his paid vacation time. It didn't matter anymore: It seemed that hard work didn't count the way it once did.

He had two sons, one 20 and in college and the other 17, who would be starting college soon. His sons were much closer to their mother than to him. He had been at work most of their waking hours when they were young, and he seldom spent time with them even now. The stress of his insecure work situation was troubling him, but when he talked to Ayako her response was cold. He sensed that she blamed him for not being more successful and could picture Ayako leaving him if he lost his job. He had accepted a gross imbalance of work and family life to show his loyalty to the company, expecting a higher salary in his middle age, lifetime employment, and a comfortable retirement. It now seemed like he was a loser both at work and at home.

For a few months he had been experiencing typical symptoms of clinical depression: trouble sleeping, worsening of his back and neck pain, loss of interest in his work and his favorite television shows, a sense of being tired and slowed down, and feeling discouraged and hopeless. His weekly dinners with Midori cheered him up, but he felt low again by the time he got home at night. A few days he felt so slow and tired in the morning he was late to work—very unusual for him. He had little appetite and began to lose weight. After participating in every company-related social event for years, he avoided several of them because he preferred to spend time with Midori. He tried to bear his depression, telling himself that every man's life is painful; but his self-reassurance stopped working, and he felt weak and ashamed that he couldn't keep his spirits up. He started thinking of suicide and how he could die in a way that would seem accidental. A death that appeared accidental, or of indeterminate intention, would spare his family the embarrassment of a suicide and avoid any problem with Ayako and his sons benefiting from his life insurance policy.

He consulted an internist about his fatigue, lack of energy, and neck and back pain. The doctor prescribed anti-inflammatory medication, told him that psychological problems were contributing to his pain, and referred him to a psychosomatic specialist. The specialist diagnosed depression, prescribed a SSRI, and offered him a letter recommending a month of medical leave. Kimura would not consider taking leave; he felt that if he did, he would surely land in the *oidashibeya*. He tried the SSRI, keeping the diagnosis and the medication a secret from his wife. After a week, he felt physically uncomfortable with the effects of the medication and, more troubling, thought of suicide much more often, even imagining specific ways he might die. He resolved to die by suicide, but he needed to say goodbye to Midori first.

The next time he saw Midori he said, "This is our last time together. Don't worry about me; be strong and have a beautiful life. If you're happy, I will know." Midori burst into tears. "If you kill yourself, I will be alone and miserable again. I wouldn't want to die with you, but if you kill yourself, I will follow you." Kimura could not bear the thought that his suicide could lead to the young woman's death. He resolved to stay strong, to live for her sake. Their friendship continued and sustained them both. Kimura resumed the antidepressant, and his symptoms gradually improved.

The prevalence of depression among middle-aged male white-collar workers in Japan rose significantly beginning in the mid-1990s when Japan's dramatic postwar economic growth came to an end. In 1960 Japan's per capita gross domestic product (GDP) in 2023 U.S. dollars was $475; in 1995 it was $44,198, 93 times higher. Japan's per capita GDP exceeded its 1995 level from 2010 to 2012, but otherwise it has been lower than it was in 1995 for the past 28 years (World Bank, 2023a). One consequence has been the gradual end of Japan's system of lifetime employment with promotions and salary determined by age, and a progressive increase in irregular employment with lower compensation and less security. During Japan's period of extraordinary growth and prosperity, large companies were growing, and they steadily and predictably promoted white-collar employees. After the slowing of Japan's growth, middle-aged employees could no longer count on promotions, or even on lifetime employment, despite 20 years or more of loyal service to their companies. The emotional consequences of this change were a reaction not only to lower financial expectations but also to the loss of the meaningful emotional connection of the employee to the employer, in which loyalty on the employee's side was rewarded by the employer's concern for their welfare.

Japan never became a welfare state like the Nordic countries; it has relatively poor publicly funded pensions and unemployment insurance, and its national health insurance requires significant cost-sharing by patients. It had relied on pay and benefits from long-term full-time employment and low unemployment rates as the basis of its people's security. Women's wages and salaries and labor force participation were relatively low, but most women were married and could rely on their spouses' compensation. Between 1960 and 2021 Japan's life expectancy at birth increased from 68 years to 85 years, the latter age significantly higher than the average of 80 years for high-income countries (World Bank, 2023b). Most large employers in Japan have had mandatory retirement, initially at age 55 and then at age 60 for most companies. Its public pensions now do not begin until age 65 for men and 64 for women, leaving a gap that most Japanese must fill by taking employment at markedly lower compensation. As the population has aged, pensions as a percentage of salary have been decreased to keep the system sustainable, and some companies give employees a lump sum at the time of retirement instead of a pension, implying for most a continually decreasing standard of living as they get older. According to the latest available statistics, Japan's poverty rate for people aged 66-75 is 16%, and the rate for those over 75 is 24%. By contrast, the poverty rate for all people over 65 in France—a country with similar average income for wage earners—is 4% for people aged 65-74 and 5% for those aged 75 and older (Organisation for Economic Co-operation and Development, 2023).

The situation for women is even worse than that for men. They are paid less, have less opportunity for high-level positions, and suffer negative consequences for their career prospects if they take leave from work after giving birth. Given the worsening prospects for men's employment, marriage can become a losing proposition economically for Japanese women: If her husband does not have well-paid employment, her standard of living probably will be lower than if she worked and continued to live with her parents. If she has children and her marriage ends in divorce, both she and her children may experience poverty. In her old age, if she is divorced, she will not receive the same income supports as if she were married or widowed but will have less savings from her working years than if her work had been undisrupted by family life.

Young Japanese men with insecure prospects are increasingly avoiding marriage. In 2020, 28.3% of 50-year-old Japanese men had never been married, up from 5.6% in 1990 and 12.6% in 2020. Between the early 1970s and 2021 the country's marriage rate per 1000 population fell from 10.0 to 4.1 (Statistics Bureau of Japan, 2023a). Because dating has traditionally been an activity related to seeking a spouse, many have given up dating as well, with a recent poll showing that 34.1% of Japanese men in their 30s had never been on a date (Nippon.com, 2022; Statistics Bureau of Japan, 2023b). Along with the decline in marriage there has been a decline in births, to well below the minimum rate for sustaining Japan's population, which has been declining since 2015.

Consequently, the population has aged. In 2020, people 65 and older constituted 28.6% of all Japanese. For comparison, the rates for the United States (U.S.) and for Sweden in the same year were 16.2% and 20.0%, respectively. In 2015, 6.72 million older Japanese people lived alone (Statistics Bureau of Japan, 2023b).

While the Japanese economy grew explosively from the end of World War II through 1995, there has been virtually no growth in Japan's inflation-adjusted per capita income since then. The flattening of economic growth has translated into an increase in precarious employment without job security or traditional benefits. Of all Japanese workers (excluding company executives) in 2022, 38.4% were non-regular employees such as part-time workers, temporary workers, or workers employed via an agency. Non-regular employment was disproportionately held by adults under 25 or over 65. Non-regular employment in Japan is highly gendered: 22.2% of employed men and 53.4% of employed women have non-regular positions (Statistics Bureau of Japan, 2023c).

Given the relationship of loneliness, disappointment, and financial insecurity to depression, one might expect an increase in Japan's prevalence of MDD to correlate with the country's demographic and economic changes. In fact, the increase in the prevalence of MDD over the past three decades has been relatively small. Over the past two decades, the largest increases in MDD prevalence in Japan have been for young adults of both genders and for middle-aged men. In 2019, Japan's age-standardized prevalence rates for MDD were 1.98% for females and 1.38% for males, significantly lower than the benchmark rates for high-income countries—3.74% for women and 2.14% for men. Yet, its age-standardized mortality rates from known suicides (20.6 for males and 7.9 for females) are the third highest among high-income countries (Institute for Health Metrics and Evaluation [IHME, 2023]). This suggests that in Japan, clinical depression without the full syndrome of MDD is more common than MDD. Furthermore, Japan's reported suicide rates are almost certainly spuriously low because its rates of "unintentional" drowning of middle-aged and older adults dwarf those of all high-income countries, including countries that are islands and ones that have similarly high reported suicide rates. The undercounting of suicides among unnatural deaths is seen in other countries, notably in mainland China; but deaths by drowning are a larger factor in Japan than anywhere else in the world. Table 11.1 shows 2019 suicide and drowning mortality rates for people aged 70 and over for Japan and five other high-income countries (IHME, 2023). We will return to the theme of death by drowning later in this chapter.

Japan's high suicide rates are not explained by correspondingly high rates of diagnosed MDD. Looking at depression in Japan through a cultural lens suggests

Table 11.1 2019 Suicide and Drowning Mortality Rates per 100,000 People Age 70+: Japan and Comparators

Country	Men ≥70 Suicide	Men ≥70 Drowning	Women ≥70 Suicide	Women ≥70 Drowning
Japan	36.7	26.0	16.9	20.6
South Korea	111.4	5.9	47.5	2.6
Taiwan	52.9	7.0	26.2	2.8
New Zealand	19.0	1.8	5.1	0.8
Iceland	42.0	2.9	8.5	0.6
Greenland	119.8	10.8	14.1	2.6

Note. Data are from the 2019 Global Burden of Disease (IHME (2023).

that many cases of clinically significant depression associated with high suicide risk do not get recognized as major depression. This is partly because many Japanese with MDD conceal their symptoms and partly because many Japanese people have forms of clinically significant depression that would not meet criteria for MDD even if their symptoms were fully disclosed. A review of selected aspects of Japan's culture helps make sense of the epidemiologic data. It suggests why Japanese people can tolerate suffering without displaying overt signs of depression, why clinical depression often expresses itself in ways not diagnosed as MDD, and why suicide rates are disproportionate to rates of MDD. Japanese culture provides reasons why depression often is unrecognized or ineffectively treated and why the country's institutions have done relatively little to change the social determinants of health and lack of effective mental health services that underlie many cases of depression and many deaths by suicide.

In Japan, there are four frequently occurring presentations of conditions meeting this book's criterion for clinical depression but not necessarily *Diagnostic and Statistical Manual of Mental Disorders* (DSM)/*International Classification of Diseases* (ICD) criteria for MDD. These are modern type depression (MTD; *shingata utsubyō*; 新型うつ病; literally "new type depression"), *karōshi* (過労死; death from overwork), *kodokushi* (孤独死; lonely death, discussed in Chapter 1), and *hikikomori* (引き籠もり; prolonged and severe social withdrawal).

Syncretism and the Yamato Spirit

Unlike many nations in Asia, Japan was never conquered and occupied by a foreign power. Rather than having a way of life or religious system imposed on it by an invader, it intentionally imported language, arts, technology, philosophy, and religion from other cultures and adapted them to its unique environment. Elements of Confucianism, Buddhism, and Daoism were merged with Shintō (神道), the indigenous religion of Japan that emphasizes the spiritual dimension of nature. The Chinese logographic system was combined with a phonetic alphabet to create the Japanese written language. Scientific and technological knowledge was imported from the West at a rapid pace beginning in the Meiji period (1868–1912).

From Confucianism, Japan adopted the principle of harmonious existence through a structure of hierarchical relationships and the principle that one should consistently display righteous, honorable behavior, even at the cost of one's public reputation and self-interest. In Japan, loyalty to superiors in a hierarchy (chūsei; 忠誠) predominates over obligations of filial piety (kōkō; 孝行), opposite to the situation in China. For example, a samurai (侍) would give his life for the shōgun (将軍) he served, but not necessarily for his father.

The importance to Japanese people of *haji* (恥), internalized shame that differs both from guilt and from external shame and loss of reputation, can be understood in relation to its valuing righteousness over external face. From classical Buddhism the Japanese developed Zen (禅), a characteristically Japanese form of the religion. Zen emphasizes simplicity, non-attachment, and appreciation of the transience of life. Zen values meditation over formal prayer and a spiritual life over the practice of rituals. From Daoism, Japan adopted the ideal of mindfully accepting life as it is. A love of nature and appreciation for its spiritually restorative properties persisted from Shintō as Japan adopted, modified, and blended the elements of other nations' religious and philosophical traditions.

Buddhist temples (*otera*; お寺) in Japan were built based on Chinese models, with pagodas containing images of the Buddha. The design of the capital city of Nara (奈良) was inspired by the Chinese capital city of Chang'an (长安), today's Xi'an (西安), which during the Tang Dynasty was the largest and most technologically advanced city in the world. In the syncretic culture of Japan, Buddhism and Shintō have coexisted; in present times, Japanese life cycle rituals draw from both traditions, with birth and marriage usually following Shintō traditions and funerals following Buddhist ones.

Between 1600 and 1868, Japan was a closed, feudal society under the leadership of the Tokugawa shōgun and his daimyō (大名), local lords who owned the land and directly ruled the subjects who lived on it. The military force that maintained the shōgun and his daimyō comprised samurai, soldiers loyally attached to a specific daimyō or directly to the shōgun. Samurai were expert in martial arts and willing without hesitation to fight and die for the one they served. A samurai was not afraid of death and would prefer a noble death to a life without honor and glory. The shōgun and his daimyō recognized an obligation of reciprocity toward the samurai who served them. They and their families were secure and enjoyed high status in their communities.

The relationship between fathers and sons differed between Japan and China in ways that made loyalty stronger and filial piety weaker in Japan compared with China. Until the mid-20th century in Japan, the firstborn son would have several sons, and the estate would be divided among them. The Japanese custom weakened the connection of younger sons to their father, while the Chinese custom favored the development of large multigenerational families where everyone descended from a single patriarch and was loyal to him. In Japan, a man's parents might "retire" at some point, live separately, and pass leadership of the family to the firstborn son, whereas in China the father would remain in place as the patriarch until his death (Hsu, 1971).

Japan's rapid modernization during the Meiji period, and its ascendance as a world economic power beginning in the 1960s, were facilitated by the rapid growth of private companies and government agencies managed by stable and efficient hierarchies of loyal employees. This was made possible by loyalty. In the Confucian tradition and especially in its Japanese adaptation, loyalty implied reciprocal obligations of care on the part of superiors toward subordinates. The breakdown of Japan's system of lifetime employment in the late 1990s was a breach of reciprocity that contributed to an increase in the prevalence of depression and the incidence of suicide. In late middle-aged men, depression usually took the form of melancholic MDD; in young men, it often took the form of MTD, which will be described below.

In the mid-19th century the Tokugawa shogunate (*Tokugawa bakufu*; 徳川幕府), which had ruled since 1600, lost power, and the merchant class got stronger. In 1868 the shōgun's regime was replaced in a "bloodless coup" by a centralized government with the emperor as head of state, Shintō as the official state religion, and political power controlled by an oligarchy. This began the Meiji period (*Meiji jidai*; 明治時代), which began with the coup and continued until the death of Emperor Meiji in 1912. The oligarchy evolved into a constitutional monarchy more authoritarian than that of the United Kingdom, with a powerful monarch, titled nobility, a ruling oligarchy, and few guaranteed civil liberties.

Japan's Meiji-period leaders wanted their country to become like the great nations of Europe. Japan industrialized with remarkable speed, building a national railroad system, an internationally competitive textile industry, a steel industry, a telegraph network, a modern banking system, and an infrastructure for entrepreneurial capitalism. It imported 3000 foreign experts to teach English, science, engineering, and military technology and sent students to Europe and America to acquire knowledge in diverse fields. Through this process Japanese culture selectively adopted styles and ideas from the American and European cultures with which it interacted. Commercial and industrial conglomerates were founded and grew rapidly. In the early 20th century Japan invaded and annexed Korea and Manchuria, mimicking the imperialistic activities of the major Western powers.

As Japan industrialized and agriculture became more labor-efficient during the Meiji period, over a million lower-class Japanese men emigrated in search of agricultural work, mainly to Hawaii (then an independent kingdom), to the U.S., and to Brazil. Most of them remained in their new countries, eventually importing brides from Japan, starting families, and ultimately becoming citizens. The descendants of these men fully adopted their new countries; by the third generation (*sansei*; 三世) most did not speak Japanese or follow a full Japanese lifestyle—though most retained some typical Japanese values and perspectives, as will be discussed below. Japanese migrants were, in general, quick to acculturate and to transfer their loyalty to their new homelands (Japanese Diaspora Portal, 2019). The modern history of Japan, and of the Japanese diaspora, is one of a historically collectivistic culture assimilating individualistic values, resulting in a culture that is less collectivistic than that of China and less individualistic than that of the West.

Wabi-Sabi, Mujō (Impermanence), and *Mono no Aware* (the Pathos of Things) in Daily Life: Japanese Aesthetics and Depression

Japanese aesthetics are part of the national consciousness, influencing not only the fine arts, the architecture of buildings and landscapes, the designs of everyday objects, and the themes of popular culture but also Japanese people's communication styles, values, social behavior, worldviews, and inner emotional lives. As such, the themes and underlying philosophy of Japanese aesthetics impact the occurrence, phenomenology, and narratives of depression in Japanese people. They can be protective or provocative, and they can make depression harder to recognize, both by the depressed person and by others in their lives. Japanese aesthetics underlie the normalization and romanticization of some types of suicide by the Japanese. At the extreme, suicidal acts within specific contexts can be perceived as beautiful.

Japan's vulnerability to natural disasters such as earthquakes and tsunamis underlies a culturally shared awareness of the transience and vulnerability of life—its impermanence (*mujō*; 無常). This awareness sensitizes the Japanese to *mono no aware* (物の哀れ; "the pathos of things"). The Japanese have "empathy toward things" and "sensitivity to ephemera." Confronted with the transience of life, many Japanese feel sadness of a gentle, wistful nature. Melancholy beauty such as that of falling cherry blossoms is a recurrent theme in Japanese art.

Because life and its experiences are ephemeral, one must be mindful and fully present for every minute of one's life and in every human interaction. The four-character phrase *ichigo ichie* (一期一会; "one opportunity, one encounter") expresses the idea that any specific interpersonal experience will happen only once in one's lifetime; even if one sees the same person again, the circumstances will be different. One should therefore regard each meeting with another person as if it were the last time that one would ever see them.

Mindfulness practice is popular in contemporary Western integrative medicine as it has been associated in empirical studies with a wide range of psychological benefits, including enhancing positive mood states, managing stress, and reducing stress-induced mood disturbances (Brown & Ryan, 2003); reducing loneliness and increasing social contact (Lindsay et al., 2019); reducing work stress (Chin et al., 2019); and improving satisfaction with romantic relationships (Kappen et al., 2018). Japanese aesthetics promote mindfulness. They are thus a double-edged sword: possibly protective against depression in stressful circumstances but potentially disguising clinical depression by romanticizing melancholy.

Wabi-sabi (侘び寂び), described as "the beauty of imperfection" or the "beauty of serene melancholy," is an aesthetic principle originally derived from Buddhist philosophy and adapted in a characteristically Japanese manner. "*Wabi-sabi* is the art of finding beauty in imperfection and profundity in earthiness, of revering authenticity above all" (Lawrence, 2004). The *wabi-sabi* aesthetic underlies the Japanese arts of *ikebana* (生花; flower arrangement) and *bonsai* (盆栽), Zen gardens, and the Japanese tea ceremony (*chadō*; 茶道).

Wabi (侘) connotes simplicity, freshness, and modest elegance. *Sabi* (寂) refers to changes in a material object with age or wear. (It is a homonym for the Japanese word for "rust"; other meanings include "loneliness" and "silence.") The *wabi-sabi* aesthetic implies a mindful engagement with the material world, finding beauty and spiritual value in a cultivated, deliberate perception of objects and scenes, including their original or acquired imperfections. *Wabi-sabi* can refer to an attribute of an object or a scene or to the mental discipline of mindful perception. A person perceiving the material world with a *wabi-sabi* approach would find beauty in simple and flawed things and would not be distracted or troubled by random thoughts. *Wabi-sabi* can be part of a repertoire of resilience. It is an antidote for perfectionism and anxiety and can help people cope with milder forms of depression.

Yūgen (幽玄), literally translatable as "deep," "profound," or "mysterious," like *wabi-sabi*, can refer to an aesthetic principle, to scenes or objects that exemplify or embody the principle, or to thoughts and feelings evoked by such scenes or objects. *Yūgen* is experienced but not explicitly described or depicted. A flock of geese disappearing over the horizon or the sun setting over a flowered field might be a *yūgen* moment. As with *wabi-sabi*, *yūgen* often alludes to transience or sadness. People become more mindful, and thus calmer and more resilient, by cultivating their perception of *yūgen*.

Because Japanese appreciate sadness and loneliness and do not necessarily try to avoid experiencing them, distinction between being in good health and being ill with depression cannot be based on the presence or even the persistence of sadness. On the other hand, young adults with MTD are not sad at all, but rather at work or school they are negative, irritable, anhedonic, and critical of other people. A Japanese person with MDD might experience anhedonia that included a loss of appreciation of *wabi-sabi*, *yūgen*, and *mono no aware*. Instead of feeling sad, they would feel *miserable* or *empty*. Instead of feeling lonely, they might feel *alienated*. Relative to Western cultures and even to other East Asian cultures, Japanese culture recognizes a broader range and greater depth of negative emotions as compatible with a satisfying and meaningful life and with normal health and function. Cross-cultural research suggests that happiness—subjective well-being—is correlated more highly with "feeling right" (feeling as one thinks one ought to feel) than with "feeling good" (experiencing pleasure in a narrow sense) (Tamir et al., 2017).

One edge of the "sword" of the *yūgen* and *wabi-sabi* aesthetic comprises resilience, endurance, and inner peace; the other edge comprises denial of clinical depression and passivity in the face of painful circumstances that could and should be changed. Japanese aesthetics and their associated mindfulness don't address suicidal ideation or prompt people to summon help when it is sorely needed. In some cases, the culture's preference for a good death over a miserable life increases the risk that a person with depression who has lost their *ikigai* (生き甲斐; reason to live) will choose to die by suicide, by drowning under questionable circumstances, or from self-neglect. Japanese aesthetics might help a person cope with mild depression, but they do not treat it; and they are of little use for severe depression.

The many deaths by drowning of older Japanese people can be understood as a reflection of their indifference to life. Approximately two thirds of the drowning deaths of Japanese take place in bathtubs (Hsieh et al., 2018a, 2018b); the remainder take place in natural bodies of water like rivers, ponds, or the ocean. In almost all cases the drowning victim would be bathing or swimming alone—a situation with an obvious risk of death in the event of a mishap. If an older person died by drowning while alone, the circumstances of the death usually would be ambiguous with respect to the person's intentions—avoiding the family shame that might accompany a definite suicide. A typical narrative would involve an older widow living alone, rarely if ever visited by her adult children, found dead by a neighbor days after her death in her bathtub, or an older widowed or divorced man washed ashore after drowning while swimming alone. In a provocative article, "Covert Suicide Among Elderly Japanese Females: Questioning Unintentional Drownings," Rockett and Smith (1993) observed that by the 1990s Japan's cultural acceptance of suicide had begun to diminish, leading suicidal people to disguise the intentionality of their deaths. They also noted that in 1970 it was unusual for older Japanese people to live apart from their families; now, over 50 years later, this is the norm. Life expectancy is higher, birth rates are lower, and even when older people have adult children, Confucian filial piety is no longer a dominant value. If a vulnerable older person living alone loses their *ikigai*, they have a choice of ambiguous ways to die, including drowning in a bathtub and a lonely death by self-neglect (*kodokushi*) as described in Chapter 1 (Rockett & Smith, 1993). The many drownings of older Japanese people cannot be explained by mere frailty or carelessness, as mortality rates from falls for those aged ≥70 are relatively low, 56.7 for men and 35.6 for women (IHME, 2023).

Modern Consequences of Samurai Culture

Prior to the Meiji period, Japan was administered locally by nobility who held most of the nation's land, governed their property with the aid of deputies, and defended their lands with samurai who had pledged loyalty to them. Samurai were expert in Japanese martial arts including swordsmanship, archery, and techniques of hand-to-hand combat such as judo, karate, and aikido. Expertise in martial arts and a relationship with a powerful lord, rather than intellectual performance tested on written examinations, was the basis of personal advancement in social class and influence. Respect for hierarchy, loyalty to superiors, self-discipline, and the avoidance of shame were emphasized in the enculturation of the Japanese people. In contrast to Chinese culture, these duties were given greater importance than family obligations. Inheriting land and becoming a samurai were essentially the only routes to upper-class status until the Meiji period, when wealth and power could be acquired through success in commerce.

The samurai tradition has been celebrated in contemporary Japan, with shrines, books, and films extolling the samurai code of unconditional loyalty and fearlessness in the face of death. It also is exemplified in Japanese culture by striking juxtapositions of finesse and cruelty. Other expressions of the samurai tradition are the Japanese love of sports and the high value placed on stoicism in the event of injury, pain, or loss. The culture celebrates bearing suffering with minimal complaint or outward signs of distress. The kanji character 忍 (*shinobi*), with meanings of "patience," "endurance," "perseverance," and "concealment," is used in phrases describing Japanese stoicism. The character consists of the radical for "knife blade" on top of the one for "heart." Clearly, if a person could walk about calmly with a blade just above their heart, they could deal with overwork, a bullying boss, or unfair treatment and could tolerate the pain of depression.

A pathological expression of the samurai tradition in modern Japan is the phenomenon of *karōshi* (death from overwork). This is the fate of an employee who works extremely long hours; experiences continual, intense job-related strain; and neglects their health, ultimately leading to death, typically from a stroke or cardiac condition, often at a relatively young age. A variant of *karōshi* is *karōjisatsu* (過労自殺; overwork suicide), in which a person experiencing overwork and unbearable job-related stress dies by suicide during a period of excessive working hours. A review of *karōshi* by the United Nations International Labour Organization (ILO, 2013) gave examples:

1. A man working at a food processing company died of a heart attack at age 34 after working overtime for many weeks, with a peak of 110 hours in a single week.
2. A bus driver died of a stroke at age 37 after working 3000 hours per year. He had been working 15 days without a day off at the time he died.
3. A 22-year-old nurse died of a heart attack after working 34 hours at a stretch, five times in a single month.

The ILO report presented data showing *karōshi* from cardiovascular and cerebrovascular disease to be twice as frequent as *karōjisatsu*.

In Japan, employees often will submit to the authority of their employers and supervisors even when their demands are excessive. There is high job strain because work demands are high and employees' control over them is low (Karasek, 1979). For example, Japanese hospital physicians are subject to overtime of as much as 2000 hours per year. Many get no more than four days off per month, have chronobiologically stressful shift work, and have on-call responsibilities in addition to working regular clinical hours ("Efforts Needed to Reduce Doctors' Working Hours," 2019). The underlying reason is the Japanese government's policy of limiting the number of physicians in Japan to control healthcare expenditures, leading to Japan's having fewer physicians per capita than most high-income nations. As Japan's population has aged and medical technology has advanced, there is much more work physicians must do and not enough physicians to do it (Hiyama & Yoshihara, 2008). At the same time, physicians have legal and moral obligations to give care to those who need it. This overwork and the conflict between professional obligations and the need for self-care is associated with depressive symptoms as well as burnout (Saijo et al., 2014).

Most Japanese workers do not fully utilize their paid vacation days for reasons including concern that doing so would convey a lack of commitment to their employers, that their absence would burden co-workers, that they would stand out among peers who did not take time off, or that they feel that no one else can do their job (Nippon.com, 2023). In an online survey of workers aged 17 to 62 conducted in July 2023, only 18.8% responded that they take all of their paid annual leave (Nippon.com, 2023). Similarly, Japanese companies are required to offer their male employees four weeks of flexible paternity leave at up to 80% of their salary, but in 2022 only 14% of male employees with newborn children used it. A likely explanation is that employers would see their employees' use of paternity leave as showing a lack of commitment to the job. The consequence for regular employees might include long term diminution of their prospects for promotion, or reassignment to a less desirable position. A non-regular employee on a fixed-term contract might fear non-renewal of their contract (Lau et al., 2023).

Women who fully utilize their year of maternity leave usually will be paid less for the remainder of their working lives than if they had not done so. The Japanese ideal of stoicism helps explain why Japanese workers have fatalistically tolerated working conditions that might precipitate strikes or other collective action in another country. Efforts to change might make conditions better for millions of workers, but they would disrupt a centuries-old tradition of loyalty to the organization and deference to authority. In the near term it would cause overt conflict between workers and employers, something that the Japanese take pains to avoid.

High job strain, including that associated with chronic overwork, has been shown to increase the risk of several chronic diseases including diabetes, hypertension, and atherosclerotic heart disease. This implies a risk of sudden death on the job from heart attack, stroke, or malignant cardiac arrhythmia—conditions that would be classified as *karōshi* if they occurred in the setting of prolonged excessive work hours. The same factors of job strain and associated sleep deprivation are associated with clinical depression, a condition that increases the risk of cardiovascular disease and stroke. It is likely that most Japanese people who die of overwork would have some form of clinical depression or a bipolar spectrum disorder but very unlikely that they would ever seek mental health care or receive a mood disorder diagnosis.

Another aspect of Japanese people's intense involvement with work is the high prevalence of sleep insufficiency and poor sleep quality. In a study of male workers at a manufacturing plant, 34% had clinically significant insomnia when screend with the Athens Insomnia Scale. Workers who reported higher job stress from subjectively excessive or inappropriate work were more likely to have insomnia (Nishitani & Sakakibara, 2010). In a survey of Japanese adults aged 20 and above, 21.7% had complaints of poor sleep quality; and such complaũints were significantly associated with worse physical and mental health status (Furihata et al., 2012). In a longitudinal study of male Japanese workers not depressed at baseline, insomnia at baseline was associated with a significantly increased risk of developing clinical depression over the next 6 years, after adjustment for age, job type, living arrangements, total sleep time, and medication usage (Nishitani et al., 2019).

Mental Health and Self-Construal

In Japanese culture, people define and experience themselves in the context of relationships; that is, their self-construal is interdependent. The term for this in Japanese is *shūdan ishiki* (集団意識; "group consciousness"). Japanese people are enculturated to be highly sensitive to the emotional states of those around them, even if they are expressed in a subtle way, and to care very much about others' feelings and reactions. *Shūdan ishiki* helps explain why Japanese are highly vulnerable to psychological bullying in the form of exclusion from a group or coordinated derision by a group. It also helps explain why in Japan social anxiety disorders often take the form of *taijin kyōfushō* (対人恐怖症; TKS; literally, fear of personal relations disorder; Suzuki et al., 2003).

People with TKS fear that aspects of their personal appearance, behavior, body odor, or facial expression will offend others or make them uncomfortable. While most people with TKS would meet the DSM criteria for social anxiety disorder, those with TKS differ in their greater focus on others' reactions rather than their own embarrassment and on issues like body odor, physical appearance, or passing intestinal gas that are only problematic because of others' reactions to them. Patients' fears are most prominent in social situations with acquaintances and are less intense when they are with intimate friends and family or with complete strangers (Maeda & Nathan, 1999). This fits with interdependent self-construal: One's sense of security and self-worth is strongly affected by the (presumed) opinions of people such as neighbors, classmates, co-workers, and members of one's broader social circle (Choy et al., 2008; Essau et al., 2012; Hinton et al., 2009).

Concerning the longer-term aspect of interdependent self-construal, Japanese people's identity and self-esteem are strongly related to their emotional ties to other people. *En* (縁; connection or tie) is a link between a person and another person or organization that is relevant and sometimes essential to their sense of self and *ikigai*. Three types of *en* are fundamental in Japanese society: *chi-en* (血縁; ties with blood relations, including spouses and first- and second-degree relatives), *chi-en* (地縁; a homonym meaning community and neighborhood ties), and *sha-en* (社縁; organizational connections, including ones between an employee and a company). For many Japanese, especially those with the expectation of lifetime employment with the same firm, *sha-en* is as personally important as family *chi-en*, and for some it is more important. For a man to leave work earlier than his colleagues because he would like to be at home might be seen very negatively as disloyalty to the company and a lack of commitment to the job. Given the extraordinary importance of *sha-en*, a person who at the same time lost both *sha-en* and family *chi-en* might lose their *ikigai* and seriously consider suicide.

Outside of Japan, Japanese people may find social support from groups of Japanese immigrants, expatriates, or international students. This also is the case for second- and third-generation Japanese Americans or Japanese Brazilians. In America, when Japanese people encounter other Japanese people they haven't met before, their initial approach usually is friendly and trusting rather than cautious and suspicious. *Bonding social capital*—social connections between people who perceive themselves to be members of the same cultural group—can buffer the effects of stress, help protect against clinical depression, and mitigate feelings of hopelessness in those who are depressed (Chen et al., 2018; Daoud et al., 2016; Murayama et al., 2013; Nakamine et al., 2017). At the state level in the U.S., increased social capital is associated with reduced suicide mortality rates even after controlling for other correlates of suicide (Smith & Kawachi, 2014).

However, Japanese Americans' connections with Japanese culture, language, and other Japanese people often weaken with successive generations. This process was accelerated for many of the offspring of the more than 110,000 Japanese Americans who were unjustly incarcerated during World War II solely by reason of their national origin. Traumatized by their experience, many parents chose to rear their children to be as "American" as possible or even to avoid social connections with other Japanese Americans (Nagata et al., 2019).

"Reading the Air" (ba no kuuki wo yomu; 場の空気を読む) and Ambiguity (aimai; 曖昧)—The Communication Code

Japanese culture emphasizes the avoidance of overt conflict in everyday social interactions. This goal is furthered by a communication style that is high-context, indirect, modest, and self-effacing, and by avoidance of direct requests and overt disagreements. Japanese do not want to give others trouble (*meiwaku*; 迷惑). When they depend on others, their needs and desires are largely unspoken. When they do communicate, they may be intentionally ambiguous, to minimize the possibility of disagreement, embarrassment, or offense. This ambiguity is called *aimai*. Specifically, Japanese people may be ambiguous or tacit in their expression of what they want or need. This often takes place in situations of *amae* (甘え).

Amae was described by the Japanese psychoanalyst Takeo Doi (1920–2009) as a fundamental characteristic of the Japanese psyche, in his book *The Anatomy of Dependence* (1973). *Amae* captures the combination of emotional dependency and reciprocal obligation common in Japanese hierarchical relationships, a combination that is integral to Japanese but not to Chinese culture. Doi described it as "a sense of helplessness and a desire to be loved," a condition in which one could "presume upon another's benevolence." In his book, he offers the following anecdote describing a superficial form of *amae*:

> For example, not long after my arrival in America I visited the house of someone to whom I had been introduced by a Japanese acquaintance, and was talking to him when he asked me, "Are you hungry? We have some ice cream if you'd like it." As I remember, I was rather hungry, but finding myself asked point-blank if I was hungry by someone whom I was visiting for the first time, I could not bring myself to admit it, and ended by denying the suggestion. I probably cherished a mild hope that he would press me again; but my host, disappointingly, said, "I see," with no further ado, leaving me regretting that I had not replied more honestly. And I found myself thinking that a Japanese would almost never ask a stranger unceremoniously if he was hungry, but would produce something to give him without asking. (p. 11)

Identifying depression and its precipitants in Japanese people and in non-assimilated, non-bicultural Japanese Americans and Japanese expatriates is complicated by the extreme context dependence of Japanese verbal communication and its reliance on paralinguistic cues. While Chinese and Korean people also utilize high-context communication, they do not do so with the scope and subtlety of the Japanese. This aspect of the Japanese communication style is amusingly illustrated in an imagined conversation between a boss (A) and a worker (B) presented on a website devoted to Japanese culture (Japan Experience, 2008). It shows why the ability to "read the air" is especially useful in Japan. In the podcast, the actor playing the part of the worker answers each of the boss's questions with the identical phrase: *so desu ne* (そうですね; "I agree with you"). The intonation and prosody are different for each answer. The script for the conversation is as follows, with the implicit meaning of each reply given in parentheses.

A. Come in, come in. It's a little cool today, isn't it?

B. *So desu ne!* (Yes, it is a bit.)

   A. Looking at the forecast I expected a bit of sun today.

   B. *So desu ne.* (Yes, guess I did too.)

   A. Pull up a chair. There's one over there.

   B. *So desu ne.* (Oh, so there is.)

   A. Now, how are the March sales figures so far?

   B. *So desu ne.* (Hmm, yes, well, erm …)

   A. What? You mean this is it?

   B. *So desu ne.* (I'm afraid so.)

   A. We'd done a lot better last year at the same point in time.

   B. *So desu ne.* (Yes, I know.)

   A. What do you think's the problem?

   B. *So desu ne.* (It's got me beat.)

   A. Well, That's it for now then. Forward me that mail you said you got from HKL, won't you.

   B. *So desu ne.* (Yep, sure thing.)

   A. See you at lunch then.

   B. *So desu ne.* (You bet.)

When a clinician interviews a Japanese patient or a surveyor questions Japanese people about their mental health, they must be conscious that the meaning of a person's words may be uninterpretable without hearing them, knowing their context, and noting how they are delivered. Even in everyday life, Japanese communication is complex, subtle, and easily misunderstood by someone unfamiliar with the culture. Knowing that the issue might exist is the first step toward resolving it.

   Understanding the distinctive nature of Japanese verbal communication can be helpful in the comprehensive medical-psychiatric care of Japanese people with strokes, traumatic brain injuries, and other neurological conditions that affect circuits in the right hemisphere of the brain associated with paralinguistic communication. Because of the extreme importance in Japanese culture of utilizing prosody, facial expressions, and other paralinguistic features of spoken communication, right hemisphere lesions can cause greater impairment of interpersonal and occupational function for Japanese people than they might for people from a culture with explicit, low-context communication. Brain dysfunction is more likely to result in depression when it is accompanied by severe functional impairment, and a patient's feeling that a "mission-critical" function has been lost forever can lead to hopelessness and suicidality. When a physician outside Japan treats a Japanese immigrant or expatriate with right hemisphere lesion, the impact of the lesion on communication should be explored fully. If a patient has both clinical depression and impaired paralinguistic communication, integrating psychiatric treatment with speech therapy and occupational therapy may be especially important to the patient's recovery.

Congruent with the Japanese aesthetic of appreciating transience and impermanence and the beauty in sadness and pathos, the words used by Japanese to describe negative emotions may not distinguish transient everyday feeling states from the more serious alterations of mood associated with a diagnosis of depression or with suicide risk. However, there are words that are rarely used to describe mundane mood states and always raise a question deserving a clinician's follow-up if used by a patient in a diagnostic interview. An example of such a word is *zetsubō-kan* (絶望感; hopeless and despairing feeling). The first two kanji characters signify "breaking off" and "desire," and the third denotes "feeling." This suggests that a person talking about their *zetsubō-kan* has lost their *ikigai*. A clinician unfamiliar with the Japanese language might ask a new Japanese patient to say words in their language would best describe their current state of mind and then ask the patient (if bilingual) or the interpreter (if monolingual) to explain how Japanese people would use those words. Other Japanese words and phrases for negative emotional states that should raise the question of depression include:

> Kanashii (悲しい; sad/sorrowful)
> Munashii (空しい; vain/futile/fruitless)
> Tsurai (つらい; painful/causing suffering [usually emotional but can be physical])
> Kurushii (苦しい; painful/difficult/bitter [usually physical but can be emotional])
> Yū-utsu (憂うつ: depression)
> Yū-utsu na kibun ga ichinichijū tsuzuite iru (憂うつな気分が一日中続いている; feel depressed all day long)
> Nayami (悩み; worries/distress/anguish)
> Fuan de iraira suru (不安でイライラする; feeling anxious and irritable)
> Munasawagi (胸騒ぎ; morbid fear/apprehension/premonition [literally "chest commotion/turmoil/disturbance"])

Jibun ni kachi ga nai sonzai ni omoeru (自分に価値がない存在に思える; feel worthless.)
Kiete shimaitai (消えてしまいたい; want to disappear [from the world])
Shini tai (死にたい; want to die)

Japanese regularly and explicitly recognize the difference between socially appropriate, conventional responses to questions in conversation and expressions of their true, deeper feelings. The polarity can be expressed as the difference between *tatemae* (建前; "built in front") and *hon'ne* (本音; "true sound"). A clinician cannot assume that the first response a person gives to a question will be their *hon'ne*. It may be necessary to ask a question a second time or phrase it in a different way if context or paralinguistic cues suggest that the person is showing their *tatemae*. Other expressions of the polarity are *omote* (表; front) versus *ura* (裏; back) and *soto* (外; outside) versus *uchi* (内; inside). A Japanese patient prescribed an antidepressant might disagree with the physician's diagnosis and treatment but be unwilling to say so. If the physician senses this is possible, they should ask the patient using different words, making clear there is an invitation for the patient to raise a concern about the prescription and to show their *hon'ne* to the doctor. In some contexts, use of the Japanese word *hon'ne* might be appropriate. The validity of Japanese people's responses to a questionnaire or a structured research interview has the same limitations as their explicit verbal responses to a clinician's questions early in a clinical relationship. A study validating the Japanese version of the PHQ-9 showed good concordance with the Mini International Neuropsychiatric Interview (MINI) in detecting MDD in a sample of primary care patients (Muramatsu et al., 2018), but this simply means that the questionnaire and the interview give similar results with respect to MDD, not that either one is sensitive to non-standard but culturally congruent expressions of clinical depression. For a given person, responses on both the PHQ-9 and the MINI might be expressions of the person's *tatemae*. There is reason to think that Japanese people might understate depressive symptoms. For example, a study of antenatal depression in Japanese women using a Japanese version of the Edinburgh Postnatal Depression Scale showed an optimal cutoff score of 12/13 points rather than the 14/15 cutoff score that was found optimal in British, Maltese, and Nigerian studies (Usuda et al., 2017). One sensitive approach to assessing depression in Japanese patients is the use of a self-rating scale for positive mental health, the Euthymia Scale. Patients who do not endorse positive items are at high risk for clinical depression (the Japanese cultural bias toward understatement apparently does not prevent depressed people from rating as false statements like "I generally feel active and vigorous" or "I do not keep thinking about negative experiences" (Sasaki et al., 2021; Sasaki & Nishi, 2023).

Japan's Alternative to Psychiatry—*Shinyrōnaika* (心療内科)

The Japanese medical profession recognizes a form of depression that is distinguishable both from ordinary sadness and from melancholia, psychotic depression, and bipolar depression. The illness causes significant distress and functional impairment and characteristically involves distressing physical symptoms. The illness is treated by a special category of medical specialist, a *shinyrōnaikai* (psychosomatic internal medicine doctor). The professional society for *shinyrōnaika* emphasizes that the specialty treats "psychosomatic disorders" rather than "mental illness" and differentiates a condition with prominent somatic symptoms and dysphoric mood as a different illness from *utsubyō* (depression). They frequently make use of psychotherapy. A *shinyrōnaikai* has an underlying medical specialty such as internal medicine, pediatrics, or psychiatry with a special interest in psychosomatic disorders and may have taken a special examination of competence in psychosomatic medicine. (*Shinyrōnaikai* may be much weaker in the aspect of psychosomatic medicine that is outside their primary specialty; for example, an internist practicing *shinyrōnaika* may lack expertise in psychopharmacology or in the management of bipolar spectrum conditions.) In 2015, there were 3300 members of the professional society for *shinyrōnaika*—less than one third of the number of psychiatrists (Murakami & Nakai, 2017). Surveys of Japanese people suggest that more than half would prefer not to see a psychiatrist for treatment of depression. Either a primary care physician, a *shinyrōnaikai*, or a psychologist would be preferred. Most prefer psychotherapy to medication (Angermeyer et al., 2017). While depression is less stigmatized in Japan than in China, it is more stigmatized than in Western countries. Seeing a *shinyrōnaikai* is less stigmatized than seeing a psychiatrist. In a wildly popular manga on depression, the treating clinician is a *shinyrōnaikai* ("Comical Psychosomatic Medicine," 2021).

Japanese people are sensitive to the names of illnesses as well as to the names of the specialties that treat them. When the official name of schizophrenia in Japan was changed from *seishin-bunretsu-byo* (精神分裂病; mind-split disease) to *tōgō-shitchō-shō* (統合失調症; comprehensive imbalance disorder), the condition was less stigmatized, physicians told more patients about their diagnoses of schizophrenia, and patients and their families had greater hope of recovery (Sartorius et al., 2014; Sato, 2006).

Manga (漫画) and anime (アニメ)—Japanese graphic novels and animated films—are among Japan's best-known cultural exports. There are manga and anime for every demographic and of many genres from science fiction to erotica. Non-verbal expressions of emotion in manga and anime are intense and exaggerated, in contrast to the understated and ambiguous expressions of real-life Japanese communication. Their intensity of expressed emotion makes these media especially powerful for addressing psychological issues.

Psychologically oriented manga have raised Japanese people's awareness of mental health issues, reduced stigma, and encouraged people to seek help. The use of manga for this purpose was pioneered by Osamu Tezuka (手塚治虫; 1928–1989). Tezuka, Japan's leading creator of manga in the 1950s and 1960s, was a physician concerned about healing the psychological wounds of trauma, including the collective trauma of World War II.

A manga series, *manga de wakaru shinyrōnaika* (マンガで分かる心療内科; "understanding psychosomatic medicine through manga"), written by psychiatrist Yuichiro Yasuda (安田雄一郎)under the pseudonym of Yuki Yu, has been a bestseller in Japan since 2010. It provides education about mental health problems through stories about a *shinyrōnaika* and his patients. Websites inspired by the book host dialogues about mental health, including depression, that people with mental health problems use to anonymously share their experiences.

Self-indulgent (*Wagamama*), Spoiled (*Amae*), or Modern Type Depression?

Makoto Kobayashi, a 24-year-old man and a native of Tokyo, was the only child of a high official in the Japanese government and his wife, a full-time homemaker. He lived with his parents. He had an undergraduate degree in marketing from Keio University in Tokyo—Japan's highest-rated and oldest private university (Times Higher Education, 2021). He was fluent in English. After graduating from college, Kobayashi was hired in a competitive process for an entry-level position at the Tokyo headquarters of a much-admired multinational pharmaceutical company. Kobayashi was hardworking, sincere, and ambitious. During his six months of new employee training, he was well liked, and his supervisors thought he had a great future with the company.

Kobayashi's initial assignment was at the company's regional office in Fukuoka, a city of 1.5 million people 1100 km from Tokyo. He noticed with disappointment that the other three new hires who had trained with him were remaining in Tokyo. He wondered why he had to go to Fukuoka rather than one of them when his credentials and ability were obviously superior. His parents persuaded him to see the assignment as an opportunity to prove himself.

Kobayashi's new boss, Ito, was a traditional Japanese manager in his 50s with limited English proficiency and an unremarkable education, who had earned his position by 30 years of dedicated, loyal service to the company. Kobayashi perceived his new co-workers to be like Ito: hardworking and loyal but basically mediocre. With his family and friends all far away in Tokyo, Kobayashi felt extremely lonely. He would call them every day to complain of his situation, feeling that he had been deceived by the executives who had overseen his initial training. He questioned the Japanese system and wished his company were more like the American tech startups he had read about. He ate alone at restaurants, spent many hours online on social media, and longed for a transfer back to Tokyo.

After a year in Fukuoka, Kobayashi began to have symptoms. He awakened each morning feeling tired, finding it effortful to get up and go to work. Sitting at his desk his mind would wander. His colleagues found his behavior unusual; Kobayashi read their facial expressions as disapproving and thought they must be gossiping about him. He imagined that his boss and some managers in Tokyo had conspired deliberately to give him an unpleasant job and destroy his future, perhaps out of envy. He thought he was wasting his time and his talent in Fukuoka, increasingly feeling isolated and discouraged. When he interacted with his co-workers, he felt headaches, dry mouth, tightness in the chest, agitated, and full of anger. His hours at work passed slowly.

When he returned to Tokyo for a weekend or holiday, he would feel happy and lighthearted, but the nights before he returned to work his heart was heavy. He ate and slept more than usual and exercised less. Over three months he gained ten pounds. Weekday mornings he was miserable physically and emotionally, sometimes calling in sick. Ito, already disappointed by Kobayashi's performance, angrily insisted that if he was sick, he must get a doctor's letter. Aware that his problems were as much emotional as physical, Kobayashi consulted a *shinyrōnaika*, saying he thought he was depressed and needed some time off work. The doctor patiently listened to his story and examined him, diagnosed depression, and gave him a prescription for an SSRI and a letter suggesting two weeks of leave. Kobayashi asked for four weeks, but the doctor required a follow-up visit in two weeks before recommending any more time. Kobayashi was pleased to get the diagnosis and by the letter authorizing medical leave. He started the prescribed SSRI. He eagerly brought the doctor's letter to his boss, who noted his happy facial expression and felt suspicious. Ito called the doctor to verify the diagnosis and recommendation; after doing so, he had no choice but to let Kobayashi take time off. Despite the doctor's letter, Ito suspected that Kobayashi was a spoiled young man from an affluent family who lacked self-discipline and the will to work hard—a *wagamama* (self-indulgent person) who wasn't truly ill.

During his two weeks of leave Kobayashi returned to Tokyo, where he was almost symptom-free and had enjoyable times with family and friends. He posted pictures on social media of his happy experiences, including pictures of dishes he had just learned how to cook and selfies taken at a karaoke bar that showed him smiling cheerfully. His boss accidentally saw his Facebook page and was outraged, feeling that Kobayashi had deceived him. Ito asked him to return to work immediately, but Kobayashi insisted on taking the full two weeks of leave. At his follow-up visit with the doctor he related what had happened, and the doctor concluded that his patient had MTD, a form of atypical, non-melancholic depression he'd been seeing more and more in his practice. He did not suggest that Kobayashi take more leave but did recommend participation in group therapy for people with MTD and referred him to a psychologist.

He came back to work after his leave, and within two days his symptoms had returned. Despite his discomfort, he decided to remain on the job, to see if the medication and the group therapy would help with his symptoms. He slowly improved, began to take interest in his work, and eventually repaired his relationship with his boss. In the process, Ito learned about MTD with some help from the company's human resources department.

MTD is the label applied to people, usually young adults, with somatic and emotional symptoms of depression that are especially severe when at work (or at school for those who are full-time students) but improve substantially or even remit completely when the person is not at work and is doing something they enjoy. The person avoids activities they find unpleasant or burdensome. Emotional symptoms can include anger, irritability, and negativity but usually not sadness. The diagnosis of depression is accepted by the patient willingly; they usually seek time off work because of the illness. The syndrome was described in the early 2000s as "a new dysthymic type of depression fostered by modern society" (Tarumi, 2005) and subsequently came to be named "new type depression" or "modern type depression" by Japanese psychiatrists (Kato & Kanba, 2017).

Kato, Hashimoto, et al. (2016) proposed basing the diagnosis of MTD on having persistent depressive mood with associated symptoms, distress, and interference with function, together with some special, almost pathognomonic symptoms. In their view, a patient with MTD would meet the criteria for MDD if their illness is severe but usually wouldn't otherwise. It is nonetheless "really" a depressive disorder, deserving of serious study and treatment, and not deserving of special stigma. The characteristic, special symptoms of MTD include the person believing that they are clinically depressed, being attached to the diagnosis, and seeking to be relieved of duties and/or responsibilities because of depression. Functioning is worse at work or school than at other times. According to Kato and colleagues, there are typical profiles of premorbid personality and behavior for people with MTD as opposed to those with melancholic depression. The person with MTD typically is not conscientious; they are averse to hierarchies, authorities, and specified social roles; they easily blame others; and they have a vague sense of omnipotence. To use an American adjective, they act "entitled." By contrast, the premorbid personality of those with melancholic depression is conscientious, conventional, and humble.

MTD shows mood reactivity like depression with mixed (bipolar) features or "atypical depression." Atypical depression is a variant of MDD with depressed mood, mood reactivity, rejection sensitivity, hypersomnia, hyperphagia, and a heavy feeling ("leaden paralysis") in the limbs. However, the extreme, setting-specific mood reactivity, the lack of sadness, and the enthusiastic embrace of the diagnosis of depression distinguish MTD from atypical depression as well as from melancholia. People with MTD do sleep more than usual, eat more than usual, and may gain weight, as occurred in Kobayashi's case. Only severe cases of MTD would meet the criteria for MDD—others would not have five out of the nine necessary symptoms. People with MTD would undoubtedly meet this book's criteria for clinical depression in the middle zone.

From a social-psychological point of view, MTD in young Japanese employed men and melancholic MDD in middle-aged and older Japanese employed men are complementary to each other. In both cases the underlying problem is the change in Japan's economy that eliminated the assured reward for years of loyal, self-sacrificing work for an employer. This sets the stage for conflict between generations of white-collar workers. An older employee who has made expected sacrifices and then loses hope of the commensurate reward is overwhelmed by feelings of loss, disappointment, and perhaps shame and self-blaming. A younger employee begins employment with the certainty that the old system is no longer applicable but may have bosses who came of age in the old system and have Japan's traditional expectations of loyalty, hard work, and unquestioning obedience to authority by younger employees. The younger employee who has studied hard to get their credentials and has begun their employment with goodwill cannot accept the disappointing reality of the job. The timetable of effort and disappointment is accelerated in young adults with MTD, covering secondary and tertiary education and initial job assignments rather than decades of service.

The prevalence of MTD is not precisely known. A defensible prevalence estimate for young adults would be 1% for MTD without MDD and 0.5% for MTD with MDD. While this estimate is imprecise, it supports the idea that clinical depression is a much larger problem in Japan than would be inferred from its reported rates of MDD. MTD has substantial impact on both the well-being and the economic productivity of those who suffer from it, and it is just one of several distinctive syndromes of clinical depression displayed by Japanese people.

The syndrome of MTD is recognized by psychiatrists outside of Japan, but psychiatrists from different cultures have a different understanding of what causes it and what influences it. Kato et al. (2011) sent case vignettes of MTD and of melancholia to psychiatrists in Australia, Bangladesh, India, Iran, Japan, South Korea, Taiwan, Thailand, and the United States, asking them to rate on a scale of 1 to 5 the prevalence of the patient's syndrome in their country, causes of the syndrome, DSM/ICD diagnosis, suicide risk, and appropriate treatment. The average rating of "commonness" of MTD was greater than 3 out of 5 for urban psychiatrists in all countries and less than 3 out of 5 for rural psychiatrists in all countries. Taiwanese psychiatrists were most likely to call MTD a common condition. Only in South Korea and in India did the psychiatrists give a substantial role to the brain (as opposed to the mind) in the etiology of the syndrome. A large role of cultural factors in shaping the syndrome was endorsed by psychiatrists in Japan, Taiwan, Thailand, the United States, and Australia. The relative causal importance given to family, work or school environment, and the economic environment differed greatly between the countries. In Japan, family relationships were given the greatest importance. Only in the U.S. was the environment of work or school given a preeminent role, with an average score of 4.10 out of 5. With respect to treatment, psychiatrists everywhere saw psychotherapy as most likely to be effective. Only in South Korea, Bangladesh, and Iran was there strong support for pharmacotherapy; and nowhere did the psychiatrists have confidence in non-pharmacologic biological treatments or alternative medicine. In Japan, Taiwan, Australia, and the United States, self-help techniques such as exercise and other lifestyle modifications were thought to be almost as effective as psychotherapy.

More recent thinking by Japanese psychiatrists has moved toward understanding MTD as a biological response to social circumstances, in which young adults (typically men) do not accept their place in Japan's social hierarchy and feel like laboratory mice forced into subordinate roles. They develop learned helplessness, anhedonia, and social avoidance—associated with altered functioning of brain circuits associated with the maintenance of social status, such as decreased activity in the ventromedial prefrontal cortex or decreased oxytocin levels in the amygdala. In mice, a loss of status by those that previously had ranked high has greater effect on the brain than a loss in competition by an established loser. Young people with elite education, indulgent parents, and expectations of high status are thus especially vulnerable to MTD if they enter a hierarchical organization in a humble position or must compete in a work environment after being in a school environment in which they excelled.

There are several clinical implications of seeing MTD as reflecting a neurobiological response to a loss of subjective social status. It prompts greater sympathy and mitigates stigma if a person with MTD is understood as suffering from an involuntary neurobiological response to conflict between traditional collectivist-hierarchical culture and a modern culture that is more individualistic and has less power distance. And if specific brain circuits mediate the maladaptive response, an intervention like transcranial direct current stimulation could be effective in treating the syndrome (Komori et al., 2019; Wang et al., 2014). The apparently greater prevalence of MTD among young men versus young women and those of the upper middle class versus those of the working class fits with the concept of MTD as the consequence of a mismatch between expectation and reality.

Heart (*Kokoro*; 心), Chest (*Mune*; 胸), Belly (*Hara*; 腹): Metaphors for Emotional States

Like the Chinese and the Koreans, Japanese people use body part metaphors to describe emotional states, with precision or ambiguity, as context requires. They were masterfully reviewed by the Japanese linguist Rie Hasada (2002). Words and metaphors useful in understanding depression in Japanese include the following:

Kokoro (心): *Kokoro* can be literally translated as "heart." The ideogram is the same as the one used in Chinese for heart, but it is pronounced differently. It can also mean "soul," "mind," "spirit," or "inner self." It is not completely knowable by another person. A conscientious person has *kokoro*; an inconsiderate one lacks *kokoro*; a generous person has a broad *kokoro*; a stingy one has a narrow *kokoro*.

In 1999, the Japanese pharmaceutical industry introduced the metaphor *kokoro no kaze* (心の風邪; "common cold of the spirit") as a new name for non-melancholic, non-psychotic clinical depression. This was done in direct-to-consumer advertising as well as in materials directed at physicians. The official diagnosis of depression, *utsubyō*, did not change. The purpose of the renaming was to destigmatize depression while retaining a sense of its importance, with the goal of getting patients and their physicians more comfortable with using medications—specifically SSRIs—to treat it. Involving the *kokoro* immediately gives a condition importance as a person's *kokoro* is precious and essential to personal identity. Comparing it to a common cold suggests it is self-limited and not potentially disabling or life-threatening, though it might have symptoms for which medical treatment would be appropriate. The comparison also differentiates it from severe mental illness with its associated stigma. The initial effect of relabeling depression as *kokoro no kaze* was to markedly increase the rate of SSRI prescriptions in Japan, but many of the patients who took them did not continue them for a full course of treatment. In a study of the issue, most Japanese patients who discontinued antidepressants did not inform their physician (Sawada et al., 2009). The concept of *kokoro no kaze* has had two unfortunate side effects. First, it has led to the overdiagnosis and unnecessary drug treatment of people with self-limited mood states—what Allen Frances (2013) has called "disease-mongering." Second, it has misled many Japanese people with depression into thinking the illness is not serious and is always self-limited and into not appreciating that depression can lead to suicide. People who understand *kokoro no kaze* in this way might avoid seeking treatment, discontinue medication as soon as they experience a side effect, or not follow a recommendation for psychotherapy.

Mune (胸): *Mune* literally means "chest." It is a site for emotions that are strongly and deeply felt, though the emotion might be transient. A person can feel anger, joy, disappointment, or worry in their *mune*. Feeling filled with warmth in the *mune* is equivalent to the English metaphor of a lump in one's throat. A person's *mune* can jump (*mune ga odoru*; 胸が躍る) when they are excited. The *kokoro* lies within the *mune*. The *kokoro* is interior, long-term, essential, abstract, and the ultimate source of feeling, thought, and action. The *mune* is a concrete, physical place where feelings are experienced every day.

Hara (腹): *Hara* is literally translated as "belly." It is the site of "gut feelings," especially of anger and firmly held opinions. An angry person's belly stands up (*hara ga tatsu*; 腹が立つ); a person who has made up their mind has set their belly (*hara wo kimeru*; 腹を決める). When a person's *hara* is set, they can tolerate life's hardships and disappointments and remain strong (Hasada, 2002).

Ki (気), a word related to the Chinese word *qì* (气), denotes "breath"; it has a broad range of metaphorical meanings including mind, spirit, intuition, mood, feelings, inclination, will, and intention. *Ki* fills the air around a person. It can radiate from a person's *kokoro*, *hara*, or *atama* (頭; head) and surround it. While a person's *kokoro* may change slowly, *ki* is subject to rapid change at any time. *Ki* is used, often with ambiguity, in everyday conversation in Japan. *Kokoro* is not part of everyday conversation, and when it is used it usually has a specific and deep meaning. Doi (1973) noted that Japanese has a panoply of metaphors involving *ki* that are used to describe emotions and behavior, much as Chinese has an abundance of such metaphors utilizing the word *xin* (心). The words *ki*, *kokoro*, *mune*, and *hara* are more likely to be found in a depression narrative than *atama* or *nō* (脳; "brain"); and when the latter are used, they will be used metaphorically rather than as implying that depression is a dysfunction of the brain. Asking a Japanese person to talk about the body part metaphors that best describe their current feelings and to explain them may open a window into their true feelings (*hon'ne*). Even if they have scientific knowledge that depression reflects dysfunction of the brain, a depressed Japanese person's illness narrative could refer to the thorax or the abdomen.

Normalization of Bullying (*Ijime;* 虐め)

In China, harsh parental discipline is a common source of normalized traumatic experiences. In Japan, bullying (*ijime*) of students by peers, and of employees by their superiors, is a widely prevalent type of trauma that is not consistently called out and acknowledged as both traumatic and inappropriate. The verb form of *ijime* literally carries the connotation of tormenting someone weaker, with the intention of causing distress. Japan's Ministry of Education, Culture, Sports, Science and Technology (文部科学省; *Monbu-kagaku-shō*) defines *ijime* in schools as an act by a student, or students, toward another student that inflicts some physical or psychological consequence, causing the receiving child mental or physical suffering (Kiwano, 2021). Causing psychological or physical injury is an essential aim of *ijime*. This makes it more malignant than a social ritual practiced without an intention to cause harm to the victim.

In Japan, bullying and the harm it causes often are minimized—and thus normalized—by people in authority such as school administrators and corporate executives. In the worst cases, teachers participate in the bullying of students, and top executives join in the bullying of junior employees. Victims of bullying in Japan rarely make formal complaints. In the school setting they fear that complaining of bullying will lead to their being bullied even more severely, by more of their classmates, as they have stood out (in a negative way) by complaining. In work settings, employees fear retribution if they complain; and in fact, many companies do not respond helpfully to employees' complaints of being bullied.

The reluctance of victims to complain is confirmed by the wide discrepancy between the rate of complaints of bullying and the rate of victimization disclosed by surveys. The Japanese Education Ministry counted 517,163 reports of bullying of elementary and secondary school students in fiscal year 2019-2020 (Kuwabata & Mishima, 2021), implying an incidence of reported bullying of less than 4%. Yet, in a 2019 study of Japanese students in the grades 4-9 that used a anonymous questionnaire to assess bullying victimization, perpetration, and witnessing, 35.8% reported that they had been bullied at least once during the past two or three months- 40.1% of boys and 31.7% of girls (Osuka et al., 2019). This strongly suggests that either children conceal signs of bullying from their parents or that parents choose not to complain to authorities for fear that it will not be helpful, or even make matters worse for their child.

Common forms of in-person bullying include verbal abuse and humiliation, threats of violence, social exclusion, hitting and kicking disguised as playing, stealing or damaging the victim's property, and extortion of money. Secondary school students are more often bullied online (Kiwano, 2021; Nippon.com, 2018). From preschool onward, but especially during the middle school years, students who are different in any way are at risk for *ijime*. An atypical physical appearance, a lower-class or immigrant family background, and having a learning disability are typical reasons for a student being bullied. A single embarrassing mistake can target a student for subsequent bullying, as can coming to the defense of another student who is bullied. Typically, *ijime* is repeated, inescapable, and persistent until the victim shows definite signs of harm.

Not surprisingly, bullying of this kind affects mental health, including causing depressive symptoms, sometimes clinical depression (Kawabata & Onishi, 2017). The effects of childhood bullying can persist for decades, into midlife, as was shown in an American study that followed subjects from their school years through age 50 (Evans-Lacko et al., 2017). Childhood bullying is predictive of poor mental health status in Japanese adolescents (Itani et al., 2018). Bullying is a common underlying or contributing cause of a suicide attempt, as it was for Midori in the case vignette (Hidaka et al., 2008). Every year in Japan several suicides are conclusively linked to bullying, and the families of perpetrators have occasionally been successfully sued for damages.

Bullying of adults in work settings is very common—similar in prevalence to bullying at school. Forms of workplace bullying—also known as *power harassment*—include repeated criticism and humiliation of an employee in front of others, assignment of excessive or inappropriate work, giving an employee work they are not qualified to do or work that is far below their education and status, conspicuously ignoring the employee, and assigning the employee to a remote or inconvenient work location requiring excessive commuting (Naito, 2013). Sexual harassment and bullying overlap in their effects, and a male boss whose sexual advances are rejected may turn to bullying the female subordinate who rejected them. Sexual harassment has been experienced by 30% of female Japanese employees; power harassment (workplace *ijime*) of some kind has been experienced by more than half of all employees (Aoki, 2017; Naito,

2013). Workers with lower status because of lesser education, lower salaries, and/or irregular employment are most likely to be the targets of bullying, consistent with the concept of *ijime* as targeting victims perceived as being weaker than the perpetrator (Tsuno et al., 2015).

Consequences of bullying and harassment of employees include poor physical and mental health, including depression and suicidal behavior (Taniguchi et al., 2016). More than 5% of suicides in working-age Japanese people may be attributable to workplace *ijime* (Meek, 2004).

Other consequences of workplace bullying include insomnia, anxiety, and somatic pain (headaches, neck and back pain, and joint pain; Takaki et al., 2013; Taniguchi et al., 2016). The association between job strain and depression in Japanese workers appears to be partly mediated by workplace bullying (Takaki et al., 2010).

In work settings a supervisor or boss can opt to repeatedly criticize or humiliate an employee either privately or in front of other people or can burden an employee with excessive work. *Ijimeru* (虐める), the verb form of *ijime*, can be translated as "to treat a weak person harshly."

The employee may have no realistic recourse when a boss arbitrarily bullies them because in many organizations a complaint to the supervisor's superior or to the company's human resources department would make the situation even worse. The employee would need to have *gaman* (我慢; literally "patience," with connotations of tolerating something almost unbearable with dignity), as well as *shinobi*. *Gaman* is another of Japan's double-edged swords: If the employee successfully practices *gaman*, they will not get depressed. If *gaman* is insufficient, the employee's lack of reasonable recourse sets the stage for depression or medical illness. If depression develops, *gaman* can interfere with their seeking treatment.

Shame (Haji; 恥) and Suicide

Japanese culture has been characterized as a shame culture rather than a guilt culture, notably in Ruth Benedict's classic *The Chrysanthemum and the Sword* (1946). As Benedict uses the word, *shame* involves "an audience or a man's fantasy of an audience." Shame can be external or an internal experience of self-shaming or anticipation of external shame. The distinction between guilt and self-shaming is less sharp than that between guilt and external shame. Though shame is their more frequent self-conscious emotion, Japanese people do have guilt feelings (Thonney et al., 2006). People can experience self-shaming without any other person knowing of the cause or expressing disapproval. The Japanese word for the painful feeling that follows failure or wrongdoing is *haji*

(恥). Japanese culture also has the concept of losing face, which can either be superficial like embarrassment or profound like *haji*. While *haji* is usually translated as "shame," it comprises both concern about others' actual or potential disapproval or rejection and a painful self-punishment that can reach the level of self-humiliation or self-condemnation. *Haji*, a condition of the *kokoro*, is deeper and more persistent than embarrassment or regret.

Haji can lead a person into clinical depression. In its most severe form, it is an unbearable feeling that drives a person to contemplate suicide to clean their name and their family's name of *haji*. However, in a depressed state a person might overestimate how shameful a situation really is or fail to see a realistic, non-suicidal way to address the problem causing the feeling of shame. Depression rather than shame would in this case be the underlying cause of suicide.

People disgraced by circumstances—even circumstances for which they do not bear complete, direct responsibility—might choose to die by suicide to resolve their *haji*. Suicide to "clean one's name" (*haji wo susugu*; 恥を雪ぐ) is normalized and accepted in Japanese culture. For example, in March 2018 an official of Japan's finance ministry committed suicide when it was about to become public that he was involved in a corrupt sale of state property. Press coverage found the corruption to be a problem but not the suicide (Yamaguchi, 2018). Another type of suicide that has been honored is "lovers' suicide" (*jōshi*; 情死; or *shinjū*; 心中), a case where lovers whose relationship is impossible for legal, moral, or family reasons opt to die by suicide together rather than accept living apart.

Both *haji wo susugu* and *shinjū* are regarded in Japanese culture as rational expressions of self-determination and not as consequences of depression, even though people committing such acts often are depressed and might not have died by suicide if their depression had been recognized and treated. The view of suicide as often rational was discussed by Russell and colleagues (2017). A 2006 study of Japanese medical students found that even students in their fifth of six years were surprisingly uninformed about the basic facts of suicide in their country. Only 57% of them knew that mental disorders were a risk factor for suicide, and only 18% knew that physical health problems were the most common cause of suicide (Sato et al., 2006). This is a significant problem if it has not resolved since 2006, and it is unknown whether it has because to date no follow-up to the study has been published. People contemplating suicide often consult physicians shortly before they take their lives. Physicians have opportunities to prevent suicide but only if they recognize them. Suicidal people usually have a rationale for their actions, but that rationale often is driven by depression, often combined with general medical illness, and will disappear if the depression remits, the person has effective medical treatment, or time passes without a suicide attempt. A physician who does not appreciate this will miss opportunities to prevent suicide. Suicide prevention in Japan is challenging because suicide is less stigmatized than the diagnosis and treatment of depression.

The Japanese outlook on life is captured by the phrase *shisei-kan* (死生観; literally "death-life-view"), in which death comes first. In the Chinese equivalent, *shēngsǐ guān* (生死观; literally, "life-death-view"), life comes first. Compared with Chinese and with most other cultures, Japanese culture is not afraid of death and does not find death extraordinary. In 1900, the Japanese public intellectual Inazō Nitobe (新渡戸 稲造; 1862–1933), the son of a samurai, published *Bushidō: The Soul of Japan* (Nitobe, 1909). It was one of the first books written in English about Japanese culture and aesthetics. Nitobe beautifully described Japanese stoicism and lack of fear of death:

> A truly brave man is ever serene; he is never taken by surprise; nothing ruffles the equanimity of his spirit. In the heat of battle, he remains cool; in the midst of catastrophes, he keeps level his mind. Earthquakes do not shake him; he laughs at storms. We admire him as truly great, who, in the menacing presence of danger or death, retains his self-possession, who, for instance, can compose a poem under impending peril or hum a strain in the face of death. (p. 34)

In his description of the Japanese spirit, he combines fearlessness with appreciation of humility and subtlety, contrasting the flashy and heavily scented rose with the cherry blossom. He dislikes the rose because it has thorns and because of

> the tenacity with which she clings to life, as though loth or afraid to die until the bitter end ... these are traits so unlike our flower, which carries no dagger or poison under its beauty, which is ever ready to depart life at the call of nature, whose colours are never gorgeous, and whose light fragrance never palls. (p. 165)

This aspect of Japanese culture combined with the concepts of *shūdan ishiki*, *en*, and *meiwaku* help explain Japan's high suicide rate in terms of the interpersonal theory of suicide. For Japanese people, belonging to a group is extraordinarily important, so thwarted belongingness, as might occur when a person is bullied or an employee is dismissed, is strongly felt. Japanese people easily perceive themselves to be burdensome (*meiwaku*) to others and make great efforts to avoid it, including the practice of *aimai* so that they will not burden people with their differences of opinion or their unmet wants and needs. The Japanese culture's relative acceptance of suicide and lack of fear of death facilitate their people's acquiring the capability to act on their suicidal impulses.

The reasons for suicide most often mentioned in Japanese suicide notes are financial problems and health problems (Russell et al., 2017). The two are related because the cost of healthcare is a common precipitant of financial distress, and chronic health problems can interfere with work and thus reduce income. In Japan, bankruptcy is stigmatized even when the cause is beyond the bankrupt person's control. Life insurance policies in Japan, if in force for more than three years, will pay beneficiaries even when the insured party dies by suicide (Kodama et al., 2017). This offers an additional reason for suicide for a middle-aged man who has gone bankrupt. He can escape *haji* and provide for his surviving family members at the same time.

This scenario has been advanced as an explanation for an increase in suicides by middle-aged men during the Japanese financial downturn of the late 1990s. Among Japanese men, the suicide mortality rate is highest in late middle age rather than in old age, whereas in China and South Korea suicide mortality rises monotonically with age.

In 2008, Junko Kitanaka, a medical anthropologist and an expert on the history of Japanese psychiatry, published an analysis of her observations of Japanese psychiatrists' care of patients who had attempted "suicides of resolve" (*kakugo no jisatsu*; 覚悟の自殺). She noted that suicide has been valued and respected in Japanese culture as an act of self-determination. Even a psychiatrist might be reluctant to raise the issue of depression if a suicidal act were apparently motivated by existential angst in a person with a strong will. A psychiatrist who saw depression as a biologically based "mental illness" might be loath to stigmatize an admired figure by blaming their suicide on depression. Kitanaka asked how psychiatrists could "persuade patients to accept the "truth" of the psychiatric account of suicide, when its fundamental premise goes against the cultural logic of suicide" (Kitanaka, 2008). She raised a concern that attributing a suicide attempt entirely to depression—"medicalizing" it—risks trivializing the meaning of the patient's suffering and discourages serious inquiry into the personal, social, and economic circumstances that might underlie the suicidal patient's despair. In her analysis she anticipated a current trend in American academic medicine to pay more attention to social determinants of health and to advise trainees to listen with curiosity and empathy to patients' illness narratives.

Kitanaka described psychiatrists' work with survivors of suicide attempts as an effort to persuade them to see their behavior—and the view of their life situation that prompted it—as pathological and due to a biological illness. Essentially, the psychiatrist's role was to persuade the patient to distance themselves from the thoughts and feelings that preceded the attempt and to adopt an external locus of control. While acknowledging that the patient had suffered emotional pain, the psychiatrist would attempt to induce the patient "*not* to regard their act as a product of personal will." Paradoxically, however, psychiatrists' labeling some suicidal acts as mere consequences of a biological disturbance could support the idea that other suicidal behavior represented an authentic suicide of resolve—autonomous, deliberate, aesthetic, and perhaps admirable. Excessive medicalization of suicide could thus impede a more comprehensive and holistic dialogue between psychiatrists and suicidal patients that included existential, circumstantial, and biomedical elements and did not require that the patient accept an entirely external locus of control.

Japan's Varied Faces of Depression

The complexities of Japanese culture and communication underlie its diverse manifestations of clinical depression—conditions that overlap with MDD but clearly include people who would meet this book's criteria for clinical depression but not satisfy DSM/ICD criteria for MDD. Bipolar spectrum disorders have distinctive aspects in a Japanese context as well. Just as there are diverse expressions of depression in Japan, there also are forms of death that are not officially classified as suicides but may be the expression of a wish to die and/or a loss of reason to live (loss of *ikigai*).

Within the category of people with MDD itself there are those with psychosomatic conditions typically seen by *shinyrōnaika*—cases of MDD with prominent somatic symptoms, typically fatigue and somatic pain together with some form of sleep disturbance. Overlapping with MDD are cases with MTD, described in detail above. Another characteristically Japanese syndrome that can be an expression of clinical depression—or a prodrome of it—is *hikikomori*.

A "Culture-Bound Syndrome" Goes Global: The Story of *Hikikomori*

Hikikomori is a syndrome of profound and prolonged social isolation, in which a person completely withdraws from society for six months or more, rarely leaving home, seldom talking face to face with anyone including family with whom they live, and limiting social interaction to online communication. The person's social isolation interferes with education and/or employment, and they are likely to be dependent on either parents or social welfare benefits. Adolescents and younger adults with this condition usually live with parents; older adults either live with parents or live alone. If the person lives with their parent(s), they will communicate infrequently. The person is not necessarily troubled by their social isolation per se, especially early in the syndrome. After many months of isolation, the person may begin to experience loneliness. Emotional distress is more often related to comorbid conditions, common ones including depression, anxiety disorders, and autism spectrum disorder. *Hikikomori* can begin as a reaction to being a victim of bullying (*ijime*) or to a physical illness like psoriasis or irritable bowel syndrome that involves a visible stigma or embarrassing symptoms (Kato, Kanba, & Teo, 2016, 2020).

People with the syndrome, who in Japanese are called *hikikomori*, were initially described as late adolescents or young adults, living with their parents but seldom interacting with them. The 1998 book by Japanese psychiatrist Tamaki Saitō that described and named the syndrome characterized it as "adolescence without end" (Saitō, 1998/2013).

Once the syndrome was described, it was found in Japanese people of all ages. A Japanese government survey in 2016 estimated there were 514,000 *hikikomori* aged 15-39, and a survey in 2019 estimated there were 613,000 aged 40-64. The rate increased during the COVID-19 pandemic, with an estimated 1.46 million working-age adults with *hikikomori* in November, 2022 (Harrison et al., 2023).

People with *hikikomori* are not necessarily distressed by their isolation per se. They usually have mental disorders such as depression (MDD, dysthymia, or bipolar depression), an anxiety disorder, an autism spectrum disorder, or post-traumatic stress disorder. Some *hikikomori* would not meet the criteria for any other mental disorder, and a minority of psychiatrists and psychologists have argued that such people are not ill but are simply expressing a choice of lifestyle.

Two Asian American psychiatrists proposed research diagnostic criteria for the disorder that included the requirement that the person with *hikikomori* perceive their social withdrawal as ego-syntonic, even though it had to interfere with their normal routine, occupational or academic functioning, and social activities and relationships (Teo & Gaw, 2010). Indeed, at the outset of the condition, a *hikikomori* may feel relieved about escaping bullying, academic or occupational pressure, or social interactions about which they feel anxious. Over time, however, a dysphoric mood or a full syndrome of MDD can ensue.

Hikikomori initially was thought to be a culture-bound syndrome rarely seen outside Japan. However, surveys of psychiatrists and published case reports established that the syndrome has been seen in a range of countries across the spectrum of income, some with collectivistic cultures and others with individualistic ones, primarily in urban areas. Countries with psychiatrists recognizing or reporting *hikikomori* include Austria, France, Italy, and Spain in Europe; Brazil in South America; Bangladesh, China (including Taiwan and Hong Kong), India, South Korea, and Thailand in Asia; Iran and Oman in the Middle East; Australia; and the United States (Kato et al., 2011, 2012). Kato and Kanba (2017) proposed that, rather than a culture-bound syndrome of Japan, the syndrome is better seen as a "modern-society-bound syndrome."

The 25-item Hikikomori Questionnaire (HQ-25), initially available in Japanese and in English, that screens for *hikikomori* and rates its severity, was published in 2018 by Alan Teo and colleagues (Teo et al., 2018). It was subsequently translated into other Asian and European languages. Translations of the HQ-25 are available for non-commercial use through a dedicated website that aims for global awareness of the syndrome (Teo, n.d.). The HQ-25 asks subjects how accurately various statements describe them over the past six months, using a five-point Likert scale ranging from *strongly disagree* to *strongly agree*. Statements can be related to one of three factors: avoidance of socialization (e.g., "I feel uncomfortable around other people"), self-isolation (e.g., "I shut myself in my room"), and lack of emotional support (e.g., "There really is not anyone with whom I can discuss matters of importance"). The HQ-25 and common depression rating scales clearly measure different syndromes.

While there have been relatively few studies of *hikikomori* outside of Japan that involved large samples, data on American patients with the syndrome suggest that they are more likely than those in Japan to have a *clinically diagnosed* mood disorder, anxiety disorder, or substance use disorder (Kato, Kanba, & Teo, 2019). In the U.S., *hikikomori* would typically appear as a feature of a well-known psychiatric disorder, rather than as a novel, discrete syndrome. Because severe social withdrawal and prolonged dependency of an adult on their parents would be less acceptable in American culture than in Japanese culture, it would be more likely that a young adult showing the syndrome would be suspected of a mental disorder and urged to seek mental health care.

Aspects of Japanese culture favoring the development of *hikikomori* include indulgent childrearing practices and the acceptance of overdependence (*amae*), the importance of avoiding shame (*haji*), and expectations of conformity with societal norms. Japanese parents, particularly those with an only child, are likely to tolerate the prolonged dependence of an adult child. People facing shame or humiliation, whether related to a personal weakness, bullying, or a mental disorder, might opt to "disappear," with *hikikomori* a less drastic option than suicide. Success in mainstream Japanese society requires conformity with demanding expectations for work and social behavior. If a person doesn't want to conform, dropping out of society might be less difficult than trying to conform and failing or openly opposing or resisting tradition.

With this cultural background, the aging of the Japanese population, the slowing of its economic growth, and the impact of globalization have put millions of young Japanese adults, especially young Japanese men, in a challenging situation. They must make extraordinary efforts for years to compete for a limited number of jobs that offer long-term security, opportunities for advancement, and relatively high income and status. Many of those who compete and conform—a much higher proportion than in Japan's postwar boom—will not "win" but will find only "irregular employment" without job security, status, or sufficient income to make a favorable marriage and begin a family. At the same time, Japanese people have increasingly been exposed to globalized Western values of individualism and consumerism, with the explosive growth of social media accelerating the process. Conformity and compliance continue to be expected by the older generation, but their rewards are rapidly decreasing. Social media invite upward comparison, depict non-conformist alternatives, and offer an alternative to demanding in-person interactions. While some young Japanese adults will live openly unconventional lives, a *hikikomori* appears to be "unable to conform yet also is unwilling to rebel" (Toivonen et al., 2011).

Across cultures, intergenerational cultural incompatibility and global economic and demographic changes can lead to social withdrawal in young adults. In other collectivistic Asian cultures, conforming to parents' expectations might be more central than fitting in with a group, but there is the same discrepancy between the effortfulness of compliance and conformity and the doubtfulness of a successful outcome. In more individualistic Western countries, the issue of a person with *hikikomori* might be discomfort with competition to "win" in a country where there is high income inequality, social status is strongly correlated with income, and competing for a good job often requires social competence as well as job-specific ability. Dropping out via social withdrawal might be more congruent with a person's self-concept than "fighting the system" and less painful than continuing to compete but not "winning."

People with *hikikomori* are over six times more likely than others of the same age, gender, education, and general health status to suffer from a concurrent mood disorder (MDD, dysthymia, or BD; Koyama et al., 2010; Toivonen et al., 2011). In Japan, however, the diagnosis of a mood disorder would be unlikely to precede the development of the syndrome of social isolation.

Depression can worsen anxiety and might tip an anxious person into *hikikomori* if their family circumstances facilitated it. On the other hand, a socially isolated person who spends very little of their time outdoors and most of their waking hours online is predisposed to develop depression because of lack of exercise, too much screen time, chronobiologic disruption, and lack of social interaction. (Vitamin D deficiency could also contribute if the person had little exposure to sunlight and did not take a vitamin supplement.) The high prevalence of undiagnosed clinical depression in people with *hikikomori* is another reason to suspect that official statistics on depression prevalence in Japan are significant underestimates.

Kodokushi (Lonely Death)—*Hikikomori*'s Elderly Relative?

As introduced in Part I, *kodokushi*, lonely deaths, and *muenshi* (無縁死), disconnected deaths are seldom labeled as suicides; and an underlying depression rarely is diagnosed. But how is it possible that a person could suffer illness, poverty, malnutrition, and profound social isolation and not have symptoms of depression? They would have difficulty qualifying for a diagnosis of MDD because of the presence of general medical conditions to which specific symptoms could be attributed rather than to depression. Through the cultural lens, however, one sees depression, and it is hard to see how someone set on *kodokushi* could be deterred from their plan to die without addressing the person's hopelessness and lack of meaning and pleasure in life.

Many Japanese people who choose *kodokushi* do so because of poverty and abjectly miserable living conditions. Japanese longevity is yet another national characteristic with opposing implications. Many people would like a long life, but in Japan the combination of longevity and the austere terms of Japan's publicly funded pensions and national health insurance lead to 17% of the population aged 66–75 and 24% of the population aged 76 and older living in poverty, with disposable household incomes less than one half of the nation's per capita median. These discouraging percentages can be contrasted with corresponding rates of 4% and 5% for France, a country with similar per capita income (Organisation for Economic Co-operation and Development, 2023). In a six-year follow-up study of a community sample of Japanese adults aged 65 and above, there were seven indicators of deprivation that, if present at baseline, predicted significantly greater mortality over the period of follow-up: 15.3% of the sample had experienced one or more of the seven indicators, which included having utilities cut off because of inability to pay, lacking a refrigerator, having no air conditioning, having no private bathroom, and being absent from family ceremonial occasions for financial reasons. The latter indicator applied to 5.3% of the sample and by itself was associated with a 65% increase in mortality risk (Saito et al., 2019). Connections are weakened when people cannot meet and socialize with others because they cannot afford the cost of public transportation or a shared activity. Many older Japanese are ashamed of their poverty, even though the reason might be medical expenses completely beyond their control.

Diagnosing MDD can be difficult if many of a depressed person's physical symptoms could alternatively be explained by the chronic general medical conditions from which they suffer or as the consequence of adverse living conditions such as food insecurity. This book's proposed criteria for clinical depression, unlike the criteria for MDD, do not rule out the diagnosis if the symptoms of depression overlap with those of one or more coincident general medical conditions. Similarly, a clinically depressed person with symptoms partly reflecting the consequences of poverty might not meet strict criteria for MDD.

To adequately address the highly prevalent but often undiagnosed depression of older Japanese adults, the definition of clinical depression in need of treatment would have to be liberated from the constraints of MDD criteria, and the definition of treatment would need to go beyond psychotherapy and psychotropic medication. Food insecurity can lead to weight loss or weight gain; noisy environments can continually disrupt sleep; poor sleep and poor nutrition can cause fatigue. Poverty and depression have a circular relationship, and it can be difficult to address clinical depression in older people living in poverty without making improvements in their food and housing. It is hard to sustain improvements in a people's living conditions if they are apathetic, hopeless, and unable or unwilling to voice their needs.

Older Japanese adults were enculturated in *gaman* and *shinobi* (patience, perseverance, and concealment of distress). Most will not identify themselves as depressed or consult a mental health professional even when they have depression that is life-threatening and addressable by a combination of psychiatric care and practical assistance.

Results of targeted and methodologically sophisticated population surveys suggest that the estimates of depression prevalence found in databases like the Global Burden of Disease (GBD) might grossly underestimate the prevalence of clinical depression in older Japanese people. Reported prevalence estimates based on diagnosed cases don't include many cases of typical MDD that would be found with comprehensive population screening, let alone cases of clinical depression presenting as syndromes common in Japan but not meeting MDD criteria.

The JAGES prospective cohort study of a representative sample of Japanese over age 65 revealed a rate of 13.9% of new-onset clinical depression over a three-year period in 10,458 people who had no significant depressive symptoms at baseline. Childhood deprivation was a significant risk factor for the development of depression in older age. Many of the people studied had experienced poverty and other adversity during their childhoods in postwar Japan. Though the collective traumas of World War II and the postwar period were widely shared and normalized, their delayed effects exist nonetheless (Tani et al., 2016). The ability of the Japanese to endure hardship does not necessarily negate the cumulative effect of stress on their mental and physical health.

A pejorative but regrettably common colloquialism that describes and stigmatizes extremely poor older Japanese is *karyu rojin* (下流老人; low-class elderly people). They experience poverty of income and wealth but often also poverty of personal relationships. An example would be a man who devoted his life to his work and then was divorced by his wife in late middle age. His relationships outside of work would have been mediated by his wife, and he would not know how to care for himself, keep house, and carefully manage his own money. Following his divorce, he would be lonely. As he aged, he would accumulate chronic medical problems and would deplete his savings. Once he became dependent on government income support (as distinct from an earned pension), he might become the target of resentment by younger taxpayers.

He ultimately would join the *karyu rojin* (Lin, 2017). It is highly likely that he would become clinically depressed but highly unlikely that he would see himself as depressed, be seen by others as depressed, or seek psychiatric treatment.

Karyu rojin are known to commit minor crimes like shoplifting so that they can spend time in jail, where they will have food, heating or cooling, and some form of social interaction, while saving the money they would otherwise need to spend on their living expenses. It is understandable that many *karyu rojin* will eventually choose *kodokushi*, withdrawing from life altogether and dying alone from malnutrition and chronic medical conditions. Conservatively estimating that one quarter of Japan's elders living in poverty suffer from clinical depression but have not sought care for it, another 1% can be added to the total prevalence of depression in Japan.

Problems in Recognition of Bipolarity

Recognition of bipolarity among Japanese people with depression can be difficult for cultural reasons. Japanese people intensely involved in their work can be sleep-deprived and hyperactive and minimize harmful aspects of their situations because of their stoicism and their loyalty to their employers. Concerning sleep deprivation, Japanese adults consistently get less sleep than people of similar age in other high-income countries. A recently published study assessed sleep habits in 28 countries using data from 226,187 users of a consumer wearable sleep and activity tracker during 2021 (Willoughby et al., 2023). Japanese people had the lowest average weekday sleep duration (6 hours, 6 minutes), the lowest average weekend sleep duration (6 hours, 25 minutes), and Japan's exceptionally low sleep time was even more striking in a regression analysis that included age, sex, and interaction terms. Japanese people also had the latest average bedtime. It can be hard to distinguish overwork driven by cultural conventions from that reflecting hyperthymia or hypomania.

Another potential cause of missed bipolar symptoms is related to pleasure-seeking behavior. Concurrent with intense dedication to work, urban, upper-middle- to high-income Japanese have had since the Edo period a culture of pleasure-seeking, of which entertainment of men by geisha is a well-known example. Two other examples of pleasure-seeking behavior are binge drinking with colleagues, sometimes leading to risky behavior, and enjoying nightclubs until early morning and going to work a few hours later. Graphic art from the Edo period depicts *Ukiyo*, the "floating world," memorializing hedonistic behavior and showing its full acceptance by Japanese society (Fiorillo, 1999). Pleasure-seeking behavior frequently entailing sleep deprivation, intoxication, and health risks would outside of Japanese culture raise a question of bipolarity; and it could provoke bipolar symptoms in a person predisposed to them. It thus makes a bipolar dimension of depression more common in a subset of adult men but at the same time makes it harder to see without awareness of cultural context.

The Japanese psychiatrist Takaaki Abe, one of the first to publish on MTD, hypothesized that about half of young adults with MTD have conditions in the bipolar spectrum (Abe, 2003). Mood reactivity and capacity for pleasure despite continual and fluctuating negative moods is a common expression of bipolar depression with mixed symptoms, as is brittle self-confidence. Their pleasure-seeking behavior when not at work, usually in the company of people unconnected with their work and broadcast on social media, contributes to the view that many people with MTD have conditions in the bipolar spectrum.

Depression in Japanese Americans

In suburban Seattle, Jane Yoshida, a 68-year-old divorced *sansei* woman, sat in the office of Dr. H. Furukawa, a general psychiatrist. Jane was a retired civil servant; she lived alone in the house left to her by her father when he died two years earlier. Dr. Furukawa was an immigrant from Japan to the United States. He came to the U.S. for medical school and psychiatric training 20 years earlier; he married a Japanese American and decided to stay. Jane had seen two other psychiatrists for her current problems of chronic depression and insomnia but did not find them helpful. This was her first encounter with a Japanese psychiatrist.

Jane grew up in Seattle, the only child of "Mike" Yoshida, a *nisei* (二世; second generation) accountant, and his wife, also *nisei*. Her mother died of cancer when she was 15. She graduated from the University of Washington. In her late 20s she married a White American man; they had no children, and they divorced after 10 years. After her divorce, she moved in with her father and has remained in her father's house since then. She got a job with the city government shortly after graduating from college and worked in the same department until her retirement. Her social network was a small group of close friends from college. Outside of work her interests were reading literature, birdwatching with the local Audubon Society, and taking classes at the local Japanese cultural center. As her father got old, she devoted several hours a day to taking care of him.

Mike was a controlling, short-tempered, and hypercritical man, who defined himself as an American and was uncomfortable with his Japanese origins. He always drove American cars and got angry at Jane when she once considered buying a Toyota. He objected to Jane's studying Japanese in high school and college, and she grudgingly respected his opinion. When Jane began dating another *sansei* Japanese American, Mike pressured her to break off the relationship before it got serious.

Jane had minor symptoms of depression throughout her life. She had prolonged grief after the death of her mother, she got moody during her periods, and she found her menopause emotionally difficult. However, she did not develop major depression until after her father's death.

After Mike died, Jane sorted through his possessions and found a box of diaries and mementos her father had never shared with her. From the contents she learned more of her father's life story. He was given the name "Mike" by an elementary school teacher who couldn't or wouldn't pronounce his Japanese name and simply gave him a random American one. He was bullied by his White classmates throughout middle school and high school. In 1942 he and his family were relocated to an internment camp in Wyoming. Feeling humiliated and eager to prove he was a true American, he enlisted in the Army when it became possible in 1943. He served in Europe with many other Japanese Americans in the 442nd Regiment. He saw much combat, many friends were killed, and he was injured twice. He had nightmares and flashbacks of combat experiences for the rest of his life.

After the war, he married a young *nisei* woman he'd met in the internment camp. He went to college and got an accounting degree, supported by the G.I. Bill (the U.S. government program for returning veterans). He and his wife settled in a predominantly White neighborhood.

Growing up, Jane had many conflicts and quarrels with her father. After his death and her discovery of his history, she felt guilty and ashamed about her struggles with him. Visiting his grave, she had thoughts of dying and joining him in the afterlife. Her chronic low-level depressive symptoms and poor-quality sleep got worse, and she frequently had headaches. She lost interest in reading and birdwatching, became indifferent to food, and lost 15 pounds. Jane loved Japanese culture and was curious about discovering her family of origin in Japan; but her father had never told her where her family was from in Japan, and she spoke only a few words of Japanese.

Jane had consulted a couple of psychiatrists suggested by her primary care physician but didn't connect with either of them. One had prescribed cognitive-behavioral therapy with a psychologist; she found the homework assignments boring and didn't follow through on them. Another had given her an SSRI antidepressant. She tried a few doses, felt nauseated, and stopped the medication without calling the psychiatrist.

One day she mentioned her situation to her tea ceremony teacher. He suggested she see a Japanese psychiatrist. At the first encounter Dr. Furukawa elicited the details of Jane's personal and family narrative. She felt his empathy and agreed with his idea that fully recovering from her depression would require her to make peace with herself and her history of conflict with her father. He encouraged her continued involvement with the Japanese cultural center, exploration of her roots, and making social connections with other *sansei*. He arranged for the treatment of her headaches and insomnia with specialists. He prescribed an antidepressant from a different class and insisted that Jane send him a daily text message reporting on her mood state and any concerns about side effects. He told her that if he didn't hear from her, she'd hear from him.

Three million people of Japanese ancestry live permanently in other countries, predominantly Brazil (1.5 million) and the United States (1.2 million). In addition, one million Japanese citizens live overseas as expatriates or international students.

The first wave of migration from Japan to other countries began with the start of the Meiji period in 1868. Immigrants from Japan to the United States settled primarily in Hawaii and in the West Coast states of California, Washington, and Oregon. Ordinary immigration from Japan to the United States was halted by law in 1924; for the next 40 years immigration was limited to family members of U.S. residents and, after 1945, to war brides. During World War II most Japanese Americans, including people of partial Japanese ancestry, were moved to internment camps away from the Pacific coast. Internment of Japanese Americans was rationalized as necessary for national security, but the internment of people of mixed ancestry and fully assimilated Americans with Japanese roots suggests that the internments were racism-related and politically motivated. Many years later, the U.S. government admitted this and compensated the internees and their families. The internment policy was ironic because Japanese Americans identified themselves as American, and almost all were appalled by the actions of Emperor Hirohito's dictatorial regime and his alliance with Hitler's Germany. Over 33,000 Japanese Americans served honorably in the U.S. military, fighting on the European front, like Mike Yoshida in the case vignette (Blakemore, 2021).

In 1965 the Immigration and Nationality Act reopened immigration to Japanese people, and from that point forward between 4000 and 7000 Japanese people each year became permanent U.S. residents. Beyond the physical migration of Japanese people to the United States, Japanese culture penetrated American culture in the late 20th century. Japanese companies made huge investments in the United States and aggressively developed and sold products for the American market. For example, by 2018 Americans bought more passenger cars made by the top three Japanese automakers than by the top three American automakers. More than 70% of these cars were manufactured in North America, mainly in the U.S. Midwest and South. Americans developed tastes for Japanese food and for manga and anime. Zen Buddhism conspicuously influenced American artists, musicians, and writers of the second half of the 20th century.

Japanese Americans are the sixth largest group of Asian Americans. The 2019 American Community Survey estimated that there were approximately 1.5 million Americans with pure or partial Japanese origin, approximately one third of whom are of mixed ethnicity (Budiman, 2021b). Despite their relatively small number, Japanese Americans have been disproportionately influential in business, government, and science. In 2019, 52% of Japanese Americans over age 25 were college graduates and 18% had graduate degrees. In 2019, the median household income of Japanese Americans born in the United States was $82,980, slightly below the median of $85,800 for all Asian Americans, but well above the national median of $61,800 for that year.

Most adult Japanese Americans now are *sansei* or *yonsei* (四世; fourth generation). More than half marry non-Japanese spouses, and most do not speak Japanese (Taylor, 2013). They live in communities where they are in the minority, even among Asian Americans. Their attitudes toward depression and suicide are like those of other Americans with similar educational and social class background. This distinguishes them from most other Asian Americans, who stigmatize depression more, and from Korean Americans, who have a much greater acceptance of suicide. As noted in Chapter 1, Japanese Americans have a significantly lower rate of suicide mortality than Korean Americans.

Even highly assimilated Japanese Americans sometimes encounter problems related to stereotyping and discrimination. *Nisei* and *sansei* Japanese Americans, most of whom are now over age 60, might have grown up with identity issues. In their childhood, America was less diverse than it is today, Japanese were once the second largest Asian American minority, and some anti-Japanese sentiment remained from World War II. Parents of today's adult Japanese Americans might have had direct, indirect, or epigenetic effects of trauma related to the Japanese American internments during World War II. In various ways the trauma of prior generations can find its way into contemporary Japanese American depression narratives.

Development and maintenance of a bicultural identity can improve the psychological well-being of older adults who in an increasingly diverse and globalized context encounter both collectivistic and individualistic cultures in their daily lives (Yamaguchi et al., 2016). People from ethnic minorities, including Japanese Americans, who cultivate a more bicultural identity often become more resistant to depression. This consideration motivated the psychiatrist's suggestions to Jane Yoshida in the case vignette.

The relevance of Japanese Americans' cultural identity to mental health was studied in a group of undergraduate students at the University of Hawaii in Honolulu. Most residents of Hawaii are Asian or of mixed race, and Japanese Americans there are viewed and treated as Japanese and not as generically Asian. In the group, 90% of the students reported experiences of "everyday discrimination" in the past year, such as being treated with less courtesy or less respect, receiving subpar service, people acting as if they were superior, or being called names, insulted, threatened, or harassed. Students' ethnic identity was assessed by a series of questions about the role of their ethnic identity in their life and their thoughts, such as whether they spent time finding out about Japanese history, traditions, and customs; whether they were active in organizations including mainly Japanese people; whether they participate in Japanese cultural practices (food, music, customs); and whether they felt proud and happy to be Japanese. The students were assessed for depressive symptoms with the Center for Epidemiologic Studies Depression Scale (CES-D). Frequent everyday discrimination and the lifetime experience of unfair or bad treatment because of their race and/or ethnicity both were associated with depressive symptoms. A strong Japanese ethnic identity was significantly protective against depression related to everyday discrimination but not against depression related to major unfair treatment (Mossakowski, 2021).

Cultural Concerns in Antidepressant Treatment

Japanese people with depression—whether in Japan or in other countries—typically are reluctant to consult mental health professionals. If they do seek help, it is most likely to be informal support from friends or family; if they consult a professional, it is more likely to be a non-psychiatric physician rather than a psychiatrist. In Japan, the physician consulted might be a *shinyrōnaika*, or a neuropsychiatrist who would emphasize their neurological identity. In the U.S., more acculturated Japanese Americans would be more likely to consult a mental health professional; and both in Japan and abroad, women would be more likely than men to seek treatment. "Mental disorders" including depression are stigmatized in Japan. Psychosomatic symptoms and anxiety are more socially acceptable.

Among psychological treatments, those that emphasize mindfulness and behavior change are more compatible with traditional Japanese culture than those involving significant self-disclosure. Non-adherence to antidepressant prescriptions—during both initial and maintenance phases—is a common problem. Common patient concerns include becoming dependent upon the medication and worries about side effects both actual and potential.

Japanese physicians often approach the risk of non-adherence by starting antidepressants at a lower dose than that recommended by practice guidelines and the drug label, to minimize side effects early in the treatment and address patients' fears. While this reduces the risk that the prescription will be rejected, it can delay the onset of therapeutic benefit and lead to early discontinuation because of lack of effect. Surveys of Japanese psychiatrists suggest that patient education and shared decision-making might be underutilized (Slingsby et al., 2007). In an internet-based survey of 1151 Japanese adults taking antidepressants for treatment of MDD, adherence to prescribed treatment was significantly better when the patient rated the doctor–patient relationship as very good, good, or somewhat good. However, 17.6% of those surveyed gave neutral or negative assessments of their relationship with their doctor (Shigemura et al., 2010). The data suggest that many doctors presume the patient's trust and adherence to treatment and that they might get better results if they did not. In mainstream Japanese culture, a patient with reservations about the physician and/or the recommended treatment would be unlikely to disclose it, though they might acknowledge it, perhaps tacitly, if the issue were raised. Proactive education can address common concerns without requiring patients to disclose them early in a therapeutic relationship. Studies of medication adherence suggest that patients will weigh their perception of the necessity for a treatment against concerns they have about adverse effects or unwanted dependence on the treatment (Horne et al., 2013). Both issues can be anticipated, so clinicians can be alert for indirect communication about them.

Considering traditional Japanese reservations about psychiatric treatment and the contemporary culture's embrace of technology, antidepressant smartphone apps would be an appealing option for depressed Japanese patients unresponsive to antidepressants alone. A smartphone app called Kokoro-App that administered cognitive-behavioral therapy for depression was tested in a randomized controlled trial in patients unresponsive to four or more weeks of an antidepressant drug at an adequate dosage. Kokoro-App used cartoon characters to deliver content on self-monitoring, behavioral activation, and cognitive restructuring. Patients who switched medications and used the app showed more improvement on the PHQ-9 over the next two months than those who only switched medications. Benefits of the combined treatment persisted when patients were reassessed after an additional two months (Mantani et al., 2017).

The use of depression symptom questionnaires to monitor treatment response at regular intervals is rapidly becoming standard practice since incomplete treatment response in MDD is associated with a high risk of non-adherence to continuing treatment and of early relapse of the full syndrome. Periodic reassessment of symptoms also can facilitate useful clinician–patient dialogue. When using common depression symptom questionnaires with Japanese patients, several culturally related issues are relevant.

Japanese culture favors the understatement of emotion—both negative and positive. For this reason, the optimal cutoff scores for predicting an MDD diagnosis and for establishing the presence of clinically relevant residual symptoms will be lower for many subgroups of Japanese people than those typically used with Western populations when using a questionnaire like the PHQ-9 that does not have questions about positive affect. For Western populations, a cutoff score of 10 is most often used for identifying probable MDD, and a score of 5 is used to identify milder depressive symptoms of potential clinical relevance. When the PHQ-9 was tested in general internal medicine clinics in rural Japan, the optimal cutoff score for MDD was 5 (Inagaki et al., 2013).

When the structure of the CES-D, a 20-item questionnaire with four positively worded items, was studied in a survey of Japanese public employees in 1986, the four positive items were not correlated with the remainder of the scale, suggesting that the reported absence of positive thoughts and feelings does not necessarily indicate depression in people identifying with traditional Japanese culture. In the same study, the factor structure of the CES-D differed by the age cohort of the subjects. In subjects born in 1936 or earlier, somatic, affective, and interpersonal symptoms grouped together as a single factor, while for those born later—thus coming of age during Japan's period of rapid growth and Westernization—some of the cognitive/affective items grouped with the somatic items and others with the interpersonal items. Throughout the age spectrum (19–63), problems with interpersonal relationships were not a separate factor but always were associated with symptoms of depression (Iwata & Roberts, 1996). This fits with the concept of interdependent self-construal: Depression often would be brought on by problems in relationships, emotional and behavioral changes of depression would impact relationships, and consciousness of the connection would be painful for the person affected. In the analysis of a predominantly male sample, crying spells and sadness were very infrequently reported, in keeping with the expectation in traditional Japanese culture that men would suppress overt expressions of sadness. As noted above, an alternate approach to screening that assesses the presence or absence of positive mental health—the Euthymia Scale—might be useful with Japanese people who would answer traditional questionnaire items with a combination of humility and understatement.

Young adults in contemporary Japan might be expected to have the most Western or globalized perspective on depression. An internet-based study of 1000 Japanese university students conducted in 2015 suggested that even in a current cohort of young adults, the PHQ-9 and the CES-D function somewhat differently than in Western populations. For the positive items "I felt that I was just as good as other people" and "I felt hopeful about the future," students who were more depressed were less likely to indicate that they never felt that way, suggesting that very depressed students were reluctant to acknowledge their most negative thoughts and feelings. For the items "I felt happy" and "I enjoyed life," very few students endorsed intermediate scores: They either indicated that these positive feelings occurred rarely or never or that they occurred almost all the time (Umegaki & Todo, 2017). Because of such patterns of item response, the CES-D would be a poor choice for detecting residual symptoms of a partially treated depression. Two hypotheses are suggested by the findings: Most of today's Japanese educated, urban young adults are comfortable expressing their feelings; but if they become depressed, they might become insecure about doing so. Alternatively, young adults retaining a traditional Japanese reticence about emotional expression might be more vulnerable to becoming depressed under the stresses of modern Japanese life.

The study's authors found that item responses on the PHQ-9 were less complex and that it was most suitable for measuring depression across the full spectrum of severity. The study data showed a mean score of 5 on the PHQ-9, and 34% of the sample reached or exceeded the standard cutoff score for a probable diagnosis of MDD. While the study did not include diagnostic interviews, it is likely that an optimal PHQ-9 cutoff score for predicting MDD in the student population would be higher than 10—a striking contrast with the rural primary care study in which a cutoff score of 5 was optimal for MDD. This is a remarkable demonstration of how multiple intersecting identities including age/generation, education, and urban/rural status, and not just nationality, influence the expression of depression in ways relevant to its clinical diagnosis and management. A clinician working with a specific population of Japanese people optimally would choose a depression rating scale and cutoff scores appropriate to the population's intersecting cultural identities.

Chapter 12

South Korea: *Han* and Passionate Intensity

South Korea (the Republic of Korea, subsequently referred to as *Korea* in this chapter when doing so would be unambiguous), a nation of 51.5 million population, currently has the highest suicide mortality rates of all high-income countries. In 2019, Korea's overall suicide rate per 100,000 population was 28.91: 40.86 for men and 16.79 for women. In the same year, suicide mortality in the United States was 23.61 for men and 6.70 for women—thus, Korean rates were 173% and 250% of the U.S. rates, respectively. For men and women over age 70, the rates in Korea were 139.79 and 50.09, 3.9 times the rate for U.S. men and 9.0 times the rate for U.S. women in the same age range. In Korea approximately 41 people die by suicide every day. Virtually every resident of the country is touched in some way by suicide, either through the death of a friend, acquaintance, or family member or through the death by suicide of a public figure personally meaningful to them. In 1990, Korea's overall suicide rate of 11.35 per 100,000 was lower than that of the United States, substantially lower for men (16.11 vs. 21.73) and slightly higher for women (6.84 vs. 5.47). In the two decades from 1990 to 2010, Korea's rate of deaths by suicide tripled at the same time as its economy thrived, transforming it into one of the world's high-income nations (Institute for Health Metrics and Evaluation [IHME], 2023; World Bank, 2021). As economic prosperity grew, human misery increased and was expressed through self-harm.

The explanation of Korea's suicide epidemic is complex. A demographic factor contributing to the increase in the nation's overall suicide mortality since 1990 is the progressive aging of its population. The latter is related to a sharply declining fertility rate, which is now the lowest in the world. Korea's registered population (native and naturalized citizens) has begun to decrease, and its decline in population is expected to continue (Korean Statistical Information Service, 2024). Because Korea's suicide rates increase with age, an increase in suicide rates not standardized for age would be expected. However, demographics do not explain why Korea's suicide rate for men over age 70 is in triple digits and why its suicide mortality rates in younger adults are the highest among high-income countries. The explanation does not lie in a high prevalence of mood disorders; Korea's prevalence rates for major depressive disorder (MDD), dysthymia, and bipolar disorder (BD) are lower than those of the United States. The estimated prevalence of the three conditions increased by less than 25% between 1990 and 2010 at the same time as its suicide rate tripled (IHME, 2023)

The 1.8 million U.S. residents with total or partial Korean ancestry constitute the fifth largest group of Asian Americans, and the United States is home to the largest Korean diaspora community. Korean Americans comprise primarily first-generation immigrants and their American-born children and grandchildren. There were two major waves of immigration from Korea to the United States. The first, between 1950 and 1964, included Korean brides of American soldiers, war orphans adopted by American families, and an assortment of students, businesspeople, and intellectuals. A second and much larger wave began in 1965 and continued through the late 1980s, consisting mainly of people who left Korea to pursue economic opportunity or to escape an oppressive military dictatorship. During the second wave, Korea was the third largest source of immigrants to the United States, surpassed only by Mexico and the Philippines (S. Chung, 2020). Since the establishment of Korea's Sixth Republic—a parliamentary democracy—there has been less immigration from Korea to the United States, and most immigrants have been middle-class or upper-middle-class people who initially came to the United States for higher education or in connection with a business or profession. Subgroups of first-generation immigrants from Korea might differ greatly in their typical socioeconomic status and their level of acculturation, but they and their offspring all have mental health issues relatable to their Korean origins. For example, Korean Americans have the highest suicide rate of all Asian American groups. Korean Americans also share Korea's distinctively high rates of suicide in women and in adults over age 70 of both genders.

Koreans and Korean Americans suffer from depression at rates higher than those of other East Asians and other Asian Americans; but they usually do not seek treatment for it, and when they do, they often do not persist. In their native country and in America, Korean people frequently express depression in culturally distinctive ways, the best known being *hwa-byung* (火病), a psychosomatic disorder that arises in a context of long-suppressed anger. The occurrence, phenomenology, and illness narratives of depression in Korean people can be related to a collectivistic and male-dominant culture of traditional Confucianism, widely shared and transgenerational historical trauma, distinctive expressions of affective illness associated with Korean culture, and characteristic coping behaviors that often work but sometimes tragically fail.

This chapter begins with a brief review of the historical context of modern Korean culture, relating it to culturally typical, depression-relevant patterns of behavior. This is followed by a description of two characteristic "national emotions," *han* (한) and *jeong* (정), that, depending on context, can be adaptive or maladaptive. This is followed by a description of two cultural syndromes of negative emotion highly prevalent among Koreans. Then, several contributors to Koreans' depression risk are described: Harmful alcohol use, harsh parenting practices, intimate partner violence (IPV), and preoccupation with "face." Korea's high suicide rate is then explained in terms of an intersection of economic and demographic factors, intergenerational conflict, a high prevalence of harmful alcohol use, histories of trauma, and normalization of suicide in an ethnically homogeneous and cohesive society.

We then turn to the issue of depression and suicide in Korean Americans and cite evidence for similarities in depression-relevant phenomena between Koreans and Americans of Korean origin. Like all immigrant groups, Korean Americans can experience depression related to acculturative stress and acculturative family distancing. Remarkably, behavior and experiences suggesting problematic acculturation also can arise in Koreans who have not emigrated. Korea's explosive economic growth and its subsequent deceleration, its plummeting fertility rate, globalization, and the impact of social media have entailed the exposure of adolescent, young adult, and early midlife Koreans to life circumstances and cultural influences differing greatly from those that shaped the attitudes and behavior of their parents. Younger Koreans often adopt a more individualistic culture than their parents, and many—especially younger women—become less accepting of traditional power relationships and gender roles. Koreans who are now students or are early in their careers do not have the same prospects as their parents did for improving their status through hard work; academic competition is intense, but doing well academically might not translate into stable and well-paid employment. Not uncommonly in contemporary Korea, a young adult woman will choose to reman single or not to have children—decisions contrary to traditional expectations. This might lead to conflict with her parents, and distancing from them. The scenario might resemble that of a second-generation Korean American making a similar decision in conflict with the expectations of her less-assimilated parents.

There are cultural reasons why many Koreans might suffer clinical depression and either do not seek treatment or fail to meet the Diagnostic and Statistical Manual of Mental Disorders (DSM)/ICD criteria for MDD, dysthymia, or the depressed phase of BD if they do. There also are aspects of the Korean culture that increase the probability that suicidal ideation will lead to a suicide attempt and the probability that an attempt will have a fatal outcome. Some of Korea's cultural reasons for alternate presentations of depression, non-treatment, and its frequency of suicidal behavior are distinctive, while others are shared with China and Japan. Risk factors shared by the three major East Asian countries include a high prevalence of overwork and sleep deprivation in working-age adults, stressful working conditions with high job strain, widespread poverty in old age, stigma of mental illness and of psychiatric treatment, and a prevailing ethos that is permissive concerning suicide.

The Historical Context of Modern Korean Culture

Historical context is useful in understanding the distinctive attributes of Korean culture. Before the 20th century, Korea was a very low-income agricultural country with much poverty and illiteracy and an essentially feudal organization of society. Members of Korea's peasant class had little opportunity to change their lot in life. The population's overall educational level was low. In 1910, Korea was annexed by Japan and subsequently ruled in a humiliating manner. During Japanese rule, Koreans were forbidden to teach Korean history and the Korean language in their schools, and youths were denied the opportunity for secondary or higher education. Koreans were forced to adopt Japanese names and to worship at Shinto shrines. Myriad historical artifacts were expropriated or destroyed. During World War II, the Japanese abducted Korean girls and young women and forced them into sexual slavery. Though there remains some controversy about the scale and details of this atrocity, the event was eventually acknowledged by Japan with an apology and compensation to survivors.

When World War II ended in 1945, the Korean peninsula was occupied by the United States in the south and by the Soviet Union in the north. Although there originally was hope for a unified country to persist after the United States and the Soviet Union departed, it was not realized. In 1948 the peninsula was divided at the 38th parallel into two ideologically opposed states, a division that split many families. From 1950 to 1953 there was a bloody war between the Republic of Korea (South Korea) and the Democratic People's Republic of Korea (North Korea), in which over three million Koreans died, most of them civilians (McGuire, 2010). Koreans faced extreme poverty and hardship during and immediately after the war. The war ended with an armistice rather than a formal peace treaty, and troops from the two nations have perennially faced each other across a narrow neutral zone. North Korea has batteries of artillery pointed at Seoul that could kill millions of Koreans in a few hours if the nations were to go to war again.

Between the end of the Korean War and 1987, South Korea had multiple changes in its system of government, with periods of martial law and thousands of its citizens killed or imprisoned in connection with political demonstrations and power struggles. Despite the country's political instability, it rapidly grew an export-oriented economy as policies directed most available capital to a small number of large industrial enterprises. Between 1960 and 2000, Korea's per capita income (adjusted for inflation) grew by 1554%. From 2000 to 2010 it grew by only 50%, and from 2010 to 2020 by only 23% (World Bank, 2023a).

Almost half of South Korea's oldest old are poor, the country having the highest old age poverty rate in the Organisation for Economic Co-operation and Development (OECD)—34.6% for people aged 66–75 and 55.1% for those aged 76 and above (OECD, 2023). Several factors contribute. Korea was not a high-income nation before the early 1990s, so many of its elders could not save enough during their working years to provide for their old age. Korea's relatively modest social welfare system does not ensure basic support for older people who do not have substantial savings or assistance from their families. An underlying expectation appears to be that an older person's children will address their financial gaps—but millions of older Koreans have no child able and willing to provide sufficient assistance.

Millions of Koreans currently in midlife had parents who grew up with poverty and deprivation and subsequently emerged from poverty through hard work in the context of a rapidly growing economy. Today's adolescents and young adults are uncertain as to whether their future will be as bright as their parents', and many have difficulty finding employment with compensation and opportunity commensurate with their education.

Implications of Korea's economic history include normalization of poverty-related trauma for older adults, transmission of the epigenetic or behavioral consequences of older adults' poverty-related trauma to their children, and intergenerational conflicts related to differences in experience and expectations. The intrapsychic and family conflicts of many young and middle-aged Korean adults are like those of second-generation immigrants whose parents emigrated from a low-income country with a collectivistic culture to a high-income country with an individualistic one.

Essentially, every Korean has some personal or family history of trauma. The consequences of national and personal traumatic history are transmitted intergenerationally through the education and enculturation of children, individual families' stories, and epigenetic mechanisms. Korea's recent history provides context for two "Korean national emotions," *han* and *jeong*, and for two cultural syndromes related to depression though distinct from MDD, *hwa-byung* and post-traumatic embitterment disorder (PTED).

Han (한) and *Jeong* (정): Korea's "National Emotions"

Scholars of Korean culture describe it as having two "national emotions"— *han* and *jeong* (P. Y. Kim, 2020). Scholars agree that *han* is untranslatable and describe it with a list of related words and phrases: *sorrow, spite, rancor, resentment, reaction to suffering, injustice, persecution, hoping and yearning for vengeance but not actively pursuing it, resignation, bitter acceptance*, and *grim determination*. It is not simply anger or sadness; it includes an element of passion, and it is not entirely unpleasant. It is a deep and persistent emotion that can be carried in a person's heart for years as they patiently wait for an opportunity for revenge that might never come. A Korean proverb states, "A woman feeling *han* freezes the ground even in Spring" (Ahn, 1987). *Han* is "sorrow and the hope to overcome it, and it is injustice and the obsession to avenge it" (Babe, 2017). *Han* has both a positive and a negative aspect; it has enabled Koreans to endure injustice and mistreatment without losing hope, but it can interfere with more practical efforts to solve problems. However, when it fails as a defense, it may leave a person utterly hopeless. The presence of *han* may explain why the syndromes of many Koreans with clinical depression might not meet DSM criteria for MDD but instead have an illness in which anger rather than sadness or anhedonia is the most salient emotion.

Jeong is a word that can be approximated by this list of words: *love, feeling, sentiment, attachment, bond, affection, heart*. At the edges of connotation there are *generosity* and *bondage*. A baby can be penetrated by its mother's *jeong*; an adult can feel *jeong* from a good friend or from a group of which they are a member. Sharing food with a friend or acquaintance, without being prompted, is another expression of *jeong*. Too little *jeong* and a Korean is lonely and blue. If a person is "addicted to *jeong*" they may get stuck in an abusive relationship (C. K. Chung & Cho, 2018). *Jeong* also can be understood in the context of Korea's traumatic history. It is the complement of *han*: another cultural resource that enables people to endure the unendurable, an expression of the relational social capital that helps people tolerate stress without becoming depressed.

Heavy drinking—or even binge drinking—together with a group of friends or colleagues can be a social bonding experience with positive aspects. In Korea, most adults with harmful drinking behavior do their heavy drinking in social situations where such drinking is normalized. If drinking episodes are associated with the experience of *jeong*, the drinker might minimize any associated health risks. Korea's high prevalence of episodic heavy drinking might thus be related to its culture of *jeong*.

Depression-Related Syndromes Reflecting Korean Culture

One expression of *han* is *hwa-byung*, "fire illness" or "anger illness," a condition that affects at approximately 5% of middle-aged Korean women, with a substantially higher prevalence in rural areas (Lee et al., 2014; Lee and Lee, 2008; Y. J. Park et al., 2002). It is seen in men with a lower prevalence. In both genders, prevalence is higher for people in their 40s and 60s than for those in their 50s. It is also seen in first- and second-generation Korean Americans (Moon, 2014). It is understood in traditional Korean or Chinese medicine as the consequence of pent-up anger, which disrupts the balance of yin and yang. It has been characterized either as a cultural syndrome highly comorbid with MDD or simply as a variant presentation of clinical depression (Suh, 2013). The question of which characterization is most valid has been argued in the literature since the syndrome was described, but there is no disagreement that *hwa-byung* looks different from melancholia and that people with *hwa-byung* may not fully meet the criteria for MDD. It has some attributes of depression variants discussed elsewhere in this book, including atypical depression, male depression, and depression with prominent somatic symptoms. Symptoms experienced by people with *hwa-byung* include anger, hopelessness, and multiple physical symptoms and worries about physical health, with feelings of heat or heat intolerance and distressing visceral sensations especially prominent (Roberts et al., 2006).

People with *hwa-byung* know they are ill and, unlike most people with somatoform disorders, recognize that emotional problems underlie their physical distress (Pang, 2000). Two American nurse practitioners with extensive experience in treating *hwa-byung* in older first-generation Korea immigrant women published recommendations for clinical interviews of patients suspected of having the illness. They advise obtaining background information about the patient via a questionnaire rather than asking a patient at a first interview to disclose information about which they might feel uncomfortable, such as their age or level of education. In a private interview, using a professional interpreter rather than a family member if the patient has limited English proficiency and the clinician does not speak Korean, the clinician would ask whether the patient thinks they have *hwa-byung* and, if so, why they think so, how long they have had it, and how it interferes with their daily life. The clinician would also ask whether the patient had talked to anyone about their symptoms and whether they had sought any treatment for them, including traditional Korean medicine or other alternative treatment (Choi & Yeom, 2011).

Hwa-byung is most often seen in midlife and it is more prevalent in people who are less educated. The syndrome comprises extreme anger and irritability combined with multiple somatic symptoms involving the autonomic nervous system and body parts related to emotional metaphors. The symptom of anger is associated with feelings of unfairness and injustice. Hopelessness is associated with fear of death. Physical symptoms include fatigue, somatic pain, shortness of breath, sighing, tachycardia, palpitations, and a feeling of heat.

Gastrointestinal symptoms include anorexia, indigestion, and the sense of a lump in the epigastric region (J. Lee et al., 2014).

At the core of *hwa-byung* is an excess of *han*. A typical cause for *hwa-byung* in women is marital conflict. A woman with *hwa-byung* might endure a domineering, abusive, unfaithful, and/or alcoholic husband, often with disagreeable or verbally abusive in-laws. Stuck in the relationship because of her financial or emotional dependence and/or because she has traditional Confucian expectations of submission to male authority, she has suppressed her anger for many years. Finally, as her children grow up or her husband's behavior gets worse, she can no longer suppress her anger and the syndrome of *hwa-byung* develops (Min, 2004). *Hwa-byung*, which can occur in men, isn't always about domination of women in Korea's patriarchal culture but it always concerns injustice of some kind. For example, a Korean man might develop *hwa-byung* after working for years in a hostile workplace with a bullying supervisor.

Hwa-byung includes symptoms like somatic pain and anger that are not included in the criteria for MDD, and people with it might not complain of depressed mood or anhedonia, and thus not be diagnosable with MDD. However, in a Korean psychiatric patient population, 60.7% of patients diagnosed with *hwa-byung* also met the DSM criteria for major depression (Min & Suh, 2010). All people with *hwa-byung*, including those who did not meet the criteria for MDD, would meet this book's criteria for clinical depression, and their depression might be severe. In a sample of Korean women over age 60 with *hwa-byung* or with MDD alone, there was greater severity of depressive symptoms in those with *hwa-byung*, whether the symptoms were rated with (the Korean version of) the Hamilton Depression Rating Scale, the Beck Depression Inventory (BDI), or the Geriatric Depression Scale (K-GDS) (Im et al., 2017). For example, the mean score on the BDI of the women with *hwa-byung* was 21, with a standard deviation of 10 points, indicating that about one third of the patients with *hwa-byung* had severe depression as indicated by a BDI score of 30 or higher.

Increased talkativeness and racing thoughts are common in *hwa-byung*. These symptoms are unusual in patients with unipolar MDD. In a patient from mainstream Western culture, they would suggest depression with mixed symptoms; but in a Korean with *hwa-byung*, they would not necessarily be indicators of bipolarity. There are insufficient published data to know whether patients with *hwa-byung* and racing thoughts would respond better to pharmacologic treatment that included a mood-stabilizing agent rather than to an antidepressant drug alone.

Though Koreans and Korean Americans understand that *hwa-byung* is an emotional as well as a physical disturbance, they rarely consult mental health professionals unless their symptoms are persistent and intolerable. If they seek treatment at all, they are more likely to consult a primary care physician for treatment of distressing physical symptoms or to see a practitioner of traditional Korean or Chinese medicine. They tend to prefer support from family, friends, or their church (if they are religious) over counseling or psychotherapy by mental health professionals. When they do consult mental health professionals, they often do not persist with treatment.

Jieun Lee and colleagues offer a useful model for understanding *hwa-byung* in context, describing nested concentric circles of Korean culture, religious community, family, and individual factors, focusing on *hwa-byung* in middle-aged women (J. Lee et al., 2014). A woman is oppressed, dominated, or abused by a husband and/or mother-in-law, developing intense anger, resentment, and a feeling of injustice. Her treatment is rationalized by traditional Korean values of male superiority and female submission. Traditional culture also forbids defiance of her husband and discourages direct expression of her anger and unhappiness. If she is religious, her church might offer support and an opportunity to share feelings with other unhappy women, or it might simply reinforce traditional values and add to a sense of isolation or hopelessness. As noted in Part I, exploring a patient's religious identification, the nature of their religious community, and the use of positive and negative religious coping can help identify both therapeutic opportunities and potential barriers to the patient's recovery.

Within the family, there often is a discrepancy between the husband's traditional Korean values and the woman's thinking. In Korea, she will have been exposed through media, including social media, to a more modern, egalitarian model of marital relations. In America, she will have begun assimilation of American views of gender relations, perhaps more rapidly than her spouse. Individual factors that increase the incidence and severity of *hwa-byung* comprise lower socioeconomic status, acculturative stress, an impatient personality, and a baseline of commitment to traditional Korean values.

Clinicians and social scientists interested in treating or studying *hwa-byung* can make use of a psychometrically validated rating scale for the syndrome, the Hwa-Byung Rating Scale, reproduced in Table 12.1 (S.-Y. Chung et al., 2015). The table matches the questionnaire items with the aspect of the illness to which each question refers. People identified by their scale scores as having *hwa-byung* were shown to have abnormalities of heart rate variability consistent with sympathetic overactivity. *Hwa-byung* is correlated not only with abnormal sympathetic–parasympathetic balance but also with abnormalities on functional brain imaging in areas involved with processing facial expressions of emotion (B. T. Lee et al., 2009). While much more work must be done to fully characterize the biology of *hwa-byung*, it appears to be a phenotype of depressive illness with distinctive biological as well as phenomenological characteristics (Chiao, 2015).

Table 12.1 Hwa-Byung Scale and Its Relationship to Personality and Symptoms

	Item	Condition
Personality-related item	I live my life without caring about my rights	Waiving of rights
	My family or colleagues do not realize my hardships	Ignored hardships
	I tend to bear malice toward someone for a long time	Bearing of malice
	I tend to conceal my emotional pain	Concealment of emotional pain
	I tend to contain my anger until it explodes	Suppression of anger
	I tend to be bashful toward others	Bashfulness
	I have difficulty in starting conversations with others	Difficulty in starting conversations
	I have difficulty conveying what I want to say	Communication challenges
	Whenever I go somewhere, I tend to choose the same route as I have chosen in the past	Tendency toward the familiar
	When I go on holiday, I tend to revisit the places that I have enjoyed in the past	Tendency to act based on past emotions
	I make an effort to forget something bad	Avoidance of negativity
	I make an effort to avoid problematic situations	Avoidance of problematic situations
	I tend to submit to others' demands	Submission to others' demands
	I make an effort to meet others' expectations	Overemphasis on others' opinions
	I tend to accept problems as fate	Fatalism
	I tend to feel guilty about things	Feelings of guilt
Symptom-related item	I am unhappy in my life	Unhappy life
	I feel frustrated	Frustration
	My life is melancholic	Melancholic life
	I feel sorrowful	Sorrow
	I feel mortified	Mortification

(continued)

Table 12.1 Continued

Item	Condition
I feel anxious due to neuroticism	Anxiety due to neuroticism
My limbs tremble when I am anxious about something	Anxiety-related trembling of the limbs
I am disappointed in myself	Disappointment in self
I have a flush on my face	Flush
My chest feels hot	Chest heat
My chest feels constricted	Chest constriction
Anger makes my hands numb or tremble	Anger-induced numbness or trembling
I have indigestion	Indigestion
I feel fatigued	Fatigue
I think that the world is unfair	Negative outlook

Note: Analysis by S.-Y. Chung et al. (2015).

Recognition that MDD comprises multiple phenotypes with different responses to specific treatments is becoming a standard of contemporary psychiatry. From the emerging perspective of personalized medicine, one would not label a depression phenotype a *cultural syndrome* simply because it was more common among people from a specific cultural group. That said, listening for characteristic illness narratives of *hwa-byung* in depressed Korean patients who display the syndrome might enhance empathy and trust, suggest fruitful lines of clinical inquiry, and enable therapeutic engagement (Choi & Yeom, 2011). In the future, the study of *hwa-byung* might yield practical biomarkers that would aid in the personalization of treatment for patients who display the syndrome. For example, a controlled study in middle-aged Korean women showed that tailoring Adlerian psychotherapy to focus on the typical conflicts and issues of *hwa-byung* yielded excellent therapeutic results in patients with the syndrome (E. Kim et al., 2020).

Another distinctive syndrome of negative affect with significant prevalence in Koreans—though acknowledged to occur in patients of many other nationalities—is PTED. Like post-traumatic stress disorder (PTSD), PTED is a reaction to a discrete traumatic event; but the response is not one of anxiety, flashbacks, nightmares, and avoidance but rather one of a bitter mood and recurrent intrusive thoughts related to the event. Criteria were proposed by Linden and colleagues (2008); they are shown in Table 12.2. In a sample of Korean adults with no history of any psychiatric diagnosis or treatment who

Table 12.2 Diagnostic Criteria for Post-traumatic Embitterment Disorder (PTED; Linden et al., 2008)

A. Development of clinically significant emotional or behavioral symptoms following a single exceptional, though normal, negative life event.
B. The traumatic event is experienced in the following ways:
1. The person knows about the event and sees it as the cause of illness.
2. The event is perceived as unjust, as an insult, and as a humiliation.
3. The person's response to the event involves feelings of embitterment, rage, and helplessness.
4. The person reacts with emotional arousal when reminded of the event.
C. Characteristic symptoms resulting from the event are intrusive memories and a persistent negative change in mental well-being.
D. No obvious mental disorder was present prior to the event that could explain the abnormal reaction.
E. Performance in daily activities and roles is impaired.
F. Symptoms persist for more than 6 months.

were screened for PTED, *hwa-byung*, and MDD, the first syndrome had a prevalence of 1.7%. There was no overlap between PTED and *hwa-byung*, and very few subjects with either diagnosis exceeded the clinical cutoff score on the BDI (Joe et al., 2017). However, in a sample of German psychiatric inpatients with PTED, the prevalence of comorbid MDD was 52.1%. Studies of comorbidity in the general population versus clinical populations suggest that while untreated patients in the community can have *hwa-byung* or PTED without a full syndrome of MDD, people with either of the two syndromes who present for psychiatric treatment are likely to meet the diagnostic criteria for a major depressive episode as well as those for the more culturally specific syndrome.

On high-resolution brain imaging (voxel-based morphometry), people with PTED do not have the abnormalities in the medial prefrontal cortex and hippocampus that are found in people with PTSD. Instead, they have increased gray matter volume in the precuneus and increased white matter volume in the uncinate fasciculus. These two structures are involved in episodic memory retrieval, and their enlargement may reflect the continual recall and reprocessing of memories of the traumatic event that induced the person's embitterment (Kühn et al., 2018). Like *hwa-byung* comorbid with depression, PTED comorbid with depression may prove to be linked with biomarkers that will support the diagnosis and assist in the selection of an effective treatment.

Many other countries around the world share Korea's history of long-standing military conflict and/or prolonged and recurrently violent periods of political instability or autocratic rule. Clinicians might consider the diagnosis of comorbid depression and PTED in immigrants from such countries, and in refugees and asylum-seekers of diverse origins from other nations with similar modern histories.

Confucianism in Korea

Confucianism is the foundation of ethics in Korea, as it is in China and Japan. It is compatible with the practice of Christianity or of Buddhism, and most Korean Christians and Buddhists are also Confucians. In the 1880s Presbyterian and Methodist missionaries proselytized throughout the nation; many Koreans were converted, and at present over 30% of Korea's citizens profess Christianity. Christian, Buddhist, or unaffiliated, many Koreans normalize forms of family violence that are more compatible with traditional Confucianism than with contemporary standards of domestic behavior—including standards encountered in other countries with a Confucian cultural heritage.

Confucianism was introduced to Korea in 108 BCE, when the Han Chinese established a colony in northern Korea, near today's Pyongyang. During the Tang Dynasty many Koreans studied at China's national academy in Chang'an (today's Xi'an) and returned to establish schools of Confucianism. Korean scholars commented upon and elaborated upon the Confucian classics. The three hierarchical relationships fundamental to Confucianism have been a foundation of Korean society for centuries: parent–child, ruler–subject (or corporate equivalent), and husband–wife—requiring of the inferior party filial piety (*xiào*; 孝), loyalty (*zhōng*; 忠), or submission (*nán zūn nǚ bēi*; 男尊女卑; literally, "males are respected, females are inferior"). Korea's strong emphasis on male superiority—like China's emphasis on filial piety and Japan's emphasis on loyalty, distinguishes its expression of the Confucian ethos. Korea scores 105th out of the 146 countries ranked by the World Economic Forum's Global Gender Gap index of gender equality. Japan is the only high-income country with a lower rank. Korea's rank is especially low—114th—for gender equality of economic participation and opportunity (World Economic Forum, 2023, pp. 225–226). There is not the same gender gap in education as there is in work. Millions of young Korean women diligently pursue higher education, only to encounter a nearly impenetrable "glass ceiling" once they begin their careers. The formidable barriers to women's careers found in Korea are rooted in its traditional Confucian culture, and they have been very slow to change (L. Miller, 2021). The Glass Ceiling Index published by the *Economist* magazine shows Korea to be persistently in last place among 29 OECD nations for gender equality in the workplace, with a large wage gap and few women in managerial positions or on company boards of directors (*Economist*, 2023). The frustrations and disappointments of young women related to occupational gender inequality undoubtedly contribute to the high suicide rate of Korean women in their 20s and 30s.

Women in Korea are paid significantly less than men for similar work; in 2021, median female wages were 69% of median male wages. Women account for only 8.7% of board members of Korea's publicly traded companies and only 15.7% of its managers, senior officials, and legislators. Korea's distribution of unpaid domestic and caregiving work is grossly unequal, with women's proportion of such unpaid work more than three times that of men's. The total number of hours of such unpaid work increased during the COVID-19 pandemic, when women took disproportionate responsibility for childcare and home schooling (World Economic Forum, 2023).

Informal socialization after work, including drinking parties, is an important way for Korean workers to build relationships useful in their advancement at work. Women are not invited to many such parties, and they may opt out of others if they have a child or are hoping to conceive one. This puts them at a disadvantage in getting favorable work assignments and in being promoted. If a woman chooses to have a child and takes maternity leave, she is likely to suffer a lifetime diminution of her prospects for promotion and her earnings from work. Not surprisingly, Korean women are increasingly choosing not to have children, and if they do have a child, they are unlikely to pursue a serious career (L. Miller, 2021). A binary choice of work opportunity versus family life sets the stage for depression if the outcome of the choice proves disappointing.

Korea's patriarchal, male-dominated Confucian ethos is also reflected in Korea's high prevalence of IPV, the usual form being psychological, sexual, or physical violence perpetrated on married women by their husbands or on women in other long-term relationships by their male partners. Concerning physical IPV specifically, a 2010 survey of Korean married couples found a 12.8% prevalence of mild physical IPV and a 2.8% prevalence of severe IPV by men against their wives, where "mild" IPV included throwing an object at the wife, pushing, shoving, grabbing, or slapping. Severe IPV was defined as beating, choking, hitting with an object, or using or threatening to use a knife or gun. Perpetration of IPV by men was more common in men with low income and with less than a high school education. Nonetheless, 10% of college-educated men had been physically violent with their wives.

When non-violent psychological IPV and non-violent sexual coercion were included in the definition, 25% of married Korean women surveyed in 2013 reported experiencing IPV in the past year. Yet, only 2.4% of those who had experienced IPV had sought assistance with the issue. Female victims of IPV who had a traditional view of gender roles were especially likely to have clinical depression. In that group the prevalence of MDD was 20.3%, and the prevalence of suicidal ideation was 9.2%. After controlling for demographics, area of residence, income, and general health status, the combination of IPV experience and a traditional view of gender relations was associated with a 4.6 times increase in the likelihood of depressive symptoms and a 7.3 times increase in the likelihood of suicidal ideation (G. R. Park et al., 2016). In a 2016 study of pregnant Korean women, 34% reported experiencing IPV at some time in their lives (S. Lee & E. Lee, 2017). The variation in rates of reported IPV between studies in Korea suggests that women's acknowledgment of IPV depends in part on the context of questioning and how questions are asked. Physically violent IPV by women against men was reported less frequently—8.7% of men reported mild violence, and 1.2% reported severe violence. However, married Korean women under age 30, who are less inclined than older Korean women to accept gender-based inferior status, had an 18.8% rate of mild violence against their husbands and a 1.7% rate of severe violence (J. Y. Kim et al., 2016).

A study of IPV in Korean college students suggests that physical violence might be more common in dating than in marriage: 15% of the subjects in a 2011 study reported committing at least one form of physical violence in the prior year and 12% reported experiencing it. Women who were victims were much more likely to become perpetrators of physical IPV: 23% of the sample reported witnessing father-to-mother violence during their childhood, and 56% reported experiencing some form of physical abuse in childhood. The students who were physically abused in childhood were more likely to perpetrate violence against a dating partner during their college years (Gover et al., 2011).

IPV by men against women is not normalized by all Koreans. Both men and women under age 40 who are college graduates and have moderate to high household incomes are less likely to blame victims and excuse perpetrators (Han et al., 2017). However, when a clinician encounters a depressed or suicidal Korean woman, the possibility of IPV as an underlying stressor should be considered. In one possible scenario, the woman would to some extent blame herself and/or excuse her husband or partner for the violence and might not mention the IPV in an initial diagnostic interview.

Korean children who grow up in families where there is repeated violence between the father and the mother can be traumatized by witnessing such violence; witnessing parental IPV is one of the adverse childhood experiences (ACEs) shown in studies in many cultural contexts to be associated with a lifetime increase in a person's risk of depression. The impact on the child is worse if the violence involves injury to the mother or is followed by the mother developing depression or another mental disorder such as *hwa-byung*.

Harsh discipline of children by their parents is another risk factor for depression in Koreans that might be partially ascribed to adverse effects of Korean Confucianism. In a study of childhood maltreatment and its consequences for young adults, Y. Lee and Kim (2011) found that 42.2% of subjects had experienced being hit or punched, kicked, beaten with an object, shaken, cut, and/or stabbed; 36.3% recalled emotional abuse, such as being told that their parent wished they were dead or threatened to hurt or kill them. More than half of the sample perceived the abuse they had suffered as discipline—sometimes reasonable and justified, sometimes not. Victims of abuse of either kind had mean BDI scores in the clinical range, even if they thought of the abuse as reasonable and justified discipline. Those who thought their emotional abuse was worse than that experienced by their peers had especially high BDI scores.

A 2012 survey of families in Seoul with above-average income and education found that 7.2% of children had been very severely abused (beaten up, choked, or deliberately burned or scalded) and that 8.4% had been injured by their parents in the past year (Emery et al., 2015). The impact of childhood physical abuse is long-lasting. In a sample of Korean women age 60 and over studied in 2010, 55% of whom had depressive symptoms on the Center for Epidemiologic Studies Depression Scale (CES-D) in the clinical range, depression scores were significantly higher in the 37% of the sample who had experienced violence in their childhood (Nam & Lincoln, 2017). Many women in the same age cohort became immigrants to the United States, and it would thus be expected that childhood abuse would be found in the personal histories of many depressed older Korean American women.

The normalization of harsh discipline of children in Korea extends to the acceptability of corporal punishment of schoolchildren. A study of Korean middle school students showed that 30.7% of students had been the victim of physical and/or emotional maltreatment by a teacher in the previous year; 24.3% had been slapped in the face or head, spanked with a cane, or struck with a blunt object like a broom. Male gender, low socioeconomic status, and poor academic performance were risk factors for maltreatment (Lee, 2015). While Korean physicians are required to report child abuse to legal authorities, this happens in less than 2% of cases. The first law against child abuse in Korea was passed only in 1998, and through the present time violence against children in Korea usually is viewed as legitimate discipline rather than as abuse. In traditional Korean culture, parents have an almost unlimited right to physically discipline their children. As in China, when people witness a parent beating a child, they are reluctant to interfere.

Korean Drinking Culture and Its Relationship to Depression and Suicide

Korea's per capita alcohol consumption is the highest in Asia and the fourth highest in the world; only Russia, Latvia, and Romania have higher rates. In a random sample of adults aged 20–64 interviewed in the country's 2014 National Health and Nutrition Examination Survey, over 95% had consumed alcohol in the month before they were interviewed (Choe et al., 2018); 22.9% of the men and 6.8% of the women met the criterion for "harmful drinking" defined as consumption of seven or more drinks by a man or five or more drinks by a woman at least twice a week. The rates of harmful drinking were highest in people working in sales or service occupations, where 30% of men and 10.6% of women engaged in harmful drinking. Married men were 14% less likely than unmarried men to engage in harmful drinking; married women were 63% more likely than single women to have a drinking problem. The peak age period for harmful drinking in Korean women is 25–34; for men it is 30–44. Occasional heavy drinking is even more prevalent in Korea: In a 2016 survey of people aged 15 and above, 47.8% of males and 13.6% of females had consumed 60 grams of alcohol (approximately four standard drinks) on at least one single occasion in the past 30 days.

In Korea, drinking usually takes place in social contexts, most often at dinners with friends or colleagues or with friends or family at home. Of those who drink at dinners with friends, 75% binge-drink in that context; and of those who drink at business dinners, 70% binge-drink. Koreans who regularly drink at dinners with friends or colleagues average five standard drinks per occasion (Ko & Sohn, 2018). Thus, drinking to intoxication on a regular basis is normalized. A Korean man or woman who consistently binge-drank twice a week but had no associated illness, violent or high-risk behavior, injury, or obvious work impairment would not be identified as having an alcohol use disorder (AUD). In 2019 the prevalence of diagnosed AUD in men peaked at 6.4% for men in their 20s, and the prevalence for women peaked at 2.5% for women in their 20s—far lower than the rates of harmful drinking revealed by a population survey (IHME, 2023).

In Korea, AUD appears to be grossly underdiagnosed because there is solid evidence that the "harmful drinking" of its people in fact causes harm: 8.9% of all deaths in the country are attributable to cirrhosis of the liver, pancreatitis, or another disease caused or exacerbated by heavy alcohol consumption; and 38.5% of road traffic fatalities are alcohol-related. Korea's fraction of total deaths attributable to alcohol exceeds that of China, Japan, and the United States (IHME, 2023; World Health Organization, 2018). Excessive drinking is associated with increased rates of depressive symptoms, increased instability of bipolar spectrum disorders, and increased suicide risk. Koreans with harmful drinking patterns and episodes of depression usually are not diagnosed with either AUD or a mood disorder. If they present after years of drinking with alcoholic liver disease, heart disease, or pancreatitis or with a cancer associated with alcohol, they might be depressed at the time of their diagnosis; but their depression is likely to be attributed to their general medical condition.

The elevated rates of harmful drinking in younger women, married women, and women working in sales and service positions are consistent with the idea that alcohol may be used to cope—albeit maladaptively—with mistreatment at home and at work. In sales and service positions women are exposed to harassment both from customers and from bosses and co-workers. Sexual harassment at work and/or IPV at home can provoke suicidal ideas; both depression and intoxication with alcohol greatly increase the risk they will be acted upon.

Alcohol use contributes to depression by direct biochemical mechanisms, and by causing general medical illness, contributing to traumatic injuries, and impairing judgment, leading to decisions and actions with destructive consequences. In people with bipolar spectrum disorders, it decreases the time spent in a normal mood. It disinhibits behavior such as IPV that can damage relationships that are important for psychological well-being. Victims of IPV are more likely to subsequently develop AUD (Ahmadabadi et al., 2019; La Flair et al. 2012; Okuda et al., 2011). The relationship of harmful drinking to MDD is similarly bidirectional: Harmful drinkers are more likely to develop MDD, and people with MDD are more likely to develop harmful drinking patterns (Boden & Fergusson, 2011; McHugh & Weiss, 2019). When a person is suicidal, with or without clinical depression, alcohol intoxication can remove inhibitions to self-injurious action. Either alcohol intoxication or alcohol withdrawal can raise physiological arousal and motivation to act on suicidal ideas. Alcohol intoxication impairs executive cognitive function, reducing the ability to solve problems, to inhibit acting on impulse, and to maintain a long-term perspective. 40% of all Koreans who die by suicide are intoxicated at the time of their deaths (Singh, 2017). In an American study, binge drinking in the past month was associated with significantly increased odds of suicidal thoughts in men and in women, and with suicide attempts in women, in the absence of a major depressive episode in the preceding year (Glasheen et al., 2015). Globally, nations' per capita alcohol consumption is statistically correlated with their age-standardized suicide rates (A. M. Kim, 2021).

Problematic drinking in Koreans has a complex relationship with social capital because drinking in group situations can reinforce social networks. In a

2020 national interview-based study of drinking and social capital, involvement of Koreans in formal or informal non-religious organizations was associated with an increased likelihood of heavy drinking as identified by the Alcohol Use Disorders Identification Test. Their involvement solely in religious organizations, however, was associated with an increased likelihood of abstinence. A higher level of trust in other people was associated with a lower rate of heavy drinking (E. Kim et al., 2020). In Korea, episodic heavy drinking with other people can increase relational social capital but not necessarily cognitive social capital. The results comport with those of a U.S. study that found a positive association of binge drinking with denser social networks but less neighborhood cohesion (Tucker et al., 2021).

Cosmetic Surgery and the Culture of "Face"

Importance of "face" is another aspect of Korea's collectivistic culture. In Korea a person's face (*chemyon*; 체면), comprises prestige and status but also honor, dignity, and "having a good name." Thus, it combines the two forms of "face" encountered in Chinese culture—*miànzi* and *liǎn*. The Korean characters for "losing face" are those for "death" and "body," and a major loss of face can be painful and traumatic and can lead to depression and/or suicide. The accomplishments and status of children are a crucial part of their parents' face. It is assumed that children's academic performance is largely a reflection of the parents' merit rather than of the children's innate aptitudes, preferences, and predispositions.

Having a good face elevates the status of one's family, so pursuing face is an expression of family loyalty and filial piety. Conversely, loss of face hurts one's family as well as oneself, thus intensifying feelings of shame and/or guilt.

In Korea, concern about face takes an unusual form known worldwide—an extraordinarily high incidence of elective facial cosmetic procedures, ranging from injections of fillers to comprehensive reshaping of facial bones. Korea has more plastic surgeons per capita than any other country and does more aesthetic surgeries per year per capita (Heidekrueger et al., 2017; International Society of Aesthetic Plastic Surgery, 2020). In a recent survey of young adult Koreans, 65% of respondents in their 20s were willing to have surgical and nonsurgical cosmetic procedures "in relation to employment and marriage" (Seo et al., 2019); and in a survey of adults aged 20–39, 47% were willing to undergo surgery to modify their appearance (Seo & Kim, 2020). Many upper-middle-class and upper-class Koreans have cosmetic procedures performed when they are in their teens (e.g., provided by their parents as a high school graduation present). Some people become preoccupied with their appearance and have repetitive cosmetic procedures, which "cause economic, physical and psychological distress to the individual concerned, and can lead to serious maladies within families and society, such as divorce and suicide" (Seo et al., 2019).

The usual aim of facial cosmetic surgery in Korea is to give a woman a face that conforms to currently prevailing standards of feminine beauty, such standards apparently representing a hybrid of Asian ideals and globalized Western ones. One common procedure aims to give the patient double eyelids and larger-appearing eyes, and another makes the nose narrower, smaller, and higher on the face. These procedures might be aimed at giving a woman a more Caucasian appearance, but they are seen by some Korean surgeons as normalizing facial features that would be burdensome if not corrected—"Asian burden lids" (Paik et al., 2020). For example, there is a procedure that narrows the jaw and makes the cheekbones less prominent, producing an oval, pixie-like face rather than a wide, square, or diamond-shaped face—facial features exhibited by the stars of K-Pop music. Surgery aimed at making the lower face round rather than square was characterized by a Chinese plastic surgeon as reflecting Asian ideals: "In contrast to Western women, East Asian women generally prefer facial features without prominent angles, because many believe it gives them a fierce and masculine appearance. ... Thus, many Asians pursue a harmonious facial contour" (Li et al., 2013, p. 1761.e1). The term 'harmonious' occurs 14 times in a relatively brief article, in the text and in the captions of patient photographs.

Surgery to narrow the lower face requires reshaping the mandible and entails a long and painful period of recovery. Korean American women sometimes fly to Seoul to get cosmetic procedures from plastic surgeons more familiar with Korean standards of beauty, whose services are priced lower than those of American surgeons with similar skill.

Shaming of overweight people or those with "ugly" faces frequently occurs on Korean television shows. Body shaming and "lookism" are normalized in the country's mass media (Tai, 2018). While some outspoken women in Korea and in the Korean American community have begun to push back, theirs remains a minority position. One source of intrafamilial conflict involves a young woman resisting the pressure of her parents to undergo cosmetic surgery to "improve" her face.

While cosmetic procedures are not covered by Korea's national health insurance and are thus a significant expense for most women and their families, cosmetic procedures may not be experienced as entirely elective by the women who undergo them. A person's physical appearance is given great weight in hiring decisions, even for jobs that do not involve interactions with the public in which it could have some functional or commercial relevance. A person might win an entry-level job in a Korean conglomerate, a financial services firm, a law office, or a biotech laboratory over a better-qualified applicant with a less appealing face or an appearance that is in some way non-conforming. Physical appearance is equally important in the marriage market. A woman seeking to marry a man with secure, high-status employment and a favorable family background will have relatively poor prospects if she does not have a conventionally attractive face.

Facial cosmetic surgery is more popular among Korean men than among men of any other country. More than 15% of the country's men have had a cosmetic procedure, and more than 40% may be considering it. A man's getting facial cosmetic surgery is not seen as effeminate. One ideal of masculine attractiveness in Korea is a slim, muscular body, with a soft, round face and no facial or body hair. Many of the singers in Korea's K-Pop "boy bands" have this appearance (Tai, 2018).

Young Korean women also have expectations of slimness. The Korean press suggests that an optimally attractive young woman would have a body mass index (BMI) <19 kg/m^2—underweight by American standards. In the 2007 Korean National Health and Nutrition Examination Survey, 15.4% of Korean women aged 25–39 had a BMI <18.5 kg/m^2, with unmarried women 1.56 times more likely than married women to be underweight, controlling for age, income, occupation, and education (S. I. Park et al., 2013). Of underweight Korean women aged 20–29, 48% perceived themselves to be normal weight, and another 2% perceived themselves to be overweight. Among underweight Korean women aged 30–39, 43% perceived themselves to be normal weight and 4% perceived themselves to be overweight (B. Park et al., 2019). Yet, just as binge drinkers in Korea usually are not diagnosed with AUD, young Korean women who are underweight and significantly overestimate their weight usually are not diagnosed with eating disorders. The combined prevalence of diagnosed anorexia nervosa and bulimia in 2019 in Korean women aged 20–29 was 1.24%—far below the 6.7% proportion of underweight women in that age cohort who overestimate their weight (IHME, 2023). For young Korean women, being underweight is normalized. Undernutrition, with or without a diagnosable eating disorder, is associated with increased risk of depression.

Altering one's face to fit a socially determined, standard definition of beauty fits with the Confucian/collectivist celebration of conformity and the association of high social status with greater "perfection" of the self. The latter comprises both elite higher education and alteration of external appearance through clothing, makeup, and cosmetic procedures. Approaching "perfection" simultaneously demonstrates one's personal status and one's acceptance of society's rules. It also enhances the family's status, much as an unconventional appearance might entail a loss of face for the family.

A person who alters their face in pursuit of conventional "beauty" can be seen in one of two ways—as expressing self-determination and empowerment or as internalizing a destructive non-acceptance of their authentic self. A woman or man who has cosmetic surgery and is satisfied with the outcome might experience greater self-confidence, and if the surgery enhances their attractiveness (or reduces their non-conformity/unattractiveness), they might enjoy benefits in seeking a job or a promotion, a date, or a mate. The risk of depression diminishes because objective circumstances improve.

If cosmetic surgery is unsuccessful, it might lead to depression and not merely disappointment. There are several potential pathways. If the surgery is complicated by pain, infection, loss of sensation, or another medical problem, depression can result as a reaction to physical distress. If the surgery does not produce the expected change in appearance, depression can result from a sense of loss of opportunity, time, and money; from conflict with the surgeon; and/or from conflict with parents or others who encouraged the person to have the surgery. If the surgery is too obvious, the person may be ridiculed or bullied, causing a combination of self-reproach and emotional pain related to social exclusion or being the target of aggression. This is a reason why the surgeons most in demand are those who deliver the most "natural"-looking results and why young women often get cosmetic surgery during the summer between high school and college, arriving at college showing their new look to people unfamiliar with their former appearance.

Months or years after the procedure, a person who has cosmetic surgery might come to realize that they did not have the occupational, social, or romantic success that was their hope for the ultimate outcome. Regret over the decision to have surgery, along with any memory of perioperative pain and suffering, can combine with other stresses and risk factors to bring on a depressive episode.

A Young Woman Who Did Not Want Cosmetic Surgery

Su-jin Park, a 25-year-old single Korean woman, was recently accepted by a leading American law school. She had graduated in the top 5% of her college class and had near-perfect scores on the Law School Admission Test and the Test of English as a Foreign Language. Her law school application essay expressed her motivation for pursuing legal education in the United States: She was angry about Korea's pervasive gender inequality. She wanted to be a change agent, representing women who had suffered such injustices as discrimination and harassment at work and violence at home. Her plan was to get a law degree and work experience in America and then return to Korea to practice law.

Su-jin is the only child of a history professor and a middle school English teacher. As she grew up, she became fluent in English and Japanese as well as Korean. An independent and strong-willed young woman, she was an excellent debater who won awards for public speaking. Physically, she is a short, small woman with a wide face, a wide nose with a low bridge, and single eyelids. While she is pleasant-looking, her appearance is unfashionable; and many young women with similar looks would have cosmetic surgery if they could afford it. In high school she was bullied for her looks. Her mother had suggested several times that she have cosmetic surgery to give her a more "Western" nose and eyelids. It would make her more attractive to potential employers and improve her prospects for marriage. Su-jin rejected her mother's advice. She felt her academic achievement, self-confidence, and intelligence were more important than the stylishness of her looks and would rather have her own face than conform to a stereotype.

In her senior year in college Su-jin applied for jobs at companies and nonprofit organizations at which her trilingual fluency would be valued. She had many interviews but was not offered jobs by companies that hired classmates whom she knew were less qualified—but better-looking. She got discouraged, but she would never consider cosmetic surgery. She eventually got an entry-level job with a financial services firm. Her male supervisor assigned her a heavy workload but gave her little respect or encouragement, disparaged her appearance in front of others, and gave her no help in moving ahead in the company.

As time went on Su-jin got more and more angry about her situation—feeling she was in a dead-end job because she was a woman judged on her looks and not her ability. She daydreamed about revenge against her boss. She began to have trouble falling asleep and had frequent nightmares and nocturnal palpitations. She lost her appetite. Already thin, she lost another 15 pounds and looked malnourished. Her periods became irregular, with painful menses every 2 or 3 months. She thought about suicide, but she would never abandon her parents.

She consulted a Korean medicine doctor (specialist in traditional Korean medicine), who found minor physical problems but thought Su-jin's symptoms were mostly due to depression. He referred her to a psychiatrist, who expressed the opinion that Su-jin was severely depressed and suggested hospitalization. Su-jin rejected the idea immediately; she knew that a history of psychiatric hospitalization would destroy her career prospects. In addition, it is well known that in Korea, a country with the most psychiatric beds per capita of all high-income countries, there are financial incentives for private psychiatric hospitals to keep patients for prolonged stays even when they are medically unnecessary and to subject patients to involuntary treatment although they are of no danger to themselves or others (A. M. Kim, 2017).

Su-jin felt she could handle her problem herself with medication and a break from work. She quit her job and started taking an antidepressant. She didn't want paid sick leave from her employer; if she disclosed her depression, it would be on her record forever, potentially interfering with employment in the future. Within 8 weeks she felt she was well—and had resolved to prepare to pursue legal education abroad and subsequently devote herself to working for change in her country.

Sexual Harassment in the Workplace and Bullying at School

The lower status of women in Korean society is also reflected in the high prevalence of sexual harassment of women in work contexts. The entertainment industry is particularly rife with sexual exploitation of young female actors and popular singers, often enforced by abusive behavior by their agents and managers. Several high-profile performers have died by suicide, leaving notes linking their suicides to their experiences of traumatic sexual abuse by managers, agents, and male stars. In March 2009, Jang Ja-Yeon, a popular television actress who had just starred in a feature film, hanged herself. She left a suicide note detailing repeated beatings and verbal abuse by her agent, whom she accused of forcing her to have sex with 31 different men prominent in business and entertainment. After her death, some of her accusations were verified, and some of the men involved faced legal consequences.

Six months earlier, in October 2008, Choi Jin-sil, an award-winning 39-year-old actress who was nicknamed "The Nation's Actress," died by suicide. She had been married to a professional athlete who abused her physically. In August 2004, Choi came out publicly and to the police as a victim of domestic violence, appearing to the press with a bruised and swollen face. Shortly afterward, she was sued by a construction company for whom she had appeared as a model in advertisements for their apartments. The company claimed that her coming out publicly as victim of domestic abuse damaged the value of their properties and sought three billion won in damages (about $2.5 million at the time), an amount greater than half of Choi's net worth. Choi initially won the suit, but ultimately, *after her death*, the Korean Supreme Court reversed the lower court's decision, finding that Choi had not maintained her "social and moral honor." The construction company pursued the star's estate for money, at the expense of her surviving children, aged 6 and 9 at the time. The case dramatically exemplifies the Korean preoccupation with face in the literal sense, as well as its tolerance of domestic abuse of women.

Just as women are poorly protected in the workplace from sexual harassment, children in Korea are highly vulnerable to bullying at school. Korea is a conformist society, and children who are different in any way are at high risk for bullying. Having a physical deformity or disability, being physically unattractive, and being an immigrant or having immigrant parents all can be reasons for victimization. In Korean middle schools, 40% of students were found to be involved in bullying, either as a perpetrator, a victim, or both (Y. S. Kim et al., 2004). Even as early as the fourth grade, over 20% of students were victims and/or perpetrators of bullying (Yang et al., 2006). As in other countries, involvement of any kind in bullying—either as a victim or as a perpetrator—is associated with an increased risk of depression and other mental health problems. Cyberbullying is equally common. In a 2019 survey of Korean students, rates of reported cyberbullying victimization were 18.8% for those in elementary school, 22.9% for those in middle school, and 15.4% for those in high school (Jun, 2020).

In a 2016 nationally representative epidemiologic survey of over 5000 Korean adults, 8.8% reported being bullied at least once while growing up; the rate was 17.2% of subjects aged 18–29. A history of being a victim of bullying by peers during their first 18 years was associated with a 12.5% prevalence of current MDD. In a multivariate model that included age, gender, years of education, area of residence, marital status, and employment status, being bullied occasionally in childhood was associated with 3.39x odds of MDD, and frequent victimization was associated with 6.43x odds. Frequent victimization was associated with a significantly higher probability of suicidal plans and attempts in adulthood, even after controlling for the presence of psychiatric disorders including mood disorders, anxiety disorders, and alcohol use disorder (Woo et al., 2019).

Suicide in Korea

A culturally informed perspective on suicide by Koreans must attempt to account for the exceptionally high rates of suicide by Koreans and Korean Americans, why suicide rates in Korea are disproportionately high for young adult women and for older people of both genders, and why rates of suicide in Korea surged between 1990 and 2010.

A common reason for suicide in Korea is financial distress, as might occur with unemployment or with old age, no pension, and insufficient savings. Evidence comes both from psychological autopsies and from epidemiology: In 1998 all of Asia was affected by an economic crisis. In Korea in 1997 the suicide rate for men aged 50–69 was 38.0; it rose to 44.5 in 1998, and by 2001 it was 55.9. The increase in rate was smaller in Taiwan and Singapore, where the crisis had a smaller effect on gross domestic product and the unemployment rate (Chang et al., 2009). The rate of suicide for men aged 50–69 in mainland China decreased over the same period (IHME, 2023).

In an online survey of adults under age 60 in Korea, Japan, and the United States with no history of mental disorders or suicide attempts, Koreans had the highest level of lifetime suicidal ideation. In the United States and in Korea, both nations with high income inequality, income had an inverse relationship to intensity of suicidal ideation. In Korea, higher education was associated with an individualistic attribution of poverty (e.g., seeing poor people as dishonest, less intelligent, and/or having inferior values) and with permissive attitudes toward suicide (H. Lee et al., 2021). Among older, poorer, and less educated Koreans, high suicide rates might be driven by misery, while among more educated Koreans in midlife, misfortune might be accompanied by self-blame and an expectation of negative judgment by one's peers. In both cases, suicide as an escape from distress or disgrace could be normalized by the prevailing culture. Most people who die by suicide in Korea would not meet criteria for major depression at the time of their deaths, though they likely would be clinically depressed as defined in this book.

Overall, the suicide mortality rate in Korean women is 40% of the rate in men; this percentage is higher than that for the United States and for Western Europe. Table 12.3 shows 2019 suicide mortality rates by age range for Korea, the United States, and Western Europe for men and for women.

The suicide rate for women over age 70 in Korea is more than 5 times as high as the rate in Western Europe and almost 10 times as high as the rate in the United States. For men over age 70, Korea's suicide rate is over 3 times the rates for the United States and for Western Europe, the latter not differing significantly. For men and women between ages 25 and 69, Korea's suicide rate is

Table 12.3 2019 Suicide Mortality by Age Band: Korea, United States, and Western Europe
(Rates per 100,000 People)

Age range	Female			Male		
	Korea	USA	Western Europe	Korea	USA	Western Europe
15–19	5.8	4.7	2.2	7.5	14.1	5.8
20–24	10.3	4.9	3.4	15.0	23.3	12.5
25–49	15.5	8.3	5.4	33.7	24.3	18.8
50–69	15.4	9.5	8.0	51.0	30.2	22.1
≥70	47.5	4.9	9.1	111.4	35.7	33.8

Note: Data from IHME (2023)

also the highest, though not as dramatically so. For late adolescents and young adults, the pattern is different, with higher suicide rates in Korea for females and higher rates in the United States for males.

The data suggest that women in Korea are more often in despair than those in the United States or Western Europe and that, when they are, they have when younger and retain when older the capacity to act on their suicidal ideation. Viewing the statistics in the context of the interpersonal-neuropsychiatric model of suicide introduced in Part I, the following issues of Korean women can be noted: (1) In Korea women are more likely to have negative consequences for employment or marriage from a non-conventional appearance than they might in many other countries (thwarted belongingness), (2) A woman who is unsuccessful or who has been stigmatized because of a psychiatric diagnosis is likely to feel guilty and/or ashamed that she has caused a painful loss of face for her parents (perceived burdensomeness), (3) High national suicide rates for women and well-publicized suicides of female celebrities tend to normalize suicide (acquired capacity for suicide), (4) There is a high prevalence of episodic drinking to intoxication by women (decreased behavioral inhibition), and (5) intense anger (*han*) is a cultural norm for women who can no longer tolerate oppressive circumstances (increased behavioral activation).

The extraordinarily high suicide mortality rates for older Koreans reflect a combination of economic and cultural factors. As noted above, over 40% of all older Koreans and more than half of those over age 75 live in poverty. According to the Confucian principle of filial piety that underlies Korean culture, responsibility to support an older person living in poverty would be taken by the son. If there is no adult child able and willing to support the older person, there would be no escape from poverty. If an adult child's supporting their older parent would decrease support for the education of a grandchild, the older person might feel like an unacceptable burden. Korea's rapidly falling fertility rate and the intense competition of younger adults for stable and well-paid employment contribute to the frequency of such circumstances.

A large longitudinal study of Koreans over age 45 showed that retirement, either voluntary or involuntary, by a man or a woman increased the risk of clinical depression. Involuntary retirement, as when a late middle-aged employee is laid off by a company during an economic slowdown, has a worse effect on mood than voluntary, planned retirement. The retirement of an older man, even if voluntary and planned, increases, his wife's risk of depression (H. Park & Kang, 2016). Many Korean women appear to be happier when their husbands are at work much of the time and bring home paychecks, rather than their being at home during the day. Because of the marked gender inequality of Korea and the male domination of households, the voluntary retirement of a husband often entails a loss of personal freedom for the wife. Furthermore, because men tend to be older than their wives and have shorter active life expectancies, a wife might face the burden of being her husband's caregiver.

Korea's extraordinarily high suicide rates among people over age 70 virtually ensure that every older adult will know of someone in their social network who died by suicide. If so, suicide cannot be "unthinkable" and remote from their realm of possibility. In a study of adults aged 20–59 in Korea, Japan, and the United States, permissive attitudes toward suicide were strongly predictive of suicidal ideation. Such attitudes were captured by subjects' endorsement of statements like "There are situations where suicide is the only reasonable solution" and "Suicide is a reasonable means of ending an incurable disease." Lifetime suicidal ideation was more prevalent in the Korean subjects than the Japanese and American ones. Among Koreans, a permissive attitude toward suicide was associated with lower income (H. Lee et al., 2021).

Approximately 60% of Koreans have no religious affiliation. Approximately 20% are Christians, 16% are Buddhists, and the remainder identify with other faiths (Statista Research, 2024). Regardless of religious affiliation, all are influenced by the nation's Confucianism-based culture. In its local context, religion does not appear to inhibit suicide as effectively as it might in other places. Confucianism does not forbid suicide. Buddhism teaches non-attachment to the world and, though it does not encourage suicide, it does not condemn it. The rightness or wrongness of suicide depends on the state of mind of the person who chooses to die. Christianity sees suicide as sinful—rejecting the gift of life and Christ's salvation—but preaches compassion and understanding for those so miserable as to consider it. A Christian's suicide might be forgiven if it were judged to be involuntary and due to a mental illness (Alonzo & Gearing, 2021).

While celebrity suicides and copycat suicides occur everywhere, Korea's ethnic homogeneity and relative lack of diversity imply broader personal relatability of prominent people's suicides—implying, as noted above, greater impact on people's acquired capacity for suicide. Korea has a large and economically important entertainment industry; popular music and films are important exports. Its stars are universally known, and news about them fills both conventional and social media. When a popular celebrity dies by suicide, there often is a measurable increase in the national suicide rate for several weeks afterward, explained mainly by a dramatic increase in the suicide rate for people of the same gender and age as the celebrity, who often use the same method of suicide. In the four weeks following the suicidal death by hanging of a 24-year-old movie star, over 200 women aged 20–30 died by suicide using the same method. Based on analysis of death certificates from the period before and after the celebrity suicide, an excess mortality of 331 people was attributed to copycat suicides (Ji, Lee, et al. 2014). In the month following the death of Choi Jin-sil, the national suicide rate rose by 70%, with excess suicides both in young women and in adults over age 65.

As in the United States, many Korean celebrity suicides occur in a context of depression, BD, and/or histories of trauma, ACEs, and IPV. Sexual harassment and exploitation frequently have been issues in the suicides of younger female celebrities.

Rating and Screening for Depression in Koreans: Culture and Psychometrics

Korean translations of the PHQ-9, CES-D, and BDI have been tested in Koreans and in Korean Americans, and all are used in both clinical and research contexts. While the scales have acceptable psychometric properties, optimal cutoff scores are not the same as for the populations on which they were developed. The optimal cutoff score for the Korean PHQ-9 will depend on the clinical or research context, but it will often be lower than the score of 10 or higher typically used with English-speaking populations to predict a diagnosis of MDD, especially for men.

In Korea's traditional Confucian culture, overt expression of strong emotions—positive or negative—and complaints about emotional issues would be discouraged, especially among men. For this reason, Koreans with significant clinical depression might not score 10 or higher on the Korean language PHQ-9, and Koreans with active suicidal ideation might not meet the criteria for a DSM/ICD depressive disorder.

For example, in a study of a community-representative sample of 1116 Korean American immigrants over age 60 in the the Washington–Baltimore area, 14.7% reported suicidal ideation in the past two weeks. Of those, 64% did not have a major or minor depressive syndrome based on applying the DSM diagnostic algorithm to their answers to the PHQ's nine questions. There were fewer people in the sample with MDD (4.6%) or a minor depressive disorder (8.5%) than there were people with suicidal ideation. Asking a single question—whether a person would rate their mental/emotional health as excellent, good, fair, or poor—was a remarkably effective way to identify people with recent thoughts of suicide (Na et al., 2017). Of those who gave their emotional health a fair or poor rating, 24% had had recent suicidal thoughts, and screening in this way would have picked up 74% of all those who had such thoughts. While 54% of those with any depression diagnosis had suicidal thoughts, focusing only on those with DSM/ICD depression diagnoses would have missed most of those with suicidal ideation and self-acknowledged mental health problems that might have been a focus for treatment.

As the case of *hwa-byung* suggests, Koreans have a cultural propensity to express depression with somatic symptoms. Factor analysis of PHQ-9 data from the general Korean population produced a two-factor model that comprised a somatic/affective factor and a cognitive factor consisting of guilt, suicidal ideation, poor concentration, and psychomotor slowing or agitation (Shin et al., 2020). A common presentation of depression in Koreans might be a somatic chief complaint like sleep disturbance, fatigue, or altered appetite and a low mood and/or anhedonia acknowledged if asked about, with the variable presence of negative thoughts like guilt and death wishes. Such thoughts might be absent (or present but denied) even in people with severe anhedonia and depression-related somatic complaints. In the Korean population study 15.8% of the men and 26.3% of the women studied had scores of 5 or higher, and 4.1% of men and 8.1% of women had scores of 10 or higher. Given Korea's high male suicide rate, it is likely that, at least for men, a clinical cutoff score of 10 is too high for identifying cases of depression deserving clinical intervention.

However, when the PHQ-9 was given to students at Woosong University, a private university in Daejeon with an emphasis on international studies and instruction in English, analysis yielded a single factor (Y. E. Kim & Lee, 2019). This suggests that among educated people in a globalized cultural context, the cognitive, affective, and somatic symptoms of depression are experienced, recognized, and acknowledged similarly.

While Korean students appear willing to disclose affective and cognitive symptoms of depression, many will experience the illness as a body–mind condition with manifold somatic symptoms. This was shown in a study in which undergraduate and graduate students were given structured clinical interviews for depression or long-form depression symptom inventories and completed the PHQ-15, a questionnaire that lists 15 common somatic symptoms and asks if one was bothered a little, a lot, or not at all by each symptom in the preceding four weeks. PHQ-15 scores correlated strongly with scores on the BDI and were highly predictive of a diagnosis of MDD. With a cutoff score of 8, The PHQ-15 predicted MDD as well as the PHQ-9 or the CES-D typically do in college student populations. Inquiry about just five somatic symptoms—stomach pain; constipation, loose bowels, or diarrhea; nausea, gas, or indigestion; feeling tired or having low energy; and trouble sleeping—gave equally strong results with an optimal cutoff score of 3 (Lyoo et al., 2014). The latter score would be attained by students who were bothered a lot by one of the five somatic symptoms and a little by another or were bothered a little by three of the five symptoms.

Korea has compulsory military service for young men. A history of mental illness would disqualify a man from service, so no soldier would enter the military with a history of depression. However, many young men develop depression under the stress of the military environment. In a sample of 1003 soldiers evaluated with the Korean version of the Mini International Neuropsychiatric Interview, the prevalence of major depression was 4.6%, and the prevalence of lifetime suicidal ideation was 9.4%. The soldiers were given the CES-D, and analysis of their responses revealed that an efficient depression screen could be created from just three items: "I had trouble keeping my mind on what I was doing" (cognitive), "I felt sad" (affective), and "I felt that everything I did was an effort" (somatic). For prediction of major depression, the area under the receiver operating characteristic curve for the three-item test was .89, and with a cutoff score of 3—attained or exceeded by 9.5% of the sample—its sensitivity was 71.7%, its specificity was 90.4%, and its positive and negative predictive values were 28.9% and 98.3%, respectively. Soldiers with such scores had a 29.5% rate of lifetime suicidality and a 1.8% rate of suicidal thoughts in the past month (Byeon et al., 2021). A soldier could get a score of 3 on the test simply by having one of the three symptoms 5–7 days in the prior week or by having each of the three for one or two days in the prior week. The data suggest that young Korean men who are depressed tend to understate their symptoms of depression but that they are willing to report them on a questionnaire if the questions are presented in language unlikely to be stigmatizing.

Studies of Korean Americans show evidence of a "lost in translation" phenomenon on tests like the CES-D or the BDI that mix positively and negatively worded questions and that include several items about positive affect that respondents must rate on a 4-point ordinal scale. Less educated people might find the changing direction of the items to be confusing. Those with a traditional orientation, regardless of their educational level, might be unwilling to strongly endorse items about happiness and hopefulness as doing so would run counter to beliefs that expressing a very positive mood conveys a lack of appropriate restraint and that excessive optimism invites bad luck. Factor analytic studies of the CES-D and BDI in East Asian populations often find their positive affect items to be a factor uncorrelated with other indicators of depression.

Older Korean immigrants, especially those who are unacculturated, might be more effectively screened for major and minor depression using the Korean Geriatric Depression Scale (K-GDS) which has only yes–no questions, does not include somatic complaints, and puts the positive items in a way such that the non-depressed option would seem more "normal" even in a traditional Confucian cultural context. For example, answering yes to "Are you basically satisfied with your life?" or "Are you in good spirits most of the time?" does not require an assertion of positivity that a traditionalist would find inappropriate. When the K-GDS was validated in a sample of depressed people and control subjects aged 50 and over from metropolitan Seoul, it was more efficient and accurate in predicting an MDD diagnosis than the CES-D, in part because the control subjects on average answered 1.4 out of 30 yes–no questions in the depressed direction, while the average score on the CES-D was over 13. The optimal cutoff score on the K-GDS for predicting MDD was lower in subjects over age 80 (J. Y. Kim et al., 2008). They would have spent more of their lives in pre-modern Korea, and thus would be more likely to minimize overt expressions of negative affect. Somatic expressions of depression would not be captured by the K-GDS as items on somatic symptoms of depression are explicitly excluded from that questionnaire.

Korean Americans—Family Acculturative Stress

Korean Americans are the fifth largest Asian American ethnic group, with a population of 1.8 million in 2015. Korean Americans comprise two major groups with socioeconomic and cultural characteristics different in ways relevant to depression. One group comprises educated, younger, high-income people with high English proficiency, who either were born in America to Korean parents (second generation), were born in Korea but emigrated with their parents as children (generation 1.5) or got degrees from American universities as international students and subsequently remained in the United States. Members of this group often are bicultural. The other group comprises older, less educated, lower-income first-generation immigrants, many of whom have limited English proficiency and have not assimilated. Twenty percent of Korean Americans live in multigenerational households, typically ones including both first-generation immigrants and children of the second generation or generation 1.5.

Adolescent Korean Americans, like their peers in Korea, have a high prevalence of alcohol use and problematic drinking—among the highest of Asian American ethnic groups. In a study of Asian Americans aged 12-17, 22.7% of Korean Americans had consumed alcohol in the past year, 5.4% had engaged in binge-drinking in the past month, and 3.4% would meet criteria for an alcohol use disorder (Kane et al., 2017). These statistics are relevant to the assessment of Korean American adolescents with depression or suicidal ideation. Problem drinking can be a cause and/or a consequence of clinical depression, and the loss of impulse control associated with alcohol intoxication can precipitate a suicidal act. In view of the high prevalence of alcohol use among Korean American teenagers, a careful assessment of alcohol use should be a routine part of assessing depression in this demographic. If it is suspected but denied by the patient, the clinician should seek collateral information and/or consider testing a blood biomarker of recent drinking like phosphatidylethanol. The context of depression in first-generation and second-generation Korean Americans reflects the gap between Korea's traditional, paternalistic, authoritarian Confucian culture and America's more open, individualistic, and gender-equal culture. An adolescent or young adult born in the United States or who arrived as a young child will be acculturated to be less deferential to their parents and to adults of the older generation than a native Korean who immigrated as an adult. An immigrant woman—regardless of her age at immigration, is likely to acculturate to become less submissive to male authority. If a male immigrant in this situation is less acculturated than his wife or his daughter, he might feel disrespected and see her as misbehaving. He might respond with violence or with emotional distancing, either of which will be painful to the woman.

Rates of different forms of IPV by men against their wives or female partners are especially high among Korean Americans—more than 6% of the wives in a study of married Korean American couples in New York and Chicago reported experiencing severe violence. When a Korean American woman in a marriage or other intimate relationship presents clinically with symptoms of depression, IPV always should be considered by the clinician as a possible cause or aggravating factor. If a female victim of IPV lives in a Korean American neighborhood and sees a primary care physician who is an unacculturated Korean immigrant, her IPV might go unrecognized and unaddressed. In a 2009 study of 20 Korean immigrant physicians practicing in Southern California, 17 denied, minimized, or rationalized their female patients' IPV, some engaging in victim blaming. Two of the immigrant physicians who were deniers of IPV or of its medical importance were women (G. H. Chung et al., 2009).

Korean Americans have the highest age-standardized suicide rate per 100,000 of all Asian American groups and especially high suicide rates for older adults. Comparative rates from 2003 to 2012 (Kung et al., 2018) are shown in Table 12.4. Several points are noteworthy. Koreans and Korean Americans have suicide rates that increase steadily with age, for both men and women. This pattern is shared with Chinese Americans but not with Japanese Americans and non-Hispanic Whites. The rates for Korean Americans are half the rates for Koreans, until age 65, when the rates for Koreans rise disproportionately. Korean Americans aged 65 and above have suicide mortality rates significantly higher than those of non-Hispanic Whites. Non-Hispanic Whites differ from all groups of Asian Americans in having a marked midlife peak in suicide mortality rates, and the rate for women is approximately one quarter of the rate for men throughout the age spectrum. In Korean Americans, as in Koreans, female

Table 12.4 2003–2012 Suicide Mortality for Koreans, Americans of East Asian Origin, and American Non-Hispanic Whites (Rates per 100,000 People)

Age Range	Koreans	Korean Americans	Non-Hispanic Whites	Chinese Americans	Japanese Americans
Male					
0–19	4.2	2.2	5.2	0.9	3.6
20–34	34.0	17.2	28.3	6.7	14.1
35–49	39.9	20.3	42.0	7.2	16.9
50–64	53.1	28.4	39.5	9.7	19.9
65+	114.5	32.9	29.0	18.3	17.9
Female					
0–19	2.1	1.0	1.3	0.5	1.4
20–34	17.1	8.0	6.9	3.7	5.5
35–49	20.1	9.4	10.2	4.0	6.6
50–64	23.7	13.3	9.6	5.3	7.8
65+	57.6	15.4	7.1	10.0	7.0

Note. Data from Kung et al. (2018).

suicide mortality rates are approximately one half of male rates—and significantly higher than those for non-Hispanic White women after age 50.

The difference in suicide rates between Korean Americans and Japanese and Chinese Americans is paralleled by a similar difference in their rates of clinical depression. A 2015 meta-analysis of studies of depression symptom prevalence in Asian Americans estimated rates of clinical depression (a score of 16 or higher on the 20-item CES-D questionnaire or equivalent) to be 33.3% in Korean Americans, 15.7% in Chinese Americans, and 20.4% in Japanese Americans. The difference between Korean Americans and Chinese Americans was statistically significant, while the difference between Japanese Americans and Chinese Americans was not.

Older Korean Americans and Chinese Americans comprise a high proportion of first-generation immigrants who came to America at a time when Korea and China were low-income countries. Many have limited English proficiency and have not fully acculturated even though they have lived in the United States for decades. People in this category have had limited ability to accumulate wealth, and Social Security income for them would be insufficient to keep them out of poverty. (e.g., average household wealth for Korean Americans in Los Angeles in 2016 was $23,400. In contrast, Japanese Americans' average household wealth was $592,000 [Asante-Muhammad & Sim, 2020].) They might not be eligible for Medicare or Medicaid health insurance, and if they had no health insurance of any kind, a single episode of severe illness could impoverish them. In the absence of substantial support from their children, such people would experience a combination of poverty and its associated negative social determinants of health, poor social support, and inadequate medical care.

If older Korean Americans are poor and have no children willing and able to assist—for example, by having their parent(s) live with them—issues of disappointment and loss of face can add to the emotional pain of their situation. A common consequence is depression, which typically will be untreated. The hopelessness of the situation, combined with relative normalization of suicide in Korean culture, sets the stage for suicide.

The harsh disciplinary practices common in Korea are not compatible with American or European norms, and in some cases they are unlawful. Similarly, purely authoritarian parenting does not help children develop the flexibility, independent thinking, and self-assertion needed for success in an individualistic culture. Empirical study of Korean American immigrant parents suggests that as they acculturate, they forgo types of corporal punishment typical in Korea (e.g., hitting their children's hands or legs with sticks) and increase their overt verbal and physical expressions of parental warmth (E. Kim et al., 2010; E. Kim, & Hong, 2007). Even so, many second-generation Korean Americans will have experienced harsh discipline from their parents—another risk factor for depression and suicidal ideation.

Stigma of Depression and Cultural Barriers to Treatment

Mental illness is highly stigmatized in Korea, and, as in China, open disclosure of mental illness can bring a loss of face not only to affected individuals but also to their families. The Korean national health insurance system fully covers psychiatric treatment and psychiatric medications, with no co-payments required for people with low incomes. Despite this, relatively few Koreans with depression seek treatment, partly because many depressed Koreans do not recognize their condition as an illness and partly because, if they do, they often experience stigma. The stigma of depression can be external, family-based, or internal—often, it is all of these.

A contributor to stigma, and perhaps a consequence of stigma, is the overutilization of psychiatric hospitalization in Korea, which has more psychiatric beds per capita and longer psychiatric hospital lengths of stay than other high-income countries. Hospitalizations several months long are not unusual, and involuntary hospitalization has frequently been used inappropriately. When a person's admitting to suicidal thoughts can lead to a prolonged involuntary hospitalization, loss of a job, and lifetime personal and family stigma, it is understandable that they will be unwilling to acknowledge thoughts of suicide. In Korea as elsewhere in the world, older age, male gender, lower socioeconomic class, and less education are associated with greater stigmatization of depression (S. Park et al., 2015).

In 2014 the Korean government, representing a nation of 50 million people that had already had the highest suicide rate in the OECD for over 10 years, devoted only $6.6 million to suicide prevention and $242,000 to "removal of prejudice toward mental disorders and improving public awareness" (Roh et al., 2016, p. 5). The government's minimal response to a globally salient epidemic of suicide contrasts dramatically with the action taken by Norway when its prime minister suffered—and publicly disclosed—a major depressive episode and subsequently led a multi-year, multibillion-dollar mental health initiative, as will be detailed in Chapter 13.

The stigma of depression found in Korea persists through acculturation to affect Korean Americans. Surveys of Korean Americans show widespread beliefs that mental illnesses, including depression, are due to some combination of genetics, bad parenting, and personal weakness—all reasons that would bring shame to one's family as well as oneself. An analysis of data from the 2015 Asian American Quality of Life Survey compared stigmatizing beliefs about depression among the various ethnic groups including Chinese Americans, Asian Indians, Koreans, Vietnamese, and Filipinos. Most of the Korean Americans surveyed had lived in the United States for 10 years or more, and 80% had at least a college education: 43% of the Korean Americans believed that depression was a sign of personal weakness, a significantly higher percentage than among Chinese Americans; 21.6% believed it would disappoint their family; 8.5% believed it brought shame to the whole family; and 51% thought antidepressant drugs are addictive—the highest percentage among all the ethnic groups. Asian Americans who were less acculturated, were less proficient in English, had been in the United States for less than 10 years, and were over age 60 were significantly more likely to hold stigmatizing beliefs. Controlling for other factors, Korean ethnicity was associated with a significantly greater likelihood of believing that depression is a sign of personal weakness (Jung et al., 2020).

Beliefs that discourage antidepressant treatment are especially prevalent among older first-generation Korean American immigrants (i.e., those now aged 65 or above). Most people in that group arrived in the United States before 1980 and tend to be less educated—and less acculturated—than younger first-generation immigrants, even though the latter as a group have lived fewer years in the United States. In a 2010 survey of immigrants aged 60 or above in greater New York City, 30% indicated that they would be unwilling to take antidepressant medication if diagnosed with depression, and 31% said they would reject mental health counseling under such circumstances. 55% of the sample thought depression was a normal part of aging, 68% thought it was a sign of personal weakness, and 26% thought that having a mentally ill family member brings shame to the whole family. Depressive symptoms—though not diagnosed clinical depression—were highly prevalent in the sample, with a mean score on the 10-item CES-D of 9.3, less than a point away from the cutoff score for prediction of MDD (N. S. Park et al., 2018). In a 2016 study of older Korean Americans in the Washington, DC metropolitan area, 22.5% of the sample had probable MDD, but only 35% of the sample saw depression as an illness (Bernstein et al., 2021).

Reluctance to utilize formal mental health care persists into the second generation. In a study of second-generation and generation 1.5 Asian American women—including many of Korean background—with moderate to severe depression and/or a lifetime history of suicidal ideation or a suicide attempt, more than 60% of those with the most severe current symptoms did not utilize any mental health care. Interviews with actively symptomatic women suggested that concerns about both family stigma and community stigma discouraged them from pursuing treatment. A third reason women gave for not seeking treatment was a mismatch between available services and their cultural identity, expressing their wishes that clinicians would better understand issues of stigma, that they would take a more holistic, mind/body approach, and that they would understand the "dual culture" expreience of growing up in the United States but being influenced by Asian family and community attitudes toward mental health (Augsberger et al., 2015).

Possibly related to stigma or to misconception of the often chronic or recurrent nature of major depression is the low level of persistence of depressed Koreans with antidepressant treatment. Jung et al. (2020) reviewed the records of 900 Korean patients treated for diagnosed MDD with a selective serotonin reuptake inhibitor (either sertraline or escitalopram), finding that the median length of time to discontinuation of treatment was 12 weeks and that 73% of patients had discontinued their treatment within 24 weeks. Thus, many patients would have been on antidepressants for too little time to get full benefit, and for those who remitted on antidepressants, most would not remain on them long enough to minimize the risk of relapse. A widely held belief among Koreans that antidepressant drugs are addictive might contribute to the problem. In a survey of Korean Americans over 60 in the Washington DC metro area, 86% believed that antidepressants can have a rapid effect on symptoms, 83% believed that people with depression should stop taking their antidepressants when they feel better, and 66% believed that antidepressants were addictive (Oh et al., 2022). When treating a depressed Korean American, especially one who is a first-generation immigrant, the clinician should explore and address the patient's pre-existing beliefs about antidepressant drugs before prescribing them.

Depression is highly prevalent among both in Korea and in the United States, and suicide mortality rates for Koreans are high in both countries. Clinical depression is frequently expressed by Koreans in forms other than typical MDD. When depression is identified, stigma is a common barrier to seeking treatment and to persistence with treatment. Appreciating the role of issues like historical trauma, "national emotions," harmful use of alcohol, intergenerational cultural conflict, gender inequality, harsh discipline of children, normalization of suicide, and the pervasiveness of stigma can enhance a clinician's understanding of a Korean patient with symptoms of depression—and might improve the outcome of the patient's treatment.

Chapter 13

Depression and Suicide in the "World's Happiest Countries"

Every year since 2010 the Center for Sustainable Development, an agency of the United Nations, has conducted a survey of life satisfaction in the nations of the world that results in the *World Happiness Report* (Helliwell et al., 2023). The five Nordic countries and Switzerland have consistently been among the top ten happiest countries. Finland has been in first place since 2018; Denmark, Norway, and Switzerland have been number one in other years. Despite being among the "world's happiest countries," all six have a substantial prevalence of depression and significant suicide mortality. Considering the occurrence of depression in the "world's happiest countries" offers insight into the relationship between happiness and depression. And, there is less confounding of cultural issues with social determinants of health when studying depression in countries with effective social welfare systems.

While the cultural differences between Nordic nations are not as broad and deep as those between China and Japan, or even those between New England and the Deep South of the United States, they are associated with surprisingly large differences in their patterns of depression and of suicide. Switzerland, a single country with a smaller population than Sweden's, has been remarkably diverse for centuries. The regions of Switzerland that predominantly speak French, German, or Italian have cultural features resembling those of France, Germany, and Italy. They are reflected in regional differences in the occurrence and expression of depression.

As discussed in detail in Chapter 11, aspects of culture can be "double-edged swords"—in some contexts protective against depression, while in others contributing to depression or concealing it. Each of the Nordic countries has cultural features that "cut both ways." They are antidepressants for the society overall but can make matters worse for individuals.

This chapter makes quantitative comparisons among the five Nordic countries, Switzerland, Western Europe as a benchmark, and the United States as an additional comparator. Unless indicated otherwise, all prevalence and mortality data are from the 2019 Global Burden of Disease (GBD) database

(Institute for Health Metrics and Evaluation [IHME], 2023). Other health-related statistics are from the World Health Organization's (WHO's) Global Health Observatory (WHO, 2023) and from the Organisation for Economic Co-operation and Development (OECD). Data on non-epidemiologic topics were obtained from the OECD, the World Economic Forum, and the World Values Survey.

Prevalence estimates from the GBD database are based on statistical synthesis of published data from sources using diverse methodologies for case-finding and diagnosis. While the analysts who curate the database attempt to make estimates comparable, some differences between countries or subgroups within them can reflect differences in measurement. Prevalence estimates for MDD will exclude people with clinical depression who do not meet the Diagnostic and Statistical Manual of Mental Disorders (DSM)/ICD criteria for MDD even though their symptoms cause severe distress or functional impairment or lead to death by suicide. Specifically, depression with a somatoform or externalizing expression often would not be diagnosed as MDD using typical screening interviews and questionnaires. In countries with high rates of effective treatment of depression, the prevalence of MDD can be low because so many cases are treated to remission. A person on maintenance antidepressant therapy with no current symptoms of depression would not count as a prevalent case of MDD. The same country might not have a low lifetime prevalence of depression, but it is difficult to get *lifetime* prevalence data suitable for meaningful comparison across countries. Similarly, rates of death by suicide will not include deaths misattributed to accidents or to illness.

Utilizing data from the 2019 Global Burden of Disease (GBD) (Institute for Health Metrics and Evaluation [IHME, 2023]) we compared MDD prevalence and suicide mortality rates for the six "happy countries" with rates for Western Europe as a whole, and with rates for the United States. Results are presented in Tables 13.1 and 13.2. Rates that differ meaningfully from those in Western Europe are highlighted using bold face if they are higher and italics if they are lower. A "peak interval" is an age range for males or females that had the country or region's highest prevalence of MDD in 2019. The rate reported for a peak interval is the average of prevalence rates for the five-year intervals that fall within that peak prevalence interval.

Denmark, Iceland, and Norway have MDD prevalence rates for both sexes that are significantly lower than the benchmark rate for Western Europe. Finland's rates are higher. Norway and Switzerland have a below-benchmark prevalence of MDD for women but not for men. Finland and Switzerland have above-benchmark rates of MDD for men but not for women. Sweden has an above-benchmark rate of MDD for women but not for men.

Table 13.1 Prevalence of Major Depressive Disorder in 2019

Country	Women Prevalence	Women Peak Age Interval(s)	Women Average Prevalence in Peak Interval(s)	Men Prevalence	Men Peak Age Interval	Men Average Prevalence in Peak Interval(s)
Denmark	4.1%	45-69	5.2%	2.0%	35+	2.4%
Finland	4.3%	20-24	6.6%	2.7%	20-24	3.9%
Iceland	2.9%	15-24; 40+	3.4%	1.5%	35+	1.8%
Norway	3.1%	20-29	4.3%	2.0%	20-24	2.8%
Sweden	5.0%	20-24; 40-59	6.5%; 6.1%	2.2%	no peak after age 20	2.6%
Switzerland	4.0%	40-59	5.1%	2.5%	35+	2.9%
Western Europe	4.5%	40-64; 85+	5.3%	2.2%	50+	3.2%
United States	4.6%	15-24	8.0%	2.5%	20-29	4.4%

Note. Data from Global Burden of Disease 2019 (IHME, 2023). The database was queried for MDD prevalence by five-year age bands, and peak intervals were determined by graphing the findings.

Table 13.2 2019 Suicide Mortality Rate per 100,000 Population by Age Band

Country	Men Age 15–49	Men Age 50–69	Men Age 70+	Women Age 15–49	Women Age 50–69	Women Age 70+
Denmark	14.7	24.0	32.5	4.5	10.0	11.5
Finland	27.0	32.1	32.6	7.7	10.7	6.5
Iceland	16.8	26.3	42.0	3.6	5.9	8.5
Norway	17.3	18.6	18.8	6.8	9.3	6.2
Sweden	18.3	26.7	29.8	8.4	12.2	10.3
Switzerland	15.6	26.9	43.2	5.7	10.9	12.5
Western Europe	16.4	22.1	33.8	4.8	8.0	9.1
United States	22.7	30.2	35.7	7.3	9.5	4.9

Note. Data from Global Burden of Disease 2019 (IHME, 2023). https://vizhub.healthdata.org/gbd-results/. The database was queried for deaths by self-harm in 2019 per 100,000 population for the designated countries and for Western Europe overall.

The age pattern of depression prevalence differs significantly among the happy countries. Both Finland and Norway show a peak prevalence of MDD in young adults and do not show the midlife peak commonly seen elsewhere, especially in women. In the other countries studied, the MDD peak in women includes the perimenopausal period. The rates of suicide mortality for the six countries show the expected high rates in Finland and Sweden, in keeping with their higher prevalence of MDD. Less expected are the relatively high rates of suicide for women in Denmark, Iceland, and Switzerland, all nations with a relatively low prevalence of MDD in women. In most countries of the world, suicide mortality rates are highest among people over age 70. In Finland and Norway, the rates for women over age 70 are significantly lower than for women in late middle age. The same remarkably low suicide rate for older women is found in the U.S.

When rates of suicide are disproportionately high relative to reported rates of MDD, potential explanations include a significant prevalence of clinical depression not captured in rates of MDD, suicides unrelated to depression, and factors that increase the likelihood that a person—with or without clinical depression—will die by suicide. The latter are especially salient in the six "happy countries," where binge drinking is widespread, most people do not have religious beliefs that enjoin suicide, and, in all but Denmark, there is a high rate of civilian gun ownership.

The peak ages for MDD prevalence have plausible explanations in terms of the typical life course. For example, women in their 40s might be dealing with physical aging and concerns about loss of attractiveness or ageism in the workplace, symptoms of menopause, challenges of midlife parenting or of accepting childlessness, and/or midlife misbehavior of a spouse. Typical issues for women in their 20s in high-income countries with secular cultures include concerns about intimate relationships, sexuality, and marriage; education and career; and negotiating an adult relationship with their parents. The cultural environment can make the concerns of a given life stage easier or harder. For example, Sweden's combination of relatively late marriage, widespread employment of women in business and professional positions, and rampant sexual harassment of women working in higher-level jobs gives rise to stressful situations that can precipitate episodes of clinical depression.

Switzerland, the only non-Nordic nation of the six happiest countries, offers a natural model of cultural diversity within a common political framework. It is a confederation of 26 semi-autonomous cantons (equivalent to states or provinces in the U.S. or Canada) that has been ethnically and religiously diverse for centuries. Its population of 8.5 million includes 25% foreign nationals (Swiss Federal Statistical Office, 2019), a mixture of immigrants and expatriates. More than half of the foreigners in Switzerland are from France, Germany, Italy, or Portugal; 63% of Swiss are German-speaking, 23% are French-speaking, and 8% are Italian-speaking. For a small, high-income country, a surprisingly high proportion of its population is rural—26% (World Bank, 2019). Religiously, 36.5% of the population identifies as Catholic and 24.5% identify as Protestant, 5.9% are "other Christian," and 5.2% are Muslim; 24.9% have no religious affiliation (Central Intelligence Agency, 2019).

In *An Almost Nearly Perfect People*, the British journalist Michael Booth provides an account of his personal investigation of the differences among the Nordic peoples. He observes that residents of the Nordic nations stereotype one another and joke about their neighbors' strange and amusing customs (Booth, 2014). Within the Nordic region, people appreciate the hedonism of the Danes, the introversion of the Finns, the arrogance of the Swedes, and the athleticism of the Norwegians. Similar self-differentiation of neighbors from one another, including stereotyping, is seen among the three Swiss sub-nations. The demographic and cultural differences among the Nordic countries, and among the three linguistic regions of Switzerland, are reflected by their epidemiology and typical narratives of depression and suicide.

Taking the Measure of Happiness and Depression

The World Happiness Survey (Helliwell et al., 2023) calculates average happiness ratings for nations by sampling 1000 residents of each country each year and asking them to evaluate their lives today on a zero to 10 scale—from dystopia to eutopia—with the worst possible life as a zero and the best possible life as a 10. Data from a three-year period are combined. Thus, 2023 scores are based on data from 2020-2022, covering the years of the COVID-19 pandemic. In the 2023 report, the scores of the Nordic nations and Switzerland fall in a narrow range: Finland leads the world at 7.804, and Switzerland, in eighth place globally, scores 7.240.

When calculating a happiness score for a country, the World Happiness Survey averages individuals' ratings. Even in a happy country, it is unusual for a person to rate their life 9 or 10 (fewer than 15% will rate their lives that way). The plurality of scores in happy countries are 7s and 8s. It is a *lack* of *low scores* that gets a country into the top 10.

What goes into a person's judgment that their life is close to or far away from the "best possible life?" On a population basis, items like per capita gross domestic product (GDP), healthy life expectancy, social capital, and personal freedom explain much of the variance. On an individual basis, it is, of course, preferable to have more pleasure and less pain; but for many people the essence of happiness is a life of goodness, meaning, and purpose. Put differently, in a "best possible life," people fulfill their *ikigai* (reason for living, as elaborated in Japanese culture), which has both a short-term and a long-term aspect, as discussed in Chapter 11. In addition, a "best possible life" usually includes a good life for loved ones. With these considerations in mind, a person could suffer from clinical depression but give their life an 8 or even a 9. Such a person would have the insight to recognize that current thoughts of hopelessness, regret, anhedonia, and alienation were the treatable and transient symptoms of an illness. For the same reason, a fundamentally happy person with recurrent MDD who was currently euthymic might regard their major depressive episodes as the only major negative aspect of a generally wonderful life.

Happier countries tend to be less rejecting and stigmatizing toward people who are non-conforming, including people with psychiatric problems. People in happier countries usually are more willing to acknowledge depression and seek help for it, thereby increasing the country's reported prevalence of depression. So, there is no contradiction in finding a relatively high prevalence of depression in a country with a high happiness rating.

Similarly, there is no contradiction in finding a high suicide mortality rate in a "happy country." If a person is depressed, lonely, and miserable or tortured by physical or emotional pain, seeing others around them looking happy and healthy and enjoying life might make their life even more unbearable. And because happy countries tend to be secular, a smaller segment of their population will have religious beliefs that enjoin suicide. Furthermore, among the "happiest countries," Finland and Switzerland have the highest rates of civilian firearm ownership, and firearm ownership rates are correlated with suicide rates, with the relationship mediated by rates of suicide by firearm (Anestis & Houtsma, 2018; Anestis et al., 2019; Knopov et al., 2019).

Values and Cultural Dimensions in the Nordic Countries and Switzerland

For the past two decades, prevailing value systems of the world's nations have been studied by social scientists in the World Values Survey (WVS) collaborative, using survey techniques like those used in the World Happiness Survey but with more extensive and wide-ranging questionnaires. Utilizing a conceptual framework developed by political scientists Ronald Inglehart and Christian Welzel, two factors (principal components) are extracted from questionnaire responses that together explain 70% of the variation between countries in 10 indicators of beliefs, values, and attitudes (World Values Survey Association, 2023.).

To create the map, each country's national means for the two factors were put on a scatterplot. The authors then drew boundaries around groups of points that combined considerations of geography, history, and religion. Thus, a formal factor analysis was followed by an informal, hypothesis-driven cluster analysis. The map is shown in Figure 13.1. Sometimes, as with the Nordic countries, geographical neighbors have similar values. However, geographically disparate countries also can have similar values, and when they do, the explanation can be a common language (e.g., English) or a common religion (e.g., Islam). On the other hand, geographic neighbors can have dramatically different values, typically because of differing histories. For example, the Philippines, despite its location in Southeast Asia, is found in the same part of the cultural map as the countries of Latin America. Their cultural similarity can be attributed to the Philippines being a Spanish possession from 1565 through 1898.

The two dimensions of values used to create the cultural map capture traditional versus secular-rational values and survival versus self-expression values (Inglehart et al., 2014). *Traditional values* emphasize religious observance, a large role for conventional family relationships, and deference to authority. People with traditional values in this sense typically are opposed to divorce, abortion, euthanasia, and suicide. *Secular-rational values* are more individualistic, rather than family-oriented or guided by religious faith. Many people with secular-rational values are atheists, agnostics, or deists; and most who do

Table 13.3 2019 Income Inequality and Poverty Rates

Country	Gini before taxes and transfers	Gini after taxes and transfers	Disposable income P90:P10 ratio	Poverty rate before taxes and transfers	Poverty rate after taxes and transfers	Poverty rate: Age 66–75	Poverty rate: Age 76+
Denmark	0.451	0.263	2.9	24.9%	5.5%	2.1%	4.8%
Finland	0.506	0.259	3.1	34.3%	5.8%	2.6%	8.5%
Iceland	0.386	0.255	3.0	19.5%	5.4%	2.4%	3.5%
Norway	0.428	0.262	3.1	25.6%	8.2%	2.3%	7.6%
Sweden	0.435	0.282	3.3	24.9%	9.1%	7.5%	16.2%
Switzerland	0.386	0.296	3.6	15.8%	9.1%	15.5%	25.0%
United States	0.507	0.391	6.1	26.6%	17.8%	19.5%	28.1%

Note. Data from the Organization for Economic Cooperation and Development [OECD] (2023). https://data-explorer.oecd.org. The database was queried for 2019 income distribution statistics for the six "happy countries" and for the United States.

identify with a religion are not observant. People with secular-rational values tend to be egalitarian, and they are more likely to accept divorce, abortion, euthanasia, and suicide. *Survival values* emphasize physical and economic security and are associated with ethnocentrism, low levels of trust, and intolerance of non-conformity. *Self-expression values* emphasize environmental protection, tolerance of "foreigners" including immigrants, acceptance of homosexuality and gender non-conformity, and broad participation of the public, including minorities, in the political process. Self-expression values are associated with high trust.

The six happy countries of this chapter all are found in the right upper quadrant of the cultural map—secular-rational countries that value self-expression. Compared with one another, Iceland and Switzerland are relatively more traditional, and Finland and Switzerland are relatively more survival-oriented. Sweden leads the six countries on both secular-rational and self-expression values. The map suggests that the Swiss French and Swiss Italians will be more traditional in their values than the Swiss Germans but that all Swiss, regardless of their primary language, will have more self-expressive values than French, Germans, or Italians. What the cultural map misses is the difference between urban and rural culture within each of the countries. The world's high-income countries are predominantly urban, so any summary assessment of a high-income country's values will give more weight to the opinions of its urban residents. Yet, the rural–urban cultural distance within a single country can be larger than the cultural distance between the urban areas of different countries.

In the Hofstede six-dimensional model of cultures, Switzerland has a "masculine" culture, while the Nordic countries have "feminine" cultures—Sweden and Norway the most and Finland the least. Denmark and Sweden are low on uncertainty avoidance; the other countries are intermediate. Switzerland has a long-term orientation, Sweden is intermediate, and the other Nordic countries have a short-term orientation. Sweden, Denmark, Switzerland, and Iceland are indulgent; Finland and Norway are intermediate (Hofstede-Insights, 2023).

The World Economic Forum conducts an annual analysis of the "global gender gap," comparing nations on their gender equality in economic participation and opportunity, educational attainment, health and survival, and political empowerment. Of the six "happy countries," Iceland, Norway, Finland, and Sweden join New Zealand in the top five for gender parity. Switzerland ranks 21st and Denmark ranks 23rd; both Switzerland and Denmark have similar, significant inequality of economic participation and opportunity for women. Denmark trails Switzerland in women's political empowerment (World Economic Forum, 2023, pp. 11, 16–18).

Gender parity in education, healthcare, and employment by no means implies that men and women are the same in their expression of clinical depression. Like men in many other parts of the world, men in Nordic countries, and in Switzerland, are more likely than women to externalize depression through anger, irritability, risk-taking, and excessive use of alcohol. This phenomenon was thoughtfully analyzed by Wålinder and Rutzt (2001), who studied depressed men in metropolitan Gothenburg, a large port city on the west coast of Sweden. They developed a new questionnaire-based rating scale, the Gotland Male Depression Scale (GMDS), specifically sensitive to externalized depression. The questionnaire has 13 items rated on a scale of 0–3, introduced by the question "During the past month, have you or others noticed that your behavior has changed, and if so, in which way?" Items not found in typical depression scales inquire about aggressiveness, indecisiveness, being "difficult to deal with," overconsumption of "alcohol and pills," self-pity, and "seeming pathetic." There is also a family history question, inquiring about abusive behavior, suicide attempts, and "proneness to behavior involving danger." (Further details of the GDMS are provided in Chapter 18 in connection with expressions of depression in truck drivers—people working in a traditionally masculine occupation.)

The GMDS was applied to men under treatment for alcoholism at a clinic in Copenhagen, where it detected probable or definite depression in 39% of the patients, compared with a 17% detection rate using a generic gender-neutral depression rating scale (Zierau et al., 2002). A study of community depression screening in Icelandic men showed that the GMDS performed better psychometrically than the Beck Depression Inventory (BDI) (Sigurdsson et al., 2015). In that study, men with symptoms of "male depression" had elevated levels of testosterone and of cortisol in the evening (i.e., biological evidence of a stress response in addition to relatively high levels of male hormone; Sigurdsson et al., 2014). Further research has shown that the syndrome of male depression can also be seen in women, who, in a culture of greater gender equality and greater social acceptance of aggression in women, may resort to externalizing defenses against depressed moods (Möller-Leimkühler & Yücel, 2010). In both men and women, childhood abuse or neglect is associated with a higher prevalence of the symptoms of male depression (Pompili et al., 2014).

Social, Economic, and Demographic Issues

Having or not having children, the circumstances of children's births, and issues in rearing children are of obvious relevance to women's narratives of depression in a cultural context. The six "happy countries" have low birth rates, and most families have one or two children. The proportion of women who reach midlife never having given birth to a child is approximately 13% in Denmark, Norway, and Sweden and approximately 20% in Finland and Switzerland (OECD, 2023a; Statistics Denmark, 2019; Statistics Norway, 2018). The Nordic countries all have high rates of birth outside of marriage. Data from 2019 and 2020 yield rates of 69.4% in Iceland (highest of all high-income countries, 57.6% in Norway, 55.2% in Sweden, 54.2% in Denmark, and 46.1% in Finland. Switzerland stands out with a rate of 27.7%, one of the lowest among high-income nations (OECD, 2023a). The difference might be related to its more traditional culture and to the higher prevalence of religious belief and engagement.

Both men and women marry relatively late by global standards. The mean age at first marriage for men in the six countries ranges from 33.1 years in Switzerland to 34.1 years in Finland; the mean age for women ranges from 30.9 in Switzerland to 32.4 in Norway. The mean age for bearing a first child falls in a narrow range between 30.9 years in Iceland to 32.4 years in Switzerland (World Population Review, 2024).

In Finland, 41.0% of all households are single-person households; the proportion of single-person households is 39.6% in Norway, 37.5% in Denmark and Switzerland, and 36.2% in Sweden. Denmark (18.7%), Finland (19.2%), Norway (20.8%), and Sweden (25.5%) have the lowest proportions in Europe of adults aged 18–34 living with their parents (Eurostat, 2019a). When a person in their 20s or early 30s living alone suffers a significant trauma, loss, or disappointment, they may have no one at hand to offer support. In both Sweden and Finland, the highest decade of MDD prevalence for women is 20–29—an age range in which most women in those countries will be single, childless, and living alone.

Poverty, limited education, and low social status are risk factors for depression, because of the social and environmental determinants of health experienced by the lower class, a high rate of adverse childhood experiences, and the higher rates of physical illness and trauma experienced by the lower class. The "happy countries" mitigate these problems by taxing their citizens to provide a very high level of public education, healthcare, childcare, and income support for disabled, unemployed, or retired people. Relatively few people are in poverty, no one is without access to healthcare, and there are extensive opportunities for individuals and families to improve their status through study and work. The World Economic Forum calculates a Social Mobility Index based on six components: the ability of an individual to move between socioeconomic classes during their lifetime, the ability of a family group to move up or down the socioeconomic ladder across one or more generations, the ability of an individual to earn more than their parents at the same age, the ability of an individual to attain a higher level of education than their parents, how much of an individual's income is determined by their parents' income, and how much an individual's education is determined by their parents' education. The index, calculated for 82 countries, was updated in 2020 (World Economic Forum, 2020). The Nordic countries are the top five nations in the world for social mobility, and Switzerland is close behind them in seventh place. The Social Mobility Index scores for the "happy countries" range from 82.1 for Switzerland to 85.2 for Denmark. For comparison, the United States is in 27th place with a score of 70.4, and China is in 45th place with a score of 61.5.

While in the "happy countries" relatively few people become depressed because of absolute poverty, they are places where a person unsuccessful in life cannot blame "the system" for their disappointments. When suffering from depression, a relatively unsuccessful person might blame themselves for lacking talent or motivation or might focus on traumatic life events, adverse childhood experiences, or problems related to their status as an immigrant or minority. A depressed woman might be troubled by experiences of gender-based discrimination or harassment—problems that occur even in countries with small gender gaps. Among the "happiest countries," Denmark has the most barriers to occupational advancement for women, and Sweden has the highest incidence of sexual harassment.

Despite the impressive socioeconomic mobility in the "happy countries," they have substantial inequality of pre-tax income and even greater inequality of wealth. Despite relative equality of income after taxes and transfers, the Nordic countries, and even moreso Switzerland, have large inequalities of socioeconomic status, based on a combination of education, occupation, pre-tax income, and wealth. In the Nordic nations, the wealthiest 10% of households own more than half of the nation's assets and the proportion of the population in 2021 with a net worth less than $10,000 was 15% in Denmark, 27% in Norway and Sweden, and 34% in Sweden (Shorrocks et al., 2022). Even when a person without a job and with low or negative net worth receives support from the government and does not face hunger or homelessness, they are not the social equal of a person with a well-paid job and/or income from savings and investments. After retirement, most people with minimal or negative net worth are totally dependent on the government, a status supported by public policy but not necessarily appreciated by those currently working and paying more than half of their income in taxes.

Table 13.3 shows 2019 statistics on income inequality in the Nordic countries and Switzerland, with a special focus on poverty in old age. In the table, the Gini coefficient refers to the overall distribution of income, where 0 would indicate total equality and 1 would indicate ownership of the country's entire assets by one person. P90:P10 refers to the ratio of the 90th percentile of disposable

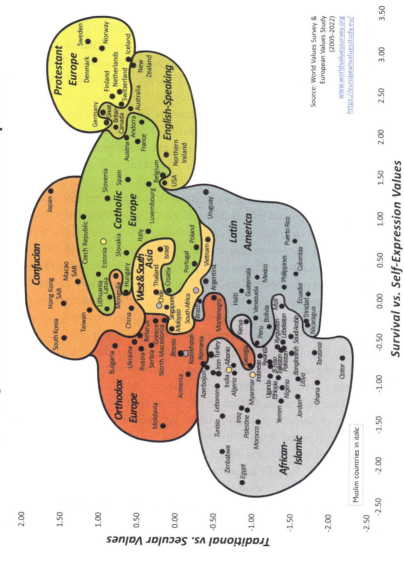

Figure 13.1 Inglehart-Welzel World Cultural Map, Wave 7

income to the 10th percentile of disposable income. *Poverty* indicates household income less than half of the national median. The poverty rates for older adults shown are net, after taxes and transfers. The income equality of the Nordic countries is the effect of an aggressive policy of taxes and transfers that redistribute income. The level of redistribution seen there could only exist in a high-trust culture with a communitarian (not collectivist) ethos, where there is general sentiment that government is not corrupt and that people in general can be trusted. Switzerland begins with less income inequality than the Nordic countries except Iceland because its working-age population is relatively well paid, and there is relatively stable employment. After taxes and transfers, its income inequality and overall poverty rate are like those of Sweden. However, Switzerland's policies, more like those of the U.S. and unlike those of the Nordic nations other than Sweden, do not ensure the economic security of its older adults. The poverty rate for Swiss aged 66-75 exceeds 15%, and the rate for those over age 75 is 25%.

In the Nordic countries and Switzerland, low socioeconomic status in later life often is accompanied by loneliness. In all six, more than 35% of women and more than 19% of men over 65 live alone (Reher & Requena, 2018). Switzerland, with a rate of old age poverty much greater than that of the Nordic countries, has the highest late-life suicide rates of the "happy countries"; and it is likely that despair and shame over poverty underlie many suicides in that country. However, Iceland's high late-life suicide rate for men is not explained by poverty.

Switzerland is placed in the secular-rational/self-expressive quadrant of the values chart, but it is nonetheless more traditional than the Nordic nations. Importantly, over one third of all Swiss residents are either immigrants or children of immigrants, almost all of whom come from countries with cultures that are more traditional and/or more survival-oriented than Swiss national culture. About half of the foreigners in Switzerland are either Italian, German, Portuguese, or French, with most of the remaining foreigners in Switzerland coming from Kosovo, Spain, Turkey, Serbia, and Macedonia. More than 60% of the population of Geneva either is foreign-born or has two foreign parents (Swissinfo, 2018). Equally important as national origin and language in determining Swiss residents' culture is rural versus urban status. Rural Switzerland is much more traditional and survival-oriented than urban Switzerland; the contrast is largest when comparing agricultural regions of the country with the sophisticated international cities of Zurich, Geneva, Bern, and Lausanne. In the framework of Hofstede's dimensions, rural Switzerland has a more collectivist culture with high uncertainty avoidance and high masculinity. Traditional norms of social behavior are more consistently observed, and non-conformity is less tolerated.

Rural–urban divides with psychiatric significance are seen in all high-income countries. They are especially salient and exemplary in Switzerland because it has a high proportion of rural residents for a high-income country. Rural Switzerland has a higher suicide mortality rate and more untreated depression than urban Switzerland and probably a higher prevalence of depression overall. There is more seasonality of depressive symptoms and of suicide in rural areas, with those working in agriculture and forestry showing the greatest seasonal variation. Suicide attempts in rural versus urban areas are more likely to be made using a firearm, and thus are more likely to be fatal.

Diet and Depression at the National Level

As discussed in detail in Chapter 9, foods have neurochemical effects that affect depression risk. Diet also strongly affects the risk of medical conditions like obesity (and its consequences of diabetes and obstructive sleep apnea) and atherosclerotic vascular disease that frequently entail secondary depression. Because other cultural, environmental, and genetic factors are involved, dietary influences on depression prevalence at the population level will be modest unless dietary differences are large, as they are with Icelanders' high consumption of seafood or Americans' high consumption of sugar-sweetened beverages. At the individual level, it is more likely in Finland than in Iceland to encounter a depressed middle-aged person with hyperlipidemia and atherosclerotic vascular disease with effects on the heart and brain that affect their health-related quality of life and have secondary consequences associated with comorbid depression. Addressing general medical problems and the lifestyle issues that relate to them is often an effective way to engage a reluctant depressed patient in a useful dialogue about health-related behavior, including habits of eating, sleeping, and exercise with significant effects on mood.

In high-income countries, diets of people not in poverty are determined by culture and personal preference rather than by the availability of foods. The patterns of food consumption of the "happy countries" differ significantly in ways relevant to health, including vulnerability to depression. This is evident from Table 13.4, which shows data from the Food and Agriculture Organization of the United Nations (2019) on national per capita annual "food balance" for various types of food, for the six "happy countries" and for the U.S.

Iceland, which has the lowest rate of MDD in the Nordic region, has by far the highest consumption of seafood, a major source of antidepressant and mood-stabilizing omega-3 fatty acids. Norway, which has the lowest overall suicide rate of the "happy countries," has the second highest seafood consumption, well ahead of Finland in third place. Denmark's high consumption of bovine

Table 13.4 Food Available for Human Consumption – (kg/capita/year) in 2020

	Seafood	Bovine meat (beef and veal)	Dairy products	Sugar and sweeteners	Fruits and vegetables
Denmark	26.5	**24.3**	249.4	**59.2**	155.3
Finland	33.5	18.4	**263.4**	49.6	155.5
Iceland	**90.6**	14.0	203.6	**89.4**	147.7
Norway	**50.2**	17.8	177.4	53.9	150.9
Sweden	32.2	**22.5**	221.6	42.1	148.5
Switzerland	16.0	19.1	**298.3**	46.8	**177.0**

Note. Data from Food and Agriculture Organization (2023). https://www.fao.org/faostat/en/#data. The database was queried for the 2020 "food balances" of the happy countries. Notably high levels are highlighted in bold face.

meat, dairy products, and sweets comports with its relatively indulgent culture and partly explains its relatively high rate of atherosclerotic vascular disease. In this connection, Denmark is an outlier in its prevalence of diabetes, most of which is Type 2 diabetes related to obesity. Its age-standardized prevalence of 8.3% for diabetes in adults over 18 is well above the unweighted average rate for the European Union. It is the only one of the happy countries with an above-average prevalence of diabetes (OECD, 2023b).

The "Nordic diet" has been promoted as an alternative to the Mediterranean diet with similar benefits for heart and brain health. It is characterized by regular consumption of fish, whole grains, berries and other fresh fruit, cruciferous and root vegetables, legumes, wild mushrooms, nuts, and low-fat dairy products. In lieu of olive oil in the Mediterranean diet, the Nordic diet features rapeseed (canola) oil, a polyunsaturated oil rich in alpha-linolenic acid, a precursor of the omega-3 fatty acids beneficial to brain health including stable mood. Consumption of red meat and sugar is minimized (Adamsson et al., 2012). It was developed in 2004 by a group of chefs and nutritionists to integrate ideas of healthy eating with preference for sustainably produced, locally sourced ingredients (Nordic Council, 2004). It was advanced as a healthier alternative to the usual diet of contemporary Nordic people, in response to the Nordic countries' increasing rates of obesity, Type 2 diabetes, and their complications. It is apparently not followed by most Nordic people, the Danes least of all.

Table 13.5 shows selected statistics about alcohol use in the happy countries. Denmark, Switzerland, and Finland consume more alcohol than the other three countries, and their increased consumption is reflected by higher death rates from liver disease, alcohol-associated cancers, and accidents involving alcohol. It is notable that Sweden and Finland have a prevalence of alcohol use disorders

Table 13.5 Alcohol Use and Its Consequences

Country	Liters of alcohol per capita per year (age ≥15 years)	15-year-olds who have been drunk at least twice in life	Prevalence of episodic heavy drinking (≥60 g of alcohol on one occasion) in past 30 days, men	Prevalence of episodic heavy drinking (≥60 g of alcohol on one occasion) in past 30 days, women	Prevalence of alcohol use disorders (age ≥15 years)	Fraction of deaths attributable to alcohol
Denmark	**9.5**	**42.0%**	46.2%	13.8%	7.5%	**5.6%**
Finland	**8.2**	25.0%	44.7%	12.6%	**9.1%**	**5.8%**
Iceland	7.7	7.0%	43.7%	12.4%	4.4%	3.8%
Norway	6.1	15.5%	**48.6%**	**18.3%**	7.2%	3.4%
Sweden	7.1	11.0%	43.7%	12.4%	**11.0%**	3.6%
Switzerland	**9.3**	13.5%	**53.4%**	**18.4%**	9.5%	4.5%

Note. Global Information System on Alcohol and Health (World Health Organization, 2018). https://www.who.int/data/gho/data/themes/global-information-system-on-alcohol-and-health. High and low values of special interest are highlighted in bold or italic type.

disproportionate to their per capita alcohol consumption, suggesting a culture that normalizes unhealthy drinking. In the countries with high rates of alcohol use disorders, alcohol use often will contribute to depression via its biochemical and/or behavioral consequences. In Denmark there is a higher likelihood that alcohol would contribute to depression via effects on general health. Iceland's remarkably low prevalence of alcohol use disorders, like its low prevalence of MDD, might reflect earlier recognition and response to developing drinking problems in a country that has a proactive mental healthcare system. Finally, it is notable that while binge drinking is far more common among males than females everywhere, Norway and Switzerland stand out for their relatively high rates of binge drinking by females aged 15 and older. The consequences of an episode of drunkenness are more likely to be part of a girl's or woman's depression narrative in those countries.

Distinctive national cultures are also expressed in the everyday mental health experiences of adolescents in the six happy countries. Table 13.6 shows differences among 15-year-olds in the six countries with respect to four indicators of mental well-being in 2021–2022. A high proportion of the teens surveyed in all six countries expressed some form of mental distress, experiencing either a low mood, trouble falling asleep, irritability, or loneliness. Remarkably, however,

Table 13.6 Mental Health Symptoms of 15-Year Olds in 2021-22 in the Happy Countries

	Girls				Boys			
	Low mood	Sleep trouble	Lonely	Irritable	Low mood	Sleep trouble	Lonely	Irritable
Denmark	29%	45%	13%	45%	7%	35%	6%	22%
Finland	42%	33%	26%	47%	13%	14%	7%	16%
Iceland	41%	36%	27%	51%	16%	23%	12%	26%
Norway	36%	35%	22%	47%	15%	29%	10%	24%
Sweden	53%	41%	24%	74%	24%	31%	13%	40%
Switzerland	43%	39%	27%	48%	13%	25%	11%	21%
England	57%	52%	40%	56%	27%	36%	18%	30%

Note. Data from Cosma et al. (2023). In 2021–2022, WHO conducted a survey of mental health issues in students aged 11, 13, and 15 in 44 countries and regions including all major European nations. Subjects were given questionnaires including items about the frequency with which they experienced symptoms including low mood, trouble getting to sleep, irritability/bad temper, and loneliness. In the table, percentages refer to the proportion of 15-year-olds who had problems with mood, sleep, or irritability more than one day per week over the past six months, and the proportion who felt lonely most of the time over the past year. Results from England are included as a comparator.

15-year-olds in the happy countries all had significantly lower overall levels of mental health symptoms that did those in England during the same period.

Differences among the countries can be correlated with their national cultures. Loneliness and low moods were least frequent in Denmark, a country with a culture that encourages people to socialize and to enjoy life. However, teenagers in Denmark were the most likely to have sleep problems, perhaps reflecting their staying up at night for social activities. In keeping with gender-specific expressions of dysphoric mood in the Nordic countries and Switzerland, boys were consistently less likely to report mental health symptoms. The gender gap in symptoms was smallest for trouble falling asleep, the only one of the four symptoms that is not explicitly emotional. Even allowing for gender-related differences in reporting, 15-year-old boys in Finland appeared to have the best mental health. Together with the peak incidence of MDD in Finnish males being in their early twenties, it raises the question of whether the transition from adolescence to young adulthood is particularly challenging for men in that country.

Sisu, Historical Trauma, and Binge Drinking: Finland

Otto M., a 40-year-old data manager, was out walking one Saturday afternoon by a small lake a few kilometers outside of town. He was contemplating suicide. His one best friend, whom he'd known since he was 10, had shot himself two years ago after his small business failed. Otto thought he had lost so much more than money, but he was still alive. However, Otto could not picture himself pulling the trigger to end his life. He thought of jumping in the lake but figured he'd reflexively swim to shore and wind up cold, wet, and even more miserable than he was already. He could picture himself taking a handful of sleeping pills and washing them down with a full bottle of *viina*; but there was nothing suitable in his medicine cabinet, and he wouldn't want to see his doctor and answer questions about how he was feeling. He was sure his 10-year-old daughter Oona, now living with his wife, would miss him if he died. Otto had taken a year off work after Oona was born to take care of her, and they had been very close ever since. When his wife Aada left him, three months before Otto's pensive walk, she took Oona with her, and Otto's heart ached every day. Oona was with him every Sunday; the time from Monday through Saturday seemed long and lonely.

As a child, Otto had shown early aptitude for mathematics and got a degree in computer science from one of the country's best technical universities. He had many job opportunities after graduation but chose to remain in the city where he'd studied, working for the university's information technology service. Otto enjoyed life outside of work and wanted a position with regular hours, job security, and low stress. His parents, father a professor and mother a schoolteacher in Helsinki, were disappointed by their only child's apparent lack of ambition and his decision not to return to his hometown. Otto felt distant from his parents. They lived several hours away by train, and he saw them only at holidays.

Otto's wife Aada was a corporate executive. Aada had always been more aggressive and ambitious than Otto, and for the last five years she'd had a much higher salary than he. Otto had begun to feel that he and Aada lived in different worlds. Otto's pleasures were hunting and fishing during the summer, cross-country skiing during the winter, drinking and taking saunas with friends from work, and, best of all, spending time with Oona. For a long time, it seemed to Otto that Aada was absorbed in her work, uninterested in him, and insufficiently engaged in their daughter's life and education. One evening about eight months ago, Otto had stopped at a bar after work and came home severely intoxicated, as he usually did when he drank. Aada complained about his drinking, and he lost his temper. Otto not only was angry about being criticized but also felt neglected and disrespected and thought that Aada had not been a good mother to Oona. He shouted and slapped her face hard. Oona saw and heard her parents' fight. Otto didn't remember all the details about what he said and did that night, but he awoke the next morning with a terrible hangover, feeling guilty and ashamed. He apologized profusely, and Aada accepted his apology. After that, Otto tried to be more attentive to Aada and keep the peace at home.

Two months later, Aada told Otto she had to be honest with him, and with herself, that her heart had changed. She had started a romantic relationship with a male co-worker at her company. They had not begun a sexual relationship—something Aada would not consider doing while still living with Otto—but they had kissed. Otto asked her to give him more time to work on their relationship. Aada agreed, but they made no progress. After several more weeks, one day she calmly told Otto that she no longer loved him. She announced her plan for their separation. The couple offered their daughter her choice about remaining with Otto or leaving with Aada. Oona opted to live with her mother.

Otto was bereft—since his best friend had died, his wife and daughter had been the only people to whom he felt truly connected. He lost interest in his usual pleasures. Fishing, skiing, saunas, drinking after work—nothing felt the same. Sundays with Oona were hard because they would always end with their separation. He felt he had no hope of different custody arrangements because Oona wanted to be with her mother and blamed him for hitting her. It was a great effort to get out of bed in the morning. He was sometimes late to work and slow and inefficient when there. Known for being meticulous, he had begun to make occasional mistakes. His supervisor had noticed, and though the feedback was discreet, Otto felt embarrassed. He continued to drink after work about twice a week, always getting drunk quickly, though he rarely enjoyed it.

After his pensive walk around the lake, Otto admitted to himself that he was depressed. He filled out an online PHQ-9 and scored 20—no surprise to him, his depression was severe. He told himself that he was a tough enough man to bear it and that depression doesn't last forever. A few weeks later he felt no better and finally went to see a psychiatrist at the university health service, who started him on an antidepressant drug and referred him to a psychologist for psychotherapy. Eight weeks later, Otto had not improved much and was feeling even more hopeless. He was given transcranial magnetic stimulation (TMS) and in a few more weeks began to emerge from his depression. He faced the painful realization that he had a problem with alcohol. Years of recovery lay ahead.

A country with high per capita alcohol consumption can display one or both of two unhealthy patterns of drinking: regular daily drinking of excessive amounts and episodic binge drinking. As previously described in connection with South Korea's drinking culture, binge drinking is alcohol consumption that rapidly brings a person to a state of intoxication, with a blood alcohol level of 0.08 g/dl or higher. While people with alcohol use disorders (AUDs) often binge-drink, the behavior is also seen in people without AUD, especially when they are part of a cultural group that normalizes the behavior. The mainstream, non-immigrant cultures of the Nordic countries accept occasional binge drinking as a normal behavior of adults; in all five countries, more than half of the adult population binge-drinks at least once a year. In Finland, regular binge drinking is normalized and socially acceptable if it does not interfere with work or lead to drunk driving. Perhaps because of Finland's binge-drinking culture, the criterion for driving while intoxicated is strict (0.05 g/dl) and the penalties for aggravated drunk driving (blood alcohol content >0.12 g/dl) are severe, with time in prison and fines based on the offender's disposable income (Daley, 2015). (A high-income drunk driver might pay a fine of over $100,000 for a single episode.) In Finland, binge drinking alone does not usually lead to a diagnosis of an AUD or to treatment for problem drinking. However, binge drinking can cause major problems even when no AUD has been diagnosed, notably motor vehicle accidents, intimate partner violence (IPV), child abuse, and suicide attempts. If the latter are made using a firearm, they are likely to be fatal.

Regular heavy drinking, with or without binge drinking, is associated with alcohol-related medical problems. Beyond conditions like alcoholic gastritis, pancreatitis, and hepatitis that are caused directly by alcohol, there are over 30 other diseases that are more likely to occur, or to have a worse outcome, if a person is a heavy drinker. Many of these medical conditions, notably several types of cancer, are commonly accompanied by depression.

Applying the Alcohol Use Disorders Identification Test (AUDIT), a standard quantity/frequency questionnaire about alcohol consumption to screen for hazardous drinking, more than 40% of Finnish men screen in with scores of 6 or higher on its 12-point scale. More than a quarter of Finnish women screen in for hazardous drinking, with their peak rate of positive screens being 32% for ages 20–34. Put simply, young Finnish women and middle-aged Finnish men are highly vulnerable to problem drinking and alcohol-related harm.

Finland has long recognized that it has a national drinking problem. It experimented briefly and unsuccessfully with prohibition of alcohol between 1919 and 1932. At the time it implemented prohibition, its national annual per capita alcohol consumption was among the lowest in Europe, but problem drinking was a salient issue because, for many Finns, drinking means binge drinking. Per capita alcohol consumption in Finland increased steadily after World War II as the country became more prosperous. It peaked in 2007. By that time, the government was making active efforts to find and treat AUDs and to discourage excessive drinking by a combination of public education and high taxes on alcoholic beverages. Though total per capita alcohol consumption has been falling since 2008, binge drinking remains so common in Finland that it is normal in the statistical sense.

Intoxication always entails risk of injury because of disinhibition and impaired judgment. Intoxication with a loaded gun at hand increases the risk of a firearm-related suicide, homicide, or accidental injury. High alcohol levels open the blood–brain barrier so that mediators of systemic inflammation (e.g., from allergy or various chronic diseases) can have greater effects on the brain and thus on mental status (Reeves et al., 2007). Problem drinking increases the risk of depression; binge drinking in a person already depressed increases suicide risk. In considering the context of a person from Finland exhibiting a depressed mood, the potential for a preexisting AUD should always be considered, as should the potential role of alcohol as a suicide risk factor.

Problem drinking and aggressive or risk-taking behavior are parts of the syndrome of "male depression," first described in Sweden and now recognized as a worldwide phenomenon. Finland is the most "masculine" of the Nordic countries, not in the sense of gender but in its valuing of stereotypically masculine virtues of toughness, stoicism, and self-reliance. A Finnish man might express clinical depression primarily through externalization rather than by verbally expressing sadness or depression. The depression will often be accompanied by problem drinking of some kind (typically frequent binge drinking). The drinking problem and the depression initially are best seen as concurrent and interacting problems. It will not necessarily emerge that one problem is primary and the other is a consequence.

Despite its many medical complications, drinking to intoxication serves an important positive function in the life of many Finns. It sets the stage for episodes of frank emotional communication in a society with norms of reticence, discretion, and modesty in expressing feelings. Intoxication with alcohol offers Finns an opportunity to say what they feel, with a potential excuse if they regret it later. Historically, when Finns got drunk at weddings, they might get into fights or have amorous encounters they would never consider when sober, and such episodes were tolerated when the same behavior would be unacceptable under other circumstances. The pattern makes sense in the context of a need for social cohesion in an often hostile environment. The sauna is a second context in which Finns communicate more freely, without the adverse health effects of alcohol.

Finland, with a population of 5.5 million, has over two million saunas. Taking saunas is a national ritual in which almost all Finns participate unless they have a medical contraindication. People taking saunas sit naked in a room heated to between 70 and 100 degrees centigrade, sweat profusely for 20–30 minutes, cool down (often by swimming or showering in cold water), and then repeat the process. Sweating rids the body of toxins and often improves complexion. The heat may relieve mild musculoskeletal discomfort such as backaches or tension headaches. Many people experience transient relief of anxiety or a mild euphoria. Finns take saunas together with friends or family, and business meetings can begin with the participants taking a sauna together before showering, dressing, and sitting down to work. Saunas are one of the few places where Finns make small talk. It is normal for Finns to talk to one another in the sauna without a utilitarian purpose.

Men and women do not take saunas together in public. Shared saunas are a healthier alternative to group binge drinking as an opportunity to build social connections and verbalize feelings. However, if a group sauna is used as a preliminary to a business meeting in a predominantly male organization, women in the organization are at a social disadvantage.

Saunas are one of the "antidepressant" aspects of Finnish culture, which along with Finns' enjoyment of nature and outdoor activity promote mental health and resilience and help Finns tolerate stress. Saunas facilitate social connections without the adverse effects of alcohol. They relieve anxiety and some forms of physical discomfort without medication. They also help people rid their bodies of environmental toxins that have potential adverse effects on the brain.

Sisu: True Grit, Finnish Style

Much as Korean culture has been shaped by its interactions with China and Japan, the culture of Finland, and its geographical boundaries, has been shaped by interactions with its neighbors, Sweden and Russia. As Korean history led to the development of its culturally characteristic emotion of *han*, Finnish history led to the development of the Finnish characteristic of *sisu*.

The Finnish people are genetically and linguistically neither Scandinavians nor Russians, but Finland was part of the Kingdom of Sweden from the 13th century through 1809; from then until 1917 it was a semi-autonomous duchy within the Russian Empire. When the Swedes and the Russians were at war from 1590 to 1595, much of the conflict took place in Finland. After the war, Finland remained under Swedish control; and, as when Ireland was under British control, its peasants paid heavy taxes and got little in return. Beginning in 1700, Russia and its allies fought against Sweden for control of the Baltic Sea, eventually leading to the occupation of most of Finland by the Russian army beginning in 1714. At the same time, Finland endured an epidemic of plague; in the year 1700, two thirds of the population of Helsinki died from the illness. The seven years of Russian occupation are known in Finland as the *Greater Wrath*, a time when thousands of Finns were killed or enslaved. Finland was occupied by the Russians again from 1741 to 1743, a period known as the *Lesser Wrath*. The Russians again fought the Swedes on Finnish territory in 1808–1809, leading to Sweden's ceding Finland to the Russians. Finland was granted autonomy within the Russian Empire. Following the Russian revolution of 1917, it became an independent republic. Immediately afterward, a civil war began between conservatives and social democrats, paralleling the conflict in Russia between the Whites and the Reds. More than 1% of Finland's population, 37,000 people, died in the civil war, from combat, terrorism, and consequences of imprisonment. Finland remained at peace for a little more than 20 years, until November 30, 1939, when it was invaded by the Russians again. Despite a vigorous defense, the small country was overwhelmed by a massive Russian force. Finland turned to Germany for support in its defense against the Russians, and consequently the United Kingdom declared war on Finland. When conflict finally ended in 1947, Finland had lost another 63,000 lives, and it was required to cede more of its territory and pay reparations to Russia equal to half of its annual GDP. While the Finns saw the requirement for reparations as unfair, they paid them off promptly, settling their debt with Russia within five years.

Following the horrors of World War II, Finland maintained neutrality in the Cold War. It urbanized, industrialized, and established a welfare state like those of the other Nordic countries. In the early 1990s the country underwent a severe economic depression, with 20% unemployment and many personal bankruptcies—yet another national trauma. Over the following 25 years, Finland not only rebounded but became one of the world's best-educated, least corrupt, most economically competitive, and most environmentally sustainable countries. The country's history is full of trauma and loss; its success reflects the national attributes of resourcefulness and resilience. The Finns are proud of their national attribute of *sisu*, a concept like "grit"—people courageously and effectively facing mentally or physically challenging situations that they might initially have thought were beyond their capacity. It is the attribute of dogged persistence that enabled Finland to thrive and remain independent when it shared a boundary, and history of hostility, with a superpower 66 times its size. It underlies the success of Finnish athletes in endurance sports.

Sisu is associated with a lack of fear of death, which increases the risk of action in a person contemplating suicide—a person full of *sisu* would have acquired capacity for suicide on a cultural basis. Finns defending their country against invaders would tell themselves they had "nothing worse than death to fear" (Wisti, 2017).

In the Finns' history they have faced environmental challenges from a harsh climate, repeated invasions, and civil conflicts. It was adaptive for Finns to repress the expression of strong emotions that might cause unnecessary conflict and to communicate pragmatically to coordinate defense. The Finnish communication style is extremely understated, avoiding small talk and confession of feelings. Even within married couples, men often say little about their feelings and rely upon their wives to discern their emotions.

The two contexts in which Finns abandon their cultural introversion and reticence are when intoxicated with alcohol, and in the sauna. The widespread acceptance of drinking to intoxication by Finns may relate to the importance of drinking with others as an occasion for emotional communication that might not otherwise occur.

In Finland, high gender equality and a secular culture make divorce easy, and more than half of marriages end in divorce. A woman can easily leave a man who is abusive or whom she no longer loves. At the same time, men in Finland may depend upon their wives to be their "emotional interpreters," understanding and helping them express feelings that they display in subtle and indirect ways and rarely talk about. A Finnish man who fits this model might feel extraordinarily lonely if his wife leaves him. Even *sisu* might not see him through his despair.

The combination of suppressed anger, externalization of male depression, and binge drinking contributes to Finland's high rate of IPV. In a 2012 survey of EU countries concerning violence against women, 27% of Finnish women reported an experience of significant physical IPV from a current partner since age 15, a significantly higher rate than the EU average of 20% (European Union Agency for Fundamental Rights, 2014).

Finland, perhaps because of its history of hunting for survival and a recurrent need for defense against invaders, has long had a high rate of weapons ownership by private citizens, overwhelmingly men. Popular weapons are knives (*puukko*) and guns. Finland has the highest rate of gun ownership in the Nordic countries, though the other Nordic nations except for Denmark also have high rates relative to the Western European average. A license for legal gun ownership requires a stated purpose such as hunting or sport shooting, and all prospective gun owners are screened by the police, with health status being one consideration. However, there are no specific medical criteria or requirements for a physician's involvement (Parker, 2011). Furthermore, Finnish gun licenses are permanent, so many men acquire their guns before they develop problems with mental health or substance use. Finland's rate of firearm suicide by men is the highest in the Nordic region, disproportionate to its already high rate of firearm ownership, though well below the rate for Switzerland and far below the rate for the United States (IHME, 2023; Karp, 2018). Firearm suicide accounts for one third of total deaths by suicide for Finnish men over age 70. Worldwide, older men are especially likely to use guns to end their lives.

Lagom, Sexual Harassment, and Cultural Conflict in an Industrial Champion: Sweden

Ebba S. was a 30-year-old junior executive in the business development department of a Swedish manufacturing company. She was an agreeable and conscientious person, reserved at first but able to relax and have a good time. She was ambitious and had always been open to new experiences, especially enjoying travel and outdoor activities. For three months she had not been herself. A year earlier, everything seemed to be right, but life had taken a downturn. Ebba was good-looking and in great physical condition, and before her current troubles she had dressed and made up with style and taste. She had worked out every morning and played tennis at a club twice a week. She had a few friends from college and business school, and she had fun with them on the weekends. She and her long-term boyfriend Liam had recently decided to wed.

Since she had been feeling low, she was waking up without energy, with no motivation to exercise and no excitement about going to work. She no longer cared about looking her best. She would wear simple, businesslike outfits instead of the more fashionable and feminine clothing she had once liked. When she was with Liam, she often felt distant from him, as if playing a role without passion. She'd had several migraine headaches since her trouble started. Migraine had been a problem for her in her teens but had seemed to resolve by the time she graduated from college.

About a year before this, Ebba's supervisor at work—an older man whom Ebba loved as a teacher and mentor—retired and was replaced by Axel T., a 48-year-old man, married with two children, and an alumnus of the same university as Ebba. At first, she liked him—he was smart and experienced, and she felt she had much to learn from him. As they got acquainted, Ebba told Axel she was engaged, described Liam, and asked Axel about his wife and children. A few months after Axel became her supervisor, things began to happen that troubled her. One evening Ebba and Axel had drinks together after work, and after a few cocktails, Axel kissed her forcibly, touching her in a way that made her uncomfortable. She attributed his behavior to intoxication and didn't make a lot of it. After that episode, she noticed him ogling her at work. When they would meet in his office, he would close the door, and sometimes she'd feel strange enough that she'd open it. He would arrange off-site meetings and business travel in a way that often put them together alone. On one business trip, when they were socializing with customers, Axel behaved as if he and Ebba were a couple, embarrassing her with his verbal and physical familiarity. Axel then started sending her romantic and sexual text messages.

Ebba knew that Axel's behavior was inappropriate but hadn't made any complaint to the company's human resources department, though she told herself she surely would if Axel ever tried to force himself on her physically. She thought that having chosen to work in a "masculine" business like manufacturing, she should be able to handle occasional male misbehavior. She criticized herself for not being able to take Axel's behavior less seriously and to defend herself with skill and humor.

One evening Liam told her that he still loved her, that he didn't want to break up, but that he wanted to delay their wedding. Ebba felt deeply shaken. She lost sleep worrying about losing her relationship with Liam and doubted her ability and her attractiveness. Sometimes she would have flashbacks of times that Axel had acted especially creepy. One evening when she and Liam had a date, she looked so miserable that he asked her what was wrong, and she broke down and told him the story of her sexual harassment at work. He responded with concern and anger. With much encouragement from him, Ebba complained to her company's human resources department. She was offered a lateral move to a position in another unit of the company, reporting to a female boss. Her new job was at a different office, much farther from her apartment. Her workday now began and ended with an hour-long commute. After Ebba's complaint was reviewed by the human resources department, Axel got a warning but faced no other consequences.

At Liam's urging, Ebba saw a psychiatrist, who diagnosed MDD. With the history suggesting that her depression was reactive to a highly stressful situation that was going to be resolved, the psychiatrist suggested beginning with psychotherapy alone rather than immediately starting medication. Two months later, with the job change, psychotherapy, and Liam's support, Ebba's depression remitted, and her headaches improved.

Sweden, the most populous Nordic country, has a Viking heritage and was a regional military power in the 17th and 18th centuries, at its peak controlling Finland, part of the Baltic States, and part of northern Germany. It was, like Switzerland, neutral in World War I and World War II and in the Cold War. It industrialized early in the 20th century, becoming a high-income nation before the World War II. After that war, it became a welfare state, with redistribution of income, universal healthcare, and strong public education. Sweden did not suffer the trauma of invasion by foreign powers or of civil war. It has for over a century been known for innovative technology, and its system of income support and national healthcare lowers the risk for people wanting to start new enterprises. Swedes are in general less introverted and more expressive than Finns; they also are more formal in their communication. Residents of neighboring Nordic countries sometimes characterize Swedes as arrogant (Booth, 2014).

Sweden ranks highest in the European Union on its Gender Equality Index, but there are signs of trouble. Sweden has the highest rate of sexual violence among the Nordic nations and a remarkably high rate of sexual harassment in workplaces and educational institutions. There is also pervasive gender stereotyping. For example, only 25% of Swedes educated in science, technology, engineering, and mathematics are women; and women have difficulty gaining promotion to management positions in technology-based companies. More generally, women in Sweden are under-represented in executive and top management positions in most sectors of the economy (Khazan, 2018; Lundeteg et al., 2017; Magnusson, 2018). Prompted by the "Me Too" movement in America, thousands of Swedish women have come forward to tell of sexual harassment in a broad range of occupations, professions, and schools (Nordberg, 2017).

In the 2012 EU survey mentioned earlier with respect to IPV in Finland, women were asked about experiences of sexual harassment, both in the past 12 months and since age 15. Sweden and Denmark led the European Union in prevalence of sexual harassment of more severe kinds, involving such behavior as unwanted touching and kissing and sending unwanted sexually explicit texts and emails. Sexual harassment was especially prevalent among women with tertiary education: In the cited survey, 83% of college-educated Swedish women and 76% of college-educated Danish women had experienced severe sexual harassment since the age of 15.

Table 13.7, based on data from this study, shows sexual harassment prevalence data for employed women in Denmark, Finland, and Sweden, with the EU average for comparison. Denmark and Sweden have exceptionally high rates of sexual harassment, while Finland's rates are closer to the EU average. More than half of employed women in Sweden have experienced sexual harassment from someone related to their employment, and 22% experienced one of the more severe forms of sexual harassment in the past 12 months. Because Iceland, Norway, and Switzerland are not in the European Union, precisely comparable data are not available. However, in a 2021 global survey, at least 45% of employed women in all five Nordic countries reported having experienced workplace sexual harassment at least once since age 16, in contrast to a rate of 29% in Switzerland (Lloyd's Register Foundation, 2023). It is possible that women in the Nordic countries are more inclined to recognize and acknowledge harassment than those from other countries, but a permissive attitude toward workplace harassment or denial of its harm appears to characterize the region.

The experience of sexual harassment at work in European countries is most prevalent among university-educated women working in management or in

Table 13.7 Sexual Harassment of Employed Women in Denmark, Finland, and Sweden—2012 Survey

Country	Experience of harassment since age 15	Experience of one of the six most severe forms of harassment since age 15	Experience of harassment by someone from employment context since age 15	Experience of harassment in past 12 months	Experience of one of the six most severe forms of harassment in past 12 months
Denmark	82%	73%	52%	34%	23%
Finland	71%	63%	37%	23%	16%
Sweden	82%	76%	54%	34%	22%
EU Average	59%	49%	37%	23%	14%

Note. Data from European Agency for Fundamental Rights (2014). Violence against women: an EU-wide survey. https://fra.europa.eu/en/publications-and-resources/data-and-maps/survey-data-explorer-violence-against-women-survey. Data were not available for Iceland, Norway, and Switzerland as they are not members of the European Union.

one of the professions, with the risk higher for younger women. In European countries overall, three-quarters of women in professional or top management positions had been harassed at least once since the age of 15, and 27% of women with university degrees reported being harassed at least once in the past 12 months (Latcheva et al., 2017). Across the European Union, 35% of women who had been harassed did not talk to anyone about the most severe harassment they had ever experienced, and the percentage was higher in Sweden. When such women were asked their reasons for not talking about it, more than half said they thought they could deal with it themselves, and about a third said it was not serious enough to talk about. However, when asked about the long-term consequences of their worst episode of sexual harassment, many women cited problems with anxiety, loss of self-confidence, difficulties in relationships, trouble sleeping, and depression (European Union Agency for Fundamental Rights, 2014). Women who experienced one or more episodes of violence in childhood were more than twice as likely to have a recent experience of sexual harassment as an adult (Latcheva, 2017). This contributes to a link between adult harassment and depression since ACEs increase a person's lifetime risk of MDD.

It would be reasonable to wonder why rates of sexual harassment and violence against women are so high in a country with a tradition of collective action to solve social problems. Severe sexual harassment by employers is against Swedish law, as is physical or sexual violence against women, whether within or outside of a marriage or domestic partnership. An important factor is the attitude of Swedish women themselves. In the same EU survey, women who had been victims of physical or sexual violence and had not called the police or made a formal report were asked why they didn't and how they coped. Their most common reason for not calling the police after an episode of violence was "too minor/not serious enough/never occurred to me" (38%). When asked what helped them overcome their most serious experience of IPV, women's most common response was "my personal strength and decisiveness" (48%). The survey results give the impression that Swedish women are tough—until they aren't.

Sweden is a largely urban (86%), wealthy, industrial country. Its manufacturing is competitive in a global economy because of its innovative designs and technology, the quality of its products, and its world-famous brands, rather than low labor costs or inexpensive raw materials. It is the third largest exporter of popular music after the United States and the United Kingdom, and it has novelists and film directors with global audiences. Most Swedes are classified as Lutheran Protestants, but only 5% regularly attend church, and when surveyed, most Swedes say they are atheists (TheLocal.se, 2015). Sweden has the largest foreign-born population of all the Nordic countries, and immigration continues. In 2016, over 18% of its population were foreign-born, 5% were born in Sweden to two foreign parents, and 7% were born in Sweden with one foreign parent. At that time, 46% of the immigrants were from other European countries; 25% were from the Middle East, North Africa, or western Asia; 11% were from eastern, western, or southern Africa; and the remainder were from assorted countries in Asia and the Americas (Statistics Sweden, 2024).

Sweden's political traditions are based on consensus-building rather than conflict. A Swedish word, *lagom*, roughly translatable as "just the right amount" or "enough but not too much," is used to characterize comfortably balanced solutions to problems. If a group were sharing a case of wine, the portion allotted to a member would be *lagom* if everyone getting that amount would exactly use up the case. Coffee of *lagom* strength would be enough to wake up the drinker without making them jittery. Sweden's solutions to its income inequality are intended to be *lagom*, reducing poverty without removing people's incentives to achieve or rewarding laziness.

There are several ways in which Sweden's *lagom* culture can contribute to its residents' mental health problems. Individuals who are hypomanic or hyperthymic and grandiose, expansive, given to boasting, or simply intense do not conform to the expectations of mainstream Swedish culture for humility and modesty and may face social distancing as a result. However, Swedes in the performing arts may, as they do in other cultures with restrained traditions, have greater license to exhibit signs of bipolarity without a social penalty. Another aspect of *lagom* culture that indirectly contributes to depression in women is Sweden's relatively moderate, *lagom*, response to its problems of sexual harassment and violence against women and to its difficulties integrating a large multicultural and multiracial immigrant population.

Sweden is characterized by cultural paradoxes. It is one of the world's leading manufacturers and exporters of weapons, but it has welcomed a disproportionate share of refugees from conflict zones. Sweden generates globally popular cultural exports, but Swedes are viewed by their Nordic neighbors as work-focused and lacking in playfulness. It ranks high on measures of gender equity, but it has high rates of physical and sexual violence against women, both by partners and by non-partners. Although its economy is strong, Sweden has a significant problem with youth unemployment. Unemployed or underemployed Swedish young adults do not lack housing, food, or medical care; but they have low status in a society that highly values work. Unemployment is stigmatized in mainstream Swedish culture, and unemployed young adults often stigmatize themselves. In a retrospective study of hospital admissions for depression, self-harm, or substance use of young adult residents of Sweden's three largest cities (aged 20-24), those neither employed nor in tertiary education had a significantly higher likelihood of hospitalization than others of their age, even after controlling for age, sex, adoption status, maternal risk factors and maternal country of origin. The odds ratios were impressively high: 2.4x for depression, 2.8x for self-harm, 3.1x for alcohol use disorders and 7.0x for drug abuse (Sellström et al., 2011). For Swedish adults of working age, the probability of a psychiatric hospitalization doubled when previously employed people lost their jobs (Hollander et al., 2013).

As noted above, Sweden has the highest proportion of immigrants among the Nordic countries. In the late 1990s, Sweden had a million foreign-born residents. Its immigrant population increased gradually until 2010; immigration accelerated rapidly after that until Sweden changed its immigration policies in 2015 in response to an unprecedented influx of 162,877 asylum seekers in that single year (Skodo, 2018). Historically, immigrants to Sweden from Europe came for employment, for education, or to join family members already in Sweden. Most recent immigrants to Sweden, more than half from outside Europe, include large numbers of refugees from Syria, Iran, Iraq, Turkey, and Afghanistan. Asylum seekers include many victims of trauma, including rape and torture, and unaccompanied children who were orphaned or traumatically separated from their families. In 2015 alone, there were 45,765 unaccompanied minors, mostly teenage boys, who came to the Nordic countries seeking asylum. Claims for asylum in Sweden are adjudicated within a year after the migrants' arrival in the country, and if they are not granted asylum, they must leave. In 2016, 77% of claims for asylum were approved; in 2017, the approval rate was 46%. Asylum seekers may live anywhere in Sweden while they await a decision. They are distributed around the country, with many in less densely populated parts of Sweden. Notwithstanding, the largest immigrant communities are in Sweden's major cities, in Stockholm, Gothenburg, and Malmö, where more than one quarter of the population is foreign-born (Statistics Sweden, 2024).

For immigrants to Sweden who are refugees fleeing war or persecution, or economic migrants from low- and middle-income countries, mental health issues are typical. Many in the refugee communities will have post-traumatic stress disorder with secondary depression. Immigrant children with early traumatic separation or loss will have lifetime vulnerability to depression.

First-generation immigrants who do not speak Swedish and have only primary education may have trouble finding regular employment. Depression can arise in a context of low-income, low-status, irregular employment and being the target of prejudice and discrimination. In some of the Muslim immigrant communities in Sweden, IPV within marriage is culturally accepted, and victim blaming is common. A woman's going outside the community for help in stopping the IPV or in dealing with depression that may result from it often is discouraged by her community. An even more disturbing phenomenon related to Sweden's influx of migrants is a disproportionate number of migrant men identified as perpetrators of rape. Many of the men convicted of rape in Sweden are natives of countries where women do not have the freedom to safely be alone in public. In addition to the trauma experienced by the victim of rape, the widespread understanding by Swedish women that they are less safe affects their emotional well-being. Migrants to Sweden from cultures with gross gender inequality must acculturate to one of the world's most gender-equal societies. Though Sweden has reduced its acceptance of migrants, it must still find a solution to facilitate the acculturation of its immigrants or suffer damage to the high trust and social cohesion of which it is justly proud. The Swedish healthcare system is working to find effective responses for the acculturation and mental health needs of its immigrant communities, but much remains to be done.

Though Sweden leads in its acceptance of immigrants, all the Nordic nations have had a significant immigrant influx in the past two decades. Mental health issues related to immigration are least prevalent in Finland, which has had the least immigration of the Nordic countries. Only 6% of its population are foreign-born, and many of the foreign-born residents of Finland are either from Sweden or from one of the Baltic nations. The cultural distance of such immigrants from native Finns obviously is far less than it is for immigrants from Asia, Africa, or the Middle East.

Hygge Culture, Indulgence, and Its Consequences: Denmark

Denmark is the oldest monarchy in Europe, dating back to the time of the Vikings. It once controlled Sweden and Norway and parts of what is now Germany and had colonies in Iceland, Greenland, the Caribbean islands, and Tranquebar on the south coast of India. Since the 17th century, Denmark progressively lost territory and international influence but at the same time became educated and industrialized. Most of the population moved to the cities, while rural Denmark became devoted to large-scale export-oriented agriculture. In World War II, Denmark was invaded and controlled by Germany, though the Danes continued to resist the Germans, an example being their rescue of most of their Jewish population by smuggling them to neutral Sweden. After the war, Denmark became a high-income welfare state with high equality after taxes and transfers and highly subsidized healthcare, education, and retirement income. The country's culture reflects its former grandeur as an imperial power; the

Danes have a sense of security and national pride atypical for a country with a relatively small area and population that shares a border with a major power. They are more indulgent and hedonistic than the Norwegians and the Finns.

Much as *sisu* is associated with Finland and *lagom* is associated with Sweden, the word *hygge* is associated with Denmark. *Hygge* refers to a pleasant feeling of coziness, safety, comfort, and quiet joy, with connotations of personal wholeness, well-being, and interpersonal harmony; "finding happiness in the little things in life"; and "finding magic in the ordinary." Several popular books by Danes offer advice to foreigners on how to make their lives more *hyggelig*. Danish author Tove Ditlevsen put it elegantly: "*Hygge* is a state of being you experience if you are at peace with yourself, your spouse, the tax authorities and your inner organs" (Goodreads.com, 2021). *Hygge* enthusiasts say the feeling makes everyday life sublime and enables Danes to fully enjoy their country's egalitarian, secure, modest, and understated lifestyle. Cynical people, minimizing its elements of mindfulness and healthy present orientation, see *hygge* culture as encouraging people to be passive and mellow when circumstances might call for decisive action and the word as a useful buzzword for sellers of handmade woolens, specialty coffees, and scented candles.

From a psychiatric perspective, *hygge* is an antidepressant. *Hygge* experience entails positivity, interpersonal connection (social capital), and mindfulness. Having more *hygge* could be an outcome of mindfulness meditation and behavioral activation therapy, both of which are sometimes effective evidence-based non-pharmacologic treatments of depression. If *hygge* is the antidepressant built into Danish life, things that disrupt it increase depression risk. IPV against women is even more prevalent in Denmark than in it is in Finland. IPV can provoke depression through trauma or the separation of a couple. In addition, it can disrupt a woman's *hyggelig* home life. A woman might have daily strain from her job, childcare, marital conflicts, and perhaps a physical condition like diabetes yet have excellent mental well-being because of frequent experiences of *hygge*. After an episode of IPV, *hygge* might be hard to find at home. If she does not find enough alternative occasions for positive thoughts and feelings, depression might ensue. In a similar way, sexual harassment at work can make it difficult to find *hygge* there.

While young Danish women (aged 20–39) have a high exposure to IPV and to sexual harassment, they do not show the high rates of MDD and suicide seen in Sweden. One hypothesis for Denmark's relatively low depression prevalence in young women is that they enjoy a high level of social capital and positive life experiences including *hygge*. The prevalence of MDD in Danish women rises as they get into their 40s. By that point in life many Danish women will have one or more chronic medical conditions, such as type 2 diabetes or obesity. Then even a life full of *hygge* might not be enough to prevent depression.

Especially relevant to depression in Denmark is its pleasure-seeking culture. Although they do not have the Finns' culture of binge drinking, the Danes have a higher annual per capita alcohol consumption than the Finns. As previously noted, the Danes consume more sugar, more meat, and less seafood than their Nordic peers, that is, a diet with relatively more depressing foods and relatively more risk of atherosclerosis. *Hygge* culture, with its cozy, indoor experiences, is associated with lower average physical activity of Danes compared to Finns or Swedes (WHO, 2023). These three lifestyle factors contribute to depression in Danish adults, both directly and via a higher prevalence of chronic cardiovascular diseases associated with depressive sequelae.

While Denmark does not report an unusually high consumption of tobacco relative to other countries in Western Europe, it has a remarkably high rate of chronic obstructive pulmonary disease (COPD) in its middle-aged and older residents (IHME, 2023). This suggests that smoking might be more widespread than reported, that Danes continue to smoke despite the early signs of lung disease, or that smoking interacts with other environmental and/or genetic factors. Whatever the explanation, COPD is associated with a high prevalence of comorbid depression, and the Danes' pleasure-seeking culture might keep people smoking when symptoms of lung disease should prompt them to quit. Similarly, Danish culture has very liberal sexual mores, with casual sex, unprotected intercourse, and marital infidelity more prevalent than in most countries of Western Europe; prostitution is legal in Denmark. Sexually transmitted diseases are epidemic. For example, 35,680 cases of chlamydia were reported in 2019, implying the highest incidence rate in the European Union (European Centre for Disease Prevention and Control, 2022). In a study of the Danish population, a single positive test for chlamydia implied significantly increased risks of future infertility and of ectopic pregnancy (Davies et al., 2016). Consequences of Danish sexual behavior that can lead to depression include sexually acquired infections and their complications, unwanted pregnancy, unwanted infertility related to sexually acquired infections, and divorce due to marital infidelity.

In sum, Denmark overall has less MDD than Finland, Sweden, or Norway. When Danes do develop MDD, the condition might arise in the context of general medical disease for which the Danes' indulgent culture puts them at greater risk. It is possible also that there is more clinical depression (using the broader definition) than the relatively low prevalence of MDD might suggest. The Danes' use of alcohol, food, sex, and *hygge* experiences might sufficiently mask or dilute depressive symptoms to the point where they would not meet

MDD criteria yet would cause people distress and impair their physical, social, and/or occupational function.

Gender Equality, Male Ambivalence, and Collective Action: Norway

Norway is remarkable for its low prevalence of MDD in women and low suicide mortality in men; both are significantly lower than the rates for Western Europe overall and for Sweden and Finland. It ranks second out of 146 nations for gender parity in World Economic Forum's *Global Gender Gap Report* (2023); only Iceland ranks higher. While Norway's gender equality partially explains its low rate of depression in women, its low rate of suicide in men suggests that other cultural factors are involved. One such factor is Norway's remarkable public investment in mental health services and its collective efforts to reduce the stigma of depression.

In 1997 the Norwegian parliament resolved that the public health system wasn't doing enough to deal with mental illness. The following year, Kjell Magne Bondevik (b. 1947), prime minister of Norway (1997–2000; 2001–2005), acutely developed MDD. He immediately disclosed his illness, took leave from his work, and was effectively treated. Upon his return a month later, he received over 1000 letters from Norwegians conveying the sentiment that his self-disclosure had enabled them to speak more freely about their issues with depression. The Norwegian parliament subsequently approved an eight-year, $4.3 billion clinical and research initiative to improve mental health services in Norway. Three years later, Bondevik was re-elected to another four-year term (Jones, 2011). Considered relative to Norway's population at the time of 4.8 million people, its $4.3 billion investment represented an incremental investment of about $112 per capita per year. Adjusting for inflation and for the size of the population, this would be equivalent to the United States making a commitment in 2023 of $66.6 billion per year in new resources for mental health services and research. For comparison, the 2023 budget for the U.S. National Institute of Mental Health was $2.2 billion.

Beginning immediately after Norway began investing in its mental health services, its prevalence of MDD began to decline. As of 2019, its prevalence of MDD was lower than that of Western Europe overall both for men and for women (See Table 3.1). Furthermore, the real improvement is probably greater than prevalence statistics suggest because fewer cases of MDD now go undiagnosed. Norway's response to its mental health needs and to its prime minister's depressive episode comports with its being a high-trust, communitarian (but not collectivistic) society.

Norway has been a leader in addressing issues of gender equality and of the treatment of women since the late 19th century. As the American social critic James Miller noted in his analysis of *Uncle Tom's Cabin* and the rise of abolitionism (J. Miller, 2008), seminal works of popular culture anticipate and help precipitate social and political change. One of Norway's literary giants was the playwright Henrik Ibsen (1828–1906). In his classic *A Doll's House* (1879/1961) Ibsen dramatized the oppressiveness of bourgeois marriage. At the end of the play, the heroine leaves her husband to find a new and independent life. This was a radical conclusion at a time in history where in most parts of the world women did not have full legal rights. In his equally famous play *Hedda Gabler* (1890/1961), the leading character is a powerful, autonomous, intellectual, and emotionally conflicted woman whose decisions change, and sometimes destroy, others' lives. Ibsen depicts women as people with full agency, often with stronger characters than the men in his plays. Admiration of strong women is part of Norway's national character, though it has competed with unwritten rules discouraging self-assertion. The following vignette from *A Doll's House* dramatizes its heroine Nora's strength and her husband Helmer's dumbfounded response to it.

HELMER: But this is disgraceful. Is this the way you neglect your most sacred duties?

NORA: What do you consider is my most sacred duty?

HELMER: Do I have to tell you that? Isn't it your duty to your husband and children?

NORA: I have another duty, just as sacred.

HELMER: You can't have. What duty do you mean?

NORA: My duty to myself.

HELMER: I would gladly work night and day for you, Nora—bear sorrow and want for your sake. But no man would sacrifice his honor for the one he loves.

NORA: It is a thing hundreds of thousands of women have done.

HELMER: To desert your home, your husband and your children! And you don't consider what people will say!

NORA: I cannot consider that at all. I only know that it is necessary for me.

Nora's self-assertion is shocking to her husband. Beyond that, he can hardly believe her lack of concern about his feelings or about the reactions of others. Today, a Norwegian might be shocked if a contemporary Helmer's feelings did make a difference to her.

While Norway has been a pioneer in feminism, male backlash against feminism has an equally long history. Changes in Norway's laws to give women the vote (1913) and to outlaw marital rape (1971) had their opponents at the time. Men as the innocent victims of feminist overreach, the "feminization" of Europe, and "replacement of patriarchy with matriarchy" are contemporary tropes and memes on Norwegian social media and alt-right websites. In a malignant variation, men complaining about Norway's feminism have asserted that men have a God-given right to sexually dominate women and that women should not control their own sexual lives or reproductive decisions. A more common yet consequential expression of antifeminism is the cyberstalking of women by men whose advances were rejected. Victims of cyberstalking can experience physical and emotional symptoms of acute stress and can develop depression if the stalking is continuing or recurrent. When a man who embraces antifeminist ideology loses to a woman in competition for a job, a promotion, or acceptance by an educational institution, he may develop feelings of angry victimhood. When a man with such feelings is in an intimate relationship with a woman, there is a high risk of IPV, with both the perpetrator and the victim at risk for poor mental health outcomes.

Norway has "cultural antidepressants" in the form of four-season outdoor activity and traditions that facilitate building and maintaining trust and social capital. Norwegians celebrate charity and community service and have a special word, *ildsjel* (literally "fire-soul") to describe people who energetically pitch in to help others. Norwegian Americans, who are concentrated in the upper Midwest, Washington State, and California, are approximately as numerous as Norwegians in Norway and have a reputation for community orientation and appreciation of volunteerism and public service.

Norwegians have a word, *kos*, with a meaning close to that of the word *hygge* in Danish. *Kos* experiences need not be literally cozy; they might just be perfect moments. Norwegians are encouraged by their culture and language to be mindful and live in the present. There is a Norwegian expression, *Glad i deg* (literally "happy in you"), which enables a person to tell another that their connection gives them happiness, without any romantic or sexual implication or presumption of excessive familiarity. Moments of meaningful connection between people are recognized and appreciated.

Like the other Nordic cultures, Norwegian culture values humility and modesty and is suspicious and/or disapproving of any behavior suggesting boasting or self-aggrandizement. This creates the risk of disapproval or social distancing for a Norwegian with a bipolar spectrum condition who has periods of hyperthymic or hypomanic expansiveness, talkativeness, and/or grandiosity. The social consequences of a bipolar person's hypomanic or mixed symptoms might accelerate the switch into a depressed phase of illness. Norwegian culture discourages individuals from talking about their mental distress. However, acknowledging that depression is a problem *for the community* and creating resources to help those who are depressed is fully compatible with Norway's ethos. As a demonstration, Norway's national health authority set up a public resource for providing immediate psychological help—in the form of cognitive-behavioral therapy—for people who presented with mental distress and had generalized anxiety or a non-psychotic, non-bipolar depression without significant suicidal ideation. When the service was utilized, it was efficacious; but many depressed people—predominantly men, people without secondary education, and immigrants—had brief contact with the service and did not follow through (Knapstad et al., 2018).

Norway's rural population benefits from substantial investments of government money in education, healthcare, and infrastructure in the country's non-metropolitan areas. Access to mental health services is relatively good in rural Norway, though many Norwegians with mental health issues do not use them because of the greater stigma of psychiatric or psychological treatment in the rural population. The prevalence of MDD in rural areas is not higher overall, but specific groups of rural residents are at especially high risk. Farmers in Norway have a high risk of depression, from a combination of factors also found in farmers in other Nordic countries and in Switzerland. These will be discussed in detail below, in connection with Switzerland's high rate of depression and suicide in the residents of its rural areas.

In northern Norway and contiguous areas of Finland and Sweden there is an indigenous population, the Sámi, sometimes also called *Lapps*, though the former term is now preferred. There are approximately 80,000 Sámi, about half of whom live in Norway. A minority now work at the traditional occupations of fishing, small-scale farming, and reindeer herding; most have assorted occupations not different from those of non-Sámi residents of northern Norway. Historically they faced prejudice, discrimination, poverty, and efforts by the Norwegian government to suppress the education of Sámi children in their native language and traditions. More recently, Norway has made efforts to improve conditions for the Sámi people. However, in all three Nordic countries, the impact of climate change on the fragile Arctic ecosystem—ironically including the environmental impact of wind farms aimed at reducing carbon emissions—is making traditional Sámi lifestyles less viable. The impact has been especially great on reindeer herding, the historical foundation of the Sámi economy (Wing, 2017). Many Sámi families both herd reindeer and have regular employment. Their herding activities are important for cultural identity (with its antidepressant effects), and the intense outdoor activity and healthy diet associated with the traditional lifestyle have benefits for both physical and mental health. As reindeer herding has declined, the prevalence of obesity, diabetes, and other lifestyle-related diseases has increased. The prevalence of symptoms of anxiety and depression now exceeds that of non-indigenous Norwegians. Stress related to work contributes significantly to their emotional symptoms (Kaiser et al., 2010).

Sámi children and teenagers living in areas where Sámi people are a minority are subject to bullying at school; this is less common in areas where they are the majority group (Kvernmo, 2004). Adults who live in majority-Sámi areas are less likely to encounter prejudice and discrimination.

Sámi people differ in their level of identification with the culture, knowledge of the Sámi language, and observance of cultural traditions. People who are bicultural—fluent in the Sámi language as well as Norwegian (or Swedish or Finnish)—have a lower rate of depression. The Norwegian Arctic Adolescent Health Study showed that the protective effect of a strong ethnic identity against common mental health problems begins well before adulthood (Bals et al., 2010).

In traditional Sámi culture, men are expected to be stoic, not to complain, and not to talk about their emotions. In the extreme, they feel that death is preferable to displaying emotional weakness. Such men would choose suicide over acknowledging depression and seeking treatment for it (Stoor et al., 2019). These attitudes have been changing as Sámi adopt more of mainstream Norwegian, Swedish, or Finnish culture.

As in Sweden with its culture of *lagom*, the norms of political and business life in Norway call for consensus and avoidance of overt conflict. This can at worst lead to the denial, minimization, or lack of response to real problems, as it does in Sweden in connection with the problem of sexual harassment. One such problem in Norway is violence against women.

Although Norway's low rate of MDD in women is encouraging, it is not explained by a lack of IPV between men and women. An estimate for Norway obtained from a random sample of women aged 20–55 gave a lifetime incidence of IPV of 26.8%, with 5.5% experiencing IPV in the past 12 months. Of the women reporting an experience of IPV in their lives, more than half had experienced moderate violence like having been kicked or beaten with fists, and 8.8% had experienced severe violence like being strangled or threatened with a knife; 9.4% had been forced to have sex. Of women who had been injured repeatedly—about 8.0% of all victims of IPV—18.2% were receiving antidepressants at the time they were interviewed (Neroien & Chei, 2008).

An internet-based study of American men's attitudes toward IPV against women provides insight into the dynamics of IPV in countries like Norway with high gender equality. Blake and Brooks (2018) gave American single men online questionnaires on their attitudes about psychologically controlling behavior of men toward their female partners of the kind known to precede IPV. (This was done rather than ask subjects directly about IPV, which the investigators thought would evoke conventional expressions of disapproval.) On a random basis, they primed the subjects with material describing either a gender-equal or a gender-unequal context. The explainable variance in responses was mainly related to an interaction between status (*mate value*— attractiveness to a potential spouse) and gender equality. In a gender-equal context, high-status men were more accepting of controlling behavior toward female partners, while low-status men were less accepting. In a gender-unequal context, the opposite was the case. The hypothesis, supported by their findings, is that in a gender-equal context high-status men would be anxious that their partners will leave them or be unfaithful to them because their financial, legal, and psychological independence makes it easy for them to separate, and their time working or studying outside the home gives them opportunities to meet other men. This would lead them to be controlling to keep their partner attached and faithful; the risk of losing their partners would be offset by their confidence in their attractiveness to other women. Lower-status men would worry about losing their spouses or partners if they were too controlling, with subsequent trouble finding new ones because of their low status and damage to their reputations. In a gender-unequal context, a low-status man would be likely to feel he had license to be controlling with his spouse or partner and that his being controlling would not make him less desirable. He would be unlikely to fear abandonment or infidelity by his spouse or partner if he were controlling because she would probably not have good options for work or study outside the home, and she might worry about damage to her reputation. On the other hand, because of her vulnerability within the gender-unequal culture, he might have strong protective feelings.

This theoretical perspective is compatible with the higher rates of IPV observed in Norway in two groups: immigrant couples from gender-unequal cultures where controlling or even violent behavior toward women is common and native Norwegian couples where both partners are of high socioeconomic status. As noted previously, IPV is strongly associated with depression, either concurrent with ongoing IPV or as a sequel to it. Among recent immigrants to Norway are refugees from war zones who have experienced torture, rape, and/ or the traumatic death or injury of loved ones. Men with such experiences are at high risk of depression. They may perpetrate IPV as an externalization of depression or as an expression of anger permitted by the culture they left behind when they fled to Norway. People who migrate to Nordic countries for work, education, or family reunification have better general mental health and less depression than refugees and asylum seekers. They are less likely to be victims or perpetrators of IPV.

Norwegian men who are poorly educated or out of work are more likely to perpetrate IPV than employed, well-educated men. This might appear contradictory to the hypothesis above but may not be, for two reasons. First, many such men are from immigrant communities, which have lower education and higher unemployment rates than native Norwegians. Second, many such men have poorly educated partners who are not able to take full advantage of Norway's gender equality. If they are not employed outside the home or have poorly paid work, and no money under their direct control, it might not be easy for them to leave an abusive or otherwise unhappy relationship.

Subarctic Warmth: Iceland

Iceland is an island nation of approximately 340,000 people in the North Atlantic Ocean just below the Arctic Circle. Formerly part of Denmark, it has been independent since 1944. It consistently ranks in the top five happiest countries and in the top five for gender equality. Its prevalence of MDD is the lowest among the Nordic countries, while its consumption of antidepressant drugs is the highest. Like Norway, Iceland has an individualistic culture but is a high-trust social welfare state accustomed to taking community action. This was illustrated during the global financial crisis of 2008, which triggered a five-year economic depression in the country. Iceland was particularly hard-hit because it had become involved in international banking, with its banks handling assets many times greater than the nation's GDP. When the banks collapsed, the Icelandic government stepped in to support them, assuming billions in debt, devaluing the nation's currency, and restricting capital flows. Icelanders accepted the painful readjustment and carried on. The government conducted an extensive investigation that found fault with its own functions of regulation and oversight and named individuals responsible for errors and omissions. Public trust was preserved. During the economic depression there was no disruption of individuals' education or healthcare. The country's prevalence of MDD and its suicide mortality rates did not change during the country's economic depression. Remarkably, suicide rates did not rise in middle-aged men, the demographic most likely to experience damage to their financial status from which they would never recover. By contrast, Japan and South Korea saw large increases in middle-aged male suicide rates beginning with the onset of the financial crisis in 1997 and continuing for more than 10 years.

More than 90% of Icelanders are of Viking and Gaelic origins; the country is remarkably homogeneous genetically and ethnically. Immigrants currently comprise approximately 11% of the population, and people born in Iceland with at least one immigrant parent comprise another 6% (Heleniak & Sigujonsdottir, 2018). Immigrants come from many countries; 65% are European, and about half of the Europeans are Poles. There is little racism in Iceland as there are no minorities large or powerful enough to pose a threat to the majority. Iceland is 94% urban, with more than half of its population located in its capital region, metropolitan Reykjavik. It has remarkable income equality, with the world's second lowest World Bank Gini coefficient, 0.256. Its wealth inequality, while greater than its income inequality, is also among the lowest of all high-income nations. Fewer than 7% of its population live in poverty. Its low inequality of income and wealth, its high-trust culture, and its relative lack of racial and ethnic conflict imply high social capital, which is protective against depression under stressful circumstances.

The dominant Icelandic culture is oriented toward enjoyment of nature. The country is a place of great physical beauty, with mountains, glaciers, geysers, and hot springs. Skiing and snowmobiling, hiking, bathing, swimming in hot springs, and other outdoor activities expose Icelanders to light, physical exercise, natural environments, and pleasant social interaction during the winter months. There are thus several antidepressant factors built into the Icelandic lifestyle.

Icelanders have cultural traditions for building and preserving social connections which buffer stress and prevent loneliness. The Icelandic language has an all-purpose word for indicating that a situation should go no further down its present road: *jæja*. If a person were joking in bad taste or were in some other way making others uncomfortable with their behavior or speech, someone might use the word *jæja*. The person speaking or behaving inappropriately would get the message and stop but would not feel insulted. Positive relations would be preserved. Implicit is the idea that if people bother or offend others without malice, they should have the opportunity to stop without losing face.

The language also has an often-used phrase to offer encouragement and reassurance when something unfortunate happens, *þetta reddast*, which is roughly translated as "everything will work out" or "life will go on." Using the phrase is not as trivial as saying "Don't worry, be happy!"—it is an invitation to be mindful of the present and not unduly focused on the future. Another indicator of the Icelandic emphasis on social connection is how people are named. Icelanders do not have family names. They have only a patronymic or occasionally matronymic in addition to their given name, for example, Sigurður Jónsson or Guðrún Jónsdóttir ("Jon's son" or "Jon's daughter") rather than a surname that might be associated with a family's status and thereby place one Icelander above another by virtue of their birth. Furthermore, a person can only have a name from an approved list of official Icelandic names. If a baby's parents want to give their child a different name, they must apply to the government for permission. This too reduces social distance between Icelanders, as well as promoting acculturation of immigrants, who must give their Iceland-born children Icelandic names.

The time Icelanders spend regularly in natural surroundings contributes to their low prevalence of MDD. Time in natural environments, exposure to natural light, and living in proximity to "green space" have been shown to reduce mental distress (Beute & deKort, 2018; Min et al., 2017; Wu et al., 2015). Because of a combination of genetic and cultural factors, Icelanders have a much lower prevalence of seasonal affective disorder (SAD) than people of other nationalities who live at the same latitude (Magnusson et al., 2000). The difference is inherent in Icelanders and not in the specifics of the island's winter sunlight. A study in the Canadian province of Manitoba demonstrated significantly lower occurrence of SAD in people of Icelandic origin than in Canadians of other ethnic origins (Axelsson et al., 2002).

The public stigma of depression, and of mental illness in general, is low in Iceland. Population samples in Iceland, Germany, and the United States participated in a survey on the stigma of mental illness (Manago et al., 2019). Subjects were read case vignettes of a person with MDD or with schizophrenia and asked a broad range of questions to probe their attitudes about the person described. While 71.7% of Icelanders thought it likely or somewhat likely that the person would do something violent to themselves, only 15.2% were concerned that the person would do something violent to others. This was dramatically lower than the proportion of Americans—45.5%—who were concerned about mentally ill people's dangerousness to others.

More than 70% of Icelanders would accept a person with depression or schizophrenia as a friend, neighbor, or co-worker; and more than half were comfortable with the idea of the person described in the case vignette as an in-law. The sole type of relationship rejected by more than half of the Icelandic subjects was having the person with depression or schizophrenia care for their child. Icelanders' level of acceptance of people with mental illness was significantly higher than that of the Germans or the Americans. These results are particularly impressive because depression and schizophrenia were considered together, and schizophrenia is more consistently seen as "mental illness" rather than as a common emotional problem. The authors of the study partially attributed the inclusive attitude of Icelanders toward people with mental illness to the sympathetic, non-sensationalistic coverage of mental health issues including suicide in the Icelandic press, contrasting such coverage with the more sensationalistic press coverage encountered in most other countries. They called special attention to the focus of the American press on the potential dangerousness of people with mental illness.

Icelanders are avid consumers of antidepressant drugs, with the highest per capita consumption in Europe in 2020 (OECD, 2023c). Several factors contribute to this statistic. First, a high proportion of cases of depression are treated as depression is widely recognized and has little public stigma. Second, because Iceland is a high-trust society, patients tend to fill their prescriptions and take medication as prescribed or let their physicians know if there is a problem with their medication. Third, medication is covered by Iceland's national health plan and psychotherapy is not.

Though Iceland is an island in the North Atlantic far from both Europe and North America, its residents are strongly connected to Western Europe and North America by the internet. High-speed internet access is available in the most remote parts of Iceland, and 98% of the adolescent and adult population is regularly online, by either smartphone or computer. This makes telemedicine available to every Icelander if needed. The median daily screen time for an Icelandic adolescent is five hours (Hrafnkelsdottir et al., 2018). In a seven-country study of internet use by adolescents aged 14–17 in seven European countries, 8% of the Icelandic subjects had dysfunctional (addiction-like) internet behavior as measured by the Internet Addiction Test (Moon et al., 2018). Those who did had more self-reported depressive symptoms. Iceland's rate was the lowest of the seven countries studied; by contrast, over 22% of Spanish teenagers showed dysfunctional internet behavior (Tsitsika et al., 2014). Human interaction, including athletic and cultural activities, remains attractive to Icelanders despite the charms of the internet, and their frequency of attendance at cultural events and visiting of cultural sites is the highest in Europe (Eurostat, 2019b). Icelanders also read books for pleasure, and one in ten Icelanders will publish a book at some time in their life (Goldsmith, 2013).

Picturesque but Sad Countryside: Switzerland

Jean-Pierre C., a 62-year-old Swiss French farmer, lives and works on a 25-hectare dairy farm near the France–Switzerland border that has been in his family for four generations. He and his wife Camille love the rural life and are attached to their 200-year-old house and their animals. In the winter, their barn is full of cows and pigs, and they have a few chickens to keep them supplied with fresh eggs. In the summer Jean-Pierre takes the cattle up into the mountains to graze. Their milk is used to make the alpine cheese that brings the farm most of the money that keeps it going. When Jean-Pierre was younger, there were milk price supports that provided his family with a better income. Since these were phased out by the Swiss government, he and Camille have been working harder because they could no longer afford to hire help. As they've aged both he and Camille have developed health issues. For Camille it's osteoarthritis; for Jean-Pierre it's mild chronic bronchitis. Camille gets achy as she works, and during summer in the mountains Jean-Pierre often stops to catch his breath. They don't know how much longer their health will permit them to continue the hard work of farming.

The couple have two children in their early 30s—a son and a daughter. Both are college graduates, and both live in cities. Their daughter had thought about returning to the family farm but married a man who had grown up in Geneva and had no interest in the rural life. Their son had worked hard alongside his parents until he went to college and continued to work summers until he graduated. He now spends part of his annual vacation time on the farm, but he really couldn't do more than that.

Last year a neighbor had died by suicide, and Jean-Pierre often thought about him. They'd gone to school together and occasionally would drink together and share complaints about changing times and the hard work of farming. Jean-Pierre always woke up early to milk the cows, but he now wakes up earlier than usual, before sunrise, and lies in bed worrying about the future. He gets impatient when Camille complains about her aches and pains and regrets it later. He gets tired more quickly, and sometimes his chest feels heavy. He had his heart checked out, and all the tests were negative. The doctor told him his chest discomfort might be due to stress and hinted at his seeing a psychologist, but Jean-Pierre had never thought of himself as someone who would need counseling. He knew how to live his life.

He recently had an offer to buy his farm. It was attractive, but he was not ready to give up the work that he'd done all his life. What would he do if he didn't have the farm? His wife noticed he seemed preoccupied and humorless. One day she saw him cleaning his gun—the one he took home in the 1980s after his military service. She thought it best to hide the ammunition.

Switzerland is a wealthy and highly developed country with picturesque rural areas of which the Swiss are proud. The Swiss Alps are magnificent. The agricultural areas, with their natural beauty, traditional architecture, and simple and delicious cuisine are a tourist attraction and part of the national identity. The government is committed to preventing the depopulation of its rural areas. For years this took the form of price supports for milk. As these were phased out in connection with liberalization of international trade policies, subsidies were initiated for sustainable and organic farming. Most Swiss farms would not be economically viable without government subsidies, which in many cases account for more than half of a farm's total revenue. Even with subsidies, farmers have had to work hard for modest incomes. In 2013 the average income for a Swiss farmer was 47,000 CHF (approximately $55,000 in late 2023), of which one third came from non-agricultural employment. This is well below the median income for Switzerland. The average workweek for a self-employed farmer is 60 hours, highest among all occupational groups. 84% of all workers on farms are family members of the farmer, and one third receive no pay for their work (Swiss Federal Statistical Office, 2015). In Switzerland, farming is hard work for relatively low pay.

The rural areas of Switzerland are more conservative and traditional than its cities, with a much lower proportion of foreigners. While the urban–rural divide in culture, demographics, and epidemiology in Switzerland is like that of the Nordic countries and other high-income nations, the high percentage of the Swiss population that is rural makes it a larger public health issue. With respect to depression, the prevalence of clinical depression might be higher in the country than the city, but the prevalence of diagnosed MDD is lower. Depression can present differently—with "male depression" or with a somatoform condition—and there is more stigma for seeking and receiving psychiatric treatment. While all Swiss have health insurance that includes coverage for psychiatric conditions, its rural residents may not have easy access to specialized mental health care. In the case of Jean-Pierre, driving to the nearest clinic would take him 45 minutes each way during the daytime, meaning that he would lose almost 3 hours of precious time for farm work in addition to the annoyance of making the drive, parking in the city, and waiting to see the doctor. He felt he ought to face his problem without professional help. Though Switzerland has more psychiatrists per capita (50 per 100,000 population) than other high-income countries, the great majority of them practice in urban areas. Telemedicine and collaborative care are not widely available, so typically MDD is treated by primary care physicians with limited expertise in psychiatric diagnosis and the many pharmacologic and non-pharmacologic alternatives for its treatment.

Changes related to technological development, urbanization, and large-scale migration have widened the cultural and economic gap between metropolitan and rural areas. At the same time as a country's large cities show economic vitality and full employment, its rural areas might be economically depressed, with unemployment and underemployment, lower wages, lower-quality educational institutions, and little opportunity for occupational advancement or entrepreneurship. Migration of educated and talented people from rural to urban areas can make urban–rural differences even greater. In urban areas a country's traditional culture often is diluted or modified by contact with other cultures or exists alongside other cultures—whether the latter are foreign or native but non-conformist. In general, urban areas show greater awareness and lesser stigma of depression and other common mental health problems. A typical pattern is of more diagnosed, typical MDD in cities and more undiagnosed depression, somatoform presentations of depression, and "male depression" in rural areas. In addition to issues of awareness and stigma, simple inconvenience contributes to less consistent treatment of depression in Switzerland's rural areas. Rural residents involved in agricultural occupations have long working hours and cannot easily take time away from work during the day even when they own their farms and control their schedules. When free outpatient care is provided at public clinics, the distance a patient must travel to see a clinician is directly and negatively correlated with receiving care (Stulz et al., 2018).

Bipolar disorder (BD) is more common in urban areas of Switzerland. Diagnoses of bipolar spectrum conditions such as cyclothymia, bipolar II disorder (BD-II), and depression with mixed features are more likely to be made by psychiatrists than by primary care physicians. The latter are trained to recognize clinical depression and anxiety but not necessarily to differentiate conditions within the full spectrum of mood disorders. Furthermore, urban areas are more likely to attract and offer opportunity for individuals with talent and conditions in the bipolar spectrum that are adaptive most of the time.

Rural areas are associated with greater seasonality of suicide, with highest rates in the late spring. The seasonality of suicide is entirely explained by rates of violent suicide; the rate of poisoning is not seasonal. Drowning and hanging have the greatest seasonality; cutting and firearm use are less seasonal. In rural areas, more people are engaged in outdoor occupations where environmental changes involving light and dark, temperature fluctuations, and presence of allergens have the greatest impact. In Switzerland, the seasonal variations in suicide rates seen in rural areas are virtually absent in Zurich, its largest city. Switzerland's decline in the seasonality of suicide over the past century has paralleled the country's progressive urbanization (Ajdacic-Gross et al., 2005).

Reported rates of clinical depression are greater in the French- and Italian-speaking cantons of Switzerland: an average 8.9% versus 5.5% in the German-speaking cantons. The difference is even greater among women: 10.9% versus 5.7% (swissinfo.ch, 2017).

Studies of urban–rural differences in mental health conditions usually conclude that mental health is worse in urban areas (Peen et al., 2010). However, the higher rates of suicide in rural areas of many countries suggest that there may be methodological issues behind the observed differences, as well as a cultural "double-edged sword." Most studies of the issue dichotomize urban–rural status, yet there is clearly a great difference between a metropolis and a city of 50,000 in both culture and access to health services. Also, rural and small-town life can offer a high level of antidepressant social capital, but when key relationships are lost or disrupted, the adverse effects may be greater as fewer alternative sources of support may be available.

In high-income countries, rural residence often is associated with socioeconomic disadvantage, another reason for depressive symptoms (though not necessarily MDD) and increased risk of suicide. The lack of consistency in how countries aggregate and report their mental health and suicide statistics can make the impact of urban–rural factors as well as those related to latitude, altitude, and climate harder to discern and disentangle. In Switzerland rurality is associated with higher altitude. In Finland, Norway, and Sweden it is associated with higher latitude. Analyzing the association of urbanicity/rurality with depression, the biggest difference may be between metropolitan areas and others. Smaller cities and towns may have depression and suicide epidemiology, and mental health service use, more like those of rural areas than like those of major cities.

The rate of civilian gun ownership in Switzerland is one of the highest in the world; the Nordic countries except for Denmark have high gun ownership rates as well. Table 13.8, based on GBD data, shows 2019 male rates of firearm suicide for Switzerland and the Nordic countries, with rates for Western Europe and for the United States as benchmarks (IHME, 2023). Widespread ownership of guns

Table 13.8 2019 Male Firearm Suicide Mortality Rate per 100,000 People

Country	Age 15–49 Suicide by firearm	Age 15–49 Percentage of all suicides	Age 50–69 Suicide by firearm	Age 50–69 Percentage of all suicides	Age 70+ Suicide by firearm	Age 70+ Percentage of all suicides
Denmark	1.3	9%	2.9	12%	4.2	*13%*
Finland	**4.4**	**16%**	**7.8**	**24%**	**9.4**	**29%**
Iceland	1.7	10%	3.1	13%	7.3	*17%*
Norway	**2.6**	**15%**	3.7	**20%**	4.3	**23%**
Sweden	1.5	8%	3.9	15%	5.9	20%
Switzerland	**2.9**	**19%**	**6.7**	**25%**	**13.8**	**32%**
United States	**11.2**	**50%**	**18.4**	**61%**	**27.4**	**77%**
Western Europe	1.3	8%	3.0	13%	6.7	20%

Note. Data from IHME (2023). Mortality rates significantly higher than the benchmark rate for Western Europe are displayed in bold; rates significantly lower are displayed in italics. Percentages are highlighted to correspond with mortality rates.

is a Swiss national characteristic that directly contributes to its high suicide rate in older men.

Switzerland has universal national military service obligation for young men (participation in a national militia), and optional military service for young women. Between training courses and during weekend militia exercises, men store their military weapons at home. After their service, men have the option of buying their military weapon for a fee, and most men do. For most of them, that weapon is the only firearm they own. Beginning in 2003, fewer men were recruited for the militia, members were discharged at age 33 rather than age 43, and the fee was increased. Beginning in 2004, the rates of firearm suicide and of all suicide in men aged 18–34 fell significantly and remained lower than they had been before the policy changes. Decreased suicide rates were not seen in women or in older men. The reduction in firearm suicides was not offset by an increase in suicides by other means (Reisch et al., 2013).

Finland and Switzerland are outliers in Western Europe, both for their high male suicide mortality rates and for the proportion of suicides by firearm. Finland and Switzerland, and other countries like them in which firearms are used in a substantial percentage of male suicides, might especially benefit from public health strategies that encourage clinicians to carefully explore firearm ownership and safe storage with men at risk for suicide because of depression or personal crises.

Switzerland, which ranks below the Nordic countries on measures of economic opportunity and political empowerment for women, has a culture that is rated 70/100 on Hofstede's dimension of masculinity. Nonetheless, it has a lower prevalence of MDD in women than Finland or Sweden. The peak interval of MDD prevalence for women is 40-59, the midlife period that that includes menopause. Switzerland does not show the especially high prevalence of MDD in women under 30 that is encountered in the Nordic countries other than Denmark (see Table 13.1).

Data on sexual harassment, violence against women, and IPV are less available for Switzerland than for countries in the European Union including Denmark, Sweden, and Finland, but available data suggest there is significantly less IPV and sexual harassment in Switzerland than in the Nordic countries. A nationwide, extensive telephone survey conducted by the Swiss government found that 10% of employed women had reported a personal experience of sexual harassment in the past year and that 28% had experienced it at some time in their working life. Rates of experienced harassment were higher in German-speaking regions of the country than in French- and Italian-speaking regions, but rates of harassment of others observed by the study subjects were not significantly different between linguistic regions (Strub & Moser, 2010). The rates were significantly lower than those of the Nordic countries, despite the latter's having more gender equality. The discrepancy between experienced and observed harassment suggests that women in the French- and Italian-speaking regions of Switzerland are more adept at managing situations of harassment or are less troubled by them. Alternatively, women in German-speaking regions of Switzerland may be less willing to challenge authority or to express negative emotion in response to harassment, so they are less able to deter it.

Higher rates of reported MDD prevalence in French- and Italian-speaking regions of Switzerland might reflect a greater willingness of their residents to talk about their symptoms and lesser stigma of getting treated for depression. The higher female-to-male depression prevalence ratio in the French- and Italian-speaking regions might reflect greater gender inequality in those areas, paralleling the much greater gender inequality prevailing in France and Italy than in Germany (World Economic Forum, 2023). The higher rate of suicide in German-speaking areas might reflect a combination of less treatment of depression, less effective prohibition of suicide by Protestant Christianity than by Catholic Christianity, and more widespread ownership of guns and ammunition.

The combination of long-term orientation and masculinity in Swiss culture might contribute to Switzerland's high rate of death by suicide for men over age 70. In a country with expectations for male independence and success and an emphasis on planning for one's future, finding oneself lonely, dependent, and poor in old age might be especially unbearable for a man.

Chapter 14

American Regional Cultures and Geography of Mood

Mainstream American culture can easily be distinguished from the cultures of other high-income countries. In terms of Geert Hofstede's dimensions, it is high on individualism and indulgence, and low on power distance and long-term orientation. Its prevalent communication style is relatively direct and low-context (Hofstede-Insights, 2023; Liu, 2016). Nuclear families are more common than extended families, and 40% of children are born to unmarried parents (U.S. Census Bureau, 2023b). The United States (U.S.) ranks 43rd for gender parity among the 156 nations ranked by the World Economic Forum, behind the major nations of Western Europe and many countries of Latin America. Women are paid less than men for the same work and have lower average earned incomes; they are underrepresented on corporate boards and in Congress and state legislatures; and, despite equal education overall, far fewer women than men have advanced education in science and technology. The U.S. lags most upper-income nations in maternity leave and resources for childcare (World Economic Forum, 2023).

Americans' trust in people in general, in government, in public education, and in the media is low compared with the nations of northern Europe. Only 70% of adults over age 18 "completely trust" their own families (Gecewicz & Rainie, 2019; Wilcox & DeRose, 2017). In a survey of American adults conducted late in 2018, before the COVID-19 pandemic, respondents were asked three questions about their trust in other Americans: 47% of respondents opined that most people cannot be trusted, 58% that most people would try to take advantage of them if they had the chance, and 62% that most of the time people just look out for themselves rather than try to help others. Only 22% answered all three questions favorably, while 35% answered all three unfavorably. Trust was associated with older age, higher income, and more education. Black and Hispanic Americans were more likely to mistrust others than non-Hispanic White Americans. Mistrust of others was associated with mistrust of scientists, professors, public school principals, journalists, business leaders, and elected officials (Rainie et al., 2019). The United States' endemic mistrust recently had fatal consequences via refusal of vaccinations and masking during the COVID-19 pandemic. During the pandemic there were further increases in mistrust, exacerbated by political polarization and disinformation about the pandemic disseminated via social media.

The United States' income and wealth inequalities are the largest among major high-income nations, and they have been increasing (Chancel et al. 2022). In 2021 the top 10% of the U.S. population had an average income of $350,440 while the bottom 50% had an average income of $20,520—a ratio of 17:1. The average annual income of adults in the top 1% was approximately $1.4 million, 70 times greater than that of those in the bottom 50%. Inequality of wealth is even greater: In 2021, the top 1% of the U.S. population had a greater share of the country's wealth than the bottom 90%, and the average wealth of an adult in the top 1% was over 1000 times greater than that of one in the bottom 50%, and over 50 times greater than that of one in the middle 40%.

In the U.S., socioeconomic classes are "worlds apart." The financial distance between a rich and a poor American is far greater than that between an average American and an average citizen of China. However, inequality of wealth and income varies greatly between regions, states, and metropolitan areas of the U.S. Large differences in wealth and income translate into significantly different epidemiology, phenomenology, and outcomes for depression and bipolar illness.

Just as differences between America's socioeconomic classes are larger than many international differences, the subcultures of American regions differ from one another more than the cultures of many nations differ from those of their neighbors. Regional cultural identity intersects with people's other identities, including those related to ethnicity and class. An especially important aspect of this intersectionality relates to the traditional category of *race/ethnicity* as it appears in thousands of publications. The likely national origin, ethnic background, socioeconomic status, and cultural identity of a person categorized as *non-Hispanic White*, *Black/African American*, *Hispanic/Latino*, *Asian*, or *American Indian* (aka *Native American*) depends greatly on geography. A Black person in the Deep South, including northern Florida, is likely to be a descendant of American slaves. A Black person in southern Florida is more likely to have a Caribbean heritage, usually Jamaican, Haitian, Trinidadian, or Dominican (Thomas, 2012). In the western U.S. states most Hispanic Americans are of Mexican ancestry (including immigrants from Mexico). In south Florida, Hispanic people are more likely to identify as Cuban (28%), Puerto Rican (19%), or South American (19%) than Mexican (16%). Median household income is significantly higher for Cuban Americans than Mexican Americans, and the former are far more likely to be U.S. citizens (U.S. Census Bureau, 2023b).

American Indians have tribal identities, and from a culturally aware perspective they are distinguished by tribe, just as Hispanic people are distinguished by their national origin. Culturally, those who live on ethnically homogeneous reservations differ significantly from those of the same tribe who reside in metropolitan areas. Almost half of the over 600,000 American Indians in Arizona and New Mexico are members of the Navajo tribe. About two thirds of the tribe's members reside in the Navajo Nation, a rural territory covering 27,413 square miles of Arizona, New Mexico, and Utah; the remainder live in cities and towns in the two states (Discover Navajo, 2018). California's approximately 800,000 American Indians comprise dozens of different tribes, and 90% of them live in urban areas. Los Angeles County has the largest concentration of people of American Indian descent in the U.S.—163,464 on the 2020 Decennial Census (U.S. Census Bureau, 2024a). Lumping metropolitan Californians of varied indigenous descent with residents of the Navajo Nation is likely to obscure more than it illuminates.

Earlier chapters of this book have detailed depression-relevant differences between Chinese, Japanese, and Korean cultures. The cultures of Southeast Asia and South Asia differ even more from those of East Asia than the East Asian cultures differ from one another. It verges on absurdity to categorize an important segment of the American population as *Asian or Pacific Islander*, throwing together Maoris with Manchurians and Hmong with Hawaiians. An exemplary distinction within the Asian category is between Indian Americans, who as a group are more highly educated and have higher incomes and wealth than non-Hispanic Whites, and Bangladeshi Americans, whose median educational attainment and household income are well below those of the non-Hispanic White population (Budiman, 2024). A detailed presentation of intra-racial economic differences correlated with ethnic origin is presented in Chapter 7.

Cultures of American states and regions are influenced by their history and geography and by the ancestries of their majority populations. Most of the U.S. was originally settled by migrants from Great Britain and their descendants, who brought with them the social structures and shared values of the regions of Britain from which they migrated (Fischer, 1989). Subsequently, in the 19th and early 20th centuries, millions of migrants from Europe settled in America, each nationality in a distinctive pattern that is reflected in the 21st century by the distributions of self-described ancestry. We explored this theme in data from the 2022 American Community Survey (U.S. Census Bureau, 2021). In America's Upper Midwest, more than one quarter of the population claim German ancestry. People with Norwegian ancestry constitute more than 10% of the population of Minnesota and the Dakotas and more than 5% in Iowa, Wisconsin, Montana, and Washington. People with Italian roots are concentrated in the Northeast and those of French background in northern New England, in the three states adjacent to Quebec. Differences in ancestry and ethnicity among the non-Hispanic White population help explain economic and epidemiologic differences between adjacent states in the same region. For example, over 22% of the residents of Minnesota claim Scandinavian ancestry. This helps explain the state's more communitarian ethos, higher trust, greater support for government services, and higher gender equality compared with neighboring Wisconsin, which has similar racial demographics but is more Germanic than Scandinavian.

The U.S. is home to more immigrants than any other country. As of 2018 there were 44.8 million foreign-born U.S. residents, making up 14.1% of the American population (Budiman, 2020). An additional 12.3% of the population are second-generation immigrants—people with at least one foreign-born parent. More than half of America's immigrants live in four states: California, Florida, New York, and Texas. In most American states, fewer than 10% of the residents are foreign-born. Of the 16 states that are the focus of this chapter, immigrants constitute 10% or more of the population in four: Arizona (13%), Massachusetts (17%), Oregon (10%), and Washington (14%). In states with relatively high immigrant populations, there will be many urban neighborhoods and small cities in which more than half of the population will be immigrants from a specific country (e.g., Mexico) or region (e.g., Southeast Asia). In states with a low proportion of immigrants, foreign-born people will be treated as minorities most places they go. In areas with a high proportion of immigrants, elements of the cultures of the largest immigrant groups can become incorporated into the predominant local/regional culture, and the most prevalent minorities can become fully accepted as part of that culture. Some immigrants maintain a strong identification with their native culture, ultimately becoming bicultural (or multicultural), while others either minimize their non-native roots or don't assimilate American culture at all and largely confine themselves to a community of other immigrants from the same country. Immigrants' response to the challenges of acculturation are influenced by the regional and local culture of their new home. Assimilation will be easier if the regional and local cultures are compatible with an immigrant's native culture, and it can be quite difficult if the regional and/or local culture is rejecting of immigrants.

Salient Categories of Immigrants to the U.S.

The U.S. is home to approximately 10.5 million undocumented (aka unauthorized or illegal) immigrants (Krogstad et al., 2019). With a few exceptions, such as those brought to the U.S. as young children and some asylum seekers, undocumented immigrants are at ongoing risk of deportation. This is a source of chronic stress but also a powerful incentive for them to work hard, obey the law, conform with local customs, and build their social capital. In 2017, 80% of undocumented immigrants had lived in the U.S. for five years or more, 66% for 10 years or more, and half for over 15 years. Undocumented immigrants with long residence in the U.S. have established occupations, families, and social connections in the U.S. and might have children who speak only English. For them, deportation would be personally catastrophic, so they make great efforts to avoid it. Undocumented immigrants often for this reason will minimize contact with the healthcare system—including avoiding mental health care even if it is needed—out of concern that their precarious immigration status will be disclosed. Among clinically depressed Hispanic/Latino non-citizens studied in a national survey between 2014 and 2017, 27% of documented non-citizens reported use of antidepressants, but only 7% of undocumented non-citizens did so (Ross et al., 2019).

Highly educated immigrants, mostly from Asia, come to the U.S. in pursuit of educational and/or professional opportunities. They often have superior talent, industriousness, health, and resilience. Depending on their nationality, they might be subject to stereotyping and discrimination, which can be especially difficult for people who feel they have earned the respect of others.

Working-class immigrants often come from countries where the lives of working people are much harder and pay is much lower than in the U.S. First-generation working-class immigrants have incomes higher than they would have had in their native countries, and immigration brings improvement in their material circumstances, including their access to healthcare. They might have access to high-quality healthcare—including mental health care—for the first time in their lives. When the U.S. is a "happier" country than the one from which they emigrated, the overall happiness of first-generation immigrants usually is higher than that of the relatives they left behind. When their native country is happier than the host country, first-generation immigrants will be less happy than residents of the country they left, despite improvement in their incomes and living conditions (Hendriks et al., 2018).

Refugees from war or persecution include both more and less resilient personalities, but all have been exposed to traumatic events, either directly as victims or witnesses or indirectly via familial or other close relationships. Post-traumatic issues such as post-traumatic stress disorder (PTSD) are their predominant mental health issues shortly after immigration. After several years, depression increases in prevalence, especially among refugees who encounter financial hardship or discrimination in the host country. There are thus two peaks of prevalence of mental health problems in refugees—one in the first year after immigration and one five or more years later (Bogic et al., 2015; Giacco et al., 2018).

First-generation immigrants tend to have better health, after adjusting for socioeconomic class and other risk factors, than either natives or second-generation immigrants—the *healthy immigrant effect*. The effect is much weaker among refugees than among those who migrate for economic reasons (Lu & Ng, 2019).

Many immigrants come to the U.S. to join family members. Having relatives who are well established in their host country usually reduces immigrants' stress through material support, social support that begins immediately after their arrival in the U.S., and help with acculturation. However, immigrants having significant conflicts with relatives who sponsored and/or supported their immigration can be especially stressful.

Describing Regional Cultures

Regional culture has attracted increasing interest over the past two decades because of the ongoing decline in America's social capital and concerns that enduring cultural differences between regions may underlie health disparities and political strife that makes such disparities more difficult to resolve. An increase in rates of suicide and death by opioid overdose and liver disease—"deaths of despair"—is seen predominantly among non-Hispanic Whites without college education, living outside of large urban areas (Case & Deaton, 2015, 2017; Stein et al., 2017). A popular explanation of the phenomenon is that the benefits of economic growth and technological advances have been distributed unevenly and that, in many places, non-Hispanic White people without higher education who had expected to find stable, well-paid employment have found it difficult or impossible. Deep disillusionment and practical challenges of low pay and few benefits, precarious employment, and poor working conditions have occurred at the same time that social capital (including interpersonal and institutional trust) has been rapidly declining. Those in emotional pain might comfort themselves with alcohol, opiates, tobacco, and overindulging in unhealthy food. The prevalence of obesity, type 2 diabetes, and chronic pulmonary and cardiovascular diseases—conditions associated with high rates of comorbid depression—has increased in demographic groups highly impacted by economic and technological changes. Among the lower and lower-middle classes, immigrant and ethnic minority populations have done better than native non-Hispanic Whites of the same income strata; their mortality rates have fallen at the same time as the rates for Whites have increased. The difference might be due in part to immigrants' and minorities' lower initial expectations, hopes for their offspring, and greater social capital among people from ethnic minorities who live in communities with a shared culture. However, notwithstanding the contrast in mortality trends between native non-Hispanic Whites and immigrants and minorities, in many parts of the U.S. epidemiologic statistics for lower socioeconomic classes favor native non-Hispanic Whites because of disparities in access to and quality of healthcare.

American regions differ greatly in their predominant industries, the health of their economies, the proportion of the population that is rural, their percentage of immigrants, and their racial/ethnic composition. States and regions that have relatively more middle-aged, less-educated, non-metropolitan non-Hispanic Whites have higher mortality rates from deaths of despair, including suicides. They also have a higher prevalence of symptoms of physical and mental distress, though not necessarily of diagnosed MDD.

American regional cultures are remarkably persistent, with several dating back to migrations of British people to America in the 17th and 18th centuries. People from four different regions of Britain migrated to four different regions of the land that would become the U.S., a process described in exquisite detail by historian David Hackett Fischer in *Albion's Seed* (1989).

In 1629–1641 English Puritans migrated from East Anglia to Massachusetts in search of religious liberty, with the agenda of creating a faith-based society. They created the New England Yankee culture, which subsequently spread across the northern tier of the U.S. as Americans migrated west.

In 1642–1675, cavaliers and indentured servants from southern England migrated to Virginia seeking better fortune and there established a hierarchical society with aristocratic leadership like the one they left behind. This became the Tidewater culture of the Delaware Bay region, eastern Virginia and North Carolina (Woodard, 2011). The Tidewater region and its culture gave birth to many of America's Founding Fathers, whose fears of mob rule led to their incorporation of anti-democratic features into the American Constitution over the objections of more egalitarian groups of colonists.

In 1675–1725, Quakers migrated from the North Midlands of England to the Delaware River region, establishing what would become Pennsylvania. They created a relatively egalitarian, tolerant society with strong moral values that was the origin of America's Midlands culture.

In 1717–1775, people from less prosperous areas of North Britain, including northern English counties, lowland and western Scotland, and northern Ireland, migrated to the Appalachian backcountry, creating a society of rugged individualists in which clan identity was more important than political boundaries and there was widespread dislike for central authority, aristocracy, and elitism. The culture accepted violence in defense of one's property, honor, and clan. What became American Appalachian culture spread westward across the mountains, ultimately becoming the predominant culture in most of Kentucky,

Tennessee, Arkansas, and Oklahoma, territory that historian Colin Woodard has called *Greater Appalachia* (Fischer, 1989; Woodard, 2011).

Culture of the Deep South

The Deep South was settled in the late 17th and 18th centuries by British people of two kinds. Wealthy entrepreneurs came to establish large plantations growing tobacco, cotton, rice, and indigo with the labor of slaves of African origin. Yeoman farmers came to acquire their own land rather than be tenant farmers in England. They grew crops for local consumption, and sometimes also for export, on smaller plots. Most yeoman farmers did not own slaves; only one third of all households did (Lumen Learning, 2019). However, the revenue from the area's agricultural exports brought prosperity to the region, so most White non-slaveholders supported the system of slavery. The founders of the Deep South states established a hierarchical, authoritarian culture.

While slaves were emancipated in 1863 and the abolition of slavery was enforced by the Union's victory in the American Civil War, the legacy of slavery and the trauma of the Civil War have a continuing role in the culture of the Deep South. After the slaves were freed, land continued to be very unequally held. Black people, though not enslaved, were oppressed economically and legally. Segregation and legal discrimination against Blacks continued until the 1960s, and some forms of structural racism (e.g., discrimination in housing) persisted for decades after the end of segregation. Now, over a half-century since the Civil Rights Act, there are still huge disparities between White and Black Southerners in wealth, income, education, employment opportunities, and treatment by the police and criminal justice system (Hardy et al., 2018).

The culture of the Deep South is more authoritarian (higher power distance), more masculine (more gender inequality), and more conservative (higher uncertainty avoidance) than generic American culture. Communication is higher-context, more indirect, and more self-effacing. Southern manners are more polite than generic American manners. The culture is relatively low-trust; family and close friends might be trusted, but business and government are regarded with suspicion. One expression of the Deep South's low-trust culture has been the mistrust of medical scientists and public health authorities during the COVID-19 pandemic. This has led to the Deep South having low vaccination rates and its political leaders actively opposing mandates for indoor masking in schools and workplaces. The people of the Deep South have less higher education than Americans in general.

They are more religious both in belief and in formal observance. In common with Appalachia and the Mountain States, the Deep South has a gun culture, with most households owning one or more firearms. Many gun owners are hunters, target shooters, or collectors; but some own guns solely for self-defense, based on a belief that violent self-defense might be required by future circumstances. Gun owners in the Deep South are significantly more likely than those in most other regions of the U.S. to keep their guns loaded and unlocked (Hamilton et al., 2018). Keeping guns in this condition increases the risk of suicide by firearm, homicide related to intimate partner violence (IPV), and accidental death related to the mishandling of firearms by children or cognitively impaired adults (Grossman et al., 2005).

Most residents of the Deep South are religious, and evangelical Protestantism is by far the most prevalent religion. Approximately three-quarters of the residents of Mississippi and Alabama, the quintessential Deep South states, say religion is very important in their lives (Cooperman et al., 2015). Family traditions, religious belief and practice, and political conservatism often go together in defining a southern identity.

Culture of the American Southwest

The American Southwest was settled by Spanish-speaking migrants, originally from Spain and subsequently from Mexico. People of European ancestry intermarried with those of indigenous background, both in Mexico and in the Southwest, creating a culture with primarily Hispanic and some indigenous elements. While other regions of America were settled mainly by Protestants of various denominations, Catholics make up the plurality of Christians in the Spanish-speaking parts of the Southwest. Overall, the residents of the Southwest are not as religious as those of the Deep South (Cooperman et al., 2015).

The Hispanic population of the Southwest is predominantly of Mexican origin. Most Mexican Americans in the Southwest either are Mexican-born or have one or more Mexican parents or grandparents. Of the Mexican-born population, approximately two thirds have limited English proficiency (Rosenbloom & Batalova, 2022). A second, much smaller segment of the Hispanic population, concentrated in New Mexico and southern Colorado, comprises people with ancestors who settled in the Southwest when it was still under Spanish rule. These people, known as Hispanos or Neomexicanos, have a distinct "non-Mexican" identity (Healy et al., 2017).

Mexican culture is known for its collectivistic ethos of *familismo* for all, *machismo* for men, and *marianismo* for women. *Familismo* (familism) values commitment to one's immediate and extended family, including adult children asking for their parents' advice on major decisions, and family members helping one another when they are in need. *Machismo* and *marianismo* describe exaggerated gender roles. Within the context of Latino culture both have positive and negative aspects with respect to depression.

Familismo differs from the Confucian concept of filial piety in several ways. While as in the Confucian ethos one's parents and grandparents—especially the males—deserve respect and deference, assistance is offered when feasible not only to parents but also to siblings, children, and even second-degree relatives. Furthermore, *familismo* does not require that children be high achievers to satisfy their parents. The core attitudes of familism were captured in an internally consistent questionnaire-based scale (Steidel & Contreras, 2003). The 18 items of the scale divided into four factors (with exemplary items): *familial support* (a person should live near their parents, aging parents should live with their relatives, children should support their parents and members of the extended family if they are in need), *familial interconnectedness* (parents and grandparents should be treated with great respect regardless of their differences in views, a person should often do activities with their immediate and extended families, a person should cherish time spent with relatives), *familial honor* (children under 18 who work should give almost all of their earnings to their parents, a person should feel ashamed if something they do dishonors the family name, a person should be prepared to defend their family's honor no matter what the cost), and *subjugation of self for family* (a person should respect their older brothers and sisters regardless of their differences in views, children should obey their parents without question even if they believe they are wrong).

In a culture of *familismo*, children's moral behavior, obedience, and loyalty to the family are more important than their academic achievements or financial success. Implicit in *familismo* is the idea that a person with a family should never be alone and unsupported. Family solidarity may be one reason that suicide rates are lower among Hispanic people throughout the U.S. than they are among non-Hispanic Whites. A meta-analysis of familism and mental health showed a significant (though relatively small) negative association between familism and depression and suicidal behavior (Valdivieso-Mora et al., 2016). Depending on a person's family situation and level of acculturation to mainstream American culture, *familismo* can buffer stress or create stress. A person with strong *familismo* might reject an opportunity to escape a depressing situation because it would violate family norms or imply separation from the family. *Familismo* might keep a woman in an abusive marriage or keep a young adult from leaving their economically depressed hometown to find a good job in another city.

Machismo is a tradition of exaggerated masculinity expressed by many Latino men and expected of them in social contexts that more frequently arise in places with a predominantly Latino population. A *macho* man is brave, proud, assertive, honorable, and chivalrous, and is committed to supporting his family— qualities comprised in the concept of *caballerismo* (Arciniega et al., 2008). *Caballerismo* can be protective against depression. However, a *macho* man can be callously sexual, court danger, be excessively violent, be emotionally constricted, and be insensitive to the needs and feelings of his wife or partner (Nuñez et al., 2016). Though he is protective of his family, he is not necessarily faithful to his wife. It is expected that if a *macho* man is sufficiently successful in life and devoted to his family, his misbehavior will be forgiven by his wife, and he will be admired by his peers. *Machismo* is associated with binge drinking and perpetrating IPV. *Machismo*-related behavior can have consequences including injury (e.g., due to fighting or reckless driving) and illness (e.g., sexually transmitted diseases or alcohol-related medical conditions) that are risk factors for depression. Depression in a *macho* man often will be partly or entirely externalized, expressed as the syndrome of "male depression" that might be missed by a clinician lacking cultural awareness.

Marianismo is a tradition of women's serving as wives and mothers, faithfully caring for their husbands, family, and homes while, if necessary, tolerating their husbands' infidelity, mistreatment, or insensitivity. It is associated with chastity in single young women and with marital fidelity. A woman living the ideal of *marianismo* would be the main source of strength, stability, and spirituality for her family; she would be sexually virtuous; she would be respectful and obedient toward the men in her life; and she would silence herself to maintain harmony in a marriage or intimate partnership with a man. If a woman can live the ideal of *marianismo* without becoming enraged or depressed, she respects herself and is respected by others in her community. Thanks to her sacrifice, her husband and her children have a better life, and she credits herself for it. The Marianismo Belief Scale (Castillo et al., 2021), has five subscales: Family Pillar, Virtuous and Chaste, Subordinate to Others (especially men), Silencing Self (to maintain family harmony), and Spiritual Pillar. Not surprisingly, the Family Pillar and Spiritual Pillar components of *marianismo* can be protective against depression, while the other components can be risk factors for depression (Cano et al., 2020; Nuñez et al., 2016). For example, a woman with *marianismo* might tolerate IPV to the point that she is severely injured or ignores physical symptoms and so delays the diagnosis of a serious illness that brings depression as a complication or comorbidity. When such a woman does seek medical care, her depression might be expressed primarily as intolerable somatic pain or other physical symptoms.

Regions with Hybrid Cultures: The Midwest, the Mountain States, and the Pacific Northwest

The American Midwest was settled primarily by people from New England, the Midlands, and Appalachia, with each group bringing its cultural traits to the region. The Midwestern states have the three cultures in varying proportions: From Pennsylvania west through Ohio, Indiana, and Illinois there is Yankee culture in the north, Appalachian culture in the South, and the culture of the Midlands in between. In the southern states and in eastern Texas, there is Appalachian culture in the highlands and Deep South culture elsewhere (Woodard, 2011). The culture of western Texas is more like that of New Mexico and Arizona.

The Mountain States (aka the *Far West*) developed a hybrid culture that incorporated the same three elements as the Midwest but was shaped by the geography of the region—vast, beautiful, and economically dominated by railroads, mining companies, and other powerful commercial entities. The residents of the region are proud, independent, and highly suspicious of government (Woodard, 2011). The citizens of Montana—a state with significant poverty and health disparities—voted to end state-subsidized healthcare (Medicaid) for people just above the poverty line, even though most of the cost would have been assumed by the federal government, and broader Medicaid coverage had helped support the state's struggling rural hospitals. Voters objected to paying any additional taxes for the Medicaid program, even though the additional funds would have come solely from new taxes on tobacco products (Ollove, 2018). Ironically, many residents of the region are remarkably submissive to large commercial interests, supporting increased mining, logging, fracking, and construction in unspoiled wilderness areas, even though they would get no personal benefit from it and might suffer financially if their income were related to tourism. Eight percent of the residents of Montana are American Indians, most of whom live on reservations isolated from the remainder of the state. The twelve tribes recognized by the State of Montana are the Assiniboine, Blackfeet, Chippewa, Cree, Crow, Gros Ventre, Kootenai, Little Shell Chippewa, Northern Cheyenne, Pend d'Oreille, Salish, and Sioux. (Montana Office of Public Instruction, 2020). Their cultures are distinct from those of White Montanans, as well as from those of the tribes that predominate in other regions of the U.S.

An additional cultural influence in the Mountain States, dominant in the state of Utah and strong in adjoining parts of neighboring states, is the Church of Jesus Christ of Latter-day Saints (whose members are variously referred to as Latter-day Saints, LDS, or Mormons, with the first of these the preferred usage of the church itself). The Latter-day Saints are a tightly organized evangelical group with an exclusively male hierarchy. Members of the Latter-Day Saints Church have been extraordinarily successful financially while maintaining high engagement with the practice and moral code of the religion. The dominance of the religion from Utah's founding to the present time has established a persistent culture emphasizing commitment to the church, industriousness, charity, family orientation, and relatively rigid gender roles. While cultural maps of the U.S. usually don't separate Utah from the other intermountain/Far West states, there are obvious distinctions between Utah and the other states where Latter-day Saints are a minority. Residents of the Far West who are not Latter-day Saints tend to be less religiously observant, and they do not share the Church's prohibition against drinking alcohol or its rigid gender roles. As noted in Chapter 1, Utah's exceptional gender inequality is associated with the nation's highest rate of MDD in young women. Young women from Latter-day Saints families throughout the Mountain States often face similar work/family conflicts and discrimination in employment, finding themselves in situations in which accepting traditional rules is intolerably stressful but rejecting them implies conflict with or distance from their families and the traditional community (Dengah et al., 2019). To its credit, the Latter-day Saints Church has recognized that depression is an issue in its young women and has begun efforts to destigmatize it and to promote mental health care (Park, 2017).

The Pacific Northwest (Washington, Oregon, and California north of the San Francisco Bay Area) was settled in the 19th century by a combination of Yankees, people with German and Irish ancestries, people of Scandinavian (especially Norwegian) background, and people of other European nationalities. The economy of the Pacific Northwest initially was based on forestry, agriculture, mining, commercial fishing, and trans-Pacific trade. East of the Cascade Mountains, the Northwest has a Mountain States culture. West of the Cascades, the regional culture is more open-minded, liberal, and ethnically diverse. Colin Woodard (2011) characterized the western parts of Washington, Oregon, northern California, and British Columbia as the "Left Coast." On both sides of the mountains there is a widespread love of nature and outdoor activity, and concern about the environment.

Additional distinctive American regional cultures are defined by large metropolitan areas with unique cultures influenced by their predominant industries and by the ethnic groups that had an important historical role in the settlement and development of the region and/or currently constitute a large fraction of the population. Such areas include Southern California, the San Francisco Bay Area/Silicon Valley, the New York metropolitan area (including parts of New Jersey and southwestern Connecticut), and the Washington, DC metropolitan area (including parts of Maryland and Virginia). The entertainment, media, and hospitality/tourism industries influence the culture of Southern California and New York City. Technology-related business and the historical counterculture of San Francisco influence the culture of the Bay Area. Government and its commercial and non-profit penumbra influence the culture of the DC area.

Three metropolitan areas of the eastern U.S. were initially settled by Europeans other than the English: greater New York City by the Dutch, greater Miami by the Spanish, and greater New Orleans by the French. Their historical roots contribute to their cultural distinctiveness. New York has always been open to diversity. The Hispanic culture of Miami is not Mexican, more resembling the culture of a prosperous South American city. New Orleans, with its French heritage, is far more liberal and far more Catholic than its Deep South location might suggest.

Region, Personality, and Mental Health

Large-scale surveys have consistently shown that average personality traits differ between regions—and probably have done so for many generations. While interindividual variation is much larger than variation due to geography, a higher or lower prevalence of traits like extraversion, openness, and conscientiousness translates into regional differences in what industries develop, what organizations are formed, and what institutions are built. In turn, the institutions of business, education, religious life, and social life cultivate and reward some traits and suppress others. If a person's personality is incompatible with a region's norms, they may choose to move to a region that fits better. For example, most highly educated people with interests in science, technology, engineering, and mathematics (STEM) are open-minded, and this is especially true for women in STEM. When a new STEM graduate seeks employment or further education, they probably will move to a region (or a major metropolitan area) with a strong technology-based economy and/or excellent universities, which is likely to be a place where the population has the trait of openness. If the graduate is a woman entering a technical field that already has issues with gender equity, she probably will move to a place with a less "masculine" culture. The continual moves of STEM graduates from regions with low average openness to ones with high average openness help maintain regional differences in the trait—and differences in the dynamism of regional economies.

Knowledge of regional culture is helpful in the clinical setting to suggest questions to ask, details to notice, and conditions for effective treatment. For example, there are regions (and demographic groups within regions) in which for generations there have been high rates of IPV and adverse childhood experiences (ACEs). IPV and ACEs have a circular relationship: Adults with traumatic childhoods are more likely to become perpetrators and/or victims of IPV. Witnessing IPV or being affected by its consequences (e.g., parental divorce, injury of the victim, or incarceration of the perpetrator) adds to a child's adverse experiences and sometimes results in lifetime psychological vulnerabilities (M. J. Brown et al., 2015; Mair et al., 2012; Willie et al., 2018). When specific types of IPV and certain types of ACEs have been highly prevalent for generations within a cultural group, they frequently are normalized and/or rationalized, and consequently might not be spontaneously mentioned in a first clinical interview—or even in response to routine screening questions. A story of ACEs or of IPV might unfold only over several encounters, as trust develops.

When, for cultural or other reasons, a clinician suspects a patient might be a victim and/or perpetrator of IPV, it is essential that the patient be interviewed outside the presence of their partner. If an assessment is done remotely via videoconference or telephone, it must be timed or otherwise arranged to ensure that the partner cannot eavesdrop on the encounter. Similarly, when there is a suspicion that a child or adolescent has been abused, neglected, or harshly disciplined, interviewing them without a parent present is especially important. In the context of suspected mistreatment by a parent or other adult, remote assessment of depression may be feasible with an adolescent but not with a younger child unable to use technology independently.

The definition of dysfunctional or unacceptable behavior can vary with regional culture. A level of hyperthymia and informality that might be common and even adaptive in the entrepreneurial culture of the San Francisco Bay Area or Southern California might be judged negatively in the conservative, authoritarian culture of the Deep South. Knowing the boundaries of acceptable behavior in a person's social context should inform clinical judgment about whether a person's symptoms suggest a diagnosis in the bipolar spectrum.

A region's relative reported prevalence of bipolar disorder (BD) versus MDD is related not only to norms for appropriate conduct in the region but also to the involvement of psychiatrists in diagnosing people with depressive symptoms and the influence of academic medical centers and psychiatric clinics and hospitals in an area. Psychiatrists and psychologists with expertise in mood disorders are more likely than primary care physicians or generic mental health professionals (e.g., "counselors") to recognize and correctly diagnose people with bipolar spectrum disorders who present with depression or mixed symptoms and have not had recorded episodes of obvious mania or hypomania. The ratio of diagnosed MDD to BD prevalence varies widely among states, tending to be higher in more rural states than more urban ones (Institute for Health Metrics and Evaluation [IHME], 2023). This supports the idea that bipolar depression is more likely to be recognized in states with more psychiatrists.

Regional Variations in Mental Health

Variation among American states in the prevalence of MDD is significantly less than the variation in rates of death by suicide. In 2019, the prevalence of MDD (both genders, all ages) in the 50 U.S. states plus the District of Columbia ranged between 2.8% in Connecticut to 5.0% in Utah; the highest rate was thus 1.81 times greater than the lowest. The 2019 suicide mortality rate per 100,000 people (both genders, all ages) ranged from 7.04 in New Jersey to 20.05 in Montana, an almost threefold difference. Interstate variations in suicide mortality are even greater for demographic groups defined by age and gender—far greater than interstate variation in diagnosed MDD or BD. The 2019 rate of death by suicide for women aged 15–49 ranged from 4.28 in the District of Columbia to 13.84 in Montana; the rate for men aged 70 and over ranged from 17.14 in the District of Columbia to 62.69 in Nevada (IHME, 2023). A clinician evaluating a dysphoric male patient from a state with a high suicide rate should be especially attentive to suicidal ideation, dangerous behavior, and suicide risk factors (e.g., firearm ownership and social isolation). A man who would not meet Diagnostic and Statistical Manual of Mental Disorders (DSM)/ICD criteria for MDD could nonetheless be clinically depressed by broader criteria and could be high-risk on most or all the criteria of the interpersonal/neuropsychiatric model of suicide.

Regional culture influences the occurrence, phenomenology, and narratives of depression through multiple pathways. It shapes personality, contributing to a person's likelihood of experiencing negative emotions, their resilience when stressed, and their ability to find social support. It includes social capital, which can buffer the effects of stress, and, on a population basis, can reduce the prevalence of depression. It defines the kinds of suffering that are normal and the prototypical idioms of distress. It influences the reasons for living and the hopefulness of the region's residents. Regional culture interacts with regional environment. Altitude (DelMastro et al., 2011; Reno et al., 2018; Basualdo-Meléndez et al., 2022), sunlight, temperature, barometric pressure, trace elements in water, and pollution of water and air have quantifiable effects on depression prevalence and suicide risk. Regionally prevalent diets can have depressant or antidepressant effects. Regional norms for smoking, drinking, and drug use affect the likelihood that an individual will use specific substances. The relative status of women, of children, of older adults, and of specific minorities varies significantly by region. Those who frequently experience stereotyping, discrimination, and/or microaggressions are stressed in ways that can precipitate depression. Regional culture, including its intersections with race/ethnicity, age/generation, gender, socioeconomic class, religion, and occupational culture, affects the likelihood that such stress will cause distress and whether such distress will be expressed in a syndrome recognizable as depression, in a somatoform condition, or in externalized behavior. Stress might not produce illness if it is mitigated by social support, collective action, and/or individual resilience—all factors to which regional culture contributes.

The availability, quality, and affordability of mental health services vary greatly by region and by state within the U.S. Access to mental health services within a state depends as much on its culture as on its economy. If a state is unappealing to people with graduate degrees because of an anti-intellectual culture, it will attract fewer mental health professionals. If a state's population is suspicious of scientific expertise and resentful of taxation, there will be little support for public sector mental health services. In states with cultures of high deference to authority and high stigma of mental illness, there is unlikely to be collective action to challenge insurance companies that do not provide parity of coverage for mental illness and general medical conditions.

Within any region or state, a place's status as rural, metropolitan, or "micropolitan" will obviously affect its culture and the fate of a person at risk for depression. A simple urban–rural distinction is not adequate when approaching mental health issues. A town of 10,000 people is not rural according to official definitions, but it will not have the same diversity of population and access to mental health services as a city of a million people. Neither a non-conformist nor a person with a serious mental illness can easily remain anonymous in a small town. Even when an "urban cluster" has mental health professionals, it may be difficult for a specific depressed person to find one who would be sufficiently compatible personally to be an effective psychotherapist. For the rural population there is a major difference between those with high-speed (broadband) internet access and those without it. Those with such access have many more educational opportunities, may be able to work from home at least some of the time, and will be able to receive psychotherapy and other clinical services online. Those without broadband access have less educational and occupational opportunity and must physically travel to receive mental health services that involve face-to-face interaction.

Cultural awareness is not only relevant to clinical work with immigrants and ethnic minorities. It is equally empowering for clinicians who treat non-Hispanic Whites immersed in a distinctive regional culture. Such people's cultural identities reflect intersectionality that includes the "culture of place." When an individual's personality and values are atypical for the region in which they live, the regional culture's response to non-conformity can add to their stress or provide resources and supports for coping with it. Regional social capital and institutions will affect what resources are available to address problems, and regional attitudes and beliefs may determine whether a person finds social support for actions they take to improve their life circumstances and mental health.

Lessons from Cultural Comparison of Eight Pairs of States

Eight pairs of neighboring states illustrate a "culture of place" perspective on depression and suicide. Each pair represents entirely or largely one of America's regional cultures. Their similarities are characteristic of the region to which the two states belong. Their differences can be understood in relation to the states' history, geography, demographics, economy, environment, and, in some cases, the effect of a secondary regional culture in part of the state.

Following are pairs of adjacent states with cultural commonalities. Each pair is followed by a name for the region to which it belongs, and a brief description of the applicable regional culture(s).

- Alabama (AL) and Mississippi (MS): Deep South (culture of descendants of slave owners, yeoman farmers, and Black slaves)
- Arizona (AZ) and New Mexico (NM): Southwest (hybrid of Mexican, American Indian, and Mountain State cultures)
- Iowa (IA) and Nebraska (NE): Central Midwest (English Midlands culture with 19th-century German influence)
- Kentucky (KY) and West Virginia (WV): Appalachia (culture with North British–Lowland Scottish roots and Irish influence)
- Massachusetts (MA) and New Hampshire (NH): New England (Yankee culture influenced by cultures of Italian and Irish immigrants of the late 19th and early 20th centuries, French culture in NH, the concentration of institutions of higher education in MA, and the cosmopolitan culture of greater Boston)
- Minnesota (MN) and Wisconsin (WI): Upper Midwest (Yankee culture as modified by German, Scandinavian, and Irish influences—more Scandinavian in MN and more German in WI)
- Montana (MT) and Wyoming (WY): Mountain States (hybrid of Yankee, Midlands and Appalachian culture, German and Irish influences, and Scandinavian influence in MT, combined with impact of distinctive geography; also, a large American Indian population in MT)
- Oregon (OR) and Washington (WA): Pacific Northwest (Yankee culture with German, Irish, and Scandinavian influences, the latter greater in WA; eastern OR and WA have a Mountain States culture, and Metropolitan Seattle has a large Asian immigrant population)

A series of tables now presents aspects of the 16 states' demographics, economy, social capital, and religious orientation, along with characterization of the average personality traits of the states' adult populations. They are followed by tables on education, health habits, IPV, and ACEs. The conclusion is a set of tables on the epidemiology of MDD and BD, suicide overall, and suicide by firearm. Epidemiologic data are organized by gender and by age ranges: 15–49, 50–69, and 70 or older. Inferences are drawn and hypotheses suggested about the context, distribution, and typical narratives of depression in the states and their region, and how those insights might inform culturally aware clinical interviews and strategies for prevention and treatment of depression and suicide.

Throughout the chapter there are tables comparing the eight pairs of states. Data for the tables are from the U.S. Census except when indicated otherwise. The 2020 Census data provide an urban–rural breakdown, but they do not separate truly urban areas from those with populations between 2000 and 50,000—areas often more typical of rural areas with respect to availability of mental health services and diversity of population and opportunity. In the data tables, states are represented by their two-character postal codes. The final three rows of each table give the 20th percentile, median, and 80th percentile values for the 50 U.S. states plus the District of Columbia. These benchmarks provide further context for the comparison of the states and regions. Values of variables above the 80th percentile for the U.S. are highlighted in bold; values below the 20th percentile are highlighted in italics. Sources of the data used to construct the tables are given in footnotes to the tables. In most cases, data were obtained by accessing an organizational website, logging in and entering a search query.

Table 14.1 shows the distributions of the states' populations. Within the eight cultural regions, interstate differences in urbanization are largest between Alabama and Mississippi, between Arizona and New Mexico, and between Massachusetts and New Hampshire. Alabama's urban population is truly urban—concentrated in the cities of Huntsville, Birmingham, Montgomery, and Mobile, all with populations around 200,000. Mississippi has only one city with a population greater than 100,000 (Jackson); much of Mississippi's "urban" population lives in small towns (urban clusters). Arizona's population is much more urban than New Mexico's. Almost 40% of the population of New Hampshire is rural, compared with less than 10% of Massachusetts' population.

In large urban areas, standards of healthcare, including mental health care, are set by major hospitals and clinics and their medical staff. Such institutions often are among the largest employers in a city, and their achievements and shortcomings are widely noted. By contrast, an urban cluster may not have its own hospital or may have one with limited capacity to handle severe illness. With no competition and a smaller community of medical professionals, a

Table 14.1 Rural–Urban Population Distribution for the 16 States

State	Population	Urban	Rural
AL	5,024,279	57.7%	42.3%
MS	2,961,279	46.3%	53.7%
AZ	7,151,502	89.3%	10.7%
NM	2,117,522	74.5%	25.5%
IA	3,190,369	63.2%	36.8%
NE	1,961504	73.0%	27.0%
KY	4,505,836	58.7%	41.3%
WV	1,793,716	44.6%	55.4%
MA	7,029,917	93.1%	8.7%
NH	1,377,529	58.3%	41.7%
MN	5,706,494	71.9%	28.1%
WI	5,893,718	67.1%	32.9%
MT	1,084,225	53.4%	46.6%
WY	576,851	62.0%	38.0%
OR	4,237,256	62.5%	19.0%
WA	7,705,281	83.4%	16.6%
20th percentile	1,377,529	61.0%	13.1%
Median	4,505,836	73.0%	27.0%
80th percentile	9,288,994	86.9%	39.0%

Note. Data from 2020 U.S. Census (U.S. Census Bureau, 2023b), Table H2 : Urban and Rural. https://data.census.gov/table/DECENNIALDHC2020.H2?q=urban+rural+2020+census.

small-city hospital can remain in operation even if its quality of care is substandard in some specialties and/or for some conditions. In a small city, a single outstanding specialist or a single unethical practitioner can have citywide impact. The quality of mental health care available at a small-city hospital might depend on the skills—and availability—of a single psychiatrist.

Throughout the U.S., mental health professionals are concentrated in larger cities. Their availability in an urban cluster depends on its size, the prevailing culture of the cluster, and the attractiveness of the location as a place for a professional to live. A small urban cluster in a remote and impoverished area might have no mental health professionals, whereas a city of 25,000 in a resort area might have 50 or more. Most people who live in rural areas and seek mental health care must either drive long distances or utilize telehealth services.

Residents of rural areas who have mild to moderate depression usually do not receive care for their conditions, for reasons including a shortage of care providers, concerns about anonymity, greater stigma of depression in rural areas, and less consistent availability of employer-based health insurance (Kitchen et al., 2013). When they do receive care, it usually is pharmacotherapy without psychotherapy, regardless of the patient's preference (Fortney et al., 2009). This pattern has begun to change with the explosive growth of telepsychiatry during the COVID-19 pandemic. However, a shortage of mental health professionals continues to limit the availability of services in most rural areas of the U.S.

Consistent delivery of timely care (including non-pharmacologic treatment) to depressed rural Americans will continue to be difficult without universal broadband internet access and telehealth services adequately covered by affordable health insurance. Clinical consequences of changes in public and private payers' telemedicine policies during the COVID-19 pandemic and a political consensus favoring universal broadband access might eventually lead to durable improvements in rural Americans' access to treatment for depression.

In the states of the Deep South, Appalachia, and the Mountain States, one third to one half of the population is truly rural. In the Midwest, the Southwest, and the Pacific Northwest, urban clusters have a greater role. The "country" culture—exemplified by the popularity of country music and enthusiasm for firearms—is strongest where more of the population is rural and where urban clusters are relatively small and better described as small towns than as cities. Arizona and New Mexico, though they are both large in area, do not have high percentages of rural residents. Both have well-respected hospital systems based in their largest cities that have outreach to urban clusters.

Table 14.2 shows regional demographic differences that underlie depression-relevant cultural differences. For example, the two Deep South states in this chapter's sample have very large Black populations, and African Americans are the only large minority group. Despite their large non-White populations, their percentages of multiracial people are in the bottom 10 nationally—reflecting a persistent cultural opposition to interracial marriages (and, historically, legal prohibition of such marriages). Even West Virginia, the "Whitest" state in the U.S., has more multiracial residents than Mississippi, the "Blackest" one. Even in more liberal states, interracial marriages, or even marriages across lines of religion or ethnicity, can cause family conflicts that precipitate depression in one or more of those involved. Nonetheless, the stakes are higher in a state like Mississippi or Alabama.

The Southwestern states have, as expected, large Mexican American populations. New Mexico, however, has a much higher proportion of Hispanic residents than Arizona, and has a distinctive Spanish-speaking population—the

Table 14.2 Race and Ethnicity of the 16 States' Populations on the 2020 Census, and Immigrant Percentage in 2022

State	White	Black	Hispanic	Asian	American Indian	Mixed Race	Immigrants
AL	63.1%	25.6%	5.3%	1.5%	0.5%	3.7%	3.6%
MS	55.4%	36.4%	3.6%	1.1%	0.5%	2.8%	2.2%
AZ	53.4%	4.4%	30.7%	3.5%	3.7%	3.7%	13.1%
NM	36.5%	1.8%	47.7%	1.7%	8.9%	2.8%	9.1%
IA	82.7%	4.1%	6.8%	2.4%	0.3%	3.4%	6.3%
NE	75.7%	4.8%	12.0%	2.7%	0.8%	3.7%	7.1%
KY	81.3%	7.9%	4.6%	1.6%	0.2%	3.9%	4.0%
WV	89.1%	3.6%	1.9%	0.8%	0.2%	4.0%	1.8%
MA	67.6%	6.5%	12.6%	7.2%	0.1%	4.7%	18.1%
NH	87.2%	1.4%	4.3%	2.6%	0.2%	4.0%	5.9%
MN	76.3%	6.9%	6.1%	5.2%	1.0%	4.1%	8.4%
WI	78.6%	6.2%	7.6%	3.0%	0.8%	3.5%	4.9%
MT	83.1%	0.5%	4.2%	0.7%	6.0%	5.0%	2.4%
WY	81.4%	0.8%	10.2%	0.9%	2.0%	4.1%	3.2%
OR	71.1%	1.9%	13.9%	4.5%	1.0%	6.1%	10.0%
WA	63.8%	3.8%	13.7%	9.4%	1.2%	6.6%	15.3%

Note. Data from U.S. Census Bureau (2023b). https://data.census.gov. Queries: distribution of race and Hispanic ethnicity on the 2020 Census, and percentage of first-generation immigrants on the 2022 American Community Survey. Data retrieved October 15, 2023.

Hispanos or Neomexicanos—whose ancestry is Spanish and to some extent American Indian. The Spanish began settling what is now New Mexico at the end of the 16th century, and many of today's Hispanos can identify at least one ancestor who came from Spain. Hispano families have substantially higher status in New Mexico than Mexican immigrant families, and they are culturally distinct, as would be indicated by a higher educational level, greater wealth and income, and more generations of residence in the U.S. Despite their status in their local communities, Hispanos can be inappropriately stereotyped by non-Hispanic White people in places where they and their families are not well known.

All American states have some degree of racial and ethnic diversity. However, an important distinction can be made between states in which there is one majority culture throughout and those in which a minority population is so concentrated in some regions that it constitutes the majority in those regions. In Arizona, New Mexico, and Montana much of the American Indian population lives on reservations where almost everyone is of the same tribe. In Arizona and New Mexico there are rural counties, urban clusters, and metropolitan neighborhoods where Mexican Americans constitute a majority. In Alabama and Mississippi, there are many counties in which Blacks are the majority.

Concentration of a racial/ethnic minority has both positives and negatives with respect to depression. On the negative side, it can concentrate economic or educational disadvantage. On the positive side, it can increase local social capital and reduce daily experiences of prejudice, discrimination, and microaggressions.

Throughout the U.S., and in most high-income and upper-middle-income countries (China is a notable example of the latter), suicide rates are higher in rural areas than in urban ones even though diagnosed depression is more prevalent in urban areas. Several factors contribute: Depression is more likely to be diagnosed in urban areas with greater availability of mental health services. Expression of depression through externalization or somatization is more common in rural areas. Crisis intervention services for suicidal people are more available in urban areas. In less prosperous rural areas, hopelessness related to poverty and lack of employment often is expressed as suicidal ideation. And, highly lethal means of suicide might be more conveniently available in rural areas than in cities—conspicuous examples being firearms in the U.S. and highly toxic pesticides in China.

Race and ethnicity affect the magnitude of urban–rural differences in depression prevalence and suicide rates and the relationship of both to education and economic status. African Americans living in majority-Black areas of the Deep South have lower rates of depression than those living in in places where Blacks are a minority, even though as a group they suffer more poverty and have worse educational opportunities (Keyes et al., 2015; Weaver et al., 2015). And, in contrast to the pattern for non-Hispanic Whites, rural Blacks in the U.S. do not have higher suicide rates than urban Blacks. For Asian Americans and Hispanic Americans, the rural-to-urban ratio of suicide rates is higher than it is for non-Hispanic Whites. For American Indians the rural suicide rate is more than twice the urban rate. When the rural suicide rate is higher, the effect of rurality is stronger for men than for women. Details are shown in Table 14.3 which is based on data from the U.S. National Vital Statistics System as analyzed by a team at the Centers for Disease Control (Ivey-Stephenson et al., 2017).

Behind the statistics are demographic and social issues. In traditional cultures, men are more defined by their occupational role and women by their role in the family. Work opportunities are greater in metropolitan areas than

Table 14.3 2013–2015 American Suicide Rates by Level of Urbanization

Population	Large metropolitan (>1,000,000)	Medium to small metropolitan (>50,000)	Non-metropolitan (rural with or without an urban cluster)	Urban to rural rate increase
All	12.7	16.8	19.7	55%
Male	20.2	26.7	31.6	57%
Female	5.9	7.5	8.1	36%
White (non-Hispanic)	17.2	20.2	22.0	27%
Black (non-Hispanic)	6.6	6.9	6.1	−7%
Hispanic (any race)	6.4	8.0	10.2	60%
Asian/Pacific Islander	6.7	8.4	9.4	40%
American Indian/Alaska Native	14.0	19.6	29.1	108%
Age 15–24	10.1	12.3	15.8	56%
Age 25–34	12.4	17.5	22.0	77%
Age 35–64	15.6	20.9	23.4	50%
Age 65+	14.5	17.3	19.7	36%
Death by firearm	5.6	8.6	11.5	106%
Death by other means	7.1	8.2	8.2	15%

Note. Data from Ivey-Stephenson et al., 2017.

in rural ones. Rural Latinos are predominantly Mexican Americans working in agriculture—physically demanding work with low pay, high risk of serious occupational injury, exposure to agricultural chemicals, poor access to healthcare, and exploitation of unauthorized immigrants (Figueroa et al., 2021). There are relatively few Asians in rural and small-town America, and those who live there frequently face stereotyping and social exclusion from the White majority. Some confront it effectively by a combination of assimilation, teaching others about their background, and allying with minorities of other nationalities (Walton, 2018). Others experience a combination of chronic stress and negative social capital that leads to depression.

The cultural differences between different European nationalities are highly relevant to depression and to suicide. U.S. Census data are available on self-reported European ancestries of Americans. Table 14.4 shows the percentage of self-reported primary ancestries of non-Hispanic White residents of the 16

Table 14.4 Self-Reported Primary Ancestry of the 16 States' Non-Hispanic White Residents

State	American	English	French	German	Irish	Italian	Norwegian	Polish
AL	18.5%	19.3%		10.0%	12.0%			
MS	17.1%	18.4%		9.0%	12.8%			
AZ	18.4%			22.5%	15.9%			
NM		21.9%		21.6%	17.5%			
IA		12.2%		36.5%	14.6%			
NE		12.0%		40.4%	15.5%			
KY	14.4%	18.2%		16.0%	13.5%			
WV	10.6%			15.6%	12.9%			
MA		13.9%	8.3%		27.1%	16.7%		
NH		20.2%	20.9%	10.2%	22.0%	10.4%		
MN	8.7%			37.6%	12.7%		15.5%	
WI		19.8%		45.8%	13.0%		8.0%	10.0%
MT	7.1%	16.0%		26.8%		16.0%	8.1%	
WY	6.9%	19.2%		26.8%	14.1%			
OR		19.4%		22.6%	14.9%			
WA		18.8%		22.1%	14.7%			

Note. Data from U.S. Census (2023). Self-Reported Ancestry on 2020 Census. https://data.census.gov/table?q=first+ancestry+by+state&g=040XX00US01,04,19,21,25,27,28,30,31,33,35,41,53,54,55,56. Retrieved October, 19, 2023.

states, for all European nationalities claimed by at least 5% of the state's residents. *American* is included as a category because some White respondents to the survey described their heritage as purely American. For most such respondents, the last immigrant in the family tree arrived in the U.S. prior to the mid-19th century.

German and Irish ancestry is common throughout the 16-state sample. Residents of the Deep South and Appalachian states take pride in their long family histories as Americans. Scandinavian influences are found in states of the nation's northern tier, and these might underlie the states' relatively high social capital. The New England states have meaningful French and Italian contributions to their gene pools and their cultures, and the combination of French, Italian, and Irish nationalities implies a significant role for the Catholic Church in many residents' religious beliefs and life narratives.

Regional Variation in Social Capital

Social capital, discussed at length in Part I as an attribute of populations usually protective against depression and suicide, varies greatly among the regions of the U.S. Interstate and inter-regional differences reflect their histories and contemporary cultures and demographics. The different types of social capital—relational, institutional, and cognitive; bonding, bridging, and linking—can vary independently of one another, creating the potential for places being well connected but highly suspicious, or disconnected yet trusting. Data from the Social Capital Project of the Joint Economic Committee of the U.S. Senate facilitates the interstate comparison of the components of social capital and the conception of regional social capital profiles. The Social Capital Project was conceived by Senator Mike Lee, a conservative LDS Christian from Utah, who favors local, private initiatives to address contemporary social, economic, and environmental challenges. He sees social capital as essential to the success of these initiatives and to a healthy relationship of citizens to their government and to one another (Joint Economic Committee, 2021).

The staff of the Social Capital Project investigated over 50 state-level quantitative indicators of social capital derived from various publicly available national data sets, assessing their psychometric properties and their correlation with outcomes of interest. They selected 25 indicators, converted numerical scores into z-scores (standard deviations above or below the national mean), and created seven sub-indices and a single composite index using principal component analysis. Each sub-index is a weighted sum of selected indicators. The composite index had high internal consistency, and a correlation of .81 with Robert Putnam's index of social capital (Joint Economic Committee, 2018). Several of the analyses and tables later in this chapter utilized the Social Capital Project database, which is in the public domain and available online for download and secondary analysis. In the definitions of the sub-indices that follow, it is self-evident which items are reverse-scored because of their negative correlations with social capital.

The Family Unity sub-index is based on 2012–2016 data from the American Community Survey. It combines scores based on the percentages of births that are to unwed mothers, of children living in single-parent families, and of women aged 35–44 who are married and not separated.

The Family Interaction sub-index is based on the 2016 National Survey of Children's Health. It is based on the percentages of children age five or under who are read to daily by a family member, children who watch television or play video games at least four hours a day, and children who use computers, mobile phones, and other electronic devices for purposes other than schoolwork at least four hours a day.

The Social Support sub-index combines data from the 2006 and the 2010 Centers for Disease Control and Prevention (CDC) Behavioral Risk Factor Surveillance System survey and the 2008 and the 2013 U.S. Census Current Population Survey (CPS). It includes the percentage of adults who "sometimes, rarely, or never" get the "social and emotional support [they] need," the percentage of adults who do favors for neighbors at least monthly, and the percentage who trust most of their neighbors or all of them. There is an additional item on the number of "close friends" adults claim to have.

The Community Health sub-index, also based on CPS data, comprises percentages of survey respondents who volunteered for an organization, those who attended a public meeting to discuss community affairs, those who worked with neighbors on a community project, those who served as an officer or committee member of a group, those who attended a public meeting where political issues were discussed, and those who participated in a march, rally, or demonstration. These data were supplemented by information from other sources on the number of non-profit organizations per capita and the number of religious congregations per capita.

The Institutional Health sub-index included the percentage of adult citizens who voted in the 2012 and 2016 presidential elections, the rate at which residents returned the 2010 mail-in U.S. Census questionnaire, and the percentages of adults who had "great confidence" or "some confidence" in corporations, in media, and in public schools to "do what is right."

There were two single-item indicators. Collective Efficacy was measured by the rate of violent crimes per 100,000 population. Philanthropic Health was measured by the percentage of adults who gave more than $25 in the past year to "charitable or religious organizations." Table 14.5, summarizing indices of social capital, shows a "north–south divide" among the 16 states compared in this chapter. Social capital is very low in the Deep South and the Southwest and below the national median in Appalachia. It is very high in the Midwest and in New Hampshire, and above the national median in the Massachusetts, the Pacific Northwest, and the Mountain States.

A Social Capital Project report noted that a north–south gradient in social capital applied to the entire nation and attributed it to "deep-seated roots in historical immigration and internal migration patterns, regional culture, and perhaps even features of climate and topography" (Joint Economic Committee, 2018). Noting the low social capital in the Deep South, the project staff tested the hypothesis that it might be related to the region's history of slavery. They found a strong correlation at the county level between the slave population in 1860 and low Family Unity 150 years later. Remarking on the finding, their

Table 14.5 Indices of Social Capital

Indices of Social Capital in the 16 States

State	State-level summary index	Family unity	Family interaction	Social support	Community health	Institutional health	Collective efficacy	Philanthropic health
AL	−0.94	−0.92	−0.82	−0.67	−0.86	−0.02	−0.35	−1.19
MS	−1.15	−2.02	−1.38	−0.27	−0.70	−0.66	0.48	−1.20
AZ	−1.33	−0.55	−1.38	−0.95	−1.20	−1.90	−0.20	−0.70
NM	−1.50	−1.35	−0.31	−0.52	−0.05	−3.46	−1.30	−1.12
IA	**1.07**	**0.87**	0.57	**1.09**	0.65	**1.30**	0.51	0.59
NE	**1.09**	**0.98**	0.69	**0.93**	0.44	**1.28**	0.47	0.82
KY	−0.63	−0.07	−1.15	−0.40	−0.78	−0.31	**0.85**	−1.10
WV	−0.45	−0.29	−0.13	0.67	−0.47	−0.74	0.35	−1.72
MA	0.38	0.45	0.55	0.21	−0.16	**1.07**	−0.15	−0.11
NH	**1.45**	0.85	**1.75**	0.78	**1.15**	**1.07**	**0.94**	**1.13**
MN	**1.81**	**1.11**	0.85	**1.62**	0.83	**2.18**	**0.76**	**2.02**
WI	**1.61**	0.50	**0.94**	**1.54**	**0.93**	**1.94**	0.41	**1.96**
MT	0.76	0.79	**1.04**	0.67	**1.34**	−1.21	0.23	**1.02**
WY	0.86	**1.15**	**1.26**	0.59	0.55	0.06	**0.94**	0.05
OR	0.79	0.43	0.56	**0.85**	**1.04**	−0.32	0.74	0.88
WA	0.73	0.87	0.33	0.29	0.73	0.52	0.44	0.72
20th percentile	−0.88	−0.55	−0.82	−0.73	−0.86	−0.71	−0.46	−0.94
Median	−0.09	−0.02	0.07	−0.15	−0.19	0.01	0.21	−0.09
80th percentile	0.98	0.85	0.72	0.78	0.83	0.81	0.74	0.82

Note. Data from the Social Capital Project (Joint Economic Committee, 2018b).

report quoted novelist William Faulkner's famous line, "The past is never dead. It's not even past" (Faulkner, 1951).

Though social capital is either positive or negative for both states in each pair of states, there are significant differences in the magnitude of positive social capital between Massachusetts and New Hampshire, Minnesota and Wisconsin, and Montana and Wyoming. The difference between Massachusetts and New Hampshire is largely attributable to very low social capital in Boston, possibly related to a diverse population that includes many transient residents. Minnesota has a much stronger Scandinavian influence than Wisconsin, which contributes to its higher social capital. Montana's lower social capital than Wyoming is due to much lower scores for Social Support, Institutional Health, and Philanthropic Health, with the dimension of Institutional Health showing the greatest difference. A large contributor is lower trust in Montana. This can be related to the state's history of problematic relationships between workers and employers and between Whites and American Indians.

There is reasonable consensus that social capital is negatively correlated with the prevalence of depression and with the rate of death by suicide. However, the relationship depends greatly on the characteristics of the population being studied, what measures of social capital are used, and whether social capital is measured at the level of the individual, the neighborhood or community, or the state or nation. For example, the Mountain States have the nation's highest suicide rates despite having above-median social capital. High altitude, rurality, gun culture, and the racial/ethnic composition of Montana and Wyoming outweigh the benefits of family unity, family interaction, and social support, at least as measured at the state level. A person might find social isolation especially unbearable in a place where most other people are socially connected, recalling the theme of "thwarted belongingness" as a risk factor for suicide. On the other hand, when the Community Health and Institutional Health dimensions of social capital are high (people are active in community organizations and trust major institutions like schools and the media), future collective action to improve public mental health might be more feasible.

The Social Capital Project team examined correlations at the state level between their index and its components with "deaths of despair," the latter including suicides, drug overdoses, and deaths due to alcoholism. They found that their composite index of social capital was not correlated at all with deaths of despair. Of the component indices, only Institutional Health (a mixture of structural and cognitive social capital) had a negative (protective) correlation. The correlation was weak, at .41 (Joint Economic Committee, 2018, p. 34).

We approached the state-level analysis of social capital and unnatural death differently, looking at suicide rates specifically (rather than all deaths of despair), analyzing male and female suicide separately, and considering individual items of the social capital index rather than multi-item scales or a summary indicator. As might be expected from the Social Capital Project's findings, the dimension of Institutional Health had the highest negative correlation with suicide for both men and women. Surprisingly, the percentage of the population with some or a great deal of trust in the media showed an extremely strong negative correlation with suicide rates. The adjusted R^2 for linear regressions predicting suicide rates from this item alone was 41.6% for women and 30.4% for men, findings significant at the level of $p < .000001$ for women and $p < .00002$ for men. As would be expected from the extraordinary p values, the statistical significance of these relationships sentiment about the credibility of the media appears to be an indirect indicator of a type of social capital that is protective against suicide. Perhaps public campaigns to destigmatize help-seeking and increase mental health literacy are effective when people trust their motives and accuracy and are of little value when they don't. Distrust of scientific expertise and suspiciousness toward physicians might be seen more often in local or regional subcultures that disparage the "elitist experts" who communicate about mental illness and suicide through ever-suspect "mainstream media."

Regional Personality

In every nation and region, individual personality varies across a wide range, but the validity of *regional personality*—significantly different mean values for major personality traits by region—is provable quantitatively and fits with the published impressions of journalists, social scientists, and novelists (Rentfrow et al., 2013; Woodard, 2011). Residents of the Midwest really are (on average) more agreeable and polite than those from New England or the Mountain States. People in California and New York, the Northeast, and the Northwest are more open to new ideas and feel less threatened by change and diversity. Table 14.6 displays rankings for the 16 states (relative to the 50 states and the District of Columbia) on mean scores on the "Big Five" personality traits. The scores are based on averaging results of web-based personality surveys weighted by gender and ethnicity to make them representative of each state's population.

The table also ranks states on the cultural dimension of "tightness–looseness"—a concept from anthropology and social psychology that captures a culture's having many strongly enforced rules and little tolerance for deviance versus having few strongly enforced rules and greater tolerance for deviance.

Table 14.6 Rank Order within the Fifty States of Average Personality Trait Scores and "Tightness–Looseness" Scores and Ranks

State	Extraversion	Agreeableness	Conscientiousness	Neuroticism	Openness	Tightness score	Tightness Rank
AL	20	36	36	30	48	75.45	2
MS	19	3	12	4	41	78.86	1
AZ	24	31	9	45	31	47.56	29
NM	22	33	1	29	23	45.43	35
IA	15	15	33	22	43	49.02	26
NE	4	10	7	44	44	49.65	24
KY	36	21	19	7	45	63.91	8
WV	23	32	32	1	22	52.48	17
MA	42	40	43	11	4	35.12	45
NH	50	30	44	14	14	36.97	42
MN	5	2	22	41	40	47.84	28
WI	2	5	20	35	47	46.81	30
MT	43	42	29	39	16	46.11	31
WY	41	49	47	38	50	51.24	19
OR	44	18	31	48	3	30.07	49
WA	48	22	25	46	5	31.06	48

Note. Based on data from Harrington and Gelfand (2014).

The tightness-looseness dimension overlaps with Hofstede's dimension of Uncertainty Avoidance.

Tightness develops in cultures that are oriented toward defense against threats. In a tight culture it is less necessary to build trust with individuals because people's behavior can be reliably predicted from their social position and organizational and family connections (Gelfand, 2018). Tighter states tend to have lower average levels of openness and higher average levels of conscientiousness. This relationship was found to be statistically significant in a study by Harrington and Gelfand (2014), who measured tightness–looseness with a composite of nine indicators: (1) legality of corporal punishment in schools, (2) the percentage of students hit in schools, (3) the rate of executions from 1976 through 2011, (4) the severity of state marijuana laws, (5) the proportion of counties in the state that do not permit sale of alcoholic beverages, (6) the legality of same-sex marriage or civil union prior to the U.S. Supreme Court decision permitting same-sex marriage nationwide, (7) the percentage of individuals for whom religion is important or very important in daily life, (8) the percentage of individuals with no religious affiliation, and (9) the percentage of the population that is foreign-born. The scale they developed was internally consistent ($\alpha = .84$), and a factor analysis showed that all items loaded on a single factor that explained 46% of the total variance.

The ten tightest states all fall entirely or partially within the Deep South or greater Appalachia. The ten loosest states are those of New England and the Pacific Northwest plus California and Hawaii. In keeping with the idea that tightness is a defense against threat, tight states have a higher incidence of natural disasters (e.g., tornadoes and floods), more environmental pollution, fewer natural resources, and a higher prevalence of chronic diseases. They also have a higher prevalence of poverty and food insecurity. The historical trauma of the American Civil War has had enduring effects on the cultures of the Deep South and of the large part of greater Appalachia that lay within slave states. Even families that did not own slaves experienced the war as a threat to their tradition, heritage, and way of life—and many 20th-century residents of the same regions have felt similarly threatened by federal initiatives to improve the status of Black Americans, to accurately memorialize the horrors of slavery, and to teach that the Civil War was fought over the preservation of slavery (Lemann, 2015; Theroux, 2015).

Tightness is associated with rurality. Residents of urban areas can keep norm-breaking behavior anonymous and/or segregated in specific neighborhoods and less troubling to those who don't want to see it. Tightness also is associated with less happiness of the population, even after adjusting for the higher rate of poverty in tight states.

The COVID-19 pandemic exposed a paradoxical correlate of tightness—during a pandemic that ultimately took more American lives than the Civil War, residents in tighter states resisted the consistent pleas of public health officials to get vaccinated, and their political leaders actively opposed vaccine mandates and requirements that masks be worn in public schools. When we compared states' vaccination rates as of July 1, 2021 (USA Facts, 2021) with their tightness scores, the Kendall rank correlation was −.75, implying a highly significant negative correlation of tightness and statewide vaccination rates ($p < 3.15 \times 10^{-10}$). Tight states' respect for authority apparently did not extend to respect for scientific or medical expertise on how to respond to a viral pandemic. This observation has implications for the willingness of tight states' residents to accept destigmatizing, scientifically based concepts of depression and BD. If certain behaviors of people with mood disorders are unacceptable within a tight state's culture, disapproval of the behavior will not reliably be reduced (at the population level) by a medical explanation—whether the latter involves genetic vulnerability, brain dysfunction, maladaptive learning, environmental toxicity, or sequelae of ACEs. The professional opinion or advice of a psychiatrist or other clinician might be received with skepticism and suspicion, with persistent stigmatization of both mood disorders and the clinicians who treat them.

Data show, as expected, that Alabama and Mississippi are the tightest states in the 16-state sample; they are the tightest in the country overall. Their levels of openness are in the lowest quintile. A person in Alabama or Mississippi who is deviant—perhaps by having an unconventional gender identity or by being an outspoken atheist or political liberal—is likely to face social ostracism and might even be rejected by their immediate family. Non-conformists from Alabama or Mississippi who don't migrate to another region of the U.S.—or to a relatively loose 'island' within the state like a university community or technological hub, are at risk for depression related to the stress of being rejected and disdained. Those who leave may suffer emotional pain related to leaving family and friends behind or to having been rebuked or rejected by loved ones.

The states of New England and the Pacific Northwest are among the loosest in the U.S., with ranks between 42 and 49 out of 51. They are high on openness and low on conscientiousness and extraversion. An important distinction is that the New England states are high on neuroticism (tendency toward negative affect and associated physical distress), and the Pacific Northwest states are low on that trait.

In a very loose and open state, depression would more likely be precipitated by the breakup of a close relationship or the failure of a new business venture than rejection by one's family and social circle because of one's political views, religious beliefs, or choice of a life partner. In the Deep South, an interracial marriage might precipitate a family crisis, while such marriages are commonplace and unremarkable in New England and the Pacific Northwest.

The relationship between the tight–loose dimension and health outcomes between nations was studied by Harrington and colleagues (2015). They found that the relationships between tightness and dysthymia (chronic depression) and tightness and suicide rate were best captured by quadratic curves; both extreme tightness and extreme looseness were associated with higher dysthymia prevalence and higher suicide mortality. They interpreted the findings as reflecting the importance of a sense of control to emotional well-being. In a very tight culture, people have relatively few options for adapting their behavior to their individual differences. In a very loose one, people are challenged to cope with excessive uncertainty and instability. While the theory is appealing, we were unable to replicate among U.S. states the mathematical relationships Harrington and colleagues showed in an international sample linking the tight–loose dimension to dysthymia and suicide. A possible explanation is that moving to another state is much easier than emigrating from one's native country. If a substantial proportion of adults with personalities or lifestyles incompatible with their regional culture leave the region, the state-level correlation of tightness and population mental health will be weaker.

One aspect of tightness seen in the Deep South and greater Appalachia is the importance of religion. A quantitative perspective on the issue from survey research was reported in the Pew Foundation Religious Landscape Study (Cooperman et al., 2015); data for the 16-state sample are presented in Table 14.7. In Alabama, Mississippi, Kentucky, and West Virginia more than 60% of the adult population said that religion was very important in their daily lives. Evangelical Protestantism is professed by at least one third of the adult population in every state of the Deep South and greater Appalachia. Evangelical Protestant communities usually are tighter than the states in which they are based, even when the state is already tight. A conformist within such a community usually can find substantial social support to buffer their stress, while an overt non-conformist is likely to experience disapproval and rejection. The looseness of New England is reflected in a greater than 12% combined proportion of self-described atheists and agnostics in Massachusetts and New Hampshire, where only one third of residents find religion very important.

Table 14.7 Religious Identification and Subjective Importance of Religion

State	Evangelical Protestant	Mainline Protestant	African American Protestant	Catholic	Latter-day Saints	Muslim	Jewish	Atheist	Agnostic	Religion very important	Religion not at all important
AL	**49%**	13%	16%	7%	1%	<1%	<1%	<1%	<1%	77%	4%
MS	**41%**	12%	24%	4%	1%	<1%	<1%	1%	3%	74%	4%
AZ	26%	12%	1%	**21%**	5%	1%	2%	3%	4%	51%	11%
NM	23%	14%	1%	**34%**	2%	<1%	<1%	3%	5%	59%	13%
IA	28%	**30%**	2%	18%	<1%	1%	<1%	4%	2%	53%	9%
NE	25%	24%	2%	23%	1%	<1%	<1%	1%	4%	54%	8%
KY	**49%**	11%	5%	10%	<1%	<1%	<1%	4%	4%	63%	7%
WV	**39%**	29%	2%	6%	2%	1%	1%	1%	1%	64%	5%
MA	9%	10%	2%	**34%**	1%	1%	3%	5%	7%	33%	20%
NH	13%	16%	1%	**26%**	1%	<1%	2%	6%	7%	33%	15%
MN	19%	**29%**	2%	22%	1%	1%	1%	3%	4%	46%	13%
WI	22%	18%	4%	**25%**	<1%	1%	1%	3%	5%	44%	12%
MT	**28%**	14%	<1%	17%	4%	<1%	<1%	4%	5%	44%	15%
WY	**27%**	16%	<1%	14%	9%	<1%	<1%	3%	3%	49%	9%
OR	**29%**	13%	1%	12%	4%	1%	2%	5%	8%	45%	17%
WA	**25%**	13%	2%	17%	3%	<1%	1%	5%	5%	44%	16%

Note. Data from the Pew Religious Landscape Study (Cooperman et al., 2015). The most prevalent denomination in each state is highlighted in bold face.

Religion, Depression, and Suicide

As noted in Chapter 4, religious belief and practice, and religion-based relationships, can protect against depression and suicide or can have an adverse effect. In areas where religion is very important to the majority, the mental health effects of local culture are partly mediated by religion. Mere affiliation with a religion—even associated with belief—does not usually bring consistent psychological benefits, and it can be problematic if one's life does not conform to the religion's norms or if a religious identity subjects one to stereotyping, discrimination, or the potential for violent attacks. Among people affiliated with an area's majority religion, religious practice (e.g., church attendance, regular prayer) often is associated with a lower incidence and prevalence of MDD. This was illustrated in a three-year longitudinal study of older adults in Utah County, in which 94% of the population identify as members of the LDS Church. Self-identified Latter-day Saints who did not attend church at least weekly had an incidence of MDD higher than those who attended services weekly or more frequently, and higher than those who did not identify with the LDS Church. The mental health effects of engagement with a religious congregation will depend on the intersection of religion with other aspects of a person's identity. For example, in one recent study, more frequent religious attendance was associated with lesser suicidal ideation among heterosexual adults, but with greater suicidal ideation among those identifying as gay, lesbian, or bisexual (Park & Hsieh, 2023).

Leaving a religion—particularly if it is the dominant faith in one's area of residence and/or one's ethnic group—is a profound life experience. People who severed—or seriously modified—their relationships with Roman Catholicism, Orthodox Judaism, or Islam have written volumes about their sometimes-agonizing spiritual journeys. An article on Utahns who left the LDS Church, entitled "The Disenchanted Self," describes their emotional distress as a distinctive cultural syndrome (Brooks, 2020, p. 194). Those who express it are preoccupied with religious and philosophical themes and experience "a loss of personal identity, debilitating bouts of loneliness and regret, and symptoms akin to clinically defined episodes of depression and anxiety." Most of the people described by Brooks would meet this book's criteria for clinical depression, if not DSM/ICD criteria for MDD. Optimal psychotherapy for their depression would need to address their religious/spiritual issues.

When a clinician assesses a depressed person from a place where religion has a prominent role, a holistic assessment would include inquiry about the patient's religious affiliation, their religious practice, and how they use—or don't use—religion to cope with their current life situation, including depressive symptoms. The Brief Religious Coping Scale described in Chapter 4 is a useful prompt for questions clinicians might ask to learn more about the potential relationship of religious beliefs to the patient's current state of mind (Pargament et al., 2011).

The relationship between religion and suicide is complex. Religious affiliation appears to be more protective against suicide in environments where religious practice is less of a social mandate. In a systematic review of ten years of publications on religion and suicide primarily based on studies in Western countries, Lawrence and colleagues (2016) found that religious affiliation and religious service attendance usually protect against suicide attempts and that the effect of regular service attendance persists after adjusting for social support. However, they noted that the effects of affiliation with a specific religion vary with its role in the ambient culture. Involvement in a minority religion can be associated with social isolation, prejudice, stereotyping, and discrimination. While Islam is thought to be protective against suicide, this may not be the case in rural America, where stereotyping, discrimination, and suspicion against Muslims by the Christian majority might outweigh the benefits of Islamic belief and practice.

An international study of university students suggests that religion has a greater protective effect against suicide in countries where there is greater freedom to be non-religious and religious practice is not normative or compulsory (Eskin et al., 2019). Most studies of religion and suicide in Western countries, including the U.S., show protective effects of religion (Lawrence et al., 2016). However, these effects are dependent on the social, cultural, and institutional contexts. Religious affiliation might be less protective in Mississippi or Utah than it is in California or Massachusetts. In a relatively non-religious place, regular participation in worship and congregational life indicates more than mere conformity with local norms—and therefore might be expected to have a stronger correlation with positive mental health outcomes.

In this chapter's 16-state sample, Catholicism is the most prevalent religion in four states: Arizona and New Mexico, reflecting their large Hispanic population, and Massachusetts and New Hampshire, reflecting their French Canadian populations and histories of large-scale immigration in the early 20th century from Ireland and Italy. As detailed in Chapter 4, Catholic belief is more often protective against suicide than Protestant belief, though "the devil is in the details."

Historically, African American Protestant churches, such as the African Methodist-Episcopal Church, retain great importance in the Deep South, where most Blacks are affiliated with one of them. African American churches offer support to their members that helps them bear poverty and discrimination.

Seeking pastoral counseling is a common initial approach to depression by African Americans in the South (Anthony et al., 2015).

Differences in Education and Their Impact

Patterns of educational attainment vary greatly among the 16 states. Table 14.8 shows their proportions of adults over age 25 at each of several educational levels: Less than high school graduate, high school graduate or GED, some college but no degree, associate degree, bachelor's degree, and graduate or professional degree.

Table 14.8 Educational Attainment of State Residents Aged 25 or Older (%)

State	No HS Diploma or GED	HS Diploma or GED	Some College	Associate degree	Bachelor's Degree	Graduate or Professional Degree
AL	**11.2**	30.4	20.6	9	*17.5*	11.3
MS	**12.4**	30.8	21.4	**10.7**	*15.2*	9.6
AZ	**10.9**	*23.8*	23	9.4	20.4	12.5
NM	12	25.7	**22.7**	9.1	*16.9*	13.5
IA	6.6	29.5	19.7	**12**	21.5	10.8
NE	7.2	25.1	21.6	**11.5**	22.6	12.1
KY	11	**32.4**	19.9	8.8	*16.5*	11.4
WV	10.8	**38.3**	*17.2*	8.8	15	9.8
MA	8.7	23	14.3	*7.4*	**25.3**	**21.3**
NH	*5.4*	27.1	*16.8*	9.3	**24.6**	**16.7**
MN	6	*23.4*	19.6	**11.9**	**25.4**	13.7
WI	*6.5*	29.6	19.5	**11.2**	21.7	11.6
MT	6	27.7	**22.3**	9.5	22.9	11.7
WY	*6.2*	27.3	**24.9**	**12**	*18*	11.6
OR	8.4	*22.7*	**23.7**	8.9	22.2	14.1
WA	7.8	*21.5*	21.2	10	**23.8**	15.7
20th percentile	6.6	23.9	17.8	8	19	10.8
Median	8.4	27	19.6	8.9	21.7	12.9
80th percentile	10.8	30.4	22.1	10.2	23.6	15.7

Note. Data from U.S. Census Bureau (2023b), American Community Survey 2022. https://data.census.gov. Queried educational attainment of adults over 25 for U.S. states and the District of Columbia. Data retrieved October 10, 2023. Rates above the 80th percentile are displayed in bold face; those below the 20th percentile are displayed in italics.

The populations of the Deep South, Appalachia, and the Southwest are less educated than those of other regions, a fact with profound economic and public health implications. Better-educated people have better physical and mental health, in part because they have higher health literacy and healthier lifestyles. Among the 16 states, graduate education is most prevalent in New England and the Pacific Northwest. Advanced degrees are associated with opportunities for work that is both personally meaningful and well compensated—a combination protective against depression. And, as became evident during the COVID-19 pandemic, many of the jobs held by people with graduate education allow them great flexibility in the times and/or places they can work. Jobs open to people without a high school education seldom permit working from home—and often are poorly paid, lack healthcare benefits, and expose the employee to health hazards.

Several features of the states' educational patterns are noteworthy regarding their potential relevance to depression and its clinical care. More than 10% of adults over 25 lack a high school education in the states of the Deep South, Greater Appalachia, and the Southwest. Everywhere, less educated people share economic disadvantages, and are likely to have unhealthy habits. However, the details of the populations are different between the regions. In the Deep South, most adults without high school education are rural, and a disproportionate number are Black. In the Southwest, most adults without high school education are Mexican immigrants with limited English proficiency. In Greater Appalachia, adults without a high school education do not have distinct ethnic origins. In West Virginia, the "Whitest" state in the U.S., low social status is more likely to be related to socioeconomic class than to race or ethnicity, and in that state, household income and educational level are highly correlated.

The proportion of adults who have attended college but not graduated varies by state, and it is unusually high in the Mountain States, Oregon, and New Mexico. Many such adults, especially those under 40, have significant educational debt, and the stress related to their debt will be greater if they lack a degree that usually would be necessary for a highly paid job. In New England, fewer than one-third of adults over 25 have not attended college. Personal and family expectations for education and subsequent employment tend to be higher than in less educated states. Narratives about education-related failures and disappointments are common among depressed New Englanders.

Lack of a high school education is a known risk factor for depression, suicide, and substance use disorders associated with depressive symptoms and unnatural deaths. Lack of education is associated with poor health literacy, poor nutrition, unhealthy lifestyles, and the development of conditions like diabetes and obesity that cause depression through direct and indirect pathways. The obese, diabetic, smoking, and chronically depressed resident of the Deep South or Appalachia is a stereotype but one that accurately represents the state of millions of poor Americans.

Another aspect of the educational difference between states is their significantly different rates of literacy and numeracy in the adult population. Literacy has obvious relevance to people's ability to understand written communications about their health and to validly respond to questionnaire-based self-ratings. However, a poorly literate adult might not call a clinician's attention to their weakness. If screening for depression or suicidal ideation in a clinical setting relies on questionnaires alone, it might miss a significant proportion of affected patients with low literacy—and there will be more such patients in places where low literacy is more prevalent. As noted in Chapter 10, with respect to depression questionnaires in poorly educated or illiterate Chinese immigrants, questionnaires that use Likert scales and/or mix positively and negatively worded questions can be problematic in such patients. Simple yes/no questions like those used in the Geriatric Depression Scale have proven more reliable and valid for assessing depression in people with low literacy.

Apart from literacy, numeracy has a significant relationship to health and well-being, perhaps because numerate people can better understand and weigh risks when making decisions about lifestyle and medical care. For example, in a sample of medical outpatients at a Veterans Administration Medical Center in Miami, Florida, higher numeracy was associated with higher trust in physicians, a lower total burden of chronic disease, a lower rate of depressive symptoms, and higher self-rated mental health (Garcia-Retamero et al., 2015). Higher numeracy was associated with greater adherence to preventive healthcare recommendations (e.g., colon cancer screening, influenza immunizations, dental checkups) by middle-aged and older Americans (Yamashita et al., 2020). In the context of the COVID-19 pandemic, more numerate people are more likely to get vaccinated (Thorpe et al., 2024).

Thus, more numerate people are less likely to develop general medical conditions associated with depression. They will be more likely to accept antidepressant drug prescriptions and not be dissuaded by anecdotes about individual bad experiences with them. They will be less likely to develop depression or anxiety based on the emotional effects of health misinformation on social media, as appeared in massive amounts during the COVID-19 pandemic. Of relevance to treatment of clinical depression, a poorly numerate person will be more likely to worry about very rare but very severe potential side effects of an antidepressant treatment. They will be less likely to grasp that the best evidence-based treatment will not work for everyone, understanding immediately that their non-response to a first prescribed treatment means neither that their doctor was wrong or that they are hopelessly ill. If a clinician hopes that a poorly numerate patient will persist through an adequate trial of an antidepressant—and perhaps more than one if the first trial does not bring a remission—some combination of acknowledging the patient's doubts, providing education compatible with the patient's literacy and numeracy, and communicating with the patient frequently will increase the odds that they will persist through the weeks that often are needed to reach a pharmacologically-based remission.

The literacy and numeracy of the adult population of the U.S. aged 16–74 is regularly assessed by the National Center for Education Statistics. The center's estimates of the population's literacy and numeracy by state and county were updated in June 2020 (National Center for Education Statistics, 2021). Separately for literacy and numeracy, three of the indicators reported are the percentage of the population with skills at Level 1 or below, the percentage of those with skills at Level 3 or above, and the average score. (Level 1 literacy comprises skills like reading a simple paragraph to extract a single piece of information or filling out a form requesting personal information. Level 3 literacy requires extracting relevant information from lengthy or complex texts, making inferences, and performing multi-step operations. Level 1 numeracy comprises skills like one-step arithmetic operations and understanding simple percentages like 50%. Level 3 numeracy includes the ability to solve mathematical problems presented in text and understanding of basic statistics.) Among the 16 states of our sample, the states in the Deep South, the Southwest, and greater Appalachia scored below the median for both literacy and numeracy on all three indicators; the remaining states scored above the median. Minnesota was at or near the top on all indicators, Mississippi was near the bottom. The differences are large and consequential: In Mississippi 43.3% of the population have numeracy at Level 1 or below, and 28.0% have literacy at Level 1 or below; the corresponding statistics for New Hampshire are 19.1% for low numeracy and 11.5% for low literacy. In both Mississippi and Alabama, there are several counties in which more than half of the adult population is at the lowest level of numeracy.

The differences among states not only have cultural and medical consequences but also have cultural roots related to the importance placed on public education in the region. Per-pupil public funding of education in grades K–12 in 2020 was $10,001 in Mississippi, $10,871 in Alabama, $18,667 in New Hampshire, and $20,581 in Massachusetts (Hanson, 2021).

While having a graduate or professional degree reduces the risk of depression via higher socioeconomic status, more opportunities for meaningful and satisfying work, and access to social capital, attaining an advanced degree involves living through a situation of increased depression risk. Graduate and professional education are associated for many students with educational debt and with family or personal imperatives to realize success after years of academic effort and expense. Graduate students have a remarkably higher prevalence of clinical depression than other adults matched for age and gender (Flaherty, 2018). International students' rates of common mental disorders are approximately the same as those of students who grew up in the U.S., but they are much less likely to seek treatment for them. Many come from countries in which mental illness and its treatment are highly stigmatized, and/or students fear that a history of psychiatric treatment would be noted on their academic record or even lead to revocation of their student visas (Redden, 2019). States like Massachusetts and California, and regions like the New York City metropolitan area, which have many universities and professional schools, have a disproportionate share of America's depressed adult students.

The Southwest's unusual combination of a relatively low high school completion rate and a relatively high percentage of adults with advanced degrees reflects economic and cultural differences between the Hispanic and American Indian populations and the non-Hispanic White population of the states. In the Southwest, almost all Hispanic residents except for the Hispanos (see above) are either of Mexican origin or are Guatemalan, Honduran, or Salvadorian. These four groups of Hispanic Americans have much lower rates of college graduation than those from the Caribbean, South America, or other nations of Central America (Musu-Gillette et al., 2017). This is related partially to economic disadvantage and partly to a culture that emphasizes hard work, family loyalty, and sharing of resources within the extended family over educational achievement (Barshay, 2018). American Indians also have a low college graduation rate, reflecting that group's chronic educational and economic disadvantage (Oliff, 2017).

The concentration of people with higher education in a minority of states reflects the geographical distribution of colleges and universities but also the net migration of people with higher education to places (states and metropolitan areas) where there is more opportunity for their occupational success and/or more advanced study. The net effect is that most American states suffer a net loss of their educated residents through outmigration exceeding immigration and that highly educated people are concentrated in the most dynamic metropolitan areas of California, Texas, Florida, the Pacific Northwest, New England, and the Mid-Atlantic, plus Chicago and Minneapolis. These migrations sustain and amplify the cultural and economic differences among American regions (Joint Economic Committee, 2018b).

Highly educated people tend to be open to psychotherapy or counseling, and most do not stigmatize themselves for seeking such help. Acceptance of a major psychiatric diagnosis and treatment with medication may be different. Two specific concerns that creative professionals have about antidepressant drug therapy, discussed in Chapter 15, are applicable to highly educated people with other occupations. A person with a cognitively intense occupation is likely to be distressed by side effects of antidepressant or mood-stabilizing medication that reduce their psychomotor speed and precision, emotional sensitivity, creativity and/or motivation. Also, in centers of innovation and elite education there is an increased concentration of people with hyperthymia or cyclothymia, who have an increased probability of developing a bipolar spectrum disorder if treated with an antidepressant without a concurrent mood stabilizer.

Income Inequality, Poverty, and the Context of Depression and Its Treatment

Poverty and income inequality importantly affect the epidemiology of depression, the themes of depression narratives, the choice of optimal treatment, and the feasibility of treatment alternatives. Both poverty rates and income inequality are high throughout the U.S., but regions differ by severity of poverty, by the relative security or insecurity of the middle class, and by the degree of inequality at the top. Table 14.9 provides statistics for the 16 states on average household income in 2022 by quintile and for the top 5%. Table 14.10 shows rates of poverty for subgroups defined by age, gender, and race/ethnicity. In 2022 the "poverty line" (Federal Poverty Level) was $13,590 for individuals, $18,030 for a household with two members, and $27,750 for a family of four. Thus, when a state's average income for the first quintile is less than $13,590, every household in the first quintile will be in poverty, and children living in households in the first quintile will be in abject poverty.

Poverty rates among the states vary greatly, from a low of 7.25% in New Hampshire to a high of 19.1% in Mississippi. Strikingly, in the five states with the highest poverty rates, those of the Deep South and Appalachia plus New Mexico, childhood poverty rates are disproportionately higher—in Mississippi and in West Viriginia, one quarter or more of all children were living in poverty in 2022. In all states, the rate of poverty is higher for females than for males, but the difference is greater in states with greater gender inequality. Late life poverty, a problem mitigated somewhat by Social Security and Medicare, still affects approximately 10% of Americans over age 65. Its prevalence is higher in states with higher poverty rates overall. With respect to race and ethnicity, poverty is greater among Black, Hispanic, and American Indian people than it is among non-Hispanic Whites everywhere in the country, while poverty among Asian Americans varies greatly according to the specific Asian nationalities

Table 14.9 Income Distribution by State: 2022 Average Household Income by Quintiles and for the Top 5%

State	First Quintile	Second Quintile	Third Quintile	Fourth Quintile	Fifth Quintile	Top Five Percent
AL	*$11,137*	*$31,534*	*$54,417*	*$87,743*	*$194,783*	*$340,996*
MS	*$9,738*	*$28,055*	*$49,085*	*$80,285*	*$173,076*	*$300,597*
AZ	$15,838	$42,333	$69,087	$105,980	$232,648	$415,144
NM	*$10,472*	*$31,865*	*$54,874*	*$89,251*	*$198,485*	*$343,386*
IA	$15,850	$40,758	$65,956	$99,447	$210,483	$372,563
NE	$15,569	$41,180	$67,248	$102,568	$219,478	$391,315
KY	*$11,356*	*$32,525*	*$56,008*	*$88,356*	*$192,927*	*$341,277*
WV	*$10,555*	*$29,853*	*$51,651*	*$83,127*	*$186,283*	*$337,547*
MA	$16,040	**$50,598**	**$90,296**	**$144,566**	**$322,443**	**$566,762**
NH	**$21,308**	**$54,067**	**$88,393**	**$131,496**	$264,274	$451,371
MN	**$18,888**	$48,551	$78,229	$119,000	$251,857	$439,236
WI	$16,220	$41,858	$67,596	$102,206	$213,641	$373,977
MT	$15,165	$38,467	$63,211	$97,681	$220,891	$399,224
WY	$14,437	$39,254	$65,707	$99,072	$216,086	$397,621
OR	$15,707	$43,105	$71,736	$110,448	$237,317	$409,985
WA	**$18,741**	**$51,434**	**$85,151**	**$131,965**	**$294,454**	**$520,392**
20th Percentile	$13,098	$36,919	$62,122	$95,573	$210,483	$372,525
Median	$14,823	$40,643	$67,081	$102,568	$226,918	$401,099
80th Percentile	$16,575	$48,551	$81,493	$126,946	$272,972	$465,118

Note. Data from U.S. Census Bureau (2023b). American Community Survey 2022, Table B19081. Mean Household Income of Quintiles. https://data.census.gov/table/ACSDT1Y2022.B19081?q=income+ine quality&g=040XX00US01,02,04,05,06,08,09,10,11,12,13,15,16,17,18,19,20,21,22,23,24,25,26,27, 28,29,30,31,32,33,34,35,36,37,38,39,40,41,42,44,45,46,47,48,49,50,51,53,54,55,56. Values above the national 80th percentile are displayed in bold face; those below the national 20th percentile are displayed in italics.

involved. For example, in West Viriginia, the poverty rate for non-Hispanic Whites was 17.1%, while the rate for Asians was 10.0%. In West Virginia many Asians are Indian Americans, an ethnic group that nationally has an average household income much higher than that of non-Hispanic Whites.

The states of the Deep South, greater Appalachia, and the Southwest all have poverty rates in the top quartile nationally, but beyond that, the *extent* of poverty is greater. An annual household income of less than $10,000 per year, as

Table 14.10 State Poverty Rates by Age and Gender, Race and Ethnicity in 2022

State	All residents	Age <18	Age ≥65	Male	Female	Non-Hispanic White	Black	Asian	Hispanic	American Indian
AL	**16.2%**	**22.0%**	12.0%	14.5%	**17.8%**	11.3%	26.8%	9.8%	**27.6%**	18.1%
MS	**19.1%**	**26.4%**	**14.7%**	**17.5%**	**20.7%**	11.9%	**29.3%**	**16.9%**	**22.4%**	**27.2%**
AZ	12.5%	15.8%	10.4%	11.5%	13.4%	9.1%	16.5%	11.8%	15.9%	**29.0%**
NM	**17.6%**	**23.5%**	**13.0%**	**15.9%**	**19.2%**	**12.1%**	18.0%	**14.0%**	19.6%	**30.9%**
IA	11.0%	12.2%	8.5%	9.8%	12.1%	9.3%	**34.0%**	**14.1%**	14.7%	**36.0%**
NE	11.2%	13.8%	9.2%	9.9%	12.6%	9.1%	**28.7%**	10.2%	16.0%	20.8%
KY	**16.5%**	**20.9%**	**13.1%**	**14.8%**	**18.1%**	**15.0%**	26.6%	10.9%	**21.1%**	**22.8%**
WV	**17.9%**	**25.0%**	12.1%	**16.6%**	**19.3%**	**17.1%**	**30.7%**	10.0%	**22.4%**	–
MA	10.4%	*11.5%*	11.2%	9.5%	11.1%	7.6%	17.4%	11.6%	19.9%	10.5%
NH	*7.2%*	*6.9%*	*7.9%*	*6.3%*	*8.2%*	*6.8%*	*11.9%*	*3.8%*	*14.8%*	–
MN	9.6%	*10.9%*	9.0%	8.8%	*10.5%*	*7.2%*	24.7%	11.8%	16.8%	**30.1%**
WI	10.7%	12.7%	9.6%	9.6%	11.9%	8.5%	26.5%	11.5%	18.6%	23.1%
MT	12.1%	13.4%	12.5%	11.4%	12.9%	10.4%	–	–	**24.2%**	**32.7%**
WY	11.8%	14.1%	9.8%	10.5%	13.2%	**11.6%**	33.9%	–	*10.2%*	22.6%
OR	12.1%	13.8%	9.9%	10.9%	13.3%	11.2%	21.8%	10.7%	*14.8%*	19.0%
WA	*10.0%*	*11.4%*	*9.3%*	*9.1%*	*10.9%*	*8.5%*	17.0%	*7.8%*	*14.8%*	16.8%
20th percentile	10.4%	12.2%	9.0%	9.4%	11.1%	7.7%	17.2%	8.9%	13.6%	16.6%
Median	12.1%	15.2%	10.2%	11.0%	13.2%	9.3%	22.5%	10.9%	17.2%	20.6%
80th percentile	14.0%	18.8%	12.1%	12.5%	15.2%	11.2%	27.2%	12.9%	20.8%	28.3%

Note. Data from U.S. Census Bureau (2023b). Estimates from 1-year American Community Survey, 2022. Table S1701 Poverty Status in the past 12 months. https://data.census.gov/table/ACSST1Y2022.S1701?q=american+community+survey+poverty+rates. Values above the national 80th percentile are displayed in bold face; those below the national 20th percentile are displayed in italics.

many Mississipians experienced in 2022, could make a parent's $5 copayment for an antidepressant prescription imply a child's malnutrition. In the states with the lowest incomes at the bottom, more than a quarter of preschool children experience a level of poverty necessarily implying adverse childhood experiences that increase their lifetime risk of depression and bipolar illness.

The dominant culture of the Deep South does not favor public assistance to poor people. Despite their states' high poverty rates, the citizens of Mississippi and Alabama chose not to expand their Medicaid programs to provide health insurance to families who were poor but not destitute. For lack of insurance, poor people in these states get much of their healthcare in emergency rooms. Non-emergent problems, including depression without acute suicidal ideation and chronic general medical conditions related to depression, frequently go untreated.

In Massachsuetts and Washington, the two most prosperous states in the 16-state sample, the average income of the top five percent is dramatically higher than that of the fifth quintile overall. The incomes of the top 1% and top 0.1%, not shown in the table, are extremely high. A similar distribution is found in metropolitan areas of California including the San Francisco Bay Area and Silicon Valley, and metropolitan New York City and Washington DC. In such locales, a person in the top quintile of income but not in the top 1%—might regard themselves as a failure or a loser if they were inclined by personality or by culture to be perfectionistic or to engage in upward comparison. In a metropolitan area with a high cost of living and many conspicuously wealthy residents, the relative socioeconomic status of a mental health professional might not be high. The income of an early-career physician or psychologist, a physician assistant or advanced practice nurse, or a psychotherapist without a doctoral degree might not make it into the area's top quintile for employed adults. In might be a challenge for a clinician in such a situation to empathize with a patient whose household income is $300,000 per year and who feels like a loser, but if the clinician succeeds, they will gain cultural awareness helpful in many other cases.

In such locales, depressed people in the top 1% of household income will have no difficulty paying for expensive treatments of depression, like intensive psychotherapy or new medications not covered by insurance. As pointed out in Chapter 6, an expensive treatment especially likely to work well for an individual might be offered earlier if the clinician knows that the cost will not be a realistic barrier.

The marked differences between states in the average household income in the third quintile—the middle of the income distribution—is relatable to the tightness of the states' cultures. We tested the correlations of the states' tightness scores with the average incomes of the five quintiles and of the top 5%. While the expected negative correlations were seen for all quintiles, the strongest correlation of tightness with lower average household income (a coefficient of −.71) was for the third quintile—the 20% of households around the state median. If a typical third-quintile household has an income less than twice the threshold for poverty, most of the state's residents will be concerned about survival issues, leading to a generally tight culture. If many third-quintile households have incomes more than three times the poverty threshold, more than half of the state's residents are likely to not be in "survival mode," and their culture will be looser.

Poverty is a cause of depression, and poverty in childhood is associated with food insecurity and nutritional deficiencies, a lack of regular pediatric care, and multiple ACEs, which, as noted elsewhere in this book, can lead to a lifetime vulnerability to clinical depression. Pathways include nutritional, toxic, and traumatic effects on brain development; educational disadvantage; chronic inflammation; and epigenetic mechanisms. Poverty in infancy and early childhood is especially harmful. For families that have been poor for generations, deprivation might be normalized, and this can create self-defeating beliefs. Depression risk is higher in people who have experienced childhood poverty even if they join the middle or upper class as adults.

A potential consequence of childhood poverty and related ACEs is the expression of depression through externalizing behavior. This can occur in both males and females, though it is more common in males. If a boy engages in delinquent behavior as an adolescent, it can prematurely end his formal education and/or lead to early incarceration, which has lifetime effects on the occupational and financial prospects of the boy and can have traumatic impact on family members.

Regions of the U.S. differ greatly in their rates of incarceration. The variance in rates of incarceration is not well explained by differences in their incidence of crimes. The likelihood and duration of imprisonment for a given criminal offense correlate with the "tightness" of the state's culture. The states of the Deep South, greater Appalachia, and the Mountain States all have above-median incarceration rates (>370 prison inmates per 100,000 population), while those of New England, the Pacific Northwest, and the central Midwest have below-median rates. The Southwest splits—Arizona has an above-median rate, while New Mexico's is below-median, as does the upper Midwest, with Minnesota's rate much lower than that of Wisconsin. Differences can be extreme, with Mississippi's incarceration rate almost 6 times the rate of Massachusetts (World Population Review, 2021).

A high incarceration rate has several implications for depression: Formerly incarcerated people have a high risk of depression, as do the family members of those currently in prison. People with histories of imprisonment have difficulty finding employment, and their unemployment often keeps them and their families in poverty. States with high per capita spending on their prison systems tend to have low per capita spending on mental health services, so more depression goes untreated. A clinician usually will know if a patient has a record of imprisonment, but the past or current incarceration of a family member might not be disclosed spontaneously. Knowing that a depressed patient comes from a state with a high incarceration rate should prompt a clinician to consider the possibility of the current or past incarceration of a patient's parent, spouse or partner, child, or other relative.

Adult poverty rates among the 16 states vary widely, but the rate for women is always higher than the rate for men, reflecting the financial trials of single motherhood and occupational gender inequality. The gap in poverty rates between men and women is largest in the Deep South and Appalachian states. Child poverty rates do not differ significantly between boys and girls, but their variability between states is even larger, reflecting differences in states' economies, percentage of births to single mothers, and level of public support for child welfare.

The highest incomes in more rural states are more often based on inheritance or on participation in a family business than on personal entrepreneurial success. For this reason, wealthy people in rural states less often serve as role models for ambitious young people born into working-class or middle-class families. Talented people often leave these states, with emotional consequences for family members left behind and the economic consequence that the state creates fewer successful new businesses. A vicious circle underlies generations of poverty, lesser learning opportunities for talented and ambitious young adults, a less educated population, and limited upward mobility.

Poverty and poor education have long been known as risk factors for depression, and it is now widely recognized that severe inequality is directly associated with worse population health. The connection is mediated both by inequality's association with lower social capital and by direct effects on the material circumstances, education, and opportunities of those with lower incomes (Pearce & Davey Smith, 2003).

Except in Massachusetts and New Hampshire, more than half of all households in the sixteen state sample have incomes less than 400% of the poverty line; and in the Deep South, the Mountain States, and the Southwest, more than 30% of the population have incomes between 125% and 300% of the poverty threshold. A person with a household income in the latter range is unlikely to have significant savings or available credit to deal with a significant unexpected problem with their home, car, job(s), health, or the health of a family member. Severe vulnerability to unexpected financial stress was evident during the COVID-19 pandemic, where a few months of income disruption brought millions of families to the brink of eviction from their homes. For people with household incomes less than 300% of the poverty line, treatments of depression that involve substantial out-of-pocket expense or significant time off work often will be unaffordable, or will seem so to a person already discouraged by their depression. Perceived unaffordability will be greater if there is culturally based doubt about depression being a real illness rather than a the result of personal weakness or an inevitable part of life to be stoically tolerated rather than expensively treated. A depressed person in a financially precarious position can be treated more effectively if financial barriers to treatment are addressed up front. This might require modifying the plan of care to better fit the patient's budget, for example, by prescribing the lowest-cost antidepressant drug or utilizing a psychotherapeutic smartphone app rather than individual psychotherapy.

In the U.S., a country without a national health system, poverty impedes access to mental health care. Access to treatment of depression by poor Americans requires a combination of public mental health services, Medicaid or other insurance coverage of the poor, parity of coverage for mental health care and general medical care, and an adequate number and distribution of mental health professionals. State-level indicators of access to mental health care, assembled by the advocacy group Mental Health America (2023), are shown in Table 14.11.

Several of the states that have high poverty rates and a high proportion of financially precarious households—Alabama, Mississippi, West Virginia, and Arizona—also have shortages of mental health professionals and poor insurance coverage for mental health services. Differences between states in the same region are of interest. The Pacific Northwest and the Mountain States have more mental health professionals per capita than most states in other regions with similar economic status and rurality, perhaps because the states are appealing places to live. However, the mental health professionals are concentrated in more prosperous areas with a higher quality of life, and states in these regions have many rural counties with no psychiatrist. New Mexico offers better access to mental health care than Arizona, and Iowans have better access to mental health care than Nebraskans. Unfortunately, even the states ranked highest by Mental Health America have unacceptably high rates of untreated and undertreated mental illness, with depression in children and adolescents especially likely to go untreated.

Culture, and not just the state's economy, plays a role in determining access to care. New Mexico and Alabama have similar distributions of income; but in Alabama, many more adults with mental illness are uninsured, and the state has an extreme shortage of mental health professionals. Alabamians' poor insurance coverage reflects a culture in which access to healthcare is seen as a

Table 14.11 Indicators of Access to Mental Health Care

State	Overall rank	Adults with mental illness who did not receive treatment	Adults with mental illness who are uninsured	Adults with mental illness with unmet needs despite seeking treatment	Youths with major depression who did not receive mental health services	Children with private insurance that did not cover mental or emotional problems	People per mental health professional
AL	47	57%	19%	19%	70%	5.9%	990
MS	49	58%	22%	24%	66%	7.5%	630
AZ	40	53%	10%	26%	60%	12.1%	750
NM	25	57%	6%	21%	63%	7.8%	260
IA	15	50%	8%	26%	53%	7.5%	640
NE	29	53%	10%	26%	55%	12.6%	380
KY	18	51%	5%	25%	49%	11.0%	440
WV	30	52%	8%	23%	59%	7.2%	770
MA	2	50%	4%	22%	61%	1.2%	160
NH	10	52%	8%	25%	60%	2.5%	330
MN	6	53%	7%	21%	55%	7.5%	400
WI	7	49%	7%	25%	47%	5.4%	490
MT	19	54%	10%	25%	56%	5.5%	330
WY	38	65%	23%	20%	57%	12.0%	300
OR	21	59%	9%	30%	54%	6.7%	190
WA	16	54%	11%	24%	48%	5.2%	270

Note. Data from Mental Health America (2023).

private concern and not a community issue. Its lack of mental health professionals reflects the lack of appeal of its "tight" culture to mental health professionals who are highly educated and tend to be open-minded. By contrast, New Mexico has a more communitarian culture, and it is an appealing place for mental health professionals to live, with great natural beauty and towns like Santa Fe, Los Alamos, and Taos with concentrations of highly educated, creative people.

However, having a mental health workforce and broad insurance coverage does not ensure that people with depression will be identified and treated. Despite differences in insurance coverage and the mental health workforce, the two states' rates of untreated mental illness are virtually the same, and in both states most children and teens with major depression go untreated. The most effective strategies to improve the public's mental health would be different between the two states. An anti-depression public health initiative in Alabama could not rely on referring depressed people to mental health professionals as there are so few of them, nor could it rely on a public education campaign as there is a low level of trust in government, public schools, and scientific expertise. It might instead focus on equipping primary care providers with more tools and support for identifying and managing depression in their patients since most people in Alabama trust their personal physicians. In New Mexico, an anti-depression public health initiative might focus on increasing telepsychiatry services (including improving high-speed internet access), enabling mental health professionals based in Santa Fe or Albuquerque to provide remote service to rural areas, and improved outreach to the state's Mexican American and American Indian populations.

For poor or near-poor people living in states with poor access to timely and adequate mental health care, mild to moderate clinical depression without suicidal ideation or bipolar features might be more effectively managed by addressing social determinants of health than by offering patients a potentially stigmatizing diagnosis and prescribing treatments that they would find impractical, unaffordable, or simply unavailable. An optimal care team for a depressed poor or near-poor patient population might include social workers dealing with living arrangements and potential income supports; nutritionists knowledgeable about antidepressant diets that would be culturally compatible, accessible, and affordable; and people to assist with employment issues.

Behavioral and Environmental Risk Factors

ACEs, including divorce, single parenthood, and IPV, are risk factors for depression that vary significantly between states and across regions. Health habits, especially those related to diet and exercise, both directly and indirectly affect mood. Household gun ownership and associated gun culture are important determinants of suicide rates as most suicides in America use firearms, suicide attempts with firearms usually are fatal, and distressed people do not necessarily find another equally lethal means of self-harm if a firearm is unavailable. A state or region's physical environment comprises risk factors for depression related to altitude, latitude, and pollution of air and water. Ownership of firearms and whether they are stored loaded and unlocked are subject to cultural norms. Whether pollution of water and air is tolerated politically, which subsets of the population normalize it, and which disadvantaged groups are involuntarily subjected to it also are reflections of regional culture. The regional distribution of selected behavioral and environment risk factors is the subject of the next set of tables, beginning with Table 14.12, which shows the percentage of children in each state who have experienced various ACEs (Joint Economic Committee, 2018b; United Health Foundation, 2020).

ACEs increase lifetime vulnerability to mental disorders, including depression and BD. Addressing ACEs with primary and secondary preventive strategies can have long-term benefits for mental health. When clinicians encounter people with depressive symptoms from populations with a high rate of ACEs (e.g., low-income and/or ethnic minority patients from a state with a high prevalence of ACEs), inquiry about ACEs should come relatively early, as it is likely to reveal history relevant to therapeutic engagement with the patient.

The percentage of children experiencing two or more ACEs before age 18 varies in the 16-state sample between 15.9% in Massachusetts and 30.6% in Arizona. Even the rate in Massachusetts is high enough to warrant exploration of the theme in virtually every patient with depression at some point in their clinical assessment. Regional differences in demographics, culture, and behavioral norms prompt place-specific considerations. Exploring the theme of incarceration of parents or other significant people is more likely to illuminate a case of depression in Kentucky, where almost 15% of children under 18 experience incarceration of a parent, than it is in Massachusetts, where only 3.5% of children under 18 have had a parent imprisoned. Domestic violence is a consideration everywhere, but it should be explored earlier in the dialogue when engaging with a patient from the Southwest, the Deep South, or another region where there is a history of cultural normalization of corporal punishment and violence within marriage. Similar considerations apply when a patient comes from a cultural group in which certain forms of domestic violence are a norm, including some Chinese and Korean populations, as discussed in Chapters 10 and 12.

Table 14.12 Prevalence of Adverse Childhood Experiences (ACEs) Among Children Aged 0–17

State	Parental divorce	Parental death	Parental incarceration	Domestic violence	Mentally ill family member	Lived with substance abuser	Witnessed neighborhood violence	Two or more ACEs
Percentage of children with ACEs								
AL	29.9%	**4.8%**	7.6%	6.2%	7.6%	10.1%	4.1%	**27.7%**
MS	**32.2%**	**4.7%**	**10.7%**	**10.7%**	8.7%	**11.7%**	2.1%	**27.2%**
AZ	**31.9%**	2.8%	**12.9%**	**10.8%**	9.9%	**15.9%**	**5.9%**	**30.6%**
NM	**31.5%**	**4.6%**	**11.8%**	**11.1%**	**11.5%**	**12.6%**	**6.2%**	**27.8%**
IA	22.9%	2.2%	5.9%	5.2%	9.6%	9.4%	5.3%	20.0%
NE	*22.1%*	2.1%	8.0%	4.6%	**10.1%**	9.5%	3.7%	*19.9%*
KY	**32.8%**	2.7%	**14.9%**	6.8%	9.9%	**12.0%**	3.3%	**26.9%**
WV	**31.1%**	**5.0%**	8.7%	7.4%	**11.5%**	11.3%	2.8%	**26.1%**
MA	*19.1%*	3.8%	*3.5%*	*2.8%*	*6.6%*	*6.2%*	2.4%	*15.9%*
NH	23.7%	3.6%	4.5%	4.1%	9.1%	9.0%	2.2%	19.7%
MN	*20.1%*	*2.1%*	6.5%	4.9%	7.5%	8.8%	4.5%	16.8%
WI	22.2%	2.6%	9.1%	5.7%	8.7%	8.5%	4.4%	20.3%
MT	28.4%	3.6%	10.4%	7.0%	**13.8%**	**13.5%**	**5.7%**	**26.1%**
WY	25.9%	3.1%	9.0%	**8.0%**	**12.1%**	11.6%	2.9%	**26.0%**
OR	24.8%	2.0%	7.0%	6.1%	10.5%	10.8%	3.0%	22.4%
WA	23.5%	*1.5%*	5.5%	4.3%	**10.7%**	10.2%	2.2%	19.3%
20th %ile	*22.0%*	*2.4%*	*5.9%*	*4.5%*	*6.9%*	*7.9%*	*2.9%*	*19.4%*
Median	25.7%	3.4%	8.6%	5.9%	8.7%	9.9%	4.1%	22.4%
80th %ile	**29.1%**	**4.5%**	**10.4%**	**7.4%**	**10.5%**	**11.6%**	**5.7%**	**26.1%**

Note. From United Health Foundation (2020). Rates above the 80th percentile are displayed in bold face; those below the 20th percentile are displayed in italics.

Children with single parents, especially those born to unmarried women, are more likely to experience ACEs. Table 14.13 shows the percentage of births in 2021 that were to single mothers. The rate of births to unmarried women is higher in "tight" states than in "loose" ones, perhaps because in tight states there is less sex education in public schools, lesser access to contraceptives and abortion, and greater gender inequality. It is higher in rural areas and thus higher in states with a more rural population. In the 16-state sample, the percentage of births to single mothers is remarkably high in the Deep South, Appalachia, and the Southwest and remarkably low in New England, the Midwest, and the Pacific Northwest. The high rate of births to unmarried women in the Southwest partly reflects the culture of *marianismo* in the states' Latina population.

Clinical encounters with unmarried women related to symptoms of depression are opportunities to address sexual and reproductive health issues. Similarly, visits by single women to obstetrician/gynecologists are opportunities to address mental health concerns. However, ob-gyn physicians usually fail to diagnose depression—even moderately severe depression—when their patients do not present with a psychological chief complaint and do not mention psychological distress, and this is the case for most ob-gyn visits of depressed women (Cerimele et al., 2013). Depression diagnoses might be made more often if there were convenient and culturally acceptable options for follow-up. For example, short-term psychoeducational groups for Latinas in the second trimester of pregnancy, led by nurse practitioners, were pilot-tested in El Paso, Texas, and in a rural area outside Austin. A six-session class reduced women's use of negative coping behaviors and resulted in clinically meaningful reduction in depressive symptoms (Ruiz et al., 2019). Pregnant low-income Black women have a high rate of trauma exposure, PTSD, and clinical depression; but few cases of either PTSD or depression are detected by routine ob-gyn care, and most are not treated (Powers et al., 2020). As the ob-gyn frequently is the only regular source of non-emergency healthcare for young low-income women, integration of culturally aware mental health services with ob-gyn practices is an obvious intervention for addressing depression on a population basis in communities where Blacks are in the majority.

Single mothers in the U.S., especially those in their late teens and early twenties and those who are non-White or poor, are at high risk for postpartum depression (Cabeza de Baca et al., 2018; Campbell-Grossman et al., 2016; Kim et al., 2012). The increased risk of single American women for PPD relates to circumstances beyond their relationship status alone. A study of postpartum depression in single women in Sweden suggests that single status might not

Table 14.13 Percentage of Births to Single Mothers in 2021

State	Percentage of births to single mothers
AL	**46.5%**
MS	**54.8%**
AZ	45.4%
NM	**52.4%**
IA	*35.1%*
NE	*34.2%*
KY	42.7%
WV	**45.7%**
MA	*32.6%*
NH	*31.0%*
MN	*31.8%*
WI	36.8%
MT	*33.0%*
WY	*32.9%*
OR	36.5%
WA	*31.6%*
20th percentile	33.2%
Median	39.4%
80th percentile	45.5%

Note. Data from Centers for Disease Control and Prevention. CDC WONDER database. Inquiry on births in 2021. https://wonder.cdc.gov. Retrieved October 13, 2023. Values above the national 80th percentile are displayed in bold face; those below the national 20th percentile are displayed in italics.

imply increased risk in places with extensive public support for single parents and lesser stigma of single motherhood (Agnafors et al., 2019).

Divorce is another contributor to ACEs and an indicator of family conflict that is sometimes expressed as IPV. It also is a major life event associated with an increase in depression risk for the adults involved. Divorce rates differ significantly among the states, reflecting local norms, the role of religion, the typical age and circumstances of marriage, and aspects of divorce laws that influence the cost of divorce and its aftermath to the party initiating the legal action.

Early marriage, which increases the risk for divorce, is common both in the Southwest and in Appalachia. Evangelical Christianity promotes earlier marriage through both individual- and community-level mechanisms. Individuals who affiliate with a conservative/evangelical Protestant denomination (e.g., Southern Baptist) are more likely to marry and have children by their mid-20s, and a young mother with an evangelical Protestant affiliation and with an employed husband is unlikely to work outside the home when her children are young. These decisions are associated with increased divorce risk. In areas where most individuals have the same religious affiliation, the religious community determines social norms and expectations for everyone in the area, with effects on the average age at first marriage and first childbirth even for women not affiliated with the predominant religious group (Glass & Levchak, 2014).

The Midwestern states have combinations of Yankee and Midlands cultures with significant Scandinavian influence in three of the four. Their divorce rates are relatively low. In Yankee and Midlands cultures, it is expected that people will stay married despite troubles and conflicts. These cultures favor family stability and reduce poverty rates for women and children. However, they increase the prevalence of depression related to the emotional strain of long-term unhappy marriages. In a zone of "secular Puritan" culture, it should not be inferred from the stability of a marriage that it is a happy one.

One expression of unhappiness in a marriage or other long-term intimate relationship is IPV. Table 14.14 displays data on the lifetime prevalence of IPV reported in the *National Intimate Partner and Sexual Violence State Report* (NISVS) for 2010–2012 (Smith et al., 2017). The table includes a contemporary Gender Inequality Index, which was calculated using a United Nations (UN) Development Programme formula based on the pregnancy-associated mortality rate, the teen birth rate, women's representation in government, women's educational attainment, and women's labor force participation (Willie & Kershaw, 2019). Across the U.S., gender inequality is significantly associated with IPV of all types against women and with psychological but not physical IPV against men. Apparently, women in states with high gender inequality are more likely to attack their partners—or defend against them—with words and aggressive behavior rather than with blows.

The authors followed up on the Willie and Kershaw analysis by exploring, for U.S. states and the District of Columbia, the relationship between overall gender inequality and the gap between men and women for each type of IPV. In the entire sample, gender inequality was significantly associated with the gender gap for sexual violence and stalking but not with the gap for physical IPV or psychological IPV. The variability in the IPV gender gap is much greater than the

Table 14.14 Lifetime Prevalence of Physical and Psychological Intimate Partner Violence (IPV)

State	Gender Inequality Index	Lifetime prevalence of victimization—Women			Lifetime prevalence of victimization—Men			Victimization Gender Gap		
		Any IPV	Physical IPV	Psychological IPV	Any IPV	Physical IPV	Psychological IPV	Any IPV	Physical IPV	Psychological IPV
AL	0.259	37.5%	32.4%	46.4%	29.5%	28.6%	44.8%	8.0%	3.8%	1.6%
MS	**0.340**	39.7%	34.8%	46.1%	31.7%	30.4%	46.9%	8.0%	4.4%	−0.8%
AZ	**0.368**	**42.6%**	38.6%	**55.4%**	33.4%	29.8%	**55.4%**	9.2%	8.8%	0.0%
NM	0.286	37.6%	31.1%	48.0%	33.3%	31.5%	49.1%	4.3%	−0.4%	−1.1%
IA	*0.183*	35.3%	28.6%	45.4%	29.3%	27.1%	42.0%	6.0%	1.5%	3.4%
NE	0.228	33.7%	30.0%	46.9%	28.0%	24.8%	45.3%	5.7%	5.2%	1.6%
KY	0.280	**45.3%**	**42.1%**	**57.2%**	**35.5%**	32.1%	47.7%	9.8%	**10.0%**	**9.5%**
WV	0.237	39.4%	36.3%	48.5%	**36.3%**	**34.0%**	50.9%	3.1%	2.3%	−2.4%
MA	0.309	33.9%	26.8%	44.1%	31.7%	30.3%	47.5%	2.2%	−3.5%	−3.4%
NH	*0.178*	34.7%	28.2%	45.1%	35.4%	31.9%	42.8%	−0.7%	−3.7%	2.3%
MN	0.311	33.9%	26.2%	42.3%	25.1%	23.5%	38.7%	8.8%	2.7%	3.6%
WI	0.219	36.3%	31.2%	48.0%	32.1%	28.7%	45.7%	4.2%	2.5%	2.3%
MT	0.287	37.2%	30.3%	47.0%	34.6%	32.5%	51.3%	2.6%	−2.2%	−4.3%
WY	**0.337**	33.9%	29.7%	51.9%	30.5%	28.2%	40.9%	3.4%	1.5%	**11.0%**
OR	*0.190*	39.8%	35.0%	**52.4%**	**36.2%**	**34.4%**	44.5%	3.6%	0.6%	**7.9%**
WA	*0.180*	**41.4%**	**37.5%**	48.7%	31.7%	28.0%	46.9%	9.7%	**9.5%**	1.8%
20th percentile	0.218	33.9%	28.6%	44.4%	27.9%	25.2%	41.9%	3.1%	0.6%	−3.4%
Median	0.253	37.4%	32.3%	46.9%	31.1%	28.6%	46.6%	6.0%	3.2%	0.8%
80th percentile	0.320	40.1%	35.1%	51.9%	34.9%	32.1%	51.4%	9.8%	7.6%	4.2%

Note. Data from a 2019 analysis of data from the 2010–2012 National Intimate Partner and Sexual Violence Survey (Willie & Kershaw, 2019). No more recent state-level analyses were available to us as of September 2023. Values above the 80th percentile are displayed in bold face; those below the 20th percentile are displayed in italics.

variability in the prevalence figures. In keeping with the less violent cultures of New England and the Midwest, the states in these regions have low rates of IPV. The highest rates of IPV in the 16-state sample are found in Appalachia and the Southwest. In our sample, victims of physical and psychological IPV are more often male than female in two states: Massachusetts and Montana. Despite its high score on the UN Gender Inequality Index, Massachusetts is a state with a high proportion of highly educated and empowered women and a cultural ideal of gender equality. Montana has a historical culture of independent, self-sufficient frontierswomen and was one of the first states to give women the right to vote. Montana's neighbor Idaho shows a similar pattern of more male than female victims of physical and psychological IPV (NISVS data show that Idaho's rates of victimization for all three types of violence are more than 5% higher for men).

Being a victim of IPV is associated with a range of adverse physical and psychological consequences, from asthma to depression (Sugg, 2015). Psychological IPV is no less damaging to mental health than physical IPV, but because there is no obvious physical injury, it is more likely to be missed or underappreciated by clinicians. Endocrine and inflammatory responses to the chronic stress of IPV are involved in mediating the relationship between IPV and adverse health outcomes (Yim & Kofman, 2018). Depression leads to decreased marital satisfaction and to increased perpetration of physical and psychological IPV in those predisposed to it (Barros-Gomes et al., 2019). The lifetime prevalence table suggests that clinicians assessing depressed people of either gender should consider the possibility that they are victims of IPV.

Regional Differences in Lifestyle Risk Factors for Depression

Lifestyle—particularly diets, alcohol consumption, smoking, and physical activity—accounts for much of the variance among regions in the prevalence of chronic health conditions, and it contributes significantly to the occurrence and persistence of depression. Table 14.15 compares four common health risk factors among the 16 states. For each factor, there is substantial interstate variation, and for each factor there are impressive outliers.

The prevalence of binge drinking is low in the states of the Deep South and Appalachia, which have cultures strongly influenced by evangelical Protestantism. On the other hand, the same states have high rates of nonmedical use of prescription opioids—a topic with which the evangelical churches have a shorter history. Physical inactivity is more common in the

Table 14.15 Selected Behavioral Health Risk Factors—Results from a 2022 Survey

State	Adult binge drinking in past 30 days	Physical inactivity when not at work	Obesity (from self reported height and weight)	Cigarette smoking by adults
AL	13.7%	**30.7%**	36.1%	**20.2%**
MS	*13.4%*	**33.2%**	**40.8%**	**20.4%**
AZ	17.2%	23.3%	31.4%	14.9%
NM	14.7%	23.7%	31.7%	16.0%
IA	**21.8%**	24.5$	33.9%	16.4%
NE	**20.8%**	24.3%	34.1%	14.7%
KY	*13.8%*	**32.5%**	36.5%	**23.6%**
WV	*13.4%*	**30.1%**	**39.7%**	**23.8%**
MA	17.6%	23.3%	*25.2%*	*12.0%*
NH	16.0%	21.5%	31.8%	15.9%
MN	**19.3%**	*21.0%*	**40.8%**	**20.4%**
WI	**23.5%**	21.9%	34.2%	15.4%
MT	**22.9%**	21.5%	*28.3%*	16.6%
WY	17.2%	23.6%	29.7%	18.4%
OR	17.2%	*20.7%*	29.0%	14.5%
WA	16.1%	*18.4%*	*28.3%*	*12.6%*
20th percentile	14.1%	21.5%	30.6%	13.5%
Median	16.8%	24.7%	33.6%	16.0%
80th percentile	19.2%	27.6%	37.7%	19.0%

Note. Data from the CDC Behavioral Risk Factor Surveillance Survey of 2022. (CDC, 2023a). Site queried October 1, 2023. https://data.cdc.gov/browse?category=Behavioral+Risk+Factors. Values above the 80th percentile are displayed in bold face; those below the 20th percentile are displayed in italics.

same states, possibly reflecting passivity and fatalism and a vicious circle in which deconditioning makes physical exercise effortful, leading to more sedentary behavior and thence to more obesity and deconditioning. Inactivity is less prevalent in the states of the Southwest, the northern Midwest, the Mountain States, the Pacific Northwest, and New Hampshire, all of which have cultures of outdoor recreation. Obesity is especially prevalent in states of the Deep South and Appalachia, places where mainstream Western diets are the norm and sugar-sweetened beverage consumption is high. Unhealthy diets combined with inactivity lead to obesity, a well-established risk factor for clinical depression (Luppino et al., 2010).

Excessive drinking, obesity and its complications of type 2 diabetes and obstructive sleep apnea (OSA), and physical inactivity (i.e., no significant physical activity apart from what is necessary for one's job) all are associated with a higher prevalence of depression. Smoking can transiently improve mood, but its long-term medical consequences, including cardiovascular diseases, chronic obstructive pulmonary disease (COPD), and cancers, are associated with high rates of comorbid depression. Obesity rates are lower in New England, the Mountain States, and the Pacific Northwest than in the other regions discussed in this chapter. New England has a historical culture of restraining gluttony and prizing industriousness. In modern times it is a relatively health-conscious region.

Undiagnosed OSA is endemic in regions with a high prevalence of obesity. It is associated with depression directly, and indirectly through obesity, type 2 diabetes, and traumatic and occupational consequences of excessive daytime sleepiness. It is less likely to be diagnosed in regions with shortages of physicians and/or where the lack of health insurance makes treatment infeasible or prohibitively expensive even when the condition is diagnosed.

Smoking is highly prevalent in the same states that have especially high rates of obesity. It is supported by regional cultures that tolerate smoking in public places—in contrast to the cultures of states like California or Massachusetts where most adults would be offended by passive exposure to others' smoke.

Smoking rates are highest in the states of the Deep South and Appalachia, where smoking continues to be normalized in much of the area. It is also prevalent in the Mountain States, where smoking is part of a persistent idealized cowboy culture, and the freedom to live as one chooses is highly valued. When smoking, physical inactivity, or obesity is highly prevalent in a region, it is likely that it will be normalized, decreasing people's motivation and social support for changing the unhealthy behavior. It is harder to quit smoking when one has daily contact with friends, family, and/or co-workers who smoke.

In areas where mental health resources are scarce and where there is a high prevalence of general medical conditions associated with depression, an attractive first step in the treatment of mild to moderate MDD, or in secondary prevention for a person with subsyndromal MDD, is for a primary care physician or their team to address under-treated medical conditions and harmful health habits. For example, the initial focus for a patient with mild depression, smoking, and COPD might be to facilitate smoking cessation with medication, perhaps using a medication like bupropion, which both diminishes symptoms of nicotine withdrawal and has an antidepressant effect. For a patient with depression and significant OSA, treating the sleep disorder is a medically necessary first step that might be enough by itself to relieve the depression. Treatment of medical conditions that contribute to depression has little or no stigma, and health plans' differential coverage and "carved out" management of mental disorders would not be a barrier. "Behavioral health" coverage for mental health services that are not fully integrated with general medical care—a common feature of insurance plans and managed care organizations—favors the initial treatment of mildly depressed people by independent non-medical mental health professionals, decreasing the likelihood that medical comorbidities contributing to the depression will be promptly addressed.

Interstate Differences in Firearm Culture

Table 14.16 shows statistics on the ownership and storage of guns in the 16 states. Data are cited from the 2002 Behavioral Risk Factors Surveillance Survey. After 2004, inclusion of gun-related content in the survey was forbidden by legislation. It shows wide variance in the rate of gun ownership and even greater variance in prevalence of guns stored unsafely—loaded and unlocked. Unsafely stored guns are more likely to be used in impulsive suicide or violence than those stored according to the standard recommendations of gun owners' organizations. Because suicidal people do not necessarily have backup suicidal plans, many suicides could be prevented by keeping guns locked up and unloaded, and storing ammunition in a separate, secure location.

Gun owners with children aged six or under at home were asked about home safety practices and about gun storage: 92% of those questioned kept poisons out of children's reach, 90% kept their children restrained when in cars, 82% had the telephone number for a poison control center, 72% kept electrical outlets capped, and 65% kept their hot tap water temperature at 120 degrees Fahrenheit or less. 56% of the study subjects kept a handgun at home. Of those that did, 46% kept the gun unlocked, 33% kept it loaded, and 12% kept it both loaded and unlocked. The overall home safety scores did not differ significantly between gun owners and non-owners, or between gun owners who stored their guns safely and those who did not (Coyne-Beasley et al., 2002).

In a nationally representative online sample of 2072 American gun owners surveyed in 2015, 29.7% kept at least one firearm loaded and unlocked. Gun owners who had had formal firearm safety training were no less likely to store at least one gun unsafely (Berrigan et al., 2019). Azrael and colleagues (2018) conducted a more detailed exploration of the determinants of unsafe gun storage in gun owners living with children under age 18. Overall, 21% of gun owners with children at home kept at least one gun loaded and unlocked. Women (31%), handgun owners (27%), and people who gave protection as their primary reason for owning a firearm (29%) were significantly more likely to keep at least

Table 14.16 Household Gun Ownership and Storage

State	Gun in Home	Loaded Gun in Home	Loaded and Unlocked Gun in Home	Homes with Guns that Keep One or More Loaded and Unlocked	2002-16 Change in Household Gun Ownership
AL	**57.2%**	**19.2%**	**12.7%**	**22.0%**	−4.4%
MS	**54.3%**	**15.9%**	**8.9%**	16.0%	−0.2%
AZ	36.2%	11.3%	**7.6%**	**21.0%**	−0.2%
NM	39.6%	10.0%	6.6%	17.0%	−3.7%
IA	44.0%	*3.9%*	*2.5%*	*6.0%*	−5.5%
NE	42.1%	4.0%	*2.0%*	*5.0%*	−2.9%
KY	**48.0%**	12.2%	6.6%	14.0%	**4.5%**
WV	**57.9%**	9.4%	5.5%	9.0%	2.1%
MA	*12.8%*	*1.6%*	*0.4%*	*3.0%*	−3.8%
NH	30.5%	*3.9%*	*2.1%*	7.0%	**15.8%**
MN	44.7%	*3.4%*	*2.3%*	*5.0%*	−5.6%
WI	44.3%	*3.4%*	*2.2%*	*5.0%*	**2.8%**
MT	**61.4%**	**12.8%**	**8.6%**	14.0%	**3.6%**
WY	**62.8%**	**12.8%**	**8.3%**	13.0%	−2.1%
OR	39.8%	10.3%	7.1%	**18.0%**	1.6%
WA	36.2%	7.1%	4.3%	12.0%	−4.1%
20th percentile	*26.0%*	*3.4%*	*2.1%*	*6.9%*	
Median	40.8%	7.0%	4.2%	12.1%	
80th percentile	**48.0%**	**12.3%**	**7.6%**	**17.3%**	

Note: Statistics on firearm ownership and storage are from the 2002 Behavioral Risk Factors Survey, analyzed by Okoro et al. (2005). Estimated change from 2002 to 2016 is based on data from Schell et al. (2020). Values at or above the 80th percentile for the 50 states and DC are highlighted in bold face; those at or below the 20th percentile are highlighted in italics.

one gun loaded and unlocked. The study also found that unsafe gun storage was more common among residents of the South (30%), those who lived in rural areas (26%), and those who described themselves as politically conservative (24%). However, the latter findings did not reach statistical significance (Azrael et al., 2018).

Rates of gun ownership and how guns are stored are attributes of regional and local culture directly relatable to the risk of impulsive suicide. Suicide attempts are made by many people who do not have the persistence of symptoms to warrant a diagnosis of clinical depression. When they are made with a gun, they are likely to have fatal outcomes. Further, estimated changes in gun ownership between 2002 and 2016 suggest that large interstate differences are persistent (Schell et al., 2020). The data from that study show that rates of gun ownership and of safe gun storage closely correspond with region and that the variability in having a gun stored loaded in an unlocked location was much greater than the variability in gun ownership per se (Hamilton et al., 2018). When two states in a region differ significantly in gun ownership, an obvious explanation is a difference in the rurality of a state, since gun ownership is higher in rural areas than urban ones, worldwide. In the Deep South and in the Mountain States most households own a gun, and often a loaded gun is kept in an unlocked location. The Appalachian States have above-median household gun ownership, with the rate in West Virginia higher than that in the Deep South; but a significantly smaller proportion of households keep their guns loaded and unlocked. The Midwestern states have above-median household gun ownership but remarkably low rates of unsafe gun storage. Interstate differences in rates of storing guns loaded and unlocked might relate to different subjective perceptions of the imminence of threats that might require self-defense with a firearm.

A state with a relatively high rate of unsafe gun storage is more likely than other states with similar gun ownership rates to have a historical culture of using violence to settle quarrels and insults to honor and a belief that one must always be prepared for violent self-defense. The Midwestern states' combination of high household gun ownership with unusually safe gun storage reflects their prudent, conservative culture. Guns are a cultural anchor in the Mountain States, Appalachia, and the Deep South, all of which initially had a rural culture, with hunting a popular sport and guns seen as essential for defense against crime and sometimes against wild animals in areas where police or neighbors would be too far away to help in a crisis.

The Deep South states have a historical memory of the American Civil War, during which every Southern man was armed to defend Dixie; and they continue to have an "honor culture," in which men who have been insulted and disrespected are motivated to respond with violence. Multiple cultural factors, including the presence and strength of a region's gun culture, lie behind the great variability between regions in rates of firearm-related suicide. In states with strong gun cultures, gun-related activities are an important part of many men's social lives, and gun ownership is associated with freedom, vigor, and masculinity. In the worst case, non-gun owners are respected less by their peers. The most common reason given for gun ownership is defense of oneself and one's family. This is the case even for gun owners who regard their own neighborhood as relatively safe (Gaffley et al., 2023; Hofstadter, 1970; Siegel & Boine, 2020; Ye et al., 2022).

Environmental Influences on Depression Risk

The physical environment of an area has direct effects on mood, impulsiveness, and suicidal behavior. Table 14.17 shows data for the 16 states on representative environmental influences on mood and on the risk of suicide. The influences listed are elevation, mean temperature, latitude, latitude, and the U.S. Environmental Protection Agency's Risk Screening Environmental Indicators (RSEI) score for the state (Joint Economic Committee, 2018b; U.S. Environmental Protection Agency, 2023). The risk score is a summary estimate of the cumulative exposure of an area's residents to toxic substances, based on data about the amount of toxic chemicals released from discrete sources, together with factors such as the chemicals' fate and transport through the environment, each chemical's relative toxicity, and potential human exposure. Adverse health effects considered include central nervous system (CNS) toxicity as well as cancer, reproductive, developmental, reproductive, and respiratory toxicity. Notably, agricultural chemicals are not included in the RSEI score.

For long-term residents of a region, their physical environment is "normal," and a person with depression and suicidal impulses would seldom consider relocating to a lower altitude or a cooler climate. Higher altitude is associated with depression and suicidality, with one hypothesized mechanism being the effect of hypoxia on serotonergic transmission and on brain bioenergetics (Kious et al., 2018; Reno et al., 2018). Higher mean temperatures, and heat waves, are associated with increases in suicide attempts and deaths by suicide, and with higher rates of psychiatric hospitalizations and emergency room visits (Thompson et al., 2023).

Seasonality of mood disorders is greater at higher latitudes. Clinicians of all disciplines can learn to recognize seasonal affective disorder (SAD) and seasonal exacerbations of MDD or BD. Light therapy often is effective for these conditions, and it also can be a valuable adjunct to antidepressants or mood-stabilizing drugs (Nussbaumer-Streit, 2019; Penders et al., 2016; Ravindran et al., 2016; Sit & Haigh, 2019).

While many people will try light therapy without medical supervision, a clinician should recommend light therapy for a depressed patient only after a thorough assessment to make a confident diagnosis, to identify medical comorbidities needing treatment, and to exclude conditions that would require psychopharmacologic treatment or active management of suicide risk. For

Table 14.17 Representative Environmental Influences on Depression

State	Enivornmental Protection Agency 2020 Risk Screening Environmental Indicators (RSEI) score in millions	Percentage of population affected by drinking water safety violations in 2021	Percentage of housing with lead risk	Average exposure of public to particulate air pollution (micrograms per cubic meter of PM2.5)	Mean elevation (feet)	Mean temperature (°F)
AL	16.810	0.2%	11.1%	7.8	500	76.8
MS	1.647	6.3%	10.7%	8.2	300	76.1
AZ	4.302	0.9%	6.6%	10.5	500	76.8
NM	0.016	2.9%	11.3%	6.7	3700	68.0
IA	2.885	0.0%	25.5%	7.8	1100	60.8
NE	1.789	0.1%	21.3%	6.2	2600	63.5
KY	4.279	0.0%	14.6%	8.3	750	66.6
WV	2.816	10.2%	20.6%	7.3	1500	62.8
MA	6.483	0.0%	29.7%	7.3	500	56.7
NH	0.063	0.2%	20.0%	4.6	1000	52.8
MN	1.358	1.1%	19.0%	7.4	1200	53.3
WI	7.289	4.4%	21.7%	7.9	1050	54.3
MT	.144	0.2%	17.4%	6.1	3400	51.7
WY	0.012	0.2%	15.2%	4.7	6700	51.6
OR	2.251	0.3%	15.7%	8.9	3300	55.2
WA	3.147	0.5%	14.1%	8.0	1700	53.7

Note. Data from United Health Foundation (2023), based on 2019–2021 U.S. Environmental Protection Agency Data.

example, if a person has BD, standard antidepressant light therapy for depression can induce hypomania if given without a mood stabilizer, and the optimal parameters for light therapy of bipolar disorders are different from those for unipolar depression (Esaki et al., 2021; Hirakawa et al., 2020). Once light therapy has been started and shown to be efficacious, it can be monitored and encouraged by a primary care provider or non-medical mental health professional. Light therapy for SAD or for MDD that is worse in winter is unlikely to be stigmatized, even in cultures that stigmatize MDD and other mental disorders. Light therapy as an adjunct to a first-line antidepressant for an incompletely remitted depression is likely to be more affordable than switching to a different antidepressant drug with a higher out-of-pocket cost or adding a second pharmacologic or psychotherapeutic treatment.

Frequently encountered pollutants of air and water have well-established effects on depression and suicide risk, and their prevalence varies greatly by region and specific location. In urban areas, a main concern is particulate matter in the air. Long-term exposure to high concentrations of $PM_{2.5}$ (particulate matter 2.5 microns or less in diameter) is associated with a higher incidence and prevalence of depression (Briathwaite et al., 2019; Gladka et al., 2022; K-N. Kim et al., 2016; Petkus et al., 2022; Qiu et al. 2023; Yang et al., 2023). Exposure to high levels of $PM_{2.5}$ at age 12 has been linked to a higher prevalence of MDD at age 18 (Roberts et al., 2019). Neighborhood social capital, especially the dimension of trusting one's neighbors, might have some protective effect against depression related to atmospheric pollution (Wang et al., 2018).

In agricultural areas, neurological and psychiatric consequences of exposure to organophosphate insecticides are a significant concern, and long-term exposure to non-organophosphate insecticides at levels commonly experienced in agricultural communities also can cause neurological and psychiatric disorders (Abreu-Villaca & Levin, 2017; Altinyazar et al., 2016; Serrano-Medina et al., 2019). Continual low-level exposure to such agents has significant CNS effects, increasing learning problems in children, the risk of conduct problems, attention deficit hyperactivity disorder (ADHD), and depression in adolescents, and increasing the risk of depression, neurocognitive disorders, and sleep apnea in adults (Baumert et al., 2018; Cassereau et al., 2017; Serrano-Medina et al., 2019; Suarez-Lopez et al., 2019a, 2019b). Prenatal exposure to organophosphates can affect children's brain development (Sagiv et al., 2019).

Organophosphate pesticide use, though obviously higher in states where agriculture is a major industry, also varies by culture, including consumers' willingness to pay more for organic food and the relative proportion of family farms versus industrial-scale agriculture. For example, the six New England states are all in the lowest quintile nationally in annual pesticide use. In the 16-state sample of this chapter, West Virginia and Wyoming also are low-using states, while Washington, Minnesota, Iowa, and Nebraska are in the highest quintile. When farm workers are poorly educated immigrants with limited English proficiency and sometimes without legal resident status, they and their families are in a weak position to address unsafe working and living conditions related to organophosphate exposure.

Within states, chemical pollution is always geographically localized to the areas where toxics are released into the environment, downstream or downwind from them, or where drinking water comes from contaminated reservoirs, steams, or aquifers. Locally increased incidence of neuropsychiatric disorders or suicide sometimes is seen in these areas. The cultural element concerns denial, normalization, rationalization, and/or tolerance of environmental pollution. Environmental pollution is less likely to be challenged by the public in states that are tight, are low on openness, and have a culture of deference to power and mistrust of science. People are more likely to find pollution acceptable if they or their neighbors depend upon polluting industries (including large-scale conventional agriculture) for their jobs.

In the states of greater Appalachia especially there is a historical dislike of the "elite," among whom scientists might be included. Americans with less scientific knowledge and more conservative political views are inclined to mistrust—or at least be highly skeptical of—scientists' direct input into matters of public policy (Funk et al., 2019). Environmental activists sometimes are lumped with "liberals" or "socialists," seen as advocating policies that will cost jobs, and generally disliked. There is a concentration of people mistrustful of scientific expertise in many of the states, and areas within states, that have America's worst environmental pollution. The same cultural factors underlying several states' low rates of COVID-19 vaccination are likely to underlie the relative passivity of those states' residents in the face of known environmental health hazards.

For each state, the counties with the highest concentrations of potentially harmful chemicals in the environment are known, with recent data available from the Environmental Protection Agency and other reliable online sources. Depending on a patient's clinical syndrome and personal situation, moving to a cleaner location might be part of a treatment recommendation. For example, a depressed, asthmatic single mother of a son in the first grade with ADHD, who lived in an area with known particulate air pollution and suspected endocrine disruptors in the public water supply, might be encouraged to move to an area with cleaner air and water and offered support in doing so if appropriate services were available to assist patients with medically necessary changes in living arrangements.

Even if a person's political views are opposed to regulation of toxic substances, they might be open to their physician's explaining the personally relevant health risk of an environmental hazard. A man who needed and appreciated his job in an industrial plant that polluted the surrounding air could still be concerned about the effect of the air pollution on his wife's asthma or his child's school performance. Though he might keep his job and resent any regulations that might affect it, he might choose to commute to his job from an area with a less toxic environment if doing so would be better for the health of his family. If the man were skeptical of science relating environmental toxins to behavior or cognition, the clinician could focus on the relationship between air pollution and asthma, a connection too obvious to dismiss.

Trust in physicians' recommendations is associated with better adherence to treatment and it may be present even when people don't trust the opinions of non-clinician scientists. While no published studies directly link American regional cultures to trust in physicians, data from the Pew Research study cited earlier in this chapter show that (on average) Americans with lower incomes, Black and Hispanic Americans, people without higher education, and those with conservative political views have less trust in physicians and in medical researchers than those without these attributes. These findings taken together with the known regional distribution of incomes, ethnicity, and political orientation imply regional differences in the prevalent levels of trust in medicine. However, many survey respondents who did not trust the medical profession in general expressed trust in their personal physicians (Funk et al., 2019).

While it is never wise for a clinician to assume uncritically that their advice will be trusted if a new or unfamiliar treatment is under consideration, initially not assuming the patient's trust is especially important when practicing within a low-trust culture. In conceiving public health interventions to prevent depression or encourage its early treatment, the wide prevalence of mistrust of scientific and other expertise should be kept in mind, with awareness that the subtexts of mistrust are different between segments of the population. Lower-income and ethnic minority patients might be concerned that a clinician's unexpected diagnosis or treatment recommendation was the result of prejudice, discrimination, and stereotyping rather than a result of a thoughtful and complete assessment and appropriate personalization of care. Patients with mistrust of science and fears that doctors are corrupted by the influence of the pharmaceutical industry or "government scientists" might doubt the validity of evidence-based treatment guidelines.

A widely-cited systematic review and network meta-analysis of randomized clinical trials of antidepressants has showed significant efficacy and excellent tolerability for several of them (Cipriani et al., 2018). However, a person inclined to mistrust authority would question the integrity of the underlying studies. In an editorial following the publication of the positive assessment of antidepressant efficacy, an eminent academic psychiatrist published an editorial titled "The Benefits of Antidepressants: News or Fake News." The term "fake news," is popular among Americans united in mistrust of "the establishment" and "the mainstream media" (Parker, 2018). The editorial thoughtfully addressed the inadequacy of the DSM diagnosis of MDD to define the population that needs treatment for clinical depression, and the still unmet need to effectively and feasibly subdivide the phenotypes of clinical depression to enable personalized treatment.

In American regions with low institutional social capital, many patients will begin with mistrust of medical science, especially in the specialty of psychiatry where diagnostic criteria usually don't involve laboratory tests or diagnostic images. A transparent and thoughtful process of characterizing a patient's unique experience of depression, and personalizing their treatment, can both build the clinician–patient relationship and address the legitimate concerns that might underlie a patient's more culturally-based mistrust. It is reassuring to know that most patients trust their personal physicians more than they trust medical science or the medical profession in the abstract.

A clinician's a priori estimate of a patient's mistrust should take the patient's cultural identity into account. The culture that determines the patient's trust in the clinician and in the relevant medical science is an intersection that includes regional culture.

A primary care physician usually is in the best position to deliver the opinion that an environmental factor contributes to a patient's illness. When reducing harmful environmental exposure is a central part of the plan for treatment of depression, a collaborative care model might work better than traditional psychiatric care. Primary care physicians who recognize pollution-related factors that might be exacerbating depression—and other medical conditions—in a specific patient sometimes can suggest practical remedies such as drinking purified water, not wearing shoes indoors, being scrupulous about handwashing after exposure to toxic chemicals, or avoiding outdoor exercise on hot days where heat would interact with air pollution to increase its harmful effects. In an effective collaborative care model, psychiatrists can assist primary care physicians in recognizing pertinent environmental issues. The process can build trust and common understanding among mental health clinicians, primary care physicians, and depressed patients.

Linking Regional Culture with the Epidemiology of MDD, Bipolar Disorder, and Suicide

The epidemiology of mood disorders and suicide can usefully be interpreted in the light of regional differences in demographics, economy, and culture. Regional effects can be appreciated by examining the gender-specific epidemiology of MDD, BD, and suicide, subdividing the population into three age bands: 15–49 (adolescence, young adulthood, early middle age), 50–69 (late middle age), and 70+ (old age). In doing the research for this book, we explored other ways to construct age groups; but for this chapter's purpose of illustrating regional culturally-related differences in epidemiology the present approach proved especially fruitful. For a finer-grained exploration of age and generational effects in multivariate models, it is best to use narrower age bands and analyze epidemiologic data aggregated over several years. The value of studying the detailed age distribution of MDD prevalence is illustrated in the comparison of Nordic countries in Chapter 13, and in the comparison of Connecticut and Utah in Chapter 1.

In Tables 14.18 and 14.19, prevalence rates for diagnosed MDD and BD by gender and age in 2019 are compared for the 16 states. Table 14.20 shows for each state the proportion of adults in a 2017–2019 survey who were ever told by a physician that they were (clinically) depressed. If such patients were evaluated psychiatrically, and most were not, their diagnoses might have been MDD, minor (subsyndromal) depression, adjustment disorder with depressed mood, complicated bereavement, dysthymia, depression with mixed features or a bipolar specifier, bipolar depression, or an unspecified depressive disorder.

New Mexico and West Virginia stand out in the 16-state sample—and in the nation—for their high prevalence of MDD in both women and men. Factors relatable to their demographics and their culture are likely to contribute. Both states have poverty rates in the top ten nationally. The population of West Virginia is predominantly rural. New Mexico has remarkably low overall social capital, and both have low "institutional health"—the type of social capital most strongly protective against depression. The educational level of both states' populations is relatively low. Both have high rates of multiple ACEs. Finally, West Virginia leads the U.S. in the prevalence of neurotic personality traits. For all these risk factors, the two states have less favorable statistics than their neighboring comparator.

The prevalence of MDD is in the lowest quintile nationally for men in Massachusetts and for women in Nebraska. Both states have low rates of poverty, and both have well-educated populations. In both, the rates of multiple

Table 14.18 2019 Prevalence of Major Depressive Disorder (MDD) and Bipolar Disorder (BD) in Women

State	MDD			Bipolar disorder		
	15–49	50–69	70+	15–49	50–69	70+
AL	6.2%	3.9%	3.3%	0.8%	0.7%	0.4%
MS	6.9%	4.7%	3.9%	0.6%	0.5%	0.3%
AZ	7.4%	4.6%	3.8%	1.0%	0.8%	0.5%
NM	7.9%	5.0%	4.2%	0.8%	0.8%	0.5%
IA	6.1%	3.8%	3.2%	0.6%	0.6%	0.3%
NE	5.6%	3.5%	3.0%	0.9%	0.7%	0.5%
KY	7.2%	4.6%	3.8%	0.9%	0.9%	0.5%
WV	7.7%	5.3%	4.4%	1.4%	1.2%	0.6%
MA	6.1%	3.8%	3.2%	1.1%	0.9%	0.5%
NH	7.0%	4.6%	4.0%	0.9%	0.8%	0.5%
MN	6.2%	3.9%	3.3%	0.6%	0.5%	0.3%
WI	6.6%	4.1%	3.4%	0.8%	0.6%	0.4%
MT	7.2%	4.3%	3.6%	1.1%	0.7%	0.5%
WY	7.5%	4.7%	4.0%	0.9%	0.7%	0.4%
OR	7.2%	4.5%	3.8%	0.9%	0.7%	0.5%
WA	7.2%	4.6%	3.9%	0.9%	0.8%	0.5%
20th percentile	6.1%	3.8%	3.2%	0.8%	0.6%	0.4%
Median	7.0%	4.5%	3.7%	0.9%	0.8%	0.5%
80th percentile	7.4%	4.7%	4.0%	1.0%	0.9%	0.5%

Note. Data from the Global Burden of Disease 2019 database (IHME, 2023). Query: 2019 prevalence of MDD and BD in females by age band and state. https://vizhub.healthdata.org/gbd-results/. Data retrieved September 1, 2023.

childhood ACEs and of births to unmarried women are low. Both are in the top quintile nationally on the Institutional Health dimension of social capital.

The relative prevalence of BD with respect to MDD varies greatly among states, from a high in Massachusetts to a low in Mississippi; it is higher in Arizona than in New Mexico and higher in Nebraska than in Iowa. Two factors deserve consideration in conceiving an explanation. Patients with depression are more likely to see psychiatrists in more urban and more educated states, and psychiatrists are more likely than non-psychiatric physicians and non-medical clinicians to diagnose bipolar depression and conditions in the bipolar spectrum that do not present as typical manic-depressive illness. States

Table 14.19 2019 Prevalence of Major Depressive Disorder (MDD) and Bipolar Disorder (BD) in Men

State	MDD			BD		
	15–49	50–69	70+	15–49	50–69	70+
AL	3.7%	2.3%	2.1%	0.6%	0.5%	0.3%
MS	3.5%	2.3%	2.1%	0.5%	0.4%	0.3%
AZ	4.1%	2.6%	2.3%	1.0%	0.7%	0.5%
NM	**4.9%**	**3.1%**	**2.8%**	0.8%	0.7%	0.4%
IA	3.7%	2.2%	2.0%	0.6%	0.5%	0.4%
NE	3.8%	2.3%	2.2%	0.8%	0.5%	0.4%
KY	4.1%	2.6%	2.4%	0.8%	0.7%	0.4%
WV	**4.5%**	**3.0%**	**2.8%**	1.1%	0.9%	0.6%
MA	3.4%	2.2%	1.8%	1.1%	1.0%	0.6%
NH	4.2%	2.8%	2.5%	0.9%	0.7%	0.5%
MN	3.7%	2.3%	2.0%	0.6%	0.5%	0.3%
WI	4.0%	2.4%	2.1%	0.8%	0.6%	0.4%
MT	4.3%	2.6%	2.3%	1.0%	0.7%	**0.5%**
WY	4.2%	2.5%	2.4%	0.7%	0.5%	0.4%
OR	4.1%	2.6%	2.3%	0.8%	0.6%	0.4%
WA	4.0%	2.5%	2.3%	0.8%	0.6%	0.4%
20th percentile	3.5%	2.2%	2.0%	0.7%	0.5%	0.4%
Median	4.0%	2.5%	2.3%	0.8%	0.6%	0.4%
80th percentile	4.2%	2.8%	2.5%	1.0%	0.8%	0.5%

Note. Data from the Global Burden of Disease 2019 database (IHME, 2023). Query: 2019 prevalence of MDD and BD in males by age band and state. https://vizhub.healthdata.org/gbd-results/. Data retrieved September 1, 2023.

with more economic opportunity will attract high-functioning hyperthymic or cyclothymic adults with creative and/or entrepreneurial talent and/or expectations. Some of those people will eventually display signs of a condition in the bipolar spectrum.

Table 14.20, based on 2017–2019 data from the CDC Behavioral Risk Factor Surveillance System, gives the percentage of adults who reported being told by a health professional that they have a depressive disorder such as "depression," major depression, minor depression, or dysthymia. The numbers are, as expected, substantially higher than the lifetime prevalence of MDD since many cases are included that would not meet the criteria for MDD. The lifetime

Table 14.20 Lifetime Prevalence of Clinical Depression in 2022

State	Adults ever told they were depressed by a health professional	
	Women	Men
AL	30.1%	17.3%
MS	26.0%	14.5%
AZ	24.4%	15.8%
NM	24.9%	16.8%
IA	25.6%	*11.2%*
NE	*23.6%*	*10.4%*
KY	**32.8%**	18.4%
WV	**33.8%**	**19.8%**
MA	26.9%	15.9%
NH	31.4%	**18.7%**
MN	29.8%	17.2%
WI	29.6	16.3%
MT	**32.3%**	16.6%
WY	29.9%	14.4%
OR	30.8%	17.0%
WA	31.8%	18.1%
20th percentile	23.7%	13.6%
Median	27.3%	15.3%
80th percentile	31.4%	18.4%

Note. Data from CDC Behavioral Risk Factor Surveillance System, (2023a). Subjects in a telephone survey were asked if they had ever been told by a health professional that they had a form of depression. Data on survey responses by women and men obtained by query at https://www.cdc.gov/brfss/annual_data/annual_data.htm. Data retrieved September 15, 2023. Rates above the 80th percentile are displayed in bold face; those below the 20th percentile are displayed in italics.

prevalence of depression for women is greatest in the states of the Deep South, Appalachia, and the Northwest, while the Southwestern states have lifetime prevalence rates well below the median. Lifetime prevalence of depression for men follows a similar pattern, though the rate in Mississippi is lower than would be expected from the 2019 MDD prevalence estimates. The table underscores the point that the reported rates of formally diagnosed MDD underestimate the true rates of clinical depression in all 16 states. "Subsyndromal" depression can be disabling or even fatal, but it is not included in MDD prevalence statistics. Depression expressed as externalizing behavior or by predominantly physical symptoms might not be recognized as a mood disorder at all. "Male depression"—the disorder of dysphoric mood and externalizing behaviors discussed at several other places in this volume—is more common as an expression of depression in cultures and subcultures that are more "masculine." Among the eight regions discussed here, masculinity as a cultural attribute is greater in the Southwest, the Deep South, Appalachia, and the Mountain States. Regions with masculine cultures also appear to accept somatic presentations of depression with relatively little stigma in men if they are related to the consequences of hard work (e.g., fatigue in a man who works long hours or low back pain in a truck driver or construction worker). The combination of a masculine culture with a high prevalence of chronic general medical conditions involving somatic pain or dyspnea (e.g., lumbar disc disease or COPD) underlies the expression of chronic depression as chronic physical disability. Table 14.21, based on data from the U.S. Social Security Administration, shows the proportion of working-age adults (ages 18–64) receiving long-term disability benefits (Social Security Disability Insurance [SSDI]), highlighting the proportions with disability attributed to a mood disorder and disability attributed to a musculoskeletal disorder. *Mood disorder* refers to diagnosed depressive disorders (MDD, dysthymia, and BD), and *musculoskeletal disorder* comprises low back pain, neck pain, and osteoarthritis (Social Security Administration, 2020).

One indicator of an area's cultural bias toward somatization of depression is its prevalence of disability among working-age adults and its attribution to a physical rather than a "mental" cause. The proportion of working-age adults claiming SSDI benefits varies greatly among the 16 states, from 3.8% in Minnesota to 8.6% in West Virginia. The Appalachian and Deep South states have the nation's highest rates of receipt of SSDI. Those states have a comparatively high proportion of their workforce in physically strenuous jobs, but their distribution of job types is insufficient to explain their unusually high disability rates.

There are structural reasons for their higher disability rates. Median incomes and costs of living are relatively low, so SSDI is more likely to adequately replace earnings from work. Educational levels are lower, and a high proportion of the population is rural, so there might be fewer alternative jobs for someone whose health ruled out physically strenuous employment. The states have a relatively high prevalence of depression, and particularly in men it might be expressed somatically by making symptoms like musculoskeletal pain or respiratory problems subjectively worse and harder to bear. Explicitly talking of depressed mood would be displaying a lack of toughness and resolve, whereas reluctantly giving in to chronic pain would be more honorable. In these regions,

Table 14.21 Long-term Disability (Social Security Disability Insurance) in Adults Aged 18–64 in December 2021

State	Percentage of adults aged 18–64 receiving SSDI	Percentage of those on SSDI with a mood disorder	Percentage of those on SSDI with a musculoskeletal or connective tissue disorder
AL	**7.2%**	9.7%	**36.2%**
MS	**7.0%**	10.9%	29.7%
AZ	*3.4%*	9.0%	29.2%
NM	4.9%	**12.7%**	31.1%
IA	4.3%	10.2%	26.6%
NE	*3.7%*	11.8%	*24.5%*
KY	**7.1%**	11.6%	**35.6%**
WV	**7.9%**	*9.4%*	**33.4%**
MA	4.3%	**20.5%**	*22.5%*
NH	5.4%	**20.8%**	*21.4%*
MN	*3.6%*	**15.0%**	*23.2%*
WI	4.6%	11.7%	27.5%
MT	4.1%	9.5%	28.8%
WY	4.0%	*9.4%*	27.5%
OR	4.0%	11.0%	29.5%
WA	*3.4%*	**12.9%**	27.3%
20th percentile	3.3%	9.8%	25.1%
Median	4.2%	11.2%	28.6%
80th percentile	5.5%	12.7%	32.4%

Note. Data from Social Security Administration (SSA) Annual Statistical Report on the Social Security Disability Insurance Program (SSA, 2020). Rates above the 80th percentile are displayed in bold face; those below the 20th percentile are displayed in italics.

the prevalence in men of endemic diseases related to lifestyle like obesity and COPD is high, creating a basis for depression-related somatic distress.

In New England overall rates of disability are lower, but the proportion explicitly attributed to mood disorders is much higher. The six New England states have, together with Minnesota, the highest percentages in the nation of SSDI claims related to mood disorders. The cultures of these regions are more permissive of the expression of negative affect by both genders, and depression may be less stigmatized. In addition, the New England states have high rates of female labor force participation, so more women are eligible to receive SSDI if they cannot work. Throughout the country, depression is a more acceptable and more frequent affliction of women than men. The cognitively intense work required in many of New England's leading industries is easily disrupted by depression. While SSDI is legally based on complete inability to work (rather than inability to work at one's usual occupation), becoming unable to do the work of one's usual occupation often is the beginning of a person's progression into long-term disability. Finally, New England has a generous supply of mental health professionals qualified to certify a psychiatrically-based work disability.

Culture and Variability in Suicide Rates

As noted earlier, interstate variability in suicide rates is greater than interstate variability in the prevalence of MDD and BD. Differences in states' physical environments affect their residents' predispositions to impulsive behavior: High altitude and high temperature both increase impulsiveness. Differences in their cultures operate on the components of the interpersonal-neuropsychiatric model of suicide introduced in Part I. In tighter cultures, non-conformists are more likely to experience thwarted belongingness and perceived burdensomeness. In looser ones, people without spiritual or religious beliefs might find suicide more acceptable, increasing their acquired capacity for suicide. In regional cultures with a high prevalence of ACEs, more adults will have impairments of their behavioral inhibition systems. In regional cultures with somatic idioms of distress, continual, unbearable pain might underlie a person's wish to end their suffering permanently. In rural areas—especially for people without broadband internet service—timely mental health care may be hard to access. In cultures low on trust, help might be hard to accept, messages about the treatability of depression might be hard to believe, and hopelessness may be hard to relieve. Regional culture can interact with a person's other cultural identities to make their reasons for living non-viable. This can happen when what means the most to a person makes them an ostracized non-conformist. Finally, gun culture, which is associated with relatively easy access to unsafely stored firearms, can make highly lethal means of suicide readily available.

Diagnoses of depression and BD are subject to clinical errors and biases, including the limitations of MDD criteria for capturing the range of syndromes of clinical depression, and to the ill-defined boundaries of the bipolar spectrum. The depressed and bipolar population is a fuzzy set (though not a "warm and fuzzy" one). The diagnosis of death by suicide would appear to be less subject to bias and error, but, as noted in Chapter 6, it also can be underestimated. When a person dies by an opioid overdose, in a car crash, by homicide related to an easily avoided fight, or by drowning without having expressed suicidal intentions or having left a note, their death usually will not be classified as a suicide. Judgment is required, and sometimes a full psychological autopsy, to make a confident inference of suicidal intent as opposed to recklessness, impaired judgment due to intoxication, etc. Further, an attitude of indifference to life and lack of a reason to live can lead to dangerous behavior like habitual use of injected opioids, swimming alone in bad weather or heavy surf, neglecting a chronic medical condition, or driving while intoxicated. Such behavior carries an obvious risk of a fatal "accident." Such deaths often would not be classified as suicide, though they might be included in a count of "deaths of despair."

The rate of overdose deaths that are not definitely suicides varies greatly between states, and there are states, including Massachusetts and New Hampshire, that have much higher rates of death by opioid overdose than their suicide mortality rate. This apparent inconsistency is also seen in Connecticut and Rhode Island. A plausible hypothesis is that treating pain aggressively, using opioids when necessary to reduce patients' self-reported pain ratings, is commonplace in most of New England. The region's leading hospitals, several of which are internationally renowned academic centers, were in the forefront of the campaign within the medical profession to address widespread under-treatment of pain, by treating pain as "the fifth vital sign" and viewing a high prevalence of persistent severe pain as an indicator of substandard quality of care. More widespread prescribing of opioids led to higher rates of opioid misuse and opioid overdoses. The "loose" culture of New England does not stigmatize the use of opioids to treat pain, and it is relatively tolerant of recreational drug use (albeit not of recreational opioid use). Many opioid overdose deaths in New England might be due not to unrecognized depression and despair but rather to a combination of good medical intentions with unwanted adverse effects and permissiveness about drug use in general. Table 14.22 displays state-level age-adjusted death rates from opioid overdoses and for all overdoses, and number of opioid prescriptions filled annually per 100 people.

The rate of opioid overdose deaths varies among states much more than their rates of opioid prescriptions, suggesting that the problem of opioid overdoses is not *primarily* iatrogenic. In the 16-state sample, opioid overdose deaths are highest in the states of the Southwest, Appalachia, and New England, and in Wisconsin. While inquiring about the medications that patients have at home is part of a complete evaluation of any depressed patient, early inquiry about opioids is especially important in states where opioid overdoses are common.

Appalachia and the Southwest share two risk factors for opioid overdoses: a high rate of drug use disorders (IHME, 2023) and a high rate of disability due to musculoskeletal disorders with pain that might be treated with opioids. These

Table 14.22 Age-adjusted Overdose Death Rates per 100,000 Population (2021) and Opioid Prescriptions Dispensed per 100 Persons (2020)

State	Drug overdose deaths in 2021 (primarily opioids)	Opioid overdose deaths in 2021	Opioid prescriptions per year per 100 persons (2020)
AL	30.1	21.2	**80.4**
MS	28.4	20.3	**64.2**
AZ	38.7	28.8	40.5
NM	**51.6**	37.2	40.5
IA	*15.3*	*8.6*	40.2
NE	*11.4*	*6.0*	48.0
KY	**55.6**	**44.8**	**68.2**
WV	**90.9**	**77.2**	53.7
MA	36.8	32.5	*33.3*
NH	32.3	28.4	*35.2*
MN	24.5	17.9	*30.2*
WI	31.6	29.5	39.6
MT	*19.5*	*11.1*	46.1
WY	*18.9*	12.4	46.7
OR	26.8	18.1	45.6
WA	30.1	20.5	39.5
20th percentile	22.1	13.7	36.5
Median	31.5	26	43.1
80th percentile	43.0	37.2	54.4

Note. Data from the National Center for Health Statistics [NCHS] (2023) and the Centers for Disease Control [CDC] (2023b). Rates above the 80th percentile are displayed in bold face; those below the 20th percentile are displayed in italics.

conditions often are associated with clinical depression, so it is always worthwhile to look for one diagnosis when the other is encountered. As will be noted in Chapter 15 with respect to the tragic deaths of star performing artists who struggled with addiction, providing "rehab" focused only on sobriety can create suicide risk if a person also has an untreated depression or bipolar spectrum condition.

The data in Table 14.22 reveal another remarkable fact—among the 16 states studied in this chapter, the rates of death by opioid overdose are lowest in Montana, Wyoming, Iowa, and Nebraska, despite their having opioid dispensing rates higher than those in the New England States. The discrepancy can be explained by two facts, both related to regional culture. The proportion of suicides by firearm is especially high in Wyoming (72%) and Montana (60%), reflecting those states robust gun culture and high rates of gun ownership. In Iowa and Nebraska, the rate of opioid use disorders is especially low. A suicidal person in the Far West would be more likely to utilize a firearm than an opioid for fatal self-harm. An Iowan or Nebraskan filling an opioid prescription would be relatively unlikely to be an abuser of the prescribed drug.

Suicides by firearm constitute more than half of the deaths by suicide in America. Tables 14.23 and 14.24 show 2019 statistics on deaths by suicide and by firearm suicide, for men and for women, by age band. Data are from the

Table 14.23 Female Death Rate per 100,000 Population by Firearm and Non-Firearm Suicide, 2019

State	Suicide—All means			Suicide by firearm			Percentage of suicides by firearm		
	15–49	50–69	70+	15–49	50–69	70+	15–49	50–69	70+
AL	8.6	10.3	5.0	**4.9**	**6.4**	**3.0**	**57%**	**62%**	**60%**
MS	7.7	8.9	4.3	**4.3**	**5.5**	2.6	**56%**	**62%**	**60%**
AZ	9.9	**14.7**	**6.9**	3.6	**5.7**	**2.8**	36%	39%	41%
NM	**12.4**	**13.9**	**6.9**	3.8	4.5	2.4	31%	32%	35%
IA	7.0	7.5	4.0	*1.4*	*1.7*	*1.0*	20%	23%	25%
NE	*6.0*	7.5	4.6	*1.4*	1.9	*1.2*	24%	26%	25%
KY	8.7	11.1	4.9	**4.0**	**5.7**	2.6	46%	51%	**52%**
WV	9.8	10.9	5.4	**4.1**	4.9	2.5	41%	45%	46%
MA	*5.5*	*7.1*	*3.8*	*0.4*	*0.6*	*0.4*	*8%*	*8%*	*10%*
NH	8.6	9.5	6.5	1.9	2.2	1.6	22%	23%	24%
MN	6.7	7.8	4.2	*1.2*	*1.4*	*0.9*	18%	*19%*	*22%*
WI	8.3	9.4	4.6	1.6	1.9	1.1	19%	20%	25%
MT	**13.8**	**13.8**	**7.8**	**4.8**	5.1	**3.0**	35%	37%	38%
WY	**10.6**	11.2	**7.2**	**4.7**	5.2	**3.4**	44%	**47%**	47%
OR	9.1	**13.2**	**7.3**	2.7	4.2	2.5	30%	31%	35%
WA	7.7	11.4	5.9	2.1	3.1	1.8	27%	27%	31%
20th percentile	6.5	8.2	4.2	1.4	1.9	1.1	15%	16%	24%
Median	8.2	9.6	5.0	2.5	3.3	1.8	30%	32%	33%
80th percentile	9.9	11.9	6.5	3.8	5.2	2.6	48%	56%	47%

Note. Data from 2019 Global Burden of Disease Study (IHME, 2023). Rates above the 80th percentile are displayed in bold face; those below the 20th percentile are displayed in italics.

Table 14.24 Male Death Rate per 100,000 Population by Firearm and Non-Firearm Suicide, 2019

State	Suicide—All means			Suicide by firearm			Percentage of suicides by firearm		
	15–49	50–69	70+	15–49	50–69	70+	15–49	50–69	70+
AL	27.2	36.8	42.1	17.9	**28.3**	36.2	**66%**	**77%**	**86%**
MS	25.4	30.9	36.0	16.7	23.5	30.3	**66%**	76%	**84%**
AZ	28.7	**41.6**	**49.8**	15.9	**28.8**	**41.6**	55%	69%	**83%**
NM	**36.0**	**40.3**	**48.4**	**19.7**	27.4	**39.3**	55%	68%	81%
IA	28.1	28.7	32.6	13.3	17.1	23.3	47%	60%	72%
NE	24.4	*26.2*	31.9	12.2	15.8	23.4	50%	60%	73%
KY	28.4	36.5	45.1	17.8	27.3	**38.6**	**63%**	**75%**	**86%**
WV	28.7	**39.5**	45.8	18.2	30.5	**39.2**	**64%**	**77%**	**86%**
MA	*17.2*	*21.8*	*19.5*	*3.9*	*6.7*	*9.9*	*23%*	*31%*	*51%*
NH	27.8	32.7	39.1	14.5	19.7	28.2	52%	60%	72%
MN	24.3	27.1	*28.8*	11.2	*15.4*	*20.6*	46%	57%	72%
WI	24.7	29.5	*31.1*	12.5	17.9	22.7	51%	61%	73%
MT	**39.7**	**45.2**	50.4	**24.6**	**32.7**	**41.1**	**62%**	**72%**	82%
WY	**37.1**	37.0	51.1	**23.4**	**27.5**	**43.0**	**63%**	**74%**	**84%**
OR	28.0	**38.9**	**49.3**	14.5	24.5	**39.6**	52%	63%	80%
WA	23.7	31.4	39.2	11.2	*18.0*	29.9	47%	57%	76%
20th percentile	21.9	27.1	31.2	11.0	15.8	22.7	44%	56%	71%
Median	25.9	32.5	37.9	14.5	21.1	30.3	53%	64%	79%
80th percentile	32.3	37.3	45.8	18.2	27.4	37.6	60%	72%	83%

Note. Data from 2019 Global Burden of Disease Study (IHME, 2023). Rates above the 80th percentile are displayed in bold face; those below the 20th percentile are displayed in italics.

Global Burden of Disease database (GBD) (IHME, 2023). The rate of suicide by firearm—and thus the total rate of suicide—is higher in states with more widespread household gun ownership. The epidemiology of firearm suicide is dramatically different between men and women. In 41 out of 50 states, men more often use a firearm for suicide than all other means put together. This is the case for women in only three states, all in the Deep South: Alabama, Mississippi, and Louisiana. The proportion of women's suicides by firearm is almost 50% in the Appalachian states and Wyoming. In New England and the Midwest, a firearm is involved in fewer than one quarter of women's suicides. Thus, only in the Deep South does the gun culture come close to gender equality.

The male rate of death by suicide rises steadily with age, with most of the increase related to firearm suicides. In the 16-state sample, 70% or more of suicidal men used a gun in every state but Massachusetts. Nationally, the only exceptions apart from Massachusetts are the District of Columbia, Hawaii, New Jersey, New York, and Rhode Island. Even in states with the lowest rates of firearm suicides, more than half of men over age 70 who died by suicide used a firearm. A possible explanation is that men over age 70 in 2019 would have been subject to the military draft. Many more men of their generation would have experience with firearms than men of subsequent generations who were not subject to compulsory military service.

Non-firearm suicides in men do not consistently rise with age. Our analysis of suicide mortality data broken down by 5-year age bands (not shown) showed a consistent pattern for non-firearm suicides in men: They rise steadily through young adulthood, peak in midlife, have a relative nadir between ages 50 and 75, and then rise steeply after age 75 (IHME, 2023; suicide mortality rates from the GBD 2019 database were queried by five-year age band for males and females). For women, the suicide rate decreases in old age, with both firearm and non-firearm suicides decreasing at approximately the same rate. Women's suicide rates peak in midlife, though the difference in rates between young adulthood and middle age usually is not large.

The numbers suggest, as does the literature on firearms and suicide, that wide availability of firearms and a strong gun culture are associated with increased rates of firearm suicide and with suicide overall. Substantial experience with firearm use, whether from hunting, sport, or military service, further increases the likelihood they will be used for self-harm. Other means of suicide do not substitute for firearms, in part because few other means of suicide can be as lethal with so little advance planning. Only the ingestion of large quantities of highly toxic pesticides, the preferred method of suicide in rural China, comes close to firearms in combining lethality and minimal need for advance planning. Jumping from a height, crashing a car, inhaling carbon monoxide, hanging, and overdosing on drugs all are highly lethal; but they require advance planning and/or offer possibilities for rescue. The greater interstate variability in suicide rates as opposed to rates of MDD is entirely due to differences in firearm suicide rates. For non-firearm suicide, interstate variability in suicide is not greater than that for depression. A clinical implication is that early inquiry about firearms at home and how they are stored is essential when assessing a depressed older man in a state with a strong gun culture and a high firearm suicide rate. Patients might find questioning them about guns to be more acceptable if the clinician has some personal experience with firearms and if issues of gun storage are framed more generally in terms of safety (e.g., regarding visiting grandchildren)—unless the patient explicitly acknowledges suicidal plans.

Variation in suicide rates and their pattern by age and gender for the 16 states can now be interpreted. The lowest suicide rates for women are encountered in the Midwest and in Massachusetts—five states with below-median rates of ACEs and female poverty, a >90% rate of high school graduation or equivalent, above-median gender equality scores, high scores on the Institutional Health sub-index of social capital, and excellent access to mental health care. The states with the highest female suicide rates—the two Mountain States and the two Southwestern states—have varying combinations of high mean altitude (New Mexico, Montana, and Wyoming), low Institutional Health (Arizona, New Mexico, and Montana), high female poverty (Arizona, New Mexico, and Montana), high physical and/or psychological IPV against women (all four), below-median gender equality scores (Arizona, New Mexico, and Wyoming), above-median rates of multiple ACEs (all four), below-median access to mental health care (Arizona, Montana, and Wyoming), and high rates of household gun ownership (Montana and Wyoming). Among the 16 states, the largest increases in suicide rates with age, between ages 15–49 and ages 50–69, are seen in the Pacific Northwest and in Arizona. Possible explanations include above-median divorce rates in the three states and the effect of immigration. Because of relatively recent immigration, the ethnic composition of Arizona, Oregon, and Washington differs by age, with a higher proportion of non-Hispanic Whites and American Indians—groups with high suicide rates—in the cohort aged 50–69 in 2019. The states' younger populations have a higher proportion of Hispanic or Asian immigrants, who have relatively lower suicide rates related both to ethnicity and to the "healthy immigrant effect."

The lowest suicide rates for men are seen in the Midwest, New England, and Washington State. The seven states have household gun ownership rates below the median for the 16 states and even lower-ranked rates of guns kept loaded and unlocked, immediately explaining much of the difference. In addition, they all have above-median scores on Institutional Health, including the item on trust in the media that is most strongly and negatively correlated with suicide rates at the state level. They have below-median rates of ACEs and below-median rates of male poverty. Except for Nebraska, 40% or more of households in the seven states have incomes >400% of the poverty line. Except for New Hampshire, the states have below-median percentages of SSDI recipients. In short, men tend to have relatively healthy work lives, adequate finances, non-violent intimate relationships, and trust in institutions. And, when they are acutely distressed, a loaded gun, stored in an unlocked location, usually is not at hand.

The highest suicide rates for men are seen in the Mountain States, Appalachia, New Mexico, and Oregon. High household gun ownership is an obvious contributor in the Mountain States and Appalachia. High altitude is significant in the Mountain States, New Mexico, and Oregon. Multiple ACEs have above-median prevalence in all six states. Except for Wyoming, male poverty rates are in the highest (worst) quintile nationally, and Institutional Health is below the national median. Oregon has the additional risk factor of an unusually high level of environmental pollution with chemicals potentially harmful to the brain or the endocrine system. Many men in the states with the highest suicide rates have experienced personal trauma or financial distress, without trusted sources of information or support to help them cope, or timely access to affordable and culturally acceptable mental health care. Suicide, usually by firearm, can be an appealing and readily available solution for such men.

In the states of the Midwest and in New England, male suicide rates do not rise significantly with age as they do in other regions. The poverty rates for older men in these states are relatively low. And, the Midwest and New England have cultures of respect for older people, along with a substantial presence of government and/or non-profit agencies that provide support to older people who are alone or functionally impaired. The latter is especially important to widowed men, who tend to do much less well than female widows after losing their spouse. "No country for old men" is less applicable in states with cultures with a communitarian ethos and openness to collective problem-solving.

Depression During the COVID-19 Pandemic

Study of depression in America during the COVID-19 pandemic offers a remarkable opportunity to observe the effects of cultural intersectionality, the role of place in modifying the relationship of cultural identity to depression, and the importance to depression of the structural factors and social determinants of health associated with cultural identity. In the final section of this chapter, we present the results of an exploratory study of data on depression from the U.S. Census Bureau's Household Pulse Survey (2023d) Wave 39—a nationwide survey of households conducted between September 29 and October 11 of 2021—approximately 21 months into the pandemic. The survey obtained data from 57,065 respondents aged 18 and above that included their demographics; racial, ethnic, and gender identity; sexual orientation; educational attainment; marital status; living arrangements; 2020 household income; current financial status; their physical, cognitive, and sensory function; and their COVID-19 vaccination status. Race is described as White, Black, Asian, or Other/Mixed, and it is indicated whether the respondent endorses

Hispanic ethnicity. Some American Indian respondents could be identified by their having insurance through the Indian Health Service. Regarding mental health, respondents were asked to complete the PHQ-2 and the two-item Generalized Anxiety Disorder questionnaire (and most did so) and to indicate whether they were receiving counseling or therapy, whether they thought they needed counseling or therapy, and whether they were taking prescription drugs for a mental health problem. The public use file indicates the state in which each respondent lived at the time of the survey. If the respondent lived in one of the nation's 15 largest metropolitan areas, the file indicates which one. More detailed localization of respondents and specification of their national origin/heritage were not provided in the public use file, to protect their confidentiality. However, the probable heritage of Asian and Hispanic respondents sometimes can be inferred from their area of residence. For example, most Asians in metropolitan San Francisco are Chinese, while this is not so for Asians in the non-metropolitan Midwest. Most Hispanics in metropolitan Miami have Caribbean heritage, while most Hispanics in Los Angeles or Phoenix have Mexican or Central American ethnicity.

We estimated the prevalence of clinical depression in various areas and populations by estimating the percentage of respondents with PHQ-2 scores of 3 or higher. The denominator was limited to survey respondents who answered the two items of the PHQ-2 and the percentage calculated using the person-level weights provided by the U.S. Census Bureau to enable adjustment for varying response rates.

In a population with a prevalence of 7% for MDD and a prevalence of 18% for any diagnosable depressive disorder, the PHQ-2 with a cutoff of 3 had a positive predictive value of 38.4% for MDD and 75.0% for any depressive disorder (i.e., clinical depression). The positive predictive value would be greater in a population with a higher base rate of MDD. In the Pulse survey population, the percentage was 20.3% for men and 23.3% for women, implying an MDD prevalence of at least 7.8% and 8.9%, respectively, and a clinical depression prevalence of 15.3% and 17.5%, respectively—all numbers well above pre-pandemic rates. For example, the 2019 prevalence of MDD in the U.S. for adults ages 20 and older was 2.94% for men and 4.93% for women (IHME, 2023).

Table 14.25 shows the rates of PHQ-2 scores of 3 or higher for American adults who responded to the Household Pulse Survey including the items of the PHQ-2, subdivided by gender and by several different determinants of cultural identity: race/ethnicity (Non-Hispanic White, Black, Asian, Other/Mixed, or Hispanic), age range, marital status, educational attainment, and 2020 household income. Another subdivision is by financial status—a count of three indicators of financial distress: somewhat difficult or very difficult to pay usual

Table 14.25 Depression and Its Treatment During the COVID-19 Pandemic: September/October 2021

	Percentage of population with depression		Percentage of those depressed taking psychiatric medication		Percentage of depressed people who got or thought they needed psychotherapy	
	Men	Women	Men	Women	Men	Women
Race/ethnicity						
Non-Hispanic White	19.6%	21.9%	36.7%	54.5%	42.0%	51.8%
Black	19.3%	25.4%	20.1%	33.5%	38.3%	46.3%
Asian	16.1%	16.1%	22.0%	19.0%	13.0%	34.3%
Other or Mixed Race	36.6%	31.5%	40.5%	38.1%	33.2%	46.3%
Hispanic	22.0%	27.1%	22.6%	30.8%	32.3%	44.7%
Age						
<30	34.0%	38.3%	21.1%	34.6%	42.3%	60.0%
30–44	25.6%	25.8%	35.3%	41.0%	42.3%	53.5%
45–64	16.0%	22.4%	33.6%	50.6%	36.2%	44.9%
≥65	11.1%	13.3%	43.4%	60.7%	22.8%	30.3%
Education						
Less than high school	30.9%	36.9%	46.9%	52.5%	42.6%	16.5%
Some high school	24.9%	29.0%	16.0%	29.1%	21.4%	32.7%
High school graduate	22.0%	24.4%	34.6%	46.2%	30.1%	42.8%
Some college	24.8%	29.2%	31.4%	44.3%	47.2%	54.6%
Associate degree	21.8%	23.8%	31.3%	47.5%	35.9%	51.1%
Bachelor's degree	15.7%	19.3%	28.0%	49.3%	44.2%	60.8%
Graduate degree	12.0%	14.2%	37.3%	45.8%	42.6%	51.0%
Financial precarity						
None	12.5%	14.0%	30.9%	45.0%	39.1%	47.4%
Mild to moderate	35.0%	35.3%	29.8%	46.3%	36.9%	49.6%
Moderate to severe	55.5%	58.8%	37.6%	46.5%	37.8%	28.1%
Very severe	73.2%	77.8%	42.9%	38.3%	37.7%	62.8%
Marital status						
Married	13.6%	17.1%	33.8%	47.6%	33.5%	44.2%
Widowed	13.5%	19.4%	41.1%	64.4%	31.1%	30.9%
Divorced	27.7%	26.1%	41.9%	54.1%	30.9%	47.9%

Table 14.25 Continued

	Percentage of population with depression		Percentage of those depressed taking psychiatric medication		Percentage of depressed people who got or thought they needed psychotherapy	
	Men	Women	Men	Women	Men	Women
Separated	34.0%	39.8%	45.6%	43.2%	49.5%	49.0%
Never married	33.2%	34.6%	27.3%	35.7%	44.0%	57.3%
2020 Household income						
<$25,000	41.5%	36.2%	38.7%	45.9%	34.1%	51.3%
$25,000 to $34,999	26.8%	31.3%	30.2%	47.3%	39.5%	42.9%
$35,000 to $50,000	29.4%	25.0%	20.8%	40.2%	34.9%	47.8%
$50,000 to $74,999	18.0%	23.0%	37.1%	46.5%	40.0%	53.2%
$75,000 to $99,999	16.8%	18.1%	33.6%	50.0%	39.3%	50.1%
$100,000 to $149,999	13.4%	14.1%	29.0%	48.5%	47.8%	57.2%
$150,000 to $199,999	9.1%	13.2%	44.4%	49.0%	40.2%	50.6%
$200,000 or higher	10.9%	10.9%	30.0%	45.9%	45.2%	48.3%

Note. Data from U.S. Census Household Pulse Survey (U.S. Census Bureau, 2023d).

household expenses over the last seven days, sometimes or often not enough to eat over the last seven days, and concern that eviction or foreclosure on one's residence in the next two months is somewhat likely or very likely. Financial distress is rated mild to moderate if there is one indicator, moderate to severe if there are two, and very severe if there are three. The table also shows the percentages, among those with PHQ-2 scores of 3 or higher, of people who were, at the time of the survey, taking psychotropic drugs and of people who had either seen a mental health professional for counseling or therapy in the past four weeks or thought they needed to but couldn't do so for some reason.

For both men and women, people of mixed or "other" race were most likely to report depression, while Asians were least likely to do so. For non-Hispanic Whites, Blacks, and Hispanic/Latino Americans, the prevalence of depression was higher in women. For Asians the prevalence was lower than in other racial/ethnic groups, but it was equal for men and women. Among people of mixed race, men were more likely to be depressed. "Cultural homelessness"—a risk for people of mixed race as it is for immigrants of generation 1.5 or 2.0—might be a bigger problem for men than for women. Hispanic/Latino people reported more depression than those of other ethnicity; this might partially reflect a greater willingness to acknowledge symptoms rather than a truly higher prevalence. The crude prevalence of depression in Black men and White men was equal, and that of Black women was slightly higher than that of White women; but after controlling for socioeconomic status and social determinants, Blacks turned out to have less depression than Whites.

In the Household Pulse Survey data, depression rates fall with increasing age, with higher education, and with greater household income. However, the details vary by racial/ethnic identity, gender, and region of residence, as we will illustrate with multivariate models. Acceptance of psychotherapy falls with age, while use of psychotropic drugs increases with age—with differences approximately twofold between men and women under age 30 and those age 65 or above. People with any post-secondary education were more accepting of psychotherapy. Single, divorced, and separated people had markedly higher rates of depression than married people, in part relatable to how the pandemic intensified the loneliness of people living alone. Depression rates in widowed people are harder to interpret because of confounding age effects. Income appears protective against depression, with a consistent correlation across the spectrum of household income. Among people deeply in poverty (household income <$25,000), men suffered more depression than women. Acceptance of treatments of depression—both pharmacologic and psychotherapeutic—was not strongly related to income.

As noted earlier in this chapter, characterization of people as *Asian* or *Hispanic* blurs distinctions between national cultures. Household Pulse Survey data allow comparison of rates of depression (PHQ-2 ≥3) in people living in each of several large metropolitan areas, from which inferences can be drawn about such distinctions.

In Southern California most Hispanic/Latino people are of Mexican origin. In the Los Angeles metropolitan area, the prevalence of depression was 26.0% in men and 21.4% in women; and in the Riverside metropolitan area, it was 41.4% in men and 32.0% in women. The rates are well above the national rates, and, unusually, the prevalence of depression is higher in men than in women.

Culture might contribute to the high male depression prevalence. In the Mexican culture of *machismo*, men are expected to support their families; but most Mexican immigrant men in Southern California are poorly paid, and the cost of living in the area is notoriously high. This can lead to men feeling unsuccessful and blaming themselves for not being good enough providers.

The situation is far different in Miami, a city where most Hispanic/Latino people are of Caribbean and South American origins, average household income does not differ between Hispanic/Latino people and non-Hispanic Whites, and there are many Hispanic/Latino families in the upper class and upper middle class. The prevalence of depression among Hispanic/Latino people in metropolitan Miami was 9.1% for men and 25.7% for women. The extreme gender disparity in depression prevalence was unique among the top 15 metropolitan areas. The contrast between Miami and Riverside offers a dramatic example of cultural intersectionality. Generalizations about depression in Hispanic Americans during the pandemic have limited validity if they don't include how the interaction of gender, social class, and national origin shape the narrative.

For Asian Americans overall, the prevalence of depression was the same in men and women—16.1%. However, in San Francisco, where 36% of the population is Asian and 62% of Asians are Chinese, the prevalence of depression was 10.9% in men and 5.9% in women, significantly lower than in the U.S. as a whole and with an unusual male preponderance. In San Francisco, with 22% the total population being Chinese, one might expect to find Chinese norms of understating negative emotion, as described in Chapter 10. Within San Francisco's large Chinese community, the pressure on young men to succeed is especially great, and pandemic-related disruption of work and study hit them especially hard. Young Chinese women have, perhaps, "more ways to win." In Los Angeles County, where only 15% of the population is Asian and only 31% of the Asian population is Chinese, the more typical female preponderance of depression was seen, with prevalence of 14.8% in men and 20.8% in women. Compared with the Asian population of San Francisco, that of Los Angeles is more diverse, with large Filipino, Korean, Vietnamese and Japanese American communities (U.S. Census Bureau, 2023e).

American regions—and their subpopulations defined by race/ethnicity, education, social class, and generation—differ greatly in their level of cognitive social capital. Trust in institutions, including government agencies, schools and colleges, the health professions, the media, and corporations, appears to reflect an intersection of cultural identities including those related to place. Residents of states with very low-trust cultures might reject medical advice that one might expect them to accept based on their education and social class alone. Regions differ also in the distribution of numeracy in their populations.

During the COVID-19 pandemic, low institutional trust found expression as rejection of vaccination and masking, and consequently in higher rates of COVID transmission, morbidity, and mortality. It also was expressed in a high prevalence of depression. People in a low-trust environment are more likely to be depressed when facing severe stress. And in an environment where COVID-19 cases are more likely to lead to hospitalization or death, the actual or potential illness of oneself, friends, and family is more stressful than it is in a highly vaccinated and consistently masked population where COVID transmission rates are low and infection rarely is life-threatening.

Concluding Comment

In this chapter American regional cultures have been characterized by integrating qualitative historical perspectives with analyses of quantitative demographic, economic, and environmental data. The epidemiology of mood disorders, their likely contexts and presentations, and considerations for prevention and treatment can be better understood with the aid of cultural awareness. This includes "structural competence"—knowledge of the social, economic, and environmental determinants of depression, bipolar spectrum disorders, and suicidal behavior. The methodology illustrated here with eight pairs of states representing eight regions can be applied to the remaining U.S. states and regions, as might be needed to address depression and/or suicide as clinical or population health issues. The data sources used to construct the tables in this chapter cover the entire country. Fischer (1989) and Woodard (2011) offer comprehensive historically-based qualitative perspectives on all American regions that relate their contemporary cultures to their historical legacies. A more encyclopedic reference on American regional cultures is the eight-volume *Greenwood Encyclopedia of American Regional Cultures* (Ferris, 2004). Synthesis of qualitative and quantitative perspectives yields an understanding of regional culture of practical value in addressing the nation's epidemic of depression and suicide, in populations and in individuals in distress.

Part III

Depression and the Cultures of Occupations

Chapter 15

The Dark Side of Creative Talent

On the afternoon of July 23, 2011, the globally acclaimed jazz/R&B singer and songwriter Amy Winehouse was found dead in bed at her home in north London. She was 27. The coroner deemed the cause of death to be accidental alcohol intoxication. Her blood alcohol level was 416 mg/dl, a level that can cause death from respiratory depression. The police found three empty bottles of vodka in her bedroom. Winehouse was under treatment for anxiety with Librium® (chlordiazepoxide), a benzodiazepine anti-anxiety drug with respiratory depressant effects that intensify those of alcohol. The drug had been prescribed by a psychiatrist who had recommended ongoing treatment that Winehouse rejected. The drug was found in her blood at autopsy.

Winehouse had been seen by her primary care physician, Dr. R., the evening before her death. Her doctor noticed that she was "tipsy," and she admitted that she had resumed drinking on July 20 after 17 days of abstinence. She had no definite plan to stop drinking. She agreed to telephone her doctor over the weekend. Her full-time bodyguard, who resided at her home, knew Winehouse was drinking that night but did not intrude upon her privacy.

According to a press interview with Dr. R. following the singer's death, Winehouse had seen a psychiatrist and a psychologist the prior year. They both had recommended treatment, but she was "opposed to any form of psychological therapy." Neither Dr. R., her bodyguard, nor her parents thought she was suicidal. Dr. R. recalled Amy's telling her that "I do not want to die" and "I have not achieved a lot of the things I want to" and discussing her plans for a 28th birthday party.

Amy Winehouse at age 24 was the first British woman to win five Grammys in a single year. In addition to winning awards for her performances, she won three awards for her songwriting from the British Academy of Songwriters, Composers and Authors, the first for the song "Stronger than Me," which she wrote at age 20. Her posthumous album *Back to Black* was one of the best sellers in UK history ("Amy Winehouse," 2019; Davies, 2011).

Winehouse had a history of bulimia nervosa (binge eating followed by self-induced vomiting accompanied by intense dissatisfaction with her body shape and weight), abuse of alcohol and illicit drugs (including crack cocaine,

3,4-methylenedioxy-methamphetamine ["ecstasy"], cannabis, and opioids), and deliberate self-injury by cutting (Hauber et al., 2019; Hughes, 2015). She was prescribed paroxetine at age 14 for treatment of depression in the context of her parents' divorce; it is not known how long she remained on the drug. She had several episodes of inpatient substance use "rehab," including at least one involuntary hospitalization, but did not receive medication-assisted treatment (MAT) for her alcoholism and had inconsistent follow-up. A heavy smoker, she had been diagnosed with early-onset emphysema. In her songs, most of which were autobiographical, she described frequent impulsive sexual behavior and drinking to intoxication to cope with unbearably intense emotion.

When she was 21, she began a mutually destructive relationship with Blake Fielder-Civil. He introduced Winehouse to heroin and other drugs and joined her in self-cutting episodes. Their relationship often was physically violent. Married to him for two years between ages 23 and 25, she could not fully end the relationship despite its obvious harm to her. After her divorce, she gave up cocaine and heroin and relied solely upon alcohol.

While the press and Winehouse's parents, who now run a charitable organization focusing on prevention of alcohol and drug abuse, have consistently focused attention on her addictions, Amy Winehouse obviously had mental health issues not caused by substance use. An illness in the bipolar spectrum is supported by her early onset of clinical depression and her intense drive, ambition, hypersexuality, harmful substance use, and impulsive risk-taking. She suffered from three mental disorders in addition to alcohol use disorder—a mood disorder in the bipolar spectrum (probably bipolar II disorder [BD-II]), bulimia nervosa, and non-suicidal self-injury disorder (NSSI). People cared about her, but at the time of her death she was receiving no psychiatric treatment, and her only psychoactive medication was an anti-anxiety drug (Milloy, 2011).

As will be discussed further below, Winehouse might have had a genetic disorder that is associated with creativity, increased risk of bipolar disorder (BD), and the early onset of emphysema—a condition that she developed at age 24.

Productive, Eminent, and "Touched by Fire"

Depression, bipolar illness, and suicide are linked in the public mind with the tumultuous careers of creative geniuses, from poets to popular musicians, novelists to painters, composers to stand-up comedians. Since ancient times, artistic genius has been linked to mental illness. Aristotle's line in his *Poetics* is frequently quoted: "There is no great genius without some touch of madness" (Aristotle, 1995; see also Chapter 9). This may be true metaphorically, but throughout history there have been geniuses of the arts and sciences with no mental disorder, let alone one so severe that it would warrant the label of "madness."

Well-known modern studies of creativity and bipolarity and mood disorder include the work of the British psychiatrist Felix Post (1996) on the careers of eminent creative people and Kay Jamison's book *Touched with Fire* (1993). They analyzed public biographies of famous creative people and searched for evidence of BD, major depressive disorder (MDD), and other mental disorders. A second line of investigation has studied life expectancy and causes of death in creative people versus controls. A third has been based on psychological tests and mental disorder screening in individuals with creative occupations and those with mood disorders. This chapter draws on all three types of studies in an attempt to synthesize modern views of mood disorders in creative professionals.

In this chapter, we will refer to creative professionals in several ways. For our purposes, the universe of creative professionals comprises creative writers (poets, novelists, short story writers, playwrights, screenwriters, writers of creative non-fiction), visual artists and designers (painters, graphic artists, illustrators, animators, sculptors, ceramicists, fashion designers), musicians (instrumentalists, composers, songwriters, singers, conductors), actors and directors (of stage, film, and broadcast media), and comedians (including stand-up comedians and actors specializing in comedy). When we mention creative disciplines in this chapter, the reference is to professionals of the discipline unless noted otherwise. The words *creator* and *artist* may refer to any discipline. *Performing artists* and *performers* comprise musicians, actors, and comedians. A *successful* creator is one who is respected in their discipline and has a relatively high personal income based on their creative work. An *eminent* creator is one likely to be familiar to anyone interested in the creator's discipline and genre. A *star*—usually a performing artist—is a creative professional who is famous and highly paid. A *celebrity* is someone widely recognized by the public because of extensive coverage by mass media.

Creativity and bipolar spectrum disorders are related on a population basis, via attributes of personality and temperament shared by people with bipolar disorders and people with either eminent or non-eminent creativity. Srivastava and Ketter (2010) reviewed studies of bipolarity (both clinical and non-clinical) and creativity (both eminent and non-eminent), relating the two attributes to assessments of personality with the Neuroticism-Extraversion-Openness Personality Inventory (NEO-PI; McCrae & Costa, 1987) and the Myers-Briggs Type Indicator (MBTI; Myers & McCaulley, 1985) and assessment of temperament with the Temperament Evaluation of Memphis, Pisa, and San Diego Autoquestionnaire (TEMPS-A; Akiskal et al., 2005). On the NEO-PI, people with BD in remission share with creative professionals the attributes of neuroticism (predisposition to experience negative emotions and physical sensations), openness to experience (e.g., curiosity, preference for novelty and variety), and decreased conscientiousness. Both bipolar people and creative people can be either introverted or extraverted. On the MBTI, both currently euthymic bipolar people and creative people showed a preference for intuition over sensation as a cognitive style: They tended to prefer abstract thinking and are concerned with meanings and relationships over focusing on objective facts and sensory input. On the TEMPS-A, both people with BD in remission and creative people scored high on cyclothymia (a temperament characterized by intense emotionality and variability in mood, sleep, energy, self-esteem, and sociability). When ill, a person with BD might be irritable or have a high or low mood, but people with BD in remission do not consistently have irritable, hyperthymic, or dysthymic temperaments. Srivastava and colleagues (2010) gave all three assessments along with a psychological test of creative thinking (the Barron-Walsh Art Scale) and confirmed the relationship of measured creativity to neuroticism, a cyclothymic temperament, and an intuitive cognitive style.

Vellante and colleagues compared affective temperaments between a group of Italian college students preparing for creative careers (music, theater, dance, or visual arts) with a comparison group of those studying law, engineering, or foreign languages. The the two groups did not differ significantly in age, sex, marital status, or socioeconomic status. Those preparing for creative careers scored higher on the hyperthymic, cyclothymic, and irritable scales of the TEMPS-A. The cyclothymic scale was specifically related to a biographical measure of creative achievement. Students who simultaneously scored high on the scales for cyclothymia, dysthymia, and anxiety—a group at risk for bipolar spectrum disorders—were highly involved in creative activities but had not achieved as much as those endorsing cyclothymia alone (Vellante et al., 2011).

Reviews and meta-analyses have found an increased lifetime prevalence of bipolar spectrum disorders among working creative professionals, and writers and visual artists are more likely to have first-degree relatives with BD than the general population. Though relatively few people with BD are employed in creative professions, as many as 80% of people clinically diagnosed with Bipolar I disorder (BD-I) or BD-II self-report engaging in creative activities when manic or hypomanic, such as writing prose or poetry, painting or drawing, or making music. Those with BD-II are more likely to succeed at their creative pursuits than those with BD-I (Klein, 2019; McCraw et al., 2013; Taylor, 2017).

Creative professionals without BD have no immunity to (unipolar) MDD, and they have the same precipitating factors for major depressive episodes (MDEs) as people in other occupations, including trauma, loss, somatic pain, and general medical illness. A common issue of writers, artists, and performers is fluctuation in the reception of their work and the market for it. If their work becomes less popular, their income will decrease, and they might face financial hardship if they do not have wealth or another source of income. Either financial problems or the blow to self-esteem associated with worsening reception of their work can precipitate an episode of depression.

Writers have a remarkably high prevalence of unipolar MDEs, well beyond what might be expected from their demographics and disproportionate to their increased prevalence of BD. In an analysis of 2005–2014 data from the National Survey on Drug Use and Health, the 12-month prevalence of MDEs among employed adults aged 18–64 was 6.6%. Among writers, the prevalence was 19.8%—triple the rate in the general employed population. Twelve-month MDE prevalence rates for other creative professions exceeded the national benchmark but were well below the rates for writers. For visual artists, the 12-month prevalence of MDEs was 10.9%; for musicians the rate was 9.0% (Woodward et al., 2017). Allowing for standard errors of approximately 2%, the difference between the benchmark prevalence of MDEs and the rates for visual artists and musicians might be attributed entirely to creative people's higher prevalence of bipolar disorders. Creative professionals other than writers do not share the latter's vulnerability to unipolar depression.

Among male writers, playwrights have the highest lifetime prevalence of major depression and poets the lowest. Playwrights and novelists both have rates of alcohol use disorders above those of the general population. Poets have the highest rates of bipolar illness among writers, but they do not have increased rates of unipolar MDD or alcohol use disorders (Post, 1996). Similar statistics by genre of writing are not available for female writers.

While BD is highly prevalent in the creative professions and unipolar MDD is a common affliction of writers, mood disorders are not "normal" in the sense of being necessary or inevitable accompaniments of a creative life. Unfortunately, clinical depression and bipolar illness frequently are minimized, rationalized, or romanticized simply because the affected person is a writer, artist, or performer. Most cases of depression and bipolar illness in working creative professionals—as in people employed in other occupations—can be understood as related to an interaction of individual vulnerabilities including those due to genetics, development, traumatic experiences, personality and temperament, personal circumstances, and the working conditions and associated hazards of their occupations. Successful writers, visual artists, and performers are admired and their works enjoyed, and it seems to many that they have enviable lives. However, they often face challenging working conditions and non-trivial occupational hazards, some related to the creative life, some to specific disciplines and genres, and some to success and celebrity.

A Spectrum of Misconception

As suggested in Chapter 3 on the bipolar spectrum, mood disorders in the creative professions are "normal," in the sense of being frequently present but not in the sense of being normative, necessary, or inevitable. Nonetheless, creators may see their own depressive or hypomanic symptoms simply as part of who they are, rather than symptoms of treatable illness, or they may self-treat specific symptoms of a mood disorder with alcohol or drugs. Audiences might be sympathetic if the performing artist suffers but do not necessarily conceive of the suffering as a symptom of a potentially treatable illness. When a depressed or otherwise mood-disordered performer is known to misuse alcohol or drugs, their audience is likely to regard the problem solely as one of addiction, to be solved simply by maintaining sobriety.

Eminent writers, artists, and performers are relatively few but have disproportionate influence on the broader culture. Eminent creators' disclosures of their experiences of depression, bipolar illness, self-destructive behavior, and suicidality have inspired members of their audiences to come forward with their own stories and, in some cases, to seek help for the first time. When they take anti-psychiatry positions or relate unhappy experiences with mental health care, they can discourage people from seeking help and can add to the stigma of psychiatry. Partially depending on how they are reported, suicides of eminent performers either prompt suicidal people to seek help or add to their sense of hopelessness. At worst, they trigger "copycat" suicides, a problem that can be worse if details are publicized of specific suicide triggers and methods.

Audiences might appreciate creative works that elegantly express their creators' experiences of depression or hypomania and not be aware of or concerned about whether the artistic expressions of mood states are confessional or vicarious. Non-psychiatrist physicians treating creative professionals who present with depression sometimes focus on the somatic symptoms such as insomnia and physical pain but discount the cognitive and affective ones, ascribing their patients' strong emotions to artistic sensibilities. Many physicians do not appreciate how even subtle cognitive impairments related to depression—or subtle emotional blunting by antidepressant medications—can make creative work more difficult. If insomnia is treated with a sedative-hypnotic or anxiolytic drug, fatigue is treated with a stimulant, or pain is treated with an opioid, a depressed patient can be provided with a means of self-harm. As in Amy Winehouse's case, a relatively benign prescription drug (a benzodiazepine anti-anxiety drug) can increase the toxicity of an abused substance (alcohol). Or, as happened with the actor Heath Ledger (1979–2008), a depressed person can obtain an array of prescriptions from multiple physicians, each relatively benign, and consume them all at once with a fatal outcome. While in the United States (U.S.), states with prescription drug monitoring programs can help identify such situations when the prescriptions involved are for controlled substances, many prescription drugs and over-the-counter products that are not controlled substances can contribute to a life-threatening multi-drug interaction.

A common diagnostic error in the clinical assessment of creative professionals is correctly diagnosing a substance use disorder but failing to diagnose a mood disorder that is comorbid with it and might have preceded it. When this happens, the person might be treated for the substance use problem with a narrow focus on abstinence. After a period of sobriety, the patient finds the symptoms of the mood disorder to be unbearable and self-medicates with one or more of the substances previously abused or with a potentially dangerous alternative. This can be especially dangerous if the person takes a high dose of a substance to which they were formerly tolerant but are no longer.

While mood disorders are frequent comorbidities of substance use disorders, they are especially prevalent in creative professionals with problematic alcohol and/or drug use. Both creators and the public often view alcohol or drug use as common problems of creative people and do not heavily stigmatize a successful writer, artist, or performer for having an addiction or for being "in recovery" or "learning to live sober." There is greater stigma attached to a diagnosis of "mental illness." As the case of Mariah Carey will illustrate, artists with truly extraordinary success might nonetheless fear public stigma and consequently stigmatize themselves for having a mood disorder.

Knowledge that a person is a successful creative professional alters the prior probabilities a clinician should consider before examining them. If a professional writer complains of insomnia or physical pain, suspicion of clinical depression (with or without a painful comorbid general medical condition) should be high; and the clinical history and mental status examination should be thorough. The clinical assessment might be supplemented with a depression screening questionnaire followed by a structured interview for depressive symptoms if the screen is positive. If a writer, artist, or musician presents with clinical depression, they deserve careful assessment for bipolarity because misdiagnosing bipolar depression as unipolar depression can have serious adverse consequences. Giving antidepressants without mood stabilizers to people with bipolar depression can cause rapid cycling or depression with mixed features, conditions associated with increased suicide risk (Phelps & James, 2017). As discussed in detail in Part I, screening for bipolarity might include administering the Hypomania Checklist (HCL-32) or the MDQ, review of medical records, and, if the patient agrees, talking with someone who knows them well about potential prior hypomanic symptoms. In the future, automated analysis of data from mobile devices is likely to supplement such history-taking, by offering data-driven insight into periods of increased activity, more frequent and diverse communication, diminished sleep, and text message content suggesting euphoria and/or irritability.

When hypomania screening tests like the HCL-32 or MDQ are used, cutoff scores may be adjusted downward to enhance the tests' sensitivity, since there will be less concern about false positives when the population being screened is known to have a high base rate of bipolarity (Phelps & Ghaemi, 2006; Zimmerman & Holst, 2018). It is not uncommon for a person to be correctly diagnosed with BD but subsequently to be incorrectly diagnosed with unipolar MDD by another clinician. A "forgotten diagnosis" of BD can result in a poor outcome of treatment for a depressive episode.

In the U.S., the average delay in diagnosing BD after the onset of symptoms—over nine years—is unacceptably long (Drancourt et al., 2013). It might be shortened for creative professionals if the association of creativity with bipolarity appropriately modifies their clinicians' prior probabilities of diagnoses in the bipolar spectrum, and thus changes their clinicians' approach to diagnostic evaluation.

Heath Ledger, whose career as an actor had begun at age 18, was nominated for the Best Actor Academy Award for his performance in Ang Lee's film *Brokeback Mountain* (2005) and soon after gave an iconic performance as the Joker in *The Dark Knight* (Nolan, 2008). At the age of 28 he died of a simultaneous overdose of the prescription opioid analgesics oxycodone and hydrocodone, the anxiolytics diazepam and alprazolam, the hypnotic drug temazepam, and the over-the-counter antihistamine doxylamine. The coroner determined that his death was accidental (Barron, 2008). It is unknown where he obtained the assortment of medications.

In a 2007 interview with the *New York Times* Ledger described severe insomnia in words strongly suggesting hypomania: "Last week I probably slept an average of two hours a night ... I couldn't stop thinking. My body was exhausted, and my mind was still going." After taking a prescription hypnotic (zolpidem), he slept for 1 hour, then awakened with his mind "still racing" (Lyall, 2007). His former fiancée recalled, "He had too much energy. His mind was turning, turning, turning—always turning" ("Remembering Heath Ledger," 2017). Other quotations from Ledger support a suspicion of undiagnosed bipolar disorder: "I'm kind of addicted to moving"; "I thought, I need to be more cautious about my choices" (AZ Quotes, 2019); "I don't feel like I have anything to lose, so I don't really understand what I'm putting at risk" (BrainyQuote, 2019).

Heath Ledger had sophisticated friends, and he had seen physicians. Did none of them raise the seemingly obvious question of BD? If no one did, one explanation is that the existence of a bipolar spectrum with milder expression than classic manic-depressive illness (BD-II) was less widely appreciated at the time. Another is that journalists' questions sometimes reveal more than those asked by busy physicians.

Mariah Carey (b. 1969), the most popular singer of the 1990s and *Billboard*'s "Artist of the Decade," was diagnosed in 2001 with BD-II. She publicly disclosed her illness only 17 years later, in 2018. In an interview with *People*, she gave the reason: "I didn't want to carry around the stigma of a lifelong disease that would define me and potentially end my career. I was so terrified of losing everything.... I convinced myself that the only way to deal with this was not to deal with this" (Bromwich, 2018). This from a singer who has sold over 200 million records, with 64 million albums sold in the U.S. alone, and whose net worth is over half a billion dollars (Ngomsi, 2018). Her case offers striking evidence that wealth and celebrity do not immunize a person against self-stigma and fear of public stigma. Inquiring about issues of stigma and shame should always be on the agenda for assessing eminent creative professionals with symptoms of depression.

The Culture of the Creative Professions

Eminent creative professionals are part of an actual or virtual community of those who practice their creative discipline—a community that appreciates the challenges of a creative occupation, including the need to work continually to connect with audiences and critics and to maintain one's reputation through changing times and shifting popular tastes. Among creative professionals, ambition, perfectionism, and competitiveness are common, as are expansiveness when new work reaches an appreciative audience and discouragement when new work is not well received. Hearing gossip or critics' opinions that one is past one's prime can be demoralizing.

Within conformist cultures, creative professionals might be allowed more freedom to be atypical in their lifestyles, appearance, language, and behavior. However, in places under authoritarian rule, a non-conformist artist or writer who is too successful can become a target of criticism and even oppression.

Because there is a relatively high prevalence of depression and bipolar illness among artists, it is likely that an artist will know peers who have been treated for these conditions. Peers' experiences of treatment, positive or negative, can influence an artist's decision to consult a psychiatrist or to accept a recommended treatment. The influence of peers is especially important when the decision involves obvious risk (e.g., electroconvulsive therapy [ECT]), great expense (e.g., psychoanalysis or private residential treatment), or "coming out" about one's psychiatric issues (e.g., seeking help for a suicidal crisis). Some celebrity performers have taken strong anti-psychiatry stances, and others have given well-publicized accounts of treatment that was unhappy and unhelpful. Superstar actor Tom Cruise, an adherent to Scientology, dismissed the entire specialty of psychiatry as without scientific basis and encouraged all psychiatric patients to discontinue their medications. His influence is unfortunate (Neill, 2005). Cruise and other celebrities have allied themselves with the Citizens Commission on Human Rights (CCHR), a fervent anti-psychiatry group. The CCHR has assembled and published a collection of stories of celebrities' adverse experiences of psychiatric treatment, including accounts of unethical behavior and financial exploitation by psychiatrists, inappropriate or excessive use of ECT, humiliating involuntary hospitalizations, severe medication toxicity, and fatal overdoses on prescribed medications (CCHR, 2019). It makes its anti-psychiatry case entirely with anecdotes, what we would call "numerators without denominators." Nonetheless, true stories of mistreatment and adverse outcomes are memorable and might worsen creative professionals' preexisting fears of treatment.

Amy Winehouse's song "Rehab" (Winehouse, 2006) was a powerful recommendation against inpatient substance abuse treatment. In the lyrics she acknowledges that she's been "black" with her troubles; but she feels too busy to take time off in a facility, and in any case her boyfriend thinks she's "fine."

Amy Winehouse's rejection of alcohol and drug rehab was not due to denial of illness; she acknowledged she had struggled with depression and believed she had BD. However, she did not want to cancel concerts and disappoint those counting on her to appear. She objected to "psychological" treatment, but it is possible that this reflected her conclusion that treatment narrowly focused on abstinence from alcohol and drugs was neglecting the underlying problems that drove her to self-medicate. Apparently, her experience with paroxetine in her teens did not make her a believer in pharmacotherapy. It might not have been helpful—selective serotonin reuptake inhibitors (SSRIs) often aren't in people with BD, especially if taken without a concurrent mood stabilizer. It is not known whether she ever received a straightforward diagnosis of BD and a prescription or recommendation for its treatment with a mood-stabilizing drug.

A reason many creative professionals reject antidepressant drug treatment, don't persist with it, or advise peers against it relates to commonly occurring emotional and cognitive side effects of SSRI and SNRI antidepressants. These medications can cause a syndrome called *emotional blunting*, one that prescribers often do not warn their patients about (Goodwin et al., 2017). Emotional blunting interferes with creativity and its expression, and a creative person whose productivity has already suffered from their depression can find additional medication-related impairment to be intolerable.

If the patient has been warned about the potential issue and lets the prescriber know promptly if it arises, the treatment can be changed, and the therapeutic relationship usually will be preserved. If a proactive approach is not taken and the patient develops emotional blunting, there are several possible negative outcomes. The patient might attribute the emotional blunting to the depression and become hopeless and suicidal. The patient might blame the blunting on the medication, be troubled that they were not warned about it, stop the medication, and terminate their relationship with the prescriber. The patient might continue the medication for several weeks, with the depression improving but emotional blunting persisting. If they don't relate the blunting to the medication and the prescriber doesn't recognize it, they might continue the medication and suffer a persistent impairment in creative productivity. If they relate the blunting to the medication, they might stop the drug too soon to prevent a relapse of depression, and no alternate treatment for maintaining remission will be started.

The keys to avoiding the problem are in the hands of clinicians who treat depressed creative professionals and others whose work or personal situation requires emotional intelligence and a full range of emotional expression. First, they should be familiar with a broad range of treatments for depression, including biological treatments other than SSRIs and SNRIs. Second, they should discuss the risk of emotional blunting with patients prior to prescribing SSRIs or SNRIs and present realistic alternatives. If they think an SSRI or SNRI is the treatment of choice and the patient concurs in a shared decision-making process, they and the patient would work out a plan for tracking positive and negative effects of treatment. Treatment would be adjusted if it had negative effects the patient found distressing or incompatible with their creative work. Third, patients can be reassured that remission of depression might reduce emotional blunting enough that remaining negative medication-related effects would be mild and acceptable—and that the clinician will collaboratively monitor the issue with the patient until it is resolved to the patient's satisfaction. If an SSRI or

SNRI produced a remission of depression with very mild emotional blunting, it might prove acceptable to the patient for maintenance treatment.

Understanding emotional blunting, eliciting the syndrome when it is present, and measuring its response to antidepressant treatment are aided by study of an instrument specifically designed for the purpose—the Oxford Questionnaire on the Emotional Side-Effects of Antidepressants (Price et al., 2012), which was later renamed the Oxford Depression Questionnaire (ODQ). While the ODQ is a proprietary instrument, its content is available publicly; and published studies of the ODQ support the validity of the concept of emotional blunting, clarify its multidimensionality, and show that it reflects an intersection of depression itself with antidepressant drug side effects (Aşçibaşi et al., 2020; Christensen et al., 2021; Goodwin et al., 2017).

The ODQ comprises 26 Likert-type items, each rated on a five-point scale: 12 items ask respondents about their experience in the past week, eight items ask about changes from before their illness to the past week, and six items ask about their attribution of experiences in the past week to effects of antidepressants. Factor analysis identified four dimensions of emotional blunting (each followed by an exemplary statement with which the respondent could agree or disagree): not caring ("Other people being upset doesn't affect me"), emotional detachment ("I feel 'spaced out' and distant from the world around me"), reduction in positive emotions ("I don't fully enjoy things that should give me pleasure, such as beautiful places or things or music"), and general reduction in emotionality ("My emotions lack intensity").

The ODQ has been used to demonstrate the beneficial effect of vortioxetine treatment in 150 patients with MDD who had not remitted after six or more weeks on an SSRI (escitalopram, paroxetine, or sertraline) or an SNRI (duloxetine or venlafaxine) and who had complaints of emotional blunting and an ODQ score ≥50. Vortioxetine, a newer antidepressant with complex actions on multiple serotonin receptor types and downstream effects on other neurotransmitters including dopamine and GABA, is less likely than an SSRI to cause emotional blunting. After eight weeks on vortioxetine, approximately half of the subjects no longer had emotional blunting, and approximately half were in remission from MDD. The patients showed improved function at work or school, in social relationships, and in family life. Mediation analysis showed that most of their functional improvement was directly related to relief of emotional blunting rather than to improvements in their core depressive symptoms (Fagiolini et al., 2021).

A reduction in positive emotions is a core symptom of clinical depression as defined in Chapter 2. It is a more inclusive concept than anhedonia, a core criterion for MDD. The other three dimensions of emotional blunting—emotional detachment, lesser intensity of emotion, and not caring—can be characterized as "impaired function." In the case of creative professionals, these symptoms often imply impaired occupational function.

Suicide and Premature Death

People in several creative occupations have significantly increased mortality rates and a disproportionate number of "unnatural deaths" (i.e., suicide, homicide, and accidents). Peterson and colleagues (2018) aggregated suicide data from the 17 U.S. states that participated in 2012 and 2015 in the National Violent Death Reporting System and reported suicide mortality data by occupational group. For women, the group with the highest rate was Arts, Design, Entertainment, Sports and Media, with an annual suicide rate of 15.6 per 100,000 in 2015. For men, the same occupational group ranked second in 2015, with a suicide rate of 39.6 per 100,000. For comparison, the U.S. national suicide rates that year for women and for men were 6.7 per 100,000 and 22.8 per 100,000, respectively. General population suicide mortality rates for women in the 17 states included in the study ranged from 3.9 in New Jersey to 12.1 in Utah; for men the general population rates ranged from 14.4 in New Jersey to 33.9 in New Mexico (Institute for Health Metrics and Evaluation [IHME], 2023). The differences between suicide rates for creative professionals and population benchmarks would probably have been larger had the study included data from states like New York and California, where most eminent creative professionals live and where population suicide mortality rates are well below the national average.

The suicides and accidental deaths of leading creative professionals are widely covered in the press and move the hearts of people who admire them and appreciate their work. Many such deaths are preventable because the underlying risk for the deaths is depression or BD—both conditions for which treatment usually is successful if the clinician is persistent and the patient remains committed and engaged. However, the suicides of creative people often are seen not as the outcome of non-treatment or ineffective treatment of a mood disorder but rather as legitimate, autonomous existential acts of thoughtful people who decided that their lives were no longer worth living. When the suicide of a creative person is associated with the use of alcohol or drugs, substance use is widely viewed as the person's primary or sole problem, when it might be a symptom of hypomanic disinhibition, depressive nihilism, or self-medication for pain or anxiety.

Apart from deaths by suicide, many creative professionals have had non-suicidal deaths linked to behavior related to an episode of a mood disorder—depressed, hypomanic, or mixed. Some such deaths have been in car crashes related to inattentive (depressed) or reckless (hypomanic) driving. Others have involved drug and/or alcohol overdoses taken without suicidal intent, related to bad judgment made worse by a depressed or hypomanic mood. In one tragic scenario, a person with a substance use disorder comorbid with a mood disorder will, with treatment, succeed in abstaining from alcohol or opioids. Their abstinence reverses the tolerance the person had developed to the substance's effects during the period of excessive or harmful use. Suffering mental distress from an untreated mood disorder and disinhibited by it, they resume drinking or consuming opioids at doses that once were tolerated but now are lethal.

Creative people with BD who live intensely and are open to novel experiences might become involved in intimate relationships with dangerous people, exposing themselves to intimate partner violence or to sexually transmitted diseases. A rich and/or famous writer, artist, or performer can be a target of seduction by a person who, if successful, can lead them into a risky or dangerous situation that ends in an unnatural death.

Finally, having ongoing symptoms of an untreated or unsuccessfully treated mood disorder is a potent risk factor for self-neglect and bad judgment about medical matters. Many creative professionals have died from general medical illnesses that could have been prevented or effectively treated but for their avoiding medical treatment, persisting in a grossly unhealthy lifestyle, not taking prescribed medications, otherwise disregarding medical advice, and/or pursuing dubious alternative treatments instead of mainstream treatments of well-established efficacy. Writers, visual artists, and others who do not perform for the public are at higher risk for the self-neglect/non-adherence scenario than celebrity performers whose deteriorating health would be noticed by fans and commented on in the press.

When eminent creative professionals die by suicide or have an accidental death under suspicious or ambiguous circumstances, fans, colleagues, and the press comment on the tragic loss and how much the person will be missed. Yet, eminent, successful writers, artists, and performers have the resources to access psychiatric treatment; and if they are celebrities, it will be widely known if their lives are troubled. Many people care about them. The high incidence of unnatural deaths of creative professionals—most of which were potentially preventable if psychiatric or general medical conditions had been effectively treated—deserves analysis as a system failure. Untreated life-threatening mood disorders reflect malfunction of the healthcare system as much as do cancers of the breast or colon that go undetected and untreated until they have metastasized.

Successful creative people have an audience, which depending on the genre and their place within it can comprise demanding and discriminating patrons or unrestrained, uncritical fans. The appreciation of an audience can be comforting to depressed performing artists, and a crowd of wildly enthusiastic fans can intensify the euphoria of hypomanic ones. They can become emotionally dependent on their audiences and suffer a form of withdrawal when they are without an audience. They can experience such withdrawal on a day off between performances or between concert tours. For writers and visual artists, withdrawal can take place if their work becomes less popular or if they are in an unproductive period in which they do not create noteworthy new work. An eminent creative professional's fans or patrons, however enthusiastic, are not personal friends; and their love of the artist's work or the artist themselves does not relieve loneliness.

If creative professionals are known for work with a depressive flavor (e.g., blues singers or writers of confessional novels or poetry) or a hypomanic edge (e.g., stand-up comedians or flamboyant rock musicians), fans may not perceive them as ill if they display behavior and moods consistent with the themes and style of their work. Fans may be disappointed if an artist known for excitement looks slowed down and sad or one known for melancholy themes produces work that is skillfully executed but not emotionally intense. Either the symptoms of depression or bipolar illness or the effects of treatment for these conditions can change the way that creative professionals appear to their audiences in ways that reduce their popularity. Though remissions of illness, whether spontaneous, due to treatment, or related to changes in life circumstances or general health, can make creative people more consistently productive, remissions sometimes are associated with significant changes in the content and/or style of their work.

An excellent example of thematic and stylistic change paralleling the long-term course of a mood disorder is the case of the Norwegian artist Edvard Munch (1863–1944). Between the start of his artistic career in 1881 and his eight-month hospitalization for psychotic depression in 1908, he lived a life of intense emotionality, frequent travel, and heavy drinking. He sometimes was self-destructive, as when he shot himself in the hand after a quarrel with a romantic partner. Following his recovery from depression, Munch settled on a farm outside Oslo and lived a much quieter life. Prior to his hospitalization, his paintings dealt with themes of intense emotion, with titles like and *The Scream* (1893), *Anxiety* (1894), and *Melancholy* (1894). His paintings had many dark colors and little empty space. *The Scream* secured Munch a permanent place in cultural history, associating him with a representation of fear and despair recognized worldwide. Following his hospitalization, he painted landscapes, pastoral scenes, and portraits of models, in a pleasing style that was far less dramatic and less deeply memorable than his earlier work (Edvardmunch.org,

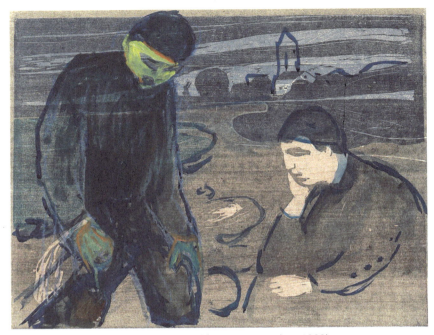

Figure 15.1 *Melancholy III* (Woodcut with Crayon Drawing, 1902)

2019). Munch's pre-treatment and post-treatment art is exemplified by two images, reproduced in Figure 15.1 and Figure 15.2 with the gracious permission of the Munch Museum.

Figure 15.1, a hand-colored version of the 1902 woodcut *Melancholy III*, depicts a sad man seated, holding his head with his right hand. To his left is a green-faced man, bending forward and looking down. His facial features are ill-defined. The image suggests that the sad man's low mood is amplified by the gloomy thoughts and images in his mind. Figure 15.2 is *Naked Woman in a Landscape*, a watercolor painted sometime between 1919 and 1925. It depicts a serene and peaceful scene, mildly erotic but not suggestive of hypomania.

Eminent writers, artists, and performers who have episodes of depression usually can find effective and personally compatible psychiatric treatment if they look for it; but many do not. There are several common reasons: non-recognition of illness, self-stigma and anticipated public stigma, pessimism about the value of treatment, mistrust of clinicians, and fear of adverse effects of treatment. Highly successful creative people might not seek treatment because they think depression is a normal part of an artistic life, to be endured and perhaps made the subject of their creative works. They might recognize that depression is an illness but fear that treatment will change them in a way that would

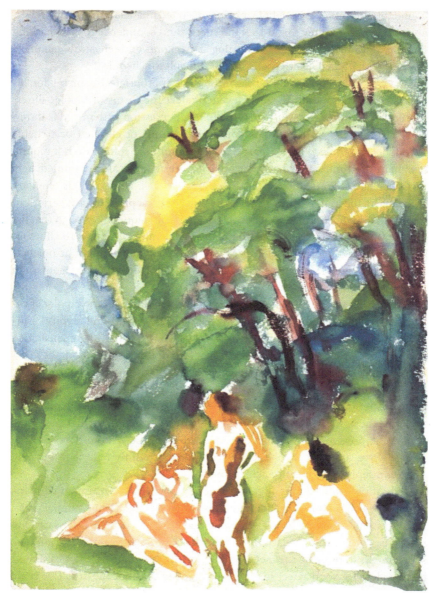

Figure 15.2 *Naked Woman in a Landscape* (Watercolor, 1919–1925)

affect the quality or authenticity of their work—their main source of meaning and purpose in life. This fear is especially common for pharmacotherapy and ECT. If they are considering psychotherapy, the trustworthiness of the therapist might be a concern. Celebrities often worry about envy, schadenfreude, and/or confidentiality; and they might fear being exploited financially by a psychotherapist. If depressed, they might lack the energy and confidence to start looking for a therapist they can trust. Performing artists' tours and rehearsals can make sessions with mental health professionals difficult to schedule.

Creative professionals' difficulties in getting appropriate treatment for bipolar spectrum conditions can be even greater. The forms of bipolar illness most often seen in successful artists are BD-II, depression with mixed features, and cyclothymia—all conditions where the periods of elevated or irritable mood, decreased need for sleep, and psychomotor acceleration do not require hospitalization and do not have psychotic features, so they are not immediately identified as a "mental illness" like the mania of BD-I. High periods often are enjoyable in the moment, and they can be times of great productivity. Periods of depression might alternate with periods of euphoria frequently enough that the bipolar writer or artist puts up with the former to enjoy the latter. The fluctuation and cycling, perhaps even more than depression alone, might be normalized as part of an artistic life or managed with alcohol, drugs, or engagement in intensely distracting activities.

Finding the right medication for an artist with an illness in the bipolar spectrum can be challenging. If an antipsychotic drug is used—and atypical antipsychotics often are used for BD-II—the artist may feel that their sensitivity, perceptiveness, or mental agility has been affected. If lithium is used, the artist may have a similar experience, though in general lithium is less problematic than an antipsychotic. However, lithium-induced tremor can be problematic for a performing artist or a painter. A mood-stabilizing antiepileptic drug might be the best tolerated of the evidence-based treatments for BD, but if it is effective at preventing hypomania, it might deprive the writer or artist of the intense drive, ambition, expansiveness, and/or speed of thought that they rely upon as a support for creative achievement.

Medication-induced weight gain frequently complicates treatment with antipsychotic drugs. This side effect can imply unacceptable changes in the physical appearance of a performer. When an antipsychotic drug is necessary, one should be chosen with a relatively low incidence of weight gain. Medication or supplements to mitigate the metabolic adverse effects of antipsychotics should be considered as soon a decision has been made to continue the drug (De et al., 2023). Pharmacologic options include metformin, GLP-1 agonists and SGLT2 inhibitors (Prasad et al., 2023; Stogios et al., 2023; Vasiliu, 2023a, 2023b). If a psychiatrist thinks that prescribing such agents is beyond their scope, they should collaborate with the patient's primary care physician or with an appropriate medical specialist. When lithium yields a positive psychiatric outcome but causes an unacceptable tremor, the clinician should find the minimum effective dose, use extended-release lithium, and consider adding a beta-blocker if the first two steps are insufficient (Baek et al., 2014; Pelacchi et al., 2022). In the shared decision-making process of medication choice, both the risk of occupationally relevant side effects and approaches to mitigating them should be discussed with the patient.

Why Depressed and Bipolar Creative Professionals Often Avoid Treatment

The myth of the tortured genius, with its associated romanticizing of mood disorders in writers, artists, and musicians, is universal and has endured since classical times. It is not restricted to the Romantic period or to Western cultures. In this myth, creative people's mental disorders are a necessary and unavoidable cost of their literary, artistic, or musical gifts. If they die by suicide, their audiences will miss them but do not usually see their deaths as preventable and rue the lack of effective psychiatric treatment. Audiences enjoy the brilliance with which the experience of depression is described or admire the determination of a creative star to excel despite emotional suffering. Some fans, including some who themselves have bipolar spectrum conditions, will vicariously enjoy their favorite writer's or performer's hypomanic escapades.

The romanticizing of depression or hypomania can discourage creative professionals from getting treatment. Even when depression is seen as an illness, if bearing depression is admired as a sign of strength of character, getting treatment for it would be a sign of weakness that would make the creator less admirable. If depression were not seen as an illness at all, a depressed man or woman who sought psychotherapy might be a neurotic complainer or a pathetic lonely person paying by the hour for a confidante. One who accepted the side effects of antidepressant medications would be a fool. The contrast between depression and cancer—both potentially life-threatening conditions—is ironic.

Stigmatization of depression can be a serious deterrent to timely treatment for early-career performing artists who do not yet have established reputations and stable incomes. They might realistically fear that if it were generally known they had been clinically depressed, it would be hard to launch a successful career. An actor might be less likely to be cast in a leading role. A musician might be passed over for membership in a successful band or prominent orchestra and might have less chance of becoming a soloist.

Well-established performers, and especially those who are eminent, in fashion, or celebrities, usually can seek treatment for depression without damage to their careers—though for performers like action movie stars with a tough persona doing so openly might affect their reputation and the roles they are offered in the future. Successful writers and visual artists can seek treatment for depression with even less concern about damaging their reputations. For eminent creative people, stigma is much less of an impediment to treatment than the romanticizing of mood disorders and fear of the effects of treatment on their creativity.

Mania in eminent writers and artists sometimes is misunderstood by the public as passionate engagement, particularly if the content of preoccupations or even delusions is compatible with a meaningful and popular theme. Writers and artists have other identities—national, religious, sexual—that can connect them with their audiences in profound ways. Some creative works are universal, while others are quintessentially American or Japanese, Catholic or Protestant, gay or bisexual. When an eminent writer or artist produces works—and makes public statements—strongly aligned with a specific identity, an audience sharing that identity sometimes embraces the art and the artist enthusiastically even if both the work and the behavior are extreme and driven by hypomania or even manic psychosis. Ernest Hemingway (1899–1961) and Yukio Mishima (三島 由紀夫; 1925–1970) are two examples of this phenomenon.

Lessons from Tragic Lives: Mishima, Hemingway, Kawabata

Yukio Mishima was an extraordinarily prolific Japanese novelist, poet, playwright, actor, and film director. His best-known works include *Confessions of a Mask* (仮面の告白; 1949/1958), *Forbidden Colors* (禁色; 1951,53/1968), *Death in Midsummer and Other Stories* (真夏の死; 1953/1966), and *The Temple of the Golden Pavilion* (金閣寺; 1956/1959). His personality was shaped by a traumatic childhood. Until age 12 he lived with his extremely controlling and disagreeable grandmother, who did not permit him to go outdoors, engage in sports, or play with other boys. Afterward he lived with his parents and suffered from their eccentricity. For example, his father once held Yukio within inches of a speeding train.

Mishima was of short stature and slight build. He dealt with his insecurity about his appearance by taking up bodybuilding and becoming a nude model. In his teens he discovered that he was bisexual. His literary works have been described as "aesthetic terrorism" (Rankin, 2018). They deal with themes of homoeroticism, bisexuality, sadomasochism, rape, vengeance, anger, and humiliation. Mishima was a right-wing ultranationalist who criticized Hirohito for his surrender in World War II and his renunciation of divine status, and wanted Japan to remilitarize. He formed a private militia of like-minded Japanese. Mishima wrote incessantly, while making many public appearances as an actor and celebrity. He displayed a grandiose attitude of self-importance, seeing his work as essential to the very survival of Japan (Piven, 2004).

Mishima was preoccupied for his entire adult life by his bisexuality, which was accompanied by episodes of erectile dysfunction in sexual encounters with women. He addressed his conflicts about his sexuality through his writing, explicitly rejecting psychotherapy as a solution. He wrote in 1949 to psychiatrist Ryūzaburō Shikiba (1898–1965), who was also a literary critic, about his situation:

> What is written in *Confessions of a Mask*, apart from adjusting some of the characters modeled on real people and conflating the two characters into one, etc., is all a faithful rendition of facts taken from my own personal experience. I think that both in this country and abroad, candid, confessional descriptions of "sexual inversion" are rare ... I suffered much more because of my physical inability to proceed in a normal direction rather than because of my innate sexual orientation and so thought confession would be the most effective means of psychotherapy. (Flanagan, 2014, pp. 98–99)

Mishima died at age 45 of a *seppuku* (切腹; literally "cutting the belly")—a samurai ritual of self-disembowelment with a sword followed by decapitation by an accomplice. The episode began with an attempted coup d'état by Mishima and three other men armed only with swords. Its aim was to restore the emperor of Japan to absolute power. Mishima's apparent BD was accepted—whether normalized, romanticized, or minimized—by his audience and his social circle in part because the content of his work and his obsession with samurai tradition were aligned with a historical culture of which many Japanese remain proud to this day and with the political outlook of the Japanese far right.

Ernest Hemingway was a bipolar alcoholic who died at age 61 of a self-inflicted gunshot wound. Hemingway wrote novels and short stories that are classics of American literature, for which he was awarded the Nobel Prize in Literature at age 55, in 1964. He had an extraordinarily colorful life, with four marriages, romantic affairs, continual international travel including visits to conflict zones and other dangerous places, and multiple traumatic injuries that led to chronic pain. He had a hereditary disease, hemochromatosis, associated with multiple organ system dysfunction and cognitive impairment later in life. His father, a brother, and a sister had died by suicide. In 1959, he had difficulty completing a journalistic assignment and became severely depressed with psychotic features, for which he was treated with two courses of ECT. His suicide followed his second course of ECT, which was discontinued before completion at the request of his family. Hemingway was admired for his literary talent and his aggressive, adventurous, hypermasculine persona, which many saw as characteristically American. His suicide, while obviously related to illness, was viewed by many as an autonomous, existential act by a man who could not bear the thought of living in a weak and debilitated state (Dearborn, 2017; Meyers, 1999).

Normalization or mischaracterization of mood disorders in creative professionals is especially likely to occur within national, regional, ethnic, or religious cultures in which mental illness is highly stigmatized. In such cultures, acknowledgment of a diagnosed mood disorder could lead to social ostracism or even a humiliating involuntary hospitalization. Simply exhibiting symptoms would not necessarily affect the social status, audience appreciation, or personal freedom of a writer, artist, or performer.

The misdiagnosis of a great writer's chronic depression as insomnia and its treatment with dangerous hypnotic drugs is exemplified by the case of Yasunari Kawabata (川端康成; 1899–1972), the first Japanese writer to receive the Nobel Prize in Literature (in 1968). His three novels that were specifically cited by the Nobel Committee were *Snow Country* (雪国; 1935-37/1956), *Thousand Cranes* (千羽鶴; 1949-51/1958), and *The Old Capital* (古都; 1962/1987). Kawabata's case demonstrates not only misdiagnosis but also how the themes of depression and hypnotic use infused his fiction. Kawabata made use of a hypnotic drug to facilitate his literary production. He died by suicide at age 72 from inhaling natural gas in his apartment. He had been troubled by the loss of his colleague Mishima in 1970. Beyond that, he was fascinated by suicide and wrote about it in connection with philosophical musings about the meaning of life and death. In his 1968 Nobel Lecture he quoted the suicide note of the short-story writer Ryunosuke Akutagawa (芥川龍之介; 1892–1927):

> It is the phrase that pulls at me with the greatest strength. Akutagawa said that he seemed to be gradually losing the animal something known as the strength to live, and continued:
> "I am living in a world of morbid nerves, clear and cold as ice.... I do not know when I will summon up the resolve to kill myself. But nature is for me more beautiful than it has ever been before. I have no doubt that you will laugh at the contradiction, for here I love nature even when I am contemplating suicide. But nature is beautiful because it comes to my eyes in their last extremity."
> Akutagawa committed suicide in 1927, at the age of 35. (Kawabata, 1968)

Kawabata had a childhood full of traumatic losses. He was orphaned at an early age and subsequently lost the remainder of his close relatives by the time he was 16. These losses were followed by romantic disappointments. This led to chronic depression with prominent insomnia. He became addicted to barbiturate sleeping pills in his 20s; after methaqualone (Quaalude® in the U.S.) became available in Japan in 1960, he became a habitual user of that drug. Methaqualone—subsequently withdrawn from the market in many countries—is known for its high incidence of tolerance and dependence and its liability for abuse. Methaqualone was used as a recreational drug for its disinhibiting and euphorigenic effects. Late in his career, Kawabata dosed himself with methaqualone prior to writing sessions, putting himself in a state of emotional analgesia and behavioral disinhibition in which he produced works with beautiful descriptions but disjointed plots. Though Kawabata was once hospitalized to be withdrawn from hypnotics, he was never treated for the chronic depression that preceded his hypnotic dependence and persisted throughout his adult life. Kawabata's literary work expresses themes of *mono no aware* (物の哀れ; "the pathos of things" or "sensitivity to ephemera"), *mujō* (無常; impermanence), and *wabi-sabi* (侘寂; "flawed beauty"), aspects of the Japanese aesthetic discussed in detail in Chapter 11. In his book *House of the Sleeping Beauties* (眠れる美女; 1961/1969), he describes a 67-year-old man who visits an establishment where patrons pay to sleep beside and non-sexually touch beautiful young women who have been drugged into unconsciousness.

Concerning *The Old Capital*, Kawabata described in the afterword to the novel how he took methaqualone prior to writing sessions:

> I have lost most of my memory of writing *The Old Capital*. It was almost spooky to me. I don't remember what I wrote. Indeed, I cannot recall. Each day, before I started working on this novel, and during the writing, I took sleeping pills. I was intoxicated with the sleeping pills and in an unreal world when I wrote this novel. I would say that *The Old Capital* is an abnormal product of mine. (authors' translation)

It is likely that, in Kawabata's time, dependence on prescription hypnotics would be less stigmatized than having a mental disorder diagnosis—even a non-psychotic one like major depression—and being treated by a psychiatrist. The non-recognition of his depression and suicide potential led to his receiving a drug that might have worsened his depression and reduced his self-control, leading him to act on a suicidal impulse.

Creative Productivity and Its Relationship to Illness

Diagnostic criteria for mood disorders require both distress and impairment of function in addition to the characteristic symptoms of depression and/or hypomania. In contrast to people in most other occupations, many creative professionals are unusually productive during periods of depression, depression with mixed features, or hypomania.

If depressed, they are productive during periods when the depression does not cause excessive apathy, emotional blunting, psychomotor retardation, or cognitive impairment or during periods when alcohol or a drug brings temporary relief. Periods of spontaneous improvement in unipolar depression can be related to diurnal variation (typically better in the evening, though better in the morning in atypical depression), to environmental influences, or to intrinsic fluctuations in symptom intensity. Periods of intense energy combined with dysphoric mood—"driven dysphoria"—are common during the depressed phase in bipolar spectrum disorders other than BD-I. Hypomanic writers, artists, and performers can be normally or even extraordinarily productive if they are able to concentrate on their work and avoid distraction. Outsiders might see only their continuing creative output and assume that they don't have a significant mental health problem.

A disproportionate number of creative professionals, writers most of all, are exposed to adverse childhood experiences (ACEs)—an overarching concept of emotionally traumatic events including abuse or neglect, being bullied, witnessing domestic violence, and having a parent be incarcerated or hospitalized for a mental illness. (The topic is discussed in depth in Chapter 5 and in several chapters in Part II.) ACEs not only leave memories that might be included in the content of creative works but also affect brain development, executive function, and epigenetics (González-Acosta et al., 2021; Lund et al., 2020; Saavedra & Salazar, 2021). They are associated with a lifetime increase in the risk of major depression, BD, alcohol use and drug use disorders, and suicidality, as well as an increased risk of chronic medical conditions with depressive comorbidity (Gloger et al., 2021; Hughes et al., 2021; Nelson et al., 2020; Robinson & Bergen, 2021; Sahle et al., 2021). An increased risk of mixed bipolar states in adulthood is another consequence of early childhood trauma (Janiri et al., 2020). The "driven dysphoria" of a mixed bipolar state is more likely to be expressed as creative work than unipolar MDD with psychomotor retardation.

Themes of trauma and loss are common in works of fiction, and authors' personal experiences often underlie their stories. Writing about past painful experiences can provide relief or resolution, can aid in forgiveness and reconciliation, or can reopen painful emotional wounds. Whatever the outcome, many writers feel compelled to express their childhood suffering in literary form.

Creative expression itself can make depression easier to bear. Writing confessional poetry or autobiographical novels has helped writers endure depression. Art therapy, music therapy, and creative writing groups sometimes help people with MDD and BD who are not in the creative professions (Chiang et al., 2019). Creative work often expresses themes related to artists' mood states and mood-related thought content. It often provides meaning of life and reason for living that can counteract suicidal impulses. Positive audience reactions can provide temporary relief from despair.

Alcohol or drugs sometimes reduce emotional pain and inhibition and transiently increase creative productivity, but this effect is unreliable and unsustainable in the long term. Alcohol and drugs can lose their benefits with time.

If tolerance develops and the dose escalates, the alcohol or drug will impair cognition and the quality of creative work.

Many eminent writers, artists, and performers, especially those who have commercial as well as critical success, have found physicians who would prescribe upon their request hypnotics, opioids, amphetamines, or other drugs with dependence and abuse liability. The drugs are then used to sustain an addiction, to cope with symptoms of an undiagnosed and untreated mood disorder, or both. A fatal or near-fatal overdose can be a tragic consequence. The decline and death of Michael Jackson (1958–2009) illustrates this phenomenon. In 2009, Jackson engaged Dr. Conrad Murray, a cardiologist, to become his exclusive personal physician who would accompany him on concert tours. Dr. Murray treated Jackson for chronic insomnia using propofol, a drug approved for use by intravenous injection to induce anesthesia. Propofol is not approved for use as a hypnotic and is sufficiently dangerous that it is rarely used without an anesthesiologist's supervision. Dr. Murray dosed Jackson with two short-acting benzodiazepines and with intravenous propofol on the night of his death. Following the injection of propofol, he had a respiratory arrest followed by a cardiac arrest (Levy, 2011). Jackson's recent drug use history included the antidepressants paroxetine and sertraline and the opioid drugs oxycodone and hydromorphone, though no opioids were found in his blood at the time of his death. The history strongly suggests that Jackson, unsuccessfully treated for a misdiagnosed bipolar spectrum disorder by a non-psychiatrist, resorted to sedative-hypnotic and opioid drugs to address the specific depressive symptoms of insomnia and pain. This is a familiar pattern when depression is misdiagnosed or mistreated. Deepak Chopra, a physician friend of Michael Jackson, criticized "this cult of drug-pushing doctors," saying "their co-dependent relationships with addicted celebrities, must be stopped. Let's hope that Michael's unnecessary death is the call for action" (Posner, 2017).

Depressive symptoms including apathy, emotional blunting, and cognitive slowing usually diminish productivity or affect the quality of creative work. Negative audience reactions to inferior work—or even self-criticism based on self-awareness of worse performance—can be devastating. When creative expression no longer works as a counter to depression, suicidal despair can rapidly follow. This phenomenon might, as might a switch from hyperthymia into depression, account for some writers' and artists' deaths by suicide shortly after they appeared to be working productively as usual. Creative productivity can deceive treating clinicians as well as family and friends about the severity of a creative person's suffering or the imminence of suicide.

Working Conditions of Creative Professionals

Creative writers, visual artists, and performing artists work on schedules different from those of more common occupations. Their work schedules have both positive and negative aspects with respect to depression and bipolar illness. Though creative writers, visual artists, composers, and songwriters can be under pressure to meet deadlines for publication, exhibition, or performance, they usually can choose their days and hours of work, helping them get rest when they need it, address personal and family concerns, and get treatment for medical problems including depression. However, if their schedule—especially their timing and duration of sleep—is inconsistent, it can exacerbate bipolar spectrum conditions. If they procrastinate and then must work very long hours to meet a deadline, sleep deprivation can trigger either depression or hypomania.

Performing artists have precise times at which they must appear for rehearsals or performances, but times for performances necessarily differ from the working hours of their audiences and might extend late into the night. Rehearsals often require long hours. Maintaining adequate sleep and healthy patterns of activity and eating can be challenging when work has shifting hours. If a performing artist is predisposed to depression or bipolar illness or is attempting to recover from an episode of depression, inconsistently timed and often inadequate sleep and exercise can make matters worse. Identifying and addressing schedule-related issues should be part of culturally aware treatment of a performing artist, just as it would be in the treatment of a truck driver, airline pilot, or physician. Bright light therapy, scheduled exercise, and sleep hygiene can mitigate the adverse chronobiological effects of work schedules; and their use is not stigmatized, nor do they have adverse effects on creativity.

The flexible schedules of creative writers, visual artists, composers, and songwriters have some positive aspects for those coping with depression or bipolar illness. When creative professionals can choose their work times, they can adapt their work schedules to accommodate the fluctuations of depressive symptoms from hour to hour or from day to day. They work when their depressed mood is less severe, cognition is more fluid, emotions are not blunted, and they are more energetic and motivated. Most people with bipolar spectrum conditions other than BD-I have significant periods when their mood—either normal, mildly hypomanic, or mixed with mild hypomanic features—is compatible with creative productivity. If such periods occur with sufficient frequency and duration, they can accomplish the goals of their work. However, the flexibility of creative writers' and artists' work schedules is a double-edged sword: Irregular sleep times, periods of overwork with inadequate sleep, and a lack of regular physical activity can easily happen when one is accountable only to oneself. Knowing the risk of disrupted chronobiology and inadequate sleep, a culturally aware clinician will include a careful assessment of sleep and activity patterns—not just the presence or absence of sleep complaints—in assessing a writer or artist with symptoms of depression or bipolar illness. Constant, 24/7 tracking of sleep and activity with a wearable device can add further insight. Many creative professionals already have a smartwatch, ring, wristband, or other wearable device for tracking activity and sleep; and if they don't, they are easily affordable by a successful writer or artist.

Musicians and stand-up comedians who must perform at fixed times, especially star performers who have demanding tour schedules, must repeatedly deliver a high standard of performance regardless of their emotional, cognitive, or physical symptoms. Many are tempted to self-medicate with alcohol or drugs if they must appear on stage when they are ill. The details of the patient's work and travel schedule, pattern of sleep and activity and how it changes day to day, and how and when the patient might use substances to manage symptoms that interfere with work are items that should be explored early in the evaluation of a performing artist with symptoms of depression or a bipolar illness.

"Stairway to Hell": The Toxicity of Pop Music Stardom

Creative professionals in general have increased rates of mood disorders and unnatural deaths. Among them, star performers in diverse genres of popular music are especially likely to have an unnatural death. Because of their celebrity, their deaths by suicide, homicide, accidents, and self-neglect claim public attention; and narratives of their deaths influence public attitudes, including public stigma.

Table 15.1, created with reference to a recent *Rolling Stone* article (Browne et al., 2017) and the Wikipedia biographies of the performers listed in the article, lists 28 pop superstars who died young. Their cases introduce themes that will be explored in the remainder of this chapter.

Star performers in all genres of popular music often die young. The causes of death are both natural (cancer, liver disease, AIDS) and unnatural (accidents, suicide, and homicide). In the general U.S. population, approximately 5% of all deaths are unnatural, including about 1.6% by suicide. Among eminent pop musicians, between 10% and 20% of deaths are unnatural, approximately 5% by suicide and 5% by homicide (Kenny & Asher, 2016). The adverse effects of popular music stardom on life expectancy and on the rate of "unnatural deaths" are greater for performers with a history of ACEs (Bellis et al., 2012) and for young women (Kenny & Asher, 2017). Dianna Kenny, author of two frequently

Table 15.1 Early (and Mainly Unnatural) Deaths of Pop Superstars

Performer	Role/genre/specialty	Age at death	Cause of death	Notes
Patsy Cline (1932–1963)	Singer (country and western)	30	Plane crash	Flew in small plane in bad weather despite warnings and a pilot without instrument training.
Sam Cooke (1931–1964)	Singer/songwriter and entrepreneur (soul and pop)	33	Homicide. Was shot by a motel manager during a fight started by Cooke while he was at the motel for a casual tryst.	Multiple extramarital affairs. Easily angered.
Otis Redding (1941–1967)	Singer/songwriter and producer (soul and R&B)	26	Plane crash	Flew in small plane in bad weather despite warnings.
Brian Jones (1942–1969)	Guitarist and founder of the Rolling Stones (rock)	27	Drowned in pool. Coroner judged death to be accidental, but this has been questioned.	Abused alcohol, cocaine, amphetamine, cannabis. Two drug-related convictions. Drowned one month after being fired from the band.
Janis Joplin (1943–1970)	Singer/songwriter (rock, soul, and blues)	27	Drug overdose	Overweight and had severe acne in her teens; bullied by peers. Abused heroin, amphetamines, and alcohol. Bisexual.
Jimi Hendrix (1942–1970)	Guitarist and singer/songwriter (rock)	27	Drug overdose with barbiturates supplied by a friend. Vomited, aspirated, and died from asphyxia.	ACEs included parents' divorce and sexual abuse. Abused alcohol, cannabis, LSD, and amphetamines. Violent when intoxicated. Sang about manic depression.
Jim Morrison (1943–1971)	Singer/songwriter/ poet and founder of The Doors (rock)	27	Found dead in a Paris hotel bathtub under obscure circumstances. No autopsy. Possible heroin overdose. Took long walks alone for weeks before his death.	Grew up in a military family; estranged from his family as young adult. Drank heavily and was unpleasant when drunk. Snorted heroin. Never married but had many relationships with women. Well-read and intellectual.

Duane Allman (1946–1971)	Guitarist and session musician; founder of the Allman Brothers Band (rock, blues, soul, and jazz)	24	Motorcycle crash	
Nick Drake (1948–1974)	Singer/songwriter (acoustic/alternative music)	26	Suicide by antidepressant (amitriptyline) overdose following breakup with girlfriend. Had been on the drug for three years before the overdose.	Son of an affluent British family; University of Cambridge dropout. Introverted and chronically depressed. Habitual cannabis user.
Phil Ochs (1940–1976)	Singer/songwriter known for topical songs and political activism. His songs were covered by many famous singers (folk)	35	Suicide by hanging, following a period of total disability due to psychotic symptoms and paranoid ideas.	Had BD like his father. Self-medicated with alcohol, benzodiazepines, and stimulants. Traveled widely with many trips to dangerous places.
Marc Bolan (1947–1977)	Singer/songwriter, guitarist, and poet. Wrote best-selling poetry book, *Warlock of Love* (glam rock)	29	Car crash; car driven by his girlfriend.	Expelled from school at 15 for bad behavior. Worked as a model.
Ronnie van Zandt (1948–1977)	Singer/lyricist; co-founder of Lynyrd Skynyrd (southern rock)	29	Plane crash	Flew on a small plane that ran out of fuel.
Keith Moon (1946–1978)	Drummer for the rock band The Who. *Rolling Stone's* "second greatest drummer in history" (rock)	32	Clomethiazole overdose. Prescribed 100 pills of a barbiturate-like drug used to treat alcohol withdrawal that is unsafe to use unsupervised. Moon took 32 of them following a quarrel with his girlfriend.	History of violence—destroying property and abusing his wife. Demanded attention continually. Accidentally killed his bodyguard. Abused alcohol and amphetamines.
John Bonham (1948–1980)	Drummer and songwriter for rock band Led Zeppelin. "Greatest drummer of all time" (rock)	32	Alcohol intoxication (had over 40 drinks in less than 24 hours)	Had stage fright and other anxieties. Drank to control them and became addicted.

(continued)

Table 15.1 Continued

Performer	Role/genre/specialty	Age at death	Cause of death	Notes
Ian Curtis (1956–1980)	Singer/songwriter (punk rock)	23	Suicide by hanging	Developed treatment-refractory epilepsy at age 22. Suicide attempt by medication overdose 2 months before suicide.
Karen Carpenter (1950–1983)	Singer and drummer (pop)	32	Heart failure due to anorexia nervosa with use of laxatives, ipecac, and thyroid hormone to lose weight.	Chronic eating disorder. Brief, unhappy marriage to an abusive husband.
Marvin Gaye (1939–1984)	Singer/songwriter and producer (soul)	44	Homicide (killed by father after he tried to protect his mother from abuse by his father)	Serious physical abuse in childhood by his father. No known mental disorder.
Freddie Mercury (1946–1991)	Singer/songwriter and producer. Lead singer for Queen (rock, metal, gospel, and disco)	45	AIDS resulting from unsafe sex	Experimented with drugs; was not addicted. Bisexual. No history of mental disorder.
Kurt Cobain (1967–1994)	Singer/songwriter. Co-founder of Nirvana (alternative rock)	27	Suicide (shot himself while intoxicated with morphine and diazepam, shortly after leaving drug rehab against medical advice. Made a suicide attempt by overdose one month earlier).	Troubled adolescence after parents' divorce. Probable BD. Abused alcohol, solvents, hallucinogens, and opioids. Bisexual identity.
Selena (1971–1995)	Singer/songwriter, actress, and fashion designer. "Queen of Tejano music" (Tejano)	23	Homicide (shot by an employee of a business she owned whom she had caught embezzling money).	No apparent mental disorder or substance use problem.
Tupac Shakur (1971–1996)	Rapper, writer, and actor. Sold over 75 million records (rap)	25	Homicide (shot in revenge after a fight)	History of violence; had been convicted of assault and rape.

Name	Description	Age	Cause of death	Notes
Notorious B.I.G. (1972–1997)	Rapper. Rated by *Billboard* as the greatest of all time (rap)	24	Homicide (murdered by an unknown assailant)	Drug dealer in his teens. Did not abuse drugs personally.
Aaliyah (1979–2001)	Singer and actress (pop)	22	Plane crash	Flew on an overloaded chartered flight. Early success. 4.0 GPA in high school. Disciplined; close to family.
Whitney Houston (1963–2012)	Singer; most awarded female recording artist; actress (pop)	49	Drowning; multiple drugs found at autopsy	Abuse of alcohol, cannabis, cocaine, prescription drugs. Possible eating disorder. Domestic abuse. Multiple stints of drug rehab.
Prince (1958–2016)	Singer, songwriter in multiple genres: funk, rock, R&B, soul, pop, psychedelic (sold over 100 million records)	58	Fentanyl overdose	Son of two musicians. Began using opioids after hip surgery in 2010 and became addicted. Had epilepsy but didn't treat it. Religious conversion.
George Michael (1963–2016)	Singer/songwriter and producer. Sold over 115 million records (pop)	53	Cardiomyopathy, myocarditis, and fatty liver	Cannabis and hypnotic drug abuse. Bisexual.
Chris Cornell (1964–2017)	Lead vocalist for Soundgarden and Audioslave (rock)	52	Suicide by hanging	Alcohol and drug use beginning in his teens. Disclosed an episode of major depressive disorder with suicidality.
Chester Bennington (1976–2017)	Songwriter. Lead vocalist for Linkin Park (rock)	41	Suicide by hanging	Childhood sexual abuse. Addicted to alcohol and drugs.

cited studies of performers' mortality, opines that "the pop music scene is toxic and needs rehabilitation," stating that it "fails to provide boundaries and to model and expect acceptable behavior. It actually does the reverse—it valorizes outrageous behavior and the acting out of aggressive, sexual and destructive impulses that most of us dare only live out in fantasy" (Kenny, 2014). Though concert promoters, managers, agents, and record company executives usually express grief or sympathy after a star dies, such feelings have not changed the working conditions of star performers who are still alive.

Excessive consumption of alcohol and the use of stimulants, sedative-hypnotic drugs, cannabis, and/or opioids are so common as to be normalized in the pop music industry. Even those without substance use disorders might engage in binge drinking (four or more drinks at one sitting for women, five or more for men) or in heavy drinking (more than seven drinks per week for women and more than 14 drinks per week for men). Alcohol is a carcinogen, and heavy drinkers are at increased risk for oral and pharyngeal cancers (5 times), laryngeal cancer (2.6 times), esophageal cancer (5 times), liver cancer (2 times), breast cancer (1.6 times), and colorectal cancer (1.5 times). And if they drink heavily and smoke, their risks of oral, pharyngeal, laryngeal, and esophageal cancer are even greater (National Cancer Institute, 2021).

Female stars often feel pressure to be slim, which might require food restriction. This has changed somewhat, with overweight female pop stars now more common than they were in the 20th century. However, unhealthy diets to maintain slimness historically have been normalized for women in show business, and it remains difficult for an overweight or obese woman to launch a successful career as a popular musician.

Touring performers usually are separated from family and friends and commonly are lonely despite being surrounded by people. They are exposed to both sexual and non-sexual seduction and have many opportunities to engage in high-risk behavior. One does not hear of stars arranging their tours to allow adequate rest, private time with family, and healthy exercise. Tight touring schedules, sometimes coupled with a desire to avoid intrusive fans or journalists, lead stars to fly on chartered private aircraft. In several cases in the table, performers died in plane crashes because they persuaded pilots to fly under unsafe conditions. The pilots (or their employers) apparently had trouble saying no to their celebrity clients.

The creative professions have an extremely skewed distribution of fame and fortune, with relatively few famous and well-paid stars and many who make a modest living or live with precarious employment, financial insecurity, and professional obscurity ("starving artists"). The time course of fame and fortune is characteristic. Most eminent writers, artists, and performers have had the experience of relatively sudden and profound changes in their circumstances related to the public's reception of their work. A novelist's first bestseller, a playwright's first sold-out show, or a musician's first platinum recording dramatically changes their status. Though the creator might have longed for such an event, it nonetheless entails stressful and often negative consequences. As an example of the latter, the mortality rate of popular musicians following their first number one recording is more than twice that of demographically matched controls, and the increased mortality rate persists for the next 25 years (Bellis et al., 2007; Kenny & Asher, 2016).

Potential side effects of sudden fame and wealth include disruption of relationships with less successful colleagues, loss of privacy, excessive spending, family conflicts, and exposure to seduction. In the case of pop stars, bodyguards might be needed to protect the star and their family members. Positive and durable relationships, professional or intimate, might be difficult to establish because of the creative star's sometimes justifiable suspiciousness of others' motives. These stresses can contribute to the onset or relapse of clinical depression or BD, and they are impediments to the performer getting reliable social support of the kind that reduces a person's risk of depression when under stress and that makes their suffering more bearable if depression does occur.

Lonely at the Top

People who write about the downside of celebrity point to loneliness as the most painful aspect of fame. Celebrities are continually approached by strangers who greet them, ask for an autograph or their appearance in a selfie, or perhaps disparage or threaten them if they object to their lifestyle or politics. They might be hounded by paparazzi and photographed when they look their worst. When they go to a restaurant or store, they risk being recognized and receiving unwanted attention. Their life is thus constrained because their appearance in public is always risky.

A star's intense periods of writing, rehearsing, or recording and weeks on tour can put stress on friendships and family relationships; and the support of a friend, spouse, or relative might be absent or impaired when it is most needed at a crucial time in the star's life. When the star needs more and has less to give, there may be no one there to meet their needs or effectively offer comfort and support. Loneliness, a risk factor for depression and for suicide, can affect successful creative people who have legions of fans.

When the creative person comes from a conformist culture, they may find social support from a bohemian counterculture of artists, writers, and performers.

The social support of peers—if the creator respects them and their work—can buffer stress and disappointment, help prevent or moderate depression, and mitigate suicide risk. Conspicuous success, however, can weaken support from fellow creators. Supportive relationships can be weakened by envy or by success-related changes in the creative person's residence or living arrangements. Dependable relationships they had before a big success and its associated wealth and celebrity might be replaced by relationships with higher-status people who are less willing or able to give support when the person needs it most.

The loneliness of success and celebrity was the subject of "Lonely at the Top," a song by Randy Newman (b. 1943) written for the legendary (and bipolar) Frank Sinatra (Newman, 1972). Newman, a singer-songwriter whose works have been covered by numerous stars, is also known for composing the scores of hit films including *Awakenings*, *Ragtime*, and the *Toy Story* films. The singer laments that despite his money, fame, popularity with audiences, and appeal to women, he's still lonely. His career is just a "crazy game," and the love of the fools who idolize him leaves him cold.

Parasocial Relationships and the Culture of Fandom

Parasocial relationships (PSRs) are defined by communication theorists as unidirectional relationships that individuals (fans) have with celebrities (star musicians or actors, media "personalities," political leaders, etc.) in which a fan feels that they are in a genuine two-way social relationship with an admired celebrity that they follow in the mass media and online. These can include a feeling of personal connection with the celebrity, that they are a "faultless soulmate." In a more pathological form of PSR, the fan might believe that they communicate with the celebrity through a secret code or that the celebrity would come to their aid in a crisis (North & Sheridan, 2009). PSRs, like genuine social relationships, can affect the mood and thinking of fans. A fan can feel that a celebrity's engaging in harmful substance use or an act of self-harm makes the action acceptable. A celebrity's death can cause intense grief in a fan with a PSR, and the suicide of a celebrity increases the risk of self-harm or suicide by avid fans. The effect is largest in fans of the same gender and similar age to the celebrity who died, and fans who attempt suicide following a celebrity's death usually use the same method of self-harm (S. A. Jang et al., 2016; Mesoudi, 2009; Niederkrotenthaler et al., 2009; Yang et al., 2013). Evidence from Korea suggests that establishment and enforcement of guidelines for media coverage of suicides reduces or eliminates the increase in deaths by suicide following the suicides of celebrities (J. Jang et al., 2022). However, in most countries, information (and misinformation) about celebrity suicides can be freely distributed on social media. Praticable and publically acceptable regulation of suicide reporting on social media is an issue yet to be addressed (Ha and Yang, 2021).

On the positive side, PSRs have the power to reduce the stigma of depression and bipolar illness and to encourage depressed and suicidal people to seek help for their conditions. The impact of a depressed creative celebrity's suicide on fans is illustrated by fans' reactions to the suicide of the comedian Robin Williams (1951–2014), which were studied via an internet survey by Hoffner and Cohen (2018). Robin Williams' fans had varying strengths of PSR with him, and they encountered media coverage of various kinds—informational, stigmatizing, and celebratory of Williams' work. Regardless of the type of coverage fans saw, those with a strong PSR prior to his death were more willing to seek treatment for depression and to reach out to others who were depressed. Exposure to informational coverage of his death made these feelings stronger. Coverage of the suicide that included negative and stigmatizing messages about depression increased fans' stigmatization of the illness but nonetheless increased their interest in reaching out to other people with depression. Media coverage that celebrated Williams' work but did not deal with his depression made fans less willing to seek treatment for depression and less willing to offer support to others with depression.

The findings of Hoffner and Cohen's study support the premise that media coverage of the suicides of beloved celebrity artists that celebrates their lives but offers little information about their mental health issues and their treatment can unintentionally normalize or stigmatize depression and discourage depressed fans from seeking treatment. Fans might think that if suicide were the deliberate act of an admired person with whom they had a PSR, it might have been a rational one. They might think that if treatment of depression didn't work for someone so accomplished and successful, what good could it do for ordinary people like them?

The concept of PSRs adds another dimension to the understanding of the popularity of literature, art, and music on themes of sadness and depression. In addition to experiencing direct neurobiological rewards for vicariously experiencing sadness (Trimble, 2012), fans who have PSRs with depressed stars or stars who have attempted suicide often feel less alone with their own sadness, depression, or suicidal thoughts. They might stigmatize themselves less, and if they see improvement or recovery in a person whom they admire, they might have more hope for themselves.

Issues of Specific Musical Genres

Creative writers, visual artists, and performers have a common culture relevant to mood disorders; and eminent ones have in addition cultural issues related to wealth, status, fame, or celebrity. Beyond that, there are cultural issues of specific creative disciplines and genres with impact on depression, BD, and suicide.

For musicians of all genres, excessive noise exposure is an important risk factor for hearing loss, tinnitus, and depression. While it is obvious that rock or metal musicians are subject to unhealthy levels of noise, the problem of acoustic trauma is equally relevant to the musicians in a classical orchestra; and it is perhaps more pernicious because it is minimized or denied by most classical musicians, who as a rule do not wear ear protection. About 26% of professional musicians suffer from tinnitus, and the rate is the same for classical and for popular/rock musicians. Rock musicians do have a higher rate of noise-induced hearing loss, with an estimated prevalence of 63.5%; but the 32.8% rate of hearing loss in classical musicians is high enough that hearing loss is clearly a major occupational health issue for them too. Unfortunately, ear protection is rarely worn by professional musicians of any genre (Di Stadio et al., 2018). Consideration of hearing loss, tinnitus, and occupational noise exposure thus should be part of the comprehensive assessment of a depressed musician.

Classical musicians need to play complex musical compositions with great precision, and there is intense competition for a small number of opportunities to be a soloist or a conductor. Performance anxiety is common among classical performers. In a survey of over 2000 orchestral musicians, 24% reported experiencing stage fright, and 17% reported depression (Matei & Ginsborg, 2017).

Classical musicians frequently are perfectionists. This can drive them to practice incessantly at the expense of adequate sleep. Sleep deprivation can precipitate hypomania in a musician with bipolar illness. Intense self-criticism can lead to depression, especially if the musician has additional risk from genetics, chronic general medical illness, trauma, or ACEs. Musical performance can be impaired by the psychomotor slowing and cognitive impairments of depression and by the cognitive and behavioral disorganization of hypomania. Prescription drugs used to treat mood disorders can cause adverse effects that impair musical performance, including decreased muscular coordination, tremors and other involuntary movements, and emotional blunting that interferes with the subtleties of musical interpretation.

Many famous classical soloists have suffered from depression. Typically, they launched their careers before they developed depression or at a time when their depression was in remission. Established soloists can build their repertoires during periods when their depression is in remission or is mild. Once pieces are mastered, they might be played well even if the performer is moderately depressed, if psychomotor retardation and cognitive symptoms are not prominent. However, severe depression is incompatible with excellent performance of classical music.

Several renowned pianists had chronic or recurrent depression that was a major challenge throughout their lives. These include Frederic Chopin (1810–1849), Sergei Rachmaninoff (1873–1943), and Artur Rubinstein (1887–1982). Clinical depression in classical performers is not normalized or romanticized, but it is not free from stigma. Disclosure of a history of depression can adversely affect the prospects of an early-career soloist. With the extreme competition for solo opportunities, a concert promoter or orchestra leader might be reluctant to engage a performer with an illness that might cause them to miss a concert or perform worse than expected.

Classical composers, whether historical or contemporary, and composers of scores for film and theater, experience the positives and negatives of a writer's flexible schedule. Their depression may find expression as sad music; but many composers have written upbeat, cheerful music at times they were depressed, and many more have written sad music after recovering from an episode of depression. Chopin, who suffered from chronic depression (dysthymia with recurrent MDEs) throughout his adult life, composed lively dances as well as pensive nocturnes. Gustav Mahler (1860–1911), often depressed, composed orchestral works expressing a broad range of emotion with no special emphasis on the melancholic.

Despite the many examples of classical composers and musicians who have suffered from mood disorders, classical musicians overall have a lower prevalence of depression than writers of prose and verse. This might be explained by the apparent antidepressant effects of classical music itself. It has been proposed. It has been proposed that musical work activates the right hemisphere of the brain in a way that protects against depression.

Unlike pop music stars, eminent classical musicians tend to have normal life spans, and many have long careers. Chronic illness need not disrupt their careers if it does not directly affect their musical skills. If a classical soloist's health allows them to keep performing, there is low risk of late-life depression based on a feeling of lost ability.

BD-I would undoubtedly disrupt the work of a classical performer, but mild illness in the bipolar spectrum might not. However, conductors of classical music can lose their jobs if poor judgment due to BD leads to personal indiscretion or professional misbehavior. As leaders of musical organizations, they face demands for consistent executive function and adherence to norms of appropriate behavior with the musicians they direct and the managers and donors to whom they report.

Across all genres of popular music, substance use and the expression of intense moods by stars are accepted. Some performers are known for, and appreciated for, their description of sad, depressed, angry, or euphoric moods. Pop performers' performances need not be as precise as those of classical musicians, and it is more feasible for a depressed or anxious pop musician to self-medicate with alcohol or drugs before a show.

Kenny and Asher (2016) studied the deaths of 13,195 American popular musicians between 1950 and 2014. They determined that compared with demographically matched controls pop musicians of all genres had excess mortality from some combination of suicide, homicide, accidents including vehicular crashes and drug overdoses without prior suicidal intent, and liver disease. The mortality rate of musicians under age 25 was more than twice that of controls.

Musicians of the country, rock, and metal genres had elevated rates of death by suicide and death from liver disease. Rap and hip-hop musicians had elevated rates of death by homicide. Accidental deaths—including those from unintentional drug overdoses and from car crashes—were increased in musicians of the jazz, folk, rock, pop, country, metal, and punk genres. The causes of excess deaths all can be linked to possible depression or hypomania, either directly or through substance abuse, intentional risk-taking, or careless behavior. However, mood disorders rarely were diagnosed during the lifetimes of the musicians who died young.

Women now constitute about one third of all popular musicians. Like male popular musicians, they have a disproportionate number of deaths due to suicide, homicide, or accidents: 20% of all deaths of female popular musicians during their working years are due to one of those three causes (Kenny & Asher, 2017).

Like Amy Winehouse, many popular musicians who destroyed their lives with alcohol and drugs continued to have hit recordings and play sold-out shows even when they showed obvious signs of mental and/or physical impairment or instability. Fans continue to buy tickets to see performers whom they know may appear on stage intoxicated. Managers and agents arrange concert tours for performers whom they know are actively abusing substances. This suggests that the medical seriousness of the substance-related problems of popular musicians is minimized. The tolerance of fans and promoters for performers' substance-related mental health and performance-quality issues can weaken the performers' resolve to undergo treatment.

In considering the substance abuse problems of popular musicians, "dual diagnosis" is the rule and not the exception. In addition to mood disorders, posttraumatic stress disorder (PTSD) is a frequent comorbidity of substance use disorders among creative professionals. Bellis et al. (2012) studied premature mortality of rock and pop stars and found that deaths due to substance use or accidents disproportionately involved stars with histories of ACEs. For female performing artists, eating disorders are an additional consideration.

Jazz musicians and others who play improvisational music have the challenge of composing music in real time, an activity fundamentally different from the performance of a previously written work. To do this they must combine mental energy and flexibility with self-monitoring executive function to refine their output and stay in synchrony and harmony with other members of their band. Hyperthymia or mild hypomania can increase improvisational output, and mild to moderate depression would not necessarily interfere with it; but depression with cognitive impairment or psychomotor slowing, or mania with executive dysfunction, would interfere. Treatment with antidepressants or mood-stabilizing drugs might restore a depressed or bipolar jazz musician's ability to perform, but many of the psychotropic drugs that might be used have potential side effects relevant to the ability to improvise. Antipsychotic drugs can slow cognitive processes and interfere with creativity, SSRI and SNRI antidepressants can cause emotional blunting that could diminish the expressiveness of a musical performance, and drugs of several classes can have subtle effects on motor coordination that can impact skill at playing an instrument and thus impair the translation of the performer's inspiration into music. While all musicians with mood disorders can face a similar balance between impairment from illness and side effects of drug treatment, the dilemma can be especially challenging for jazz musicians, who are simultaneously composers and performers.

Like popular musicians, jazz musicians work late at night and frequently travel. On the side of stability, jazz musicians once established can have long careers. This contrasts with the case of popular musicians who might enjoy a few years of stardom followed by many years of lesser repute or even cultural irrelevance. Also, jazz is a collaborative medium in which accomplished and gifted musicians can find a community of peers with whom they engage creatively and personally, thereby creating bonding social capital that can protect against depression.

Rap and hip-hop are inseparable from the experience and identity of urban Blacks. Mortality from homicide, especially firearm homicide, is high for all young men of this demographic (Riddell et al., 2018). It is reflected in the disproportionate number of young rap stars who have died by homicide.

Country music is linked to the ethnic identities of specific American regions, comprising greater Appalachia, the Midwest Midlands, the Deep South, and the Far West. Cultural dimensions of depression, bipolar illness, and suicide in country musicians often involve the intersection of identity as a musician with regional cultural identity. The stigma of mental disorders is greater in the regions from which country music originates than in other regions of the U.S., and relatively few eminent country musicians have been open about their treatment for depression or bipolar illness.

Rock musicians have the greatest exposure to noise as a risk factor for depression. More than half of rock musicians develop hearing loss, and more than a quarter develop tinnitus, both risk factors for depression. Tinnitus can contribute to insomnia that can exacerbate a bipolar condition or lead to the use of dangerous substances to induce sleep. Famous rock musicians with hearing loss and tinnitus from occupational noise exposure include Sting, Pete Townshend, Ozzy Osbourne, Neal Young, Eric Clapton, and Jeff Beck (Cavan Project, 2019). Despite the significant risk of acoustic trauma, few rock musicians wear ear protection. The rock musician who does protect their hearing and thus promote their mental health is an outlier (De Stadio et al., 2018; Halevi-Katz et al., 2015; Størmer et al., 2015, 2017).

Young and successful rock musicians can deny the need to protect their ears when performing, just as they deny or minimize other threats to their physical and mental health in the excitement of their creative work. Clinicians working with rock musicians with complaints of depression, insomnia, or pain should always assess their patients' hearing and encourage their patients' use of ear protection.

Comedians' Lives: Not So Funny

Comedians deserve special attention in a discussion of depression in creative professionals because of their special qualities as performers and the association of their discipline with mood disorders and with specific temperaments. Many comedians have well-publicized histories of depression, BD, or substance use disorders. Many have had miserable, traumatic childhoods. Many comedians with histories of trauma or depression have built comic routines on their own unhappy experiences.

Systematic analysis of comedians' psychological profiles confirms that, as a group, they are unlike other kinds of performing artists. In a questionnaire-based study of 523 comedians compared with 364 actors and 831 controls, Ando et al. (2014) showed that comedians as a group displayed a combination of impulsive non-conformity, cognitive disorganization, and introverted anhedonia. (Of course, there were individual comedians in their sample who had totally normal personality profiles and no symptoms of a mood disorder.) Taken together the symptoms described in the study of Ando and colleagues suggest a mixed bipolar state, though individual comedians with bipolar spectrum conditions might alternate between depressed, anhedonic, and emotionally isolated states of mind and outwardly focused, "wild and crazy" periods. By contrast, male actors were not significantly different from controls on the dimensions of conformity, cognitive organization, and extraversion. Female actors were lower than controls on the dimension of introverted anhedonia but did show a tendency toward impulsive non-conformity and cognitive disorganization. In first-person accounts, many comedians have described themselves as joking and clowning externally to win the audience's laughter and love and thus alleviate their internal emotional distress. When such comedians are more severely depressed, they require more laughs and audience attention to relieve their suffering, and the relief lasts for a shorter time.

Some critics have proposed that most comedians suffer from depression or bipolar illness and that their mood disorders and their work as comedians are related. From this viewpoint, the comedian's depression and/or hypomania, as well as their perceptions of the world and of life from the perspective of a depressed or hypomanic person, provide material for comic routines, scripts, or imagined characters. A depressed comedian can find comfort and/or distraction in transforming their unhappy situation into a context for humor. The laughs of the audience soothe the comedian's heartache and calm the comedian's jagged nerves.

It is hard to know the precise prevalence of depression and BD in elite comedians because many do not seek treatment or publicly disclose their psychiatric status. Furthermore, depression and hypomania can be obscured by the comedian's public persona.

Comedians, like popular musicians, have relatively short life spans. A recent study of eminent male British comedians showed that the funniest of them had shorter lives than those who were less funny. When a comedy act was based on a funny man–straight man duo, the funny man was more than three times as likely to die prematurely than his partner (Stewart & Thompson, 2015).

The American comedian Sarah Silverman (b. 1970), who has suffered from recurrent depression (and probably a bipolar spectrum disorder) since age 13, has delivered both one-liners and introspective comments about her illness. Once asked by her stepfather what depression feels like, she said, "It feels like I'm desperately homesick, but I'm home."

In 2015, she described the relationship between her illness, her treatment, and her work:

> I'm on a small dose of Zoloft® [sertraline], which, combined with therapy, keeps me healthy but still lets me feel the highs and lows. The dark years and those ups and downs—chemical and otherwise—have always informed my work; I believe that being a comedian is about exposing yourself, warts and all. (Field, 2015)

With the aid of an ongoing therapeutic relationship, she found a way to prevent severe depression while preserving the cyclothymic temperament that underlies her creativity. She apparently does not expect to be "cured" of her mood disorder and appreciates the value of emotional intensity for creative productivity. Silverman is clear that depression should not be romanticized: "I don't think people really understand the value of happiness until they know what it's like to be in that very, very dark, place. It's not romantic. Not even a little." (Silverman, 2010).

The Role of Undiagnosed Medical Problems

Eminent and successful writers, artists, and performers with mood disorders can have general medical conditions related to their creativity and/or to their mood symptoms that are undiagnosed or not optimally treated. Two will be mentioned here—one recognized since ancient times and the other recognized very recently.

Temporal lobe epilepsy (TLE) is associated with increased rates of depression, bipolar spectrum disorders, emotional intensity (e.g., cyclothymia and dysthymic, hyperthymic, or irritable temperament), and the *Geschwind syndrome* of hypergraphia (compulsive writing), religious/spiritual preoccupation, atypical sexuality, circumstantiality, and an intensified mental life (Devinsky & Schachter, 2009). Historical writers and artists with TLE include Vincent Van Gogh (1853–1890), Fyodor Dostoyevsky (1821–1881), Gustave Flaubert (1821–1880), Lewis Carroll (1832–1898), Edgar Allan Poe (1809–1849), and Edward Lear (1812–1888). The pop musician Prince (1958–2016), an extraordinarily prolific songwriter with atypical sexuality and religious preoccupations, suffered from the condition, as does Neil Young (b. 1945), an immensely popular singer-songwriter well known for spiritual themes in his songs.

TLE is associated with a high rate of suicide, and death by suicide is a more common cause of premature mortality in people with TLE than sudden death due to generalized seizures. It also is associated with a higher proportion of bipolar relative to unipolar depression. The Geschwind syndrome does not reverse when seizures are fully controlled with antiepileptic drugs. Some notable creative professionals with mild TLE have chosen not to take medication for their epilepsy, perhaps concerned that treatment of their epilepsy will adversely affect their creativity.

A more recently recognized medical correlate of creativity and mood disorders is having a recessive gene for alpha-1 antitrypsin (A1AT) deficiency. People with A1AT deficiency develop emphysema and cirrhosis of the liver as young adults, even if they do not drink alcohol or smoke tobacco (Silverman, 2016). People with a single gene for A1AT deficiency will not develop emphysema unless they smoke (or are chronically exposed to smoke), but if they do, they can develop emphysema by their 20s. Remarkably, having a single gene for A1AT deficiency is associated with creativity, especially writing and musical performance. Most people with the condition pursue a creative activity as an avocation, and many do so professionally. A few attain eminence in their disciplines, becoming prominent writers, artists, or performers. People with a gene for A1AT deficiency also have an increased risk of BD (Schmechel, 2007; Schmechel & Edwards, 2012). Physicians cited in popular media after her death suggested that Amy Winehouse had an abnormal gene for A1AT given her early-onset emphysema, her impressive creativity, and her apparent BD. Similar speculations can be found in medical journals concerning performing artists from Frederic Chopin to Michael Jackson (Erlinger, 2010; Kuzemko, 1994). If Amy Winehouse indeed had A1AT deficiency and her genetic condition had been identified early, she might have been assisted in quitting smoking before she developed severe emphysema, and she might have been appropriately treated for bipolar depression. Instead, she received antidepressants without mood stabilization as an adolescent and treatment for a substance use disorder without concurrent treatment of her mood disorder as an adult.

A related problem frequently seen in midlife or older creative professionals with mood disorders is adverse effects on their mental state from medications used to treat comorbid general medical disorders. For example, propranolol and metoprolol, beta-blockers used to treat angina pectoris and certain cardiac arrhythmias, readily cross the blood–brain barrier and can cause or worsen a depressed mood.

Recognizing comorbid general medical conditions in creative professionals with mood disorders—with or without substance use issues—can help redefine a creative professional's mood disorder as a medical problem rather than as an accompaniment to their personality, an elective lifestyle choice, or solely a consequence of substance use. Adopting a biomedical perspective sometimes can counteract the various combinations of denial, minimization, normalization, romanticization, and stigmatization of mood disorders and substance use disorders when they occur in writers, artists, and performers.

Bipolar Illness and the Creative Biography

People with bipolar conditions have life narratives and courses of illness covering a spectrum from the hopeful to the tragic. Some people will have cyclothymia that occasionally crosses the line into distressing and dysfunctional depression or into hypomania with risky or self-destructive behavior—but never attempt suicide or suffer prolonged periods of disability. Others will begin with a productive hyperthymic or cyclothymic temperament in their youth and then develop a progressive and severe psychiatric illness like BD-I with psychotic features, frequent relapses, occupational incapacity, and suicidal behavior.

In a typical worst-case scenario, the course of illness starts with cyclothymia, mild hypomania, or mild clinical depression (possibly with mixed symptoms) and moves on to BD-II, then to BD-I. The person suffers periods of disabling depression accompanied by suicide attempts and/or psychotic symptoms and eventually dies by suicide, homicide, an accident, self-neglect, or sequelae of substance use. If they live, the illness leads to a burnt-out, unproductive state. To avoid such tragic outcomes, clinical interventions should begin no later than the first appearance of functional impairment, self-harm, or substance misuse. At that point, however, the person's symptoms might be normalized as part of the life of a writer, visual artist, or performing artist or erroneously be attributed solely to a general medical problem like chronic pain following an injury, to grief after a loss or to suffering after a traumatic event. Even when their depression or bipolar condition is recognized, the usual barriers of stigma, mistrust, and fears of treatment often interfere with their seeking treatment and following through with it. Clinicians who take a holistic, longitudinal, and empathetic view of the creative professional's illness—including their barriers to acceptance of treatment—are more likely to establish a durable and effective therapeutic relationship.

For performing artists, whose reputation requires continuous maintenance of excellence and for already eminent creative professionals who expect their work to equal the quality of their past work, a decline in function due to progressive bipolar illness can be personally devastating. If a decline in the quality of their creative work is concurrent with depression and/or substance misuse, creative professionals are at risk for suicidal despair. The risk is greater if it is accompanied by financial insecurity. A writer with a tenured faculty position at a university or a film director or songwriter with residual income from past hits is at less risk than a creative professional who relies solely upon income from their current work.

Another dangerous situation is that of writers, artists, or performers who have become famous for specific works and are not able to equal their quality, because of either illness, substance use, personal difficulties, age-related physical or cognitive changes, or simply a lack of inspiration. Even when they enjoy the admiration of fans and people pay for their work, they are painfully self-critical; and at worst, their reason to live is gone. If they are depressed, a creative professional in this situation may be unable to see the end of a problem that is in fact transient and, if simply past their prime, can be unable to accept the situation and find other sources of meaning and purpose in life. The creator's depression reduces not only their productivity and/or the quality of their work but also their cognitive flexibility and resilience. They can be intensely self-critical and hopeless, seeing no path forward to an alternative source of meaning and purpose in life or an alternative realistic basis for self-esteem.

Older creative professionals who are in an unproductive period, whether temporary or long-term, can find meaning in mentoring and encouraging younger people in their field; in relationships with family, friends, and colleagues; and/or in the pursuit of an avocation, philanthropy, or involvement in an organization. A writer suffering from survival guilt after living through war, persecution, or a natural disaster might feel undeserving of success, high repute, and life itself if their creative work declines. Depression can trigger a vicious circle of guilt if a writer's creative work is the basis of forgiving themselves. This phenomenon might have had a role in the suicide of Primo Levi (1919–1987), an Italian chemist and writer in multiple genres who survived Auschwitz and subsequently wrote about his experience. Levi suffered from dysthymia for most of his adult life, with recurrent MDEs as he got older that impaired his ability to write. During one such episode, he died by falling down the well of the spiral stairway of his apartment building. His death was ruled a suicide (Thomson, 2004). An alternative explanation proposed by critics is that, while looking over the railing of the stairway, he fainted from medication-induced hypotension. Levi's antidepressant medication was prescribed by a physician cousin (Gambetta, 1999). Despite his fame, wealth, and extraordinary intelligence, he did not receive the psychiatric care that might have prevented his traumatic death.

Some creative professionals with symptoms of depression or the bipolar spectrum beginning in adolescence can have a benign life narrative. In this scenario, the adolescence and young adulthood of the person is a time of Sturm und Drang, which gradually transitions to a calmer and more emotionally stable but still productive state. Although the creative person has a biological disposition to BD or recurrent major depression, it is mitigated by the resolution of childhood trauma, the completion of grief, the attainment of professional success, the resolution of conflicts with family, and/or the maturation of the brain. In some cases, effective psychiatric treatment has a role. In engaging a talented but emotionally turbulent young writer, artist, or performer in treatment, an effective clinician will appreciate that the patient might have unfinished business related to trauma, loss, or family conflicts. If so, taking a narrowly biological approach or one using solely manual-based cognitive-behavioral or interpersonal psychotherapy might leave the patient feeling misunderstood and feed into suspicion of psychiatry. It is also common for a young creative professional to fear that psychiatric treatment will diminish their personal uniqueness and creativity—and it is important for the clinician to see if this is the case and what specific concerns the patient might have. Fear of psychiatry is an especially poignant issue for creative professionals in places where psychiatric and psychological treatments sometimes are misused as tools for enforcing conformity with an authoritarian regime or intolerant culture.

Later in their careers, the work of creative professionals might become less popular or be less appreciated by critics. Even those who have had consistent success can fear a decline in their popularity and reputation with age. If this happens and is accompanied by financial insecurity, they might lose relationships that were based in part on their wealth and status and/or might need to make residential moves or changes in their lifestyle that add to their feelings of depression, loneliness, or discouragement. Eminent writers, artists, or performers who once could afford to indulge in an expansive, grandiose, and expensive lifestyle might no longer be able to do so, and thus might newly need to acknowledge past mistakes and cope with their consequences.

The Promise of Personalized Treatment

When an eminent creative professional or celebrity performer seeks treatment for a neuropsychiatric condition, they might have an expectation of "special treatment." The expectation might be reasonable or unreasonable and the clinician's response appropriate or inappropriate. It is a reasonable expectation that a clinician, to the extent feasible, will arrange the timing of in-person visits or secure teleconferences to accommodate the "special" patient's work and travel schedule. It is unreasonable to expect a clinician to be on call 24/7 to talk whenever the patient feels distressed. It is appropriate for a clinician to allow extra time for clinical encounters and for coordinating care with providers of general medical care or substance abuse rehab services and to charge the patient for all professional time involved in their care. It is inappropriate to charge a higher-than-usual fee or to schedule more time than clinically necessary. The clinician should avoid having a non-professional personal relationship with the patient, even if the patient seeks one, and should not accept expensive gifts if they are offered.

Creative stars, especially if they are celebrities, often have realistic concerns about privacy. Addressing them might require going beyond usual confidentiality protections, but two responses are not appropriate. One is seeing a patient at their home when a home visit would not be clinically justifiable. The other is to avoid documenting important points of history because of fears that leaks could lead to a scandal. If there is a concern about keeping the patient's records secure and confidential, it should be addressed directly. For example, many hospital systems have a policy requiring a clinician to "break the glass" to see a celebrity's medical records, recording their reason for needing access to the records, and facing termination of their employment or clinical privileges for misrepresentation or inappropriate disclosure.

Personalization of treatment for depression and BD and their common comorbidities (e.g., substance use disorders) is likely to improve clinical outcomes for eminent creative professionals. Such personalization would consider their distinctive lifestyles and working conditions; their increased base rates of bipolar spectrum disorders, substance use disorders, and unnatural deaths; genre-specific mortality risks; and potential adverse medical and psychological consequences of wealth and fame. It would recognize that despite easy access to medical care, people absorbed in creative careers often neglect general medical problems or health maintenance activities. It would acknowledge that writers, artists, and performers can have realistic concerns that biological treatments for a mood disorder might adversely affect their creative work.

For the many successful creative professionals who travel in connection with their work or maintain more than one home, consistent treatment will be a hybrid of in-person and remote visits. While remote appointments might sometimes need to be outside of the clinician's usual office hours, the clinician should minimize "as-needed" phone calls, providing accessibility without cultivating unhealthy dependency or raising a suspicion that the clinician desires personal intimacy with the patient. Scheduled phone calls and text interchanges, however, fall within the scope of contemporary, post-pandemic psychiatric practice.

To begin a therapeutic relationship with a creative professional and set the stage for effective, personalized care, the initial assessment should not be rushed. It should include identification of working conditions, occupational hazards, and lifestyle; screening for undiagnosed or inadequately treated comorbidities; exploration of substance use; and exploring issues of fear of treatment, stigma, and/or mistrust of clinicians. If the history or screening questions suggest relationship problems or a history of trauma, these also deserve follow-up. Eliciting the patient's illness narrative is an important part of the process, and doing it goes far beyond a structured interview and mental status examination, completing a checklist of diagnostic criteria, and assigning ICD and CPT codes to the encounter. When the relationship begins with an emergency like a suicide attempt, eliciting the narrative might need to wait; but it should not wait too long. A comprehensive and holistic evaluation of the kind recommended here will take considerably more than an hour and usually will require two or more visits.

As a basis for personalized treatment, the clinician needs to know what specific fears and concerns the patient might have that are most likely to complicate or disrupt treatment before there is time for it to be effective. Is the patient worried about confidentiality? Medication side effects? Being hospitalized? Receiving a diagnosis that might be problematic in a custody dispute?

The clinician should begin with as few assumptions as possible about the details of the patient's life and working conditions. The patient's travel, work schedule, and sleeping and eating habits should be explored, as well as any environmental hazards like exposure to noise or to physical danger. An accurate picture of the patient's diet is important: Depending on the patient's age, gender, creative discipline, genre, and other cultural identities, there might be issues of unhealthy eating (empty calories with nutritional gaps), anorexia or bulimia, consuming fad diets, or use of potent nutritional supplements. A substance use history is critical, and some patients may not be ready to be honest about it on a first visit. Questions about sensitive issues might need to be asked—or repeated—at a second or third visit, and the patient might be asked to allow questioning of a significant other. Identification of comorbid general medical conditions is essential and might require laboratory tests, imaging, or physical examination. Creative professionals intensely engaged in their work and star performers frequently on tour often take poor care of themselves physically, neglecting health maintenance activities, not adhering to treatment of general medical problems, or not getting persistent symptoms properly diagnosed and treated.

Psychiatric comorbidities relevant to the choice of the type and focus of psychotherapy such as PTSD, specific phobias, or borderline personality, should be identified. Over several visits the clinician will form an opinion about whether the patient needs an open-ended long-term supportive psychotherapeutic relationship, whether there is a circumscribed problem addressable by short-term counseling, or whether a biomedically oriented, chronic illness management/health maintenance/secondary prevention concept of a therapeutic relationship fits the patient best. If the patient is already involved with some form of alternative medicine, the clinician should learn enough about it to know whether it is helping the patient or having adverse effects. If alternative treatment has had positive results, the potential for integrating alternative and conventional treatment should be explored.

Current suicidality, past suicidal thoughts and behavior, and current reasons to live/meaning of life (*ikigai*) must be assessed, with the recognition that the meaning of life is multidimensional, with long-term and short-term aspects, related to the patient's creative work and independent from it. Initial screening for suicidality is part of any comprehensive clinical assessment. However, even when there is no suicidal ideation, subsequently exploring the patient's meaning of life often yields information helpful in personalizing treatment. When the patient has multiple risk factors for future self-harm, the clinician should, if feasible, assess all elements of the interpersonal-neuropsychiatric model of suicide discussed in Chapter 6.

Lifestyle modification should be presented as a foundation of recovery from the present problem, prevention of future acute problems, long-term mental health, and preservation or even enhancement of creative productivity. Lifestyle changes for mental health might include changes in diet, learning a meditative practice, physical exercise, sleep hygiene, wearing ear protection in noisy environments, using light therapy to address chronobiological stress, and taking targeted nutritional supplements of established purity. If the patient is already interested in a specific diet, exercise regime, nutritional supplement, and/or meditative practice, the clinician's role may be one of making suggestions, gently challenging the patient's questionable or potentially harmful choices, and monitoring the effects of any deliberate change the patient makes in their lifestyle.

Any biologic therapy—usually pharmacotherapy but sometimes brain stimulation with transcranial magnetic stimulation (TMS), light, transcranial alternating current or direct current stimulation, or near-infrared photobiomodulation—should be given with a focus on the patient's most distressing symptoms and attempting to avoid potential side effects that would interfere with the patient's creative work. Emerging pharmacological therapies to be considered include ketamine infusions or intranasal esketamine, as they act quickly, reduce suicidal ideation, appear less likely to precipitate hypomania in bipolar patients than monoaminergic antidepressant drugs, and do not have the high incidence of emotional blunting and sexual dysfunction seen with SSRIs (Alnefeesi et al., 2022; d'Andrea et al., 2023; Feeney & Papakostas, 2023; Jawad et al., 2023; J. W. Kim et al., 2023; Lullau et al., 2023). Ketamine and esketamine are now used primarily for treatment-resistant depression, defined as a failure to respond to two or more consecutive treatments. In the case of creative professionals, failure to respond might partially reflect intolerance of emotional blunting, sexual dysfunction, and/or antidepressant-induced induction of a dysphoric mixed state in the context of an undiagnosed condition in the bipolar spectrum.

Follow-up of treatment should include not only measurement of change in the primary symptoms of the patient's illness but also systematic inquiry about side effects, especially emotional and cognitive effects. The latter can be assessed using an instrument like the ODQ or using items from the ODQ to suggest relevant interview questions. Exploration of possible sexual side effects would be especially important in patients for whom intimacy is central to their meaning of life and/or whose creative work regularly incorporates sexual themes. Follow-up should be especially close, with frequent in-person visits, remote visits, or scheduled email, text messages, or phone calls until the patient is clearly improving. It is useful early on to find out if there is someone the patient fully trusts and to get the patient's permission to talk with that person if there is a concern about the patient's risk of self-harm, a need for a significant other's support, or concern that the patient is withholding or denying critically important information.

If there is a substance use disorder, MAT should always be a serious consideration. Overall, MAT has a better prognosis than abstinence alone both for alcohol use disorder and for opioid use disorder (Connery, 2015; Fairley et al., 2021; Nissly & Levy, 2018; Varenbut et al., 2017). MAT can be more effective if supported by telemedicine visits (Eibl et al., 2017). The approach might be successfully adapted to the treatment of opioid use disorder in a musician or stand-up comedian who frequently goes on tour.

A patient receiving MAT should be re-evaluated for general medical and psychiatric comorbidity after several weeks of abstinence. If there is any sense that the patient denies or minimizes their level of substance use, the magnitude of ongoing use or confirmation of abstinence should be assessed by regular blood and/or urine testing.

The patient should be charged for all time spent on their case. This includes time spent interacting with the patient in person or via videoconferencing or phone calls; engaging in written exchanges via email or text; interviewing family, friends, or co-workers with the patient's consent; reviewing medical records, laboratory data and wearable device output; and coordinating care with other clinicians. A consistent message of "no exploitation and no favors" conveys respect and helps allay suspicion. The aim is for the patient to feel that the clinician's rewards are seeing the patient recover from their illness and stay well and being paid fairly for their time, including the substantial extra time often needed to address issues related directly or indirectly to the patient's occupation.

Finally, documentation of treatment that is accessible and comprehensible to the patient is important. It helps with patient empowerment and continuity of care and underscores the clinician's professionalism, respect for the patient, and expectation that clinician and patient will work together.

The approach described is time-consuming and expensive, but for eminent creative professionals, cost per se is rarely a realistic issue. Mistrust, fear, and concerns about compatibility of treatment with their creative work are much bigger issues for most who consider treatment for depression or illness in the bipolar spectrum. Addressing the genuinely special needs of an eminent creative professional or celebrity performer requires a holistic perspective, transparency, respect, scrupulous conduct, personalization of treatment, empathetic listening to the illness narrative, understanding atypical working conditions and identifying occupational hazards, and taking the extra time that is almost always needed for an optimal outcome.

Chapter 16

Physicians in Pain: Depression in the Medical Profession

On April 26, 2020, Dr. Lorna Breen, chief of emergency medicine at New York-Presbyterian Allen Hospital, died by suicide at age 49. She had been working overtime caring for patients with COVID-19, many of whom would arrive at the hospital in respiratory failure and die shortly thereafter, sometimes even before they could be removed from the ambulance, or while waiting in a hallway because all hospital beds were full. The hospital had a shortage of personal protective equipment, and vaccines were not yet available. Breen contracted COVID-19 herself. Despite suffering continuing symptoms, she attempted to return to work less than two weeks later. Directed by the hospital to return home to recover further, she went to her parents' home in Virginia and died by self-inflicted injuries a few days later (Moutier et al., 2021).

In the *Washington Post* article reporting her suicide, emergency medicine specialists with a special interest in suicide opined on why Breen did not seek help for her mental distress. They noted physicians' culture of stoicism, fears of their colleagues' seeing them as incompetent or of burdening them, and the stigmatization of treatment by state medical boards and hospitals that require physicians to disclose prior treatment for depression (Iati & Bellware, 2020).

The pandemic brought public attention to the widespread preexisting problem of burnout and depression in physicians and to the vulnerability of physicians to suicide. While in the pandemic context physicians getting counseling for burnout or moral injury was encouraged and was not stigmatized, it remains to be seen whether the diagnosis and treatment of major depression in physicians now will be normalized and destigmatized and whether the organizations that employ physicians will—appropriately—see depression as an occupational health issue.

A systematic review and meta-analysis of depression and anxiety among doctors during the COVID-19 pandemic, which included all studies published through March 3, 2021, calculated a pooled prevalence of moderate or severe depression of 20.5%—based on 26 studies with low to medium risk of bias that comprised 31,447 participants. Standard questionnaires like the PHQ-9 and the Hospital Anxiety and Depression Scale (HADS) were used in the studies, usually with cutoff scores indicating moderately severe clinical depression likely to meet the criteria for MDD (Johns et al., 2022). Women physicians' mental health was especially impacted by the pandemic; their work–family conflicts were exacerbated by increased demands both at work and at home (Sriharan et al., 2020). Reviews and meta-analyses of depression in physicians and medical students prior to the pandemic show similar findings: The rate in resident physicians has been estimated via meta-analysis at 28.8% (Mata et al., 2015) and the rate in medical students at 27.3% (Rotenstein et al., 2016).

Several categories of physicians are more likely to die by suicide than people of the same age and gender with other white-collar occupations:

- Female physicians (Duarte et al., 2023; Dutheil et al., 2019; Lindeman et al, 1996; Schernhammer & Colditz, 2004; Ye et al., 2021)
- Male physicians over age 45 (Petersen & Burnett, 2008)
- Physicians in the specialties of anesthesiology, emergency medicine, psychiatry, general practice, and general surgery (Duarte et al., 2023)

Physicians appear more likely than the general population to have suicidal ideation, though they are less likely to make suicide attempts. In a meta-analysis of studies comprising 70,368 physicians, the lifetime prevalence of suicidal ideation was 17.4%, and the one-month prevalence was 8.6%. However, the lifetime prevalence of suicide attempts was only 1.8%, and the one-year prevalence was 0.3%. By contrast, the worldwide lifetime prevalence of suicide attempts is 2.7%, and in the U.S. it is 4.6%. The one-year prevalence and lifetime prevalence of suicidal ideation were greater in European than American physicians and greater in female than in male physicians (Dong et al., 2020). However, death by suicide appears more common in American then European physicians (Dutheil et al., 2019).

Much of the recent literature on physician mental health has focused on the phenomenon of *burnout*, a psychological syndrome with primary symptoms of emotional exhaustion, alienation, depersonalization and/or cynicism, and a decreased sense of personal accomplishment. The syndrome is distinct from that of major depression; but most burnt-out physicians would meet this book's criteria for clinical depression, and many will develop Major Depressive Episodes (MDEs) if their burnout persists. In a survey of Austrian physicians, more than half of respondents experienced burnout. Criteria for MDD were met by 20% of those with moderate burnout, and 54% of those with severe burnout. Symptoms of emotional exhaustion correlated most strongly with symptoms of major depression (Wurm et al., 2016).

While an individual physician's depression can of course be unrelated to their work, problematic working conditions and occupational hazards underlie many cases of depression and are aggravating factors in others. Incompatibility between physicians' long-established professional culture and their objective working conditions contributes to the strain of their jobs and thereby to their risk of depression. In the pandemic setting, physicians witnessing tragic outcomes they were powerless to prevent suffered moral injury and its psychological consequences including depression and post-traumatic stress disorder (PTSD; Amsalem et al., 2021).

Worldwide, physicians have high social status—though it is somewhat lower in China, a country in which public policy has made most medical jobs unsatisfying or even dangerous. In most countries, they are relatively well paid. They practice a profession with glorious historical roots, informed by findings from the latest biomedical science. Most physicians begin their careers feeling it is a privilege to be a doctor, and they are self-critical if they do not enjoy their work and/or do not perform up to their own high standards. They will continue to work when they feel ill or fatigued, putting their patients' needs ahead of their own. At the beginning of the pandemic, when personal protective equipment was insufficient and vaccines were not yet available, physicians cared for patients with COVID-19 despite the risk to their own health and the health of their families.

If physicians have emotional difficulties related to their work, they are likely to blame themselves for a lack of grit or resilience. Most are slow to seek a new job or leave the profession, even when it would be feasible for them to do so. An occupational culture of stoicism underlies the self-stigma most physicians feel if they become depressed. While public stigma and institutional stigma of depression in physicians vary between communities, self-stigmatization by depressed physicians is found everywhere.

The vulnerability of physicians to depression and to suicide is remarkable since higher education, high socioeconomic status, and stable employment usually are protective against depression and since young people with severe preexisting problems with mental illness or substance use are unlikely to be admitted to medical school. Individual physicians can, of course, have other vulnerabilities to depression—a family history of depression or bipolar disorder (BD), a history of adverse childhood events, general medical conditions associated with depression, or having an intersecting cultural identity that can make them a target of prejudice, discrimination, microaggressions, or even violence. That said, depression in physicians frequently is triggered or exacerbated by a combination of work-related factors: (1) Work schedules, working environment, and work–life conflict; (2) Job stress associated with imbalances of demand and control and/

or effort and reward, the burden of "illegitimate tasks," and/or organizational injustice; (3) Workplace harassment or bullying related to gender, status as a medical student or resident physician, and/or other cultural identity; and (4) Moral injury from circumstances in which they are unable to live up to their ideals. Because these issues are ubiquitous among practicing physicians and physicians in training, they deserve identification and exploration routinely in the clinical evaluation of a depressed physician or medical student.

The historical occupational culture of the medical profession conflicts with the modern reality of healthcare as a service delivered by organizations with cultures of their own, often having norms and values inconsistent with those of a traditional physician. The ideals of a physician who is a "knowledgeable humanitarian" are not those of a corporate employer for whom excellence is defined by the bottom line on a financial statement (Clark, 2018). Specific aspects of physicians' professional culture and their employers' organizational cultures interfere with efforts to address the conflict.

Although physicians are more health-conscious than the general population, their mortality rates from medical complications of depression and its behavioral expressions—as well as from suicide—are relatively high (Agerbo et al., 2007; Albuquerque & Tulk, 2019; Center et al., 2003; Schernhammer & Colditz, 2004). Physicians' risk of suicide, and the newsworthiness of physicians' suicides, was evident in the English-language medical literature in the mid-19th century (Bucknill & Tuke, 1858) and has been a recurrent topic ever since. An editorial in the *Philadelphia Medical and Surgical Reporter* in 1897 cited 151 physician suicides in the United States in the prior three years. Stating, perhaps erroneously, that medicine was the most suicide-prone profession, it noted that physicians had "special reasons for discontent." The anonymous editorialist continued,

> The practice of medicine affords little in return for the demands which it makes. The doctor, like the teacher, lacks the stimulation of men's society, but unlike the teacher, he has no compensation of short hours and holidays. Like the minister, he has many ethical and moral burdens to bear but without the loyal support which the latter enjoys if his work is performed well. (Legha, 2012)

Elevated rates of depression in physicians have been reported for high-income and middle-income countries in Europe, Asia, the Middle East, and North and South America. They are seen in countries with comprehensive public healthcare systems, in those with a predominantly private practice model, and in those with hybrid systems. A survey of physicians in five European countries completed before the COVID-19 pandemic assessed their self-reported rates of depressive symptoms and of clinical depression. Clinical depression was common in four of the five: Germany (33%), France (20%), the United Kingdom (14%), and Portugal (12%). Spain was the outlier, with a 7% prevalence (Locke, 2019). The circumstances of the pandemic led to an increase in depression among physicians, with the magnitude of change depending on doctors' specialties, setting of practice, stage of career, and non-occupational aspects of their identities.

Depression is widespread among medical students and resident physicians. In a global meta-analysis of 167 cross-sectional studies ($n = 116,628$) and 16 longitudinal studies ($n = 5728$) from 43 countries, the pooled prevalence of diagnosed depression or clinically significant depressive symptoms (i.e., clinical depression) in medical students was 27.2%. Pooling data from the nine longitudinal studies of students before and after entering medical school (time intervals differing among the studies), the increase in the prevalence of clinical depression during medical school was 13.5%, implying a powerful adverse effect (on a population basis) of medical education on students' mental health. In the 24 studies that measured suicidal ideation ($N = 21,002$), the pooled prevalence was 11.1% (Rotenstein et al., 2016).

Despite the high prevalence of depression among medical students, few seek treatment—in the global meta-analysis just cited, only 15.7% of those with moderate to severe depression did so (Rotenstein et al., 2016). Another meta-analysis of depression in medical students (77 studies, $n = 62,728$) reached similar conclusions: Pooled prevalence rates were 28.0% for depression and 5.8% for suicidal ideation, but only 12.8% of the depressed students sought treatment (Puthran et al., 2016).

In a meta-analysis of 54 studies of depression in resident physicians from 17 countries, comprising a full range of specialties, the prevalence of significant depressive symptoms was 28.8%. In the four studies that used the PHQ-9 with a cutoff score of 10, the pooled prevalence was 20.2% (Mata et al., 2015). Given the 88% sensitivity and specificity of the PHQ-9, the results suggest that more than 18% of resident physicians would meet the diagnostic criteria for major depression. Sen and colleagues (2010) conducted a longitudinal study of depression in medical interns (i.e., first-year resident physicians) at 13 U.S. hospitals, having them complete a PHQ-9 quarterly. Forty percent of the sample had a score of 10 or higher on at least one assessment. At least in the U.S., depression in medical interns is normalized in physicians' professional culture. The internship year is especially stressful for several reasons, including very long working hours, first experience of direct personal responsibility for patient care and its outcomes, and a high prevalence of bullying and shame-based education (Bynum & Goodie, 2014; Kost & Chen, 2015; Vogel, 2016).

At the University of California, Davis Medical Center, 1800 residents, fellows, and faculty were sent questionnaires screening for depression and suicide risk and offering confidential follow-up mental health care to those at moderate or high risk. The response rate was 14.4%, with 98% of those who did respond in the moderate- or high-risk category; 28% of those at high risk and 16% of those at moderate risk were already receiving treatment. Of those not already receiving treatment who were invited to talk with a counselor about a possible referral for mental health care, only 40% did so. Of those who subsequently talked with a counselor, only 8% provided requested follow-up information. Both the non-response rate and the lack of follow-up suggest a combination of normalization of depression (including suicidal ideation) and stigmatization of acknowledging depression and seeking mental health care.

A "suicide prevention and depression awareness program" at the University of California, San Diego School of Medicine launched a similar anonymous web-based screening and referral process that included medical students, residents, and faculty (Haskins et al., 2016). Remarkably low rates of response at each stage of the process provide further evidence for structural stigma (adverse cultural norms and institutional policies) of depression among physicians that begins in medical school and is continually reinforced (Hatzenbuehler, 2016).

The chief wellness officer of the University of Michigan Medical School has explicitly opined that medical students are acculturated by a "hidden curriculum" that, contrary to the explicit content of their psychiatry classes and rotations, teaches them that depression is shameful and should be concealed (Brower, 2021). His hypothesis is supported by descriptions of the positive effects of faculty members' self-disclosure of their own treatment on resident physicians' willingness to acknowledge depression and seek treatment (Vaa Stelling & West, 2021).

In the United States and in many other countries, the surge in prevalence of clinical depression in the general population during the COVID-19 pandemic normalized the condition in a way that enabled its disclosure, notably by young and middle-aged men. One reflection of this is the relatively high response rates to depression items on health surveys conducted in the U.S. in 2020 and 2021, a fact noted in Chapter 14. This phenomenon has not been seen consistently in surveys of physicians. For example, in a survey of residents, fellows, and attending physicians at SUNY Stony Brook University Hospital in April and May of 2020, the response rate was only 16.3%, of whom 6.2% scored 10 or higher on the PHQ-9. The response rate among orthopedic surgery residents and fellows was highest, at 52%, perhaps related to the study's principal investigator being an orthopedic surgeon. None of them had scores in the depressed range on the PHQ-9, a highly unlikely finding if survey respondents were representative of the full population. The highest percentage of respondents with depression was found in the anesthesia department, where 14.3% scored 10 or higher.

However, the response rate for the anesthesiology department was only 9.2% (Al-Humadi et al., 2021).

Physicians' Complex Cultural Identities

All physicians have multiple identities related to gender, age and generational cohort, race/ethnicity, socioeconomic class background, and religion/spirituality or its absence. Physicians are enculturated during their training to put their professional identity ahead of their other ones, and often the primacy of professional identity is supported by significant others in the physician's life. When there is a conflict between professional duties and family life, physicians usually put their work first, and their spouses and children usually support them in doing so. Faiths that otherwise forbid work on the Sabbath or on religious holidays will permit physicians to practice on those days and to do what is necessary to save lives and relieve the suffering of the sick. For most physicians, their profession is a vocation—an essential part of their meaning of life and sense of purpose. This can make the loss of their professional work an existential crisis, whether it be brought on by illness, injury, loss of license, or even planned retirement. Especially when a physician's career is interrupted suddenly or unexpectedly, depression is a common emotional reaction. Many physicians' suicides have apparently been precipitated by a loss of their ability—or their license—to practice medicine.

Common elements of the professional culture of physicians include commitment to patients' welfare, empathy for patients' suffering, dedication to lifelong learning, a tradition of collegial support of physicians by one another, willingness to make personal sacrifices to serve patients and support colleagues, and respect for patients' confidentiality. As noted, there is an expectation of toughness and resilience in the face of adversity. Neither self-care nor social activism is part of physicians' usual professional culture.

Critically, the traditional culture of physicians does not conceive of medical care as a service delivered by a complex system of which physicians are but a part and that they do not control. One cannot find the concept of the physician as an employee anywhere in the writings of either the ancient or the contemporary icons of medical practice and philosophy. It would be absurd to picture Hippocrates or Galen, Zhāng Zhòngjǐng or Sun Simiao, Avicenna or Maimonides (see Chapter 9), the legendary internist Sir William Osler (1849–1919), or the pioneering neurosurgeon Harvey Cushing (1869–1939) describing himself as a "healthcare provider," a "supplier of healthcare services," or an employee occupying a rectangle on an organizational chart.

Fewer than 15% of American physicians are in solo practice, and two thirds are in practices of five or more physicians supported by sundry clinical and non-clinical staff. More than half are employees or contractors with no ownership of the practice that employs them (C. K. Kane, 2019). For those physicians, decisions concerning their duties and responsibilities, scope of authority, and working conditions are made by others, often without due consideration of their input. Nonetheless, patients and their families will hold a physician accountable for unsatisfactory encounters or adverse outcomes, even when critical elements of their care were not under the physician's control. Physicians often blame themselves for outcomes not under their control, as many did when their patients died of COVID-19 or when they transmitted the infection to members of their families. Such events were widespread in early 2020 when there were shortages of ventilators, ICU beds, and personal protective equipment, and vaccines had not yet become available.

Independently of the pandemic, many physicians fear being blamed, sued (in America), or physically attacked (in China and some other middle-income countries) when a patient has a bad outcome. The extent and nature of fear, and of self-blame, vary according to physicians' cultural identities, as well as their personalities and the facts of each case. Even when there are no dire events like malpractice suits or physical attacks, physicians' jobs are stressful. Several specific aspects of doctors' jobs known to cause potentially unhealthy stress are described in detail later in this chapter.

Physicians' responses to the conflict of professional culture with organizational culture and to job stress and adverse working conditions seldom involve organized efforts to change their organizational culture or working conditions. At best, physicians make changes to improve their personal lives, become more efficient at their work, seek support from colleagues, and develop their resilience. At worst, they become burnt out, disillusioned, and/or alienated, sometimes to the point of clinical depression. Some will resort to substance use to cope with their stress. When physicians respond maladaptively to their job strain and adverse working conditions they have less empathy for their patients; and they sometimes have increased troubles at home. Many physicians' self-defeating reactions to their occupational hazards can be understood better with consideration of the reasons why people choose the medical profession, physicians' "career anchors," and the gendered nature of specific medical specialties.

Physicians' Motives and Career Anchors

People choose medicine as a profession for a combination of reasons, of which the most important varies among physicians. Reasons for choosing medicine include a desire to be of service to others, interest in one or more of the relevant sciences, enjoyment of technical mastery, family tradition or family aspiration, a wish for a secure job with no risk of unemployment, a relatively high income, social status, flexibility in choice of residence, feasibility of part-time work, and the potential for occupational autonomy as one might have in a solo practice. When a representative sample of 19,328 American physicians across 30 specialties was asked to state the most rewarding aspect of their jobs, the top three reasons offered were relationships with patients (including patients' gratitude), satisfaction from their technical competence (finding answers, making diagnoses, etc.), and knowing they were making the world a better place. Making good money doing a job they liked was in fourth place and was the primary reward of practice for only 12% of the physicians surveyed (L. Kane, 2019a). Similar motives apply in other countries, though the relative importance of the various motives differs for both cultural and practical reasons. Primary care physicians in middle-income countries with socialized medical systems often are poorly paid. For example, the income of a family practitioner in a small Chinese city might not even put them in the upper- middle class. Intrinsic satisfaction from the work, social status, and job security would be more common motives than pay in that situation. In countries like the Nordic nations with high per capita income and a strong social welfare system, part-time work is very common for physicians with young children. In those places, many people are attracted to the medical profession as one with an option of part-time work that is intellectually challenging, emotionally satisfying, well paid, and not precarious.

Physicians, like other professionals, have *career anchors*—self-perceived areas of competence, motivation, and values that guide and constrain their career choices. If the attributes of a specific position don't fit with an individual's career anchors, it is unlikely that the person will be happy in their work. When a person persists in work incompatible with their career anchors, there will be an imbalance of effort and subjective reward, a situation of job strain that predisposes to burnout and to depression.

Career anchors comprise technical/functional competence, general managerial competence, autonomy/independence, security/stability, creativity/entrepreneurship, service/dedication to a cause, pure challenge, and lifestyle integration including the harmonization of work and family life (Schein & Van Maanen, 2013). Career anchors for physicians vary by specialty, setting of practice, and the physician's other cultural identities. A physician opting for solo practice in an underserved rural area is likely to have service to others as a career anchor. If not, they are likely to drown in the ocean of the community's unmet clinical needs. A neuroradiologist is likely to have technical competence as a career anchor. Physicians whose work comprises an assortment of short-term locum tenens contracts are likely to have autonomy and/or lifestyle as career anchors.

Career anchors were studied systematically in a group of 1159 Chinese physicians working as general practitioners at community health centers (J. Wang et al., 2019). Job security was the principal career anchor for most of them (71.6%), followed by technical competence (12.2%). General practitioners aged 40 and above scored higher on the anchor of service and lower on the importance of autonomy and lifestyle. The findings of the study demonstrate the relevance of intersecting identities—in this case nationality and age/generation—in defining the context for understanding depression in physicians.

Career anchors tend to evolve over a professional's first ten years of work and then remain stable. Physicians sometimes discover their career anchors by taking jobs they turn out to greatly dislike. A physician's choice of a first job following residency or subspecialty training might be influenced by a trusted mentor or by colleagues with whom they have trained; in some cases, it is driven by financial need or, in the case of immigrants, by visa considerations. Compatibility of the job with the young physician's career anchors might never be considered. When a physician-patient presents with symptoms of depression, the issues of job satisfaction and job strain usually will arise spontaneously, but if they don't, the clinician should consider them. For many early-career physicians, a change in job might be the most effective way to prevent a recurrence of depression. However, a physician's appraisal of their job and its challenges and rewards can change significantly when clinical depression is successfully treated. Whether an apparent mismatch of a physician with their job is a cause of depression or its effect is a question requiring the clinician's insight and judgment, and sometimes it cannot be settled until the physician's depression has improved with medical treatment.

In the United States, educational debt is a serious concern for a high proportion of early-career physicians and of mid-career physicians in less well-compensated specialties. Approximately 80% of American physicians graduate from medical school with educational debt, typically between $200,000 and $250,000; and 45% of medical students say their ability to pay off their educational debt is one of their primary personal concerns. Black and first-generation immigrant physicians have the highest average debt at medical school graduation (Hanson, 2021a). If a newly graduated physician with typical educational debt chooses a specialty with relatively low compensation, full repayment might take as long as 20 years if they devoted 10% of their income to loan payments (Hanson 2021b). If an indebted physician had a life event or encountered a life situation that involved unexpected expenses or necessarily reduced their work hours, financial distress or anxiety about it might quickly develop. Financial distress can easily precipitate emotional distress. If a physician is anxious about money and their depression is making that anxiety worse, they might be reluctant to spend money on psychiatric treatment or take time off work if needed to get effective treatment or to fully recover from their illness. Inner conflict over the cost of treatment can be especially great if the treatment that best fits the physician-patient's individual circumstances is an expensive one like intensive psychotherapy or a biological therapy (e.g., transcranial magnetic stimulation) that is poorly covered by their health insurance.

Patients sometimes find questions about their personal finances as sensitive and potentially embarrassing as questions about their sexual lives. Clinicians evaluating depressed physicians should not avoid the subject of their physician-patients' compensation and financial status. If the clinician is a non-medical therapist unfamiliar with the financial dimension of medical careers, they might incorrectly assume that a depressed physician is unlikely to be in financial distress. Many of the life circumstances that can precipitate an episode of depression—including divorce; illness of a spouse, parent, or child; and disruption of one's professional practice—also can rapidly cause financial hardship in a person who begins with a substantial debt burden.

Gender-Related Challenges

While in many countries most new medical school graduates now are women, medicine has been a male profession, and many medical specialties remain highly masculine (i.e., with marked gender inequality and expectation or acceptance of stereotypically masculine behavior). At the time in the 19th century when several women's medical colleges were founded in the U.S., the nation's leading medical schools did not accept women at all. Elizabeth Blackwell (1821–1910), America's first woman physician, received her MD degree in 1849. A century later, in 1950, only 6% of American doctors were women. By 2019, 30% of physicians and half of medical students were female, but men continued to predominate in the leadership of medical schools, hospital departments, and specialty societies. While there now is no apparent discrimination against women for admission to American medical schools, the medical profession continues to have gender inequality in other forms. For example, U.S. women physicians are paid less than male physicians of the same specialties (L. Kane, 2022). They are less likely to become deans or department chairs or full professors at medical schools (Jena et al., 2015).

Gender inequality in the medical profession is especially severe in countries with 'masculine' cultures. For example, at a time when 66.2% of Japanese obstetrician-gynecologists were female, only 1.9% of the leadership positions in the Japanese Society of Obstetrics and Gynecology were women. In Hungary, where there are high expectations for women in their traditional roles as wives and mothers, few women physicians have the option of part-time employment, leading to a high rate of burnout related to work-family conflict. This situation persists despite more than half of practicing physicians being female (Ramakrishnan et al., 2014).Women medical students and physicians working in predominantly male academic and clinical settings often experience sexual harassment, sometimes by male physicians and sometimes by patients or non-physician staff (Jagsi, 2018; Mathews & Bismarck, 2015). A global meta-analysis of 51 surveys of 38,353 medical students and resident physicians found that the majority of trainees experienced sexual harassment (Fnais et al., 2014).

Gender inequality is apparent in medical research as well as in clinical practice. Women medical researchers' first grants from the National Institutes of Health are significantly smaller than those awarded to men (Oliveira et al., 2019). Women joining medical school faculties tend to receive smaller startup packages than men with similar credentials (Sege et al., 2015). Women researchers are more likely than men to report inadequate access to grants and statistical support to make their proposals more competitive (Holliday et al., 2015). In an analysis of the compensation of physician researchers, men's salaries were significantly higher than women's, after controlling for relevant covariates (Jagsi et al., 2012).

The choice of specialty by American senior medical students has shown strong gender-based differences. In 2018, the five most "feminine" specialties (with the percentage of new residents who were women) were obstetrics/gynecology (82.7%), pediatrics (73%), allergy and immunology (70.4%), medical genetics (67.1%), and dermatology (64.4%). The five most "masculine" specialties (with the percentage of new residents who were men) were orthopedic surgery (85.1%), neurological surgery (82.5%), thoracic surgery (73.8%), radiology (73.8%), and vascular surgery (67%). The organizational culture of a training program in orthopedic surgery or of an orthopedic surgery clinic is likely to reflect masculine attitudes. A female orthopedic surgeon would have to accept some casual sexism to be comfortable in the daily working environment of the specialty, much as would a female airline pilot or truck driver. Conversely, a male pediatrician or obstetrician would be in continual contact with female colleagues, who, being in the majority, would set the standards for acceptable speech and behavior. Women who choose not to apply for training in masculine specialties often cite reasons like inflexible schedules, a poor work–life balance, and a procedural rather than a personal orientation. Other reasons, less often volunteered by female medical school graduates, include a lack of female role models and mentors in the masculine specialties and concerns about discrimination and sexual harassment (Jagsi et al., 2016; Murphy, 2018).

Gender inequality in the medical profession, and the gendered aspect of the masculine medical specialties, is even more evident in countries with especially large occupational "gender gaps," such as China, Japan, South Korea, and the Arabic nations. In Japan, it is difficult for women physicians to arrange maternity leave or to make suitable arrangements for childcare. Few hospitals offer on-site or conveniently located care for the young children of their staff physicians, a particular problem for women physicians working weekends or night shifts or having a sick child at home (Fujimaki et al., 2016). In Japan, women physicians are expected by others to be the primary caregivers for their children, and most expect it of themselves. The culture of the procedural specialties is not conducive to a physician's modifying her work schedule to be more compatible with her role as a mother (Izumi et al., 2013; Nomura et al., 2015; Yamazaki et al., 2011). Japanese female neurosurgeons appear to address the issue by avoiding marriage and motherhood altogether. In a survey by the Japan Neurosurgical Society, only half of the women neurosurgeons were married, and only 39.2% had a child (usually only one). Half of the women neurosurgeons, even those single or married without children, reported difficulty maintaining a work–life balance. Work–life conflicts are a challenge for all physicians, but they are worse for women physicians and for physicians of either gender working in a masculine specialty.

Gender-related challenges for female physicians—and their mental health consequences—reach an extreme with female resident physicians in Saudi Arabia, a country with high gender inequality, a masculine culture, and a state religion that mandates a subordinate status for women. In a 2021 study of 133 female resident physicians in Jeddah, 52% reported gender discrimination, and 40% reported regularly experiencing harassment; 53% were severely depressed, 14% had suicidal thoughts, and five had already made suicide attempts. Only eight of the 53 regularly experiencing sexual harassment had reported it to their superiors in the hospital hierarchy (Yaghmour et al., 2017). Apparently, the harassment of young women physicians was normalized, and complaining about it would be more likely to elicit retribution than positive change.

An exception to the trend for gendered specialties is found in the Nordic countries—the world's leaders in gender equality. Except for a special interest of women in obstetrics and gynecology, male versus female medical students in those countries show no significant difference in specialty preference (Kristoffersson et al., 2018). In Sweden, where there is high income equality, public funding of higher education (no educational debt), publicly funded childcare, and liberal paid parental leave, 54% of female and 36% of male medical students surveyed in 2012 intended to work part-time following graduation. For those intending to enter family medicine, 80% of the women and 68% of the men planned to work part-time (Diderichsen et al., 2013). Men and women had somewhat different career anchors, with lifestyle (work–life balance) being relatively more important to the women and technical competence being relatively more important to the men. While Swedish women physicians sometimes get depressed, work–life conflict is far less likely to be a cause or contributor than it is in countries like the United States with greater gender inequality, no publicly funded childcare, and a high prevalence of large educational debts among young physicians.

Cultural Conflict, Working Conditions, and the Commodification of Healthcare

Medical practice has always been stressful at times, and most physicians encounter traumatized patients or deal with the deaths of patients and the grief of their loved ones. Emergency physicians and trauma surgeons see severe trauma continually and unnatural deaths regularly. Pediatric oncologists frequently must deliver the news to parents that their child is dying of cancer. Stress, emotional demands, and exposure to trauma do not necessarily cause depression, however, if a physician is prepared for them, is psychologically resilient, and has emotional support from colleagues, family, and/or close friends. Depression risk rises when the stressful demands of practice are combined with a lack of autonomy and control (job strain); insufficient positive experiences and interactions; and/or bullying, harassment, or verbal or physical hostility from patients. Patients' direct or indirect expressions of mistrust, if they occur frequently, also can affect physicians' job satisfaction, morale, and depression risk. These concerns have increased over the past 25 years due to changes in the organization of medical care in most high-income and many upper-middle-income countries.

Commodification (commercialization) of healthcare can be defined as financing of healthcare by individual payment or private insurance, rendering of services with the primary aim of cash income or profit, and distribution of healthcare services and related goods through the market according to ability to pay (Mackintosh & Kovalev, 2006). Commodification can take place even in countries that have national health systems and universal coverage, if the national system is based on public subsidies for private insurance, if it operates under a hybrid model with both public and private hospitals and clinics, and/or the national health system pays relatively little for "units of service." In the last case, the hospitals and clinics that employ physicians press them to maximize their number of patient encounters and to do procedures or prescribe medications or other treatments for which they will receive additional reimbursement. Patients offering gifts and gratuities to get extra time and attention from overworked physicians is another face of commodification seen in countries with national health systems that underpay physicians for their time.

Healthcare in China, Germany, and the United States is highly commodified. Healthcare in in Japan, Norway, and the United Kingdom is not. Australia, Denmark, and South Korea show an intermediate level of commodifiation (E. C. Huang et al., 2018; Yan, 2018). Patients' trust in physicians generally is lower in countries in which healthcare is more commodified, though Switzerland and Denmark, both unusually high-trust countries, are places where trust in physicians is high despite moderate commodification of healthcare. And, in Germany—another high-trust country—trust in physicians, while not high, is greater than it is in Japan or South Korea (Heymann, 2018; Huang, Pu, et al., 2018). Commodification appears to interact with other aspects of a country's culture influencing patients' trust in their physicians.

When healthcare is commodified, many patients will deal with a physician's care as a consumer service rather than as an essentially personal encounter between a patient and a learned and dedicated professional. The effect of commodification on patient–physician relationships has become larger as costs of care have increased, healthcare organizations have gotten larger, health plans and hospital systems have merged, solo or small-group private practice has declined, and health-related information of variable quality has been disseminated over the internet along with direct-to-consumer advertising of medical centers and pharmaceuticals. These changes have put physicians in positions with less control, treated more as employees than as autonomous professionals. Where in the past physicians might have perceived hospitals and other medical institutions as serving and supporting them, most physicians now feel that they are serving and supporting the institutions that employ them.

Electronic medical records (EMRs, or *electronic health records*) have become since the mid-1990s the standard of medical practice in all high-income nations. While EMRs have many benefits, they have greatly increased the amount of time doctors spend in front of a computer screen rather than face to face with their patients. This has happened not only in countries like the United States with its cumbersome system of multiple payers but also in countries like Norway with a national healthcare system and relatively little commodification of care (Rosta & Aasland, 2016). Administrative requirements for documentation have increased so that physicians must generate more text and check more boxes on screens for the same amount of personal interaction with patients. Reduction of time spent in face-to-face interaction reduces the satisfaction that both the doctor and the patient get from the clinical encounter. This can lead to a reduced sense of accomplishment and to depersonalization and cynicism, two of the three components of professional burnout.

If, to have less screen time and more face time with their patients in the clinic, a physician completes their documentation while sitting in front of a computer screen at home in the evening, a price often is paid in the form of increased work–family conflict and/or disrupted sleep. In addition, prolonged periods of sitting looking at a screen while dealing with the EMR can contribute to musculoskeletal problems and their associated pain and effects on mood, to the adverse health effects of a sedentary lifestyle, and to disruption of the circadian rhythm if the physician's screen time is late in the evening.

Measurement and benchmarking of care processes and outcomes using quantitative methodology has become a focus for healthcare regulators, payers, specialty societies, and health system executives. These quality measures are greatly facilitated by EMRs and by the ubiquity of computers and internet access, but they can add to an already great burden of documentation. Furthermore, most of the quantitative performance measures have limitations that inevitably will result in poor scores for some physicians who give excellent care. Specifically, those who work with patients with high comorbidity and adverse social determinants of health might appear to have worse outcomes of care than physicians who treat patients with better general health, more resources, and fewer economic and environmental barriers to healthy behavior and adherence to prescribed treatment. They might need to deviate from published practice guidelines to effectively adapt their patients' care to deal with their cultural, environmental, and practical constraints. The challenges faced by physicians treating underserved populations are not all recognized by the risk adjustment methodologies used in calculating quality measures and benchmarking physicians' performance. Consequently, physicians making personal sacrifices to treat underserved populations might find themselves criticized, given low ratings on public websites, or even financially penalized for poor performance when they might have "gone the extra mile" to serve their patients.

Evidence-based practice guidelines have become a global standard that physicians are expected to follow in non-exceptional cases. These are directives for how to diagnose or treat conditions based on an expert synthesis of published clinical trials and retrospective outcome studies. The implementation of these guidelines implies additional study obligations for physicians and often involves additional documentation. Patients might be dissatisfied if care that follows standard practice guidelines does not jibe with their preferences or meet their expectations. Flexibility might be required to adapt care planning to allow not only for patient preferences but also for comorbid conditions, social determinants of health, and individual differences. Securing support from an employer or from third-party payers for appropriate deviations from guidelines can require substantial extra work for the physician.

Many recently approved, efficacious treatments are very expensive. Getting insurance to pay for them or getting a national health system to approve them requires additional work from physicians and can involve difficult conversations with patients and/or their families. The outcome of the physician's efforts with insurance companies or government agencies might be disappointing, leaving the physician to come up with a next-best alternative. If the outcome of the second-choice treatment is poor, the situation is painful both for the patient and for a compassionate physician. If the outcome is death or disability that might have been prevented, the physician can suffer *moral injury*.

Demand for medical services has increased disproportionately to the growth in population. There are physician shortages in many areas and in many specialties. More conditions are treatable and/or preventable than 25 years ago, and, thanks to the internet, there is far broader awareness of diseases and their treatments by the public. Patients need more service, but there is less time to spend with them because of more patients needing care and requirements for physicians to spend time on activities not involving direct patient interaction, including electronic documentation and compliance with practice guidelines and with organizational and regulatory policies.

The physician workforce of most high-income countries has become more diverse, with many more female physicians and more immigrant, expatriate, and/or ethnic minority physicians in most high-income countries. In a situation of diversity, patients frequently are seen by physicians with cultural backgrounds or identities they ordinarily would avoid and would be disinclined to trust. Patients or their families might stereotype, discriminate against, or harass physicians. The physician might have no choice but to tolerate a patient's aggression or disrespect and persist in delivering care, but the experience of being disrespected, devalued, mistrusted, or otherwise ill-treated takes a psychological toll. In some cases, a physician will have a realistic fear of violence, especially if the treatment outcome is disappointing.

In many countries, across the spectrum of per capita GNP, physicians are at significant risk from violent attacks by patients or their families, for example, India (Ghosh, 2018), China (Sun et al., 2017; "Violence Against Doctors," 2014), South Korea (Hong, 2019), Germany (Vorderwülbecke et al., 2015), and Norway (Johansen et al., 2017). Workplace violence against physicians, both verbal and physical, has long been recognized as a problem in the United States, with emergency medicine, psychiatry, and the primary care specialties at the highest risk (Phillips, 2016; Pompeii et al., 2015). In areas of the United States with a high prevalence of opioid abuse, primary care physicians are at risk of attacks from people—either patients or not—attempting to extort medically inappropriate opioid prescriptions. More than half of physicians specializing in treating chronic pain report having been threatened with violence by patients seeking inappropriate prescriptions. Seven percent of the cases reported involved a firearm (David et al., 2015). An ongoing risk of workplace violence is a known occupational risk factor for depression.

In addition to facing interpersonal issues and conflicts between physicians' professional culture and workplace realities, physicians may work in physically hazardous environments. Pathologists work with toxic chemicals, and anesthesiologists might be exposed daily to hazardous concentrations of anesthetic gases. Physicians working in inner-city hospitals might be exposed to toxic levels of air pollution. Military physicians have the same exposure to noise, explosive blasts, etc. as combat troops in the same locations. Finally, emergency physicians and trauma surgeons are continually exposed to victimized people—an experience that can be cumulatively traumatic.

For physicians of all ages there often is a stressful conflict between the realities of their work and the ideals and principles they learned during their training and might have admired in their teachers and mentors. For older ones, there might also be a conflict between the past and the present. A physician who was successful and happy at work when the practice of medicine was different might be less successful and much less happy now. Older physicians who have not adapted to contemporary expectations can be the target of patient complaints or organizational disapproval. Complaints filed with hospitals, health plans, or the state medical board can damage a physician's reputation, as can disparaging online reviews, even ones of dubious validity. If complaints and negative reviews spread widely online or lead to a formal investigation, they raise the risk that a physician will develop clinical depression or even suicidal ideation (Hawton, 2015).

Trials of Physicians in Training

Physicians in training (interns, residents, and fellows) are part of a hierarchy, with more senior trainees above them and attending physicians or surgeons supervising all. As in other hierarchical work situations, there is the potential for harassment, bullying, or otherwise humiliating treatment by a trainee's superiors. Estimates vary by country, setting, and methodology; but at least a third of physicians in training, and a similar proportion of early-career physicians in hierarchical settings, will experience humiliating treatment or harassment—usually by a superior but sometimes by a peer—on an ongoing basis. In a study of suicidal ideation in Italian and Swedish surgeons, harassment and humiliating treatment were the external factors most strongly linked to suicidal ideation (Wall et al., 2014).

Depending on the institutional culture of the hospital or medical school, mistreated trainees may have little alternative but to tolerate the mistreatment if they want to complete their training and launch their medical careers. Women physicians and those from racial/ethnic minorities can face prejudice, discrimination, and/or disrespect from patients and sometimes from colleagues. The norms of the profession call for junior physicians and trainees to treat their superiors respectfully and for all physicians to treat patients with courtesy and empathy even when patients behave badly. Even for physicians who have learned to cope with mistreatment, recurrent experiences of victimization contribute to burnout and depression. Physicians, including trainees, who are mistreated by superiors or peers typically are reluctant to make formal complaints. They might criticize themselves for not being strong enough to tolerate their situation. They might have realistic concerns about retribution or loss of opportunity. If they anticipate working long-term in a locality or clinical setting, they must find a way to get along with their colleagues. For example, a younger physician might expect to rely on referrals of patients from established physicians. Open criticism or disparagement by a powerful physician of their specialty could cause long-term damage to their professional reputation—and raising even a valid complaint about the behavior of a well-established practitioner might lead to such an outcome. In a strongly stated case in the *Canadian Medical Association Journal*, Amitha Kalaichandran, a resident physician, and Daniel Lakoff, an emergency medicine assistant residency training director, argue that a change in organizational culture is essential for effectively addressing the mental health problems—and suicides—of physicians in training. They point out problems of bullying and harassment of residents, their fear of reprisal if they report concerns, and conflicts of interest involving directors of physician health programs (PHPs)—who cannot most effectively serve physicians in training if they owe their primary allegiance to a medical school or another organization (Kalaichandran & Lakoff, 2019).

Physicians undergo training at a time in their lives when many people start families. In the United States, women physicians in training might not be given adequate time for prenatal care, and they might have very little time off around the time of giving birth. Options for paternal leave in the United States are even less adequate. In many training programs, a resident physician who takes more than six weeks of parental leave can be required to take another full year of training to be eligible for certification in their specialty (Varda & Glover, 2018). Resident physicians who take leave apart from scheduled vacations know they are burdening their colleagues with additional coverage responsibilities, a fact that either deters them from taking as much parental leave as they would like or adds to feelings of conflict and discomfort if they do take additional time off.

The problem of adapting one's work schedule to address the requirements of motherhood is less challenging in the Nordic countries, where a year of parental leave is built into all jobs, and most severe in countries like Japan, which make essentially no accommodations for working parents of infants. In Japan, the expectation is that a woman physician will stop practicing medicine for several years following the birth of a child. When she does—and not all will—she is likely to find that her career opportunities and compensation will forever be worse, reflecting her time away from working in her specialty.

The physical stress of a pregnant woman's working during pregnancy as a resident physician in a surgical specialty has been associated with preterm labor, miscarriage, pre-eclampsia, and intrauterine growth retardation. Furthermore, most female resident physicians believe that having children will negatively impact their careers (Kin et al., 2018). The paid parental leave policies of America's leading medical schools fall far short of the 12-week minimum recommended by the American Academy of Pediatrics (Riano et al., 2018). Before a change in policies limited resident physicians' duty hours, pregnant residents in obstetrics and gynecology would routinely work more than 80 hours per week until the week of giving birth, a striking example of a stoic, self-sacrificing culture that persists among American physicians. Higher than expected rates of prematurity and pre-eclampsia were observed in pregnant female ob/gyn residents working such extreme hours (Gabbe et al., 2003). The emotional consequences of a major pregnancy complication related to overwork cannot be overstated— and a physician would be painfully aware of the potential lifetime implications of a pregnancy complication for the health of her newborn child.

If a resident physician develops a medical condition that requires time off from work, any time they take away from work will increase the demand on their fellow residents and perhaps impact the care of some especially meaningful patients. There is thus great pressure on residents to work when they are ill, a phenomenon known as *sickness presenteeism*. Working hard while feeling ill, perhaps not performing at one's best, is a depressing circumstance, especially for physicians who are conscious that others' welfare depends on the quality of their work and who tend to be perfectionistic and self-critical. The phenomenon was in evidence during the early months of the COVID-19 pandemic, when physicians caring for critically ill patients would contract the disease themselves. They would take off only the minimum time needed for quarantine and then return to work even though they had not fully recovered from their illness. This was the case for Dr. Lorna Breen, whose case was discussed earlier in this chapter.

Professional Burnout

An Italian psychiatrist recently published a poem, "The Cry Into the Darkness of a Burned Out Physician" (Maffoni, 2021).

> I began my path as a star full of light, as a rushing unstoppable river.
> I dreamed to change the world; it changed me.
> Overwhelmed by the pounding torrent of unavoidable deaths, I succumbed.
> I couldn't accept so much sickness, neither bear the overflowing grief.
> Now I'm empty, dark as a sky without its moon.

The work lives of physicians are demanding and stressful. Physicians often develop stress-related symptoms, notably the syndrome of professional burnout that was first described in 1974 by the psychologist Herbert Freudenberger (Freudenberger, 1974). Burnout of clinical severity is significantly correlated with medical errors, malpractice claims, conflicts with co-workers, job turnover, and early retirement. Potential personal consequences include depression, alcohol abuse, motor vehicle accidents, marital and family conflict, and suicidal ideas and behavior (Kumar, 2016). The adverse behavioral and professional consequences of burnout can occur in the absence of depression; but depression is a frequent consequence of burnout and burnout-related behavior, and it is a frequent mediator between burnout and its worst consequences. In addition, a physician who becomes depressed for reasons unrelated to their job is more likely to become burned out. Burnout without depression does not necessarily cause a measurable decline in quality of care, even when physicians feel their performance is worse than usual. A burnt-out physician can be unreasonably self-critical. In a professional culture in which patients' welfare is put ahead of one's own, an exhausted physician might preserve clinical performance at the expense of their family life and personal health (Mangory et al., 2021; Rathert et al., 2018). The lack of impact of burnout (at least as measured by the Maslach Burnout Inventory [MBI]) on standard quality measures might underlie healthcare institutions' relative neglect of physician burnout in their organizational goals, plans, and performance metrics.

While burnout and depression are not the same, their symptoms overlap, they often are comorbid, and either can precede and contribute to the other. Because burnout is less stigmatized than depression, physicians are more likely to accept that they are burnt out than to accept that they are depressed. But misdiagnosing clinical depression as professional burnout can be harmful to a physician-patient as it can delay their getting effective treatment (Oquendo et al., 2019). A depressed physician might indeed be burned out; but effectively treating their depression might end the burnout, and when both conditions are present, focusing on the burnout alone might be ineffective. A clinically depressed physician might be unwilling or unable to make behavioral changes that would improve their work experience or, if they are employed, to address problematic working conditions with their employer. When a burned-out, depressed physician recovers from depression and is still burned out, focusing on the burnout can be essential to preventing a relapse of the depression.

Mild professional burnout is easily distinguished from severe MDD, but there is a large middle zone of syndromes that would meet criteria both for moderate to severe professional burnout and for mild to moderate clinical depression as this book has defined it. In states where physicians are mandated to disclose treatment for any mental disorder, a clinician seeing a physician-patient with such a syndrome faces a dilemma. The patient might do best with antidepressant treatment, but recording a diagnosis of a depressive disorder might subject the patient to involuntary disclosure and a risk of institutional stigma and intrusive, expensive, embarrassing, and unnecessary monitoring by a Physician Health Program (PHP). Labeling the condition as *professional burnout* rather than a *mental disorder* would allow the physician-patient to get help without the penalty of institutional stigma but might discourage the appropriate use of effective biological treatments for depression and might unintentionally encourage the physician-patient to deny that they have a medical illness that might have serious consequences if not treated.

The syndrome of physician burnout has been the subject of thousands of journal articles, with the number increasing every year. There is no definitive consensus on whether burnout is a unidimensional construct or a multidimensional one, and the prevalence of burnout among physicians varies significantly depending on the questionnaire used to assess it and the cutoff point for making a binary judgment that a physician is indeed burnt out.

There is consensus that the one essential element of burnout is physical and emotional exhaustion that is not necessarily associated with other features of clinical depression like anhedonia, changes in sleep or appetite, or negative thoughts. In the original concept of burnout, exhaustion was specifically associated with paid interpersonal work like teaching, social work, or clinical care. The concept was later extended to cover other types of work, ultimately including unpaid work like caring for one's own children.

Research on burnout relies on questionnaire-based instruments to measure the construct. The concept of burnout differs among commonly used measures. Consequently, the relationship of burnout to depression depends on how burnout is measured. All published burnout questionnaires are lists of Likert-type items—statements to which the respondent assigns an ordinal value based either on the frequency with which the situations described by the item are experienced, on how much the item applies to the respondent, on how strongly the respondent agrees with the item, or on how intensely the respondent has a feeling described by the item. Publications on professional burnout will variably refer to respondents as *subjects* or *patients* and the people with whom the professional works as *clients* or *patients*. When standard questionnaires are used in surveys or in clinical settings, language is adapted to the profession and setting of the respondent. In the discussion below, we will consistently use the terms *physician* to refer to the respondent to a questionnaire and *patients* to refer to those the physician serves.

Most publications on burnout in healthcare providers use the MBI to measure burnout (Maslach & Jackson, 1981). Burnout as captured by the MBI has three dimensions: emotional exhaustion (EE), attributed to work; depersonalization (DP), a category comprising alienation from patients and colleagues, cynicism, and lack of empathy; and (a reduced sense of) personal accomplishment (PA). While any burnt-out physician will be exhausted, people with equal levels of exhaustion can vary greatly in their extent of depersonalization. A sense that one's work is meaningful and effective and that one is good at it—elements of PA—is a psychological resource that helps a physician cope with EE, minimize DP, and avoid depression. Many physicians with severe EE do not have a diminished sense of personal accomplishment. Resident physicians, highly prone to EE because of their long work hours and subordinate positions, are relatively unlikely to have a poor sense of professional accomplishment. Most are proud to have come far down the road to mastering their chosen profession and look forward to a rewarding practice when their training is complete. They can ascribe their exhaustion to their circumstances as trainees.

The EE and DP scales of the MBI can be validly approximated for clinical purposes by two single items. The subject is asked "How often do the following statements describe the way you feel about working as a doctor?" Possible responses are *every day* (6), *a few times a week* (5), *once a week* (4), *a few times a month* (3), *once a month or less* (2), *a few times a year* (1), and *never* (0). The two statements are

- I feel burned out from my work.
- I have become more callous toward people since I took this job.

To estimate the score on the EE and DP scales of the MBI, the score on the first of these two items is multiplied by 9 and the score on the second item is multiplied by 5 (West et al., 2009). The correlation of the one-item scores with the scores from the MBI is strong enough that the vast literature on the association of MBI scores with working conditions and the professionals' health and function can be tapped for understanding burnout in a specific organizational context.

Burnout is highly prevalent among physicians in the U.S. (Ford, 2019). In a survey of 9,175 U.S. physicians in 2022, 53% reported being burned out, 23% reported depressed mood, and 4% self-reported clinical depression. Rates of burnout were 63% in women and 46% in men (L. Kane, 2023) Primary care specialties—emergency medicine, internal medicine, pediatrics, ob/gyn, and family medicine, had the highest rates of burnout, while surgical specialties all had burnout prevalence less than 50%. The two specialties with the lowest rates of burnout were pathology and public health. The main causes of burnout in the respondents' opinion were having too many bureaucratic tasks, feeling a lack of respect from coworkers, working too many hours, receiving insufficient compensation, lacking control and autonomy, and dealing with electronic medical records.

A survey of physicians in rural British Columbia using the MBI found that 80% suffered from moderate to severe EE, 61% had moderate to severe DP, and 44% had diminished PA. The European General Practice Research Network Study Group found that 43% of European general practitioners surveyed had high EE, 35% had high DP, and 32% had low PA (Soler et al., 2008; Thommasen et al., 2001). One third of colorectal surgeons in the United Kingdom had a high score on at least one of the three dimensions of burnout (Sharma et al., 2008). The syndrome is ubiquitous, but the prevalence of the full syndrome and of its three components varies across countries and specialties (Lee et al., 2013).

If a person has high scores on EE and DP and has low PA, they are likely to meet the criteria for major depression. However, it is possible for a person to be severely burned out and not depressed. There is a published case report of a burnt-out physician who satisfied criteria for moderately severe burnout on the MBI but had a score of zero on the PHQ-9. The patient, a 50-year-old medical specialist, felt entirely well, without negative thoughts or unhappy feelings, when he was away from work. He had a happy family life and a serious avocation (Messias & Flynn, 2018). The situation recalls the profile of young Japanese salarymen with "modern type depression," who appear to be well when away from work but truly suffer from multiple depressive symptoms when on the job or when anticipating return to work. Modern type depression is described in detail in Chapter 11.

Much more typical of burnt-out physicians than zero on the PHQ-9 are scores of 5 to 9, which suggest mild clinical depression but probably not an MDE. Bianchi et al. (2015) did a comprehensive review of 92 studies of the burnout–depression overlap and concluded that distinction between the two is "conceptually fragile"—one might call burnout "work-related depression" and not be too far off. Both burnout and depression are multidimensional, not categorical.

Most cases of moderate or severe burnout would easily fit the more inclusive definition of clinical depression proposed in Chapter 2.

An overlapping but different perspective on physician burnout is offered by the Oldenburg Burnout Inventory (OBI), also a public domain scale. It has 16 questions, all rated on a scale of 1 (*strongly agree*) to 4 (*strongly disagree*), with half the items reverse-scored to minimize response bias. There are two scales, one measuring work-related exhaustion and the other measuring disengagement. Questions about exhaustion emphasize the relationship to work, such as "I can tolerate the pressure of my work very well" (reverse-scored) and "After my work, I usually feel worn out and weary." Questions about disengagement touch on the meaning of work in a way the questions on the Copenhagen Burnout Inventory (CBI) do not: "This is the only type of work I can imagine myself doing" and "I always find new and interesting aspects in my work" and "It happens more and more often that I talk about my work in a negative way" (reverse-scored). The disengagement scale appears to combine elements of the MBI's concepts of depersonalization and personal accomplishment. The OBI would not accurately measure exhaustion in a physician that was mainly related to demands outside of work like those of childcare. It might also underestimate the suffering of a physician who was dedicated to medicine and scientifically curious but oppressed by their working conditions.

The CBI (Kristensen et al., 2005) was designed to avoid the psychometric weaknesses of the MBI and other preexisting burnout instruments, to focus more narrowly on emotional exhaustion and fatigue, and to be easily translated into different languages and adapted for non-Western cultures. It focuses on measuring the frequency of exhaustion and fatigue and on determining how much they are specifically related to work and how much they affect the physician's relationships with patients. There is no content related to cynicism or loss of empathy or to a diminished sense of PA. In a comparative review of different burnout measures, the CBI got the highest marks for psychometrics (Shoman et al., 2021). However, it has been much less utilized than the MBI in published studies of burnout.

The CBI has respondents rate burnout on a 5-point Likert scale. Frequency questions are rated as *always, often, sometimes, seldom,* or *never/almost never*. Intensity questions are rated as *to a very high degree, to a high degree, somewhat, to a low degree,* and *to a very low degree*. There are three scales—personal burnout, work-related burnout, and client (i.e., patient)–related burnout. The score on each scale is the average of the item scores rather than their sum, so scoring is not disrupted if a respondent leaves an item blank.

Personal burnout is assessed with six frequency-rated items, such as "How often do you feel tired?" and "How often are you physically exhausted?" and

"How often are you emotionally exhausted?" Work-related burnout is assessed with four frequency-rated items and three intensity-rated items. Examples of frequency-rated items are "Do you feel worn out at the end of the working day?" and "Are you exhausted in the morning at the thought of another day at work?" and "Do you have enough energy for family and friends during leisure time?" (reverse-scored). Examples of intensity-related items are "Is your work emotionally exhausting?" and "Does your work frustrate you?" Patient-related burnout is assessed with five frequency-rated items and two intensity-rated items. Examples of the frequency-rated items are "Does it drain your energy to work with patients?" and "Do you feel that you give more than you get back when you work with patients?" The two intensity-rated questions are "Are you tired of working with patients?" and "Do you sometimes wonder how long you will be able to continue working with patients?" Notably, the CBI does not ask whether a physician is treating patients or colleagues insensitively or without empathy or whether they have become cynical about the profession of medicine.

The value of the CBI in distinguishing professional burnout from patient-related burnout was evident in a study of 300 resident physicians at a public sector hospital in Delhi, India. The residents worked an average of 88 hours per week, and two thirds of them reported personal burnout (i.e., exhaustion and fatigue). However, only one sixth had patient-related burnout. As tired as they were, most of the burnt-out residents were energized and rewarded by their work with patients (Dhusia et al., 2019). Medical students doing clinical rotations, even if burnt out by their work, are unlikely to experience patient-related burnout (Armstrong & Reynolds, 2020). A similar dissociation of work-related burnout and patient-related burnout was seen in a survey of 52 child and adolescent psychiatric consultants in Ireland. Thirty-nine of them (75%) had work-related burnout but only 14 (27%) experienced patient-related burnout. Thirty-seven (71%) indicated they would retrain in child psychiatry if they once again had a choice of specialty (McNicholas et al., 2020).

Physicians with a greater workload are, as one would expect, more likely to get exhausted; but they do not necessarily feel tired of working with patients. Positive experiences with patients, including patients' expressions of gratitude, are protective against work-related burnout, as are opportunities for professional development (Scheepers et al., 2020).

Internationally, there is a gender effect on the flavor of physician burnout. Women are more likely than men to be emotionally exhausted but less likely than men to experience patient-related burnout (as described by the CBI) or depersonalization (as described by the MBI) (La Torre et al., 2021).

When a physician-patient (or a medical student-patient) has work-related burnout but not patient-related burnout, it is a good sign that with some combination of changes in work arrangements, treatment of depression if present, and learning new coping strategies will enable them to enjoy their clinical work. When there is prominent patient-related burnout, there is likely to be moderate or severe depression and/or a major career issue like an inappropriate choice of specialty.

Physicians with major demands on their time and energy outside of work can be personally burned out but not have work-related burnout. Likewise, physicians with happy and pleasant lives outside of work can score relatively low on personal burnout but have significant work-related burnout. Physicians who hate aspects of their work that don't involve patient contact—like dealing with administrative issues and documentation—might love their time with patients and have virtually no patient-related burnout. The CBI, or questions extracted from it and asked in a clinical interview, offers insights into the nature of a physician's burnout that are not readily available from the MBI. Also, because it uses both frequency- and intensity-rated questions, it is less sensitive to people's differing communication styles. If a patient scores frequency-rated questions differently from intensity-rated questions about the same construct, they can be asked to explain why. This can give insight into the patient's preferred way to communicate about their emotional experience and inform a choice of a rating scale for measuring response to an antidepressant treatment, resilience training, or modification in working conditions.

Biomarkers of Burnout

Published studies of biomarkers in burnout show its association with altered physiology, but the abnormalities seen vary between studies, with differences partially attributable to characteristics of the populations studied—such as whether they included subjects with comorbid MDD—and partly to how burnout was measured and diagnosed. One study found elevated levels of serum and saliva cortisol, adrenocorticotropic hormone, fasting blood glucose, and hemoglobin A1c in a group of burnt-out medical professionals, suggesting an adrenal stress response with associated glucose intolerance (Deneva et al., 2019; Jonsdottir & Sjörs Dahlman, 2019). Another found elevated hair cortisol in about two thirds of a group of burnt-out parents—but noted that the remainder had normal or even low levels of that biomarker (Brianda et al., 2020). In a study of 25 female ob/gyn clinicians at the Massachusetts General Hospital that used the two-item MBI and assessed hair cortisol and urinary oxytocin as potential biomarkers of burnout, greater EE was significantly correlated with higher hair cortisol levels, while greater DP was significantly correlated with lower hair cortisol levels. Clinicians with a greater sense of engagement in their work and those with a greater sense of connection and community with their colleagues had higher urinary oxytocin levels (Begin et al., 2021). The work suggests that exhausted and stressed physicians can alleviate their stress negatively by DP (lowering a previously elevated cortisol level) or positively, becoming more engaged at work and more connected with their colleagues (raising their oxytocin level). In a group of burned-out physicians who began with elevated salivary cortisol levels mid-day and at the 24-hour nadir, those whose burnout had improved after 4 months of combined psychological and pharmacological treatment showed significantly lower levels than those whose burnout didn't (Pilger et al., 2018). A high-cortisol and low-cortisol type of physician burnout parallels the recognized dichotomy of high-cortisol and low-cortisol MDD.

The Dresden Burnout Study took a longitudinal view of burnout and its biomarkers in healthcare professionals including physicians. Subjects with low vagally mediated heart rate variability at baseline were significantly more likely to have high scores on the EE scale of the MBI one year later, after adjusting for demographics and for both burnout and depressive symptoms at baseline (Wekenborg et al., 2019).

Neuroendocrine and physiologic differences between and among burnt-out people and depressed people suggest it might eventually be feasible to define, using biomarkers, discrete phenotypes of burnout with and without comorbid depression. This would be helpful in conceptualizing and studying treatments for both conditions. Data on sleep architecture and heart rate variability from wearable devices, and self-administered point-of-care biochemical tests, might then facilitate the self-recognition of burnout phenotypes by physicians on the frontlines of care.

Treatment of Physician Burnout

Because burnout often precedes clinical depression, effectively addressing burnout reduces an individual physician's risk of depression and reduces the incidence and prevalence of depression among the physicians in a healthcare organization. Typical but often ineffective organizational responses to burnout have been to provide optional "counseling" and "support" for stressed physicians, encouraging them to take up yoga or meditation, etc. Unsurprisingly, these are not used by most burnt-out doctors. Burnt-out physicians usually feel their schedules are already overloaded and think that their adding another time commitment for participation in a burnout support group or "physician wellness" program will further increase their work–life conflicts. They might also feel embarrassed or inadequate if they publicly acknowledge a need for help by getting counseling, support, or psychoeducation from a source at their home institution. Furthermore, when a hospital or clinic provides counseling and support but does not show any serious concern about improving physicians' working conditions, physicians can feel blamed for a problem that is in large part caused by job strain and other addressable occupational risk factors. A physician's practicing yoga and mindfulness will not resolve work–life conflicts if they have young children and an inflexible clinic schedule, nor will it reverse the emotional effects of a gross mismatch of their expectations of work as a physician and the realities of employment in a clinic that values "productivity" and obsessive documentation in a user-unfriendly EMR system at the expense of face time with patients and work schedules that allow physicians sufficient time for relaxation, recreation, and enjoyable interactions with family, friends, and professional colleagues. Meditation and regular physical exercise can make working under depressing circumstances more bearable, but by themselves they are unlikely to make a job sustainable in the long term if there are unhealthy working conditions and a mismatch of the position with the physician's personal situation and career anchors. In this situation, many physicians—especially younger ones—will ultimately change jobs. Older ones might retire early. Others will opt to practice part-time or give up clinical medicine.

The most successful organizational programs for reducing burnout begin with the leadership of a hospital or clinic adopting burnout as a key performance indicator, measuring it systematically, and making the reduction of burnout a priority (Olson, 2017; Shanafelt & Noseworthy, 2017). In the absence of commitment to a meaningful change in working conditions by the leadership of an organization that employs physicians, the organization's expressed concern about physician well-being is unconvincing.

When the management of the Mayo Clinic made burnout and depression in its physicians a key performance indicator for its executives, it led to management decisions that gave physicians much more control over their daily clinical schedules and disconnected physicians' salaries from the number of patients seen or procedures completed. When physicians could adjust their schedules to address personal and family needs and were explicitly trusted to work efficiently and effectively, they had better work–life balance and felt more respected by clinic managers and more in control of their work lives. These changes led to less burnout and ultimately to less depression (Shanafelt & Noseworthy, 2017). Engaging scribes to document clinical encounters in EMRs and having consistent support for physicians by advanced-practice nurses or physician assistants has been shown to decrease burnout, as has increasing the amount of time physicians have with each of their patients. The extra cost of such efforts can be offset by decreased costs related to physician turnover. The resignation—or disability—of a single full-time physician can cost a clinic a million dollars, after accounting for lost clinical revenue, recruitment costs, and decreased productivity during the orientation and onboarding of a new member of the medical staff (Shanafelt et al., 2017). Perhaps more awareness of the bottom-line impact of physician burnout might eventually move the issue to the "front burner" for financially focused decision makers at hospitals, clinics, and health systems.

Because physicians, especially those in "masculine" specialties, generally do not wish to acknowledge weakness, more of them will participate in anti-burnout/antidepressant activities if they are compulsory for all physicians in their group (e.g., all residents in a subspecialty training program or all physicians in a specialty clinic). Another strategy for addressing burnout at the individual level while minimizing stigma is to have anti-burnout education bundled with non-psychological activities like continuing medical education conferences or financial education seminars.

A Toxic Tetrad of Job Stress: Demand–Control Imbalance, Effort–Reward Imbalance, Organizational Injustice, and Illegitimate Tasks

Whether a distressed physician is simply burnt out, has clinical depression but not major depression, or has a major depressive episode, job stress is a likely contributor. In treating a depressed physician or attempting to prevent depression in a burnt-out physician, it is almost always helpful to understand the sources of the physician's job stress, to what extent they can be modified, and the resources—both external and internal—they might have for managing and coping with the stress.

Social and behavioral sciences have generated three widely cited characterizations of job stress. Each has been linked to an increased risk of incident depression in workers experiencing the stress (Harvey et al., 2017; Siegrist & Wege, 2020). The first, *demand–control imbalance* (DCI) (Karasek, 1979; Karesek, 1998), characterizes jobs in which the worker experiences high psychological demands but does not have sufficient autonomy and decision-making authority to do the work in the most efficient, effective, and sustainable way. The second, *effort–reward imbalance* (ERI), characterizes jobs in which the worker has substantial responsibility, has a high volume and rapid pace of work, and must deal with interruptions and distractions but does not have a commensurate reward in the form of salary, job security, opportunities for promotion, and/or esteem and recognition (Rugulies et al., 2017; Siegrist, 1996; Siegrist & Li, 2016). As illustrated by the 1897 editorial on physician suicide cited above (Legha, 2012), ERI as an attribute of medical practice was described long before the concept was described in the social sciences literature. The third, *organizational injustice*, comprises inequity and unfairness in how authorities within an organization (e.g., managers, supervisors, senior colleagues) treat workers. It includes issues like not including workers in major decisions that affect them, not providing them with timely information, not addressing their legitimate complaints, and not fairly evaluating their performance (Ndjaboué et al., 2012). To these three major categories of job stress can be added a fourth, *illegitimate tasks—* unnecessary or unreasonable work demands that divert workers' time and energy from activities more essential to their jobs (Anskår et al., 2019; Kilponen et al., 2021; Semmer et al., 2015). Workers burdened with illegitimate tasks might need to work overtime to adequately complete the essential tasks of their jobs or might be unable to perform essential tasks at the high standard they expect of themselves. Illegitimate tasks have been associated with increased burnout symptoms in physicians, and the issue is far from trivial. In a survey of Norwegian internists, one in 12 indicated they spent more than 30% of their work time on unreasonable illegitimate tasks (Thun et al., 2018).

Much of the published research on job stress and its consequences concerns employees of large hierarchical organizations like government agencies and multinational corporations. Though historically physicians have been thought of as autonomous professionals and have a corresponding culture, contemporary physicians virtually all practice within an organizational context. Most are now employees of hospitals, clinics, or medium to large group practices; and even those who are not must deal with insurance companies, government agencies, hospital staff leadership, and other entities that can make non-trivial demands on their time and in various ways limit their professional autonomy.

Job stress is almost always relevant in understanding a depressed physician. Even if it is not the cause of the physician's depression, excessive and unhealthy job stress can make it worse, and addressing it can aid the depressed physician's recovery. Analysis of the stress faced by a depressed or burnt-out physician can be aided by the theoretical perspectives of occupational health. Standard questionnaires and ratings of job stress will work—perhaps with minor modification—for assessing job stress in physicians employed in hierarchical organizations like academic medical centers or large clinics. For physicians in other settings, content from job stress questionnaires can be adapted to suggest useful questions for clinical interviews. In the following pages we present examples of the different types of work stress a physician might face and questions from standard job stress questionnaires of evident applicability to medical practice.

Demand–control imbalance (DCI) in medical practice is illustrated by the following two examples:

A primary care physician works in a clinic in a poor urban neighborhood, where he is responsible for the care of hundreds of complex patients with challenging social determinants of health (high demand). He has little say over the length of patient appointments, the availability and qualifications of support staff, documentation procedures, and his personal work schedule (low control).

A pulmonary medicine specialist is called upon by her hospital to work many extra shifts caring for COVID-19 patients in respiratory failure (high demand). She is frequently asked to work overtime with little notice. The hospital has too few ventilators, and there are intermittent shortages of personal protective equipment (low control).

ERI in medical practice is illustrated by the following two examples:

A newly hired academic physician in an internal medicine subspecialty works at a famous teaching hospital in a city with a high cost of living. He has many patients, substantial teaching and supervision duties, new patient appointments too short for optimal patient assessment, and interruptions of office visits by phone calls and pages, and must work after hours to complete EMR documentation tasks. He is expected to compete successfully for research grants and to generate a steady stream of publications in peer-reviewed journals (high effort). As an instructor at the medical school, he has a relatively low salary that is barely adequate to sustain a middle-class lifestyle after he pays high rent for an apartment near the hospital and makes payments on his large educational debt. He feels little respect from senior faculty, unnoticed by colleagues, unsupported by his department chair, and uncertain about ever being promoted. His wife is disappointed by how often his work interferes with their time together (low reward).

An ob/gyn works at a small, poorly funded rural hospital, caring for a large panel of high-risk pregnant women, mostly low-income and lacking insurance or covered by Medicaid. She makes consistent efforts to engage patients in optimal prenatal care and healthy eating habits, encouraging them to keep regular appointments and communicate promptly with her about emerging problems. She makes timely diagnoses of pregnancy complications and quick but wise decisions about interventions and often must carry out urgent procedures like emergency C-sections on short notice (high effort). Her difficult work schedule disrupts her sleep and her plans for recreation on her time off. Medicaid reimbursement for ob/gyn care in her state is low, and some patients cannot pay at all, so her salary from the hospital is much lower than that of a colleague from residency who had joined a group practice in an affluent suburb. Support by nurses, social workers, and dietitians sometimes is unreliable. She feels that the hospital's chief executive officer and colleagues from other specialties don't appreciate how hard she works. Her patients sometimes have poor clinical outcomes despite her best efforts. This is reflected by mediocre scores on standard quality measures that don't adjust for social determinants. The chief of the medical staff has criticized her performance (low reward).

Organizational injustice related to medical practice is illustrated by the following example:

A behavioral neurologist who has worked at a teaching hospital for 20 years has built up a large practice of patients with chronic neurological diseases, while every week evaluating several new patients with cognitive impairment who usually have complex psychosocial and family issues in addition to needing a neurological diagnosis. She is informed suddenly that the clinic administrator has reduced the time allotted for new patient visits from 90 minutes to 60 minutes and the time for follow-up visits from 30 minutes to 20 minutes. In addition, the social worker she has relied on for assistance has been reassigned to a different clinic, and his replacement is a new hire from another city who is not yet familiar with local resources for supporting cognitively impaired patients and their families. Her opinion was not sought before the changes in scheduling and staffing were made, and she was not informed of them in advance of their implementation. Though the changes in visit length implied that she would be seeing a larger volume of patients and would probably need to do documentation at home in the evenings, there was no evident prospect of an increase in salary.

Work–family conflict, an important contributor to depression particularly salient to female physicians with an unequal share of domestic responsibilities in most cultures, was for many women physicians aggravated by new pandemic-related demands at work and at home (Frank et al., 2021; Sriharan et al., 2020). They were, depending on the details of the physician's work, related to all three forms of job stress. For example, a woman's lack of control over her schedule and perhaps of her exposure to COVID-19 contrasted with increased demands for her time and attention at work and at home. Her increased efforts at work and at home were not accompanied by increased pay, access to convenient and free or inexpensive childcare, a more flexible schedule, or special recognition by her supervisors. Hospital administrators making decisions about its COVID-19 response without staff physician input or planning for support of physicians with young children reflected organizational injustice.

Unnecessary illegitimate tasks are exemplified by burdensome documentation that—if truly necessary at all—could be done efficiently by a scribe (or perhaps a robot or an artificial intelligence application) and interactions with pharmaceutical benefit administrators that could easily be handled by a pharmacy assistant serving all the physicians in the same clinic. Another typical unreasonable illegitimate task would be created when, without prior notice or the junior resident's agreement, a senior resident physician signed out early to a junior resident, who in addition to their other activities would have to take on hours of clinical work that the senior resident should have done before leaving the hospital.

Questions for Characterizing Physicians' Job Stress

For research on each of the four types of stressful working conditions, psychometrically validated questionnaires have been developed, and stress identified using them has been linked to depression and other health issues. However, the comprehensive, definitive questionnaires used in social science research usually are impractical for daily use in the clinic. For routine clinical purposes, useful options are asking patients to fill out abbreviated questionnaires with a handful of items or, more typically, using such questionnaires as a source of content for the part of the clinical interview dealing with the physician-patient's working conditions. Often, a clinician can accurately predict the physician-patient's responses to questionnaire items from information in an ordinary clinical interview.

Physician-patients can be screened for DCI with questions adapted from the Demand–Control–Support Questionnaire (Theorell et al., 1988). In the 17-item questionnaire the first five items deal with psychological demands, the next six with decision latitude (skill discretion and decision authority), and the last six with social support at work, a factor that can mitigate the stress associated with DCI. Patients respond to items on a four-point scale, rating frequency for the demand and control items and agreement or disagreement for the social support items. The demand and control items are as follows:

1. Do you have to work very quickly?
2. Do you have to work very intensively?
3. Does your work demand too much effort?
4. Do you have enough time to do everything you need to do?
5. Does your work often involve conflicting demands?
6. Does your work offer you the possibility of learning new things?
7. Does your work demand a high level of skill?
8. Does your work require ingenuity?
9. Is your work boringly repetitive?
10. Do you have a choice in how you do your work?
11. Do you have a choice in deciding what you do at work?

The social support items are as follows:

12. Is there a calm and pleasant atmosphere where you work?
13. Is there good spirit of unity?
14. Are your colleagues there for you?
15. Do your coworkers understand that you can have a bad day?
16. Do you get on well with your superiors?
17. Do you get on well with your colleagues?

Screening for ERI can be done with (or using questions from) a work-stress questionnaire developed by Siegrist, the originator of the ERI model together with German and American colleagues (Siegrist et al., 2010). Each of nine statements is evaluated by the patient, who would indicate if they agreed or disagreed with the statement and, if their answer implied job stress, whether they were not at all distressed, somewhat distressed, distressed, or very distressed by it. Converting the patient's responses to a number from 1 to 5 (the direction of scoring is obvious) and averaging the numbers yields a practical numerical score for ERI.

1. I have constant time pressure due to a heavy workload.
2. I have a lot of responsibility in my job.
3. I have many interruptions and disturbances in my job.
4. Over the past few years, my job has become more and more demanding.
5. The prospects of my future job development are poor.
6. I have experienced or I expect to experience an undesirable change in my work situation.
7. My job security is poor.
8. Considering all my efforts and achievements, I receive the respect and prestige I deserve for my work.
9. Considering all my efforts and achievements, my income is adequate.

While ERI is common among physicians, not all who experience it become burnt out or depressed (Weigl et al., 2015). As with DCI, the psychological effects of ERI can be mitigated by social support and personal resilience. However, pursuing change in one's working conditions or one's job might be called for if ERI has an important role in causing clinical depression.

Questions about organizational justice were assembled by Ndjaboué et al. (2012) from several questionnaires on the theme. In the questions that follow, adapted from their article, there are references to *management* and *supervisors*. In physicians' working environments, the relevant authority might have another name, such as *department chair*, *practice manager*, or *chief resident*. The essential point is that practicing physicians usually are part of a hierarchy—or part of more than one hierarchy. It might be painfully obvious to them, or they might deny or minimize it. Questions about organizational justice deal with relational justice (including justice in sharing information), procedural justice, and distributive justice. If the questions were part of a formal questionnaire, they would be scored on an ordinal scale.

1. Do you get consistent, sufficient, and timely information from management?
2. When you have difficulties at work, is your supervisor usually willing to listen to your problem? Does your supervisor consider your viewpoint?
3. Does your supervisor give you timely feedback on your work? Do you ever get praised for your work? Unfairly criticized?
4. Is your supervisor honest with you?

5. Are procedures for decision-making at your workplace designed to:
   a. Hear the concerns of all who will be affected?
   b. Consider the interests of all who will be affected?
   c. Provide opportunities for decisions to be appealed or challenged?
6. Are procedures designed to promote the consistency of decisions with one another?
7. Do procedures include providing workers with explanations of what was decided and why?
8. Has your employer (hospital, clinic, medical school, group practice) been fair in rewarding you considering:
   a. The amount of education and training you've had?
   b. Your job responsibilities?
   c. The work you've done and the efforts it's required?
   d. The stresses and strains of your job?
9. Considering the volume and difficulty of the work you do compared with that of your colleagues, do you think your salary is fair? Do you feel adequately appreciated for the work you do?

The overlap in content with questions about ERI is clear. One perspective emphasizes the result, the other the process for getting there.

Illegitimate tasks can be assessed with the eight questions of the Bern Illegitimate Tasks Scale, four about unnecessary tasks and four about unreasonable ones (Semmer et al., 2015). They would be answered on an ordinal scale measuring the frequency with which the tasks are required. The questions can be paraphrased as follows:

1. Do you have work tasks to take care of about which you question:
   a. If they need to be done at all?
   b. If they make sense at all?
   c. If they wouldn't exist, or could be done with less effort, if work were organized differently?
   d. If they wouldn't exist, or could be done with less effort, if some other people made fewer mistakes?
2. Do you have work tasks to take care of that:
   a. You think should be done by someone else?
   b. You feel should not be expected of you?
   c. Put you in an awkward position?
   d. It is unfair to expect you to do?

If a depressed physician-patient is dealing with severe job stress, the clinical context will determine whether it should be an explicit focus of their initial treatment and whether the emphasis will be on modifying or changing their job or on adapting in a healthier way to their working conditions. In the case of a physician in training, a theme in psychotherapy might be evaluating post-training work opportunities with their mental health in mind.

Moral Injury on the Clinical Battlefield

An additional occupational hazard of medical practice—also associated with emotional distress and with clinical depression—is *moral injury*. The concept of moral injury was initially introduced to describe the emotional suffering of soldiers who had been forced by their superiors' orders or the circumstances of combat to participate in or to witness actions that violated their standards of righteous conduct. Two phrases that capture the idea are "perpetrating, failing to prevent, bearing witness to, or learning about acts that transgress deeply held moral beliefs and expectations" (Litz et al., 2009) and "betrayal by a leader or trusted authority" (Shay, 2014). The concept of moral injury was subsequently extended to other professions with responsibility for the life and welfare of others—including physicians (Day et al., 2022).

Early in the COVID-19 pandemic in the U.S. there were shortages of ventilators and of personal protective equipment. Physicians had to deny ventilatory support to patients who would have received it under normal conditions, and when some of those patients died many of the doctors involved felt guilty and ashamed of their decisions. When there was insufficient personal protective equipment in hospitals, physicians would be exposed to SARS-CoV-2 in the hospital, then return home to family members and put them at risk for infection. If their family members did fall ill with COVID-19, physicians might be unable to forgive themselves for having harmed their loved ones.

Moral injury also can occur in the context of a physician's giving a patient a treatment other than their first choice because of financial or administrative constraints or to avoid a burdensome process of seeking a third party's authorization of the treatment they would prefer. If the patient rejects the treatment, doesn't adhere to it, or can't tolerate it and the outcome is life-threatening or disabling, the physician might feel painfully guilty or ashamed. Representative examples would be the suicide of a patient who did not receive an expensive antidepressant treatment more likely to be effective, the death from metastatic cancer of a patient who did not receive a potentially life-saving immunotherapy, or the long-term disability of an injury victim who was denied a trial of intensive inpatient rehabilitation.

In a more mundane way, physicians can experience moral injury when they become so caught up in administrative duties, record-keeping, and managing an overwhelming case load that they don't give their patients the time, attention, and empathy they feel they should. If their patients recurrently miss appointments, don't fill prescriptions, and have many potentially preventable emergency department visits and hospitalizations, they can lose faith in the basic rightness of their clinical work.

As there are rating scales for the different dimensions of job stress, there is a rating scale for moral injury in health professionals, The Moral Injury Symptoms Scale of Health Professionals (MISS-HP; Mantri et al., 2020). When it uncovers moral injury as a major issue for a physician with symptoms of depression, the issues identified should be addressed in psychotherapy. There might be a potentially remediable occupational situation related to the moral injury, and dealing with it can be a healing experience for the physician involved. Moral injury is strongly associated with burnout and thus with depression, but the three concepts are different and can exist independently of each other. Dealing with moral injury, like dealing with burnout, can prevent subclinical depression from getting worse. Generic measures for reducing burnout do not address moral injury and are unlikely to help a physician for whom the latter is the main issue.

The MISS-HP has 10 statements, each rated on a scale of 1 to 10—*strongly disagree* to *strongly agree*—with 5 and 6 being neutral scores. These are followed by a question about the relationship of the symptoms of moral injury to distress and/or impairment in occupational function, social functioning, and/or taking care of business at home, rated on a five-point scale from *not at all* to *extremely*. If a physician feels moderate or worse distress or impairment, the inference is that moral injury is a problem in need of attention. The items with which the physician agrees most strongly can be the point of departure for psychotherapeutic treatment of a depressed physician-patient. The last two questions touch on negative versus positive religious coping and are especially relevant to physician-patients for whom religion is an important dimension of personal identity.

The MISS-HP (Mantri et al., 2020):

1. I feel betrayed by other health professionals whom I once trusted.
2. I feel guilt over failing to save someone from being seriously injured or dying.
3. I feel ashamed about what I've done or not done when providing care to my patients.
4. I am troubled by having acted in ways that violated my own morals or values.
5. Most people with whom I work as a health professional are trustworthy. (reverse-scored)

6. I have a good sense of what makes my life meaningful as a health professional. (reverse-scored)
7. I have forgiven myself for what's happened to me or to others whom I have cared for. (reverse-scored)
8. All in all, I am inclined to feel I'm a failure in my work as a health professional.
9. I sometimes feel God is punishing me for what I've done or not done while caring for patients.
10. Compared to before I went through these experiences, my religious/spiritual faith has strengthened. (reverse-scored)

Like burnout, moral injury can occur concurrently with clinical depression, and when this occurs, the patient will do best with simultaneous treatment—addressing the issue of moral injury with a psychotherapeutic or spiritual intervention, while treating the depression medically. To do this, moral injury should be distinguished from burnout (Kopacz et al., 2019). Furthermore, efforts toward organizational change will have a different focus if preventing moral injury, rather than preventing or mitigating burnout, is the object. Day et al. (2021), in an exploration of physician moral injury that criticized *burnout* as an often facile description of physicians' distress, noted the sobering conclusion of a meta-analysis of resiliency training to address physician burnout: "a small to moderate effect," with "low confidence" (Leppin et al., 2014).

Two reasons for disappointing results of resiliency training are that burnout is fundamentally a problem of healthcare organizations rather than one of individual physicians and that suffering due to moral injury is misattributed to burnout. Optimally addressing moral injury requires the clinician's treating the physician's depression and/or PTSD if present, the morally injured physician's finding support in a social network that shares similar moral values, and the organization(s) involved addressing the circumstances that led to the event or events causing the moral injury.

Physicians and Financial Stress

In the United States, debt related to higher education is becoming a national crisis. Early-career physicians are especially likely to have a high debt burden because most have had eight or more years of higher education. Those who borrowed money to finance their education thus might combine undergraduate debt with medical school debt, with undergraduate debt accumulating interest as additional debt was added. Of the 16,657 respondents to a 2019 survey of 19,933 graduating medical students (83.6% response rate) conducted by the American Association of Medical Colleges, 73% reported graduating with debt.

Of those who owed, the median amount was $200,000, and students in the top third owed $247,000 or more. Debt burden was lowest for Asian Americans, of whom 61% had education debt with a median amount of $180,000. It was highest for Black Americans, of whom 91% had education debt with a median amount of $230,000. The difference in part reflected Asian students having a higher contribution by family members to the financing of their medical education. In this respect, early-career Asian physicians tend to have greater interpersonal indebtedness, while early career Black physicians have greater financial indebtedness. Among the 8% of medical school graduates with dependents, 79% had educational debt and 38% had non-mortgage, non-educational debt; 48% of the graduating students endorsed income expectations as a moderate or strong influence on their choice of specialty, and 22% endorsed their education debt as a moderate or strong influence on their choice (Youngclaus & Fresne, 2020).

If a new physician with $200,000 in debt at graduation chose to defer payment on their education debt until completing residency, debt repayment after beginning practice would be $3000 per month or more, depending on the length of post-MD training. The total repayment with interest might be $400,000 or more, and repayment would take at least 10 years. Thus, many U.S. physicians will be spending more than 10% of their income on education debt repayments, well into their 40s.

An early-career physician who is starting a family while living comfortably—but not luxuriously—in an area with a high cost of living and/or high state and local taxes might struggle to service their debts. They might opt to work more hours and see more patients in their practice or to take a secondary job like moonlighting in an emergency room or being a physician on call to a hospital inpatient service on weekends and holidays. Doing this can lead to severe work–life imbalance and/or to sleep deprivation with its well-known adverse effects on cognitive performance, mood, and driving safety as well as patient care. In the setting of the COVID-19 pandemic, it might have entailed additional exposure to the coronavirus. Because of financial insecurity, early-career physicians might choose to delay having children for additional years beyond delays made to accommodate their medical education and specialty training. When their debt is paid off, or their salaries make their debt less consequential, they might face problems with infertility. The issue of debt can become especially distressing if a physician requires time off work or must reduce work hours because of their own physical or mental health issues or the illness of a family member. Separation or divorce greatly increases the risk of depression and often is expensive. For a resident or early-career physician with substantial debt, the added financial stress associated with the dissolution of a marriage can be overwhelming.

Physicians sometimes lack financial literacy commensurate with their salaries and educational attainment. This can lead to their making inadequate provision for retirement. A physician of late middle age who is burnt out, declining in skill, or simply tired of practice might find that retirement is not a financially feasible option. Depression is a likely consequence. Some medical centers offer seminars for their staff physicians that provide information and advice about personal finance, including managing debt, planning for retirement, and saving and investment strategy. Because there is no stigma in attending them, they are appropriate venues for introducing other issues related to physicians' well-being.

Inquiring about financial concerns if they are not brought up spontaneously by a physician-patient can reveal an important issue to be addressed in psychotherapy and sometimes by a referral for financial counseling. For many people, talking about money matters is more difficult than talking about once-taboo topics like their sexual lives. It is sometimes useful to normalize the topic by noting that many physicians have financial concerns that contribute to their stress. For example, early in the COVID-19 pandemic many physicians in private practice experienced a decrease in patient volume, some independent private practices closed, surgeons in specialties like cosmetic surgery performed fewer elective procedures, and many employed physicians experienced reductions in their salaries.

Stigma and Its Consequences

Many physicians suffer from persistent low mood or clinical depression and recognize it, but most of them do not seek help from a psychiatrist, psychotherapist, or non-psychiatrist physician. In a 2018 anonymous survey of 15,069 American physicians concerning burnout and depression, fewer than half of those with depression reported seeking help (L. Kane, 2019a). In the six countries of the Medscape international survey, fewer than 20% of physicians with burnout or depression sought professional help or planned to do so. Physicians' most frequent reasons for not seeking help were thinking their symptoms weren't severe enough and thinking they could handle the situation themselves. Except in Spain, 30% or more of the depressed and/or burnt-out physicians thought they didn't have the time for treatment. Risk of disclosure of their condition was a significant concern in the United States and the United Kingdom. Despite their reluctance to seek treatment, most of the depressed physicians saw depression as a medical problem. In all countries but the United Kingdom, psychiatrists were the preferred source of help (Locke, 2019).

These responses reflect the high prevalence among practicing physicians of three ideas about depression. The first is that depression, apart from cases of severe, disabling melancholia, psychotic depression, and obvious "mental illness," is a condition for which treatment is optional and for which delaying treatment is not harmful. The second is that physicians with mild to moderate depression ought to be able to tolerate its symptoms and not need any treatment. The third is that one's reputation might be damaged if it were known that they were diagnosed with MDD or a related condition and treated for it by a psychiatrist. Some physicians in the Medscape survey reported traveling an hour or more to see a psychiatrist outside the community in which they practice and paying cash for treatment so that their health insurance company would not know they had been depressed. In a 2005 study, 5000 physicians in Michigan were sent the PHQ-9 along with additional questions about their attitudes toward depression and its treatment. Of the 1154 who replied, 11.3% had moderate to severe depression (PHQ-9 ≥10). Although 57.7% of those with moderate to severe depression thought their condition decreased their work productivity and 90.8% thought it reduced their work satisfaction, fewer than half were willing to seek treatment: 50.7% had concerns about confidentiality, and 30.0% would consider self-prescribing antidepressants (Schwenk et al., 2008). In the 2018 Medscape survey, 7% of those who received mental health care pursued "secret treatment," for example, by seeing a therapist in a different town, or by seeking care under a different name (L. Kane, 2019a).

The stigma of depression might be worse among physicians than in the general population despite their having learned about depression as an illness during medical school and perhaps again during their residency. Stigma is widespread among medical students of the millennial generation, despite their exposure to anti-stigma messaging on social media. A 2009 survey on depression and its stigma in students at the University of Michigan medical school provides evidence. A web-based survey on depression was sent to 769 students, of whom 505 responded, constituting a sample representative of the overall student body with respect to ethnic background, class year, and standing in their class. 14.3% of subjects had a PHQ-9 score ≥10, 5.0% of the entire sample had a current diagnosis of depression, and 7.0% were currently receiving treatment for depression. Thus, most students with moderate to severe depressive symptoms—and thus an 88% probability of major depression—were not diagnosed and not treated. The lifetime rates of depression diagnosis and antidepressant treatment reported by respondents were 14.7% and 18.2%, respectively. These numbers imply that many medical students had received antidepressants but denied that they had been diagnosed with depression. While it is possible they had received antidepressants for a different indication than depression, it is likely that the students reporting treatment without diagnosis were simply uncomfortable labeling themselves as depressed—even in the past.

Survey respondents answered 27 questions about depression and its stigma: 95% of respondents agreed that depression is a "real medical illness," and only 2.6% thought a medical student with depression could "snap out of it if they wanted to do so." Nonetheless, 7.9% of the respondents saw depression as "a sign of personal weakness," and another 16% neither agreed nor disagreed with that view. 15.8% agreed with the statement that a medical student's seeing a counselor is admitting that they are unable to handle the stress of medical school; 67.5% agreed that "If I were depressed, I would be unable to complete medical school tasks and responsibilities as well as other students"; and 16.2% agreed or strongly agreed with the statement that "Medical students with depression are dangerous to their patients." Only half of the sample agreed with the statement that "Medical students with depression are not to blame for their problems" (Schwenk et al., 2010).

Expectations of public stigma were widespread: Many respondents who personally had no negative views about depressed medical students endorsed statements about negative consequences of being open about a diagnosis or treatment of depression. More than half of the sample agreed with the following statements: "Most people believe that depressed medical students would provide inferior treatment to their patients"; "If I were depressed, I would worry that I would miss out on educational opportunities"; "If I were depressed and applying to a residency, my application would be less competitive than that of a student who does not have depression"; and "If I were depressed, it would be risky to reveal my depression on my residency application." Only 30.3% agreed that "If I were depressed, I would tell my medical student friends." Medical students who themselves had moderate or severe current symptoms of depression were significantly more likely to endorse items describing expected public stigma.

The survey results convey a sense of a profession still in the process of adopting a modern view of depression. While students said—reflecting either belief or knowledge of what they ought to believe—that depression was a real illness for which a person was not to blame, most would feel ashamed or embarrassed if they were depressed, and most would expect to face discrimination from other medical students, teachers, patients, and selection committees of residency training programs. More than two thirds would be reluctant to let a friend know that they were depressed. A depressed medical student who had such expectations would be unlikely to get either treatment or emotional support from classmates.

Medical students are exposed not only to formal teaching about psychiatric illness but also to a "hidden curriculum" of casual and often inappropriate comments made by resident physicians, attending physicians, and faculty. Disparagement and devaluation of psychiatrists, psychiatry, and patients with mental disorders is a common component of that hidden curriculum (Dyrbye et al., 2015; Lawrence et al., 2018; Mahood, 2011). In a US–UK survey, most medical students reported hearing residents and academic physicians making negative comments about psychiatrists (Ajaz et al., 2016). The lessons of the hidden curriculum often discourage medical students with an interest in psychiatry from pursuing training in the specialty. The broad knowledge and competencies of well-trained psychiatrists, the rigors of psychiatric residency education, and the scientific accomplishments of leading psychiatrists are ignored.

Another source of self-stigma and cause for avoidance of treatment in depressed physicians is emotional difficulty in accepting the patient role. Doctors' difficulty in becoming patients applies not only to psychiatric conditions but to illness in general. Complaining of symptoms or functional limitations is contrary to the physician culture of stoicism and persistence in serving patients despite personal adversity. Furthermore, being a patient implies a loss of autonomy and control. Physician-patients might need to accept inconvenient times for appointments, wait to be seen, receive a diagnosis other than the one they expect, or adhere to a treatment other than the one they might prescribe for one of their patients. If the treating doctor lacks empathy, a physician-patient might feel humiliated by the disappointing behavior of their professional colleague.

Stigmatizing Policies of Medical Licensing Boards and PHPs

With respect to institutional stigma, two thirds of U.S. states (including the District of Columbia) require that physicians seeking initial licensure and/or renewal of licensure disclose to the state's medical licensing board (MLB) any history of treatment for mental illness, even if the condition did not cause impairment of the physician's ability to practice and/or the condition is currently remitted or resolved. Such questions are non-compliant with the Americans with Disabilities Act (Lawson & Boyd, 2018a). Several states' MLBs publish guidelines for identifying physicians potentially impaired by mental disorders and in need of treatment supervised by a PHP that reports to the board. They recommend that physicians report to the MLB the names of colleagues who display symptoms and signs of concern. Unfortunately, the criteria published by some state boards are shocking in their breadth and non-specificity, such as encouraging physicians to report a colleague to the MLB if their spouse is receiving therapy or taking psychoactive drugs or if their documentation is often late (Gold et al., 2017; Jones et al., 2018).

In a study with provocative conclusions, members of the general population employed full-time were given 25 descriptions of potential impairment taken from state MLB websites and asked whether the statements applied to them. Even when the statements were worded narrowly, 70.9% of respondents endorsed at least one description of impairment, and 59.2% endorsed more than one (Lawson & Boyd, 2018b). An appendix to the paper presents actual items from 23 state MLB websites, showing the extraordinary breadth of many MLBs' reasons for "concern." A physician's complaining to a colleague of fatigue, insomnia, or low mood is among the triggers for potential referral in some states.

Over-inclusive referral guidelines and intrusive monitoring programs have effects opposite to their intentions. By increasing institutional stigma, they exacerbate internalized stigma, making depressed physicians even more miserable at the same time as making them extremely reluctant to openly seek help or disclose their diagnoses and treatment. Forty percent of American physicians surveyed in 2014 said they would be reluctant to seek formal medical care for a mental health condition because of concerns about negative effects on their medical licensure. Physicians from states with licensing applications non-compliant with the Americans with Disabilities Act were significantly more likely to have such concerns (Dyrbye et al., 2017). In a 2016 survey on a closed Facebook group of women physicians who also were mothers, 47% of respondents had been diagnosed and/or treated for a mental disorder, but only 6% of those had reported their illness to a state MLB. Of those who were diagnosed but not treated, 44% gave licensing requirements as a reason for not seeking treatment (Gold et al., 2016).

America's MLBs have a history of prejudice against physicians with mental disorders. A 2007 survey of MLB executive directors received responses from 35 states; 13 (37%) of the executive directors answered yes to the questions "Is the diagnosis of mental illness sufficient for sanctioning by the board?" and "Does the state medical board deal differently with physicians receiving psychiatric vs. medical care?" Follow-up interviews with MLB directors established that a physician who was impaired by their illness would "eventually be allowed to have an unrestricted license." However, the physician might be expected to refrain from practice during the investigation, to disclose highly personal information, and/or to pay substantial fees for evaluations duplicative of those they had already had in connection with their clinical care. The process not only can cause distress for the physicians who experience it but can "diffuse fear of seeking treatment throughout the profession, even in states that have no such policies" (Hendin et al., 2007). The concerns identified in the 2007 study have persisted to the present.

If a physician acknowledged a history of treatment for depression or BD, some states would require them, as a condition of licensure, to have ongoing re-evaluations separate from whatever treatment they were getting for the condition. The physician might have no say in the choice of the examining psychiatrist, might be assessed a large fee not covered by insurance, and might have no right to challenge the official evaluation even if it were discrepant with a well-established psychiatric and medical history (Lenzer, 2016). The physician would be required to consent to full disclosure of all medical and psychotherapy records to a review panel that might include physicians with no psychiatric expertise. Such expensive, embarrassing, and unnecessary requirements discourage physicians from getting treatment for depression in the first place. Ironically, many of the states with non-compliant MLB policies have shortages of physicians, but their policies would discourage a highly skilled physician with a history of psychiatric treatment—even far in the past—from practicing there.

PHPs are organizations entrusted by states' medical licensing authorities to address physician impairment or incompetence due to substance abuse or other health problems. They began with an exclusive focus on physicians impaired by substance abuse but now deal with a broader range of problems, including major psychiatric illness. They are empowered by MLBs. They can be independent organizations (usually, but not always, non-profit) or units of state medical societies. PHPs overall have a success rate of approximately 75% in helping physicians of various specialties with substance use disorders remain abstinent and continue in practice in the long term (five years or more; Domino et al., 2005; DuPont et al., 2009; McLellan et al., 2008; Weenink et al., 2017). Their success probably derives from the combination of intensive and persistent treatment and a requirement that the physician adhere to treatment if they want to continue practicing medicine. PHPs are less consistently successful with physicians who have problems other than substance use disorders. Further, the rigid policies and intrusive interventions developed for functionally impaired physicians under investigation by MLBs often are inappropriate for a physician who voluntarily presents to the PHP seeking help for depression or suicidality, for whom there had never been a question of their practicing while impaired. While few depressed physicians would report themselves to a PHP, the potential for official humiliation is a powerful deterrent to their openly seeking treatment—one that contributes to both public and internalized stigma.

There are many accounts in the press and social media of physicians with histories of depression whose careers were severely disrupted by PHPs and

MLBs, despite their mood disorders being well treated and their having no impairment of professional performance (Miller, 2017; Randhawa, 2019; Wible, 2015). Once the physician engaged with the PHP, they would be deemed "noncompliant" if they did not agree with the PHP on the plan of care. The PHP would inform the state MLB, putting the physician's license and livelihood at risk. For example, the PHP could require five years of drug testing and monitoring visits for a physician with depression who had never had a substance use problem. It could require that a depressed physician have a month of costly inpatient care not covered by insurance, rather than the outpatient treatment that was recommended by the physician's treating psychiatrist, preferred by the physician, covered by insurance, and delivered at times that did not interfere with the physician's own clinical practice.

Several MLBs do not permit physicians with histories of depression or bipolar illness to speak for themselves in front of the review panels, even though the PHP might have erred in its appraisal of their mental health and demanded inappropriate or unnecessary treatment. Because of the special relationship of PHPs to MLBs, a physician's conflicting with the state PHP can cause lifetime career issues. Actions of state MLBs are entered into a national database that is accessible by all other states' licensing boards and all potential employers. Many physicians are afraid to defy a PHP, right or wrong, because of potentially dire professional and financial consequences.

Emerging concerns about PHPs, including those related to confidentiality and potential conflicts of interest, were addressed in depth in 2017 in a resource document on recommended best practices authored by a work group of the American Psychiatric Association's Council on Psychiatry and the Law (Recupero et al., 2017). The work group emphasized that physicians voluntarily seeking help for depression (or other mental disorders unrelated to substance use) differ in important ways from those mandated by a state MLB to receive treatment for substance use disorders with associated functional impairment. Physicians who turn to a PHP—or are referred to one by a colleague—for help in managing depression should not be required by the PHP to undergo clinically unnecessary hospitalizations at substance abuse treatment facilities, as some have been obliged to do. The PHP should not share information about the depressed physician with the state MLB unless the physician is unable to practice competently because of their depression and refuses to voluntarily refrain from practicing until their health has improved and full professional competence is regained. When the PHP recommends sources of clinical treatment, the depressed physician should be offered multiple options, outpatient whenever possible, located in places the physician finds suitable, and covered by the physician's health insurance if possible. Any evaluations conducted by the PHP should be fully and immediately available to the physician for review, and if the PHP communicates with the MLB, the physician should have the opportunity to see the communication in advance and comment upon it if they disagree. Any referral the PHP makes for a professional service of any kind should be free from conflicts of interest—or even the appearance of such conflicts. Essentially, the PHP would provide confidential referrals, care coordination, and encouragement for the depressed physician to persist with treatment, rather than deliver coercive monitoring on behalf of the state MLB.

Substance Abuse

Many depressed, burnt-out, sleepless or otherwise distressed physicians self-medicate with alcohol or, less commonly, other psychoactive substances like opioids or cannabis. The rate of alcohol use disorders in practicing physicians exceeds 10%. In a survey of 7288 American physicians of all specialties, 12.9% of male physicians and 21.4% of female physicians met the diagnostic criteria for an alcohol use disorder (Oreskovich et al., 2015). The higher prevalence of substance use disorders in female physicians is remarkable because in the general population the age-standardized prevalence of alcohol use disorders is 1.79 times higher for men than for women (IHME, 2023). Women who were married or partnered but without children had an especially high risk of alcohol abuse or dependence. Physicians working 40 to 60 hours per week had higher risk than those working less than 40 or more than 60. Dermatology, orthopedic surgery, and emergency medicine were associated with a higher prevalence of alcohol use disorders, while neurology, pediatrics, and subspecialties of internal medicine had lower rates. Anesthesiologists have a unique vulnerability to abuse of legal drugs including opioids (Bryson, 2018).

Physicians identified as having substance use disorders usually do not lose their practice privileges but are required, as a condition of licensure, to abstain from alcohol and drugs of abuse, to appear for counseling or support groups, and to submit to testing to ensure abstinence. Some states impose mandatory inpatient alcohol and drug rehabilitation. The stigma associated with substance use disorders in physicians is not necessarily greater than the stigma associated with depression—and in some communities it might be lesser.

In the U.S., most states' PHPs focus on doctors with substance use disorders rather than those with primary depression or BD without comorbid substance abuse. This is the main reason many depressed physicians referred to such programs feel out of place. When a physician with both a substance use problem and a mood disorder is treated by a clinician or facility focused on treating substance abuse, the mood disorder might be undiagnosed, misattributed, or inadequately treated. In this situation a physician now abstaining from alcohol or drugs might experience severe depressive symptoms that could lead to suicidal despair.

A disclosed history of diagnosed and treated depression might also be a disadvantage for a physician applying for a competitive position as a subspecialty trainee or as a junior member of (and future partner in) a prominent and successful private practice. When fictional medical students' résumés were sent to residency training directors that were similar except for one's mentioning a history of "psychological counseling," the applicant with the counseling history was significantly less likely to be invited for an interview. Thus, there was institutional stigma even when there was no formal psychiatric diagnosis recorded, no impairment documented, and no medication involved. Women physicians who become mothers during their residency training might develop postpartum depression but be reluctant to obtain treatment for it because of concern about damage to their subsequent careers.

Clinical Care of Physicians with Depression or Bipolar Disorder

While physicians worldwide have increased rates of depression and of death by suicide, it is not clear that they are especially vulnerable to BD. Uncontrolled bipolar I disorder (BD-I) is incompatible with the safe and competent practice of the medical profession, but BD-I well controlled on medication might not be disabling. As with eminent creative professionals, physicians having bipolar II disorder (BD-II) and other disorders in the bipolar spectrum might have acceptable professional performance even if their moods are not completely stabilized with treatment. A hyperthymic physician without impaired judgment might be extraordinarily productive, treating a high volume of patients, publishing prolifically in medical journals, and/or making significant scientific discoveries. The greatest risks for medical practice by bipolar physicians are impaired function, accompanied by a lack of insight into the impairment, and comorbid substance use.

The percentage of people with recurrent depression who have an illness in the bipolar spectrum is not known; but there is general agreement that it is at least 5%, and it is likely that the percentage is substantially higher for depressed patients who see psychiatrists, as such patients are more likely to have illnesses that are either recurrent, severe, atypical in some way, or poorly responsive to first-line treatments (Angst et al., 2011). Bipolar patients spend more time in depressed and euthymic states than they do in manic or hypomanic states, and they usually present with depression or a mixed state with prominent depressive features.

The standard of practice in psychiatry is to carefully question new patients with depression about past symptoms suggestive of hypomania. In the case of physicians, hyperactivity with diminished sleep is an occupational requirement at times during their training. The overlap of symptoms with occupational experiences can make a bipolar diagnosis difficult in less severe cases.

The use of questionnaires like the 32-item Hypomania Checklist (HCL-32) can be especially helpful in screening a depressed physician for evidence of bipolarity. Numerous questions on the HCL-32 relate to behavior not easily linked to the physician's occupational circumstances and activities. However, because a physician-patient will understand the purpose of the HCL-32 and will be aware of the stigma of bipolar illness, they might deny or minimize symptoms. The clinician treating the physician-patient can minimize the problem by introducing the concept of a bipolar spectrum with milder, non-disabling symptoms far from "mental illness" but highly relevant to the choice of treatment for depression and to protecting the patient from serious and preventable side effects of antidepressant treatment. The physician-patient can be told that antidepressant-induced hypomania can have serious personal and professional consequences for a physician, and it can be avoided by using a mood stabilizer first in treating a patient with bipolar depression or depression with mixed features.

While it is unknown whether physicians have more BD than the general population, it is a reasonable hypothesis because the rate of depression is elevated in physicians, and there is little reason to think that the proportion of depressed patients who are bipolar is lower among depressed physicians. Avoidance of psychiatric care is especially problematic when a depressed physician is bipolar because a hypomanic episode can have serious professional consequences and because untreated BD is a risk factor for substance use disorders and for suicide. Physicians who present for care with symptoms of depression or of bipolar spectrum disorders will virtually always have job-related stress. Job stress should be considered by the treating clinician even when a major life event unrelated to work preceded the onset of the depression and even when the physician-patient has a predisposition to depression based on genetics or a personal history of early loss or trauma. Listening for references to job-related stressors and symptoms of burnout, acknowledging them, asking for details, and not normalizing them helps a psychiatrist establish an empathetic relationship with a physician-patient and begins to address a physician's self-stigma if it is present. A psychiatrist can make clear that even a strong, stoic, and adaptable person can develop symptoms if a job combines toxic working conditions, high demand, a lack of control, an imbalance of effort and reward, a lack of social support, and perhaps the burden of illegitimate tasks. It should not be assumed that if the physician were resilient enough, they would be symptom-free with no change in the objective circumstances of their work. Sometimes it is feasible for a burnt-out physician, perhaps together with colleagues, to directly pursue organizational change or report mistreatment such as bullying or harassment. When organizational change isn't feasible, and individual coping strategies aren't enough to manage job strain, it might be appropriate for the physician to consider changing or modifying their job. This would not necessarily involve changing employers or moving geographically. A simple example would be a physician changing their work schedule from five days to four days per week.

When depressive symptoms are job-related, the physician-patient's career anchors should be assessed informally, and the question should be asked whether their current job description is compatible with them. This might open a fruitful discussion of possible job modification or job change. Work–life conflicts might be addressed similarly. A physician (usually, but not always, female) might have unrealistic expectations for equally outstanding performance at work and at home. There might be too much expected at work and not enough support at home, and the imbalance might be addressable by practical changes, for example, making different childcare arrangements, hiring domestic help, or negotiating changes in the division of household responsibilities within a couple. Regarding the last point, the cultural background of the patient and her spouse or partner might constrain the options for change unless cultural gender role issues are identified and discussed. Substance abuse, binge eating, compulsive overwork with insufficient sleep, and other risky or unhealthy coping strategies should be identified. Because the dominant culture of physicians puts patients' welfare ahead of one's own, it should not be assumed that a physician-patient's having a reputation for excellent clinical work rules out an unhealthy lifestyle, self-destructive behavior, or neglect of their personal general medical problems.

A physician, despite their medical education, might not fully understand and accept the concept of depression as an illness. Some depressed non-psychiatric physicians need to be taught about depression. Medical school psychiatry courses do not successfully destigmatize depression for all students. If medical students were not interested in psychiatry in medical school, they might persist in having major misconceptions about the causes, consequences, treatment, and prognosis of depression and/or BD. If a depressed physician-patient has misconceptions about the illness, these should be addressed systematically. Knowledge gaps and misconceptions might be framed as getting up to date on a field of medicine in which there has been much recent progress.

Depressed physicians also should be carefully screened for chronic general medical conditions, and the status of known or newly diagnosed diseases should be reviewed. Because the dominant culture of physicians supports their working despite being ill themselves, depressed physicians might ignore or minimize the symptoms of general medical illness. They might lack diligence in caring for their own chronic diseases, either because they minimize them or because they don't feel they have the time. The scenario of general medical illness presenting with depression is common in midlife, and physicians are not immune to it.

In some cases, chronically depressed physicians pointedly neglect their own healthcare despite continual reminders of the potential consequences of doing so. A dysthymic pathologist working at a cancer specialty hospital might forgo mammograms, Pap smears, and screening colonoscopy; or a surgeon with BD-II might not adhere to treatment of high low-density lipoprotein cholesterol and mild hypertension. Part of a comprehensive clinical assessment of a depressed physician includes inquiry about the patient's health maintenance, including cancer screening and the identification and management of cardiovascular risk factors like hypertension, hyperlipidemia, and glucose intolerance. Self-neglect despite expert knowledge can be evidence of depression-related impairment in judgment. Attention to their neglected medical issues might help engage a physician in a therapeutic relationship. Effectively treating previously neglected medical problems sometimes helps the patient's mood or augments the effect of biologic and/or psychotherapeutic treatment for depression.

Surgical specialists, of either gender, working in a masculine profession that values toughness and stoicism and tends to accept bullying of subordinates by superiors, might display the syndrome of "male depression," in which irritability, anger, risk-taking behavior, and substance abuse are more frequent symptoms than sad or depressed mood (Cavanagh et al., 2017; Martin et al., 2013). In such cases, initially focusing on issues like self-control, avoiding embarrassment, and preserving or enhancing function can be more effective than beginning treatment with an emphasis on mood symptoms.

If depression or BD is diagnosed in a physician, its treatment should respect the physician's clinical responsibilities and associated work schedule. If the physician-patient is too ill to maintain a high standard of clinical work, they should be strongly encouraged to take leave and not risk a medical error that might harm a patient. If they would do better with a temporary reduction in hours or change in schedule (e.g., elimination of shift work or reduction in night call), the clinician should encourage them to ask for the change and not be ashamed about it. If there is a concurrent general medical condition that can also be cited as a reason for the change, the clinician might suggest that the physician-patient mention it if it would help them avoid embarrassment or be more persuasive to an employer or their partners in a group practice.

Whenever optimal treatment of a physician's depression includes special attention to general medical issues, there is special value in a psychiatrist being the treating clinician. A physician-patient is more likely to heed general medical advice from another physician than from a non-medical mental health professional. Psychiatrists with dual credentials that include a second specialty like internal medicine, neurology, or ob/gyn sometimes can break through a physician-patient's denial when psychiatrists without dual training cannot.

Appointments for psychiatric care (including psychotherapy) should be scheduled so that they can be kept consistently without disrupting the physician-patient's work. As with many other occupations involving demanding schedules, working on call, or frequent travel—ranging from performing artists to journalists to long-haul pilots and truck drivers—consistent treatment might require frequent sessions via secure videoconferencing, sometimes outside of the treating psychiatrist's usual clinical hours. Frequent checking in by email or text messaging should be considered as well, with the goal of treatment being emotionally salient while interfering as little as feasible with the physician-patient's clinical work. Smartphone apps that deliver cognitive-behavioral psychotherapy are another tool for making treatment sufficiently intense but non-disruptive to the physician-patient's work. An approach to treatment that combines optimal intensity with flexibility conveys empathy and a realistic appreciation of the many demands on a practicing physician's time. This increases the likelihood of long-term adherence to the plan of treatment.

Pharmacologic Treatment

Given the range of treatments available for depression and bipolar illness, personalization of treatment is important for all patients with depression; but, as with eminent writers, artists, and performers, it is especially important when patients are people with busy lives who do cognitively intense work. Medications should be selected to avoid side effects that might interfere with the physician-patient's performance at their specialty. A drug-induced tremor could greatly interfere with a surgeon's performance; for such a physician who had a bipolar spectrum disorder, lamotrigine usually would be a better choice than lithium or an atypical antipsychotic drug. An emergency medicine physician working nights would be greatly impaired by drowsiness. If they required an antidepressant, one with minimal sedative effects would be selected. If drowsiness were an issue with an antidepressant that otherwise was effective, the patient might be prescribed modafinil, armodafinil, methylphenidate, or an amphetamine to be taken before evening or night shifts. A physician-patient who was a psychiatrist would function worse professionally if they had the side effect of emotional blunting from a SSRI or a SNRI. An antidepressant of a different class, e. g., vortioxetine, or a non-pharmacologic therapy might be a better initial choice for treatment of a depressed psychiatrist. Emotional blunting would not be obvious from a typical depression rating scale or a routine inquiry about physical side effects, but it can be identified using a structured instrument like the Oxford Depression Questionnaire (ODQ; Christensen et al., 2021) or by asking questions focusing on the same content as the ODQ. The issue of emotional blunting is discussed in detail in Chapter 15.

Assessment and Management of Suicidal Physicians

Depressed physicians, like all depressed patients, require careful and systematic assessment of suicide risk. When a depressed physician mentions or acknowledges suicidal thoughts or plans or has a history of suicide attempts or serious self-harm, a comprehensive assessment of suicide risk is especially important because all physicians know which methods of self-harm are most lethal, and most will have ready access to some of them (Agerbo et al., 2007; Albuquerque & Tulk, 2019; Center et al., 2003; Schernhammer & Colditz, 2004). A transient mood of hopelessness and despair is more likely to be fatal when the depressed person has a highly lethal method of self-harm at hand.

In the framework of the interpersonal-neuropsychiatric model of suicide, the stigma of depression in physicians can contribute to thwarted belongingness. An excessive, inflexible, or unpredictable work schedule can cause work–family conflicts that contribute to perceived burdensomeness; during the COVID-19 pandemic this problem often was aggravated by a physician's fears of bringing infection home to their family or by guilt feelings related to moral injury. In many specialties, physicians regularly experience the deaths of patients or of patients' family members, so death might be less frightening and "abnormal" to them. Sleep deprivation or substance use can impair behavioral inhibition. If the physician-patient's depression has mixed features, either initially or due to antidepressant treatment (which might be self-prescribed), there will be increased behavioral activation. Chronic medical problems worsened by self-neglect can cause pain or discomfort that makes life less bearable.

Each of the above contributors to suicide risk is potentially addressable in the physician-patient's treatment. Early in the process, risk can be reduced by asking the physician to remove potentially lethal drugs from their home or to otherwise control their access to them. The clinician should ascertain whether the physician has firearms at home, and if so, the physician-patient should be encouraged to store their gun(s) unloaded and locked up.

With respect to preventing suicide, it is important for the psychiatrist to know how the practice of medicine relates to the physician's self-esteem and meaning of life, how the physician's work has contributed to the depression, and how the depression is affecting their work. Positive feelings about their professional work can sustain a physician through a difficult period. Many physicians find great meaning in clinical work despite its stresses and adversities. A psychiatrist treating a depressed physician often can help them identify and remove impediments to their satisfaction from caring for patients and help them rediscover a sense of vocation.

Sometimes a physician's depression is precipitated by an event—an illness, injury, legal issue, or job loss—that temporarily prevents them from practicing medicine long before they intend to retire. It also might develop in connection with a physician's retirement. In both cases, a critical issue for the physician can be the loss of meaning and purpose in life. Full and sustained recovery from depression usually requires dealing with this issue explicitly. Sometimes there is a meaningful and appropriate way the physician-patient can remain involved with medicine, such as involvement with a health-related philanthropy or doing part-time teaching of a subject related to medicine. When there isn't, and the patient does not have a serious avocation or a well-developed agenda for life after retirement, the patient might benefit from psychotherapy specifically addressing their search for meaning and perhaps from encouragement to take up a new avocation or renew involvement in a former one.

A Psychiatrist Is the Clinician of Choice for a Depressed Physician

Throughout this chapter, we frequently refer to the treating clinician as a psychiatrist, though we are aware that it will sometimes be a psychologist or a non-psychiatrist prescriber working collaboratively with a non-physician mental health professional. Our opinion, however, is that, whenever feasible, a depressed physician should be treated by a psychiatrist—either alone or in active collaboration with a non-physician psychotherapist who regularly works with them. A 2017 Medscape survey showed that more than half of U.S. physicians who considered seeing a mental health professional for depression or burnout indicated a preference to see a psychiatrist (Peckham, 2018). The treatment of a depressed physician by a psychiatrist powerfully communicates that depression is a serious medical condition and that a depressed physician deserves respectful treatment by a medical colleague with specialized expertise. Once a depressed physician has overcome their internal barriers to acknowledging their illness and seeking help for it, a collegial, culturally aware, and personalized approach to psychiatric treatment can help keep a physician-patient engaged in treatment, persisting until a full remission is attained, and continuing a long-term clinical relationship to prevent a relapse.

In many ways, the optimal treatment of depressed physicians requires similar knowledge, skills, and attitudes as the treatment of eminent creative professionals. In both cases, psychiatrists begin with capacities that can be developed to provide personalized and culturally aware treatment of physicians. They are more likely than non-psychiatrist physicians to know about alternative biologic treatments for depression, about presentations of the bipolar spectrum in high-functioning patients, and about side effects of medications especially relevant to a physician's professional function.

Ideal personalization of a treatment plan might not be compatible with the physician-patient's organizational context, job demands, and working conditions; but treatment can come closer to the ideal when the psychiatrist has a clear vision of what the ideal would be. A psychiatrist with a special interest in treating depressed or bipolar physicians can engage in dialogue with representatives of health insurance plans, hospital or clinic administrators, PHP leaders, and other stakeholders about the value of personalized treatment, how such treatment might be supported, and how institutional stigma might be mitigated. Even when third parties are inflexible, a physician-patient is likely to appreciate their psychiatrist's efforts.

When a depressed or bipolar physician without other causes for persistent impairment of professional function recovers fully from their illness, they may be able to provide better medical care than before. They may be quicker to recognize mood disorders as comorbidities in their patients and may have greater empathy for depressed people. If they are willing to disclose their depression and recovery to colleagues, they will by example help counteract the stigma of depression that keeps so many depressed physicians from seeking treatment.

Psychiatrists' advocacy for depressed physicians can contribute to organizational change and reduction in stigma. Some state PHPs have been responsive to the suggestions of the American Psychiatric Association's work group on PHPs and impaired physicians. As experts in the diagnosis and treatment of mood disorders who see the destructive and occasionally fatal impact of institutional stigma on depressed or bipolar physicians and medical students, psychiatrists are well positioned to work for change in the medical profession, healthcare organizations, PHPs, and MLBs, taking a stand against institutional stigma and adverse working conditions in the medical profession. Beyond that, a depressed physician may find it easier to confide in and accept help from a psychiatrist who is visibly engaged in challenging institutional stigma and in fighting the epidemic of burnout and depression in physicians. If a physician's own treating psychiatrist is known to be actively addressing stigma as a systemic problem, it can help the physician-patient reduce their own self-stigma.

Chapter 17

Flying High, Feeling Low: Depression in Airline Pilots

For each of us is created to die,
And within me I know,
I was born to fly.
From "Impressions of a Pilot" (Stoker, 2019)

Flying is a passion. Piloting is a vocation. Airline pilots are responsible for the lives of their passengers, who may number in the hundreds. While pilots are self-selected for health and vigor, and further screened for mental disorders and general medical illness, they are not immune to disease and impairment. The public fears impaired pilots—and even more so those both impaired and malign—and the strict, inflexible regulations concerning health certification for air transport pilots (ATPs; pilots of scheduled passenger flights) are responsive to those fears. A pilot who is diagnosed with depression and treated with an SSRI antidepressant will be grounded for at least six months, even if the treatment produces a full remission of symptoms and has no adverse effects relevant to their performance as an aviator. They will then be required to undergo periodic official psychiatric and neuropsychological examinations at personal expense if they wish to resume flying professionally. Yet, undiagnosed or untreated depression is much more likely than effectively treated depression to underlie incidents of pilot error. Depression can be a presenting symptom of a general medical condition like obstructive sleep apnea (OSA) that can seriously impact flying performance. But if a pilot conceals their depression, underlying medical causes might go undetected.

Pilots have occupation-specific stresses and environmental hazards that raise their risk of depression. Many stressors, like pressure to meet schedules and exposure to noise and air pollution, are shared with other transport workers. The profession is highly masculine, over 95% of ATPs being men. Female pilots face gender-related challenges like those encountered by women truck drivers, firefighters, or orthopedic surgeons, including dismissive treatment, microaggressions, and occasionally sexual harassment. Male pilots, like men in other masculine professions, often express depression through externalization.

Like the cultures of other masculine occupations, the culture of airline pilots encourages them to deny, minimize, and/or conceal symptoms of depression and other mental disorders. Norms of pilot culture are amplified by the severe institutional stigma of depression in airline pilots. A consequence is that few pilots with clinical depression—including those with the syndromes of MDD, dysthymia, bipolar depression, adjustment disorder with depressed mood, and depression secondary to a general medical illness—seldom seek or receive treatment unless they are obviously impaired. In many cases, the impaired flying performance of a depressed pilot might have been prevented by more timely treatment. As will be detailed below, anonymous web surveys reveal a much higher prevalence of clinical depression in actively working ATPs than shown by official statistics on pilots' diagnoses and treatments. The point prevalence rate cannot be estimated precisely because of the lack of reliable data, but it is almost certainly greater than 10%, and thus greater than that seen in working people of other occupations matched on demographics, education, and salary.

When airplane crashes—including those of scheduled passenger airline flights—are entirely or partially due to pilot error, the pilot rarely has a diagnosed psychiatric disorder and seldom has been taking an antidepressant drug. When legal prescription or over-the-counter (OTC) drugs are involved in the causation of plane crashes, the most common culprits are sedating OTC antihistamines (e.g., diphenhydramine) rather than antidepressants (Canfield et al., 2012; McKay & Groff, 2016). Alcohol use disorders are a more important risk factor for dangerous pilot errors than depression. Between 2008 and 2012 in general aviation crashes in which the pilot was killed, 5.3% of the pilots autopsied had antidepressants in their blood. By contrast, blood alcohol testing of 233 pilots fatally injured in general aviation crashes revealed that 25 (11%) had blood alcohol concentrations of 20 mg/dl or higher. Among those, the mean level was 75 mg/dl—above the threshold for impairing automobile driving, let alone piloting a plane.

Fatal crashes of scheduled passenger flights are extraordinarily rare, and crashes due to deliberate actions of pilots—essentially murder–suicides—are even rarer: 13 were reported worldwide in the 40 years ending in 2015. In only three of the 13 did the pilot have any formal psychiatric history. In the other ten cases, legal, financial, relationship, and/or occupational conflicts were the apparent proximate cause of the event (Kenedi et al., 2016).

Nonetheless, the extensive and disturbing publicity surrounding crashes of airliners with mentally ill pilots raises public anxiety, leading to pressure on regulators to "do something" about pilots' mental health problems. Published accounts of a deliberate airline crash by a disturbed pilot typically emphasize the pilot's known or inferred psychiatric diagnosis (e.g., depression) rather than their obvious immorality and evil intent (e.g., pathological narcissism or "destructive entitlement"). Depressed people are much more likely to be suicidal than homicidal, and homicidal ideation in depressed people is almost never attributable to depression per se. A depressed person with paranoid delusions might be homicidal based on a belief that they are acting in self-defense. When depressed people have homicidal intent toward people and blame them for causing their misery, it is immorality, amorality, and/or pathological narcissism—not depression—that would provide them with a "license to kill." When people have preexisting homicidal intent, agitated depression (including bipolar spectrum conditions with mixed features) can entail a combination of increased behavioral activation, decreased behavioral inhibition, and impaired executive function that increases the probability that their intent will turn into action.

The two most recent examples of murder-suicide via deliberate crashing of a scheduled airline flight occurred in 2014 and 2015. In one, the pilot had a diagnosed depression with psychotic features. In the other, there was no formal psychiatric diagnosis, but the pilot's history suggested both bipolar disorder (BD) and habitual immoral conduct.

On March 24, 2015, Andreas Lubitz, a 27-year-old pilot with a history of recurrent major depression with psychotic features, intentionally crashed Germanwings Flight 9525 into a mountainside in the French Alps, instantly killing 150 passengers and crew. Official investigation following the crash determined that Lubitz had a psychotic depressive episode that began in 2014 and continued through the day of the accident (Bureau d'Enquêtes et d'Analyses, 2016). Despite Lubitz both having psychotic symptoms and being on medications that often affect flying performance, he did not inform the airline or aviation authorities. Apparently, flying was Lubitz's reason for living, and he preferred to die rather than give it up. His lack of concern for the lives of others, however, cannot be blamed on his depression. Two weeks before the crash, Lubitz's psychotherapist had recommended inpatient treatment of his depression, but respecting his patient's confidentiality, he did not inform the airline of his patient's condition (P. Brown et al., 2015). The therapist's decision reflected Germany's extremely rigid medical confidentiality laws. In most other countries, a clinician would have been obliged to notify authorities if an actively psychotic patient intended to pilot a passenger flight.

On March 4, 2014, Zaharie Amad Shah deliberately ditched Malaysia Airlines Flight 370 into the South Indian Ocean off Western Australia, killing the 239 people on board. Shah had no history of psychiatric illness or treatment, but his Facebook postings over the prior year raise the question of whether he had been hypomanic for several months of the year preceding the event. In one month of 2013, Shah posted 119 comments attacking the Malaysian government, including one in which he called the prime minister "a moron," thereby risking his job with Malaysia's national airline. In the year before the incident, the 53-year-old Shah, who was married with two children, posted 97 messages, several sexually suggestive, to Lan Qi Min and Lan Qihui, 21-year-old twin celebrity fashion models. At the time of the tragic event, Shah recently had been left by his wife because of his marital infidelity (Chapman, 2018; Langewiesche, 2019). Shah's public and apparently hypomanic behavior on social media did not trigger an assessment of his fitness to fly. Ironically, if he had sought treatment for BD, he would have been permanently grounded even if his treatment led to a long-term remission of symptoms with no impairment of occupational function.

Regulations and Institutional Stigma

In the United States, an applicant for certification or recertification as an ATP must present a first-class medical certificate, which indicates that they have no medical condition that could interfere with safe operation of an aircraft. The application for the medical certificate requires disclosure of any psychiatric diagnosis or treatment the patient has ever received, even for conditions not currently symptomatic, and a complete list of all current and recently discontinued medications. If the applicant has ever had treatment for a mental health problem—even in the remote past—they must provide detailed information about the treatment. An aviation medical examiner (AME) may not issue a medical certificate if the applicant has a history of depression or BD of any kind but must refer the case for evaluation by a specialized examiner with expertise in evaluating pilots with mental health issues—a sometimes-costly evaluation that is done at the pilot's personal expense. That examiner can authorize "special issuance" of a first-class medical certificate to a pilot with a history of depression and no lifetime history of psychosis or suicide attempts if the pilot meets narrowly defined criteria (Federal Aviation Administration (FAA), 2023): Either they have been off medication for at least 60 days with a stable mood as reported by the treating physician or they are in a stable remission of depression while being treated with one of five permitted antidepressants at a dosage that has not changed for six months or more, with no occupationally relevant side effects.

The five permitted antidepressants are four SSRIs—fluoxetine, citalopram, escitalopram, and sertraline—and bupropion in either an extended-release or sustained-release formulation. If the pilot is under treatment with any other psychotropic medication, either as an alternative or in combination with a permitted antidepressant, they will be denied a special issuance. Thus, a treating psychiatrist is not free to personalize the pilot's care by finding a more effective and/or better tolerated antidepressant if they do not do well on an SSRI or bupropion, or to augment an approved antidepressant with a second medication that would enable a fuller remission of symptoms. Any change in dosage—increase or decrease—in the past six months would delay issuance of certification. Establishing for the purpose of a special issuance that there are no adverse effects of the SSRI on cognition, perception, or reaction time requires that the pilot take a computerized cognitive assessment. This is required even if the pilot has no cognitive symptoms or cognitive signs on clinical mental status examination. The pilot must undergo a comprehensive neuropsychological examination if performance on the computerized assessment does not meet or exceed quantitative norms for aviators. A pilot successfully treated for MDD strictly according to evidence-based practice guidelines, with a complete and stable remission of symptoms, could be denied a first-class medical certificate for administrative reasons of no clinical relevance. Once a special issuance has been denied, it is difficult and expensive (though not totally impossible) for a pilot to get one in the future.

Criteria for medical certification of airline pilots treated for depression vary remarkably among high-income English-speaking nations. The United Kingdom's criteria are similar to those of the United States and in some areas are stricter. SSRIs are the exclusive pharmacologic treatment option, and testing in a flight simulator is required if a pilot plans to remain on antidepressants. A pilot receiving treatment must be formally reassessed every three months, and if their medication is discontinued, they might not fly for a minimum of two months if on fluoxetine and one month if on another SSRI (UK Civil Aviation Authority, 2023). By contrast, Canada's guidelines for medical certification of airline pilots treated for depression explicitly note that various antidepressants have similar efficacy, but that a specific antidepressant might be better for an individual pilot. It does not restrict the choice of antidepressants to SSRIs alone, it requires only four months of remission on a stable dose, and it requires follow-up assessments only twice a year. In its information sheets for pilots, Transport Canada points out the high frequency of untreated, secretly treated, or self-treated depression, and encourages depressed pilots to disclose their condition and seek treatment (Transport Canada, 2023). Its guidelines aim to normalize rather than stigmatize depression.

Australia goes even further to normalize depression, promote depressed pilots' self disclosure, and facilitate their treatment. In its "Depression and anxiety safety fact sheet," the Australian Civil Aviation Safety Authority (2023) begins by explaining how conditions associated with aviation can "exacerbate the symptoms of people suffering from, or with a history of, depression or anxiety." The fact sheet mentions fatigue, sleep deprivation, time zone changes, social isolation, and irregular access to medical care as contributors to depression, and then points out how depression can cause either overt or subtle incapacitation. It tells pilots they must report depressive symptoms to their designated aviation medical examiner, and states that any changes in medication will require grounding for *two to four weeks*—a remarkably more flexible policy than that of the other three countries. It recommends specific SSRI and SNRI antidepressants and suggests that pilots take only one medication, but it does not absolutely rule out certification for pilots successfully being treated with drugs of other classes, or even with a combination of medications. The fact sheet concludes with a remarkable paragraph that begins: "You are unique. Every case of depression is different. We make aeromedical decisions on a case-by-case basis."

The European Union Aviation Safety Agency, (EASA), like the Australian agency, has a flexible and sophisticated approach to assessing whether a pilot under treatment for depression should receive medical certification. The requirement is that the pilot has had a "full recovery"; this is followed by "full consideration of the individual case." (EASA, 2020).

The U.S. FAA's rigid rule against issuing a first-class medical certificate to a pilot with a BD diagnosis collides with modern psychiatric thinking about a bipolar spectrum that includes conditions milder than Bipolar II disorder (BD-II) and the relatively high frequency of mixed features or a history of subsyndromal hypomania in people who present for treatment of depression. Patients with "soft bipolarity" can be made worse—and sometimes become suicidal—when treated with an antidepressant without concurrent mood stabilization. Sometimes a patient who once showed some symptoms of hypomania (not necessarily the full syndrome) when treated with an antidepressant drug—but has no history of spontaneous hypomania or affective instability—will receive a bipolar spectrum diagnosis (e.g., bipolar III disorder (BD-III) or depressive disorder with bipolar specifier). The bipolar label can be helpful clinically, in that it alerts (or reminds) subsequent physicians not to prescribe antidepressants to the patient without a concurrent mood stabilizer and/or close monitoring for treatment-emergent symptoms of hypomania. If such a patient were treated with psychotherapy and lifestyle modification alone, they would have a low risk of hypomania, but the appearance of the adjective *bipolar* in the medical record would probably—and perhaps unnecessarily—end a career the pilot spent many years to build.

Depressed Pilots Often Conceal Their Illness

In the United States, ATPs under age 40 undergo annual medical examinations for fitness to fly; for pilots over age 40, semi-annual examinations are required.

AMEs are not required to perform any standardized mental status examination or screening for depression. Depressed pilots who avoid treatment or have secret treatment and deny symptoms of depression on their annual or semiannual medical examinations will have much less difficulty getting an ATP medical certificate than those who acknowledge their illness and are appropriately, effectively, and openly treated for the condition. Since much can happen medically between scheduled examinations, pilots are on the "honor system": A pilot is expected to stop flying immediately and seek medical care if they develop a new condition or start a new medication with potential effects on their flying performance. If the condition is other than a mild, transient problem like a respiratory infection, they must notify an AME and be recertified before returning to work. Since a pilot who is honest about a problem with depression will suffer damage to their career, many pilots will not report their problems and will do their best to cope without formal treatment.

Two studies of ATPs that had subjects anonymously answer web-based questionnaires both showed a point prevalence of clinical depression much higher than 5%—the proportion of pilots who are temporarily or permanently grounded because of a formal diagnosis of depression. An estimate of depression prevalence based on a survey of active ATPs depends not only on the actual prevalence of depression in the group but also on their cultural identity, the ostensible purpose of the survey, and the instrument used to detect and measure depressive symptoms. In some locales, the underreporting of depression by commercial airline pilots is extreme.

Aljurf et al. (2018) reported on 324 commercial pilots from three airlines in the Persian Gulf region, whom they screened for excessive daytime sleepiness and fatigue using standard questionnaires and for depression using the Hospital Anxiety and Depression Scale (HADS): 34.5% of the pilots screened had HADS depression scores of 8 or higher. According to a recent meta-analysis, the HADS with a cutoff score of 8 and a stringent criterion for MDD diagnosis has a sensitivity of 66% and specificity of 86% (Y. Wu et al., 2021). In this context, a 20% prevalence of MDD among the pilots surveyed is a reasonable estimate.

The age-adjusted prevalence of clinical depression in male pilots probably is more than the prevalence for employed men overall. (There is no reliable information available about depression in female airline pilots as there have been no studies of sufficiently large, representative samples of them.) The reported prevalence of depression in published studies of pilots ranges from 1.9% to 12.6%. The lower number is more likely to reflect denial or concealment of symptoms rather than a true low prevalence (Pasha & Stokes, 2018).

Anonymous web-based surveys of depressive symptoms, including questions about suicidal ideation, support the hypothesis of an elevated prevalence of depression in pilots (A. C. Wu et al., 2016). Between April and December of 2015, A. C. Wu and colleagues obtained complete nine-item PHQ-9 responses from 1848 commercial airline pilots, of whom 1430 had flown in the week preceding their completion of the survey. Pilots were from over 50 countries around the world, approximately 58% from the United States or Canada, 11% from Australia, and 12% each from European countries and from Asian countries. 13.5% of the respondents had scores of 10 or higher, implying a depressive syndrome of at least moderate severity, though not necessarily a diagnosis of MDD, and 4.2% of the sample had had suicidal thoughts more than one day in the preceding week. However, only 3.1% of the sample had ever been diagnosed with depression. Depression was significantly more prevalent among male pilots from Asian and Middle Eastern countries, of whom 22.5% met the threshold of 10 on the PHQ-9. Depression prevalence was remarkably high—over 30%—among pilots of either gender who had flown in the past 30 days and had experienced either sexual harassment (3.3% of the sample) or verbal harassment (8.9%) twice or more in the prior year. Depressive symptoms were more prevalent in pilots under age 50—both for pilots who had flown in the past seven days and for those who had not.

On the PHQ-9, anhedonia ("little interest or pleasure in doing things") was much more common among the pilots in the survey than having a depressed mood ("feeling down, depressed, or hopeless"); 32.6% of respondents had anhedonia several days in the prior two weeks, 6.1% had anhedonia more than half the days, and 3.3% had anhedonia nearly every day. By contrast, only 19.1% had a depressed mood several days in the prior two weeks, 3.9% had a depressed mood more than half the days, and 1.7% had a depressed mood almost every day. The predominance of anhedonia over depressed mood among airline pilots is partly due to a "masculine" occupational culture in which a depressed mood, sadness, or hopelessness might not be acknowledged to another person, or even to oneself, but physical complaints or a loss of interest or pleasure could be admitted. In addition, loss of interest and pleasure can be related to the chronic sleep insufficiency and chronobiologic disruption that are occupational hazards of airline pilots. Inadequate or frequently disrupted sleep is a risk factor for the full syndrome of major depression, and it also can cause apathy, anhedonia, and fatigue without a depressed mood. The other primarily emotional symptom of depression on the PHQ-9, "feeling bad about yourself—or that you are a failure and have let yourself or your family down," was relatively uncommon among the pilots, with 75.6% of the sample saying they had not felt that way at all in the prior two weeks. By contrast, 74.6% of the sample felt tired or lacking in energy at least several days in the prior two weeks, and 69.6% had sleep problems several days in the prior two weeks: trouble falling asleep, staying asleep, or sleeping too much. 48.2% of the respondents thought the problems they described on the PHQ-9 made it at least somewhat difficult for them to do their work, take care of things at home, or get along with people.

In the previously cited online survey of airline pilots from countries in the Gulf Cooperation Council (Aljurf et al., 2018), a conservative interpretation of HADS depression scale scores would imply that more than 15% of the pilots surveyed would have been diagnosed with a Diagnostic and Statistical Manual of Mental Disorders (DSM)/ICD depressive disorder if they had been examined by a psychiatrist and had responded honestly and fully to the examiner's questions. A 15% prevalence of depression would be remarkably high for a group of relatively young, well-paid men with no chronic medical conditions that would have made them ineligible to fly professionally.

Even 15% is probably an underestimate of clinical depression prevalence in male pilots. An estimate of depression prevalence in a highly masculine occupation is likely to be falsely low if it is based on a standard depression screening instrument like the PHQ-9, the Center for Epidemiologic Studies Depression Scale (CES-D), or the HADS. As noted with respect to truck drivers, men with a strong stereotypically masculine identity are prone to expressing depression with externalizing symptoms like drinking, drug use, angry and argumentative behavior, and impulsive risk-taking—all symptoms not mentioned on either the PHQ-9 or the HADS.

Financial and Psychological Impact of Pilots' Health Conditions

Airlines in the United States have different policies concerning income support for pilots temporarily or permanently grounded for a medical condition. Major airlines might offer 50% of salary for as long as a pilot is not able to fly, up to age 65—the mandatory retirement age for pilots. Smaller regional and commuter airlines usually provide less or no income support at all. Currently certified pilots can purchase "loss of license" insurance that provides income support if a medical condition prevents their certification. It differs from temporary disability insurance in that the pilot need not be incapable of other employment—just not certifiable to fly. If the insurance is additive to that supplied by the employer, the combination of the two streams of replacement income might be adequate to support the pilot (and their family, if applicable). However, many of the more affordable policies reduce their payments if the grounded pilot has income from other employment or from other disability insurance. Some, though not necessarily all, underwriters of loss of license insurance limit the income benefit to 12 or 24 months if the reason for the loss of license is a mental illness or substance use disorder.

There is a baseline 5% probability that a pilot without a known chronic disease will be temporarily grounded by illness at some time in the next year. It would seem an easy decision for a pilot to buy loss of license coverage. However, a young pilot beginning their career as a poorly paid co-pilot at a regional airline, worried about paying off educational debt, might feel such insurance is unaffordable.

Even when loss of first-class medical certification is not financially ruinous for a pilot, the loss of their life's work can be emotionally difficult. Some grounded pilots find other work in a non-flying job related to aviation, while others find it easier to leave the industry completely. A pilot who loses their ATP certification because of depression and subsequently remains depressed might find it particularly difficult to move on to a different occupation. Grief over the loss of their chosen life's work could be a barrier to recovery if not effectively addressed in psychotherapy.

Developing a general medical condition or having a traumatic injury with impact on aviation performance can be difficult, but most pilots are realistic about such situations. Depression and BD are different. A depressed pilot might not see their problem as a medical condition at all, thinking of it in terms of "stress" or "fatigue" obviously attributable to demanding working conditions. The pilot's depression might be expressed primarily as somatic symptoms or externalizing behavior, perhaps as the syndrome of "male depression." They might minimize any adverse effect of the depression on flying performance if one were present. A pilot with hypomania might lack awareness that anything was abnormal about their mental state but hear comments from other crew members or from family members about changes in their behavior related to hypomania, such as anger/irritability, loquaciousness, or intemperate drinking. However, whether their mood was low, high, or mixed, the pilot would know that seeking any form of mental health care could endanger the career they had worked for years to establish.

Stigma and Choice of Treatment

The issue of institutional stigma looms so large that optimal treatment of depressed airline pilots must be tailored to minimize inappropriate stigma while still keeping pilots unable to fly safely out of the cockpit. A depressed pilot is more likely to seek help if they are not afraid of losing their career unnecessarily. If a pilot develops a mental condition or requires a treatment that would cause long-term impairment in their ability to fly safely, the clinician's task will include helping the pilot face that unhappy reality and cope with their disappointment.

The regulatory bias against treating pilots with antidepressant medication makes it especially important for clinicians treating pilots to be familiar with a broad range of non-pharmacologic therapies for treating mild to moderate clinical depression and to utilize them preferentially if the pilot's depression per se does not compromise their capacity to fly safely. If the pilot must be temporarily grounded because of depression-related cognitive, psychomotor, or other functional impairment, there is no reason to avoid antidepressants if they are an otherwise attractive option given the details of the patient's case. If a pilot's depression improved but did not remit on an approved antidepressant, adding a non-pharmacologic treatment such as a nutritional supplement or bright light therapy would leave open the option that the pilot could return to flying if a remission were attained. In the United States, augmenting the SSRI with a second psychotropic drug could end the pilot's flying career.

In choosing which non-pharmacologic treatment(s) to recommend, the clinician should aim for compatibility of the treatment with the pilot's work. Weekly face-to-face psychotherapy would be difficult for a pilot who was usually away from home and on a variable schedule. A combination of in-person psychotherapy and telepsychiatry sessions and/or smartphone apps for cognitive-behavioral therapy (CBT) would be more feasible. Mental health care via videoconference was normalized during the COVID-19 pandemic. Non-pharmacologic somatic treatment options for mild to moderate clinical depression include nutritional supplements (omega-3 fatty acids, *N*-acetylcysteine, and *S*-adenosylmethionine [SAMe]), bright light therapy, and transcranial alternating current stimulation. Although non-pharmacologic somatic treatments are not stigmatized as much as prescription psychotropics, they are not placebos; and if they were used, the prescriber would need to monitor their effects closely and advise the pilot not to fly until their potential impact on flying performance was assessed.

Suicide in Active and Retired Pilots

Suicide mortality has increased in White male American airline pilots, especially after their mandatory retirement age of 65. The National Institute for Occupational Safety and Health (NIOSH) National Occupational Mortality Surveillance (NOMS) system counts and compares rates of deaths from various causes by principal occupation (current at the time of death or most recent prior to retirement), based on death certificates from 26 American states. The most recent available NOMS statistics are based on aggregated demographic, occupational, and cause-of-death data from 5.8 million deaths from the years 1999, 2003–2004, and 2007–2014. NOMS calculates proportional mortality ratios (PMRs)—the proportion of individuals with a given occupation who die of a specified cause divided by the proportion of people of all occupations who die of that cause, adjusting for age. The occupational category of "airline pilots and navigators" has a PMR of 1.39 for death by suicide for White males aged 18–64 ($p < .01$) and a PMR of 2.00 for White males aged 65–90 ($p < .01$). The sample did not have enough female or non-White pilots at risk to reliably estimate their PMRs (NIOSH, 2019b).

The higher PMR for suicide in pilots over age 65 is not a general age effect; it signifies a disproportionate increase in suicide mortality in retired pilots over age 65 compared with people over age 65 retired from other occupations. One contributor to suicide in retired pilots might be the loss of an occupation that is central to their meaning of life.

The Culture of Airline Pilots

Airline pilots all over the world have a similar cockpit culture, with ideals of resourcefulness, decisiveness under pressure, respect for the authority of the captain, stoicism, and loyalty to one's team. Airline pilots' personal identities emphasize their occupation. While a pilot has a nationality, ethnic identity, generational membership, gender, religion (or lack of it), etc., these identities typically are less important than their occupational identity when the pilot is in the cockpit. For example, pilots are required to communicate in English with an air traffic controller if the latter does not speak the pilot's native language.

Pilots from different countries do show patterns of behavior reflecting the intersection of their occupational culture with national culture and other identities. Merritt (2000) analyzed questionnaire data from 9417 pilots from 26 airlines representing 19 countries, focusing on Hofstede's six dimensions, comparing national culture with occupational culture, and quantitatively analyzing the interaction of the cultures. Regarding power distance (PD), half of the variance among pilots was explained by national culture. However, pilots' mean PD scores were higher than national means in 17 of the 19 countries. Whether national culture is egalitarian or hierarchical, the captain is the boss in the cockpit, though the co-pilot is expected to tell the pilot if they disagree on navigation or operation of the plane. Compared with working people of other occupations from the same country, pilots were significantly more likely to be afraid to disagree with superiors. The threshold for a co-pilot questioning a captain varied according to national culture, higher in more authoritarian cultures with higher PD. Pilots from all 19 countries were more likely than other civilian workers to see their leadership as autocratic and directive. The pilots surveyed felt they were expected to get along with other crew members with few conditions, tolerating bullying or arbitrariness by the captain if it occurred.

Pilots tend to score high on uncertainty avoidance—reflecting their working in an environment where standard operating procedures and checklists are the rule. In the multinational survey of Merritt (2000), pilots from English-speaking countries and from Western Europe were more tolerant of uncertainty and more willing to deviate from standard procedure than those from other parts of the world. Pilots had relatively high masculinity scores even when they came from countries like the Nordic nations with high gender equality. For most pilots, work would take precedence in a work–family conflict.

On an airline flight, the pilot and co-pilot (captain and first officer) share the work of piloting the plane. If there is a flight engineer (second officer), they will fly the plane when both the pilot and co-pilot are not available. On long flights, piloting duties are divided by plan so that everyone on the crew has time to rest. In addition to scheduled rest periods, co-pilots and flight engineers sometimes take over when the pilot or co-pilot scheduled to fly is too sleepy to perform well; in some cases, the pilot will fall asleep at the controls of the plane and be relieved on an urgent basis. In the above-cited study of Gulf Cooperation Council pilots, 45.1% of the pilots surveyed reported unexpectedly falling asleep at the controls at least once, and 67.4% recalled making mistakes in the cockpit on account of fatigue (Aljurf et al., 2018). When pilots make mistakes because of fatigue, sleepiness, or distraction and another crew member steps in to correct the error, it is rarely reported to the airline. The culture of pilots is one of supporting and defending fellow crew members against criticism by the airline and regulators. It is unusual for another crew member to raise issues about a pilot's mental health or behavior. A problem would have to be extreme to outweigh the culture of solidarity and confidentiality. The fact that pilots have co-pilots dramatically improves the safety of air travel, but it also enables problems to persist that would immediately demand attention if a pilot were flying solo.

Special Issues of Female Pilots

In 2018 the United States had 162,145 certified ATPs, of whom 7136 (4.4%) were women. Female pilots face challenges typical of women in highly masculine occupations. To thrive in the profession, they must tolerate everyday harassment, discrimination, and stereotyping, handling them with grace and humor. On the other hand, they must be willing to report and challenge the most severe forms of male misbehavior such as physical harassment, sexual coercion, or being passed over for deserved and expected promotion (Davey & Davidson, 2000). Female pilots must tread a thin line between violating norms of the occupational culture and masochistically tolerating behavior by superiors and colleagues that ideally would be grossly unacceptable to everyone. In the words of one female captain, "The cockpit is a very small, cozy place. You have to spend hours and hours with a person sitting 18 inches from you. It's very difficult to say to somebody, 'That was offensive'" (Kaye, 1993).

Cristofich (2015) did in-depth interviews of 10 successful female airline pilots and analyzed the common elements of their experiences. She concluded that two characteristics were especially important to the women persevering and thriving in a highly masculine profession. The first was psychological resilience, a characteristic shared by men and women who thrive and remain physically and mentally healthy in high-stress occupations. The second was their wholehearted adoption of the social role and identity of "airline pilot," which superseded other cultural identities such as those related to age and gender. Women who truly love to fly will try to accept the unwritten rules of the occupation.

Those who do it successfully build their competence and self-confidence. Those who don't are at risk for emotional distress that can lead to clinical depression. Those who are depressed for a reason unrelated to occupational gender issues might find it harder to negotiate the challenges of being a woman in a highly masculine occupation.

Being an airline pilot is hard work under difficult working conditions, and usually there are several years of less desirable assignments at lower pay before a pilot becomes a captain. Because of these negatives, people rarely become professional airline pilots unless they truly love to fly. Surveys of senior pilots show that few of them would want a managerial job at their airline even if it paid more and was easier work. They would prefer to spend their workdays flying an airplane. For both male and female pilots, a sense of vocation and love of flying makes them willing to work hard under stressful conditions. The same sense of being "born to fly" can make it psychologically devastating for a pilot to lose their career because of a physical or mental health issue.

Financial Aspects of Pilots' Careers

The FAA annually publishes demographic data on the distribution of ATPs by geography, gender, and age (FAA, 2018). These aid in understanding the culture and the economics of the occupation in America.

Geographically, American ATPs are not distributed proportionally to the population: 55% of ATPs reside in the South, the Southwest, the Mountain States, or states with an Appalachian culture (Arkansas, Kentucky, Missouri,

Oklahoma, Tennessee, and West Virginia). Pilot culture is more likely to intersect with those regions' cultures than with those of the Pacific Coast, the Midwest, New England, or the Mid-Atlantic. Regarding the age distribution of ATPs, 55% are aged 45–65, while only 31% are 25–44; 13% of certified ATPs are over 65 and thus not permitted to work as airline pilots. For female pilots, the proportions are 51% aged 45–64 and 43% aged 25–44. The average age of active male ATPs is 51.0 years; for active female ATPs the average age is 46.4 years. Thus, as older pilots retire, the net number of pilots is likely to decrease, worsening the pilot shortage. However, at present, younger pilots' prospects for promotion are limited by the large number of more senior pilots still in the workforce. Female pilots are younger overall, and their age distribution is more even. It is remarkable that 13% of ATPs maintain their certification after they are no longer permitted to work as airline pilots, suggesting that they feel their occupational identity is worth the cost and inconvenience of maintaining their credentials.

The age distribution of pilots and the current pilot shortage in the United States reflect the economics of the occupation. ATPs typically start their careers as first officers (co-pilots) for smaller regional airlines and end their careers as captains for major national or international airlines. The regional airlines pay less, have worse benefits, and have less job security than the major carriers; and co-pilots have less pay, control, and status than captains. With middle-aged and older pilots holding the prime positions as captains at major airlines, it may take many years for a pilot to advance to the job of their dreams. In the meantime, they may have financial pressures and job strain due to imbalances of demand and control, effort and reward.

Historically, many airline pilots entered the profession after serving as military pilots. Currently, most take a civilian path, getting an undergraduate degree in a field related to aviation and getting the required hours of supervised flying experience at their own expense either during college or afterward. The cost of private, civilian flight training to qualify as an ATP is over $100,000 (ATP Flight School, 2023). If a pilot borrows money for their aviation training, they will need to fly for years to repay the debt. Physical or mental health problems that prevent the pilot from flying can lead to financial distress for young pilots with large educational debts unless they have insurance for loss of license.

Experienced airline pilots working as captains for major U.S. airlines can earn well over $300,000 per year. However, salaries vary greatly between airlines, with regional airlines and some nations' major airlines paying much less. For example, in 2023, at the regional airline Air Wisconsin, the annual salary of a new first officer was $60,000 per year and the salary of a new captain was $102,000. Emirates Airlines paid a new first officer $67,956 per year, and a new captain $97,008 (Epic Flight Academy, 2023). In effect, regional airlines function like minor league baseball teams, with remarkably low pay for playing the same game. If a new ATP has significant debt from college and flight school, they can have distressing worries over personal finance despite the superficial glamor of their job. A newly licensed ATP typically begins their career as a first officer at a regional airline, then becomes a captain at a regional airline, then a first officer at a major airline, and finally a captain at a major airline. From start to finish the process can take ten years or more, and since seniority is accrued at a specific airline in a specific position, a pilot's losing their job at a regional airline because of illness—or financial problems of their employer—can significantly set back their career development timetable. Loss of a job with a regional airline because of the pilot's illness or the airline's business problems can set back the timetable for promotion because seniority is accrued at a specific airline. Airlines' corporate business problems have been directly related to pilots' stress (Little et al., 1990). An American pilot who is frustrated with their lack of upward progress can become an expatriate and work for a carrier in a country with a rapidly growing airline sector and a shortage of experienced pilots. The pilot will have a higher-level and better-paid job, but their emotional well-being and general health status will depend on their adaptation to life abroad. Furthermore, the national airlines of middle-income countries often have working conditions even worse than those of airlines in the United States, with difficult work schedules and poor-quality accommodations when the pilot is away from their home base.

In the past two decades the airline industry has been unstable, with mergers, changes of ownership, and bankruptcies. Corporate instability of airlines can entail adverse changes in pilots' terms of employment, compensation, working conditions, and job security. In the worst cases, airlines have skimped on maintenance of airplanes and other equipment or have not rigorously trained pilots on technological changes in the planes they fly. A dramatic example is the story of the Boeing 737 Max. Boeing made changes in the control systems of its most popular short- to medium-range airplane, to accommodate larger engines that increased the plane's payload. However, Boeing did not mandate flight simulator training on the modified plane, and it made certain "fail-safe" technology optional for the airlines. Several airlines did not buy the add-on technology or provide additional training for their pilots. This led to two crashes in which hundreds of passengers and crew members died (Gelles, 2019). It can be extremely stressful for a pilot to doubt the safety of their airplane and to have a positive relationship with an employer that appears to risk the lives of pilots and passengers to cut costs.

Health Hazards—Generic and Specific

Many of the occupational hazards of pilots are shared with long-haul truckers including exposure to noise, exposure to polluted air, disruption of sleep and chronobiology, work–family conflicts, loneliness, temptation to engage in risky behavior when away from home, and lifestyles that often combine insufficient exercise with poor-quality food. Pilots have in addition two job-specific environmental exposures that can affect their physical and mental health. One is the exposure to cosmic rays and, variably, ultraviolet-A radiation while flying at high altitudes (Cadilhac et al., 2017). These exposures give pilots approximately twice the population risk of melanoma and other skin cancers (Miura et al., 2019; Sanlorenzo et al., 2015).

Pilots also are exposed to hypoxia since the air in cabins and cockpits may be pressurized to as low as the equivalent of 8000 feet above sea level (Bagshaw, 2007). Hypoxia can worsen mood and increase the probability of suicidal ideation in people vulnerable to its effects. As noted in relation to Switzerland and the American Far West, high altitude is associated with increased suicide rates (Kious et al., 2018).

Understanding pilots' occupational hazards is one key to successful nonpharmacologic intervention to treat their clinical depression and/or to help maintain a remission that might initially have been attained using an SSRI. While cosmic rays cannot be avoided, many of the occupational hazards of pilots can be mitigated. In addition, addressing occupational hazards can be done with a focus on enhancing health, function, safe flying, and quality of life, rather than on depression alone. This can reduce self-stigma and reluctance to engage in treatment.

Sleep disturbance and chronobiologic stress can result from on-call work schedules (typical of early-career pilots), early-morning flights, and flights across multiple time zones. These sometimes can be mitigated by sleep hygiene; strategic planning of bedtimes, naps, and exercise; and light therapy.

Noise exposure of airline pilots—ambient noise in the cockpit between 74 and 80 dB(A) and sound pressure under the pilot's headset of 84 to 88 dB(A)—is high enough to lead to hearing loss and tinnitus if active noise reduction is not employed (Müller & Schneider, 2017). Active noise reduction is protective, as demonstrated by helicopter pilots: They routinely utilize active noise reduction and do not have more hearing loss than airplane pilots, even though helicopters have significantly higher ambient noise than airplanes (Wagstaff & Arva, 2009).

Airline pilots have an increased prevalence of tinnitus and noise-related hearing problems. For example, tinnitus at some time during the prior year was reported by 40% of a sample of Swedish pilots; 18% had constant or severe tinnitus, and 12% of the sampled pilots had sought medical consultation for the symptom. Pilots with more noise exposure during their leisure time were more likely to have tinnitus (Lindgren et al., 2009).

Tinnitus is associated with depression; more than 25% of people with tinnitus have depressive symptoms (Bhatt et al., 2017). Hearing loss also affects quality of life and thus increases the prevalence of depression. A pilot may have the option to use a headset with more effective active noise reduction. Even if they cannot do so on the job, they can reduce noise exposure when not working, giving the auditory system more time to recover. Many pilots live close to airports, with the consequence that they have substantial aircraft (and sometimes highway) noise exposure when they are not at work. These exposures can be reduced by soundproofing their residence or by moving to a quieter neighborhood. Pilots also can reduce exposure to noise during their leisure activities.

Obesity and sedentary lifestyle both increase depression risk, and both are very common in pilots. An online survey of male Brazilian airline pilots showed a 53.7% prevalence of overweight ($25 \leq$ body mass index [BMI] < 30) and a 14.6% prevalence of obesity (BMI ≥ 30) (de Souza Palmeira & Marqueze, 2016). In the previously cited survey of Gulf Cooperation Council pilots, there was a 23.9% prevalence of obesity (Aljurf et al., 2018).

OSA is common among airline pilots. The study of Gulf Cooperation Council pilots found that 29.3% of the sample had histories suggesting a high probability of OSA. More than half of the pilots had multiple occasions on which they felt too tired to be at the controls of the plane, and 48.8% of the pilots would not trust their colleagues to be alone in the cockpit of the plane. OSA was assessed via home sleep testing in a sample of 41 Saudi Arabian short- to medium-haul pilots and first officers; the study found mild OSA (apnea–hypopnea index [AHI] of 5–14) in 64% of the sample and identified one pilot with moderate OSA (AHI of 15–30) and one with severe OSA (AHI >30). Notwithstanding, only two pilots in the sample scored in the high-risk range on the Berlin Questionnaire, a standard OSA screening tool. The study's authors speculated that the pilots underreported symptoms like snoring, fatigue, and daytime sleepiness to "avoid jeopardizing their job if they admit or report having sleep issues" (Alhejaili et al., 2021). Han et al. (2021) studied the issue in a sample of 103 pilots, performing daytime polysomnography after the pilot had flown a long-haul nighttime flight. 73 of the pilots, none with a prior history of OSA, had moderate-to-severe OSA with an AHI of 15 or higher. Most of the pilots would have been classified as low risk on the Berlin Questionnaire, and most had scores on the Epworth Sleepiness Scale below the threshold for identifying a probable sleep disorder. Their findings further suggest an occupational culture of denying or minimizing health problems—even those that might affect job performance.

OSA is a non-stigmatized condition readily treated without medication. Even mild OSA, if accompanied by excessive daytime sleepiness, was associated in an Australian population study with an increased risk of clinical depression, even after controlling for gender, age, waist circumference, financial strain, current smoking, and sexual dysfunction (Lang et al., 2017). Addressing mild OSA offers an opportunity to prevent clinical depression in airline pilots without stigma and with direct benefits for aviation safety.

Evidence thus suggests that pilots are aware of the risks posed by fatigue and sleepiness but do not feel empowered to act to reduce the risks. Many have untreated medical conditions that could potentially impair their capacity to fly safely. Pilots can be aware of these conditions yet continue to fly, making their best efforts and pushing themselves to perform in the face of fatigue, sleepiness, and/or depression. This reflects both a culture of self-reliance as well as pilots' realistic concerns over losing their livelihood if they openly seek help for their problems. It also reflects the normalization among pilots of conditions like obesity and OSA, despite the conditions being treatable and affecting pilots' active life expectancies. Treatment of OSA reduces the symptoms of depression that are commonly associated with the condition and helps prevent the development of clinical depression. It can be done using a continuous positive airway pressure (CPAP) device a pilot could easily pack in a carry-on bag. Some people with OSA will be treatable without the inconvenience of CPAP, for example by wearing a device that prompts them to sleep on their side rather than supine.

Fatigue is a highly prevalent complaint of airline pilots. A 2015 study of daytime sleepiness and fatigue in Portuguese airline pilots analyzed data from 435 pilots, 225 captains and 210 first officers (Reis et al., 2016a): 394 (90.6%) had significant fatigue, as defined by an average score of four or higher on a nine-item, seven-point self-rating scale. They found that 201 (46.2%) showed pathological sleepiness (scores of 10 or higher on the Epworth Sleepiness Scale) and that 152 (34.9%) had frequent poor sleep quality or trouble falling asleep. Fatigue, excessive daytime sleepiness, and sleep complaints were all correlated with one another. Fatigue can be a symptom of depression, a general medical condition, or simply a consequence of insufficient or poor-quality sleep. Engaging with a pilot around improving fatigue, initially targeting sleep habits, exercise, diet, sleep and wake times, and other lifestyle interventions, is another route to preventing the worsening of a mild depression and to preserving remission after moderate depression has been successfully treated. The sleep and fatigue study of Reis and colleagues showed significantly worse symptoms in short- to medium-haul pilots as opposed to long-haul pilots (Reis et al., 2016b). Short- to medium-haul pilots are especially vulnerable to depression because more frequent, shorter flights usually are assigned to more junior pilots, who are paid less, have less status, and often have more unstable employment.

Self-medication with alcohol is a common way for pilots, and for many others working in masculine occupations, to handle negative emotions. An alcohol use disorder could ground an airline pilot until they regained and maintained sobriety, but unlike a bipolar diagnosis, it would not imply the end of their flying career. The hazard of drinking is especially great for pilots who fly long hauls and spend many nights away from their homes and loved ones. Identifying and addressing alcohol problems is yet another way to therapeutically engage with a pilot at risk for major depression. Regulations require that a pilot's last drink be at least ten hours before they report to work. However, this is compatible with heavy drinking the day and evening before a flight, and it is possible for a pilot to comply with regulations while having a diagnosable alcohol use disorder or medically significant "harmful drinking." If an alcohol use disorder is suspected, blood alcohol levels at work have always been negative, and the pilot is not forthcoming about their drinking, checking biomarkers of longer-term alcohol exposure might establish that there is a problem and provide the basis for opening a dialogue about it. Options include urine testing for ethyl sulfate and ethyl glucuronide, blood testing for phosphatidylethanol, and hair testing for ethyl glucuronide and fatty acid ethyl esters (Nanau & Neuman, 2015).

Working Around Stigma and Denial

An attractive option for reducing depression in airline pilots is the approach of secondary prevention—instituting non-pharmacologic antidepressant interventions at a time that the pilot has symptoms of fatigue, insomnia, or "stress" but would not meet criteria for MDD. The approach is like one that is used with physicians who are "burned out" but not clinically depressed or students on the verge of clinical depression who are, for cultural reasons, unwilling to seek treatment from a psychiatrist or psychologist. Intervention might be framed as building the pilot's resilience so that they could deal better with stress and modifying their lifestyle to prevent depression, reduce long-term disease risks, and improve well-being (Sarris et al., 2014). Another stigma-avoiding descriptor for antidepressant lifestyle changes and cognitive-behavioral interventions is "strategy for enhancing aviation performance, safety, and reliability."

For a pilot who acknowledges a problem with depression, non-pharmacologic treatment for depression can be described as the best way to minimize time away from flying. If the pilot is too depressed to fly safely, takes temporary sick leave, and then recovers with non-pharmacologic treatment, there is no fixed waiting period before they can be recertified to fly (FAA, 2018). The pilot's actual symptoms of depression and side effects, if any, of non-pharmacologic treatment would be the basis of the FAA's decision. Following are some options for which there is supportive evidence, albeit not specifically focused on airline pilots.

Pilots can be taught how to better manage their sleep, including principles of sleep hygiene and the use of wearable sleep trackers and/or mHealth apps to support consistent change. Low-dose melatonin or light therapy could be considered for sleep phase problems. These treatments would not disqualify a pilot from flying unless they had unusual side effects that affected cognitive or motor function.

They can receive nutritional counseling, helping them find a healthy diet tailored to their tastes, cultural background, and the realities of the places to which they fly. In Chapter 9 there is a detailed listing of "depressing" and "antidepressant" foods, with references. Having the pilot consult with an expert dietitian with a compatible personality and communication style can help them plan a diet that would be feasible for them to follow consistently. If the pilot is obese or overweight with metabolic complications (metabolic syndrome or diabetes), pharmacologic or surgical treatment of the obesity might reduce depression risk as well as improve general health and might lead to improvement or remission of OSA.

More generally, comprehensive lifestyle improvement that includes nutrition, exercise, and sleep is beneficial in treating current depression and in preventing recurrence of a prior episode of depression (Bayes et al, 2023; Hwang et al., 2023; Mrozek et al., 2023; Scott et al., 2021; Wang et al., 2023) Interventions to help pilots achieve healthier lifestyles are feasible. In 2020, during a period of decreased airline activity related to the COVID-19 pandemic, a group of New Zealand airline pilots participated in a controlled 17-week trial of guided change in lifestyle (Wilson et al., 2021): 38 of 79 pilots received a personalized program for improving sleep, diet, and physical activity; and the remainder received only follow-up. The intervention group started with a 60-minute one-on-one session with a health coach. This was followed by the development of an individualized health program, weekly emails, and a phone call after about two months. The pilots were rated on the processes and outcomes that were the objectives of the intervention. After 17 weeks, 92% of the intervention group reached seven hours or more of sleep per night, 92% reached five or more servings of fruit and vegetables per day, and 87% reached 150 minutes or more of moderately vigorous physical activity per week. Mental health ratings on the 12-item Short Form Health Survey (SF-12) improved significantly. Similar changes were not seen in the control group. A focus on wellness and an emphasis on well-defined processes and measurable goals fit well with pilots' occupational culture.

Nutritional supplements such as omega-3 fatty acids (especially eicosapentaenoic acid (EPA); Sarris et al. 2016), L-methylfolate (but not folic acid; Sarris et al. 2016), vitamin D_3 (Jamilian et al., 2019; Sarris et al., 2016), SAMe (Sarris et al. 2016), vitamin C, magnesium, and zinc (Sarris et al., 2016; Szewczul et al., 2018), and antidepressant probiotics might be considered. Supplements are appealing for several reasons. Their use is not stigmatized. They can have benefits for general health as omega-3 fatty acid supplementation can reduce cardiovascular risk related to lipid profiles. Pilots who eat many of their meals at hotels and restaurants away from home often have unhealthy diets. Nutritional supplements are not restricted by the FAA, and the ones mentioned here are not known to have side effects relevant to flying performance. (However, omega-3 fatty acids and SAMe on occasion will provoke hypomania in a patient with occult bipolar illness.) They can help prevent depression from developing in stressful conditions and reduce the risk that mild depression will worsen. A recommendation for supplements would be based on a dietary history, perhaps supported by screening laboratory tests such as a fasting lipid profile and serum levels of 25-OH Vitamin D, magnesium, vitamin B12, RBC folate, and homocysteine.

At this time, SAMe, regulated in Europe as a prescription antidepressant drug, is classified as a nutritional supplement in the United States. Since it is not a prescription drug, it could be used by a pilot without an explicit legal requirement to report it to the AME. However, in a general medical evaluation of any kind there is an expectation that the patient will disclose any nutritional supplements they are taking. And if MDD were the indication for use of SAMe, a pilot or AME would need to report it because of their obligation to report the depression itself.

Practicing a form of meditation or systematic relaxation, such as mindfulness meditation, yoga, breathing exercises, or biofeedback, can enhance psychological well-being, increase resilience, and reduce stress-related symptoms (Lurie, 2018; Sathyanarayanan et al., 2019; Zou et al., 2018). A website, the Mindful Aviator (n.d.) is dedicated to introducing aviators to mindfulness for mental health. Carl Eisen, the founder of the website and both a pilot and a psychologist, writes about the problem of disclosing mental symptoms when one is an airline pilot: "Fear of having the 'difficult conversation' about anxiety and stress was a significant source of (you guessed it), my anxiety and stress!" He encourages people with mild to moderate symptoms of "stress" to learn mindfulness and related coping strategies, which may in themselves be enough to prevent clinical depression or an anxiety disorder. However, he cautions pilots with more severe symptoms to refrain from flying and to be honest with the FAA, posting a warning in italics on his website: "The Administrator [FAA] has made it very clear that they will prosecute any individual who 'knowingly and willingly falsifies' an application for a medical certificate."

Learning mindful relaxation can be supported by electroencephalographic biofeedback using a FDA–cleared device such as the Muse (Muse, 2023). The technical, "instrument panel" aspect of a biofeedback device might have an intrinsic appeal to a professional aviator. Similarly, a pilot might be motivated to improve their sleep and exercise habits by using a wearable device that continuously tracks their sleep and activity. Quantitative data and graphical representations generated from the data fit with pilots' cognitive style. They can help a pilot relate symptoms of fatigue, low mood, and cognitive inefficiency to controllable aspects of their lifestyle.

Non-invasive brain stimulation (NIBS), including transcranial magnetic stimulation (TMS) and transcranial direct current stimulation (Liu et al., 2017; Moffa et al., 2017; Mutz et al., 2018), transcranial alternating current and potentially light therapy (Asher et al., 2017; Elyamany et al., 2021; Perera et al., 2016), and photobiomodulation with near infrared light (Caldieraro & Cassano, 2019; Cassano et al., 2018) are non-pharmacologic biologic therapies for MDD with empirical support. When it is effective for a person's depression, NIBS can produce noticeable improvement in as little as one or two weeks. NIBS can complement and add to the benefit of CBT or other psychotherapy (Sathappan et al., 2019) or can be used to augment the therapeutic effect of an SSRI (Penders et al., 2016). CBT can be delivered in a form compatible with a pilot's lifestyle, utilizing a combination of psychotherapy apps and remote therapy appointments.

Psychotherapy can be continued after an episode of clinical depression remits with biological therapy, to decrease the probability of a relapse or recurrence without the use of maintenance medication. Since an ATP with a history of treatment for depression is required by regulations to have periodic psychiatric follow-up, mandatory clinical visits can provide a structure for supporting ongoing psychotherapy, lifestyle changes, or other non-pharmacologic treatments.

Except for TMS, the NIBS treatments listed are ones a pilot could continue at home or away to maintain a remission of depression, once it was established that the treatment had no adverse effect on the pilot's aviation-related cognitive or motor performance and there was concern about bipolarity. Adverse cognitive and motor effects of these treatments are rare, though if there were any question about such effects in a pilot being treated for depression, cognitive testing and/or evaluation in a flight simulator would be indicated.

The FAA does not provide any explicit guidance about treatment of depression by NIBS. The treating psychiatrist would need to work with a psychiatric AME to document the process and outcome of care in a way that would facilitate the pilot's first-class medical certification without entailing medically unnecessary time away from work. While a pilot with MDD obviously should not be flying while undergoing a trial of a new biological treatment, trials of brain stimulation modalities and adjustment of stimulation intensity, frequency, and duration to find parameters that are efficacious and well tolerated do not have the same institutional stigma as multiple trials of antidepressant medications. The latter would make it very difficult for a pilot to get a first-class medical certificate even if the ultimate result were a full remission of depression. Similarly, augmenting an SSRI with light therapy would not automatically disqualify a pilot from flying, unlike augmenting an SSRI with a second psychotropic drug.

Psychotherapy or counseling of some kind—whether formal CBT, the use of a psychotherapeutic mHealth app, interpersonal psychotherapy, or peer counseling by another pilot—is an important component of a treatment that has the goal of long-term, stable remission without reliance on medication. A pilot can have an initial experience of peer counseling prior to a formal diagnosis of depression. They are not obliged to report peer counseling per se to the FAA if they are not aware of any diagnosis or condition likely to affect their ability to fly safely.

Electronic communication by text, phone, or email and remote visits via a secure videoconferencing application will almost always be needed for a pilot being treated for depression while still actively flying on long-haul routes. A pilot is more likely to engage fully in treatment if they know that treatment can continue undisrupted after they resume flying.

Ongoing peer counseling can be especially helpful for pilots and others with masculine occupations in which seeking help for depression is stigmatized. It addresses both personal and institutional stigma, and it is intrinsically confidential because it does not entail formal clinical encounters that must be reported when the pilot applies for medical recertification (Mulder & de Rooy, 2018). There are websites and organizations dedicated to the provision of professionally supervised peer counseling to distressed pilots. LiftAffect (www.liftaffect.com) is a for-profit organization founded by pilots that offers consultation and counseling to help pilots deal with stress, anxiety, depression, relationship problems, and post-traumatic symptoms. It also provides coaching to help pilots build positive mental health and resilience and to reach their own goals for change. It explicitly acknowledges that mental health treatment, especially if documented without awareness of the FAA's certification process, can needlessly endanger the license of a pilot who can fly safely. Reporting to the

FAA is required if consultation leads to a formal psychiatric diagnosis, psychotropic medication is used, or there is a potential safety risk in the pilot's continuing to fly. A pilot is unlikely to consult the employee assistance programs of the airlines for which they work because of concern that a mental health professional without special expertise in treating pilots could unwittingly damage their career with a single progress note.

Pilots' challenge of getting timely medical treatment while keeping their first-class certification is not limited to psychiatric conditions. Another for-profit organization, the Aviation Medicine Advisory Service (AMAS; www.aviationmedicine.com) uses a team of AMEs and case managers to help pilots get the medical care they need while optimizing documentation so that pilots with conditions that do not entail safety risks are not grounded unnecessarily. Depression is just one of the conditions that AMAS advertises as a specialty.

In the FAA's formal guidance on medical certification, it strongly advises that pilots with mental/emotional issues be examined by (and presumably treated by) "a psychiatrist with experience in aerospace psychiatry and/or familiarity with aviation standards. Using a psychiatrist without this background may limit the usefulness of the report" (FAA, 2023). Similarly, if a pilot seeks treatment for depression, there will be less unnecessary risk to their medical certification and pilot's license if treatment comes from a psychiatrist or psychologist familiar with FAA regulations. When a pilot is seen by a consulting psychiatrist in connection with care for a general medical condition, a consultant unfamiliar with FAA policies and procedures should consider getting timely advice from a psychiatrist or psychologist with expertise in the regulatory dimension of pilots' mental health care. Details of treatment plans that would be of little consequence in other contexts (e.g., using paroxetine rather than sertraline as an SSRI to treat depression) could have costly, career-disrupting consequences for a pilot.

A self-aware and ethical airline pilot would not want to fly if they were in any way impaired. Recurrent or treatment-refractory MDD, BD, general medical conditions accompanied by secondary depression, or adverse cognitive and motor side effects of treatment needed to resolve a depression might make it necessary for a pilot to stop flying—or at least stop flying professionally as an ATP. If so, the pilot might need assistance in navigating between denial and catastrophic thinking. One year after an episode of MDD, some pilots are back in the air, while others have moved on to other work. Because of the all-or-nothing nature of ATP medical certification, an episode of depression in an airline pilot will always be a major life event. With a clinician's help it can become an opportunity for psychological growth and development.

Chapter 18

Truck-Driving Blues

"Got a low down feelin' truck driver's blues."

In country music legend Merle Haggard's classic song "Truck Driver's Blues," the singer describes a low mood, fatigue, and pressure to make a delivery on time. He turns to drinking and casual sex to ease his emotional pain. Whether or not he would meet Diagnostic and Statistical Manual of Mental Disorders (DSM) criteria for MDD, he certainly would satisfy this book's criteria for clinical depression, and he would meet the suggested criteria for "male depression" (Rice, Oliffe et al., 2018).

In the United States, commercial truck-driving is the occupation of more than 3.5 million people, of whom approximately two million drive heavy trucks or tractor-trailers (aka *18-wheelers*; Bureau of Labor Statistics, 2021a; Day & Hait, 2019). In 29 U.S. states, it is the most prevalent occupation (Bui, 2015). A career in truck-driving offers secure employment with an above-median income even in less prosperous areas of the country, and it does not require a college education or prolonged and costly training. It offers drivers the opportunity to travel widely and to work semi-autonomously, not under the continual supervision of a boss. Truck driving has a distinctive occupational culture, celebrated in country music, associated with strength, stamina, stoicism, and stereotypical masculinity.

American truck-driving culture evolved at a time when most truck drivers enjoyed relatively high wages and benefits, due to a combination of national regulation of interstate trucking and the political and economic power of the Teamsters' Union. In the late 1970s, the industry was deregulated. Following deregulation, the working conditions of truckers were overseen by the Department of Transportation (DOT) rather than the Department of Labor.

The DOT proved more responsive to the interests of business owners than those of employees. The compensation and working conditions of drivers deteriorated. In 1980 truck drivers' average pay (in 2016 dollars) was $110,000 per year; in 2020 median long-haul truckers' pay was less than half of that amount, despite a nearly fivefold growth in national per capita gross domestic product over the same period (Bureau of Labor Statistics, 2021a; Viscelli, 2016). In some areas of the U.S., the mean wage of heavy truck drivers in 2020 was less than $40,000 per year (Bureau of Labor Statistics, 2021b).

About 15% of American truckers do not have health insurance, a significantly higher proportion than the 10% of all American workers who are uninsured (Day & Hait, 2019). Truckers without health insurance either are employed by small companies that are not required by law to provide insurance to employees, are independent contractors, or are owner-operators who choose not to purchase insurance. In addition, even when truckers have health insurance, it often does not provide parity of coverage for mental disorders. Despite federal legislation mandating such parity, many employers work around the requirement by "carving out" mental health care from general medical care and then making mental health care difficult to access. Barriers include burdensome and repetitive requirements for prior authorization of treatment, high co-payments for visits to mental health professionals, and a small network of "preferred providers" who often have long waiting lists and appointment times that are inconvenient and sometimes infeasible for working people. Ensuring parity of coverage requires state laws that reinforce federal regulations and fill their gaps. Most U.S. states do not have laws adequate to do this—including most of the states in which truck-driving is the most prevalent occupation (ParityTrack.org, 2021).

Job characteristics can increase the risk of clinical depression and chronic medical conditions including ischemic heart disease through mechanisms including effort–reward imbalance (ERI), and demand–control imbalance (DCI), long working hours, job insecurity, and bullying on the job. The adverse effects of these "psychosocial work factors" on mental and physical health have been shown across nations and occupations (Burgel & Elshatarat, 2019; Li et al., 2019; Mo et al., 2020; Niedhammer et al., 2021b; Shields et al., 2021; Siegrist, 2021; Siegrist & Wege, 2020; Zhuo et al., 2020). In the 2015 European Working Conditions Study of 35 countries, the fraction of depression prevalence attributable to psychosocial work factors ranged from 17% to 35%.

While some owner-operators might be exceptions, employed truckers in America, and in many other countries without strong labor laws or empowered labor unions, tend to have little control over their work schedules and demands (DCI) and are poorly paid relative to the physical demands of their work (ERI). Drivers have long working hours, and most have variable and chronobiologically challenging schedules. Long-haul drivers must deal with days to weeks at a time away from their homes and loved ones.

Though the occupationally related physical and mental health problems of truck drivers have been known for decades, truck drivers' culture of stoic "masculinity" has led them to tolerate the working conditions that contribute to them. Truck drivers' culture combines with the practical contingencies of their work to explain their underutilization of healthcare of all kinds. Truck drivers have excess morbidity from heart and lung diseases, obesity (often contributing to type 2 diabetes or obstructive sleep apnea [OSA]), chronic musculoskeletal disorders, and depression. They have excess mortality not only from chronic diseases but also from accidents and suicide. While truck drivers comprise 2.2% of the U.S. working population, they account for over 17% of all occupationally related deaths (Chen et al., 2014), and that number does not include the attributable percentage of deaths from chronic diseases that are more prevalent in truck drivers. The 2015 suicide rate for men working in "transportation and material moving" was 30.9 per 100,000, well above the national rate for all working adults and fourth highest of all major occupational groups (Peterson et al. 2018).

In 2018 in the U.S., there were 4415 fatal crashes of large trucks. The driver's distraction/inattention or impairment from drugs, alcohol, or illness was implicated in approximately 10% of the fatal crashes. (Federal Motor Carrier Safety Administration [FMCSA], 2021). Truck drivers' neuropsychiatric issues—including depression, substance use disorders, and brain dysfunction related to chronic medical problems—not only affect truck drivers and their families but also touch the public in tragic ways since the victims of large truck crashes typically are pedestrians or drivers or passengers of cars and other small vehicles. Severely depressed drivers of heavy vehicles are over 4.5 times more likely to have an accident or a near miss than truckers with normal mood—equivalent to their driving with a blood alcohol concentration of 80 mg/dl, the legal criterion for intoxication in many states (Hilton et al., 2009).

The frequency of crashes of large trucks makes it likely that a long-haul truck driver will witness one or more crashes in their working life, and frightening near-miss experiences are commonplace. In a 2010 National Institute for Occupational Safety and Health (NIOSH) survey that interviewed 1265 long-haul drivers recruited from truck stops, 35% of those interviewed had at least one crash during their careers, and 24% had at least one near miss in the previous seven days. Despite the substantial risk of crashes, 4.5% of the drivers admitted to often driving 10 mph or more above the speed limit, 6.0% to never wearing a seatbelt, and 24% to often driving in situations where fatigue, bad weather, or heavy traffic increased their crash risk. 15% of the drivers thought that safety of workers was not a high priority with their employer (Chen et al.,

2014). The normalization and acceptance of hazardous working conditions are typical of the occupation, and many drivers engage in behavior that increases the risk of a crash and an injury.

An additional risk of the job is moral injury. In most crashes of heavy trucks, the other vehicle is a car or lighter truck, so the occupant of that vehicle is far more likely than the driver to suffer a serious or fatal injury. Awareness that a potentially avoidable crash for which one was entirely or partially responsible killed or disabled another person can be a moral injury sufficient to provoke depression. If a depressed trucker has had a moral injury, addressing it can be essential to their full recovery from depression.

Fatality rates from large truck and bus crashes, in deaths per 100 million miles, vary strikingly by region of the U.S., suggesting an interaction of regional culture and economy, drivers' working conditions, and typical drivers' styles of life and work. For example, the average of the large truck and bus crash fatality rates for the five states of greater Appalachia (Arkansas, Kentucky, Oklahoma, Tennessee, and West Virginia) is 0.23 deaths per 100 million miles, while the average of the rate for the six New England states is 0.10. Corroboration of an inter-regional cultural difference potentially relevant to truck crash risk is found in measures of social capital, regionally different rates of suicide and deaths from interpersonal violence, and rates of vaccination for COVID-19. A driver who respects safety rules, trusts legitimate authorities, is serious about prevention of illness or injury, and values self-control is less likely than one who doesn't to speed, to drive when sleepy or under the influence of drugs, or to display "road rage."

For men under age 70, combined mortality rates from suicide and interpersonal violence are lower in every one of the six New England states than in any of the greater Appalachian states. The 2019 suicide or violence–related mortality rates per 100,000 males aged 20–54 range from 25.3 to 35.1 among the New England states and from 42.0 to 53.2 among the states of greater Appalachia (IHME, 2023). The percentage of the population age 18 or over who were vaccinated against COVID-19 by April 2024 ranged from 84.5% to 92.5% in the New England states, and more than 30% had received a booster in 2023 or 2024. In the states of Greater Appalachia vaccination rates ranged from 70.8% to 76.8%., and in all states fewer than 20% had received boosters (CDC, 2024). State-level social capital in 2018 was above the national median in every state of New England and below the median in every state of greater Appalachia (Social Capital Project, 2018).

The prevalence of MDD in U.S. truck drivers is not known with certainty, but it probably is significantly higher than 10%. Depression in truck drivers was studied in a secondary analysis of data from the state of Washington's Behavioral Risk Factor Surveillance Survey, which contrasted rates of mental and behavioral conditions among different occupations. In that data set, truck drivers showed a prevalence of clinical depression of 14.6%, where the latter was defined by PHQ-8 score of 10 or higher. Though truck drivers have a high rate of general health conditions and lifestyle factors that predispose them to depression, the association of truck-driving with depression is not entirely explained by comorbidities and social determinants of health. In a logistic regression model that included age, gender, income, education, race and ethnicity, marital status, obesity, smoking, binge drinking, physical inactivity, common chronic diseases, and health insurance coverage, truck drivers were 6.18 times more likely to be clinically depressed than the reference group of managerial personnel (Fan et al., 2012). In a random sample of 316 male truck drivers surveyed at a truck stop in North Carolina, the self-reported lifetime prevalence of depression was 26.7%. In the same survey, 27.9% reported loneliness, and 20.6% had chronic sleep problems (Shattell et al., 2012). In a sample of truck drivers recruited from truck stops in western Canada, 44% reported feeling depressed in the past 12 months (Crizzle et al., 2020).

Depression as an occupational hazard of long-haul truck drivers is an international problem. Age- and gender-adjusted depression prevalence rates significantly greater for truck drivers than for the general working population have been reported in studies from Australia (Rice, Aucote et al., 2018), Brazil (da Silva-Junior et al., 2009), Canada (Crizzle et al., 2020), China (Shen et al., 2013), Hong Kong (Wong et al., 2007), Kenya (Romo et al., 2019), South Africa (Wadley et al., 2020), and the United Kingdom (Longman et al., 2021). The prevalence of depression in truck drivers might be greater in middle-income countries than it is in the U.S. In a sample of 441 employed male drivers recruited from trucking companies in mainland China, more than half (53.7%) were identified as having clinical depression, with approximately half of those having moderate to severe symptoms (Shen et al., 2013).

As noted above, depression in truck drivers is associated with a significantly increased risk of crashes (Alavi et al., 2017). In studies from Africa and from China, the incidence of high-risk sexual behavior among male long-haul truck drivers was higher among drivers with mental health issues including depression (Romo et al., 2019; Wong et al., 2007). Male truck drivers with sufficient conventional depressive symptoms to meet the diagnostic criteria for MDD frequently also display externalizing behavior including irritability, aggression and anger, risk-taking, and substance misuse—the syndrome of "male depression" (Rice, Oliffe et al., 2018).

To have safer roads and prevent thousands of deaths, severe depression in truck drivers should be addressed both by primary prevention and by early identification and effective treatment of milder forms of clinical depression.

Comprehensively addressing the problem in the U.S. would require improvement in truckers' working conditions and in their health insurance coverage and reduction of the stigma of depression and of seeking and receiving mental health care (Apostolopoulos et al., 2014). Adaptation of treatment to the occupational culture of truck-driving and to drivers' working conditions would be a necessary part of an optimal solution.

The Work of Long-Haul Truck Drivers

About half of the nation's truck drivers are *long-haul* truck drivers—people who drive hundreds of miles a day and spend most of their nights away from home—sometimes on the road for weeks at a time. More than 90% of truck drivers are men, typically high school graduates without college degrees (Bureau of Labor Statistics, 2021a). Their annual incomes, though much lower after inflation adjustment than those of truckers of past generations, place them well above the median for men with similar education. Drivers with specialized skills or credentials for transporting hazardous materials, for operating tanker trucks, for moving fragile objects, or for driving on ice can earn substantially higher incomes. Some large companies (e.g., Walmart) seeking to retain experienced, safe drivers in a situation of shortage offer significantly higher salaries and provide health insurance and retirement benefits (Nassauer, 2022). However, these are the exception in the industry.

Owner-operators—drivers who own and operate their own rigs and contract with transport companies to haul goods—can earn six-figure incomes but are vulnerable to unexpected large expenses if their trucks require costly repairs. Some owner-operators (who might be called *debtor-operators*) are recent employees of transport companies who were persuaded to purchase trucks with money borrowed from the company. Typical contracts require the former employee to repay the loan in full if they stop contracting with their former employer, and if they do not pay in full, the company retains all payments made to date. Even if the former employee needs time off for illness or a family emergency, they will forfeit ownership of the truck and will lose whatever was paid to the transport company before the break in their service. The transport company can underpay and exploit a debtor-operator, who, though ostensibly independent, cannot afford to change jobs.

The most common form of compensation for employed truckers is a fixed fee per mile driven rather than an hourly wage or monthly salary. Under this system, drivers do not receive overtime pay no matter how many hours per day or per week are spent on the job. Compensation by mileage implies that when the driver must slow down because of traffic or weather, their effective hourly wage will fall precisely at a time when the work becomes more effortful and dangerous. Because American drivers have been limited by federal regulation to driving no more than 11 hours in a 24-hour period, the stress of driving in heavy traffic or bad weather is compounded by their knowing they will be paid less for the day's work. Drivers paid by the mile rather than a fixed salary work more hours, have worse sleep, and consequently have worse health. Truck drivers paid by the mile usually do not receive any compensation for the hours they spend loading and unloading the truck or waiting for access to a loading dock. Loading, unloading, and waiting time count against the daily hour limit, so they represent a loss of earning opportunity.

Culturally, employed truck drivers are in the working class, while owner-operators (other than debtor-operators) are in the middle or upper-middle class. Owner-operators are significantly less likely to suffer from depression than employed truck drivers, as are drivers who are over age 45 and drivers with post-secondary education (da Silva-Junior et al., 2009). Owner-operators also have better physical health, with a lower prevalence of the chronic diseases commonly seen in employed truckers. Education, experience, and ownership of one's own truck(s) all improve the balance of demand and control and the balance of effort and reward.

While truck-driving is not characterized as a high-status occupation in standard classifications of socioeconomic status, truck drivers are proud of their work and expect others to appreciate their role in the nation's economy. Drivers are resentful if they are treated disrespectfully by dispatchers or are stereotyped by the public as obese, unkempt, and vulgar. Truck drivers' work is essential to the American economy and to the economies of virtually all other middle- and high-income countries. It cannot be outsourced to another country with lower wages. The importance of truck drivers' work was especially salient during the COVID-19 pandemic, although renewed appreciation for the essential nature of their work usually has not translated into better compensation or health benefits. During the pandemic, truck drivers being recognized as "essential workers" did not imply that they would be provided with safe working conditions. Early in the pandemic, most truckers were not furnished with personal protective equipment and thus were at significant risk of exposure to SARS-CoV-2 every time they picked up or delivered goods.

Truck driving is physically strenuous work. Drivers feel proud of having the strength and stamina to do the job day after day. Many people who start driving trucks as young adults do not continue in the occupation. Those who are still driving by middle age have accepted the hardships of the job, have acquired valuable experience, and tend to be safer drivers than younger ones with less experience. Age-related changes in health and function typically do not begin to increase older truckers' crash risk until they are in their mid-60s (Duke et al., 2010). Experienced middle-aged drivers are likely to get jobs with better pay and benefits or to become owner-operators. The health issues of some, but not all, older truck drivers that increase crash risk, including OSA, depression, and substance misuse, are not accompaniments of aging per se but relate more to affected drivers' unhealthy lifestyles and working conditions.

To become a truck driver in the U.S., one needs a clean criminal record and several weeks of training, followed by an examination to obtain a commercial driver's license (CDL). Though most truckers are high school graduates, a high school diploma or GED is not a requirement for a CDL. Drivers must pass a screening medical examination before beginning interstate trucking and must pass a new medical examination every two years. CDL training typically costs between $3000 and $10,000 (Schneiderjobs.co, 2023). A trucker can recoup the cost of their training in several months, rather than in the years that might be needed to recoup the cost of a college education or pilot training. The occupation would seem an appealing choice for a person without a college education and even more appealing for one who had not completed high school. However, the work is physically difficult, and the working conditions are challenging and sometimes oppressive.

The working conditions of long-haul truckers are those of an intensely competitive, deregulated industry in which the well-being of workers has been—and continues to be—a low priority. Demands for "just in time" deliveries put drivers in a situation of high demand and low control. DCI is a known risk factor for depression and other stress-related disorders. In a survey of 260 long-haul truck drivers at a North Carolina truck stop, 70.4% reported working over 11 hours per day (Hege et al., 2017). Workweeks of 60 to 70 hours are common. Driving hours can change frequently because of varying times for picking up or dropping off loads; contingencies of traffic, weather, or road conditions; or the need to make up miles not driven as previously planned. The consequence is a high prevalence of short sleep duration and poor sleep quality, also well-known risk factors for depression (Garbarino et al., 2018; Guglielmi et al., 2018; Khurshid, 2018). Inadequate sleep causes fatigue that diminishes the desire for physical exercise and increases blood levels of leptin, leading to increased appetite. A sedentary lifestyle and eating large amounts of unhealthy food add further to depression risk. Truckers might be required by employers or by circumstances to drive on schedules that disrupt their chronobiology, a problem shared by shift workers and people whose work requires them to frequently fly across time zones. Long-haul drivers take breaks at truck stops and rest areas where opportunities for exercise may be lacking. Many truck stop parking areas are poorly lit and unsafe, but a truck driver hoping to park long enough for a nap or overnight sleep might have no convenient alternative.

Health Consequences of the Truck-Driving Lifestyle

Approximately 80% of long-haul truck drivers are overweight or obese, and more than a quarter are morbidly obese, with a body mass index (BMI) ≥35 (Apostolopoulos, Sönmez, et al., 2013; Thiese et al., 2015). Obesity is a risk factor for depression, with two common mediators being OSA and systemic inflammation. Sometimes trauma is the link between obesity and depression in truck drivers since obese truck drivers have 1.5 times the crash risk of their non-obese peers (Anderson et al., 2012).

While more than 80% of American truck drivers have significant general health issues—either chronic diseases or high risk for developing them—the occupational culture is one that normalizes or minimizes serious health problems. In a national survey sample of 316 long-haul drivers, 73% described their health as good, very good, or excellent. In the same sample, 53.4% of drivers were obese (BMI ≥30), 56.3% had chronic fatigue, 57.9% had sleep disorders, and 42.3% had chronic back and neck pain (Apostolopoulos, Sönmez, et al., 2013).

The drivers in the national survey mentioned many barriers to getting healthcare, including lack of health insurance, no paid sick leave, and no access to medical services other than an emergency room or urgent care clinic during the weeks they are on the road and away from home. 71.1% of the drivers reported having no regular healthcare visits. One quarter said it was difficult for them to keep medical appointments, and a similar proportion said they simply could not afford medical care. More than half said they had no interest in receiving health information, and 70% got no regular exercise.

In the U.S., truck drivers' culture of toughness and independence, and of denial and minimization of occupational hazards and health risks, makes them unlikely to organize to advocate for better working conditions. Owners and executives of most American transport companies pursue their short-term financial interest by spending relatively little to improve their employees' health and safety, while at the same time bemoaning the shortage of qualified truck drivers.

The U.S. is not alone in encountering a shortage of heavy truck drivers, worse since the COVID-19 pandemic. There is unsatisfied demand throughout the world, with as many as 25% of all driving jobs unfilled in some countries. Compared with other blue-collar jobs, truck driving attracts and retains fewer men under age 40 (Fleming, 2021). Turnover is the main reason for the shortage. Many young men try truck driving for a year or two, then move on to another job.

The American trucking industry's proposed solutions include autonomous self-driving trucks and permitting teenagers to obtain CDLs despite the evidence that teenage drivers have more crashes than adults. Improving drivers' compensation, health benefits, schedules, and working conditions is not high on the industry's list of options. In the U.S., truck drivers have not effectively advocated for meaningful changes in their working conditions that might improve their health, safety, and longevity. In many U.S. states where trucking is the leading occupation, there is antipathy and mistrust toward labor unions, reflected by strong support for right-to-work laws (laws that prohibit employers contracting with labor unions to require non-union employees to pay union dues). Of the 29 states in which truck driving is the most common occupation, 19 have right-to-work laws ("Right to Work Law," 2021; Bui, 2015).

There is also mistrust of the federal government and fear that well-intentioned regulations will make their lives worse. Federal regulations have not protected drivers' health to the extent regulators had intended. Interstate truck drivers, paid by the mile driven, are subject to complex "hours of service" (HOS) rules that limit driving to 11 hours per day, limit weekly hours, and require periodic 30-minute breaks from driving. Drivers are required to have devices in their truck cabs that track their time on the road. The rules don't protect drivers from overwork because the limits apply only to driving per se, and drivers often must do other work including loading and unloading, record-keeping, and maintaining their vehicles. Furthermore, many drivers find that HOS rules can prohibit their driving at times when there is less traffic and better weather, which would enable them to rack up more miles with fewer hours behind the wheel and less stress. For example, a driver foreseeing heavy traffic and a snowstorm on a Monday morning might prefer to drive 24 hours between Friday evening and Sunday evening and take a 24-hour break after that, but HOS rules would not allow them to do so.

It probably is more likely that an American truck driver would complain about the inflexibility of "government regulations" regarding driving schedules than they would hold employers accountable for unsafe or unhealthy working conditions. Low social capital, including mistrust of institutions, is an aspect of regional culture seen in most of the states in which truck driving is the most common occupation. Favoring personal independence and freedom of choice over health and safety is a common attribute of the "masculine" regional cultures characteristic of most states where truck driving is the most common occupation. However, there are numerous exceptions, and the decisions of any individual driver can be influenced by accurate information delivered in a culturally aware clinical context.

Truck driving entails an increased risk of painful musculoskeletal conditions, many of which are caused or exacerbated by occupational injuries, which occur 3.5 times more frequently in truck drivers than in the general employed population (Combs et al., 2018). Driving involves hours of work in a sitting posture, with no opportunity to stand or move around, a situation that increases the risk of back and neck strain as well as cardiovascular disease. Truck drivers whose jobs include assisting with loading and unloading the truck—the case for many long-haul drivers as well as virtually all drivers of local delivery trucks—are at risk for muscle strain and sprains related to heavy lifting, awkward postures, contact with heavy objects or equipment, or falls—the last of these most likely to occur during loading or unloading a truck on an uneven or slippery surface.

The risk of injury during loading or unloading is accompanied by a high incidence of insult. Many employers do not pay truck drivers for their work loading and unloading because drivers' compensation is based solely on miles driven. Further, some sites receiving goods would not allow a truck driver making a delivery to enter their premises to use the restroom.

Additional Health Risks: Vibration, Noise, and Poor Air Quality

The driver's seat of a large truck vibrates, and the amplitude of the induced whole-body vibration (WBV) can be high enough to cause or aggravate low back pain or other spinal problems (Bovenzi, 2009; Lan et al., 2016). The adverse health effects of WBV can combine with those related to awkward postures associated with loading and unloading activities (Raffler et al., 2017). WBV also contributes to fatigue and consequently can add to crash risk (Troxel et al., 2016). Muscle strain injuries cause pain that can precipitate or exacerbate depression.

Some of the more injurious types of WBV can be reduced by installing seating designed to attenuate it and by replacing and updating seating that becomes so worn with age that it transmits more vibration (Blood et al., 2015; Johnson et al., 2018; Kim et al., 2016, Kim et al., 2018). Drivers find vibration-attenuating seating more comfortable, and such seating not only can improve subjective physical and mental health status but also can improve drivers' vigilance and reaction times (Du et al., 2018; Nazerian et al., 2020). However, an employed driver has no control over how the truck they drive will be equipped. If a driver develops painful symptoms due to an occupational vibration exposure that could have been prevented, their negative emotional reaction to the physical symptoms might be stronger. As with health insurance and other expenses related to drivers' health, owner-operators and small trucking companies can be tempted to skimp on expenditures for seating improvements because of their impact on profit margins.

In addition to financial considerations, truckers' culture can be a barrier to improving seating to reduce harmful WBV. For example, *cabover* (cab over engine) designs that put the driver's seat of the truck cab over the engine and the front axle are associated with substantially greater WBV (Blood et al., 2011). They also require the driver's assuming awkward positions as they enter and exit the truck or reach for an item in the back of the cab. The cabover design was a response to regulations in force in the U.S. between 1956 and 1976—and still applicable in Europe, Australia, and Japan—that limit the total length of a tractor-trailer combination. By reducing the length of the tractor, the cabover design permits the use of a longer trailer with a larger payload.

In a sentimental online article at a truckers' website reminiscing about the glory days of cabover trucks in the U.S., the article's author offers quotes from veteran drivers about their experience with cabovers (MacMillan, 2020). Overall, the drivers quoted acknowledged the uncomfortable, unhealthy, and potentially dangerous aspects of the cabovers; but many still longed for them, perhaps feeling themselves personally immune to serious harm. The following quotes are representative:

> Man, those old cabover trucks were "back busters."
>
> Drove these trucks for years. But no more please, too uncomfortable. My Dad drove so many of these, his knees still rattle and shake!
>
> They were also louder than long hood rigs, as the driver was sitting right above the engine!
>
> A cabover rig isn't as safe as a long hood rig, in the event of an accident, as there just isn't any protection for the driver.
>
> The cabover truck is an icon. It represents the days of trucking we all long for, in today's world of trucking, that is so muddled up and complex with it's [sic] mounds of unnecessary rules, regs and guidelines.
>
> Aahhhh yes, I spent many a day in these. Heck, it reminds me of the good old days when there were way less laws and regs.
>
> My Grandpa and my Dad owned several of them. The best trucks ever.
>
> Just love the old school rigs.
>
> They were quite safe if they were driven with respect. Drivers didn't worry about "head on" collisions.

Noise exposure is a health risk for truck drivers, as it is for airline pilots and rock musicians. Truckers are exposed for many hours per day to noise near and sometimes above the 85 dB threshold that NIOSH cites as likely to be harmful if exposure is regular and prolonged. When long-haul drivers sleep in their trucks near interstate highways—and many do—they can still be exposed to over

80 dB of noise, so they have no opportunity to recover from the noise exposure they had while driving (Seshagiri, 1998). Prolonged noise exposure can precipitate depression directly (Leijssen et al., 2019; Orban et al., 2016). It can lead to tinnitus, a condition associated both with insomnia and with depression (Salazar et al., 2019.). It can also cause hearing loss, which is associated with late-life depression in men and with cognitive decline in both men and women (Amieva et al., 2018; Blazer & Tucci, 2019 Karimi et al., 2010).

Truck drivers' noise exposure can in many cases be reduced, though it seldom is. Modifications in the cabin—easily made using aftermarket sound-absorbing linings for the cabin floor and doors—can reduce the transmission of engine and road noise to the cabin. In many U.S. states, truck drivers are not legally permitted to wear earplug or noise-reduction headsets because they must be alert to the warning sounds of car horns, train whistles, and shouting people. However, there are active noise-reduction earphones that offer protection from many kinds of harmful background noise without preventing the wearer from hearing audible signals, and if it is documented that a patient has tinnitus or mild to moderate high-frequency hearing loss, a physician's note of a medical reason the driver needs ear protection—or amplification that includes noise reduction—might address the legal issue.

Drivers can be exposed to medically significant air pollution—including particulates, volatile organic compounds, sulfur dioxide, nitrogen dioxide, and ozone—from diesel and gasoline engine exhaust and from industrial plants near truck loading areas. If a long-haul driver is on the road for three weeks per month and sleeps near the highway (in their truck at a truck stop or rest area or at a roadside motel), they will be exposed to air pollution to at least the same extent as people who live close to major highways—a group known to suffer adverse health effects. If the driver is a smoker, asthmatic, or otherwise vulnerable to pulmonary symptoms, exposure to polluted air can cause shortness of breath, a distressing and often depressing condition that further reduces beneficial physical exercise. Diesel fumes can directly affect the driver's mood. People who live in areas with elevated levels of sulfur dioxide and particulate matter of 2.5 μm diameter or less from diesel emissions have increased rates of depression and suicidal behavior (Ali & Khoja, 2019; Gladka et al., 2018; Zeng et al., 2019).

Like WBV and excessive noise, dangerously polluted air is a remediable risk. Available air filtration systems for vehicle cabins can dramatically reduce levels of particulates and of toxic gases. The most effective cabin air filters combine particulate filtration with gas absorption (e.g., by activated charcoal). To be most effective, filters must be replaced regularly. In keeping with the occupational culture of normalization, denial, and fierce independence, this often doesn't happen. Drivers don't insist on it (or would find it useless to do so), and they would be likely to resent any regulations dealing with the issue.

Thus, three major occupational health hazards of long-haul truck drivers are potentially remediable by existing technologies, and solutions continue to improve. Nonetheless, interventions to reduce these hazards are seldom implemented. In the U.S., reasons for inaction to reduce identified occupational health hazards include truckers' culture of stoicism and mistrust of regulators, transport companies' pursuit of maximum profit with relatively little concern about their drivers' health, and lack of political consensus on the proper roles of government and of organized labor in addressing matters of occupational health. Owner-operators might be reluctant to invest in preventive technologies because they normalize the noxious aspects of their work environment, minimize the potential harm to themselves, and don't want to reduce the profit from their small business. Debtor-operators might be struggling with financial precarity and see the additional expense as infeasible, much as many will see routine primary care as unaffordable.

The low life expectancy (Lemke & Apostolopoulos, 2015) and general poor health of truck drivers, as well as the relationship of truckers' chronic health problems to remediable environmental exposures and other adverse working conditions, are not widely appreciated by the public. Potentially preventable occupational health issues contribute to crashes in which thousands of people are killed annually in the U.S. alone, but the cost of such crashes typically is paid through insurance and is not borne directly by a transport company or owner-operator. And when a trucker develops a potentially preventable disease or disability after years of harmful occupational exposures, the party paying for their care is unlikely to be one of the trucker's employers during the years of the most harmful occupational exposures.

Executives of trucking companies in the U.S. are aware of their labor shortages and of the implications of drivers' illnesses to employee turnover, absenteeism, diminished productivity, and safety. They are aware of the high cost of accidents and the relationship of driver fatigue and sleepiness to accident risk. Several of the largest companies have employee health programs and employee assistance programs for drivers with personal and emotional problems, but none has a comprehensive health promotion strategy that includes prevention and treatment of depression; aggressive screening for OSA, a condition strongly associated both with depression and with crash risk; and serious attention to the occupational hazards of noise, WBV, air pollution, and chronobiologic disruption. Not only do long-haul truckers have a culture that prizes self-reliance, but most of them must rely on themselves to stay safe and healthy because most employers do very little to improve their drivers' working conditions or to provide them with health coverage that would remove the financial disincentive for seeking care.

The story of heavy truck drivers' relationship with regulation suggests that population health initiatives aimed at truckers should focus on enhancing truckers' independence, self-reliance, and autonomy, rather than relying on regulations to minimize drivers' exposure to harmful aspects of their work. It would be helpful to drivers' physical and mental health for truck stops to offer healthy food options and safe, attractive spaces for exercise. However, regulations to require these and other health-oriented features at truck stops on interstate highways probably would be opposed by many truck drivers. Any increase in truck stops' prices of food, drink, or fuel probably would be blamed on the new regulations. To get truck stops to be safer for women and men, to offer exercise options, and to offer healthy food at affordable prices, demands for change must come from truckers themselves.

If trucking companies were financially at risk for their employees' healthcare costs, it would be in their interest to facilitate or pay for measures that would reduce those costs. The relatively few trucking companies that do offer health promotion programs for their employees are large firms that must provide health insurance for their drivers and are at risk for higher costs if their drivers' health is poor. Paradoxically, even requirements for smaller trucking companies to provide health insurance for their employees might be resented by truckers who would blame their low take-home pay on their employers' cost of mandated health coverage and on deductions from their gross wages to pay the employee's share of insurance premiums. Such coverage might be perceived as optional by drivers who perceived their health to be "good, very good, or excellent" despite the likely presence of significant health problems. Furthermore, most drivers would want the freedom to choose between health coverage and higher take-home pay.

Measures to improve drivers' health need not be expensive or offensive to drivers. Requirements for truck drivers' seating to be designed and maintained to reduce WBV, for cabins to be lined to reduce noise, and for cabin air filters to be of high quality and changed regularly might be acceptable to drivers. If long-haul truck cabs were routinely outfitted with refrigerators and microwave ovens, truckers could—if they chose—prepare their own healthy food and not patronize truck stop restaurants or convenience stores with poor-quality food and/or non-competitive pricing.

Loneliness of the Long-Distance Trucker

Most long-haul truckers drive alone, and they are vulnerable to loneliness—a risk factor for clinical depression, suicidal ideation, and chronic medical conditions associated with depression (Beutel et al., 2017; Erzen & Cikrikci, 2018; Ge et al., 2017; Jaremka et al., 2014). Many lonely truckers feel tempted to engage in risky behavior during their breaks from driving, such as having casual and unprotected sex (Apostolopoulos, Sönmez, & Massengale, 2013), binge drinking, or using recreational drugs (Girotto et al., 2014). Bragazzi et al. (2018) estimated, from a literature review and meta-analysis, that 19% of truck drivers engage in binge drinking, 9.4% drink alcohol daily, and 22.7% have responses to the Alcohol Use Disorders Identification Test (AUDIT; Higgins-Biddle & Babor, 2018) or CAGE questionnaire (Dhalla & Kopec, 2007) that suggest an alcohol use disorder. The proportional mortality rate of truck drivers from hepatitis C, a condition transmitted by unprotected sex and by abuse of injected drugs with non-sterile needles, is significantly elevated (National Occupational Mortality Surveillance, 2019b). Both loneliness itself and the adverse interpersonal, health-related, and/or legal consequences of high-risk behavior provoked by loneliness can lead to depression.

Long-haul truckers with families or in committed intimate relationships might be separated from their loved ones for weeks at a time as they do not necessarily return home between loads. When they return home after weeks on the road there usually is a backlog of family concerns and housekeeping activities. Spouses/partners and children have emotional needs to be met, and there might be differences to work out concerning childrearing or family finances. The family's home or car might need repairs awaiting the trucker's personal involvement. Depending on the trucker's work arrangements, they may be called upon to haul another load before the end of the time they were expecting to be at home. Work–family conflict, and more generally work–life conflict, is the norm for long-haul truckers. This is yet another risk factor for depression, both because of its direct effects on emotional well-being and because it can lead to marital conflict, legal separation or divorce, or the breakup of an unmarried couple in a committed long-term relationship.

Long-haul truck drivers' loneliness can be mitigated in several healthy ways. Having a co-driver prevents loneliness and improves driving safety. Driving with a canine companion relieves loneliness, and walking their dog ensures that a driver will have regular daily exercise.

Transport companies vary greatly in their attitudes toward drivers taking dogs on the road. Some welcome it, others prohibit it, and many require drivers to pay substantial, non-refundable cleaning fees or make long-term cash security deposits if they wish to drive with a dog. Notwithstanding, taking a dog on the road can make a meaningful contribution to a driver's mental health, and it should be considered as a potential lifestyle change a clinician might propose to a depressed driver. If the driver wanted to bring a dog on the road and their employer would not allow it, there would be good reason for the driver to consider changing employers.

Masculine Occupational Culture and "Male Depression"

The culture of truck drivers values traditional masculinity, with physical strength, endurance, and toughness in the face of adversity. Though this has begun to change in the U.S., the occupational culture defines trucking as an essentially male occupation. Truck driving offers a working man a secure identity. This is reflected in country songs that describe men as born to drive and attached to their trucks until the day they die (Eastman et al., 2013).

If a male truck driver becomes depressed, he is likely to display externalizing symptoms, with or without acknowledging a mood of sadness or depression (Rice, Oliffe et al., 2018). Such symptoms include anger, irritability, risk-taking, and self-medication with alcohol and drugs. In addition to externalizing symptoms, stereotypically masculine men with depression might complain of pain and/or fatigue that has become less tolerable since they became depressed. Various combinations of internalizing, externalizing, and somatic symptoms all are compatible with the definition of clinical depression proposed in this book.

As noted previously with respect to the cultures of places, the prevalence of "male depression" relative to typical DSM/ICD major depression is determined largely by cultural context. It is more common in places higher on the cultural dimension of masculinity and in more gendered occupations—truck driving and air transport piloting being prototypical examples. In many of the American states in which truck driving is the most prevalent occupation, the regional culture is more masculine than American culture overall. Clinical assessment of depression in truck drivers can be made more sensitive by using self-rating questionnaires for male depression and/or by incorporating the content of a male depression questionnaire into a clinical diagnostic interview. This is an especially important consideration when a patient's self-concept and/or social presentation is stereotypically masculine.

The concept of male depression is mentioned in several other chapters; its greater recognition is part of the contemporary trend toward appreciating the phenotypic heterogeneity of clinical depression. Several dimensions of cultural identity, including not only those related to gender but also those related to place, occupation, generation, and education influence the relative prevalence of the syndrome among people with clinical depression.

The three best validated questionnaire-based ratings for male depression are the Gotland Male Depression Scale (GMDS; Zierau et al., 2002), the Masculine

Depression Risk Scale (MDRS-22; Rice et al., 2013), and the Masculine Depression Scale (MDS; Magovcevic & Addis, 2008). The questionnaires can be used in evaluating a truck driver with suspected depression, or they can be used as a source of content for the clinical interview. The scales all comprise Likert-type items on which patients rate how much or how frequently a description of feelings or behavior applies to them.

The GMDS does not include terms like *depression* or *sadness* but instead uses words and phrases like *self-pity, complaining*, and *seeming pathetic*. Other items refer to aggressiveness, difficulties keeping self-control, feeling burned out and empty, and being "more irritable, restless and frustrated." Respondents are asked if others have perceived them as having such feelings—leaving room for patients to acknowledge symptoms they would not complain of spontaneously.

The MDRS measures six discrete dimensions of externalized depression. Respondents are asked to look back on the past month and rate on a scale of 0 (*not at all*) to 7 (*25+ days*) how frequently each of 22 statements applied to them. The dimensions of the MDRS and their representative statements are reproduced in Table 18.1. The GMDS is displayed in Table 18.2.

The MDS has 44 items, of which 11 concern externalizing symptoms and the remaining 33 cover typical internalizing symptoms of depression—emotional, cognitive, motivational, and somatic. The questions about externalizing symptoms mention yelling at people or things; having a short fuse; getting angry to the point of smashing or punching something; getting "mad, not sad"; using recreational drugs or alcohol "a lot" and to feel better; and needing more sex than usual to feel good. Subjects are asked if they feel under constant pressure, if they feel like they need to handle their problems on their own, and if they feel that it's been easier to focus on work or school than the rest of their life.

Subjects, male or female, who regard themselves as having stereotypically masculine attributes, and men who have a traditional concept of the masculine role, show relatively more externalizing symptoms of depression. However, men with clinical levels of depressive symptoms usually will acknowledge conventional (internalizing) symptoms of depression if asked about them explicitly (Magovcevic and Addis, 2008; Price et al., 2018). Men and women with a more "masculine" identity might experience the internalizing symptoms of depression like less masculine men and more feminine women, but they will express those symptoms differently and respond to them differently. Truckers of either gender might display the "male depression" syndrome when they become depressed. Because scores on generic depression rating scales like the PHQ-9, BDI and CES-D and scores on male depression rating scales are only partially correlated, a person's score on a male depression rating scale

Table 18.1 Content of the Male Depression Risk Scale

Symptom Domain	Representative Statements
Emotion suppression	I bottled up my negative feelings.
	I tried to ignore feeling down.
	I covered up my difficulties.
	I had to work things out by myself.
Drug use	I used drugs to cope.
	Using drugs provided temporary relief.
	I sought out drugs.
Alcohol use	I needed alcohol to help me unwind.
	I needed to have easy access to alcohol.
	I drank more alcohol than usual.
	I stopped feeling so bad while drinking.
Anger and aggression	I was verbally aggressive to others.
	I verbally lashed out at others without being provoked.
	It was difficult to manage my anger.
	I overreacted to situations with aggressive behavior.
Somatic symptoms	I had unexplained aches and pains.
	I had stomach pains.
	I had regular headaches.
	I had more heartburn than usual.
Risk-taking	I drove dangerously or aggressively.
	I stopped caring about the consequences of my actions.
	I took unnecessary risks.

Note. From Rice et al. (2013).

might reveal a more severe depression with greater functional impairment and higher suicidal risk than their score on a generic rating scale. Similarly, a clinical interview that explored the externalizing symptoms of a patient with suspected depression might reveal a level of suicide risk or functional impairment that would not be evident from one that asked only about the nine criterion symptoms of MDD. Exploring externalizing symptoms is especially important when assessing patients of either gender who have "masculine" occupations like truck driving.

Table 18.2 Gotland Scale for Male Depression: "During the past month, have you or others noticed that your behavior has changed, and if so, in which way?" (0 [not at all]; 1 [to some extent]; 2 [very true]; 3 [extremely so])

Change in Behavior	0	1	2	3
Lower stress threshold/more stressed out than usual				
More aggressive, outward-reacting, difficulties keeping self-control				
Feeling of being burned out and empty				
Constant, inexplicable tiredness				
More irritable, restless, and frustrated				
Difficulty making ordinary everyday decisions				
Sleep problems: sleeping too much/too little/restlessly, difficulty falling asleep/waking up early				
In the morning especially, having a feeling of disquiet/anxiety/uneasiness				
Overconsumption of alcohol and pills in order to achieve a calming and relaxing effect. Being hyperactive or blowing off steam by working hard and restlessly, jogging or other exercise, over- or undereating				
Do you feel your behavior has altered in such a way that neither you yourself nor others can recognize you and that you are difficult to deal with?				
Have you felt or have others perceived you as being gloomy, negative, or characterized by a state of hopelessness in which everything looks bleak?				
Have you or others noticed that you have a greater tendency to self-pity, to be complaining, or to seem "pathetic"?				
In your biological family, is there any tendency toward abuse, depression/dejection, suicide attempts, or proneness to behavior involving danger?				

Note. From Zierau et al. (2002). (Swedish version: Wolfgang Rutz, Zoltán Rihmer, and Arne Dalteg. English version: Per Bech, Lis Raabæk Olsen, and Vibeke Nørholm.)

Drivers' Relationships with Their Jobs

US truck-driving culture was explored in a series of 42 qualitative interviews with drivers of various backgrounds from 15 states. The researcher, Julia Wenger (2008), interviewed them about their reasons for choosing the occupation, their main concerns about their jobs, and what they liked most and least about their jobs.

Drivers' reasons for choosing the occupation included (relatively) good pay, a short training period, the opportunity to travel around the country and have adventures and memorable experiences, enjoying driving as an activity, independence, and the opportunity to work without being directly observed by a supervisor. Drivers voiced a long list of negatives and concerns, including lack of sleep, long periods away from their families, excessive demands from employers, and feeling that their important work was disrespected and that many people condescended to them. Many drivers were afraid of being victims of crime. Physical health problems mentioned included obesity and its complication of sleep apnea, aggravated by the poor quality of food at truck stops and lack of opportunity to exercise. Others noted frequent minor injuries. Many had no health insurance or had some health insurance coverage but were worried about the affordability of co-payments for doctor visits and medications.

Employed drivers often felt abused by their bosses, who would press them to drive unsafely to deliver a load more quickly. Some felt treated like slaves or pieces of equipment, and that their employers had no understanding of how factors beyond their control might slow down a trip. Owner-operators worried about the high cost of diesel fuel, repairs, and other expenses of operating large trucks.

Both employed drivers and owner-operators had mixed feelings about regulations. Many drivers were annoyed by the inflexibility of regulations concerning their record-keeping, the precise way their truck's load was distributed, and restrictions on HOS that sometimes prevented them from delivering a load on time. Others, however, wished that regulations would require longer periods of rest between long trips so that their employers would not press them to take on too much work, leading to fatigue and, in the worst case, a crash or an injury. Drivers were generally negative about electronic recording and tracking devices on their trucks, resenting them as an intrusion on their privacy.

Wenger concluded her qualitative study with a reflection that many of the truck drivers she interviewed spoke of their work as one might talk about an abusive relationship with a beloved spouse. They were aware of working conditions that were harmful to their physical and mental health but simultaneously loved the adventure of the open road, their occupational identity, and their camaraderie with other drivers.

Truck-Driving Women

In the song "Truck Driving Woman" (music and lyrics by Johnny Wilson and Roland Pike; first recorded by Norma Jean and covered a generation later by Patricia Maguire), the female singer claims that when driving her truck, she can outrun any man who tries to compete with her. Her truck driver father wanted a son and not a daughter, but she's sure she can "fill her daddy's shoes." She knows every legend of the road, and when she drives, she goes as fast as she can to make big money.

Worldwide, about 2% of heavy truck drivers are women; the female share of the occupation is small even in countries with high occupational gender equality. The percentage in the U.S., now approximately 9%, is likely to increase. Because there is a shortage of heavy truck drivers, anyone with a CDL and a clean record can find a job; and many employers are actively recruiting female drivers. Male and female truck drivers are paid equally even in parts of the country where there is especially high gender-based income inequality for workers in other service occupations. Some women truckers follow a family tradition, as described in the song lyrics above. Notwithstanding, a woman working in a highly masculine occupation like long-haul truck driving is likely to encounter gender-related occupational stresses.

Truck stops often are poorly suited for female drivers. Many have no women's shower, and many have parking areas that are poorly lit and dangerous for a woman walking alone (Connley, 2018). Female long-haul drivers blogging about their work describe their realistic fear that a man will break into their truck cab and assault them while they are asleep at a truck stop. Several describe the self-protective tactic of looping seat belts through the cab's door handles and fastening them to obstruct an attempted break-in. If someone tried to break into her truck, this would give a driver a few extra seconds to blow the truck horn to attract attention and help. In a recent survey of American female truckers, women were asked to rate on a scale of 1 to 10 how safe they felt on the job. The mean score was 4.4 (Woodyard, 2019). At Truck Drivers Jobs, one of many industry-sponsored websites encouraging people to become commercial truck drivers, future female truck drivers are advised to take a self-defense class and consider traveling with a "trucker dog" who will be their "faithful protector" (Truck Drivers Jobs, 2023).

Though women who drive heavy trucks might co-drive with a spouse or partner, most drive alone. Those who do require substantial physical strength and must have situational awareness and self-defense skills to stay safe at truck stops. Two distinct types of women long-haul truck drivers are described in American popular culture, on websites and in country music lyrics. One is a woman who is not typically feminine in appearance or style; she is tough and earns the respect of male truckers by displaying strength, stamina, driving skill, and willingness to help others. (Images of tough women drivers can be found online at realwomenintrucking.com.) The other is a woman who dresses and presents herself in a conventionally feminine way and earns respect by showing she can at once be a competent driver and an attractive woman. The feminine trucker image can be found in an photograph-filled article in a truckers' online magazine describing how "beautiful truck drivers are changing the stereotype," beginning with a seductively-dressed "Big Rig Barbie" posing in front of a truck cab with bright purple trim (Smith, 2020). Both the tough and the hyperfeminine descriptions are stereotypes, but they describe dimensions of a female trucker's persona that can aid in understanding the context of a depressive episode, its presenting symptoms, and its associated illness narrative.

A woman long-haul trucker who drives with a co-driver will spend weeks at a time sharing a small space and will have few breaks from her interaction with them. Any conflict between the two can escalate and become a cause for emotional distress and, at worst, interpersonal violence. A clinician assessing a depressed female truck driver in this situation must explore relationship issues and, if they are present, discern whether they are a cause of the patient's depression, a consequence of it, or unrelated—and whether and how the co-driver should be included in the treatment process. Specific inquiry about violence would be part of the assessment.

When a female trucker who drives alone has symptoms of depression, the syndrome of male depression should be considered despite her gender and should be assessed in the usual way, with a male depression questionnaire or with interview questions suggested by it. Externalizing symptoms, such as anger, irritability, violence, risky behavior, and substance use are common expressions of depression in women who have a more "masculine" identity. If the driver's persona is more conventionally feminine, circumstances (e.g., injury, significant weight gain) that make her less attractive can alter her interactions with male drivers in a way she finds discouraging. Regardless of the driver's presentation of herself, she is at risk for sexual harassment—sometimes violent—and the issue should be explored in a clinical evaluation as it would be for any woman working in a "masculine" occupation. If an employed female truck driver complains to her employer about harassment and her complaints are dismissed and/or the employer retaliates, depression can result. She would not be alone in her experience, and she might find it helpful to connect with other women truckers through websites or social media.

If a female long-haul truck driver sticks with the occupation, she might eventually become an owner-operator, which would give her much greater control over her working conditions. She might then face an occupational hazard for owner-operators—underinvestment in making the truck cabin a healthy environment in pursuit of a higher profit margin.

A female driver who eventually finds long-haul driving too exhausting, dangerous, or disruptive to her family life might find a solution by remaining in the transportation industry with a different role, such as becoming a short-haul driver or working as a dispatcher. Such a job would pay less, but the reduction in work–life conflict, stress, and risk might make it a better option for a woman with depression caused or exacerbated by the circumstances of her work. Making such a change would be more challenging for a woman who had been a long-haul trucker for years and had become accustomed to the lifestyle and relatively high income attached to her occupational identity.

In the occupational culture of heavy truck drivers, a woman's admitting to depression—like a man's doing so—suggests moderate to severe illness since one with mild depression would be unlikely to seek help and might not view her problem as an illness at all. If a female truck driver seeks clinical care, her clinical assessment should include careful assessment of issues more prevalent in heavy truck drivers than in the general working population, including unrecognized or inadequately treated chronic medical conditions, post-traumatic stress disorder or moral injury related to involvement in (or witnessing of) a crash in which someone was killed or seriously injured, and substance use or risky behavior related to long, lonely times on the road.

Female truckers, like male truckers, have a high prevalence of painful musculoskeletal conditions and a high prevalence of obesity and its consequences including OSA and atherosclerotic vascular disease. In addition, they have an elevated prevalence of migraine (Reed & Cronin, 2003). Migraine is associated with an increased prevalence of bipolar disorders (Galli & Gambini, 2019), so a depressed patient with migraine deserves especially careful screening for bipolar symptoms that might fall short of the full criteria for BD-II. The lifestyle of a long-haul truck driver includes chronobiological disruptions that can worsen the course of a bipolar condition.

If a female truck-driving patient has frequent or chronic migraines, it is unlikely that she will have had a trial of a standard-of-practice preventive treatment because she would be unlikely to see a neurologist or other headache specialist about her headaches. The combination of frequent severe headaches with pressure to deliver truckloads on time can be truly depressing, and in many cases, it can be prevented by treatments still not widely known by the public. A psychiatrist or psychologist seeing the patient for symptoms of depression might be the first clinician to focus her attention on the potential for preventing her migraines, and to make a referral to an appropriate specialist. In a 2020 survey of women's primary healthcare providers, only 6.3% were familiar with practice guidelines for migraine prevention, and only 17.3% were familiar with current recommendations for migraine treatment (Verhaak et al., 2021). A specialist consultation usually is necessary to get a prescription for a migraine preventive, and to get health insurance to pay for it.

Curiously, there are virtually no published data on the mental health of female truck drivers. There is little to suggest that women truck drivers have a higher prevalence of depression than truck-driving men, and it is possible that truck-driving women have a lower prevalence of depression. If so, it might reflect self-selection by the women who choose to enter a stereotypically masculine profession that requires substantial physical strength and stamina. Also, women who become truck drivers tend to do so in midlife, without young children who would be left at home when they are on the road. They thus might have less work–life conflict than male truckers who start driving earlier and leave young families behind when they are on a long haul.

Women in trucking, including employed drivers, owner-operators, and women in management at trucking companies, have established websites and social media groups offering education and support that include content on recognizing, treating, and preventing depression. Representative examples are Real Women in Trucking (www.realwomenintrucking.com), the Women in Trucking Foundation (www.womenintruckingfoundation.org), and the Facebook group @truckdrivingwomen.

Institutional and Personal Stigma

The FMCSA requires that interstate truck drivers undergo a medical evaluation and be recertified for fitness to drive every two years (FMCSA, 2022). FMCSA-certified examiners, who may be physicians of any specialty, advanced practice nurses, or physician assistants, review medical history forms and conduct a brief physical examination. There is no requirement for depression screening or cognitive assessment. If an applicant for certification has a history of a mental disorder (including depression), they must submit a letter from the physician treating the disorder, which will be reviewed by the examiner. If the treating physician states that neither the applicant's current mental state nor any medication side effects make them unfit to drive, it is unlikely that the examiner will challenge the treating physician's opinion. This is in marked contrast to the procedure for air transport pilot certification, where any diagnosis of depression or a bipolar spectrum disorder is automatic grounds for an initial denial of certification and the requirement for an elaborate and expensive appeal process if the pilot wishes to continue flying.

Even though it is relatively easy for a truck driver who has been successfully treated for depression to pass the medical examination, some depressed drivers will fail the examination and be told to return in three to six months for re-examination. This entails a major disruption of the driver's life and might even precipitate bankruptcy if the driver lacks savings, is in debt, and has no alternate source of income. Few truck drivers have meaningful paid sick leave or temporary disability coverage that would apply to this situation. It could be even more catastrophic for a debtor-operator who had paid tens of thousands of dollars to purchase a truck and would lose it all if they stopped working for even a few weeks.

A driver's fear of failing the medical examination for their CDL is potentially a significant deterrent to their seeking treatment for depression. Because of widespread concerns by truckers about the potential effect of seeing a psychiatrist on maintaining their CDL, a clinician assessing a truck driver for depression should assure them at the outset that relatively few drivers with depression are unfit to drive safely and that if there is no relevant functional impairment, a positive letter will be provided that the driver can take to their official medical evaluation. It is sometimes helpful to point out that by seeking treatment sooner rather than later and by adhering consistently to treatment, the driver has a better outlook for full recovery and for remaining well afterward, with little or no disruption to their work.

Fear of institutional stigma deters some depressed truckers from seeking treatment, but self-stigma probably is a bigger issue. In an occupational culture that values toughness and stoicism, seeking help for emotional distress can feel like a sign of weakness. Drivers who bear their emotional pain without seeking help can comfort themselves that they are still strong enough to tough it out. Drivers who stigmatize themselves for having sad or depressed feelings and wanting help for them can express their need through somatic symptoms or externalizing behaviors or comfort themselves transiently in unhealthy or risky ways. Somatic symptoms or the adverse consequences of externalizing behavior might bring a depressed driver to a non-psychiatric physician who might not recognize the underlying or concurrent depression.

Websites for depressed truckers—and for depressed men in general—offer forums for anonymous disclosure of depressive symptoms and are sources of advice, encouragement, and mental health education. A closed Facebook group, Truckers for Truckers, which was started by drivers who had lost friends to suicide, invited depressed truckers to anonymously tell their personal stories (Ashe, 2016). Headsupguys.org is an open website that appeals to men of all occupations to recognize depression, assess themselves for it, and deal with it (McKinnon, 2017). A trucker might visit such a site out of curiosity and become engaged in the online community, eventually seeking professional help as self-stigma decreased. Features about recognizing and dealing with depression can now be found at most of the major trucking industry news sites—sources of information that can be visited with no taint of help-seeking for a "mental" or "emotional" problem.

The high prevalence among truck drivers of distressing and treatable medical problems such as musculoskeletal pain, fatigue, and sleep disorders points to another opportunity for overcoming depressed drivers' self-stigma. If antidepressant treatment is ancillary to addressing a medical problem a driver readily acknowledges, it might be more easily accepted. Measuring and demonstrating improvement in the driver's presenting physical symptoms can be used to reinforce adherence to an antidepressant program. If this approach is taken, a collaborative care model might be best so that most of the truck driver's visits would be to a non-psychiatric physician rather than to a "mental health care" provider.

Prevention and Treatment

The very low rate of treatment for depression in truck drivers has multiple causes related to truckers' working conditions and truckers' culture. In the study of Shattell and colleagues (2012) only 8.4% of truckers with mental health problems received treatment for them. Reasons given included care being unaffordable (with or without insurance coverage), incompatibility of medical appointments with their often unpredictable driving schedules, feelings that their problems did not require a doctor's care, and opinions that professional mental health care could not be trusted to be effective. Engaging depressed truck drivers in effective treatment for depression is more likely to be successful with an approach that is culturally aware and appropriately adapted. Consistent treatment will reduce the risk of mild depression becoming more severe, at worst leading to the trucker's risk of death and/or injury to others from an accidental crash or to the driver's death by suicide or as a consequence of risky behavior.

As truck-driving is a masculine profession, enhancement of function might be a more appealing proposition to the patient than mere relief of symptoms that the driver feels should be borne without external help. There is no implication of weakness in an athlete's engaging a coach or personal trainer. A good trainer will be concerned about preventing injuries and avoiding impairments that could put the athlete on the bench. With enhancement of function as a priority, a clinician would at a first or second encounter review areas of function—whether related to work, sports or hobbies, family relationships, or sexual performance—in which the patient was concerned about an actual or potential decline or impairment.

Clinical Evaluation of Truckers with Suspected Depression

The initial clinical evaluation of a trucker suspected of clinical depression should be adapted to the patient's occupational culture, with awareness of the patient's working conditions. Unless the patient begins with a basic understanding of depression and is relatively free of self-stigma, goals and expectations for treatment can be framed in terms of improved function, well-being, and general health; safer driving; prevention of illness or injury; and dealing more effectively with demanding and sometimes difficult working conditions.

In taking the patient's history of the present illness, the clinician should systematically elicit information about externalizing symptoms and somatic symptoms of depression in addition to checking for the usual diagnostic criteria for MDD and the bipolar spectrum. Self-completed questionnaires can supplement the interview so that this can be done within realistic time constraints. The interview, or questionnaires, should screen for common medical issues of heavy truck drivers, including neck or back pain, fatigue, sleep problems (especially OSA), and hearing loss/tinnitus. If the clinician concludes that the patient has clinical depression, they can, with the patient's input, select a rating scale to follow the patient's progress that will be most sensitive to change in the symptoms that trouble the patient the most—for example, a "male depression" scale might be used for drivers with prominent externalizing symptoms. In some cases, a composite of items from more than one scale will be the most sensitive to change in the patient's depression. Items concerning road safety issues such as near-miss crashes and sleepiness at the wheel can be added, as well as items related to personal safety such as high-risk behavior. If the patient feels that every item on a questionnaire is personally relevant, they will be more likely to fill it out weekly and transmit the result to the clinician by text or email.

The patient's social and occupational history should not be as perfunctory as it often is in time-pressured primary care settings. It is important to know the details of the patient's work assignments and times away from home, the condition of their truck cabin and how it is outfitted for long hauls, the driver's sleep schedule and diet when on the road, and whether they get regular physical exercise other than that intrinsic to work. In the case of a female driver, any concerns about safety at truck stops, potential sexual harassment, and IPV should be elicited. The effect of drivers' times away on family and other important relationships should be explored, as should the issue of loneliness. The patient should be screened for potentially harmful use of alcohol. A combination of interview questions and self-completed questionnaires is the most efficient way to cover the full spectrum of relevant content. A questionnaire on a given topic like alcohol use or sleep apnea risk might be given to the patient after a topic is introduced in an interview so that the patient will understand why their answers to the questionnaire might matter to addressing their current problem of mood, behavior, and/or somatic symptoms.

Focusing on function, somatic complaints (e.g., pain, fatigue), and risks that are of greatest concern to the patient enhances the patient's engagement by linking the treatment of their depression to the outcomes that matter most to them. It parallels the approach a clinician might take with a successful performing artist who must continue to give outstanding performances or with a physician who wants to get over their burnout and continue to take excellent care of their patients.

Screening for OSA is essential because it is highly prevalent in truck drivers (most of whom are male and many of whom are obese), is easily treated, and can cause depression that improves with treatment of the OSA alone, thus not requiring antidepressants. Screening for OSA can be facilitated by questionnaires and decision rules that identify patients at the highest risk for the condition. These include the Epworth Sleepiness Scale (NIOSH, 2019a) and the STOP-BANG questionnaire for OSA (Chung et al., 2012, 2014). The latter comprises eight yes/no questions for which the test name is a mnemonic; a score of three or higher suggests the diagnosis of OSA, with especially high risk if the patient answers five or more total questions positively or answers two or more of the STOP questions positively and is male, is morbidly obese (BMI >35), or has a high neck circumference (17 inches [43 cm] or more for a man or 16 inches [41 cm] or more for a woman). The STOP questions ask about *snoring* loudly (so that it can be heard through a door or keeps a bed partner awake); *tiredness* and sleepiness during the day (including falling asleep while driving or during a conversation); being *observed* to stop breathing, choke, or gasp during sleep; and treatment for high blood *pressure*. The BANG questions ask about *BMI* >35, *age* >50; *neck size* ≥17 inches in men or ≥16 inches in women, and male *gender*. A diagnosis of OSA can be confirmed by a home-based test that does not require a visit to a sleep laboratory in a hospital or clinic.

Screening for alcohol use disorder or a pattern of harmful drinking should be done in every case because alcohol-related issues are also highly prevalent among heavy truck drivers. It is better done with the AUDIT than the CAGE since the former is more sensitive to binge drinking or consumption of unhealthy amounts of alcohol in people who are not alcohol-dependent. If a driver has musculoskeletal pain, their use of opioids, benzodiazepines, and muscle relaxants should be explored specifically, beyond asking general questions about what medications they are taking. If the driver suffers from fatigue, has very long work hours, and/or often drives at night, they should be questioned about the use of prescribed and non-prescribed simulants.

A careful review of medical conditions and a thorough physical examination and screening laboratory tests are needed even if the patient has a primary care physician and even more if they do not. Most truck drivers do not visit a primary care physician regularly for health maintenance, and even those who do may have depression-relevant general medical conditions that are undiagnosed or poorly managed. For example, screening for hypothyroidism is not part of a usual health maintenance visit, but it should be part of the general medical assessment of any patient who presented with depression and prominent fatigue. The examination of a depressed trucker should include adequate screening for hearing loss and for chronic lung disease that might be aggravated by continual exposure to polluted air.

Assessment of suicidal risk should take account of suicidal and self-destructive thoughts and behavior, easy availability of lethal means, and the patient's reason to live. Many truck drivers come from cultural groups with high rates of gun ownership, especially among men; and suicide rates are elevated in many of the states where truck-driving is the most common occupation for men. A clinically depressed, gun-owning truck driver might be encouraged, after a therapeutic relationship is established, to keep their guns unloaded, locked up, and with ammunition stored separately, to minimize the risk of an impulsive firearm suicide. Framing safe gun storage in terms of protecting children or grandchildren from accidental firearm injury sometimes is persuasive for patients who would reject advice that they would perceive as anti-gun moralizing or as implying they are "mentally ill." Depressed truck drivers who take prescription medications that are potentially lethal in overdose should be encouraged to store them in a way that reduces the risk of an impulsive overdose.

Concerning reasons to live, two issues are salient. If a truck driver feels that they were "born to drive," a medical condition that would end their driving career could be especially distressing. If a driver is attached to their family or to a romantic partner and the relationship is strained by long absences and brief, frustrating reunions, there is an ongoing risk of a breakup that leaves hopelessness in its wake.

The details of the truck driver's job and working environment are important. It is far from enough to know the patient's occupation and employer. Terms of compensation including health coverage are highly variable. Jobs differ greatly in the amount of night driving they require and in the predictability of the work schedule. Some involve the driver's participation in loading and unloading the truck, with the associated risk of back injury. Drivers' eating and sleeping arrangements on long trips are highly variable.

Of critical importance is how the trucker's work schedule influences their availability for in-person visits to a clinician for follow-up and treatment, whether the latter be psychotherapeutic or pharmacologic. If the trucker's schedule is incompatible with regularly scheduled, in-person visits, telepsychiatry and mHealth apps, and regular text and/or email exchanges might be needed to ensure adequate frequency of contact. Fortunately, these options are becoming more widely available and more likely to be covered by health insurance. The COVID-19 pandemic accelerated this trend. Monitoring of the patient's sleep and activity with a wearable device can facilitate follow-up. For some patients, having ongoing objective data on their sleep and activity can motivate and reinforce lifestyle changes with antidepressant benefits.

In some cases, it will be appropriate for the clinician to initiate a dialogue with a depressed truck driver about changing employers in pursuit of working conditions that would be healthier. With a shortage of heavy truck drivers in the U.S. and most other high-income countries, a trucker struggling with unhealthy working conditions might have a choice of feasible alternative employers. Or if the trucker is an owner-operator, the clinician might raise the issue of healthy working conditions and invite the patient to consider changes in their work schedule and/or modifications of the truck cabin that would mitigate health risk factors.

Personalized Treatment

Drivers with severe depression will require aggressive biological treatment and should refrain from work until their condition improves, given the markedly elevated crash risk associated with severe depression. Mild to moderate depression can be compatible with safe driving, depending on the driver's other medical conditions.

The foundation of the treatment of career heavy truck drivers with mild to moderate clinical depression combines several elements: Addressing unhealthy working conditions to the extent feasible; lifestyle modification including issues of sleep hygiene and an antidepressant diet; dealing with major interpersonal issues like IPV, family conflicts, and stress of frequent separations; assessing and treating substance use disorders; and non-pharmacologic treatments. If the driver's depression does not improve with these interventions, perhaps supplemented with antidepressant medication if it is accepted and tolerated, the clinician should raise the issue of whether the patient might need to change jobs—or even change career—to enjoy a long and healthy life.

The culture of the occupation works against long-term reliance on medications to remain mentally healthy. And, while most trucking jobs are stressful and entail health risks, they are not all problematic in the same way. If a trucker's main emotional issue is loneliness and time away from family, a local trucking job, while perhaps paying less, might give the trucker and their family a better quality of life. If a trucker is harassed or bullied by a boss or is continually asked to keep unrealistic schedules, they will be healthier with a different employer. If a female driver regularly encounters sexual harassment, she should be encouraged to confront it actively rather than tolerate it at the expense of her mental health.

Lifestyle modification comprises changes in diet, exercise, and sleep habits; addressing loneliness; and increasing the frequency of pleasant experiences. All of these can be challenging—but not impossible—given the working conditions of long-haul truck drivers. A clinician can engage the patient in finding ways they can modify their lifestyle that are realistic in the context of their work. A driver who has overcome reluctance to see a psychiatrist or other mental health care provider is likely to be motivated to make changes but can easily become discouraged if it is too difficult to make them within the constraints of their occupation.

For enhancement of pleasant life events and positive interactions, the driver should be encouraged to use video chat daily to stay connected with family and friends when on the road. If there are types of music or specific recordings that lift the driver's spirits, they should be encouraged to listen to them often when on the road, rather than to whatever might be on the radio. Audiobooks can help relieve the boredom of driving for hours at a stretch. They can provide health and mental health education as well as entertainment.

If a male driver is not too stereotypically masculine, he might be open to trying antidepressant aromatherapy in the cabin of his truck. Essential oils for inhalation are low risk, relatively inexpensive, and non-stigmatized. There is evidence for antidepressant effects of the essential oils of lavender, chamomile, bergamot, rose, and sweet orange, among others (Cheong et al., 2021; Ebrahimi et al., 2021; Sánchez-Vidaña et al., 2017; Xiong et al., 2018).

Hobbies compatible with the trucker's working conditions and interests should be identified, and they should be encouraged to engage in one of them. Outdoor recreation like hiking, fishing, and hunting fits well with a masculine lifestyle; and it might have been part of a driver's life before they got too busy—or too depressed—to enjoy it. In a recent study in the United Kingdom, long-haul truck drivers who spent time in a natural setting as infrequently as once a week had less acute and chronic fatigue than drivers who didn't (Longman et al., 2021). Fatigue leads to reduced participation in healthy and enjoyable activities and is associated with a higher risk of driving accidents and near misses. Long-haul drivers pass by natural settings every day. While pressure to deliver a load on time can work against it, a clinician can encourage a truck-driving to stop occasionally to enjoy nature. Finally, a depressed truck driver might consider the companionship of a dog. Having a dog can improve mood by several mechanisms—relief of loneliness, promotion of regular exercise, and providing occasions for positive social interactions with other humans.

Non-pharmacologic somatic treatments for depression worth considering include light therapy (especially if there are concurrent chronobiologic problems), transcranial electrical stimulation, and nutritional supplements like vitamin D3, magnesium, omega-3 fatty acids, or *S*-adenosylmethionine. Supplements often have a second medical indication like vitamin D insufficiency, osteoporosis, arthritis or another inflammatory condition, or an elevated low-density lipoprotein cholesterol level. Decreasing noxious elements in the driver's environment may also be useful; this is almost always feasible for an owner-operator and sometimes feasible for an employed trucker. Identifying medical comorbidities like chronic lung disease, tinnitus or hearing loss, or low back pain can aid in persuading an owner-operator or a driver's employer to take remedial action.

Adapting therapeutic dialogue to the truck-driving patient's culture can enhance the patient's engagement in treatment and adherence to a personalized treatment plan. The respect and empathy conveyed by a culturally aware approach can help in establishing a healing relationship. In shaping a treatment plan, the clinician ideally would know the role of truck driving in the patient's life, the financial feasibility of their taking time off work, the patient's work schedule, the details of the patient's working conditions, and what treatments for depression would be feasible if the patient continued to work. Realistic assessment of the feasibility of health-promoting modifications in the patient's job is part of a culturally aware approach to depression in heavy truck drivers—people with an occupation in which unhealthy working conditions and their harmful consequences are the norm.

Despite the patient's and clinician's best efforts, it might become clear that the patient's work as a truck driver is a barrier to their recovery from depression or even to their having a normal life span. If this is the case, supporting the patient in considering and seeking different work, and in preparing the patient for a career transition, might be the best course.

Afterword

As we completed our work on this book, we reached the end of a long journey—years of searching literature, reading narratives, translating texts, analyzing data, conversations and interviews. As we dug into the subject, we found our own interest in it became deeper and broader, and we noticed additional cultural dimensions of literary narratives and patients' stories. Initially we aimed our book toward clinicians, students, policy makers and researchers. However, as we had conversations with people of diverse backgrounds, demographics, and occupations, we were struck by their immediate interest in the subject of our book, their eagerness to talk about their experiences and opinions, and their intention to read our work. This led to our re-envisioning our book as one for a much larger and more diverse audience.

The COVID-19 pandemic slowed down our work but enabled us to add some analysis of new data and discussion of new publications related to the impact of the pandemic on the prevalence, context and expressions of depression. These show great variation between groups with different cultural identities. Data on the pandemic's impact continue to emerge, and much more will be learned as they are analyzed.

Over the years we worked on this book, biomedical psychiatry has been moving toward individualized precision treatment of depression. A cultural lens can enhance precision treatment by enabling a more nuanced choice among treatments of likely efficacy, pointing towards those most compatible with a patient's deeply held beliefs, hopes, fears, and circumstances.

We see our book as just the start of a much bigger project. Much remains to be done to build a knowledge base that supports a valid and broadly applicable cultural lens focusing on depression, the bipolar spectrum, and suicide. It will always be a challenge to raise cultural awareness while avoiding stereotyping. People ranging from epidemiologists, social scientists, clinicians, and policy makers to educators and literary critics can meaningfully contribute to a useful knowledge base. Cultural awareness can and should be cultivated in higher education and in clinicians in training. Working together we can bring new hope to diverse populations—for more timely diagnosis and effective treatment for depression, for reduction in the stigma of depression, for a lower incidence of depression in populations at risk, and for many fewer deaths by suicide.

Barry S. Fogel, MD
Xiaoling Jiang, PhD
Boston, Massachusetts
October 2024

Acknowledgments

We appreciate the support of family and friends during our years of work on the book. We especially thank our editors at Oxford University Press for their commitment and their patience: Craig Panner, David Lipp, Andrea Knobloch, Michelle Kelley, and Chloe Layman. We appreciate the tireless efforts of Vani Christi at Newgen KnowledgeWorks in preparing our manuscript for production. And we gratefully acknowledge colleagues who inspired us, offered helpful suggestions, made provocative comments, and encouraged us to pursue the topic. Among them are the following (in alphabetical order):

Eugene Beresin—Harvard Medical School/Massachusetts General Hospital

Kirk Daffner—Harvard Medical School/Brigham and Women's Hospital

Susanna Fogel —Film director

Melissa Frumin—Harvard Medical School/Brigham and Women's Hospital

Patrick Hanan (d. April 26, 2014)—Harvard University

Kaisa Hartikainen—University of Helsinki, Finland

Robin Hurley—Wake Forest University School of Medicine

Yutori Iizuka—Chuo University, Japan

Takeshi Kamatani—Kobe University, Japan

Ed Kovachy—Psychiatrist, Menlo Park, CA

Jin Li—Renmin University, China

Xiaohua Li—Poet, China

Kyohei Mizuta—Kobe University, Japan

Masayuki Nakagawa—Ritsumeikan University, Japan

Janet Rich-Edwards—Harvard School of Public Health/Brigham and Women's Hospital

Shirlene Sampson—Mayo Clinic, Rochester, MN

Edgar Schein (d. January 26, 2023)—MIT Sloan School of Management

Charles Silberstein—Psychiatrist, Martha's Vineyard, MA

Rose Styron—Poet and Human Rights Activist

Michael Trimble—University College London/National Hospital Queen Square

Weiming Tu—Harvard University and Beijing University, China
Valerie Voon—University of Cambridge, England and Fudan University, China
Keizo Yamada—Kobe University, Japan
Hyun-Sik Yang—Harvard Medical School/Brigham and Women's Hospital
Albert Yeung—Harvard Medical School/Massachusetts General Hospital

References

Aas, M., Henry, C., Andreassen, O. A., Bellivier, F., Melle, I., & Etain, B. (2016). The role of childhood trauma in bipolar disorders. *International Journal of Bipolar Disorders, 4*, Article 2. https://doi.org/10.1186/s40345-015-0042-0

Abbott, R., Chang, D. D., Eyre, H., & Lavretskyk, H. (2017). Mind–body practices tai chi and qìgong in the treatment and prevention of psychiatric disorders. In P. L. Gerbarg, P. R. Muskin, & R. P. Brown (Eds.), *Complementary and Integrative Treatments in Psychiatric Practice* (pp. 261–280). American Psychiatric Association.

Abe, T. (2003). 日本におけるうつ病の増加とその社会文化的背景 Increased incidence of depression and its socio-cultural background in Japan). *Seishin Shinkeigaku Zasshi, 105*(1), 36–42.

Abreu-Villaça, Y., & Levin, E. D. (2017). Developmental neurotoxicity of succeeding generations of insecticides. Environment International, 99, 55 -77. https://doi.org/10.1016/j.envint.2016.11.019

Acculturation (2019, October 9). In *Wikipedia*. https://en.wikipedia.org/wiki/Acculturation

Adams, L. B., Farrell, M., Mall, S., Mahlalela, N., & Berkman, L. (2020). Dimensionality and differential item endorsement of depressive symptoms among aging Black populations in South Africa: Findings from the HAALSI study. *Journal of Affective Disorders, 277*, 850–856. https://doi.org/10.1016/j.jad.2020.08.073

Adamsson, V., Reumark, A., Cederholm, T., Vessby, B., Risérus, U., & Johansson, G. (2012). What is a healthy Nordic diet? Foods and nutrients in the NORDIET study. *Food & Nutrition Research, 56*, 10.3402/fnr.v56i0.18189. https://doi.org/10.3402/fnr.v56i0.18189.

Agerbo, E., Gunnell, D., Bonde, J., Mortensen, P. B., & Nordencroft, M. (2007). Suicide and occupation: The impact of socio-economic, demographic and psychiatric differences. *Psychological Medicine, 37*(8), 1131–1140. https://doi.org/10.1017/S0033291707000487

Agnafors, S., Bladh, M., Svedin, C. G., & Sydsjö, G. (2019). Mental health in young mothers, single mothers and their children. BMC Psychiatry, 19(1), 112. https://doi.org/10.1186/s12888-019-2082-y

Ahmad, F., Maule, C., Wang, J., & Fung, W. L. A. (2018). Symptoms and experience of depression among Chinese communities in the West: A scoping review. *Harvard Review of Psychiatry, 26*(6), 340–351. https://doi.org/10.1097/HRP.0000000000000202

Ahmadabadi, Z., Najman, J. M., Williams, G. M., Clavarino, A. M., d'Abbs, P., & Smirnov, A. (2019). Intimate partner violence in emerging adulthood and subsequent substance use disorders: Findings from a longitudinal study. *Addiction (Abingdon, England), 114*(7), 1264–1273. https://doi.org/10.1111/add.14592

Ahmedani, B. K., Stewart, C., Simon, G. E., Lynch, F., Lu, C. Y., Waitzfelder, B. E., Solberg, L. I., Owen-Smith, A. A., Beck, A., Copeland, L. A., Hunkeler, E. M., Rossom, R. C., & Williams, K. (2015). Racial/ethnic differences in health care visits made before suicide attempt across the United States. *Medical Care, 53*(5), 430–435. https://doi.org/10.1097/MLR.0000000000000335

Ahn, B. S. (1987). Humor in Korean film. *East-West Film Journal, 2*(1), 90–98.

Ajaz, A., David, R., Brown, D., Smuk, M., & Korszun, A. (2016). BASH: Badmouthing, attitudes and stigmatisation in healthcare as experienced by medical students. *BJPsych Bulletin, 40*(2), 97–102. https://doi.org/10.1192/pb.bp.115.053140

Ajdacic-Gross, V., Bopp, M., Sansossio, R., Lauber, C., Gostynski, M., Eich, D., Gutzwiller, F., & Rossler, W. (2005). Diversity and change in suicide seasonality over 125 years. *Journal of Epidemiology and Community Health, 59*(11), 967–972.

Akbaraly, T. N., Brunner, E. J., Ferrie, J. E., Marmot, M. G., Kivimaki, M., & Singh-Manoux, A. (2009). Dietary pattern and depressive symptoms in middle age. *The British Journal of Psychiatry, 195*(5), 408–413. https://doi.org/10.1192/bjp.bp.108.058925

Akiskal, H. S., Mendlowicz, M. V., Jean-Louis, G., Rapaport, M. H., Kelsoe, J. R., Gillen, J. C., & Smith, T. L. (2005). TEMPS-A: Validation of a short version of a self-rated instrument designed to measure variations in temperament. *Journal of Affective Disorders, 85*(1–2), 45–52. https://doi.org/10.1016/j.jad.2003.10.012

Alarcão, A. C., Dell' Agnolo, C. M., Vissoci, J. R., Carvalho, E. C. A., Staton, C. A., de Andrade, L., Fontes, K. B., Pelloso, S. M., Nievola, J. C., & Carvalho, M. D. (2020). Suicide mortality among youth in southern Brazil: A spatiotemporal evaluation of socioeconomic vulnerability. Revista Brasileira de Psiquiatria 42(1), 46–53. https://doi.org/10.1590/1516-4446-2018-0352.

Alavi, S. S., Mohammadi, M. R., Souri, H., Kalhori, S. M., Jannatifard, F., & Sepahbodi, G. (2017). Personality, driving behavior and mental disorders factors as predictors of road traffic accidents based on logistic regression. *Iranian Journal of Medical Sciences, 42*(1), 24–31.

Albuquerque, J., & Tulk, S. (2019). Physician suicide. *Canadian Medical Association Journal, 191*(8), Article E505. https://doi.org/10.1503/cmaj.181687

Al-Darmaki, F., Thomas, J., & Yaaqeib, S. (2016). Mental health beliefs amongst Emirati female college students. *Community Mental Health Journal, 52*, 233–238. https://doi.org/10.1007/s10597-015-9918-9

Alhejaili, F., Hafez, A., Wali, S., Alshumrani, R., Alzehairi, A. M., Balkhyour, M., & Pandi-Perumal, S. R. (2021). Prevalence of obstructive sleep apnea among Saudi pilots. *Nature and Science of Sleep, 13*, 537–545. https://doi.org/10.2147/NSS.S299382

Al-Humadi, S., Bronson, B., Muhlrad, S., Paulus, M., Hong, H., & Cáceda, R. (2021). Depression, suicidal thoughts, and burnout among physicians during the COVID-19 pandemic: A survey-based dross-sectional study. *Academic Psychiatry: the Journal of the American Association of Directors of Psychiatric Residency Training and the Association for Academic Psychiatry, 1*(5), 557–565. https://doi.org/10.1007/s40596-021-01490-3

Ali, A., Yu, L., Kousar, S., Khalid, W., Maqbool, Z., Aziz, A., Arshad, M. S., Aadil, R. M., Trif, M., Riaz, S., Shaukat, H., Manzoor, M. F., & Qin, H. (2022). Crocin: Functional characteristics, extraction, food applications and efficacy against brain related disorders. *Frontiers in Nutrition, 9*, 1009807. https://doi.org/10.3389/fnut.2022.1009807

Ali, N. A., & Khoja, A. (2019). Growing evidence for the impact of air pollution on depression. *The Ochsner Journal, 19*(1), 4. https://doi.org/10.31486/toj.19.0011

Aljurf, T. M., Olaish, A. H., & BaHammam, A. S. (2018). Assessment of sleepiness, fatigue, and depression among Gulf Cooperation Council commercial airline pilots. *Sleep and Breathing, 22*(2), 411–419. https://doi.org/10.1007/s11325-017-1565-7

Allaert, F. A., Demais, H., & Collén, P. N. (2018). A randomized controlled double-blind clinical trial comparing versus placebo the effect of an edible algal extract (*Ulva lactuca*) on the component of depression in healthy volunteers with anhedonia. *BMC Psychiatry, 18*(1), Article 215. https://doi.org/10.1186/s12888-018-1784-x

Almroth, M., Hemmingsson, T., Sörberg Wallin, A., Kjellberg, K., Burström, B., & Falkstedt, D. (2021). Psychosocial working conditions and the risk of diagnosed depression: A Swedish register-based study. *Psychological Medicine, 52*(15), 3730–3738. https://doi.org/10.1017/S003329172100060X

Alnefeesi, Y., Chen-Li, D., Krane, E., Jawad, M. Y., Rodrigues, N. B., Ceban, F., Di Vincenzo, J. D., Meshkat, S., Ho, R. C. M., Gill, H., Teopiz, K. M., Cao, B., Lee, Y., McIntyre, R. S., & Rosenblat, J. D. (2022). Real-world effectiveness of ketamine in treatment-resistant depression: A systematic review & meta-analysis. *Journal of Psychiatric Research, 151*, 693–709. https://doi.org/10.1016/j.jpsychires.2022.04.037

Alonzo, D., & Gearing, R. E. (2021). Culture, intersectionality, and suicide. In E. P. Congress & M. J. González (Eds.), Multicultural perspectives in working with families: A handbook for the helping professions (4th ed., pp. 385–417). Springer Publishing Company.

Altinyazar, V., Sirin, F. B., Sutcu, R., Eren, I., & Omurlu, I. K. (2016). The red blood cell acetylcholinesterace levels of depressive patients with suicidal behavior in an agricultural area. Indian Journal of Clinical Biochemistry: 31(4), 473–479. https://doi.org/10.1007/s12291-016-0558-9

Amagai, H., & Okayama, M. (2006). *Yamato monogatari* [Tales of Yamato—Translation and annotation] (Vols. 1 and 2). Kodansha gakujutsu bunko.

American Psychiatric Association (2013). *Diagnostic and Manual of Mental Disorders* (5th ed.).

American Psychiatric Association (2022). *Depressive Diagnostic and Statistical Manual of Mental Disorders, Fifth Edition, Text Revision (DSM-5-TR)*. American Psychiatric Press. https://dsm.psychiatryonline.org/doi/book/10.1176/appi.books.9780890425787

Amieva, H., Ouvrard, C., Meillon, C., Rullier, L., & Dartigues, J. F. (2018). Death, depression, disability and dementia associated with self-reported hearing problems: A 25-year study. *The Journals of Gerontology, Series A: Biological Sciences and Medical Sciences, 73*(1), 1383–1389. https://doi.org/10.1093/gerona/glx250

Amsalem, D., Lazarov, A., Markowitz, J. C., Naiman, A., Smith, T. E., Dixon, L. B., & Neria, Y. (2021). Psychiatric symptoms and moral injury among US healthcare workers in the COVID-19 era. *BMC Psychiatry, 21*(1), 546. https://doi.org/10.1186/s12888-021-03565-9

Amy Winehouse (2019, June 23). In *Wikipedia*. https://en.wikipedia.org/wiki/Amy_Winehouse

An, D., Hong, K. S., & Kim, J. H. (2011). Exploratory factor analysis and confirmatory factor analysis of the Korean version of Hypomania Checklist-32. *Psychiatry Investigation, 8*(4), 334–339. https://doi.org/10.4306/pi.2011.8.4.334

Anderson, J. E., Govada, M., Steffen, T. K., Thorne, C. P., Varvarigou, V., Kales, S. N., & Burks, S. V. (2012). Obesity is associated with the future risk of heavy truck crashes among newly recruited commercial drivers. *Accident Analysis and Prevention, 49*, 378–384. https://doi.org/10.1016/j.aap.2012.02.018

Anderson, L. A., & Dedrick, R. F. (1990). Development of the Trust in Physician scale: A measure to assess interpersonal trust in patient-physician relationships. *Psychological Reports, 67*(3, Part 2), 1091–1100. https://doi.org/10.2466/pr0.1990.67.3f.1091

Ando, V., Claridge, G., & Clark, K. (2014). Psychotic traits in comedians. *British Journal of Psychiatry, 204*, 341–345. https://doi.org/10.1192/bjp.bp.113.134569

Anestis, M. D., & Houtsma, C. (2018). The association between gun ownership and statewide overall suicide rates. *Suicide & Life-threatening Behavior, 48*(2), 204–217. https://doi.org/10.1111/sltb.12346

Anestis, M. D., Houtsma, C., Daruwala, S. E., & Butterworth, S. E. (2019). Firearm legislation and statewide suicide rates: The moderating role of household firearm ownership levels. *Behavioral Sciences & the Law, 37*(3), 270–280. https://doi.org/10.1002/bsl.2408

Angermeyer, M. C., van der Auwera, S., Carta, M. G., & Schomerus, G. (2017). Public attitudes towards psychiatry and psychiatric treatments at the beginning of the 21st century: A systematic review and meta-analysis of population surveys. *World Psychiatry, 16*, 50–61.

Angst, J., Adolfsson, R., Benazzi, F., Gamma, A., Hantouche, E., Meyer, T. D., Skeppar, P., Vieta, E., & Scott, J. (2005). The HCL-32: Towards a self-assessment tool for hypomanic symptoms in outpatients. Journal of Affective Disorders, 88(2), 217–233. https://doi.org/10.1016/j.jad.2005.05.011

Angst, J., Azorin, J. M., Bowden, C. L., Perugi, G., Vieta, E., Gamma, A., Young, A. H., & BRIDGE Study Group (2011). Prevalence and characteristics of undiagnosed bipolar disorders in patients with a major depressive episode: The BRIDGE study. *Archives of General Psychiatry, 68*(8), 791–798. https://doi.org/10.1001/archgenpsychiatry.2011.87

Angst, J., & Marneros, A. (2001). Bipolarity from ancient to modern times: Conception, birth and rebirth. *Journal of Affective Disorders, 67*, 3–19. https://doi.org/10.1016/S0165-0327(01)00429-3

Anskär, E., Lindberg, M., Falk, M., & Andersson, A. (2019). Legitimacy of work tasks, psychosocial work environment, and time utilization among primary care staff in Sweden. *Scandinavian Journal of Primary Health Care, 37*(4), 476–483. https://doi.org/10.1080/02813432.2019.1684014

Anthony, J. S., Johnson, A., & Schafer, J. (2015). African American clergy and depression: What they know; what they want to know. *Journal of Cultural Diversity, 22*(4), 118–126.

Antonijevic I. (2008). HPA axis and sleep: Identifying subtypes of major depression. *Stress, 11*(1), 15–27. https://doi.org/10.1080/10253890701378967

Aoki, M. (2017, May 1). Rising "power harassment" scourge now affects 33% of workforce: Survey. *Japan Times*. https://www.japantimes.co.jp/news/2017/05/01/national/social-issues/rising-power-harassment-scourge-now-affects-33-workforce-survey/#.XMBvt6QpDb0

Apostolopoulos, Y., Lemke, M., & Sönmez, S. (2014). Risks endemic to long-haul trucking in North America: Strategies to protect and promote driver well-being. *New Solutions, 24*(1), 57–81. https://doi.org/10.2190/NS.24.1.c

Apostolopoulos, Y., Sönmez, S., & Massengale, K. (2013). Sexual mixing, drug exchanges and infection risk among long-haul truck drivers. *Journal of Community Health, 38*, 385–391. https://doi.org/10.1007/s10900-012-9628-y

Apostolopoulos, Y., Sönmez, S., Shattell, M. M., & Belzer, M. (2010). Worksite-induced morbidities among truck drivers in the United States. *AAOHN Journal, 58*(7), 285–296. https://doi.org/10.1177/216507991005800703

Apostolopoulos, Y., Sönmez, S., Shattell, M. M., Gonzales, C., & Fehrenbacher, C. (2013). Health survey of U.S. long-haul truck drivers: Work environment, physical health, and healthcare access. *Work, 46*(1), 113–123. https://doi.org/10.3233/wor-121553

Arab, L., Guo, R., & Elashoff, D. (2019). Lower depression scores among walnut consumers in NHANES. *Nutrients, 11*(2), Article 275. https://doi.org/10.3390/nu11020275

Araj-Khodaei, M., Noorbala, A. A., Parsian, Z., Targhi, S. T., Emadi, F., Alijaniha, F., Naseri, M., & Zargaran, A. (2017). Avicenna (980–1032 CE): The pioneer in treatment of depression. *Transylvanian Review, 25*(17), 4377–4389.

Arango, C., Dragioti, E., Solmi, M., Cortese, S., Domschke, K., Murray, R. M., Jones, P. B., Uher, R., Carvalho, A. F., Reichenberg, A., Shin, J. I., Andreassen, O. A., Correll, C. U., & Fusar-Poli, P. (2021). Risk and protective factors for mental disorders beyond genetics: An evidence-based atlas. *World Psychiatry, 20*(3), 417–436. https://doi.org/10.1002/wps.20894

Arango, T. (2012, June 6). Where arranged marriages are customary, suicides grow more common. *The New York Times*. https://www.nytimes.com/2012/06/07/world/middleeast/more-suicides-in-iraq-region-where-arranged-marriage-is-common.html

Araya, R., Montero-Marin, J., Barroilhet, S., Fritsch, R., Gaete, J., & Montgomery, A. (2013). Detecting depression among adolescents in Santiago, Chile: Sex differences. *BMC Psychiatry, 13*, Article 122. https://doi.org/10.1186/1471-244X-13-122

Arciniega, G. M., Anderson, T. C., Tovar-Blank, Z. G., & Tracey, T. J. G. (2008). Toward a fuller conception of machismo: Development of a traditional machismo and caballerismo scale. *Journal of Counseling Psychology, 55*(1), 19–33.

Areba, E. M., Duckett, L., Robertson, C., & Savik, K. (2018). Religious coping, symptoms of depression and anxiety, and well-being among Somali college students. *Journal of Religion and Health, 57*(1), 94–109. https://doi.org/10.1007/s10943-017-0359-3

Aretaeus of Cappadocia (1972). *De causis et signis acutorum morborum* [Of causes and signs of acute illness], book 3 (F. Adams, Trans.). Milford House. http://www.perseus.tufts.edu/hopper/text?doc=Perseus%3Atext%3A1999.01.0254%3Atext%3DSD%3Apage%3D302

Aristotle (1965). *Problemata* (W. S. Hett, Trans.). Harvard University Press.

Aristotle (1995). *Poetics* (S. Halliwell, W. H. Fyfe, D. C. Innes, & W. R. Roberts, Trans.). Harvard University Press.

Aristotle (2023). *Nicomachean Ethics* (H. Rackham, Trans.). Chapter VII. Harvard University Press.

Armenta, B. E., Lee, R. M., Pituc, S. T., Jung, K.-R., Park, I. J. K., Soto, J. A., Kim, S. Y., & Schwartz, S. J. (2013). Where are you from? A validation of the Foreigner Objectification Scale and the psychological correlates of foreigner objectification among Asian Americans and Latinos. *Cultural Diversity and Ethnic Minority Psychology, 19*(2), 131–142. https://doi.org/10.1037/a0031547

Armstrong, M., & Reynolds, K. (2020). Assessing burnout and associated risk factors in medical students. *Journal of the National Medical Association, 112*(6), 597–601. https://doi.org/10.1016/j.jnma.2020.05.019

Arshad, H., Head, J., Jacka, F. N., Lane, M. M., Kivimaki, M., & Akbaraly, T. (2024). Association between ultra-processed foods and recurrence of depressive symptoms: The Whitehall II cohort study. Nutritional Neuroscience, 27(1), 42–54. https://doi.org/10.1080/1028415X.2022.2157927.

Asante-Muhammad, D., & Sim, S. (2020, May 14). *Racial wealth snapshot: Asian Americans and the racial wealth divide*. National Community Reinvestment Coalition. https://ncrc.org/racial-wealth-snapshot-asian-americans-and-the-racial-wealth-divide/

Aşçibaşi, K., Çökmüş, F. P., Dikici, D. S., Özkan, H. M., Alçi, D., Altunsoy, N., Kuru, E., Yüzeren, S., & Aydemir, Ö. (2020). Evaluation of emotional adverse effects of antidepressants: A follow-up study. *Journal of Clinical Psychopharmacology, 40*(6), 594–598. https://doi.org/10.1097/JCP.0000000000001300

Ashe, A. (2016, July 12). Trucker creates Facebook group to open dialogue on depression. *Transport Topics*. Retrieved July 17, 2019, from https://www.ttnews.com/articles/trucker-creates-facebook-group-open-dialogue-depression

Asher, G. N., Gerkin, J., & Gaynes, B. N. (2017). Complementary therapies for mental health disorders. *Medical Clinics of North America, 101*(5), 847–864. https://doi.org/10.1016/j.mcna.2017.04.004

Assche, E., Antoni Ramos-Quiroga, J., Pariante, C. M., Sforzini, L., Young, A. H., Flossbach, Y., Gold, S. M., Hoogendijk, W. J. G., Baune, B. T., & Maron, E. (2022). Digital tools for the assessment of pharmacological treatment for depressive disorder: State of the art. *European Neuropsychopharmacology, 60*, 100–116. https://doi.org/10.1016/j.euroneuro.2022.05.007

ATP Flight School (2023). How much does it cost to become a pilot? Retrieved September 1, 2023 from https://atpflightschool.com/become-a-pilot/flight-training/pilot-training-cost.html

Attum, B., & Shamoon, Z. (2019, March 19). Cultural competence in the care of Muslim patients and their families. *StatPearls*. https://www.statpearls.com/articlelibrary/viewarticle/40656/

Augsberger, A., Yeung, A., Dougher, M., & Hahm, H. C. (2015). Factors influencing the underutilization of mental health services among Asian American women with a history of depression and suicide. *BMC Health Services Research, 15*, Article 542. https://doi.org/10.1186/s12913-015-1191-7

Australian Government Civil Aviation Safety Authority (2021). Depression. *Guidance for Medical Examiners*. https://www.casa.gov.au/licences-and-certificates/medical-professionals/dames-clinical-practice-guidelines/depression#. Retrieved August 1, 2024

Australian Government Civil Aviation Safety Authority (2023). *Depression and anxiety safety fact sheet*. Retrieved September 1, 2023 from https://www.casa.gov.au/resources-and-education/publications-and-resources/aviation-medicine-fact-sheets-and-case-studies/depression-and-anxiety-safety-fact-sheet#Effectsofflyingondepression

Axelsson, J., Stefánsson, J. G., Magnússon, A., Sigvaldason, H., & Karlsson, M. M. (2002). Seasonal affective disorders: Relevance of Icelandic and Icelandic–Canadian evidence to etiologic hypotheses. *Canadian Journal of Psychiatry, 47*(2), 153–158.

AZ Quotes (2019). *Heath Ledger quotes*. https://www.azquotes.com/author/8638-Heath_Ledger

Azrael, D., Cohen, J., Salhi, C., & Miller, M. (2018). Firearm storage in gun-owning households with children: Results of a 2015 national survey. Journal of Urban Health, 95(3), 295–304. https://doi.org/10.1007/s11524-018-0261-7

Baasher, T. A. (2001). Islam and mental health. *Eastern Mediterranean Health Journal, 7*(3), 372–376.

Babe, A. (2017, April 4). Han & jeong: Korea's sadness and love. *Anthony Bourdain Parts Unknown*. https://explorepartsunknown.com/korea/han-jeong/

Bae, M., Lee, K., Baek, J. H., Kim, J. S., Cho, Y., Ryu, S., Ha, K., & Hong, K. S. (2014). Lifetime experiences of hypomanic symptoms are associated with delayed and irregular sleep–wake cycle and seasonality in non-clinical adult samples. *Comprehensive Psychiatry*, 55(5), 1111–1115. https://doi.org/10.1016/j.comppsych.2014.02.012

Baek, J. H., Kinrys, G., & Nierenberg, A. A. (2014). Lithium tremor revisited: Pathophysiology and treatment. *Acta Psychiatrica Scandinavica*, 129(1), 17–23. https://doi.org/10.1111/acps.12171

Bagshaw, M. (2007). Commercial aircraft cabin altitude. *Journal of the Royal Society of Medicine*, 100(2), 64. https://doi.org/10.1177/01410Austr7680710000207

Bals, M., Turi, A. L., Skre, I., & Kvernmo, S. (2010). Internalization symptoms, perceived discrimination, and ethnic identity in Indigenous Sami and non-Sami youth in Arctic Norway. *Ethnicity & Health*, 15(2), 165–179. https://doi.org/10.1080/13557851003615545

Barbosa-Leiker, C., Burduli, E., Arias-Losado, R., Muller, C., Noonan, C., Suchy-Dicey, A., Nelson, L., Verney, S. P., Montine, T. J., & Buchwald, D. (2021). Gender differences in the assessment of depression in American Indian older adults: The Strong Heart Study. *Psychological Assessment*, 33(6), 574–579. https://doi.org/10.1037/pas0001024

Barrigon, M. L., & Cegla-Schvartzman, F. (2020). Sex, gender, and suicidal behavior. *Current Topics in Behavioral Neurosciences*, 46, 89–115. https://doi.org/10.1007/7854_2020_165

Barron, J. (2008, February 7). Medical examiner rules Ledger's death accidental. *New York Times*. https://www.nytimes.com/2008/02/07/nyregion/07ledger.html

Barros-Gomes, P., Kimmes, J., Smith, E., Cafferky, B., Stith, S., Durtschi, J., & McCollum, E. (2019). The role of depression in the relationship between psychological and physical intimate partner violence. *Journal of Interpersonal Violence*, 34(18), 3936–3960. https://doi.org/10.1177/0886260516673628

Barshay, J. (2018, June 18). Behind the Latino college degree gap. *Hechinger Report*. https://hechingerreport.org/behind-the-latino-college-degree-gap/

Basualdo-Meléndez, G. W., Hernández-Vásquez, A., Barón-Lozada, F. A., & Vargas-Fernández, R. (2022). Prevalence of depression and depressive symptoms at high altitudes: A systematic review and meta-analysis. Journal of Affective Disorders, 317, 388–396. https://doi.org/10.1016/j.jad.2022.08.079

Baumert, B. O., Carnes, M. U., Hoppin, J. A., Jackson, C. L., Sandler, D. P., Freeman, L. B., Henneberger, P. K., Umbach, D. M., Shrestha, S., Long, S., & London, S. J. (2018). Sleep apnea and pesticide exposure in a study of US farmers. Sleep Health, 4(1), 20–26. https://doi.org/10.1016/j.sleh.2017.08.006

Bauwelinck, M., Deboosere, P., Willaert, D., & Vandenheede, H. (2017). Suicide mortality in Belgium at the beginning of the 21st century: Differences according to migrant background. *European Journal of Public Health*, 27(1), 111–116. https://doi.org/10.1093/eurpub/ckw159

Bayes, J., Schloss, J., & Sibbritt, D. (2023). The use of diet for preventing and treating depression in young men: Current evidence and existing challenges. *The British Journal of Nutrition*, 1–5. Advance online publication. https://doi.org/10.1017/S000711452300168X

Beck, A. T., Steer, R. A., & Brown, G. K. (1996). *Manual for the Beck Depression Inventory.* San Antonio, TX: Psychological Corporation.

Begin, A. S., Hata, S., Berkowitz, L. R., Plessow, F., Lawson, E. A., Emptage, N., & Armstrong, K. (2021). Biomarkers of clinician burnout. *Journal of General Internal Medicine, 37,* 478–479. https://doi.org/10.1007/s11606-021-06757-x

Bellis, M. A., Hennell, T., Lushey, C., Hughes, K., Tocque, K., & Ashton, J. R. (2007). Elvis to Eminem: Quantifying the price of fame through early mortality of European and North American rock and pop stars. *Journal of Epidemiology and Community Health, 61,* 896–901. https://doi.org/10.1136/jech.2007.059915

Bellis, M. A., Hughes, K., Sharples, O., Hennell, T., & Hardcastle, K. A. (2012). Dying to be famous: Retrospective cohort study of rock and pop star mortality and its association with adverse childhood experiences. *BMJ Open, 2,* Article e002089. https://doi.org/10.1136/bmjopen-2012-002089

Bendik, I., Friedel, A., Roos, F. F., Weber, P., & Eggersdorfer, M. (2014). Vitamin D: A critical and essential micronutrient for human health. *Frontiers in Physiology, 5,* Article 248. https://doi.org/10.3389/fphys.2014.00248

Benedict, R. (1946). *The Chrysanthemum and the Sword—Patterns of Japanese Culture.* Houghton Mifflin.

Benuto, L. T., Zimmermann, M., Casas, J., Gonzalez, F., Newlands, R., & Segovia, F. R. (2021). ¡No me duele cuando me deprimo!: An examination of ethnic differences in depression symptoms among Latinx and non-Latinx primary care patients. *Journal of Immigrant and Minority Health, 23,* 917–925. https://doi.org/10.1007/s10903-021-01238-z

Berman-Vaporis, I., Parker, L., & Wardley, R. (2020). *The Best and Worst States to Be a Woman: Introducing the U.S. Women, Peace, and Security Index 2020.* Georgetown Institute for Women, Peace, and Security. https://giwps.georgetown.edu/wp-content/uploads/2021/03/US-Index-Summary.pdf

Bernert, R. A., Hom, M. A., Iwata, N. G., & Joiner, T. E. (2017). Objectively assessed sleep variability as an acute warning sign of suicidal ideation in a longitudinal evaluation of young adults at high suicide risk. *The Journal of Clinical Psychiatry, 78*(6), e678–e687. https://doi.org/10.4088/JCP.16m11193

Bernert, R. A., Luckenbaugh, D. A., Duncan, W. C., Iwata, N. G., Ballard, E. D., & Zarate, C. A. (2017). Sleep architecture parameters as a putative biomarker of suicidal ideation in treatment-resistant depression. *Journal of Affective Disorders, 208,* 309–315. https://doi.org/10.1016/j.jad.2016.08.050

Bernstein, K., Lee, Y. M., Gona, P. N., Han, S., Kim, S., & Kim, S. S. (2021). Depression, depression literacy, and sociodemographic characteristics of Korean Americans: A preliminary investigation. *Journal of Immigrant and Minority Health, 23*(3), 547–557. https://doi.org/10.1007/s10903-020-01092-5

Berrigan, J., Azrael, D., Hemenway, D., & Miller, M. (2019). Firearms training and storage practices among US gun owners: a nationally representative study. *Injury Prevention: Journal of the International Society for Child and Adolescent Injury Prevention, 25*(Suppl 1), i31–i38. https://doi.org/10.1136/injuryprev-2018-043126

Bertossi Urzua, C., Ruiz, M. A., Pajak, A., Kozela, M., Kubinova, R., Malyutina, S., Peasey, A., Pikhart, H., Marmot, M., & Bobak, M. (2019). The prospective relationship between social cohesion and depressive symptoms among older adults from central and eastern Europe. *Journal of Epidemiology and Community Health, 73*(2), 117–122. https://doi.org/10.1136/jech-2018-211063

Bertrand, L., d'Ortho, M. P., Reynaud, E., Lejoyeux, M., Bourgin, P., & Geoffroy, P. A. (2021). Polysomnography in seasonal affective disorder: A systematic review and meta-analysis. *Journal of Affective Disorders, 292*, 405–415. https://doi.org/10.1016/j.jad.2021.05.080

Beute, F., & de Kort, Y. A. W. (2018). The natural context of wellbeing: Ecological momentary assessment of the influence of nature and daylight on affect and stress for individuals with depression levels varying from none to clinical. *Health and Place, 49*, 7–18. https://doi.org/10.1016/j.healthplace.2017.11.005

Beutel, M. E., Klein, E. M., Brähler, E., Reiner, I., Jünger, C., Michal, M., Wiltink, J., Wild, P. S., Münzel, T., Lackner, K. J., & Tibubos, A. N. (2017). Loneliness in the general population: Prevalence, determinants and relations to mental health. *BMC Psychiatry, 17*(1), Article 97. https://doi.org/10.1186/s12888-017-1262-x

Bhatt, J. M., Bhattacharyya, N., & Lin, H. W. (2017). Relationships between tinnitus and the prevalence of anxiety and depression. *The Laryngoscope, 127*(2), 466–469. https://doi.org/10.1002/lary.26107

Bhattacharya, A., & Drevets, W. C. (2017). Role of neuro-immunological factors in the pathophysiology of mood disorders: Implications for novel therapeutics for treatment resistant depression. *Current Topics in Behavioral Neurosciences, 31*, 339–356. https://doi.org/10.1007/7854_2016_43

Bi, K., Yeoh, D., Jiang, Q., Wienk, M. N. A., & Chen, S. (2023). Psychological distress and everyday discrimination among Chinese international students one year into COVID-19: A preregistered comparative study. *Anxiety, Stress, and Coping, 36*(6), 727–742. https://doi.org/10.1080/10615806.2022.2130268

Bianchi, R., Schonfeld, I. S., & Laurent, E. (2015). Burnout–depression overlap: A review. *Clinical Psychology Review, 36*, 28–41. https://doi.org/10.1016/j.cpr.2015.01.004

Biltoft-Jensen, A., Damsgaard, C. T., Andersen, R., Ygil, K. H., Andersen, E. W., Ege, M., Christensen, T., Sørensen, L. B., Stark, K. D., Tetens, I., & Thorsen, A. V. (2015). Accuracy of self-reported intake of signature foods in a school meal intervention study: comparison between control and intervention period. *The British Journal of Nutrition* 114(4): 635–644. https://doi.org/10.1017/S0007114515002020

Blake, K. R., & Brooks, R. C. (2018). High mate value men become more accepting of intimate partner abuse when primed with gender equality. *Frontiers in Sociology, 3*, Article 28. https://doi.org/10.3389/fsoc.2018.00028

Blakemore, E. (2021, May 18). The Nisei soldiers who fought WWII enemies abroad—and were seen as enemies back home. *National Geographic* https://www.nationalgeographic.com/history/article/the-nisei-soldiers-who-fought-wwii-enemies-abroad-seen-as-enemies-back-home.

Blanco, C., Okuda, M., Wright, C., Hasin, D. S., Grant, B. F., Liu, S. M., & Olfson, M. (2008). Mental health of college students and their non-college-attending peers: Results from the National Epidemiologic Study on Alcohol and Related Conditions. *Archives of General Psychiatry, 65*(12), 1429–1437. https://doi.org/10.1001/archpsyc.65.12.1429

Blazer, D. G., & Tucci, D. L. (2019). Hearing loss and psychiatric disorders: A review. *Psychological Medicine, 49*(6), 891–897. https://doi.org/10.1017/S0033291718003409

Blodgett, J. M., Lachance, C. C., Stubbs, B., Co, M., Wu, Y. T., Prina, M., Tsang, V. W. L., & Cosco, T. D. (2021). A systematic review of the latent structure of the Center for Epidemiologic Studies Depression Scale (CES-D) amongst adolescents. *BMC Psychiatry, 21*(1), Article 197. https://doi.org/10.1186/s12888-021-03206-1

Blood, R. P., Rynell, P. W., & Johnson, P. W. (2011). Vehicle design influences whole body vibration exposures: Effect of the location of the front axle relative to the cab. *Journal of Occupational and Environmental Hygiene, 8*(6), 364–374. https://doi.org/10.1080/15459624.2011.583150

Blood, R. P., Yost, M. G., Camp, J. E., & Ching, R. P. (2015). Whole-body vibration exposure intervention among professional bus and truck drivers: A laboratory evaluation of seat-suspension designs. *Journal of Occupational and Environmental Hygiene, 12*(6), 351–362. https://doi.org/10.1080/15459624.2014.989357

Boden, J. M., & Fergusson, D. M. (2011). Alcohol and depression. *Addiction, 106*(5), 906–914. https://doi.org/10.1111/j.1360-0443.2010.03351.x

Bogic, M., Njoku, A., & Priebe, S. (2015). Long-term mental health of war-refugees: A systematic literature review. *BMC International Health and Human Rights, 15*, Article 29. https://doi.org/10.1186/s12914-015-0064-9

Booth, M. (2014). *An Almost Nearly Perfect People*. Jonathan Cape.

Bosworth, H. B., Park, K. S., McQuoid, D. R., Hays, J. C., & Steffens, D. C. (2003). The impact of religious practice and religious coping on geriatric depression. *International Journal of Geriatric Psychiatry, 18*(10), 905–914. https://doi.org/10.1002/gps.945

Bourdieu, P. (1997). *Outline of a theory of practice* (R. Nice, Trans.). Cambridge University Press.

Bovenzi, M. (2009). Metrics of whole-body vibration and exposure–response relationship for low back pain in professional drivers: A prospective cohort study. *International Archives of Occupational and Environmental Health, 82*(7), 893–917. https://doi.org/10.1007/s00420-008-0376-3

Bragazzi, N. L., Dini, G., Toletone, A., Rahmai, A., Montecucco, A., Massa, E., Manca, A., Guglielmi, O., Garbarino, S., Debarbieri, N., & Durando, P. (2018). Patterns of harmful alcohol consumption among truck drivers: Implications for occupational health and work safety from a systematic review and meta-analysis. *International Journal of Environmental Research and Public Health, 15*(6), Article 1121. https://doi.org/10.3390/ijerph15061121

BrainyQuote (2019). *Heath Ledger quotes*. https://www.brainyquote.com/authors/heath_ledger

Braithwaite, I., Zhang, S., Kirkbride, J. B., Osborn, D. P. J., & Hayes, J. F. (2019). Air pollution (particulate matter) exposure and associations with depression, anxiety, bipolar, psychosis and suicide risk: A systematic review and meta-analysis. *Environmental Health Perspectives, 127*(12), 126002. https://doi.org/10.1289/EHP4595

Brennan, D. (2018, March 19). Muslim teen and her Hindu boyfriend die in suicide pact after parents reject their love. *Newsweek*. https://www.newsweek.com/teenage-lovers-suicide-pact-after-parents-rejected-their-interfaith-love-851494

Brianda, M. E., Roskam, I., & Mikolajczak, M. (2020). Hair cortisol concentration as a biomarker of parental burnout. *Psychoneuroendocrinology, 117*, Article 104681. https://doi.org/10.1016/j.psyneuen.2020.104681

Briggs, R., McCarroll, K., O'Halloran, A., Healy, M., Kenny, R. A., & Laird, E. (2019). Vitamin D deficiency is associated with an increased likelihood of incident depression in community-dwelling older adults. *Journal of the American Medical Directors Association, 20*(5), 517–523. https://doi.org/10.1016/j.jamda.2018.10.006

Brink, A. (1979). Depression and loss: A theme in Robert Burton's "Anatomy of melancholy" (1621). *Canadian Journal of Psychiatry, 24*(8), 767–772. https://doi.org/10.1177/070674377902400811

Brody, G. H., Yu, T., Chen, E., Miller, G. E., Kogan, S. M., & Beach, S. R. (2013). Is resilience only skin deep? Rural African Americans' socioeconomic status–related risk and competence in preadolescence and psychological adjustment and allostatic load at age 19. *Psychological Science*, *24*(7), 1285–1293. https://doi.org/10.1177/0956797612471954

Bromwich, J. E. (2018, April 11). Mariah Carey opens up about bipolar disorder. *New York Times*. https://www.nytimes.com/2018/04/11/style/mariah-carey-bipolar-disorder.html

Brooks, E. M. (2020). The disenchanted self: Anthropological notes on existential distress and ontological insecurity among ex-Mormons in Utah. *Cultural Medicine and Psychiatry*, *44*, 193–213. https://doi.org/10.1007/s11013-019-09646-5

Brower, K. J. (2021). Professional stigma of mental health issues: Physicians are both the cause and solution. *Academic Medicine*, *96*(5), 635–640. https://doi.org/10.1097/ACM.0000000000003998

Brown, K. W., & Ryan, R. M. (2003). The benefits of being present: Mindfulness and its role in psychological well-being. *Journal of Personality and Social Psychology*, *84*(4), 822–848.

Brown, M. J., Perera, R. A., Masho, S. W., Mezuk, B., & Cohen, S. A. (2015). Adverse childhood experiences and intimate partner aggression in the US: Sex differences and similarities in psychosocial mediation. *Social Science & Medicine*, *131*, 48–57. https://doi.org/10.1016/j.socscimed.2015.02.044

Brown, P., Pleitgen, F., & Shoichet, C. E. (2015, April 25). Germanwings co-pilot reported depression during training. *CNN*. Retrieved September 1, 2019, from https://www.cnn.com/2015/03/31/europe/france-germanwings-plane-crash-main/index.html

Browne, D., Dolan, J., Spanos, B., Exposito, S., Betts, S., Reeves, M., Grow, K., Greene, A., Hermes, W., & Ravitz, J. (2017, August 14). Celebrity deaths that changed music history. *Rolling Stone*. https://www.rollingstone.com/music/music-lists/celebrity-deaths-that-changed-music-history-gone-too-soon-195319/buddy-holly-7-195434/

Bryson, E. O. (2018). The opioid epidemic and the current prevalence of substance use disorder in anesthesiologists. *Current Opinion in Anesthesiology*, *313*, 388–392. https://doi.org/10.1097/ACO.0000000000000589

Bucknill, J. C., & Tuke, D. H. (1858). *A Manual of Psychological Medicine*. John Churchill.

Budiman, A. (2021a). *Chinese in the U.S. Fact Sheet*. Pew Research Center, April 29, 2021. https://www.pewresearch.org/social-trends/fact-sheet/asian-americans-chinese-in-the-u-s/

Budiman, A. (2020). How many people in the US are immigrants—And where do they come from? *World Economic Forum*. Retrieved August 26, 2020, from https://www.weforum.org/stories/2020/08/united-states-immigration-migration-research/

Budiman, A. (2021b). *Japanese in the U.S. Fact Sheet*. Pew Research Center, April 29, 2021. https://www.pewresearch.org/social-trends/fact-sheet/asian-americans-japanese-in-the-u-s/. Retrieved October 1, 2013.

Budiman, A. (2024). Income inequality is greater among Chinese Americans than any other Asian origin group in the U.S. *Pew Research Center Short Reads*, May 31, 2024. Https://www.pewresearch.org/short-reads/2024/05/31/income-inequality-is-greater-among-chinese-americans-than-any-other-asian-origin-group-in-the-us/. Accessed August 1, 2024.

Bui, Q. (2015, February 5). Map: The most common job in every state. *Planet Money.* https://www.npr.org/sections/money/2015/02/05/382664837/map-the-most-com mon-job-in-every-state

Bureau d'Enquêtes et d'Analyses (2016). *Final report–Accident on 24 March 2015 at Prads-Haute-Bléone (Alpes-de-Haute-Provence, France) to the Airbus A320-211 registered D-AIPX) operated by Germanwings.* Retrieved August 5, 2017, from https://www.bea.aero/uploads/tx_elydbrapports/BEA2015-0125.en-LR.pdf

Bureau of Labor Statistics (2021a). *Occupational Outlook Handbook: Heavy and Tractor-trailer Truck Drivers.* Retrieved September 1, 2021, from https://www.bls.gov/ooh/tra nsportation-and-material-moving/heavy-and-tractor-trailer-truck-drivers.htm

Bureau of Labor Statistics (2021b). *Occupational Employment and Wages, May 2020: 53-3032 Heavy and Tractor-Trailer Truck Drivers.* Retrieved September 1, 2021, from https://www.bls.gov/oes/current/oes533032.htm#(9)

Burgel, B. J., & Elshatarat, R. A. (2019). Associations between daily-on-the job hassles with perceived mental exertion and depression symptoms in taxi drivers. *American Journal of Industrial Medicine, 62*(9), 791–802. https://doi,org/10.1002/ajim.23019

Burton, R. (2001). *Anatomy of Melancholy* (H. Jackson, Ed.). New York Review of Books. (Original work published 1620)

Byeon, G., Jo, S. J., Lee, H. W., Yim, H. W., & Park, J. I. (2021). Development of a short form depression screening questionnaire for Korean soldiers. *Journal of Korean Medical Science, 36*(27), Article e185. https://doi.org/10.3346/jkms.2021.36.e185

Bynum, W. E., 4th, & Goodie, F. M. (2014). Shame, guilt and the medical learner: Ignored connections and why we should care. *Medical Education, 48*(11), 1045–1054. https://doi.org/10.1111/medu.12521

Cabeza de Baca, T., Wojcicki, J. M., Epel, E. S., & Adler, N. E. (2018). Lack of partner impacts newborn health through maternal depression: A pilot study of low-income immigrant Latina women. *Midwifery, 64,* 63–68. https://doi.org/10.1016/j.midw.2018.05.014

Cadilhac, P., Bouton. M. C., Cantegril, M., Cardines, C., Gisquet, A., Kaufman, N., & Klerlein, M. (2017). In-flight ultraviolet radiation on commercial airplanes. *Aerospace Medicine and Human Performance, 88*(10), 947–951. https://doi.org/10.3357/AMHP.4852.2017

Cai, W., Wei, X. F., Zhang, J. R., Hu, C., & Shen, W. D. (2023). Does acupuncture treatment have satisfactory clinical efficacy for late-life depression? A systematic review and meta-analysis. *Geriatric Nursing, 51,* 215–221. https://doi.org/10.1016/j.gerinu rse.2023.03.008

Caldieraro, M. A., & Cassano, P. (2019). Transcranial and systemic photobiomodulation for major depressive disorder: A systematic review of efficacy, tolerability and biological mechanisms. *Journal of Affective Disorders, 243,* 262–273. https://doi.org/10.1016/j.jad.2018.09.048

Camacho, M., Almeida, S., Moura, A. R., Fernandes, A. B., Ribeiro, G., da Silva, J. A., Barahona-Corrêa, J. B., & Oliveira-Maia, A. J. (2018). Hypomania symptoms across psychiatric disorders: Screening use of the Hypomania Check-List 32 at admission to an outpatient psychiatry clinic. *Frontiers in Psychiatry, 9,* Article 527. https://doi.org/10.3389/fpsyt.2018.00527

Campbell-Grossman, C., Hudson, D. B., Kupzyk, K. A., Brown, S. E., Hanna, K. M., & Yates, B. C. (2016). Low-income, African American, adolescent, mothers' depressive symptoms, perceived stress, and social support. *Journal of Child and Family Studies*, 25(7), 2306–2314. https://doi.org/10.1007/s10826-016-0386-9

Canfield, D. V., Dubowski, K. M., Chaturvedi, A. K., & Whinnery, J. E. (2012). Drug and alcohol found in all civil aviation accident fatalities from 2004–2008. *Aviation, Space and Environmental Medicine*, 83(8), 764–770.

Cano, M. Á., Rojas, P., Ramírez-Ortiz, D., Sánchez, M., & De La Rosa, M. (2020). Depression and gender roles among Hispanic immigrant women: Examining associations of gender egalitarianism, marianismo, and self-silencing. *Journal of Health Care for the Poor and Underserved*, 31(2), 713–723. https://doi.org/10.1353/hpu.2020.0056

Cao, C., & Brown, B. (2020). Understanding Chinese medicine and Western medicine to reach the maximum treatment benefit. *Journal of Translational Science*, 6, 1–2. https://doi.org./10.15761/JTS.1000334.

Cao, J., Wei, J., Fritzsche, K., Toussaint, A. C., Li, T., Jiang, Y., Zhang, L., Zhang, Y., Chen, H., Wu, H., Ma, X., Li, W., Ren, J., Lu, W., Müller, A. M., & Leonhart, R. (2020). Prevalence of DSM-5 somatic symptom disorder in Chinese outpatients from general hospital care. *General Hospital Psychiatry*, 62, 63–71. https://doi.org/10.1016/j.genhosppsych.2019.11.010

Carrera, S. G., & Wei, M. (2014). Bicultural competence, acculturative family distancing, and future depression in Latino/a college students: A moderated mediation model. *Journal of Counseling Psychology*, 61(3), 427–436. https://doi.org/10.1037/cou0000023

Carroll, J. E., Gruenewald, T. L., Taylor, S. E., Janicki-Deverts, D., Matthews, K. A., & Seeman, T. E. (2013). Childhood abuse, parental warmth, and adult multisystem biological risk in the Coronary Artery Risk Development in Young Adults study. *Proceedings of the National Academy of Sciences of the United States of America*, 110(42), 17149–17153. https://doi.org/10.1073/pnas.1315458110

Case, A., & Deaton, A. (2015). Rising morbidity and mortality in midlife among White non-Hispanic Americans in the 21st century. *Proceedings of the National Academy of Sciences of the United States of America*, 112(49), 15078–15083. https://doi.org/10.1073/pnas.1518393112

Case, A., & Deaton, A. (2017). Mortality and morbidity in the 21st century. *Brookings Papers on Economic Activity*, (Spring), 397–476.

Cassano, P., Petrie, S. R., Mischoulon, D., Cusin, C., Katnani, H., Yeung, A., De Taboada, L., Archibald, A., Bui, E., Baer, L., Chang, T., Chen, J., Pedrelli, P., Fisher, L., Farabaugh, A., Hamblin, M. R., Alpert, J. E., Fava, M., & Iosifescu, D. V. (2018). Transcranial photobiomodulation for the treatment of major depressive disorder. The ELATED-2 pilot trial. *Photomedicine and Laser Surgery*, 2018, 634–646. https://doi.org/10.1089/pho.2018.4490

Cassereau, J., Ferré, M., Chevrollier, A., Codron, P., Verny, C., Homedan, C., Lenaers, G., Procaccio, V., May-Panloup, P., & Reynier, P. (2017). Neurotoxicity of Insecticides. *Current Medicinal Chemistry*, 24(27), 2988–3001. https://doi.org/10.2174/0929867324666170526122654

Castillo, L. G., González, P., Merz, E. L., Nuñez, A., Castañeda, S. F., Buelna, C., Ojeda, L., Giachello, A. L., Womack, V. Y., Garcia, K. A., Penedo, F. J., Talavera, G. A., & Gallo, L. C. (2021). Factorial invariance of the Marianismo Beliefs Scale among Latinos in the Hispanic Community Health Study/Study of Latinos Sociocultural Ancillary Study. *Journal of Clinical Psychology*, 77(1), 312–328. https://doi.org/10.1002/jclp.23031

Cavan Project (2019). *37 Musicians with Hearing Loss*. http://www.thecavanproject.com/musicians-hearing-loss/

Cavanagh, A., Wilson, C. J., Kavanagh, D. J., & Caputi, P. (2017). Differences in the expression of symptoms in men versus women with depression: A systematic review and meta-analysis. *Harvard Review of Psychiatry, 25*(1), 29–38. https://doi.org/10.1097/HRP.0000000000000128

CDC (2019). *National Occupational Mortality Surveillance: PMR Query System for Occupation (1999, 2003–2004, 2007–2014)*. Retrieved July 4, 2019, from https://wwwn.cdc.gov/niosh-noms/occupation2.aspx

CDC (2023a). *2022 BRFSS Survey Data and Documentation*. Centers for Disease Control and Prevention. Retrieved October 10, 2023. https://www.cdc.gov/brfss/annual_data/annual_2022.html

CDC (2023b). *Opioid Dispensing Rate Maps*. Retrieved October 15, 2023. https://www.cdc.gov/drugoverdose/rxrate-maps/opioid.html

CDC (2024). National Center for Immunization and Respiratory Diseases, U.S. Centers for Disease Control and Prevention. National Immunization Survey Adult COVID Module (NIS-ACM): COVIDVaxViews, United States. https://data.cdc.gov/Vaccinations/National-Immunization-Survey-Adult-COVID-Module-NI/uc4z-hbsd/about_data. Accessed August 10, 2024.

Celsus (1935/1971). *De Medicina* (W. G. Spencer, Trans.). Harvard University Press.

Center, C., Davis, M., Detre, T., Ford, D. E., Hansbrough, W., Hendin, H., Laszlo, J., Litts, D. A., Mann, J., Mansky, P. A., Michels, R., Miles, S. H., Proujansky, R., Reynolds, C. F., III, & Silverman, M. M. (2003). Confronting depression and suicide in physicians: A consensus statement. *Journal of the American Medical Association, 289*(23), 3161–3166. https://doi.org/10.1001/jama.289.23.3161

Central Intelligence Agency (2019). Switzerland. *The World Factbook*. https://www.cia.gov/the-world-factbook/geos/sz.html. Accessed January 10, 2020.

Cerimele, J. M., Vanderlip, E. R., Croicu, C. A., Melville, J. L., Russo, J., Reed, S. D., & DCDW. (2013). Presenting symptoms of women with depression in an obstetrics and gynecology setting. *Obstetrics and Gynecology, 122*(2, Pt. 1), 313–318. https://doi.org/10.1097/AOG.0b013e31829999ee

Chakravorty, S., Grandner, M. A., Mavandadi, S., Perlis, M. L., Sturgis, E. B., & Oslin, D. W. (2014). Suicidal ideation in veterans misusing alcohol: Relationships with insomnia symptoms and sleep duration. *Addictive Behaviors, 39*(2), 399–405. https://doi.org/10.1016/j.addbeh.2013.09.022

Chan, E., Tan, M., Xin, J., Sudarsanam, S., & Johnson, D. E. (2010). Interactions between traditional Chinese medicines and Western therapeutics. *Current Opinion in Drug Discovery and Development, 13*(1), 50–65.

Chancel, L., Piketty, T., Saez, E., & Zucman, G. (2022). *World Inequality Report 2022*, p. 229. Retrieved October 15, 2023, from https://wir2022.wid.world/www-site/uploads/2023/03/D_FINAL_WIL_RIM_RAPPORT_2303.pdf

Chancellor, S., & De Choudhury, M. (2020). Methods in predictive techniques for mental health status on social media: A critical review. *NPJ Digital Medicine, 3*, Article 43. https://doi.org/10.1038/s41746-020-0233-7

Chang, S. S., Gunnell, D., Sterne, J. A., Lu, T. H., & Cheng, A. T. (2009). Was the economic crisis 1997-1998 responsible for rising suicide rates in East/Southeast Asia?

A time-trend analysis for Japan, Hong Kong, South Korea, Taiwan, Singapore and Thailand. *Social Science & Medicine, 68*(7), 1322–1331. https://doi.org/10.1016/j.socscimed.2009.01.010

Chang, X., Jiang, X., Mkandarwire, T., & Shen, M. (2019). Associations between adverse childhood experiences and health outcomes in adults aged 18–59 years. *PLOS One, 14*(2), Article e0211850. https://doi.org/10.1371/journal.pone.0211850

Chao, Y. Y., You, E., Chang, Y. P., & Dong, X. (2020). Anxiety symptoms, depressive symptoms, and Traditional Chinese Medicine use in U.S. Chinese older adults. *Journal of Immigrant and Minority Health, 22*(4), 746–753. https://doi.org/10.1007/s10903-019-00935-0

Chapman, A. (2018, September 24). The MH370 captain, the twin sister models and some VERY creepy messages: How 53-year-old married pilot of doomed Malaysia Airlines flight bombarded young Instagram stars with Facebook posts. *MSN News*. Retrieved September 1, 2019, from https://www.msn.com/en-au/news/world/the-mh370-captain-the-twin-sister-models-and-some-very-creepy-messages-how-53-year-old-married-pilot-of-doomed-malaysia-airlines-flight-bombarded-young-instagram-stars-with-facebook-posts/ar-AAAAqXq

Chee, N. I. Y. N., Ghorbani, S., Golkashani, H. A., Leong, R. L. F., Ong, J. L., & Chee, M. W. L. (2021). Multi-night validation of a sleep tracking ring in adolescents compared with a research actigraph and polysomnography. *Nature and Science of Sleep, 13*, 177–190. https://doi.org/10.2147/NSS.S286070

Chen, G. X., Amandus, H. E., & Wu, N. (2014). Occupational fatalities among driver/sales workers and truck drivers in the United States, 2003–2008. *American Journal of Industrial Medicine, 57*(7), 800–809. https://doi.org/10.1002/ajim.22320

Chen, J. A., Hung, G. C., Parkin, S., Fava, M., & Yeung, A. S. (2015). Illness beliefs of Chinese American immigrants with major depressive disorder in a primary care setting. *Asian Journal of Psychiatry, 13*, 16–22. https://doi.org/10.1016/j.ajp.2014.12.005

Chen, J. A., Liu, L., Zhao, X., & Yeung, A. S. (2015). Chinese international students: An emerging mental health crisis. *Journal of the American Academy of Child and Adolescent Psychiatry, 54*(11), 879–880. https://doi.org/10.1016/j.jaac.2015.06.022

Chen, M., & Chan, K. L. (2016). Parental absence, child victimization, and psychological well-being in rural China. *Child Abuse & Neglect, 59*, 45–54. https://doi.org/10.1016/j.chiabu.2016.07.009

Chen, S., Chiu, H., Xu, B., Ma, Y., Jin, T., Wu, M., & Conwell, Y. (2010). Reliability and validity of the PHQ-9 for screening late-life depression in Chinese primary care. *International Journal of Geriatric Psychiatry, 25*(11), 1127–1133. https://doi.org/10.1002/gps.2442

Chen, S., Fang, Y., Chiu, H., Fan, H., Jin, T., & Conwell, Y. (2013). Validation of the nine-item Patient Health Questionnaire to screen for major depression in a Chinese primary care population. *Asia-Pacific Psychiatry, 5*(2), 61–68. https://doi.org/10.1111/appy.12063

Chen, W. L., & Chen, J. H. (2019). Consequences of inadequate sleep during the college years: Sleep deprivation, grade point average, and college graduation. *Preventive Medicine, 124*, 23–28. https://doi.org/10.1016/j.ypmed.2019.04.017

Chen, X., Gao, M., Xu, Y., Wang, Y., & Li, S. (2018). Associations between personal social capital and depressive symptoms: Evidence from a probability sample of urban residents in China. *The International Journal of Social Psychiatry, 64*(7), 668–678. https://doi.org/10.1177/0020764018803123

Cheng, H. Y., Shi, Y. X., Yu, F. N., Zhao, H. Z., Zhang, J. H., & Song, M. (2019). Association between vegetables and fruits consumption and depressive symptoms in a middle-aged Chinese population: An observational study. *Medicine, 98*(18), Article e15374. https://doi.org/10.1097/MD.0000000000015374

Cheng, Q., Li, T. M., Kwok, C. L., Zhu, T., & Yip, P. S. (2017). Assessing suicide risk and emotional distress in Chinese social media: A text mining and machine learning study. *Journal of Medical Internet Research, 19*(7), Article e243. https://doi.org/10.2196/jmir.7276

Cheong, M. J., Kim, S., Kim, J. S., Lee, H., Lyu, Y. S., Lee, Y. R., Jeon, B., & Kang, H. W. (2021). A systematic literature review and meta-analysis of the clinical effects of aroma inhalation therapy on sleep problems. *Medicine, 100*(9), Article e24652. https://doi.org/10.1097/MD.0000000000024652

Chetty, R., Stepner, M., Abraham, S., Lin, S., Scuderi, B., Turner, N., Bergeron, A., & Cutler, D. (2016). The association between income and life expectancy in the United States, 2001–2014. *JAMA, 315*(16), 1750–1766. https://doi.org/10.1001/jama.2016.4226

Chi, S., & Lee, M. S. (2021). Personalized medicine using neuroimmunological biomarkers in depressive disorders. *Journal of Personalized Medicine, 11*(2), 114. https://doi.org/10.3390/jpm11020114

Chi, X., Wang, S., Baloch, Z., Zhang, H., Li, X., Zhang, Z., Zhang, H., Dong, Z., Lu, Y., Yu, H., & Ma, K. (2019). Research progress on classical traditional Chinese medicine formula lily bulb and *Rehmannia* decoction in the treatment of depression. *Biomedicine & Pharmacotherapy, 112*, Article 108616. https://doi.org/10.1016/j.biopha.2019.108616

Chiang, M., Reid-Varley, W. B., & Fan, X. (2019). Creative art therapy for mental illness. *Psychiatry Research, 275*, 125–136. https://doi.org/10.1016/j.psychres.2019.03.025

Chiao, J. Y. (2015). Current emotion research in cultural neuroscience. *Emotion Review, 7*(3), 280–293. https://doi.org/10.1177/1754073914546389

Chin, B., Slutsky, J., Raye, J., & Creswell, J. D. (2019). Mindfulness training reduces stress at work: Randomized controlled trial. *Mindfulness, 10*(4), 627–638. https://doi.org/10.1007/s12671-018-1022-0

Chin, W. Y., Choi, E. P., Chan, K. T., & Wong, C. K. (2015). The psychometric properties of the Center for Epidemiologic Studies Depression Scale in Chinese primary care patients: Factor structure, construct validity, reliability, sensitivity and responsiveness. *PLOS One, 10*(8), Article e0135131. https://doi.org/10.1371/journal.pone.0135131

China wakes up to its mental health problems. (2017, January 28). *Economist*. https://www.economist.com/china/2017/01/28/china-wakes-up-to-its-mental-health-problems

China's migrant workers and their children. (2019, May). *China Labour Bulletin*. Retrieved May 25, 2019, from https://clb.org.hk/content/migrant-workers-and-their-children

Chinese Ministry of Education (2018). *2018 College Entrance Examination Outline Release*. Retrieved May 24, 2019, from http://gaokao.eol.cn/gkdg/yw/201712/t20171215_1573574.shtml

Choe, S.-A., Yoo, S., JeKarl, J., & Kim, K. K. (2018). Recent trend and associated factors of harmful alcohol use based on age and gender in Korea. *Journal of Korean Medical Science, 33*(4), Article e(23). https://doi.org/10.3346/jkms.2018.33.e23

Choi, I., Sharpe, L., Li, S., & Hunt, C. (2015). Acceptability of psychological treatment to Chinese- and Caucasian-Australians: Internet treatment reduces barriers but face-to-face care is preferred. *Social Psychiatry and Psychiatric Epidemiology, 50*(1), 77–87. https://doi.org/10.1007/s00127-014-0921-1

Choi, I., Zou, J., Titov, N., Dear, B. F., Li, S., Johnston, L., Andrews, G., & Hunt, C. (2012). Culturally attuned internet treatment for depression amongst Chinese Australians: A randomised controlled trial. *Journal of Affective Disorders, 136*(3), 459–468.

Choi, M., & Yeom, H. (2011). Identifying and treating the culture-bound syndrome of *hwa-byung* among older Korean immigrant women: Recommendations for practitioners. *Journal of the American Academy of Nurse Practitioners, 23*(5), 226–232. https://doi.org/10.1111/j.1745-7599.2011.00607.x

Choo, C. C., Harris, K. M., Chew, P., & Ho, R. C. (2017). Does ethnicity matter in risk and protective factors for suicide attempts and suicide lethality? *PLOS ONE, 12*(4), Article e0175752. https://doi.org/10.1371/journal.pone.0175752

Chow, S. K., Francis, B., Ng, Y. H., Naim, N., Beh, H. C., Ariffin, M., Yusuf, M. H. M, Lee, J. W., & Sulaiman, A. H. (2021). Religious coping, depression and anxiety among healthcare workers during the COVID-19 pandemic: A Malaysian perspective. *Healthcare, 9*(1), Article 79. https://doi.org/10.3390/healthcare9010079

Choy, Y., Schneier, F. R., Heimberg, R. G., Oh, K. S., & Liebowitz, M. R. (2008). Features of the offensive subtype of *taijin-kyofu-sho* in US and Korean patients with DSM-IV social anxiety disorder. *Depression and Anxiety, 25*(3), 230–240. https://doi.org/10.1002/da.20295

Christensen, H., Griffiths, K. M., & Jorm, A. F. (2004). Delivering interventions for depression by using the internet: Randomised controlled trial. *BMJ (Clinical research ed.), 328*(7434), 265. https://doi.org/10.1136/bmj.37945.566632.EE

Christensen, J., Vestergaard, M., Mortensen, P. B., Sidenius, P., & Agerbo, E. (2007). Epilepsy and risk of suicide: A population-based case-control study. *Lancet Neurology, 6*(8), 693–698.

Christensen, M. C., Fagiolini, A., Florea, I., Loft, H., Cuomo, A., & Goodwin, G. M. (2021). Validation of the Oxford Depression Questionnaire: Sensitivity to change, minimal clinically important difference, and response threshold for the assessment of emotional blunting. *Journal of Affective Disorders, 294*, 924–931. https://doi.org/10.1016/j.jad.2021.07.099

Chu, C., Buchman-Schmitt, J. M., Stanley, I. H., Hom, M. A., Tucker, R. P., Hagan, C. R., Rogers, M. L., Podlogar, M. C., Chiurliza, B., Ringer, F. B., Michaels, M. S., Patros, C. H. G., & Joiner, T. E., Jr. (2017). The interpersonal theory of suicide: A systematic review and meta-analysis of a decade of cross-national research. *Psychological Bulletin, 143*(12), 1313–1345. https://doi.org/10.1037/bul0000123

Chung, C. K., & Cho, S. (2018). Significance of "jeong" in Korean culture and psychotherapy. *Pacific Rim College of Psychiatrists*. Retrieved May 4, 2019, from http://www.prcp.org/publications/sig.pdf

Chung, F., Subramanyam, R., Liao, P., Sasaki, E., Shapiro, C., & Sun, Y. (2012). High STOP-Bang score indicates a high probability of obstructive sleep apnoea. *British Journal of Anaesthesia, 108*(5), 768–775. https://doi.org/10.1093/bja/aes022

Chung, F., Yang, Y., Brown, R., & Liao, P. (2014). Alternative scoring models of STOP-Bang questionnaire improve specificity to detect undiagnosed obstructive sleep apnea. *Journal of Clinical Sleep Medicine, 10*(9), 951–958. https://doi.org/10.5664/jcsm.4022

Chung, G. H., Oswald, R. F., & Hardesty, J. L. (2009). Enculturation as a condition impacting Korean American physicians' responses to Korean immigrant women suffering intimate partner violence. *Health Care for Women International, 30*(1-2), 41–63. https://doi.org/10.1080/07399330802523568

Chung, R. H. (2001). Gender, ethnicity, and acculturation in intergenerational conflict of Asian American college students. *Cultural Diversity & Ethnic Minority Psychology, 7*(4), 376–386. https://doi.org/10.1037/1099-9809.7.4.376

Chung, S. (2020). *History of Korean Immigration to America, from 1903 to Present*. Boston University School of Theology, Boston Korean Diaspora Project. Retrieved July 23, 2021, from https://sites.bu.edu/koreandiaspora/issues/history-of-korean-immigration-to-america-from-1903-to-present/

Chung, S.-Y., Park, Y.-J., Kim, J.-W., & Park, Y.-B. (2015). Validation of the Hwa-Byung Scale and its relationship with cardiovascular autonomic function. *European Journal of Integrative Medicine, 7*(4), 409–416.

Citizens Commission on Human Rights (2019). *Harming Artists: Psychiatry Ruins Creativity*. https://www.cchr.org/cchr-reports/harming-artists/introduction.html

Claman H. N. (2012). The anatomy of melancholy: Burton and Osler. The Pharos of Alpha Omega Alpha-Honor Medical Society 75(2): 20–27.

Clark, E. M., Williams, R. M., Schulz, E., Williams, B. R., & Holt, C. L. (2018). Personality, social capital, and depressive symptomatology among African Americans. *The Journal of Black Psychology, 44*(5), 422–449. https://doi.org/10.1177/0095798418780771

Clark, S. A. (2018). The impact of the Hippocratic Oath in 2018: The conflict of the ideal of the physician, the knowledgeable humanitarian, versus the corporate medical allegiance to financial models contributes to burnout. *Cureus, 10*(7), Article e3076. https://doi.org/10.7759/cureus.3076

Clark, T. T., Salas-Wright, C. P., Vaughn, M. G., & Whitfield, K. E. (2015). Everyday discrimination and mood and substance use disorders: A latent profile analysis with African Americans and Caribbean Blacks. *Addictive Behaviors, 40*, 119–125. https://doi.org/10.1016/j.addbeh.2014.08.006

Coghlan, M. L., Maker, G., Crighton, E., Haile, J., Murry, D. C., White, N. E., Byard, R. W., Bellgard, M. I., Mullaney, I., Trengove, R., Allcock, R. J. N., Nash, C., Hoban, C., Jarrett, K., Edwards, R., Musgrave, I. F., & Bunce, M. (2015). Combined DNA, toxicological and heavy metal analyses provide an auditing toolkit to improve pharmacovigilance of traditional Chinese medicine (TCM). *Scientific Reports, 5*, Article 17475. https://doi.org/10.1038/srep17475

Cohn, A., Maréchal, M. A., Tannenbaum, D., & Zünd, C. L. (2019). Civic honesty around the globe. *Science, 365*(6448), 70–73. https://doi.org/10.1126/science.aau8712

Combs, B., Heaton, K., Raju, D., Vance, D. E., & Sieber, W. K. (2018). A descriptive study of musculoskeletal injuries in long- haul truck drivers: A NIOSH national survey. *Workplace Health & Safety, 66*(10), 475–481. https://doi.org/10.1177/2165079917750935

Comical psychosomatic medicine. (2021). In *Wikipedia*. Retrieved May 15, 2021, from https://en.wikipedia.org/wiki/Comical_Psychosomatic_Medicine

Congressional-Executive Commission on China (2023). *Criminal Law of the People's Republic of China, Article 260*. https://www.cecc.gov/resources/legal-provisions/criminal-law-of-the-peoples-republic-of-china

Connery, H. S. (2015). Medication-assisted treatment of opioid use disorder: Review of the evidence and future directions. *Harvard Review of Psychiatry, 23*(2), 63–75. https://doi.org/10.1097/HRP.0000000000000075

Connley, C. (2018). *Just 6 percent of America's truck drivers are women—Here's what it's like.* CNBC. Retrieved July 17, 2019, from https://www.cnbc.com/2018/06/13/heres-what-its-like-to-be-a-woman-truck-driver.html

Cook, T. M., & Wang, J. (2011). Causation beliefs and stigma against depression: results from a population-based study. Journal of Affective Disorders,133(1–2): 86–92. https://doi.org/10.1016/j.jad.2011.03.030

Cooperman, A., Smith, G., & Ritchey, K. (2015). *America's Changing Religious Landscape.* Pew Research Center. Retrieved September 28, 2019, from https://www.pewforum.org/2015/05/12/americas-changing-religious-landscape/

Coppersmith, G., Ngo, K., Leary, R., & Wood, A. (2016). Exploratory analysis of social media prior to a suicide attempt. In *Proceedings of the Third Workshop on Computational Linguistics and Clinical Psychology*, pp. 106–117. Association for Computational Linguistics. https://pdfs.semanticscholar.org/3bb2/1a197b29e2b25fe8befbe6ac5cec66d25413.pdf

Corrigan, M., O'Rourke, A. M., Moran, B., Fletcher, J. M., & Harkin, A. (2023). Inflammation in the pathogenesis of depression: A disorder of neuroimmune origin. *Neuronal Signaling, 7*(2), NS20220054. https://doi.org/10.1042/NS20220054

Cosma A., Abdrakhmanova S., Taut D., Schrijvers K., Catunda C., & Schnohr C. (2023). *A focus on adolescent mental health and well-being in Europe, central Asia and Canada. Health Behaviour in School-aged Children international report from the 2021/2022 survey.* Volume 1. WHO Regional Office for Europe, pp. 42, 46, 50, 56.

Covassin, N., & Singh, P. (2016). Sleep duration and cardiovascular disease risk: Epidemiologic and experimental evidence. *Sleep Medicine Clinics, 11*(1), 81–89. https://doi.org/10.1016/j.jsmc.2015.10.007

Cox, J. L., Holden, J. M., & Sagovsky, R. (1987). Detection of postnatal depression. Development of the 10-item Edinburgh Postnatal Depression Scale. *The British Journal of Psychiatry, 150*, 782–786. https://doi.org/10.1192/bjp.150.6.782

Coyne-Beasley, T., McGee, K. S., Johnson, R. M., & Bordley, W. C. (2002). The association of handgun ownership and storage practices with safety consciousness. *Archives of Pediatrics & Adolescent Medicine, 156*(8), 763–768. https://doi.org/10.1001/archpedi.156.8.763

Cristofich, L. A. (2015). *A qualitative study of female airline pilots and how they achieved their goals* [Doctoral dissertation, Capella University]. *Dissertation Abstracts International.* Retrieved September 2, 2019, from http://search.ebscohost.com.ezp-prod1.hul.harvard.edu/login.aspx?direct=true&db=psyh&AN=2015-99090-200&site=ehost-live&scope=site

Crizzle, A. M. (2022). Health and safety practices and perceptions of COVID-19 in long-haul truck drivers. *Journal of Occupational and Environmental Medicine, 64*(2), 173–178. https://doi.org/10.1097/JOM.0000000000002426

Crizzle, A. M., McLean, M., & Malkin, J. (2020). Risk factors for depressive symptoms in long-haul truck drivers. *International Journal of Environmental Research and Public Health, 17*(11), Article 3764.

Cronholm, P. F., Forke, C. M., Wade, R., Bair-Merritt, M. H., Davis, M., Harkins-Schwarz, M., Pachter, L. M., & Fein, J. A. (2015). Adverse childhood experiences: Expanding the concept of adversity. *American Journal of Preventive Medicine, 49*(3): 354–361. https://doi.org/10.1016/j.amepre.2015.02.001

Cruwys, T., & Gunaseelan, S. (2016). "Depression is who I am": Mental illness identity, stigma and wellbeing. *Journal of Affective Disorders, 189,* 36–42. https://doi.org/10.1016/j.jad.2015.09.012

Cui, L., Li, S., Wang, S., Wu, X., Liu, Y., Yu, W., Wang, Y., Tang, Y., Xia, M., & Li, B. (2024). Major depressive disorder: Hypothesis, mechanism, prevention and treatment. *Signal Transduction and Targeted Therapy, 9*(1), 30. https://doi.org/10.1038/s41392-024-01738-y

Cuomo, A., Carmellini, P., Garo, M. L., Barillà, G., Libri, C., Spiti, A., Goracci, A., Bolognesi, S., & Fagiolini, A. (2023). Effectiveness of light therapy as adjunctive treatment in bipolar depression: A pilot study. *Journal of Affective Disorders, 321,* 102–107. https://doi.org/10.1016/j.jad.2022.10.009

Cutler, J. B. R., Pane, O., Panesar, S. K., Updike, W., & Moore, T. R. (2023). Treatment of mood and depressive disorders with complementary and alternative medicine: Efficacy review. Journal of Midwifery & Women's Health 68(4): 421–429. https://doi.org/10.1111/jmwh.13527

Dabboussi, N., Debs, E., Bouji, M., Rafei, R., & Fares, N. (2024). Balancing the mind: Toward a complete picture of the interplay between gut microbiota, inflammation and major depressive disorder. *Brain Research Bulletin, 216,* 111056. https://doi.org/10.1016/j.brainresbull.2024.111056

Daido, K. (2013). Treating emotion-related disorders in Japanese traditional medicine: Language, patients and doctors. *Culture, Medicine & Psychiatry, 37*(1), 59–80. https://doi.org/10.1007/s11013-012-9297-4

Daley, S. (2015, April 25). Speeding in Finland can cost you a fortune, if you already have one. *New York Times.* https://www.nytimes.com/2015/04/26/world/europe/speeding-in-finland-can-cost-a-fortune-if-you-already-have-one.html

Dallaspezia, S., & Benedetti, F. (2020). Antidepressant light therapy for bipolar patients: A meta-analysis. *Journal of Affective Disorders, 274,* 943–948. https://doi.org/10.1016/j.jad.2020.05.104

d'Andrea, G., Pettorruso, M., Lorenzo, G. D., Mancusi, G., McIntyre, R. S., & Martinotti, G. (2023). Rethinking ketamine and esketamine action: Are they antidepressants with mood-stabilizing properties? *European Neuropsychopharmacology, 70,* 49–55. https://doi.org/10.1016/j.euroneuro.2023.02.010

Dang, C., Wang, Q., Li, Q., Xiong, Y., & Lu, Y. (2024). Chinese herbal medicines for the treatment of depression: a systematic review and network meta-analysis. Frontiers in Pharmacology, 15, 1295564. https://doi.org/10.3389/fphar.2024.1295564

Daoud, N., Haque, N., Gao, M., Nisenbaum, R., Muntaner, C., & O'Campo, P. (2016). Neighborhood settings, types of social capital and depression among immigrants in Toronto. *Social Psychiatry and Psychiatric Epidemiology, 51*(4), 529–538. https://doi.org/10.1007/s00127-016-1173-z

da Silva-Junior, F. P., de Pinho, R. S. N., de Mello, M. T., de Bruin, V. M. S., & De Bruin, P. F. C. (2009). Risk factors for depression in truck drivers. *Social Psychiatry and Psychiatric Epidemiology, 44,* 125–129. https://doi.org/10.1007/s00127-008-0412-3

Davey, C. L., & Davidson, M. J. (2000). The right of passage? The experiences of female pilots in commercial aviation. *Feminism and Psychology, 10*(2), 195–225. https://doi.org/10.1177/0959353500010002002

David, K., Anuj, D., & Nabil, S. (2015). Violence toward chronic pain care providers: A national survey. *Pain Medicine, 16*(10), 1882–1896. https://doi.org/10.1111/pme.12794

Davies, C. (2011, October 26). Amy Winehouse inquest records verdict of misadventure. The Guardian. https://web.archive.org/web/20111027211038/http://www.guardian.co.uk/music/2011/oct/26/amy-winehouse-verdict-misadventure

Davies, B., Turner, K. M. E., Frølund, M., Ward, H., May, M. T., Rasmussen, S., Benfield, T., Westh, H., & Danish Chlamydia Study Group (2016). Risk of reproductive complications following chlamydia testing: a population-based retrospective cohort study in Denmark. *The Lancet. Infectious diseases, 16*(9), 1057–1064. https://doi.org/10.1016/S1473-3099(16)30092-5

Davis, C., Bryan, J., Hodgson, J, & Murphy, K. (2015). Definition of the Mediterranean diet: A literature review. *Nutrients, 7*(11), 9139–9153. https://doi.org/10.3390/nu7115459

Day, J. C., & Hait, H. W. (2019, June 6). *Number of truckers at all-time high.* https://www.census.gov/library/stories/2019/06/america-keeps-on-trucking.html

Day, P., Lawson, J., Mantri, S., Jain, A., Rabago, D., & Lennon, R. (2022). Physician moral injury in the context of moral, ethical and legal codes. *Journal of Medical Ethics, 48*(10), 746–752. https://doi.org/10.1136/medethics-2021-107225

Daydaynews (2019, November 9). Let the children win at the starting line? The documentary "No Starting Line" tells you how hard education in Hong Kong is. *Day Day News.* https://daydaynews.cc/en/baby/213374.html

De, R., Prasad, F., Stogios, N., Burin, L., Ebdrup, B. H., Knop, F. K., Hahn, M. K., & Agarwal, S. M. (2023). Promising translatable pharmacological interventions for body weight management in individuals with severe mental illness - a narrative review. *Expert Opinion on Pharmacotherapy, 24*(16), 1823–1832. https://doi.org/10.1080/14656566.2023.2254698

Dearborn, M. (2017). *Ernest Hemingway: A biography.* Knopf.

De Ayala, R. J. (2008). *The Theory and Practice of Item Response Theory.* Guilford Press.

De Berardis, D., Olivieri, L., Rapini, G., Serroni, N., Fornaro, M., Valchera, A., Carano, A., Vellante, F., Bustini, M., Serafini, G., Pompili, M., Ventriglio, A., Perna, G., Fraticelli, S., Martinotti, G., & Di Giannantonio, M. (2020). Religious coping, hopelessness, and suicide ideation in subjects with first-episode major depression: An exploratory study in the real world clinical practice. *Brain Sciences, 10*(12), Article 912. https://doi.org/10.3390/brainsci10120912

Deif, R., & Salama, M. (2021). Depression from a precision mental health perspective: Utilizing personalized conceptualizations to guide personalized treatments. *Frontiers in Psychiatry, 12,* Article 650318. https://doi.org/10.3389/fpsyt.2021.650318

DelMastro, K., Hellem, T., Kim, N., Kondo, D., Sung, Y. H., & Renshaw, P. F. (2011). Incidence of major depressive episode correlates with elevation of substate region of residence. Journal of Affective Disorders, 129(1-3), 376–379. https://doi.org/10.1016/j.jad.2010.10.001

Deneva, T., Ianakiev, Y., & Keskinova, D. (2019). Burnout syndrome in physicians—Psychological assessment and biomarker research. *Medicina (Kaunas, Lithuania), 55*(5), Article 209. https://doi.org/10.3390/medicina55050209

Dengah, H. J. F., 2nd, Bingham Thomas, E., Hawvermale, E., & Temple, E. (2019). "Find that balance:" The impact of cultural consonance and dissonance on mental health among Utah and Mormon women. Medical Anthropology Quarterly, 33(3), 439–458. https://doi.org/10.1111/maq.12527

de Souza Palmeira, M. L., & Marqueze, E. C. (2016). Excess weight in regular aviation pilots associated with work and sleep characteristics. *Sleep Science*, *9*(4), 266–271. https://doi.org/10.1016/j.slsci.2016.12.001

Devinsky, J., & Schachter, S. (2009). Norman Geschwind's contribution to the understanding of behavioral changes in temporal lobe epilepsy: The February 1974 lecture. *Epilepsy & Behavior*, *15*(4), 417–424. https://doi.org/10.1016/j.yebeh.2009.06.006

Dhalla, S., & Kopec, J. A. (2007). The CAGE questionnaire for alcohol misuse: A review of reliability and validity studies. *Clinical and Investigative Medicine*, *30*(1), 33–41. https://doi.org/10.25011/cim.v30i1.447

Dhusia, A. H., Dhaimade, P. A., Jain, A. A., Shemna, S. S., & Dubey, P. N. (2019). Prevalence of occupational burnout among resident doctors working in public sector hospitals in Mumbai. *Indian Journal of Community Medicine: Official Publication of Indian Association of Preventive & Social Medicine*, *44*(4), 352–356. https://doi.org/10.4103/ijcm.IJCM_78_19

Dickerson, F., Stallings, C., Origoni, A., Katsafanas, E., Sweeney, K., Khushalani, S., & Yolken, R. (2019). Nitrated meat products are associated with suicide behavior in psychiatric patients. *Psychiatry Research*, *275*, 283–286.

Diderichsen, S., Johansson, E. E., Verdonk, P., Lagro-Janssen, T., & Hamberg, K. (2013). Few gender differences in specialty preferences and motivational factors: A cross-sectional Swedish study on last-year medical students. *BMC Medical Education*, *13*, Article 39. https://doi.org/10.1186/1472-6920-13-39

Ding, W., Wang, L., Li, L., Li, H., Wu, J., Zhang, J., & Wang, J. (2024). Pathogenesis of depression and the potential for traditional Chinese medicine treatment. *Frontiers in Pharmacology*, *15*, 1407869. https://doi.org/10.3389/fphar.2024.1407869

Discover Navajo (2018). *Discover Navajo Fact Sheet*. Retrieved August 16, 2019, from http://www.discovernavajo.com/fact-sheet.aspx

Di Stadio, A., Dipietro, L., Ricci, G., Della Volpe, A., Minni, A., Greco, A., De Vincentiis, M., & Ralli, M. (2018). Hearing loss, tinnitus, hyperacusis, and diplacusis in professional musicians: A systematic review. *International Journal of Environmental Research and Public Health*, *15*(10), Article 2120. https://doi.org/10.3390/ijerph15102120

Di Thiene, D., Alexanderson, K., Tinghög, P., La Torre, G., & Mittendorfer-Rutz, E. (2015). Suicide among first-generation and second-generation immigrants in Sweden: Association with labour market marginalisation and morbidity. *Journal of Epidemiology and Community Health*, *69*(5), 467–473. https://doi.org/10.1136/jech-2014-204648

Doerr-Zegers, O. (2003). Phenomenology of genius and psychopathology. *Seishin Shinkeigaku Zasshi*, *105*(3), 277–286.

Doi, T. (1973). *The Anatomy of Dependence (甘えの構造; Amae no Kōzō; J. Bester, trans)*. Kodansha America. (1971).

Dolan, A. (2007). "That's just the cesspool where they dump all the trash": Exploring working class men's perceptions and experiences of social capital and health. *Health*, *11*(4), 475–495. https://doi.org/10.1177/1363459307080869

Dols, M. W., & Immisch, D. E. (1992). Galen and mental illness. In Dols, M. W. (ed). *Majnūn: The Madman in Medieval Islamic Society* (pp. 17–37). Oxford Academic. https://doi.org/10.1093/acprof:oso/9780198202219.001.0001

Domino, K. B., Hornbein, T. F., Polissar, N. L., Renner, G., Johnson, J., Alberti, S., & Hankes, L. (2005). Risk factors for relapse in health care professionals with substance use disorders. *Journal of the American Medical Association, 293*(12), 1453–1460. https://doi.org/10.1001/jama.293.12.1453

Dong, M., Zhou, F. C., Xu, S. W., Zhang, Q., Ng, C. H., Ungvari, G. S., & Xiàng, Y. T. (2020). Prevalence of suicide-related behaviors among physicians: A systematic review and meta-analysis. *Suicide & Life-Threatening Behavior, 50*(6), 1264–1275. https://doi.org/10.1111/sltb.12690

Dong, X., Bergren, S., & Simon, M. A. (2017). Cross-sectional and longitudinal association between trust in physician and depressive symptoms among US community-dwelling Chinese older adults. *The Journals of Gerontology. Series A: Biological Sciences and Medical Sciences, 72*(S1), S125–S130. https://doi.org/10.1093/gerona/glx036

Dong, X., Chen, R., Wu, B., Zhang, N. J., Mui, A. C., & Chi, I. (2015). Association between elder mistreatment and suicidal ideation among community-dwelling Chinese older adults in the USA. *Gerontology, 62*(1), 71–80. https://doi.org/10.1159/000437420

Dong, X., Yang, C., Cao, S., Gan, Y., Sun, H., Gong, Y., Yang, H., Yin, X., & Lu, Z. (2015). Tea consumption and the risk of depression: A meta-analysis of observational studies. *Australia and New Zealand Journal of Psychiatry, 49*(4), 334–345. https://doi.org/10.1177/0004867414567759

DQYDJ.com. (n.d.). *Income by City Calculator and Statistics by City*. Retrieved November 20, 2021, https://dqydj.com/income-by-city/

Drancourt, N., Etain, B., Lajnef, M., Henry, C., Raust, A., Cochet, B., Mathieu, F., Gard, S., Mbailara, K., Zanouy, L., Kahn, J. P., Cohen, R. F., Wajsbrot-Elgrabli, O., Leboyer, M., Scott, J., & Bellivier, F. (2013). Duration of untreated bipolar disorder: Missed opportunities on the long road to optimal treatment. *Acta Psychiatrica Scandinavica, 127*(2), 136–144. https://doi.org/10.1111/j.1600-0447.2012.01917.x

Du, B. B., Bigelow, P. L., Wells, R. P., Davies, H. W., Hall, P., & Johnson, P. W. (2018). The impact of different seats and whole-body vibration exposure on truck driver vigilance and discomfort. *Ergonomics, 61*(4), 528–537. https://doi.org/10.1080/00140139.2017.1372638

Du, Y. L., Hu, J. B., Huang, T. T., Lai, J. B., Ng, C. H., Zhang, W. H., Li, C., Xu, Z.-y., Zhou, H.-t., Ruan, L.-m., Xu, Y., & Hu, S.-h. (2021). Psychometric properties of the Clinically Useful Depression Outcome Scale supplemented with DSM-5 mixed subtype questionnaire in Chinese patients with mood disorders. *Journal of Affective Disorders, 279*, 53–58. https://doi.org/10.1016/j.jad.2020.09.117

Dua, D., Padhy, S., & Grover, S. (2021). Comparison of religiosity and spirituality in patients of depression with and without suicidal attempts. *Indian Journal of Psychiatry, 63*(3), 258–269. https://doi.org/10.4103/psychiatry.IndianJPsychiatry_246_20

Duarte, D., El-Hagrassy, M. M., Couto, T., Gurgel, W., Minuzzi, L., Saperson, K., & Corrêa, H. (2023). Challenges and potential solutions for physician suicide risk factors in the COVID-19 era: psychiatric comorbidities, judicialization of medicine, and burnout. *Trends in Psychiatry and Psychotherapy, 45*, 1–9. https://doi.org/10.47626/2237-6089-2021-0293

Ducasse, D., Loas, G., Dassa, D., Gramaglia, C., Zeppegn, P. Guillaume, S., Olié, E., & Courtet, P. (2018). Anhedonia is associated with suicidal ideation independently of depression: A meta-analysis. *Depression and Anxiety*, 35(5), 382–392. https://doi.org/10.1002/da.22709

Duchaine, C. S., Brisson, C., Talbot, D., Gilbert-Ouimet, M., Trudel, X., Vézina, M., Milot, A., Diorio, C., Ndjaboué, R., Giguère, Y., Mâsse, B., Dionne, C. E., Maunsell, E., & Laurin, D. (2021). Psychosocial stressors at work and inflammatory biomarkers: PROspective Quebec Study on Work and Health. *Psychoneuroendocrinology*, 133, 105400. https://doi.org/10.1016/j.psyneuen.2021.105400

Duke, J., Guest, M., & Boggess, M. (2010). Age-related safety in professional heavy vehicle drivers: A literature review. *Accident Analysis and Prevention*, 42, 364–371. https://doi.org/10.1016/j.aap.2009.09.026

DuPont, R. L., McLellan, A. T., Carr, G., Gendel, M., & Skipper, G. E. (2009). How are addicted physicians treated? A national survey of physician health programs. *Journal of Substance Abuse Treatment*, 37(1), 1–7. https://doi.org/10.1016/j.jsat.2009.03.010

Durkee, T., Hadlaczky, G., Westerlund, M., & Carli, V. (2011). Internet pathways in suicidality: A review of the evidence. *International Journal of Environmental Research and Public Health*, 8(10), 3938–3952. https://doi.org/10.3390/ijerph8103938

Durkheim, E. (1951). *Suicide*. Free Press. (Original work published 1897)

Dutheil, F., Aubert, C., Pereira, B., Dambrun, M., Moustafa, F., Mermillod, M., Baker, J. S., Trousselard, M., Lesage, F.-X., & Navel, V. (2019). Suicide among physicians and health-care workers: A systematic review and meta-analysis. *PLOS ONE*, 14(12), Article e0226361. https://doi.org/10.1371/journal.pone.0226361

Dyrbye, L. N., Eacker, A., Durning, S. J., Brazeau, C., Moutier, C., Massie, F. S., Satele, D., Sloan, J. A., & Shanafelt, T. D. (2015). The impact of stigma and personal experiences on the help-seeking behaviors of medical students with burnout. *Academic Medicine*, 90(7), 961–969. https://doi.org/10.1097/ACM.0000000000000655

Dyrbye, L. N., West, C. P., Sinsky, C. A., Goeders, L. E., Satele, D. V., & Shanafelt, T. D. (2017). Medical licensure questions and physician reluctance to seek care for mental health conditions. *Mayo Clinic Proceedings*, 92(1), 1486–1493. https://doi.org/10.1016/j.mayocp.2017.06.020

Eastman, J. T., Danaher, W. F., & Schrock, D. (2013). Gendering truck driving songs: The cultural masculinization of an occupation. *Sociological Spectrum*, 33(5), 416–432. https://doi.org/10.1080/02732173.2013.818508

Eaton, W. W., Smith, C., Ybarra, M., Muntaner, C., & Tien, A. (2004). Center for Epidemiologic Studies Depression Scale: Review and revision (CESD and CESD-R). In M. E. Maruish (Ed.), *The Use of Psychological Testing for Treatment Panning and Outcomes Assessment: Instruments for Adults* (pp. 363–377). Lawrence Erlbaum Associates.

Ebrahimi, H., Mardani, A., Basirinezhad, M. H., Hamidzadeh, A., & Eskandari, F. (2021). The effects of lavender and chamomile essential oil inhalation aromatherapy on depression, anxiety and stress in older community-dwelling people: A randomized controlled trial. *Explore*, 18(3), 272–278. https://doi.org/10.1016/j.explore.2020.12.012

Economist (2023, March 6). The Economist's glass-ceiling index. Retrieved October 1, 2023, from https://www.economist.com/graphic-detail/glass-ceiling-index

Edvardmunch.org. (2019). *Edvard Munch biography*. https://www.edvardmunch.org/biography.jsp

Efforts needed to reduce doctors' working hours. (2019, January 31). *Japan Times*. Retrieved June 1, 2021, from https://www.japantimes.co.jp/opinion/2019/01/31/editorials/efforts-needed-reduce-doctors-working-hours/

Eibl, J. K., Gauthier, G., Pellegrini, D., Daiter, J., Varenbut, M., Hogenbirk, J. C., & Marsh, D. C. (2017). The effectiveness of telemedicine-delivered opioid agonist therapy in a supervised clinical setting. *Drug and Alcohol Dependence, 176*, 133–138. https://doi.org/10.1016/j.drugalcdep.2017.01.048

Ekstein, R. & Motto, R. L. (1969). *From Learning for Love to Love of Learning; Essays on Psychoanalysis and Education*. New York: Brunner/Mazel.

Eltgeest, L. E. M., Visser, M., Penninx, B. W. J. H., Colpo, M., Bandinelli, S., & Brouwer, I. A. (2019). Bidirectional associations between food groups and depressive symptoms: Longitudinal findings from the Invecchiare in Chianti (InCHIANTI) study. *British Journal of Nutrition, 121*(4), 439–450. https://doi.org/10.1017/S0007114518003203

Elyamany, O., Leicht, G., Herrmann, C. S., & Mulert, C. (2021). Transcranial alternating current stimulation (tACS): From basic mechanisms towards first applications in psychiatry. *European Archives of Psychiatry and Clinical Neuroscience, 271*(1), 135–156. https://doi.org/10.1007/s00406-020-01209-9

Emery, C. R., Eremina, T., Yang, H. L., Yoo, C., Yoo, J., & Jang, J. K. (2015). Protective informal social control of child maltreatment and child abuse injury in Seoul. *Journal of Interpersonal Violence, 30*(18), 3324–3339. https://doi.org/10.1177/0886260514554422

Epic Flight Academy (2023). *Airline pilot salary: Comprehensive breakdown & industry comparison*. Retrieved September 1, 2023 from https://epicflightacademy.com/airline-pilot-salary/

Erlinger, S. (2010). Frederic Chopin and Michael Jackson: What could they have in common? *Gastroenterologie Clinique et Biologique, 34*(4–5), 246–249. https://doi.org/10.1016/j.gcb.2010.03.001

Erzen, E., & Cikrikci, Ö. (2018). The effect of loneliness on depression: A meta-analysis. *International Journal of Social Psychiatry, 64*(5), 427–435. https://doi.org/10.1177/0020764018776349

Esaki, Y., Obayashi, K., Saeki, K., Fujita, K., Iwata, N., & Kitajima, T. (2021). Preventive effect of morning light exposure on relapse into depressive episode in bipolar disorder. *Acta Psychiatrica Scandinavica, 143*(4), 328–338. https://doi.org/10.1111/acps.13287

Eskin, M., Poyrazil, S., Janghorbani, M., Bakshi, S., Carta, M. G., Moro, M. F., Tran, U. S., Voracek, M., Mechri, A., Aidoudi, K., Hamdan, M., Nawafleh, H., Sun, J.-M., Flood, C., Phillips, L., Yoshimasu, K., Tsuno, K., Kujan, O., Harlak, H., ... Taifour, S. (2019). The role of religion in suicidal behavior, attitudes and psychological distress among university students: A multinational study. *Transcultural Psychiatry, 58*(5), 853–877. https://doi.org/10.1177/1363461518823933

Esmaealzadeh, D., Moodi Ghalibaf, A., Shariati Rad, M., Rezaee, R., Razavi, B. M., & Hosseinzadeh, H. (2023). Pharmacological effects of Safranal: An updated review. *Iranian Journal of Basic Medical Sciences, 26*(10), 1131–1143. https://doi.org/10.22038/IJBMS.2023.69824.15197

Essau, C. A., Sasagawa, S., Ishikawa, S., Okajima, I., O'Callaghan, J., & Bray, D. (2012). A Japanese form of social anxiety (*taijin kyofusho*): Frequency and correlates in two generations of the same family. *International Journal of Social Psychiatry, 58*(6), 635–642.

European Centre for Disease Prevention and Control (2022). *Chlamydia infection. Annual Epidemiological Report for 2019.* https://www.ecdc.europa.eu/sites/default/files/docume nts/chlamydia-annual-epidemiological-report-2019.pdf

European Union Agency for Fundamental Rights (2014). *Violence Against Women: An EU-Wide Survey. Main Results Report.* https://fra.europa.eu/en/publication/2014/viole nce-against-women-eu-wide-survey-main-results-report

European Union Aviation Safety Agency (2020). *Easy Access Rules for Medical Requirements.* p. 91.

Eurostat (2019a). Share of young adults aged 18–34 living with their parents, by age and sex. appsso.eurostat.ec.europa.eu

Eurostat (2019b). Frequency of participation in cultural or sport activities in the last 12 months by income quintile, household type, degree of urbanisation and activity type. appsso.eurostat.ec.europa.eu

Evans, G. W. (2016). Childhood poverty and adult psychological well-being. *Proceedings of the National Academy of Sciences of the United States of America, 113*(52), 14949–14952. https://doi.com/10.1073/pnas.1604756114

Evans-Lacko, S., Takizawa, R., Brimblecombe, N., King, D., Knapp, M., Maughan, B., & Arseneault, L. (2017). Childhood bullying victimization is associated with use of mental health services over five decades: A longitudinal nationally representative cohort study. *Psychological Medicine, 47*(1), 127–135. https://doi.org/10.1017/S0033291716001719

Fagiolini, A., Florea, I., Loft, H., & Christensen, M. C. (2021). Effectiveness of vortioxetine on emotional blunting in patients with major depressive disorder with inadequate response to SSRI/SNRI treatment. *Journal of Affective Disorders, 283,* 472–479. https://doi.org/10.1016/j.jad.2020.11.106

Fairley, M., Humphreys, K., Joyce, V. R., Bounthavong, M., Trafton, J., Combs, A., Oliva, E. M., Goldhaber-Fiebert, J. D., Asch, S. M., Brandeau, M. L., & Owens, D. K. (2021). Cost-effectiveness of treatments for opioid use disorder. *JAMA Psychiatry, 78*(7), 767–777. https://doi.org/10.1001/jamapsychiatry.2021.0247

Fan, B., Wang, T., Wang, W., Zhang, S., Gong, M., Li, W., Lu, C., & Guo, L. (2019). Long-term exposure to ambient fine particulate pollution, sleep disturbance and their interaction effects on suicide attempts among Chinese adolescents. *Journal of Affective Disorders, 258,* 89–95. https://doi.org/10.1016/j.jad.2019.08.004

Fan, Z. J., Bonauto, D. K., Foley, M. P., Anderson, N. J., Yraqui, N. L., & Silverstein, B. A. (2012). Occupation and the prevalence of current depression and frequent mental distress, WA BRFSS 2006 and 2008. *American Journal of Industrial Medicine, 55*(10), 8934–8903. https://doi.org/10.1002/ajim.22094

Fangfang, M. A., Hewei, Z., Bingxue, L. I., Peiyu, C., Mingwei, Y. U., & Xiaomin, W. (2023). Acupuncture and moxibustion for malignant tumor patients with psychological symptoms of insomnia, anxiety and depression: a systematic review and meta-analysis. *Journal of Traditional Chinese Medicine, 43*(3), 441–456. https://doi.org/10.19852/j.cnki. jtcm.20230313.001

Faulkner, W. (1951). *Requiem for a Nun.* Random House.

Federal Aviation Administration (2018). *U.S. Civil Airman Statistics.* Retrieved September 2, 2019, from https://www.faa.gov/data_research/aviation_data_statistics/civil_airmen _statistics/

Federal Aviation Administration (2023). Decision considerations—aerospace medical dispositions item 47. Psychiatric conditions—Use of antidepressant medications. *Guide for Aviation Medical Examiners.* https://www.faa.gov/ame_guide/app_process/exam_tech/item47/amd/antidepressants

Federal Motor Carrier Safety Administration (FCMSA) (2019). *Large Truck and Bus Crash Facts 2017.* Retrieved July 11, 2019, from www.fmcsa.dot.gov/safety/data-and-statistics/large-truck-and-bus-crash-facts-2017

Federal Motor Carrier Safety Administration (FCMSA) (2021). 2020 *Pocket Guide to Large Truck and Bus Statistics.* https://www.fmcsa.dot.gov/safety/data-and-statistics/commercial-motor-vehicle-facts

Feeney, A., & Papakostas, G. I. (2023). Pharmacotherapy: Ketamine and esketamine. *The Psychiatric Clinics of North America, 46*(2), 277–290. https://doi.org/10.1016/j.psc.2023.02.003

Feng, Y., Huang, W., Tian, T. F., Wang, G., Hu, C., Chiu, H. F., Ungvari, G. S., Kilbourne, A. M., & Xiàng, Y. T. (2016). The psychometric properties of the Quick Inventory of Depressive Symptomatology-Self-Report (QIDS-SR) and the Patient Health Questionnaire-9 (PHQ-9) in depressed inpatients in China. *Psychiatry Research, 243,* 92–96. https://doi.org/10.1016/j.psychres.2016.06.021

Ferris, W. (Ed.). (2004). *The Greenwood Encyclopedia of American Regional Cultures.* ABC-CLIO Greenwood.

Field, G. (2015). Sarah Silverman opens up about her battle with depression and her gutsiest career move yet. *Glamour.* https://www.glamour.com/story/sarah-silverman-on-i-smile-back-and-battle-with-depression

Figueroa, C. M., Medvin, A., Phrathep, B. D., Thomas, C. W., Ortiz, J., & Bushy, A. (2021). Healthcare needs of U.S. rural Latinos: A growing, multicultural population. Online Journal of Rural Nursing and Health Care, 21(1), 24–48. https://doi.org/10.14574/ojrnhc.v21i1.658

Fiorillo, J. (1999). What was the "floating world?" *Viewing Japanese Prints.* Retrieved April 26, 2019, from https://www.viewingjapaneseprints.net/texts/topics_faq/faq_floatingworld.html

Fiorillo, J. (n.d.). *Ukiyo-e "Pictures of the Floating World."* Viewing Japanese prints. Retrieved October 9, 2019, from https://www.viewingjapaneseprints.net/texts/ukiyoe/intro_ukiyoe.html

First, M. B., Williams, J. B. W., Karg, R. S., & Spitzer, R. L. (2015). *Structured Clinical Interview for DSM-5—Research Version (SCID-5 for DSM-5, Research Version; SCID-5-RV).* American Psychiatric Association.

Fischer, D. H. (1989). *Albion's Seed: Four British Folkways in America.* Oxford University Press.

Flaherty, C. (2018, December 6). A very mixed record on mental health. *Inside Higher Ed.* Retrieved September 29, 2019, from https://www.insidehighered.com/news/2018/12/06/new-research-graduate-student-mental-well-being-says-departments-have-important

Flanagan, D. (2014). *Yukio Mishima.* Reaktion Books.

Fleming, S. (2021, June 10). Can a TikTok star or autonomous trucks reverse the global shortage of commercial drivers? *World Economic Forum.* https://www.weforum.org/agenda/2021/06/global-shortage-commercial-truck-drivers/

Fnais, N., Soobiah, C., Chen, M. H., Lillie, E., Perrier, L., Tashkhandi, M., Straus, S. E., Mamdani, M., Al-Omran, M., & Tricco, A. C. (2014). Harassment and discrimination in medical training: A systematic review and meta-analysis. *Academic Medicine, 89*, 817–827. https://doi.org/10.1097/ACM.0000000000000200

Fontanella, C. A., Saman, D. M., Campo, J. V., Hiance-Steelesmith, D. L., Bridge, J. A., Sweeney, H. A., & Root, E. D. (2018). Mapping suicide mortality in Ohio: A spatial epidemiological analysis of suicide clusters and area level correlates. *Preventive Medicine, 106*, 177–184. https://doi.org/10.1016/j.ypmed.2017.10.033

Food and Agriculture Organization of the United Nations (2019). *FAOStat:* Selected indicators. http://www.fao.org/faostat/en/#country

Ford, E. W. (2019). Stress, burnout, and moral injury: The state of the healthcare workforce. *Journal of Healthcare Management, 64*, 125–127.

Fornaro, M., Clementi, N., & Fornaro, P. (2009). Medicine and psychiatry in Western culture: Ancient Greek myths and modern prejudices. *Annals of General Psychiatry, 8*, 21. https://doi.org/10.1186/1744-859X-8-21

Fortney, J. C., Harman, J. S., Xu, S., & Dong, F. (2009). *Rural-Urban Differences in Depression Care* [Working paper]. Wiche Center for Rural Mental Health Research. Retrieved September 29, 2019, from https://www.ruralhealthresearch.org/publications/770

Frances, A. (2013). *Saving Normal: An Insider's Revolt Against Out-of-Control Psychiatric Diagnosis, DSM-5, Big Pharma, and the Medicalization of Ordinary Life.* William Morrow.

Francesca, M. M., Efisia, L. M., Alessandra, G. M., Marianna, A., & Giovanni, C. M. (2014). Misdiagnosed hypomanic symptoms in patients with treatment-resistant major depressive disorder in Italy: Results from the IMPROVE study. *Clinical Practice and Epidemiology in Mental Health, 10*, 42–47. https://doi.org/10.2174/1745017901410010042

Francis, H. M., Stevenson, R. J., Chambers, J. R., Gupta, D., Newey, B., & Lim, C. K. (2019). A brief diet intervention can reduce symptoms of depression in young adults—A randomised controlled trial. *PLOS ONE, 14*(10), Article e0222768. https://doi.org/10.1371/journal.pone.0222768

Frank, E., Zhao, Z., Fang, Y., Rotenstein, L. S., Sen, S., & Guille, C. (2021). Experiences of work–family conflict and mental symptoms by gender among physician parents during the COVID-19 pandemic. *JAMA Network Open, 4*(11), Article e2134315. https://doi.org/10.1001/jamanetworkopen.2021.34315

Fregna, L., Attanasio, F., & Colombo, C. (2023). The effect of bright light therapy on irritability in bipolar depression: A single-blind randomised control trial. *International Journal of Psychiatry in Clinical Practice, 27*(4), 416–418. https://doi.org/10.1080/13651501.2023.2221286

Frésan, U., Bes-Rastrollo, M., Segovia-Siapco, G., Sanchez-Villegas, A., Lahortica, F., de la Rosa, P. A., & Martinez-Gonzalez, M. A. (2019). Does the MIND diet decrease depression risk? A comparison with Mediterranean diet in the SUN cohort. *European Journal of Nutrition, 58*(3), 1271–1282. https://doi.org/10.1007/s00394-018-1653-x

Freudenberger, H. J. (1974). Staff burnout. *Journal of Social Issues, 30*, 159–165. https://doi.org/10.1111/j.1540-4560.1974.tb00706.x

Friedman, E., Hazlehurst, M. F., Loftus, C., Karr, C., McDonald, K. N., & Suarez-Lopez, J. R. (2020). Residential proximity to greenhouse agriculture and neurobehavioral performance in Ecuadorian children. International Journal of Hygiene and Environmental Health, 223(1), 220–227. https://doi.org/10.1016/j.ijheh.2019.08.009

Fujimaki, T., Shibui, S., Kato, Y., Matsumura, A., Yamasaki, M., Date, I., Hongo, K., Kuroda, S., Matsumae, M., Nakao, N., Sakurada, K., Shimokowa, S., & Kayama, T.; on behalf of the Gender Equality Committee of the Japan Neurosurgical Society. (2016). Working conditions and lifestyle of female surgeons affiliated to the Japan Neurosurgical Society: Findings of individual and institutional surveys. Neurologia Medico-Chirurgica, 56(11), 704–708. https://doi.org/10.2176/nmc.oa.2016-0119

Fujimoto, K. A., & Hwang, W. C. (2014). Acculturative family distancing: Psychometric analysis with the extended two-tier item response theory. Psychological Assessment, 26(2), 493–512. https://doi.org/10.1037/a0035757

Fukazawa, S. (1956). 楢山節考 Narayama Bushikō [The ballad of Narayama]. Chūō Kōron.

Fukuyama, F. (1995). Trust: The Social Virtues and the Creation of Prosperity. Free Press.

Funk, C., Hefferon, M., Kennedy, B., & Johnson, C. (2019). Trust and mistrust in Americans' views of scientific experts. Pew Research Center, August 2019. https://www.pewresearch.org/science/wp-content/uploads/sites/16/2019/08/PS_08.02.19_trust.in_.scientists_FULLREPORT-1.pdf. Accessed August 1, 2024

Furihata, R., Uchiyama, M., Takahashi, S., Suzuki, M., Konno, C., Osaki, K., Konno, M., Kaneita, Y., Ohida, T., Akahoshi, T., Hashimoto, S., & Akashiba, T. (2012). The association between sleep problems and perceived health status: A Japanese nationwide general population survey. Sleep Medicine, 13(7), 831–837. https://doi.org/10.1016/j.sleep.2012.03.011

Gabbe, S. G., Morgan, M. A., Power, M. L., Schulkin, J., & Williams, S. B. (2003). Duty hours and pregnancy outcome among residents in obstetrics and gynecology. Obstetrics and Gynecology, 102(5, Pt. 1), 948–951.

Gadad, B. S., Jha, M. K., Czysz, A., Furman, J. L., Mayes, T. L., Emslie, M. P., & Trivedi, M. H. (2018). Peripheral biomarkers of major depression and antidepressant treatment response: Current knowledge and future outlooks. Journal of Affective Disorders, 233, 3–14. https://doi.org/10.1016/j.jad.2017.07.001

Gaffley, M., Rauh, J. L., Gardner, A., Palmer, R., Haberman, C., Petty, J. K., & Neff, L. P. (2023). Storage practices, devices, and presence of children among owners of firearms: Informing pediatric firearm safety. The American Surgeon, 89(12), 5891–5896. https://doi.org/10.1177/00031348231180932

Gallagher, H. C., Block, K., Gibbs, L., Forbes, D., Lusher, D., Molyneaux, R., Richardson, J., Pattison, P., MacDougall, C., & Bryant, R. A. (2019). The effect of group involvement on post-disaster mental health: A longitudinal multilevel analysis. Social Science & Medicine, 220, 167–175. https://doi.org/10.1016/j.socscimed.2018.11.006

Galli, F., & Gambini, O. (2019). Psychopharmacology of headache and its psychiatric comorbidities. In V. I. Reus & D. Lindqvist (Eds.), Handbook of Clinical Neurology (Vol. 165, pp. 339–344). Elsevier. https://doi.org/10.1016/B978-0-444-64012-3.00020-4

Gambetta, D. (1999, June 1). Primo Levi's last moments. Boston Review. https://bostonreview.net/diego-gambetta-primo-levi-last-moments

Gamma, A., Angst, J., Azorin, J. M., Bowden, C. L., Perugi, G., Vieta, E., & Young, A. H (2013). Transcultural validity of the Hypomania Checklist-32 (HCL-32) in patients with major depressive episodes. *Bipolar Disorders, 15*(6), 701–712. https://doi.org/10.1111/bdi.12101

Gao, Y. (2005). 人生设计在童年-哈佛爸爸有话说 [*Life Design in Childhood: A Harvard Dad Has Something to Say*]. Guangxi University Press.

Gao, Y. (2015). 人生设计线路图—美国升学与前途 [*Life Design Roadmap—Higher Education and Future in the United States*] (6th ed.). Guangxi University Press.

Garbarino, S., Guglielmi, O., Sannita, W. G., Magnavita, N., & Lanteri, P. (2018). Sleep and mental health in truck drivers: Descriptive review of the current evidence and proposal of strategies for primary prevention. *International Journal of Environmental Research and Public Health, 15*(9), Article 1852. https://doi.org/10.3390/ijerph15091852

García-Cortés, M., Robles-Díaz, M., Ortega-Alonso, A., Medina-Caliz, I., & Andrade, R. J. (2016). Hepatotoxicity by dietary supplements: A tabular listing and clinical characteristics. *International Journal of Molecular Sciences, 17*(4), Article 537. https://doi.org/10.3390/ijms17040537

Garcia-Retamero, R., Andrade, A., Sharit, J., & Ruiz, J. G. (2015). Is patients' numeracy related to physical and mental health? *Medical Decision Making, 35*(4), 501–511. https://doi.org/10.1177/0272989X15578126

Gaydosh, L., Schorpp, K. M., Chen, E., Miller, G. E., & Harris, K. M. (2018). College completion predicts lower depression but higher metabolic syndrome among disadvantaged minorities in young adulthood. *Proceedings of the National Academy of Sciences of the United States of America, 115*(1), 109–114. https://doi.org/10.1073/pnas.1714616114

Ge, L., Yap, C. W., Ong, R., & Heng, B. H. (2017). Social isolation, loneliness and their relationships with depressive symptoms: A population-based study. *PLOS ONE, 12*(8), Article e0182145. https://doi.org/10.1371/journal.pone.0182145

Gecewicz, C., & Rainie, L. (2019, September 19). *Why Americans Don't Fully Trust Many Who Hold Positions of Power and Responsibility*. Pew Research Center. Retrieved October 2, 2019, from https://www.people-press.org/2019/09/19/why-americans-dont-fully-trust-many-who-hold-positions-of-power-and-responsibility/

Gelles, D. (2019, August 7). Boeing 737 Max needs full F.A.A. review, crash families say. *New York Times*. Retrieved September 2, 2019, from https://www.nytimes.com/2019/08/07/business/boeing-737-max-faa-recertification-stumo.html

Gelfand, M. (2018). *Rule makers, rule breakers: How tight and loose cultures wire our world*. New York: Scribner.

Generaal, E., Hoogendijk, E. O., Stam, M., Henke, C. E., Rutters, F., Oosterman, M., Huisman, M., Kramer, S. E., Elders, P. J. M., Timmermans, E. J., Lakerveld, J., Koomen, E., ten Have, M., de Graaf, R., Snijder, M. B., Stronks, K., Willemsen, G., Boomsma, D. I., Smit, J. H., & Penninx, B. W. J. H. (2019). Neighbourhood characteristics and prevalence and severity of depression: Pooled analysis of eight Dutch cohort studies. *British Journal of Psychiatry, 215*(2), 468–475. https://doi.org/10.1192/bjp.2019.100

Geoffroy, P. A., & Palagini, L. (2021). Biological rhythms and chronotherapeutics in depression. *Progress in Neuro-psychopharmacology and Biological Psychiatry, 106*, Article 110158. https://doi.org/10.1016/j.pnpbp.2020.110158

Gerbarg, P. L., Muskin, P. R., & Brown, R. P. (Eds.) (2017). *Complementary and Integrative Treatments in Psychiatric Practice*. American Psychiatric Association.

Gesundheit, B., Or, R., Gamliel, C., Rosner, F., & Steinberg, A. (2008). Treatment of depression by Maimonides (1138–1204): Rabbi, physician, and philosopher. *American Journal of Psychiatry, 165*, 425–442.

Getting It Right Collaborative Group (2019). Getting it right: Validating a culturally specific screening tool for depression (aPHQ-9) in Aboriginal and Torres Strait Islander Australians. *The Medical Journal of Australia, 211*(1), 24–30. https://doi.org/10.5694/mja2.50212

Ghaffari, F., Naseri, M., Jafari Hajati, R., & Zargaran, A. (2017). Rhazes, a pioneer in contribution to trials in medical practice. *Acta Medico-historica Adriatica, 15*(2), 261–270. https://doi.org/10.31952/amha.15.2.4

Ghosh, K. (2018). Violence against doctors: A wake-up call. *The Indian Journal of Medical Research, 148*(2), 130–133. https://doi.org/10.4103/ijmr.IJMR_1299_17

Giacco, D., Laxhman, N., & Priebe, S. (2018). Prevalence of and risk factors for mental disorders in refugees. *Seminars in Cell & Developmental Biology, 77*, 144–152. https://doi.org/10.1016/j.semcdb.2017.11.030

Gibson-Smith, D., Bot, M., Brouwer, I. A., Visser, M., Giltay, E. J., & Penninx, B. W. J. H. (2020). Association of food groups with depression and anxiety disorders. *European Journal of Nutrition, 59*(2), 767–778. https://doi.org/10.1007/s00394-019-01943-4

Gilliam, F. G., Barry, J. J., Hermann, B. P., Meador, K. J., Vahle, V., & Kanner, A. M. (2006). Rapid detection of major depression in epilepsy: A multicentre study. *Lancet Neurology, 5*(5), 399–405. https://doi.org/10.1016/S1474-4422(06)70415-X

Girotto, E., Mesas, A. E., de Andrade, S. M., & Birolim, M. M. (2014). Psychoactive substance abuse by truck drivers: A systematic review. *Occupational and Environmental Medicine, 71*, 71–76. https://doi.org/10.1136/oemed-2013-101791

Gładka, A., Rymaszewska, J., & Zatoński, T. (2018). Impact of air pollution on depression and suicide. *International Journal of Occupational Medicine and Environmental Health, 31*(6), 711–721. https://doi.org/10.13075/ijomeh.1896.01277

Gładka, A., Zatoński, T., & Rymaszewska, J. (2022). Association between the long-term exposure to air pollution and depression. *Advances in Clinical and Experimental Medicine 31*(10), 1139–1152. https://doi.org/10.17219/acem/149988

Glasheen, C., Pemberton, M. R., Lipari, R., Copello, E. A., & Mattson, M. E. (2015). Binge drinking and the risk of suicidal thoughts, plans, and attempts. *Addictive Behavior, 43*, 42–49. https://doi.org/10.1016/j.addbeh.2014.12.005

Glass, J., & Levchak, P. (2014). Red states, blue states, and divorce: Understanding the impact of conservative Protestantism on regional variation in divorce. *American Journal of Sociology, 119*(4), 1002–1046. https://doi.org/10.1086/674703

Glaus, J., Van Meter, A., Cui, L., Marangoni, C., & Merikangas, K. R. (2018). Factorial structure and familial aggregation of the Hypomania Checklist-32 (HCL-32): Results of the NIMH Family Study of Affective Spectrum Disorders. *Comprehensive Psychiatry, 84*, 7–14. https://doi.org/10.1016/j.comppsych.2018.03.010

Gloger, S., Martínez, P., Behn, A., Chacón, M. V., Cottin, M., Diez de Medina, D., & Vöhringer, P. A. (2021). Population-attributable risk of adverse childhood experiences for high suicide risk, psychiatric admissions, and recurrent depression, in depressed outpatients. *European Journal of Psychotraumatology, 12*(1), Article 874600. https://doi.org/10.1080/20008198.2021.1874600

Gold, K. J., Andrew, L. B., Goldman, E. B., & Schwenk, T. L. (2016). "I would never want to have a mental health diagnosis on my record": A survey of female physicians on diagnosis, treatment and reporting. *General Hospital Psychiatry, 43*, 51–57. https://doi.org/10.1016/j.genhosppsych.2016.09.004

Gold, K. J., Shih, E. R., Goldman, E. B., & Schwenk, T. L. (2017). Do US medical licensing applications treat mental and physical illness equivalently? *Family Medicine, 49*(6), 464–467.

Goldsmith, R. (2013, October 14). Iceland: Where one in 10 people will publish a book. *BBC News*. https://www.bbc.com/news/magazine-24399599

González-Acosta, C. A., Rojas-Cerón, C. A., & Buriticá, E. (2021). Functional alterations and cerebral variations in humans exposed to early life stress. *Frontiers in Public Health, 8*, Article 536188. https://doi.org/10.3389/fpubh.2020.536188

Goodreads.com (2021). https://www.goodreads.com/quotes/9440678-hygge-is-a-state-of-being-you-experience-if-you#

Goodwin, G. M., Price, J., De Bodinat, C., & Laredo, J. (2017). Emotional blunting with antidepressant treatment: A survey among depressed patients. *Journal of Affective Disorders, 221*, 31–35. https://doi.org/10.1016/j.jad.2017.05.048

Gottlieb, J. F., Benedetti, F., Geoffroy, P. A., Henriksen, T., Lam, R. W., Murray, G., Phelps, J., Sit, D., Swartz, H. A., Crowe, M., Etain, B., Frank, E., Goel, N., Haarman, B. C. M., Inder, M., Kallestad, H., Kim, S. J., Martiny, K., Meesters, Y., ... Chen, S. (2019). The chronotherapeutic treatment of bipolar disorders: A systematic review and practice recommendations from the ISBD task force on chronotherapy and chronobiology. *Bipolar Disorders, 21*(8), 741–773. https://doi.org/10.1111/bdi.12847

Gottlieb, J. F., Goel, N., Chen, S., & Young, M. A. (2021). Meta-analysis of sleep deprivation in the acute treatment of bipolar depression. *Acta Psychiatrica Scandinavica, 143*(4), 319–327. https://doi.org/10.1111/acps.13255

Gover, A. R., Jennings, W. G., Tomsich, E. A., Park, M., & Rennison, C. M. (2011). The influence of childhood maltreatment and self-control on dating violence: A comparison of college students in the United States and Korea. *Violence and Victims, 26*(3), 296–318. https://doi.org/10.1891/0886-6708.26.3.296

Grande, I., Berk, M., Birmaher, B., & Vieta, E. (2016). Bipolar disorder. *Lancet, 387*(10027), 1561–1572. https://doi.org/10.1016/S0140-6736(15)00241-X

Grandner, M. A. (2017). Sleep and obesity risk in adults: Possible mechanisms; contextual factors; and implications for research, intervention, and policy. *Sleep Health, 3*(5), 393–400. https://doi.org/10.1016/j.sleh.2017.07.014

Grases, G., Colom, M. A., Sanchis, P., & Grases, F. (2019). Possible relation between consumption of different food groups and depression. *BMC Psychology, 7*(1), Article 14. https://doi.org/10.1186/s40359-019-0292-1

Gresenz, C. R., Sturm, R., & Tang L. (2001). Income and mental health: Unraveling community and individual level relationships. *Journal of Mental Health Policy and Economics, 4*(4), 197–203.

Grossman, D. C., Mueller, B. A., Riedy, C., Dowd, M. D., Villaveces, A., Prodzinski, J., Nakagawara, J., Howard, J., Thiersch, N., & Harruff, R. (2005). Gun storage practices and risk of youth suicide and unintentional firearm injuries. *JAMA, 293*(6), 707–714. https://doi.org/10.1001/jama.293.6.707

Gross, C. G. (1999). "Psychosurgery" in Renaissance art. *Trends in Neurosciences, 10*, 429–431. https://doi.org/10.1016/S0166-2236(99)01488-5

Gross, M. (2018). Between party, people, and profession: The many faces of the "doctor" during the Cultural Revolution. *Medical History, 62*(3), 333–359. https://doi.org/10.1017/mdh.2018.23

Gu, M., & Magaziner, J. (2016, May 2). The *Gaokao*: History, reform, and rising international significance of China's National College Entrance Examination. *World Education News & Reviews.* Retrieved May 24, 2019, from https://wenr.wes.org/2016/05/the-gaokao-history-reform-and-international-significance-of-chinas-national-college-entrance-examination

Guglielmi, O., Magnavita, N., & Garbarino, S. (2018). Sleep quality, obstructive sleep apnea and psychological distress in truck drivers: A cross-sectional study. *Social Psychiatry and Psychiatric Epidemiology, 53*(5), 531–536. https://doi.org/10.1007/s00127-017-1474-x

Gundersen, C., & Ziliak, J. P. (2015). Food insecurity and health outcomes. *Health Affairs, 34*(11), 1830–1839. https://doi.org/10.1377/hlthaff.2015.0645

Gunier, R. B., Bradman, A., Harley, K. G., Kogut, K., & Eskenazi, B. (2017). Prenatal residential prroximity to agricultural pesticide use and IQ in 7-year-old children. Environmental Health Perspectives 125(5): 057002. https://doi.org/10.1289/EHP504

Guo, X., & Jiang, K. (2017). Is depression the result of immune system abnormalities? *Shanghai Archives of Psychiatry, 29*(3), 171–173. https://doi.org/10.11919/j.issn.1002-0829.217015

Ha, J., & Yang, H. S. (2021). The Werther effect of celebrity suicides: Evidence from South Korea. *PloS One, 16*(4), e0249896. https://doi.org/10.1371/journal.pone.0249896

Hacimusalar, Y., & Eşel, E. (2018). Suggested biomarkers for major depressive disorder. *Nöropsikiyatri Arşivi, 55*(3), 280–290. https://doi.org/10.5152/npa.2017.19482

Haghighi, M., Bajoghli, H., Angst, J., Holsboer-Trachsler, E., & Brand, S. (2011). The Farsi version of the Hypomania Check-List 32 (HCL-32): Applicability and indication of a four-factorial solution. *BMC Psychiatry, 11*, Article 14. https://doi.org/10.1186/1471-244X-11-14

Hagquist, C., & Andrich, D. (2017). Recent advances in analysis of differential item functioning in health research using the Rasch model. *Health and Quality of Life Outcomes, 15*(1), Article 181. https://doi.org/10.1186/s12955-017-0755-0

Halevi-Katz, D. N., Yaakobi, E., & Putter-Katz, H. (2015). Exposure to music and noise-induced hearing loss (NIHL) among professional pop/rock/jazz musicians. *Noise & Health, 17*(76), 158–164. https://doi.org/10.4103/1463-1741.155848

Hall, B. J., Pangan, C. A. C., Chan, E. W. W., & Huang, R. L. (2019). The effect of discrimination on depression and anxiety symptoms and the buffering role of social capital among female domestic workers in Macao, China. *Psychiatry Research, 271*, 200–207. https://doi.org/10.1016/j.psychres.2018.11.050

Hall, E. T. (1976). *Beyond Culture.* Random House.

Haller, H., Anheyer, D., Cramer, H., & Dobos, G. (2019). Complementary therapies for clinical depression: an overview of systematic reviews. BMJ Open,9(8): e028527. https://doi.org/10.1136/bmjopen-2018-028527

Hamilton, D., Lemeshow, S., Saleska, J. L., Brewer, B., & Strobino, K. (2018). Who owns guns and how do they keep them? The influence of household characteristics on firearms ownership and storage practices in the United States. *Preventive Medicine, 116*, 134–112. https://doi.org/10.1016/j.ypmed.2018.07.013

Han, S. H., Lee, G. Y., Hyun, W., Kim, Y., & Jang, J. S. (2021). Obstructive sleep apnea in airline pilots during daytime sleep following overnight flights. *Journal of Sleep Research, 30*(6), e13375. https://doi.org/10.1111/jsr.13375

Han, X., Han, X., Luo, Q., Jacobs, S., & Jean-Baptiste, M. (2013). Report of a mental health survey among Chinese international students at Yale University. *Journal of American College Health: J of ACH, 61*(1), 1–8. Https://doi.org/10.1080/07448481.2012.738267

Han, Y. R., Jeong, G. H., & Kim, S. J. (2017). Factors influencing beliefs about intimate partner violence among adults in Korea. *Public Health Nursing, 34*(5), 412–421. https://doi.org/10.1111/phn.12326

Hanely, J., & Brown, A. (2014). Cultural variations in interpretation of postnatal illness: Jinn possession amongst Muslim communities. *Community Mental Health Journal, 50*, 348–353. https://doi.org/10.1007/s10597-013-9640-4

Hanson, M. (2021). *U.S. public education statistics*. Retrieved July 4, 2021, from https://educationdata.org/public-education-spending-statistics

Hanson, M. (2021a). Average medical school debt. *Education Data Initiative*. Retrieved August 23, 2021, from https://educationdata.org/average-medical-school-debt

Hanson, M. (2021b). Average time to repay student loans. *Education Data Initiative*. Retrieved August 23, 2021, from https://educationdata.org/average-time-to-repay-student-loans

Hardy, B. L., Logan, T. D., & Parman, J. (2018). The historical role of race and policy for regional inequality. *The Hamilton Project*. https://www.hamiltonproject.org/papers/the_historical_role_of_race_and_policy_for_regional_inequality?_ga=2.1149041.1761033316.1569703717-1619433303.1569703717

Harrington, J. R., & Gelfand, M. J. (2014). Tightness–looseness across the 50 United States. *Proceedings of the National Academy of Sciences of the United States of America, 111*(22), 7990–7995. https://doi.org/10.1073/pnas.1317937111

Harrington, J. R., Boski, P., & Gelfand, M. J. (2015). Culture and national well-being: Should societies emphasize freedom or constraint?. *PloS One, 10*(6), e0127173. https://doi.org/10.1371/journal.pone.0127173

Harrison, S., Sakudo, M., Eom, T. Y., & Jeong, S. (2023). 2% of Japanese labour force could be 'modern-day recluses': Government survey. *Insight: Northeast Asia*, April 18. Published online: https://www.asiapacific.ca/sites/default/files/publication-pdf/Insight_NEA_Apr18_V2.pdf.

Harvey, S. B., Modini, M., Joyce, S., Milligan-Saville, J. S., Tan, L., Mykletun, A., Bryant, R. A., Christensen, H., & Mitchell, P. B. (2017). Can work make you mentally ill? A systematic meta-review of work-related risk factors for common mental health problems. *Occupational and Environmental Medicine, 74*(4), 301–310. https://doi.org/10.1136/oemed-2016-104015

Hasada, R. (2002). "Body part" terms and emotion in Japanese. *Pragmatics & Cognition, 10*(1–2), 107–128. https://doi.org/10.1075/pc.10.12.06has

Hashimoto, K. (2018). Metabolomics of major depressive disorder and bipolar disorder: Overview and future perspective. *Advances in Clinical Chemistry, 84*, 81–99. https://doi.org/10.1016/bs.acc.2017.12.005

Haskins, J., Carson, J. G., Chang, C. H., Kirshnit, C., Link, D. P., Navarra, L., Scher, L. M., Sciolla, A. F., Uppington, J., & Yellowlees, P. (2016). The suicide prevention, depression awareness, and clinical engagement program for faculty and residents at the University of California, Davis Health System. *Academic Psychiatry, 40*(1), 23–29. https://doi.org/10.1007/s40596-015-0359-0

Hatzenbuehler, M. L. (2016). Structural stigma: Research evidence and implications for psychological science. *The American Psychologist, 71*(8), 742–751. https://doi.org/10.1037/amp0000068

Hauber, K., Boon, A., & Vermeiren, R. (2019). Non-suicidal self-injury in clinical practice. *Frontiers in Psychology, 10*, Article 502. https://doi.org/10.3389/fpsyg.2019.00502

Hausmann-Stabile, C., & Guarnaccia, P. J. (2015). Clinical encounters with immigrants: What matters for U.S. psychiatrists. *Focus, 13*(4), 409–418. https://doi.org/10.1176/appi.focus.20150020

Have Tang, D., Li, H., & Chen, L. (2019). Advances in understanding, diagnosis, and treatment of tinnitus. *Advances in Experimental Medicine and Biology, 1130*, 109–128. https://doi.org/10.1007/978-981-13-6123-4_7

Hawton, K. (2015). Suicide in doctors while under fitness to practise investigation. *BMJ, 350*, Article h813. https://doi.org/10.1136/bmj.h813

He, G., Xie, J. F., Zhou, J. D., Zhong, Z. Q., Qin, C. X., & Ding, S. Q. (2016). Depression in left-behind elderly in rural China: Prevalence and associated factors. Geriatrics & Gerontology International 16(5): 638–643. https://doi.org/10.1111/ggi.12518

Healy, M. E., Hill, D., Berwick, M., Edgar, H., Gross, J., & Hunley, K. (2017). Social-group identity and population substructure in admixed populations in New Mexico and Latin America. *PLOS ONE, 12*(10), Article e0185503. https://doi.org/10.1371/journal.pone.0185503

Hege, A., Lemke, M. K., Apostolopoulos, Y., Perko, M., Sönmez, S., & Strack, R. (2017). US long-haul truck driver work organization and the association with cardiometabolic disease risk. *Archives of Environmental & Occupational Health, 72*(5), 303–310. https://doi.org/10.1080/19338244.2016.1242468

Heidekrueger, P. I., Juran, S., Ehrl, D., Aung, T., Tanna, N., & Broer, P. N. (2017). Global aesthetic surgery statistics: A closer look. *Journal of Plastic Surgery and Hand Surgery, 51*(4), 270–274. https://doi.org/10.1080/2000656X.2016.1248842

Heleniak, T., & Sigujonsdottir, H. R. (2018, April 18). Once homogeneous, tiny Iceland opens its doors to immigrants. *Migration Information Source.* https://www.migrationpolicy.org/article/once-homogenous-tiny-iceland-opens-its-doors-immigrants

Helliwell, J. F., Layard, R., Sachs, J. D., De Neve, J.-E., Aknin, L. B., & Wan, S. (2023). *World Happiness Report 2023.* Sustainable Development Solutions Network.

Hendin, H., Reynolds, C., Fox, D., Altschuler, S. I., Rodgers, P., Rothstein, L., Rothstein, M., Mansky, P., Schneidman, B., Sanchez, L., & Thompson, J. N. (2007). Licensing and physician mental health: Problems and possibilities. *Journal of Medical Licensure and Discipline, 93*(2), 6–11.

Hendriks, M., Burger, M., Ray, J., & Esipova, N. (2018). Do international migrants increase their happiness and that of their families by migrating? In Helliwell, J., Ledyard, R., & Sachs, J. (Eds.), *World Happiness Report, 2018* (Chapter 3, pp. 44–65). New York: Sustainable Development Solutions Network. Chapter 3, p. 44–65.

Heng, T. T. (2018). Different is not deficient: Contradicting stereotypes of Chinese international students in US higher education. *Studies in Higher Education, 43*, 22–36. https://doi.org/10.1080/03075079.2016.1152466

Henry, S. K., Grant, M. M., & Cropsey, K. L. (2018). Determining the optimal clinical cutoff on the CES-D for depression in a community corrections sample. *Journal of Affective Disorders, 234*, 270–275. https://doi.org/10.1016/j.jad.2018.02.071

Hesdorffer, D. C., Ishihara, L., Mynepalli, L., Webb, D. J., Weil, J., & Hauser, W. A. (2012). Epilepsy, suicidality, and psychiatric disorders: A bidirectional association. *Annals of Neurology, 72*(2), 184–191.

Heyadri, M., Hashempur, M. H., Ayati, M. H., Quintern, D., Nimrouzi, M., & Heyadri, M. (2015). The use of Chinese herbal drugs in Islamic medicine. *Journal of Integrative Medicine, 13*(6), 363–367. https://doi.org/10.1016/S2095-4964(15)60205-9

Heymann, A. (2018). A paradigm shift: From doctor–patient to payer–patient relationship. *The British Journal of General Practice, 68*(674), 438–439. https://www.ncbi.nlm.nih.gov/pmc/articles/PMC6104854/

Hidaka, Y., Operario, D., Takenaka, M., Omori, S., Ichikawa, S., & Shirasaka, T. (2008). Attempted suicide and associated risk factors among youth in urban Japan. *Social Psychiatry and Psychiatric Epidemiology, 43*(9), 752–757. https://doi.org/10.1007/s00127-008-0352-y

Hidese, S., Ota, M., Wakabayashi, C., Noda, T., Ozawa, H., Okubo, T., & Kunugi, H. (2017). Effects of chronic l-theanine administration in patients with major depressive disorder: An open-label study. *Acta Neuropsychiatrica, 29*(2), 72–79. https://doi.org/10.1017/neu.2016.33

Higgins-Biddle, J. C., & Babor, T. F. (2018). A review of the Alcohol Use Disorders Identification Test (AUDIT), AUDIT-C, and USAUDIT for screening in the United States: Past issues and future directions. *The American Journal of Drug and Alcohol Abuse, 44*(6), 578–586. https://doi.org/10.1080/00952990.2018.1456545

Hilton, M. F., Staddon, Z., Sheridan, J., & Whiteford, H. A. (2009). The impact of mental health symptoms on heavy goods vehicle drivers' performance. *Accident Analysis and Prevention, 41*, 453–461. https://doi.org/10.1016/j.aap.2009.01.012

Hinton, D. E., Park, L., Hsia, C., Hofmann, S., & Pollack, M. H. (2009). Anxiety disorder presentations in Asian populations: A review. *CNS Neuroscience & Therapeutics, 15*(3), 295–303. https://doi.org/10.1111/j.1755-5949.2009.00095.x

Hippocrates (2023). The sacred disease. In *Hippocrates, Volume II.* (P. Potter, Trans.) Harvard University Press.

Hirakawa, H., Terao, T., Muronaga, M., & Ishii, N. (2020). Adjunctive bright light therapy for treating bipolar depression: A systematic review and meta-analysis of randomized controlled trials. *Brain and Behavior, 10*(12), Article e01876. https://doi.org/10.1002/brb3.1876

Hirschfeld, R. M., Williams, J. B., Spitzer, R. L., Calabrese, J. R., Flynn, L., Keck, P. E., Lewis, L., McElroy, S. L., Post, R. M., Rapport, D. J., Russell, J. M., Sachs, G. S., & Zajecka, J. (2000). Development and validation of a screening instrument for bipolar spectrum disorder: The Mood Disorder Questionnaire. *American Journal of Psychiatry, 157*(11), 1873–1875. https://doi.org/10.1176/appi.ajp.157.11.1873

Hiyama, T., & Yoshihara, M. (2008). New occupational threats to Japanese physicians: *Karōshi* (death due to overwork) and *karojisatsu* (suicide due to overwork). *Occupational and Environmental Medicine, 65*(6), 428–429. https://doi.org/10.1136/oem.2007.037473

Hoebel, J., Maske, U. E., Zeeb, H., & Lampert, T. (2017). Social inequalities and depressive symptoms in adults: The role of objective and subjective socioeconomic status. *PLOS ONE, 12*(1), e0169764. https://doi.org/10.1371/journal.pone.0169764

Hoffner, C. A., & Cohen, E. L. (2018). Mental health–related outcomes of Robin Williams' death: The role of parasocial relations and media exposure in stigma, help-seeking, and outreach. *Health Communication, 33*(12), 1573–1582. https://doi.org/10.1080/10410 236.2017.1384348

Hofstadter, R. (1970). *America as a gun culture*. American Heritage. October 1970. https://www.americanheritage.com/america-gun-culture

Hofstede, G. (2011). Dimensionalizing cultures: The Hofstede model in context. *Online Readings in Psychology and Culture, 2*(1). https://doi.org/10.9707/2307-0919.1014

Hofstede, G., Hofstede, G., & Minkov M. (2010). *Cultures and Organizations: Software of the Mind*. McGraw-Hill Professional.

Hofstede Insights (2023). *Country Comparison Tool: United States*. Https://www.hofstede-insights.com/country-comparison-tool?countries=united+states. Accessed August 1, 2024.

Hofstede-Insights (n.d.). Comparison of Denmark, Finland, Iceland, Norway, Sweden and Switzerland. https://www.hofstede-insights.com/product/compare-countries

Hollander, A. C., Bruce, D., Ekberg, J., Burström, B., & Ekblad S. (2013). Hospitalisation for depressive disorder following unemployment—Differentials by gender and immigrant status: A population-based cohort study in Sweden. *Journal of Epidemiology and Community Health, 67*(10), 875–881.

Holliday, E., Griffith, K. A., De Castro, R., Stewart, A., Ubel, P., & Jagsi, R. (2015). Gender differences in resources and negotiation among highly motivated physician-scientists. *Journal of General Internal Medicine, 30*(4), 401–407. https://doi.org/10.1007/s11 606-014-2988-5

Hong, S. T. (2019). Increasing violent attacks against physicians and healthcare workers are threats to the Korean society. *Journal of Korean Medical Science, 34*(1), Article e13. https://doi.org/10.3346/jkms.2019.34.e13

Hoogasian, R., & Lijtmaer, R. (2010). Integrating Curanderismo into counselling and psychotherapy. *Counselling Psychology Quarterly, 23*(3), 297–307. https://doi.org/ 10.1080/09515070.2010.505752

Hoppe, C. (2019). Citing Hippocrates on depression in epilepsy. *Epilepsy and Behavior, 90*, 31–36. https://doi.org/10.1016/j.yebeh.2018.10.041

Hopton, A., MacPherson, H., Keding, A., & Morley, S. (2014). Acupuncture, counselling or usual care for depression and comorbid pain: Secondary analysis of a randomised controlled trial. *BMJ Open, 4*, Article e004964. https://doi.org/10.1136/bmjopen-2014-004964

Horne, R., Chapman, S. C., Parham, R., Freemantle, N., Forbes, A., & Cooper, V. (2013). Understanding patients' adherence-related beliefs about medicines prescribed for long-term conditions: a meta-analytic review of the Necessity-Concerns Framework. *PLOS ONE, 8*(12), e80633. https://doi.org/10.1371/journal.pone.0080633

Horne, R., Graupner, L., Frost, S., Weinman, J., Wright, S. M., & Hankins, M. (2004). Medicine in a multi-cultural society: the effect of cultural background on beliefs about medications. *Social Science & Medicine, 59*(6), 1307–1313. https://doi.org/10.1016/j.socscimed.2004.01.009

Horne, R., Weinman, J., & Hankins, M. (1999). The Beliefs about Medicines Questionnaire: The development and evaluation of a new method for assessing the cognitive representation of medication. *Psychology & Health, 14*(1), 1–24. https://doi.org/10.1080/08870449908407311

Horwitz, A., Wakefield, J. C., & Lorenzo-Luaces, L. (2016). History of depression. In R. J. DeRubeis & D. R. Strunk (Eds.), *The Oxford Handbook of Mood Disorders* (p. 7). Oxford University Press.

Hoskins, D., & Padrón, E. (2018). The practice of Curanderismo: A qualitative study from the perspectives of Curandera/os. *Journal of Latina/o Psychology, 6*(2), 79–93. https://doi.org/10.1037/lat0000081

Hrafnkelsdottir, S. M., Brychta, R. J., Rognvaldsdottir, V., Gestsdottir, S., Chen, K. Y., Johannsson, E., Gudmundsdottir, S. L., & Arngrimsson, S. A. (2018). Less screen time and more frequent vigorous physical activity is associated with lower risk of reporting negative mental health symptoms among Icelandic adolescents. *PLOS ONE, 13*(4), Article e0196286. https://doi.org/10.1371/journal.pone.0196286

HRSA (2024). *Area Health Resources Files.* https://data.hrsa.gov/topics/health-workforce/ahrf. Query: Psychiatrists and population by state, 2021-2022. Accessed August 1, 2024.

Hsieh, W.-H., Wang, C. H., & Lu, T. H. (2018a). Bathtub drowning mortality among older adults in Japan. *International Journal of Injury Control and Safety Promotion, 26*(2), 151–155. https://doi.org/10.1080/17457300.2018.1515231

Hsieh, W.-H., Wang, C.-H., & Lu, T.-H. (2018b). Drowning mortality by intent: A population-based cross-sectional study of 32 OECD countries, 2012–2014. *BMJ Open, 8*(7), Article e021501. https://doi.org/10.1136/bmjopen-2018-021501

Hsu, E. (2008). The history of Chinese medicine in the People's Republic of China and its globalization, April 4. *East Asian Science, Technology and Society, 2*(4), 465–484. https://doi.org/10.1215/s12280-009-9072-y

Hsu, F. L. K. (1971). Filial piety in Japan and China: Borrowing, variation and significance. *Journal of Comparative Family Studies, 2*(1), 67–74. https://www.stat.go.jp/english/data/handbook/pdf/2023half_1.pdf

Hu, H., Lu, S., & Huang, C.-C. (2014). The psychological and behavioral outcomes of migrant and left-behind children in China. *Children and Youth Services Review, 46*, 1–10.

Hu, Y. (2017). "Hukou," and what birthplace can still mean for marriage in China. *The Conversation.* http://theconversation.com/hukou-and-what-birthplace-can-still-mean-for-marriage-in-china-75032

Hu, Y., & Scott, J. (2016). Family and gender values in China: Generational, geographic, and gender differences. *Journal of Family Issues, 37*(9), 1267–1293. https://doi.org/10.1177/0192513X14528710

Hu, X., Rohrbaugh, R., Deng, Q., He, Q., Munger, K. F., & Liu, Z. (2017). Expanding the mental health workforce in China: Narrowing the mental health service gap. *Psychiatric Services, 68*(10), 987–989. https://doi.org/10.1176/appi.ps.201700002

Hua, L. W. (2009). 哈佛女孩刘亦婷 *[Harvard Girl Liu Yiting]* (Anniversary Edition). Beijing: Writers Publishing House.

Huang, E. C., Pu, C., Chou, Y. J., & Huang, N. (2018). Public trust in physicians–health care commodification as a possible deteriorating factor: Cross-sectional analysis of 23 countries. *Inquiry, 55.* https://doi.org/10.1177/0046958018759174

Huang, H. C., Liu, S. I., Hwang, L. C., Sun, F. J., Tjung, J. J., Huang, C. R., Li, T. C., Huang, Y. P., & Yeung, A. (2018). The effectiveness of culturally sensitive collaborative treatment of depressed Chinese in family medicine clinics: A randomized controlled trial. *General Hospital Psychiatry, 50,* 96–103. https://doi.org/10.1016/j.genhosppsych.2017.10.002

Huang, J., Yuan, C. M., Xu, X. R., Wang, Y., Hong, W., Wang, Z. W., Su, Y.-s., Hu, Y. Y., Cao, L., Wang, Y., Chen, J., & Fang, Y. R. (2018). The relationship between lifestyle factors and clinical symptoms of bipolar disorder patients in a Chinese population. *Psychiatry Research, 266,* 97–102. https://doi.org/10.1016/j.psychres.2018.04.059

Hughes, K. (2015, August 6). We need to talk about Amy Winehouse's eating disorder and its role in her death. *Pitchfork.* https://pitchfork.com/thepitch/861-we-need-to-talk-about-amy-winehouses-eating-disorder-and-its-role-in-her-death/

Hughes, K., Ford, K., Bellis, M. A., Glendinning, F., Harrison, E., & Passmore, J. (2021). Health and financial costs of adverse childhood experiences in 28 European countries: A systematic review and meta-analysis. *The Lancet Public Health, 6*(11), e848–e857. https://doi.org/10.1016/S2468-2667(21)00232-2

Hutka, P., Krivosova, M., Muchova, Z., Tonhajzerova, I., Hamrakova, A., Mlyncekova, Z., Mokry, J., & Ondrejka, I. (2021). Association of sleep architecture and physiology with depressive disorder and antidepressants treatment. *International Journal of Molecular Sciences, 22*(3), 1333. https://doi.org/10.3390/ijms22031333

Hwang, D. J., Koo, J. H., Kim, T. K., Jang, Y. C., Hyun, A. H., Yook, J. S., Yoon, C. S., & Cho, J. Y. (2023). Exercise as an antidepressant: exploring its therapeutic potential. *Frontiers in Psychiatry, 14,* 1259711. https://doi.org/10.3389/fpsyt.2023.1259711

Hwang W.-C. (2006). Acculturative family distancing: Theory, research, and clinical practice. *Psychotherapy, 43*(4), 397–409. https://doi.org/10.1037/0033-3204.43.4.397

Hwang, W.-C., & Wood, J. J. (2009). Acculturative family distancing: Links with self-reported symptomatology among Asian Americans and Latinos. *Child Psychiatry and Human Development, 40,* 123–138. https://doi.org/10.1007/s10578-008-0115-8

Hwang, W.-C., Wood, J. J., & Fujimoto, K. (2010). Acculturative family distancing (AFD) and depression in Chinese American families. *Journal of Consulting and Clinical Psychology, 78*(5), 655–667. https://doi.org/10.1037/a0020542

Iakimova, G., Dimitrova, S., & Burté, T. (2017). Peut-on faire une TCC sans thérapeute? Composantes actives des TCC informatisées pour la dépression [Can we do therapy without a therapist? Active components of computer-based CBT for depression]. *L'Encephale, 43*(6), 582–593. https://doi.org/10.1016/j.encep.2016.08.006

Iati, M., & Bellware, K. (2020, April 28). NYC emergency doctor dies by suicide, underscoring a secondary danger of the pandemic. *Washington Post.* https://www.washingtonpost.com/nation/2020/04/28/nyc-doctor-lorna-breen-coronavirus/

Ibsen, H. (1961). A Doll's House. In *Hedda Gabler and Other Plays* (U. Ellis-Fermor, Trans.). Penguin. (Original work published 1879.)

Ibsen, H. (1961). Hedda Gabler. In *Hedda Gabler and Other Plays* (U. Ellis-Fermor, Trans.). Penguin. (Original work published 1890)

Ide, N., Kõlves, K., Cassaniti, M., & De Leo, D. (2012). Suicide of first-generation immigrants in Australia, 1974–2006. *Social Psychiatry and Psychiatric Epidemiology* 47(12), 1917–1927. https://doi.org/10.1007/s00127-012-0499-4

IHME (2023). *Global Burden of Disease 2019*. https://ghdx.healthdata.org/gbd-results-tool.

Im, C. S., Baeg, S., Choi, J. H., Lee, M., Kim, H. J., Chee, I. S., Ahn, S.-H., & Kim, J. L. (2017). Comparative analysis of emotional symptoms in elderly Koreans with *hwa-byung* and depression. *Psychiatry Investigations*, 14(6), 864–870. https://doi.org/10.4306/pi.2017.14.6.864

Imamura, S. (Director). (1983). *The Ballad of Narayama* [Film]. Toei Company.

Inagaki, M., Ohtsuki, T., Yonemoto, N., Kawashima, Y., Saitoh, A., Oikawa, Y., Kurosawa, M., Muramatsu, K., Furukawa, T. A., & Yamada, M. (2013). Validity of the Patient Health Questionnaire (PHQ)-9 and PHQ-2 in general internal medicine primary care at a Japanese rural hospital: A cross-sectional study. *General Hospital Psychiatry*, 35(6), 592–597. https://doi.org/10.1016/j.genhosppsych.2013.08.001

Inglehart, R., C. Haerpfer, A. Moreno, C. Welzel, K. Kizilova, J. Diez-Medrano, M. Lagos, P. Norris, E. Ponarin & B. Puranen et al. (eds.). (2018). *World Values Survey: Round Six - Country-Pooled Datafile*. Madrid, Spain & Vienna, Austria: JD Systems Institute & WVSA Secretariat. https://doi.org/10.14281/18241.8

Inoue, T., Tanaka, T., Nakagawa, S., Nakato, Y., Kameyama, R., Boku, S., Toda, H., Kurita, T., & Koyama, T. (2012). Utility and limitations of PHQ-9 in a clinic specializing in psychiatric care. *BMC Psychiatry*, 12, Article 73. https://doi.org/10.1186/1471-244X-12-73

International Labour Organization (2013). *Case Study: Karoshi: Death from Overwork*. https://www.ilo.org/safework/info/publications/WCMS_211571/lang--en/index.htm

International Labour Organization (2023). *Criminal Law of the People's Republic of China*. English translation published online at https://www.ilo.org/dyn/natlex/docs/ELECTRONIC/5375/108071/F-78796243/CHN5375%20Eng3.pdf. Accessed July 24, 2023.

International Society of Aesthetic Plastic Surgery (2020). *International Survey on Aesthetic/Cosmetic Procedures Performed in 2019*. Retrieved January 2, 2024 from https://www.iasps.org/media/pubgf4jc/global-survey-full-report-2019-english.pdf

Islam, F., & Campbell, R. A. (2014). "Satan has afflicted me!" Jinn-possession and mental illness in the Qur'an. *Journal of Religion and Health*, 53, 229–243. https://doi.org/10.1007/s10943-012-9626-5

Ismail, A. A., Rohlman, D. S., Abdel Rasoul, G. M., Abou Salem, M. E., & Hendy, O. M. (2010). Clinical and biochemical parameters of children and adolescents applying pesticides. *The International Journal of Occupational and Environmental Medicine* 1(3): 132–143.

Itani, O., Kaneita, Y., Doi, K., Tokiya, M., Jike, M., Nakagome, S., Otsuka, Y., & Ohida, T. (2018). Longitudinal epidemiologic study of poor mental health status in Japanese adolescents: Incidence of predictive lifestyle factors. *Journal of Clinical Psychiatry*, 79(4), Article 17m11516. https://doi.org/10.4088/JCP.17m11516

Ivey-Stephenson, A. Z., Crosby, A. E., Jack, S. P. D., Haileyesus, T., & Kresnow-Sedacca, M. J. (2017). Suicide trends among and within urbanization levels by sex, race/ethnicity, age group, and mechanism of death - United States, 2001-2015. Morbidity and Mortality Weekly Report. Surveillance Summaries, 66(18), 1–16. https://doi.org/10.15585/mmwr.ss6618a1

Iwasaki, S., Miura, K., Abe, M., Otaka, T., Uehata, S., Shimoyama, D., Takano, M., Tando, Y., Manabu, T., Nakamura, T., Matsunaga, K., Yasuda, M., Yanagi, N., Yamamoto, T., & Wakamatsu, S. (2023). *Japanese Literature Collection for High School*. [Book in Japanese] Sanseido Textbook.

Iwata, N., & Roberts, R. E. (1996). Age differences among Japanese on the Center for Epidemiologic Studies Depression Scale: An ethnocultural perspective on somatization. *Social Science & Medicine, 43*(6), 967–974. https://doi.org/10.1016/0277-9536(96)00005-6

Izumi, M., Nomura, K., Higaki, Y., Akaishi, Y., Seki, M., Kobayashi, S., Komoda, T., & Otaki, J. (2013). Gender role stereotype and poor working condition pose obstacles for female doctors to stay in full-time employment: alumnae survey from two private medical schools in Japan. The Tohoku Journal of Experimental Medicine, 29(3): 233–237. https://doi.org/10.1620/tjem.229.233

Jacka, F. N., O'Neil, A., Opie, R., Itsiopoulos, C., Cotton, S., Mohebbi, M., Castle, D., Dash, S., Mihalopoulos, C., Chatterton, M. L., Brazionis, L., Dean, O. M., Hodge, A. M., & Berk, M. (2017). A randomised controlled trial of dietary improvement for adults with major depression (the "SMILES" trial). *BMC Medicine, 15*(1), Article 23. https://doi.org/10.1186/s12916-017-0791-y

Jacka, F. N., Pasco, J. A., Mykletun, A., Williams, L. J., Hodge, A. M., O'Reilly, S. L., Nicholson, G. C., Kotowicz, M. A., & Berk, M. (2010). Association of Western and traditional diets with depression and anxiety in women. *American Journal of Psychiatry, 167*(3), 305–311. https://doi.org/10.1176/appi.ajp.2009.09060881

Jackson, J. S., Abelson, J. M., Berglund, P. A., Mezuk, B., Torres, M., & Zhang, R. (2011). Ethnicity, immigration, and cultural influences on the nature and distribution of mental disorders: An examination of major depression. In D. Regier, W. Narrow, E. Kuhl, & D. Kupfer (Eds.), *Conceptual Evolution of DSM-5* (pp. 267–285). American Psychiatric Publishing.

Jacobs, A., & Century, A. (2012). As China ages, Beijing turns to morality tales to spur filial devotion. New York Times, September 5. https://www.nytimes.com/2012/09/06/world/asia/beijing-updates-parables-the-24-paragons-of-filial-piety.html.

Jagsi, R. (2018). Sexual harassment in medicine—#MeToo. *New England Journal of Medicine, 378*(3), 209–211. https://doi.org/10.1056/NEJMp1715962

Jagsi, R., Griffith, K. A., Jones, R., Perumalswami, C. R., Ubel, P., & Stewart, A. (2016). Sexual harassment and discrimination experiences of academic medical faculty. *JAMA, 315*, 2120–2121. https://doi.org/10.1001/jama.2016.2188

Jagsi, R., Griffith, K. A., Stewart, A., Sambuco, D., DeCastro, R., & Ubel, P. A. (2012). Gender differences in the salaries of physician researchers. *JAMA, 307*(22), 2410–2417. https://doi.org/10.1001/jama.2012.6183

Jamilian, H., Amirani, E., Milajerdi, A., Kolahdooz, F., Mirzaei, H., Zaroudi, M., Ghaderi, A., & Asemi, Z. (2019). The effects of vitamin D supplementation on mental health, and biomarkers of inflammation and oxidative stress in patients with psychiatric disorders: A systematic review and meta-analysis of randomized controlled trials. *Progress in Neuropsychopharmcology and Biological Psychiatry, 94*, Article 109651. https://doi.org/10.1016/j.pnpbp.2019.109651

Jamison, K. R. (1993). *Touched with Fire: Manic-Depressive Illness and the Artistic Temperament*. Free Press.

Jang, J., Myung, W., Kim, S., Han, M., Yook, V., Kim, E. J., & Jeon, H. J. (2022). Effect of suicide prevention law and media guidelines on copycat suicide of general population following celebrity suicides in South Korea, 2005–2017. *The Australian and New Zealand Journal of Psychiatry*, *56*(5), 542–550. https://doi.org/10.1177/00048674211025701

Jang, S. A., Sung, J. M., Park, J. Y., & Jeon, W. T. (2016). Copycat suicide induced by entertainment celebrity suicides in South Korea. *Psychiatry Investigation*, *13*(1), 74–81. https://doi.org/10.4306/pi.2016.13.1.74

Janiri, D., Kotzalidis, G. D., De Chiara, L., Koukopoulos, A. E., Aas, M., & Sani, G. (2020). The ring of fire: Childhood trauma, emotional reactivity, and mixed states in mood disorders. *The Psychiatric Clinics of North America*, *43*(1), 69–82. https://doi.org/10.1016/j.psc.2019.10.007

Japan Experience (2008, June 3). *so desu ne: How & When To Use It*. https://www.japan-experience.com/plan-your-trip/to-know/japanese-language/so-desu-ne

Japanese Diaspora Portal (2019). http://www.bu.edu/library/japanese-diaspora-portal/

Jaremka, L. M., Andridge, R. R., Fagundes, C. P., Alfano, C. M., Povoski, S. P., Lipari, A. M., Agnese, D. M., Arnold, M. W., Farrar, W. B., Yee, L. D., Carson, W. E., III, Bekaii-Saab, T., Martin, E. W., Jr., Schmidt, C. R., & Kiecolt-Glaser, J. K. (2014). Pain, depression, and fatigue: Loneliness as a longitudinal risk factor. *Health Psychology*, *33*(9), 948–957. https://doi.org/10.1037/a0034012

Jawad, M. Y., Qasim, S., Ni, M., Guo, Z., Di Vincenzo, J. D., d'Andrea, G., Tabassum, A., Mckenzie, A., Badulescu, S., Grande, I., & McIntyre, R. S. (2023). The role of ketamine in the treatment of bipolar depression: A scoping review. *Brain Sciences*, *13*(6), 909. https://doi.org/10.3390/brainsci13060909

Jena, A. B., Khullar, D., Ho, O., Olenski, A. R., & Blumenthal, D. M. (2015). Sex differences in academic rank in US medical schools in 2014. *JAMA*, *314*(11), 1149–1158. https://doi.org/10.1001/jama.2015.10680

Jennings, K. S., Cheung, J. H., Britt, T. W., Goguen, K. N., Jeffirs, S. M., Peasley, A. L., & Lee, A. C. (2015). How are perceived stigma, self-stigma, and self-reliance related to treatment-seeking? A three-path model. *Psychiatric Rehabilitation Journal*, *38*(2), 109–116. https://doi.org/10.1037/prj0000138

Ji, J., Kleinman, A., & Becker, A. E. (2001). Suicide in contemporary China: A review of China's distinctive suicide demographics in their sociocultural context. *Harvard Review of Psychiatry*, *9*(1), 1–12.

Ji, N.-J., Hong, Y.-P., Stack, S. J., & Lee, W.-Y. (2014). Trends and risk factors of the epidemic of charcoal burning suicide in a recent decade among Korean people. *Journal of Korean Medical Science*, *29*, 1174–1177.

Ji, N. J., Lee, W. Y., Noh, M. S., & Yip, P. S. F. (2014). The impact of indiscriminate media coverage of a celebrity suicide on a society with a high suicide rate: Epidemiological findings on copycat suicides from Korea. *Journal of Affective Disorders*, *156*, 56–61. https://doi.org/10.1016/j.jad.2013.11.015

Jia, C. X., & Zhang, J. (2012). Global functioning and suicide among Chinese rural population aged 15–34 years: A psychological autopsy case-control study. *Journal of Forensic Sciences*, *57*(2), 391–397. https://doi.org/10.1111/j.1556-4029.2011.01978.x

Jiang, F., Hu, L., Rakofsky, J., Liu, T., Wu, S., Zhao, P., Hu, G., Wan, X., Liu, H., Liu, Y., & Tang, Y. L. (2018). Sociodemographic characteristics and job satisfaction of psychiatrists in China: Results from the first nationwide survey. *Psychiatric Services* 69(12): 1245–1251. https://doi.org/10.1176/appi.ps.201800197

Jiang, J., & Kang, R. (2019). Temporal heterogeneity of the association between social capital and health: An age-period-cohort analysis in China. *Public Health, 172,* 61–69. https://doi.org/10.1016/j.puhe.2019.04.018

Jiang, L., Sun, F., Zhang, W., Wu, B., & Dong, X. (2019). Health service use among Chinese American older adults: Is there a somatization effect? *Journal of the American Geriatrics Society, 67*(S3), S584–S589. https://doi.org/10.1111/jgs.15734

Jiang, L., Wang, Y., Zhang, Y., Li, R., Wu, H., Li, C., Wu, Y., & Tao, Q. (2019). The reliability and validity of the Center for Epidemiologic Studies Depression Scale (CES-D) for Chinese university students. *Frontiers in Psychiatry, 10,* Article 315. https://doi.org/10.3389/fpsyt.2019.00315

Jiang, W., Jiang, X., Yu, T., Gao, Y., & Sun, Y. (2023). Efficacy and safety of scalp acupuncture for poststroke depression: A meta-analysis and systematic review. *Medicine, 102*(31), e34561. https://doi.org/10.1097/MD.0000000000034561

Jin, H. M., Khazem, L. R., & Anestis, M. D. (2016). Recent advances in means safety as a suicide prevention strategy. *Current Psychiatry Reports, 18,* Article 96. https://doi.org/10.1007/s11920-016-0731-0

Joe, S., Lee, J. S., Kim, S. Y., Won, S.-h., Lim, J. S., & Ha, K. S. (2017). Posttraumatic embitterment disorder and *hwa-byung* in the general Korean population. *Psychiatry Investigation, 14*(4), 392–399. https://doi.org/10.4306/pi.2017.14.4.392

Johansen, I. H., Baste, V., Rosta, J., Aasland, O. G., & Morken, T. (2017). Changes in prevalence of workplace violence against doctors in all medical specialties in Norway between 1993 and 2014: A repeated cross-sectional survey. *BMJ Open, 7*(8), Article e017757. https://doi.org/10.1136/bmjopen-2017-017757

Johns, G., Samuel, V., Freemantle, L., Lewis, J., & Waddington, L. (2022). The global prevalence of depression and anxiety among doctors during the covid-19 pandemic: Systematic review and meta-analysis. *Journal of Affective Disorders, 298*(Pt A), 431–441. https://doi.org/10.1016/j.jad.2021.11.026

Johnson, P. W., Zigman, M., Ibbotson, J., Dennerlein, J. T., & Kim, J. H. (2018). A randomized controlled trial of a truck seat intervention: Part 1—Assessment of whole body vibration exposures. *Annals of Work Exposures and Health, 62*(8), 990–999. https://doi.org/10.1093/annweh/wxy062

Joint Economic Committee (2018). *The Geography of Social Capital in America*. SCP Report No. 1–18. https://www.lee.senate.gov/services/files/DA64FDB7-3B2E-40D4-B9E3-07001B81EC31

Joint Economic Committee (2021). *An Overview of Social Capital in America*. https://www.jec.senate.gov/public/_cache/files/8cb559c4-3764-4706-9009-b4d8565ec820/scp-volume-1-digital-final.pdf

Joint Economic Committee (2018b). *The Geography of Social Capital in America Database*. https://www.lee.senate.gov/public/index.cfm/2018/4/the-geography-of-social-capital-in-america

Jones, B. (2011). Fighting stigma with openness. *Bulletin of the World Health Organization, 89,* 862–863. https://doi.org/10.2471/BLT.11.041211

Jones, J. T. R., North, C. S., Vogel-Scibilia, S., Myers, M. F., & Owen, R. R. (2018). Medical licensure questions about mental illness and compliance with the Americans with

Disabilities Act. *Journal of the American Academy of Psychiatry and the Law Online* 46(4), 458–471. https://doi.org/10.29158/jaapl.003789-18

Jones, P. (2005). *Doctors as Patients*. Radcliffe Publishing.

Jonsdottir, I. H., & Sjörs Dahlman, A. (2019). Mechanisms in endocrinology: Endocrine and immunological aspects of burnout: A narrative review. *European Journal of Endocrinology*, 180(3), R147–R158. https://doi.org/10.1530/EJE-18-0741

Jordan, D. K. (2016). *The 24 Filial Exemplars*. Retrieved August 21, 2018, from http://pages.ucsd.edu/~dkjordan/chin/shiaw/shiawcontents.html

Jouanna, J., & Allies, N. (2012). *Greek Medicine from Hippocrates to Galen: Selected Papers* (P. van der Eijk, Ed.). Brill. http://www.jstor.org/stable/10.1163/j.ctt1w76vxr

Juang, L. P., Syed, M., & Takagi, M. (2007). Intergenerational discrepancies of parental control among Chinese American families: Links to family conflict and adolescent depressive symptoms. *Journal of Adolescence*, 30(6), 965–975. https://doi.org/10.1016/j.adolescence.2007.01.004

Judd, S. R. (2017). Uncovering common sleep disorders and their impacts on occupational performance. *Workplace Health and Safety*, 65(5), 232. https://doi.org/10.1177/2165079917702911

Jun, W. (2020). A study on the cause analysis of cyberbullying in Korean Adolescents. *International Journal of Environmental Research and Public Health*, 17(13), 4648. https://doi.org/10.3390/ijerph17134648

Jung, H., Cho, Y. J., Rhee, M. K., & Jang, Y. (2020). Stigmatizing beliefs about depression in diverse ethnic groups of Asian Americans. *Community Mental Health Journal*, 56(1), 79–87. https://doi.org/10.1007/s10597-019-00481-x

Kadakia, A., Dembek, C., Heller, V., Singh, R., Uyei, J., Hagi, K., Nosaka, T., & Loebel, A. (2021). Efficacy and tolerability of atypical antipsychotics for acute bipolar depression: A network meta-analysis. *BMC Psychiatry*, 21(1), Article 249. https://doi.org/10.1186/s12888-021-03220-3

Kaiser Family Foundation (2021). *State Health Facts*. Retrieved November 1, 2021, from https://www.kff.org/statedata/

Kaiser, N., Sjölander, P., Liljegren, A. E., Jacobsson, L., & Renberg, E. S. (2010). Depression and anxiety in the reindeer-herding Sami population of Sweden. *International Journal of Circumpolar Health*, 69(4), 383–393. https://doi.org/10.3402/ijch.v69i4.17674

Kajta, M., & Wójtowicz, A. K. (2013). Impact of endocrine-disrupting chemicals on neural development and the onset of neurological disorders. *Pharmacological Reports*, 65(6), 1632–1639.

Kalaichandran, A., & Lakoff, D. (2019). We must also think about trainees and the role of culture in physician mental health. *CMAJ*, 191(36), Article E1009. https://doi.org/10.1503/cmaj.72749

Kamali, M., Reilly-Harrington, N. A., Chang, W. C., McInnis, M., McElroy, S. L., Ketter, T. A., Shelton, R. C., Deckersbach, T., Tohen, M., Kocsis, J. H., Calabrese, J. R., Gao, K., Thase, M. E., Bowden, C. L., Kinrys, G., Bobo, W. V., Brody, B. D., Sylvia, L. G., Rabideau, D. J., & Nierenberg, A. A. (2019). Bipolar depression and suicidal ideation: Moderators and mediators of a complex relationship. *Journal of Affective Disorders*, 259, 164–172. https://doi.org/10.1016/j.jad.2019.08.032

Kane, C. K. (2019). *American Medical Association Policy Research Perspectives: Updated Data on Physician Practice Arrangements*. Retrieved July 9, 2023, from https://www.ama-assn.org/system/files/2019-07/prp-fewer-owners-benchmark-survey-2018.pdf.

Kane, J. C., Damian, A. J., Fairman, B., Bass, J. K., Iwamoto, D. K., & Johnson, R. M. (2017). Differences in alcohol use patterns between adolescent Asian American ethnic groups: Representative estimates from the National Survey on Drug Use and Health 2002–2013. *Addictive Behavior, 64*, 154–158. https://doi.org/10.1016/j.addbeh.2016.08.045

Kane, L. (2019a). *Medscape National Physician Burnout, Depression & Suicide Report 2019*. https://www.medscape.com/slideshow/2019-lifestyle-burnout-depression-6011056

Kane, L. (2019b). *Medscape Physician Compensation Report 2019*. https://www.medscape.com/slideshow/2019-compensation-overview-6011286

Kane, L. (2022). *Medscape Physician Compensation Report 2022: Incomes Gain, Pay Gaps Remain*. https://www.medscape.com/slideshow/2022-compensation-overview-6015043.

Kane L. (2023). *'I Cry but No One Cares': Physician Burnout & Depression Report 2023*. https://www.medscape.com/slideshow/2023-lifestyle-burnout-6016058

Kappen, G., Karremans, J. C., Burk, W. J., & Buyukcan-Tetik, A. (2018). On the association between mindfulness and romantic relationship satisfaction: The role of partner acceptance. *Mindfulness, 9*(5), 1543–1556. https://doi.org/10.1007/s12671-018-0902-7

Karasek, R. (1979). Job demands, job decision latitude, and mental strain: Implications for job redesign. *Administrative Science Quarterly, 24*(2), 285–308. https://doi.org/10.2307/2392498

Karasek, R. (1998). Demand/Control Model: A Social, Emotional, and Physiological Approach to Stress Risk and Active Behaviour Development. In: Stellman, J.M., Ed., *Encyclopaedia of Occupational Health and Safety*, International Labour Office, Geneva, 34.6-34.14.

Karchmer, E. I. (2010). Chinese medicine in action: On the postcoloniality of medical practice in China. *Medical Anthropology, 29*(3), 226–252. https://doi.org/10.1080/01459740.2010.488665

Karchmer, E. I. (2013). The excitations and suppressions of the times: Locating the emotions in the liver in modern Chinese medicine. *Culture, Medicine and Psychiatry, 37*(1), 8–29. https://doi.org/10.1007/s11013-012-9289-4

Karimi, A., Nasiri, S., Kazerooni, F. K., & Oliaei, M. (2010). Noise induced hearing loss risk assessment in truck drivers. *Noise & Health, 12*(46), 49–55. https://doi.org/10.4103/1463-1741.59999

Karp, A. (2018). *Estimating Global Civilian-held Firearms Numbers Small*. Graduate Institute of International and Development Studies. http://www.smallarmssurvey.org/fileadmin/docs/T-Briefing-Papers/SAS-BP-Civilian-Firearms-Numbers.pdf

Karyotaki, E., Cuijpers, P., Albor, Y., Alonso, J., Auerbach, R. P., Bantjes, J., Bruffaerts, R., Ebert, D. D., Hasking, P., Kiekens, G., Lee, S., McLafferty, M., Mak, A., Mortier, P., Sampson, N. A., Stein, D. J., Vilagut, G., & Kessler, R. C. (2020). Sources of stress and their associations with mental disorders among college students: Results of the World Health Organization World Mental Health Surveys International College Student Initiative. *Frontiers in Psychology, 11*, Article 1759. https://doi.org/10.3389/fpsyg.2020.01759

Kashino, I., Kochi, T., Imamura, F., Eguchi, M., Kuwahara, K., Nanri, A., Kurotani, K., Akter, S., Hu, H., Miki, T., Kabe, I., & Mizoue, T. (2021). Prospective association of soft drink consumption with depressive symptoms. *Nutrition, 81,* 110860. https://doi.org/10.1016/j.nut.2020.110860

Kasim Mohamad, M. H., & Younis, M. S. (2018). Psychiatry in the Arab Islamic civilization: Historical perspective. *Arab Journal of Psychiatry, 29*(2), 175–181.

Kato, T. (2021). Measurement invariance in the Center for Epidemiologic Studies-Depression (CES-D) scale among English-speaking Whites and Asians. *International Journal of Environmental Research and Public Health, 18*(10), Article 5298. https://doi.org/10.3390/ijerph18105298

Kato, T. A., Hashimoto, R., Hayakawa, K., Kubo, H., Watabe, M., Teo, A. R., & Kanba, S. (2016). Multidimensional anatomy of "modern type depression" in Japan: A proposal for a different diagnostic approach to depression beyond the DSM-5. *Psychiatry and Clinical Neurosciences, 70*(1), 7–23. https://doi.org/10.1111/pcn.12360

Kato, T. A., & Kanba, S. (2017). Modern-type depression as an "adjustment" disorder in Japan: The intersection of collectivistic society encountering an individualistic performance-based system. *American Journal of Psychiatry, 174*(11), 1051–1053. https://doi.org/10.1176/appi.ajp.2017.17010059

Kato, T. A., Kanba, S., & Teo, A. R. (2016). A 39-year old "adultolescent": Understanding social withdrawal in Japan. *American Journal of Psychiatry, 173*(2), 112–114. https://doi.org/10.1176/appi.ajp.2015.15081034

Kato, T. A., Kanba, S., & Teo, A. R. (2019). Hikikomori: Multidimensional understanding, assessment, and future international perspectives. *Psychiatry and Clinical Neurosciences, 73(8),* 427–440. https://doi.org/10.1111/pcn.12895.

Kato, T. A., Kanba, S., & Teo, A. R. (2020). Defining pathological social withdrawal: proposed diagnostic criteria for hikikomori. World Psychiatry: *Official Journal of the World Psychiatric Association (WPA), 19(1),* 116–117. https://doi.org/10.1002/wps.20705.

Kato, T. A., Shinfuku, N., Fujisawa, D., Tateno, M., Ishida, T., Akiyama, T., Sartorius, N., Teo, A. R., Choi, T. Y., Wand, A. P. F., Balhara, Y. P. S., Chang, J. P.-C., Chang, R. Y.-F., Shadloo, B., Ahmed, H. U., Lerthattasilp, T., Umene-Nakano, W., Horikawa, H., Matsumoto, R., ... Kanba, S. (2011). Introducing the concept of modern depression in Japan; an international case vignette survey. *Journal of Affective Disorders, 135*(1–3), 66–76. https://doi.org/10.1016/j.jad.2011.06.030

Kato, T. A., Tateno, M., Shinfuku, N., Fujisawa, D., Teo, A. R., Sartorius, N., Akiyama, T., Ishida, T., Choi, T. Y., Balhara, Y. P., Matsumoto, R., Umene-Nakano, W., Fujimura, Y., Wand, A., Chang, J. P., Chang, R. Y., Shadloo, B., Ahmed, H. U., Lerthattasilp, T., & Kanba, S. (2012). Does the 'hikikomori' syndrome of social withdrawal exist outside Japan? A preliminary international investigation. Social Psychiatry and Psychiatric Epidemiology, 47(7), 1061–1075. https://doi.org/10.1007/s00127-011-0411-7

Kawabata, Y. (1956). *Snow Country* (E. G. Seidensticker, Trans.). Secker and Warburg. (Original work published 1935-37 as a series in a periodical.)

Kawabata, Y. (1958). *Thousand Cranes* (E. G. Seidensticker, Trans.). Alfred A. Knopf. (Original work published 1949-1951 as a series in a periodical.)

Kawabata, Y. (1968, December 12). *Japan, the Beautiful and Myself* [Nobel lecture]. https://www.nobelprize.org/prizes/literature/1968/kawabata/lecture/

Kawabata, Y. (1969). *House of the Sleeping Beauties and Other Stories* (E. G. Seidensticker, Trans.). Quadriga. (Original work published 1961.)

Kawabata, Y. (1987). *The Old Capital* (J. M. Holman, Trans.). North Point. (Original work published 1962.)

Kawabata, Y., & Onishi, A. (2017). Moderating effects of relational interdependence on the association between peer victimization and depressive symptoms. *Child Psychiatry and Human Development, 48*(2), 214–224. https://doi.org/10.1007/s10578-016-0634-7

Kaye, K. (1993, April 18). Women pilots fight sexual harassment. *Sun-Sentinel.* Retrieved September 1, 2019, from https://www.sun-sentinel.com/news/fl-xpm-1993-04-18-9302060762-story.html

Ke, T., Li, W., Sanci, L., Reavley, N., Williams, I., & Russell, M. A. (2023). The mental health of international university students from China during the COVID-19 pandemic and the protective effect of social support: A longitudinal study. *Journal of Affective Disorders, 328,* 13–21. https://doi.org/10.1016/j.jad.2023.02.014

Ke, Y., Jiang, J., & Chen, Y. (2019). Social capital and the health of left-behind older adults in rural China: A cross-sectional study. *BMJ Open, 9*(11), Article e030804. https://doi.org/10.1136/bmjopen-2019-030804

Kenedi, C., Friedman, S. H., Watson, D., & Preitner, C. (2016). Suicide and murder–suicide involving aircraft. *Aerospace Medicine and Human Performance, 87*(4), 388–396. https://doi.org/10.3357/AMHP.4474.2016

Kenny, D. (2014, October 26). Stairway to hell: Life and death in the pop music industry. *The Conversation.* https://theconversation.com/stairway-to-hell-life-and-death-in-the-pop-music-industry-32735

Kenny, D. T., & Asher, A. (2016). Life expectancy and cause of death in popular musicians: Is the popular musician lifestyle the road to ruin? *Medical Problems of Performing Artists, 31*(1), 37–44. https://doi.org/10.21091/mppa.2016.1007

Kenny, D. T., & Asher, A. (2017). Gender differences in mortality and morbidity patterns in popular musicians across the lifespan. *Medical Problems of Performing Artists, 32*(1), 13–19. https://doi.org/10.21091/mppa.2017.1004

Kessler, R. C., & Bromet, E. J. (2013). The epidemiology of depression across cultures. *Annual Review of Public Health, 34,* 119–138. https://doi.org/10.1146/annurev-publhealth-031912-114409

Keyes, K. M., Barnes, D. M., & Bates, L. M. (2015). Depression and mood disorder among African American and White women. *JAMA Psychiatry, 72*(12), 1256–1257. https://doi.org/10.1001/jamapsychiatry.2015.1902

KFF. (2023). Opioid overdose death rates and all drug overdose death rates per 100,000 population. *State Health Facts.* Retrieved October 15, 2023, from https://www.kff.org/other/state-indicator/opioid-overdose-death-rates/?currentTimeframe=0&sortModel=%7B%22colId%22:%22Location%22,%22sort%22:%22asc%22%7D

Khambadkone, S. G., Cordner, Z. A., Dickerson, R., Severance, E. G., Prandovsky, E., Pletnikov, M., Xiao, J., Li, Y., Boersma, G. J., Talbot, C. C., Jr., Campbell, W. W., Wright, C. S., Siple, C. E., Moran, T. H., Tamashiro, K. L., & Yolken, R. H. (2020). Nitrated meat products are associated with mania in humans and altered behavior and brain gene expression in rats. *Molecular Psychiatry, 25,* 560–571. https://doi.org/10.1038/s41380-018-0105-6

Khanna, P., Chattu, V. K., & Aeri, B. T. (2019). Nutritional aspects of depression in adolescents—A systematic review. *International Journal of Preventive Medicine, 10,* Article 42. https://doi.org/10.4103/ijpvm.IJPVM_400_18

Khazan, O. (2018, February 18). The more gender equality, the fewer women in STEM. *The Atlantic*. www.theatlantic.com/science/archive/2018/02/the-more-gender-equality-the-fewer-women-in-stem/553592

Khurshid, K. A. (2018). Comorbid insomnia and psychiatric disorders: An update. *Innovations in Clinical Neuroscience*, *15*(3–4), 28–32.

Kidwell, M., & Ellenbroek, B. A. (2018). Heart and soul: Heart rate variability and major depression. *Behavioral Pharmacology*, *29*(2–3), 152–164. https://doi.org/10.1097/FBP.0000000000000387

Kiely, K. M., & Butterworth, P. (2015). Validation of four measures of mental health against depression and generalized anxiety in a community-based sample. *Psychiatry Research*, *225*(3), 291–298. https://doi.org/10.1016/j.psychres.2014.12.023

Kilponen, K., Huhtala, M., Kinnunen, U., Mauno, S., & Feldt, T. (2021). Illegitimate tasks in health care: Illegitimate task types and associations with occupational well-being. *Journal of Clinical Nursing*, *30*(13–14), 2093–2106. https://doi.org/10.1111/jocn.15767

Kim, A. M. (2017). Why do psychiatric patients in Korea stay longer in hospital? *International Journal of Mental Health Systems 11*(2). https://doi.org/10.1186/s13033-016-0110-6

Kim, A. M. (2021). Alcohol consumption and suicide rate: A cross-sectional analysis in 183 countries. *Psychiatry Research*, *295*, Article 113553. https://doi.org/10.1016/j.psychres.2020.113553

Kim, E., Guo, Y., Koh, C., & Cain, K. C. (2010). Korean immigrant discipline and children's social competence and behavior problems. *Journal of Pediatric Nursing*, *25*(6), 490–499. https://doi.org/10.1016/j.pedn.2009.05.002

Kim, E., & Hong, S. (2007). First-generation Korean American parents' perceptions of discipline. *Journal of Professional Nursing*, *23*(1), 60–68. https://doi.org/10.1016/j.profnurs.2006.12.002

Kim, E., Seo, J., Paik, H., & Sohn, S. (2020). The effectiveness of Adlerian therapy for *hwa-byung* in middle-aged Korean women. *The Counseling Psychologist*, *48*(8), 1082–1108. https://doi.org/10.1177/0011000020946799

Kim, J., & Kim, J. (2018). Green tea, coffee, and caffeine consumption are inversely associated with self-report lifetime depression in the Korean population. *Nutrients*, *10*(9), Article 1201. https://doi.org/10.3390/nu10091201

Kim, J., Lee, D., & Park, E. (2021). Machine learning for mental health in social media: A bibliometric study. *Journal of Medical Internet Research*, *23*(3), Article e24870. https://doi.org/10.2196/24870

Kim, J. E., Saw, A., & Zane, N. (2015). The influence of psychological symptoms on mental health literacy of college students. *The American Journal of Orthopsychiatry*, *85*(6), 620–630. https://doi.org/10.1037/ort0000074

Kim, J. H., Zigman, M., Aulck, L. S., Ibbotson, J. A., Dennerlein, J. T., & Johnson, P. W. (2016). Whole body vibration exposures and health status among professional truck drivers: A cross-sectional analysis. *The Annals of Occupational Hygiene*, *60*(8), 936–948. https://doi.org/10.1093/annhyg/mew040

Kim, J. H., Zigman, M., Dennerlein, J. T., & Johnson, P. W. (2018). A randomized controlled trial of a truck seat intervention: Part 2—Associations between whole-body vibration exposures and health outcomes. *Annals of Work Exposures and Health*, *62*(8), 1000–1011. https://doi.org/10.1093/annweh/wxy063

Kim, J. S., Kim, S., Jung, W., Im, C. H., & Lee, S. H. (2016). Auditory evoked potential could reflect emotional sensitivity and impulsivity. *Scientific Reports, 6,* Article 37683. https://doi.org/10.1038/srep37683

Kim, J. W., Suzuki, K., Kavalali, E. T., & Monteggia, L. M. (2023). Ketamine: Mechanisms and relevance to treatment of depression. *Annual Review of Medicine,* 10.1146/annurev-med-051322-120608. Advance online publication. https://doi.org/10.1146/annurev-med-051322-120608

Kim, J. Y., Oh, S., & Nam, S. I. (2016). Prevalence and trends in domestic violence in Korea: Findings from national surveys. *Journal of Interpersonal Violence, 31*(8), 1554–1576. https://doi.org/10.1177/0886260514567960

Kim, J. Y., Park, J. H., Lee, J. J., Huh, Y., Lee, S. B., Han, S. K., Choi, S. W., Lee, D. Y., Kim, K. W., & Woo, J. I. (2008). Standardization of the Korean version of the Geriatric Depression Scale: Reliability, validity, and factor structure. *Psychiatry Investigation, 5*(4), 232–238. https://doi.org/10.4306/pi.2008.5.4.232

Kim, N., Cho, S. J., Kim, H., Kim, S. H., Lee, H. J., Park, C., Rhee, S. J., Kim, D., Yang, B. R., Choi, S.-H., Choi, G., Koh, M., & Ahn, Y. M. (2019). Epidemiology of pharmaceutically treated depression and treatment resistant depression in South Korea. *PLOS ONE, 14*(8), Article e0221552. https://doi.org/10.1371/journal.pone.0221552

Kim, P. Y. (2020). Teaching Korean cultural constructs to American students: Examples from a Korea study abroad course. *Psychology Teaching Review, 26*(2), 5–11.

Kim, S.-S., Chung, Y., Perry, M. J., Kawachi, I., & Subramanian, S. V. (2012). Association between interpersonal trust, reciprocity and depression in South Korea: A prospective analysis. *PLOS ONE, 7*(1), Article e30602. https://doi.org/10.1371/journal.pone.0030602

Kim, S. Y., Chen, Q., Li, J., Huang, X., & Moon, U. J. (2009). Parent–child acculturation, parenting, and adolescent depressive symptoms in Chinese immigrant families. *Journal of Family Psychology, 23,* 426–437. https://doi.org/10.1037/a0016019

Kim, S. Y., Chen, Q., Wang, Y., Shen, Y., & Orozco-Lapray, D. (2013). Longitudinal linkages among parent–child acculturation discrepancy, parenting, parent–child sense of alienation, and adolescent adjustment in Chinese immigrant families. *Developmental Psychology, 49*(5), 900–912. https://doi.org/10.1037/a0029169

Kim, S. Y., Wang, Y., Deng, S., Alvarez, R., & Li, J. (2011). Accent, perpetual foreigner stereotype, and perceived discrimination as indirect links between English proficiency and depressive symptoms in Chinese American adolescents. *Developmental Psychology, 47*(1), 289–301. https://doi.org/10.1037/a0020712

Kim, K. N., Lim, Y. H., Bae, H. J., Kim, M., Jung, K., & Hong, Y. C. (2016). Long-term fine particulate matter exposure and Major Depressive Disorder in a community-based urban cohort. *Environmental Health Perspectives, 124*(10), 1547–1553. https://doi.org/10.1289/EHP192

Kim, Y. E., & Lee, B. (2019). The psychometric properties of the Patient Health Questionnaire-9 in a sample of Korean university students. *Psychiatry Investigation, 16*(12), 904–910. https://doi.org/10.30773/pi.2019.0226

Kim, Y. S., Koh, Y. J., & Leventhal, B. L. (2004). Prevalence of school bullying in Korean middle school students. *Archives of Pediatrics & Adolescent Medicine, 158*(8), 737–741. https://doi.org/10.1001/archpedi.158.8.737

Kin, C., Yang, R., Desai, P., Mueller, C., & Girod, S. (2018). Female trainees believe that having children will negatively impact their careers: Results of a quantitative survey of trainees at an academic medical center. *BMC Medical Education, 18*(1), 260. https://doi.org/10.1186/s12909-018-1373-1

Kinoshita, K. (Director). (1958). *The Ballad of Narayama* [Film]. Shochiku Company.

Kious, B. M., Kondo, D. G., & Renshaw, P. F. (2018). Living high and feeling low: Altitude, suicide, and depression. *Harvard Review of Psychiatry, 26*(2), 43–56. https://doi.org/10.1097/HRP.0000000000000158

Kishi, T., Yoshimura, R., Sakuma, K., Okuya, M., & Iwata, N. (2020). Lurasidone, olanzapine, and quetiapine extended-release for bipolar depression: A systematic review and network meta-analysis of phase 3 trials in Japan. *Neuropsychopharmacology Reports, 40*(4), 417–422. https://doi.org/10.1002/npr2.12137

Kitanaka, J. (2008). Diagnosing suicides of resolve: Psychiatric practice in contemporary Japan. *Culture, Medicine and Psychiatry, 32*(2), 152–176. https://doi.org/10.1007/s11013-008-9087-1

Kitchen, K. A., McKibbin, C. L., Wykes, T. L., Lee, A. A., Carrico, C. P., & McConnell, K. A. (2013). Depression treatment among rural older adults: Preferences and factors influencing future service use. *Clinical Gerontologist, 36*(3), 241–259. https://doi.org/10.1080/07317115.2013.767872

Kiwano, K. (2021). Bullying in Japanese schools. *Savvy Tokyo*, May 7. https://savvytokyo.com/bullying-japanese-schools/. Accessed Augustr 1, 2024.

Kizilhan, J. I. (2014). Religious and cultural aspects of psychotherapy in Muslim patients from tradition-oriented societies. *International Review of Psychiatry, 26*(3), 335–343. https://doi.org/10.3109/09540261.2014.899203

Klein, J. (2019). The mechanisms of hypomanic creativity in bipolar II disorder. *Applied Psychology OPUS*. https://wp.nyu.edu/steinhardt-appsych_opus/the-mechanisms-of-hypomanic-creativity-in-bipolar-ii-disorder/

Klitzman, R. (2008). *When Doctors Become Patients*. Oxford University Press.

Knapstad, M., Nordgreen, T., & Smith, O. R. F. (2018). Prompt mental health care, the Norwegian version of IAPT: Clinical outcomes and predictors of change in a multicenter cohort study. *BMC Psychiatry, 18*, Article 260. https://doi.org/10.1186/s12888-018-1838-0

Knittle, K., Gellert, P., Moore, C., Bourke, N., & Hull, V. (2019). Goal achievement and goal-related cognitions in behavioral activation treatment for depression. *Behavior Therapy, 50*(5), 898–909. https://doi.org/10.1016/j.beth.2019.01.005

Knopov, A., Sherman, R. J., Raifman, J. R., Larson, E., & Siegel, M. B. (2019). Household gun ownership and youth suicide rates at the state level, 2005–2015. *American Journal of Preventive Medicine, 56*(3), 335–342. https://doi.org/10.1016/j.amepre.2018.10.027

Ko, S., & Sohn, A. (2018). Behaviors and culture of drinking among Korean people. *Iranian Journal of Public Health, 47*(Suppl 1), 47–56.

Kodama, T., Fujimoto, H., Tamura, Y., & Kataoka, M. (2017). Suicide for the purpose of gaining insurance payouts in Japan. *Open Journal of Social Sciences 5(11)*: 189–197. DOI: 10.4236/jss.2017.511014.

Kohyama, J. (2011). Sleep, serotonin, and suicide in Japan. *Journal of Physiological Anthropology, 30*(1), 1–8. https://doi.org/10.2114/jpa2.30.1

Komori, T., Makinodan, M., & Kishimoto, T. (2019). Social status and modern-type depression: A review. *Brain and Behavior, 9*(12), Article e01464. https://doi.org/10.1002/brb3.1464

Kong, Y., & Zhang, J. (2010). Access to farming pesticides and risk for suicide in Chinese rural young people. *Psychiatry Research, 179*(2), 217–221. https://doi.org/10.1016/j.psychres.2009.12.005

Kontogianni, M. D., Vijayakumar, A., Rooney, C., Noad, R. L., Appleton, K. M., McCarthy, D., Donnelly, M., Young, I. S., McKinley, M. C., McKeown, P. P., & Woodside, J. V. (2020). A high polyphenol diet improves psychological well-being: The Polyphenol Intervention Trial (PPhIT). *Nutrients, 12*(8), Article 2445. https://doi.org/10.3390/nu12082445

Kopacz, M. S., Ames, D., & Koenig, H. G. (2019). It's time to talk about physician burnout and moral injury. *The Lancet Psychiatry, 6*(11), e28. https://doi.org/10.1016/S2215-0366(19)30385-2

Kopacz, M. S., Crean, H. F., Park, C. L., & Hoff, R. A. (2017). Religious coping and suicide risk in a sample of recently returned veterans. *Archives of Suicide Research, 22*(4), 615–627. https://doi.org/10.1080/13811118.2017.1390513

Kopera, A. F., Khiew, Y. C., Amer Alsamman, M., Mattar, M. C., Olsen, R. S., & Doman, D. B. (2024). Depression and the aberrant intestinal microbiome. *Gastroenterology & Hepatology, 20*(1), 30–40.

Korean Statistical Information Service (2024). Population projections and summary indicators (Korea). https://kosis.kr/statHtml/statHtml.do?orgId=101&tblId=DT_1BPA002&vw_cd=MT_ETITLE&list_id=A41_10&scrId=&language=en&seqNo=&lang_mode=en&obj_var_id=&itm_id=&conn_path=MT_ETITLE&path=%252Feng%252FstatisticsList%252FstatisticsListIndex.do. Retrieved August 20, 2024.

Korous, K. M., Causadias, J. M., Bradley, R. H., Levy, R., Cahill, K. M., Li, L., & Luthar, S. S. (2023). "More is better" or "better near the middle"? A U.S.-based individual participant data meta-analysis of socioeconomic status and depressive symptoms. *The American Psychologist, 78*(3), 305–320. https://doi.org/10.1037/amp0001076

Kost, A., & Chen, F. M. (2015). Socrates was not a pimp: Changing the paradigm of questioning in medical education. *Academic Medicine, 90*(1), 20–24. https://doi.org/10.1097/ACM.0000000000000446

Kouba, B. R., de Araujo Borba, L., Borges de Souza, P., Gil-Mohapel, J., & Rodrigues, A. L. S. (2024). Role of inflammatory mechanisms in Major Depressive Disorder: From etiology to potential pharmacological targets. *Cells, 13*(5), 423. https://doi.org/10.3390/cells13050423

Koyama, A., Miyake, Y., Kawakami, N., Tsuchiya, M., Tachimori, H., & Takeshima, T.; World Mental Health Japan Survey Group, 2002–2006. (2010). Lifetime prevalence, psychiatric comorbidity, and demographic correlates of "hikikomori" in a community population in Japan. *Psychiatry Research, 176*(1), 69–74.

Koyama, F., Yoda, T., & Hirao, T. (2017). Insomnia and depression: Japanese hospital workers questionnaire survey. *Open Medicine, 12*, 391–398. https://doi.org/10.1515/med-2017-0056

Kraus, C., Kadriu, B., Lanzenberger, R., Zarate, C. A., Jr., & Kasper, S. (2019). Prognosis and improved outcomes in major depression: A review. *Translational Psychiatry, 9*(1), Article 127. https://doi.org/10.1038/s41398-019-0460-3

Kristensen, T., Borritz, M., Villadsen, E., & Christensen, K. (2005). The Copenhagen Burnout Inventory: A new tool for the assessment of burnout. *Work and Stress, 19*, 192–207. https://doi.org/10.1080/02678370500297720

Kristoffersson, E., Diderichsen, S., Verdonk, P., Lagro-Janssen, T., Hamberg, K., & Andersson, J. (2018). To select or be selected—Gendered experiences in clinical training affect medical students' specialty preferences. *BMC Medical Education, 18*(1), Article 268. https://doi.org/10.1186/s12909-018-1361-5

Kroenke, K., Spitzer, R. L., & Williams, J. B. (2001). The PHQ-9: Validity of a brief depression severity measure. *Journal of General Internal Medicine, 16*(9), 606–613. https://doi.org/10.1046/j.1525-1497.2001.016009606.x

Krogstad, J. M., Passel, J. S., & Cohn, D. (2019). *5 facts about illegal immigration in the U.S.* Pew Research Center. Retrieved September 28, 2019, from https://www.pewresearch.org/fact-tank/2019/06/12/5-facts-about-illegal-immigration-in-the-u-s/

Kühn, S., Düzel, S., Drewelies, J., Gerstorf, D., Lindenberger, U., & Gallinat, J. (2018). Psychological and neural correlates of embitterment in old age. *Psychological Trauma: Theory, Research, Practice, and Policy, 10*(1), 51–57. https://doi.org/10.1037/tra0000287

Kumar, S. (2016). Burnout and doctors: Prevalence, prevention and intervention. *Healthcare, 4*(3), Article 37. https://doi.org/10.3390/healthcare4030037

Kumar, V. (2003). Burnt wives—A study of suicides. *Burns, 29*(1), 31–35. https://doi.org/10.1016/S0305-4179(02)00235-8

Kung, A., Hastings, K. G., Kapphahn, K. I., Wang, E. J., Cullen, M. R., Ivey, S. L., Palaniappan, L. P., & Chung, S. (2018). Cross-national comparisons of increasing suicidal mortality rates for Koreans in the Republic of Korea and Korean Americans in the USA, 2003–2012. *Epidemiology and Psychiatric Sciences, 27*(1), 62–73. https://doi.org/10.1017/S2045796016000792

Kuwabata & Mishima (2021, November 9). Schools across nation fighting rampant surge of online bullying. *The Asahi Shinbun*. https://www.asahi.com/ajw/articles/14467739

Kuzemko, J. A. (1994). Chopin's illnesses. *Journal of the Royal Society of Medicine, 87*(12), 769–772.

Kvernmo S. (2004). Mental health of Sami youth. International Journal of Circumpolar Health 63(3): 221–234. https://doi.org/10.3402/ijch.v63i3.17716

La Flair, L. N., Bradshaw, C. P., Storr, C. L., Green, K. M., Alvanzo, A. A., & Crum, R. M. (2012). Intimate partner violence and patterns of alcohol abuse and dependence criteria among women: A latent class analysis. *Journal of Studies on Alcohol and Drugs, 73*(3), 351–360. https://doi.org/10.15288/jsad.2012.73.351

Lai, B. P., Tang, A. K., Lee, D. T., Yip, A. S., & Chung, T. K. (2010). Detecting postnatal depression in Chinese men: A comparison of three instruments. *Psychiatry Research, 180*(2–3), 80–85. https://doi.org/10.1016/j.psychres.2009.07.015

Lai, J. S., Hiles, S., Bisquera, A., Hure, A. J., McEvoy, M., & Attia, J. (2014). A systematic review and meta-analysis of dietary patterns and depression in community-dwelling adults. *American Journal of Clinical Nutrition, 99*(1), 181–197. https://doi.org/10.3945/ajcn.113.069880

LaiTimes. (2022, February 26). Anxious mothers treat their children like this, and even make 2 and a half years old children bald! *LaiTimes*. https://www.laitimes.com/en/article/376b3_3nvr9.html

Lam Ching, W., Li, H. J., Guo, J., Yao, L., Chau, J., Lo, S., Yuen, C. S., Ng, B. F. L., Chau-Leung Yu, E., Bian, Z., Lau, A. Y., & Zhong, L. L. (2023). Acupuncture for post-stroke depression: A systematic review and network meta-analysis. BMC Psychiatry 23(1): 314. https://doi.org/10.1186/s12888-023-04749-1

Lan, F. Y., Liou, Y. W., Huang, K. Y., Guo, H. R., & Wang, J. D. (2016). An investigation of a cluster of cervical herniated discs among container truck drivers with occupational exposure to whole-body vibration. *Journal of Occupational Health*, *58*(1), 118–127. https://doi.org/10.1539/joh.15-0050-FS

Lang, C. J., Appleton, S. L., Vakulin, A., McEvoy, R. D., Vincent, A. D., Wittert, G. A., Martin, S. A., Grant, J. F., Taylor, A. W., Antic, N., Catcheside, P. G., & Adams, R. J. (2017). Associations of undiagnosed obstructive sleep apnea and excessive daytime sleepiness with depression: An Australian population study. *Journal of Clinical Sleep Medicine*, *13*(4), 575–582. https://doi.org/10.5664/jcsm.6546

Langewiesche, W. (2019, June 17). What really happened to Malaysia's missing airplane? *The Atlantic*. Retrieved September 1, 2019, from https://www.theatlantic.com/magazine/archive/2019/07/mh370-malaysia-airlines/590653/

Latcheva, R. (2017). Sexual harassment in the European Union: A pervasive but still hidden form of gender-based violence. *Journal of Interpersonal Violence*, *32*(12), 1821–1852. https://doi.org/10.1177/0886260517698948

La Torre, G., Sestili, C., Imeshtari, V., Masciullo, C., Rizzo, F., Guida, G., Pagano, L., & Mannocci, A. (2021). Association of health status, sociodemographic factors and burnout in healthcare professionals: Results from a multicentre observational study in Italy. *Public Health*, *195*, 15–17. https://doi.org/10.1016/j.puhe.2021.04.004

Lau, C. (2023, March 26). Japan wants 85% of male workers to take paternity leave. But fathers are too afraid to take it. *CNN World*. https://www.cnn.com/2023/03/26/asia/japan-paternity-leave-policy-challenges-intl-hnk-dst/index.html

Lawrence, C., Mhlaba, T., Stewart, K. A., Moletsane, R., Gaede, B., & Moshabela, M. (2018). The hidden curricula of medical education: A scoping review. *Academic Medicine*, *93*(4), 648–656. https://doi.org/10.1097/ACM.0000000000002004

Lawrence, R. E., Oquendo, M. A., & Stanley, B. (2016). Religion and suicide risk: A systematic review. *Archives of Suicide Research*, *20*(1), 1–21. https://doi.org/10.1080/13811118.2015.1004494

Lawrence, R. G. (2004). *The Wabi-Sabi House: The Japanese Art of Imperfect Beauty*. Clarkson Potter.

Lawson, N. D., & Boyd, J. W. (2018a). Do state physician health programs encourage referrals that violate the Americans with Disabilities Act? *International Journal of Law and Psychiatry*, *56*, 65–70. https://doi.org/10.1016/j.ijlp.2017.12.004

Lawson, N. D., & Boyd, J. W. (2018b). How broad are state physician health program descriptions of physician impairment? *Substance Abuse Treatment, Prevention, and Policy*, *13*(1), Article 30. https://doi.org/10.1186/s13011-018-0168-z

Lazur, J., Hnatyk, K., Kała, K., Sułkowska-Ziaja, K., & Muszyńska, B. (2023). Discovering the potential mechanisms of medicinal mushrooms antidepressant activity: A review. *Antioxidants*, *12*(3), 623. https://doi.org/10.3390/antiox12030623

Lee, A. (Director) (2005). *Brokeback Mountain* [Film]. River Road Entertainment.

Lee, B. T., Paik, J. W., Kang, R. H., Chung, S. Y., Kwon, H. I., Khang, H. S., Lyoo, I. K., Chae, J.-H., Kwon, J.-H., Kim, J.-W., Lee, M.-S., & Ham, B.-J. (2009). The neural substrates of affective face recognition in patients with *hwa-byung* and healthy individuals in Korea. *World Journal of Biological Psychiatry*, *10*(4, Pt. 2), 552–559. https://doi.org/10.1080/15622970802087130

Lee, D., Baek, J. H., Cho, Y. J., & Hong, K. S. (2021). Association of resting heart rate and heart rate variability with proximal suicidal risk in patients with diverse psychiatric diagnoses. *Frontiers in Psychiatry*, *12*, Article 652340. https://doi.org/10.3389/fpsyt.2021.652340

Lee, H., Park, C., Rhee, S. J., Kim, J., Kim, B., Lee, S. S., Ha, K., Baik, C. J., & Ahn, Y. M. (2021). An integrated model for the relationship between socio-cultural factors, attitudes toward suicide, and intensity of suicidal ideation in Korean, Japanese, and American populations. *Journal of Affective Disorders*, *280*(Pt. A), 203–210. https://doi.org/10.1016/j.jad.2020.10.042

Lee, H. Y., Oh, J., Kawachi, I., Heo, J., Kim, S., Lee, J. K., & Kang, D. (2019). Positive and negative social support and depressive symptoms according to economic status among adults in Korea: Cross-sectional results from the Health Examinees-Gem Study. *BMJ Open*, *9*(4), Article e023036. https://doi.org/10.1136/bmjopen-2018-023036

Lee, J., Wachholtz, A., & Choi, K. H. (2014). A review of the Korean cultural syndrome *hwa-byung*: Suggestions for theory and intervention. *Asia T'aep'yongyang Sangdam Yon'gu*, *4*(1), 49–64. https://doi.org/10.18401/2014.4.1.4

Lee, J-G., & Lee, J-H. (2008). [Study on the prevalence of hwa-byung diagnosed by HBDIS in the general population in Kang-won Province] (article in Korean). *Journal of Oriental Neuropsychiatry*, *19*(2), 133–139.

Lee J. H. (2015). Prevalence and predictors of self-reported student maltreatment by teachers in South Korea. *Child Abuse & Neglect*, *46*, 113–120. https://doi.org/10.1016/j.chiabu.2015.03.009

Lee, K. S., Lee, H., Myung, W., Song, G. Y., Lee, K., Kim, H., Carroll, B. J., & Kim, D. K. (2018). Advanced daily prediction model for national suicide numbers with social media data. *Psychiatry Investigation*, *15*(4), 344–354. https://doi.org/10.30773/pi.2017.10.15

Lee, R. M., Choe, J., Kim, G., & Ngo, V. (2000). Construction of the Asian American Family Conflict Scale. *Journal of Counseling Psychology*, *47*, 211–222.

Lee, R. T., Seo, B., Hladkyj, S., Lovell, B. L., & Schwartzmann, L. (2013). Correlates of physician burnout across regions and specialties: A meta-analysis. *Human Resources for Health*, *11*, Article 48. https://doi.org/10.1186/1478-4491-11-48

Lee, S., Kim, H., Park, M. J., & Jeon, H. J. (2021). Current advances in wearable devices and their sensors in patients with depression. *Frontiers in Psychiatry*, *12*, Article 672347. https://doi.org/10.3389/fpsyt.2021.672347

Lee, S., & Lee, E. (2018). Predictors of intimate partner violence among pregnant women. *International Journal of Gyynaecology and Obstetrics*, *140*(2), 159–163. https://doi.org/10.1002/ijgo.12365

Lee, S. W., Stewart, S. M., Byrne, B. M., Wong, J. P., Ho, S. Y., Lee, P. W., & Lam, T. H. (2008). Factor structure of the Center for Epidemiological Studies Depression Scale in Hong Kong adolescents. *Journal of Personality Assessment*, *90*(2), 175–184. https://doi.org/10.1080/00223890701845385

Lee, S. Y., & Kwon, Y. (2018). Twitter as a place where people meet to make suicide pacts. *Public Health*, *159*, 21–26. https://doi.org/10.1016/j.puhe.2018.03.001

Lee, Y., & Kim, S. (2011). Childhood maltreatment in Korea: Retrospective study. *Child Abuse & Neglect*, *35*(12), 1037–1044. https://doi.org/10.1016/j.chiabu.2011.09.005

Legha, R. K. (2012). A history of physician suicide in America. *Journal of Medical Humanities*, *33*, 219–244. https://doi.org/10.1007/s10912-012-9182-8

Lei, H., Zhang, Q., Wang, Z., & Shao, J. (2021). A longitudinal study of depressive symptoms and delinquency among Chinese left-behind children. *Psychiatry Research, 301*, Article 113955. https://doi.org/10.1016/j.psychres.2021.113955

Leijssen, J. B., Snijder, M. B., Timmermans, E. J. Generaal, E., Stronks, K., & Kunst, A. E. (2019). The association between road traffic noise and depressed mood among different ethnic and socioeconomic groups. The HELIUS study. *International Journal of Hygiene and Environmental Health, 222*(2), 221–229. https://doi.org/10.1016/j.ijheh.2018.10.002

Lemann, N. (2015, October 26). The price of union. *The New Yorker*. https://www.newyorker.com/magazine/2015/11/02/the-price-of-union

Lemke, M., & Apostolopoulos, Y. (2015). Health and wellness programs for commercial motor-vehicle drivers. *Workplace Health & Safety, 63*, 71–80. https://doi.org/10.1177/2165079915569740

LeMoult, J., Humphreys, K. L., Tracy, A., Hoffmeister, J. A., Ip, E., & Gotlib, I. H. (2020). Meta-analysis: Exposure to early life stress and risk for depression in childhood and adolescence. *Journal of the American Academy of Child and Adolescent Psychiatry, 59*(7), 842–855. https://doi.org/10.1016/j.jaac.2019.10.011

Lenzer, J. (2016). Physician health programs under fire. *BMJ, 353*, Article i3568. https://doi.org/10.1136/bmj.i3658

Leppin, A. L., Bora, P. R., Tilburt, J. C., Gionfriddo, M. R., Zeballos-Palacios, C., Dulohery, M. M., Sood, A., Erwin, P. J., Brito, J. P., Boehmer, K. R., & Montori, V. M. (2014). The efficacy of resiliency training programs: A systematic review and meta-analysis of randomized trials. *PLOS ONE, 9*(10), Article e111420.

Leung, C. W., Epel, E. S., Willett, W. C., Rimm, E. B., & Laraia, B. A. (2015). Household food insecurity is positively associated with depression among low-income supplemental nutrition assistance program participants and income-eligible nonparticipants. *Journal of Nutrition, 145*(3), 622–627. https://doi.org/10.3945/jn.114.199414

Levy, M., Boulle, F., Steinbusch, H. W., van den Hove, D., Kenis, G., & Lanfumey, L. (2018). Neurotrophic factors and neuroplasticity pathways in the pathophysiology and treatment of depression. *Psychopharmacology, 235*(8), 2195–2220. https://doi.org/10.1007/s00213-018-4950-4

Levy, R. J. (2011). The Michael Jackson autopsy: Insights provided by a forensic anesthesiologist. *Journal of Forensic Research, 2*, Article 138. https://doi.org/10.4172/2157-7145.1000138

Li, F. D., He, F., Ye, X. J., Shen, W., Wu, Y. P., Zhai, Y. J., Wang, X. Y., & Lin, J. F. (2016). Tea consumption is inversely associated with depressive symptoms in the elderly: A cross-sectional study in eastern China. *Journal of Affective Disorders, 199*, 157–162. https://doi.org/10.1016/j.jad.2016.04.005

Li, J., Lineweber, C., Nyberg, A., & Siegrist, J. (2019). Cost, gain and health: Theoretical clarification and psychometric validation of a work stress model with data from two national studies. *Journal of Occupational and Environmental Medicine, 61*(11), 898–904. https://doi.org/10.1097/JOM.0000000000001696

Li, K., Guang, Y., Ren, L., Zhan, X., Tan, X., Luo, X., & Feng, Z. (2021). Network analysis of the relationship between negative life events and depressive symptoms in the left-behind children. *BMC Psychiatry, 21*(1), Article 429. https://doi.org/10.1186/s12888-021-03445-2

Li, M., & Katikireddi, S. V. (2019). Urban–rural inequalities in suicide among elderly people in China: A systematic review and meta-analysis. *International Journal for Equity in Health, 18*(1), Article 2. https://doi.org/10.1186/s12939-018-0881-2

Li, X., Coid, J. W., Tang, W., Lv, Q., Zhang, Y., Yu, H., Wang, Q., Deng, W., Zhao, L., Ma, X., Meng, Y., Li, M., Wang, H., Chen, T., Guo, W., & Li, T. (2020). Sustained effects of left-behind experience during childhood on mental health in Chinese university undergraduates. *European Child & Adolescent Psychiatry, 30*, 1949–1957. https://doi.org/10.1007/s00787-020-01666-6

Li, X., Hsu, Y., Hu, J., Khadka, A., Chen, T., & Li, J. (2013). Comprehensive consideration and design for treatment of square face. *Journal of Oral and Maxillofacial Surgery, 71*(10), 1761.e1–1761.e14. https://doi.org/10.1016/j.joms.2013.04.024

Li, Y., Lv, M. R., Wei, Y. J., Sun, L., Zhang, J. X., Zhang, H. G., & Li, B. (2017). Dietary patterns and depression risk: A meta-analysis. *Psychiatry Research, 253*, 373–382. https://doi.org/10.1016/j.psychres.2017.04.020

Li, Z., Feng, J., Yin, S., Chen, X., Yang, Q., Gao, X., Che, D., Zhou, L., Yan, H., Zhong, Y., & Zhu, F. (2023). Effects of acupuncture on mental health of migraine patients: a systematic review and meta-analysis. *BMC Complementary Medicine and Therapies, 23*(1), 278. https://doi.org/10.1186/s12906-023-04103-8

Li, Z., Heath, M. A., Jackson, A. P., Allen, G. E. K., Fischer, L., & Chan, P. (2017). Acculturation experiences of Chinese international students who attend American universities. *Professional Psychology: Research and Practice, 48*(1), 11–21. http://dx.doi.org/10.1037/pro0000117

Lian, Z., & Wallace, B. C. (2020). Prevalence of past-year mental disorders and its correlates among Chinese international students in US higher education. *Journal of American College Health, 68*(2), 176–184. https://doi.org/10.1080/07448481.2018.1538147

Liang, D., Mays, V. M. & Hwang, W-C. (2018). Integrated mental health services in China: Challenges and planning for the future. *Health Policy and Planning 33* (1): 107–122. https://doi.org/10.1093/heapol/czx137

Lim, A., Hoek, H. W., Ghane, S., Deen, M., & Blom, J. D. (2018). The attribution of mental health problems to jinn: An explorative study in a transcultural psychiatric outpatient clinic. *Frontiers in Psychiatry, 9*, Article 89. https://doi.org/10.3389/fpsyt.2018.00089

Lim, S.-L., Yeh, M., Liang, J., Lau, A. S., & McCabe, K. (2008). Acculturation gap, intergenerational conflict, parenting style, and youth distress in immigrant Chinese American families. *Marriage and Family Review, 45*, 84–106. https://doi.org/10.1080/01494920802537530

Lin, C., Tong, Y., Bai, Y., Zhao, Z., Quan, W., Liu, Z., Wang, J., Song, Y., Tian, J., & Dong, W. (2022). Prevalence and correlates of depression and anxiety among Chinese international students in US colleges during the COVID-19 pandemic: A cross-sectional study. *PLOS ONE, 17*(4), e0267081. https://doi.org/10.1371/journal.pone.0267081

Lin, Y. (2017, October 20). Indifferent to life, ready to die. *Commonwealth Magazine.* https://english.cw.com.tw/article/article.action?id=1698

Linde, K., Berner, M. M., & Kriston, L. (2008). St. John's wort for major depression. *Cochrane Database of Systematic Reviews.* https://doi.org/10.1002/14651858.CD000448.pub3

Lindeman, S., Laara, E., Hakko, H., & Lonnqvist, J. (1996). A systematic review on gender-specific suicide mortality in medical doctors. *British Journal of Psychiatry, 168*, 274–279. https://doi.org/10.1192/bjp.168.3.274

Linden, M., Baumann, K., Rotter, M., & Schippan, B. (2008). Diagnostic criteria and the standardized diagnostic interview for posttraumatic embitterment disorder (PTED).

International Journal of Psychiatry in Clinical Practice, 12(2), 93–96. https://doi.org/10.1080/13651500701580478

Lindgren, T., Wieslander, G., Dammström, B. G., & Norbäck, D. (2009). Tinnitus among airline pilots: Prevalence and effects of age, flight experience, and other noise. *Aviation, Space and Environmental Medicine, 80*(2), 112–116.

Lindsay, E. K., Young, S., Brown, K. W., Smyth, J. M., & Creswell, J. D. (2019). Mindfulness training reduces loneliness and increases social contact in a randomized controlled trial. *Proceedings of the National Academy of Sciences of the United States of America, 116*(9), 3488–3493. https://doi.org/10.1073/pnas.1813588116

Little, L. F., Gaffney, I. C., Rosen, K. H., & Bender, M. M. (1990). Corporate instability is related to airline pilots' stress symptoms. *Aviation, Space, and Environmental Medicine, 61*(11), 977–982.

Litz, B. T., Stein, N., Delaney, E., Lebowitz, L., Nash, W. P., Silva, C., & Maguen, S. (2009). Moral injury and moral repair in war veterans: A preliminary model and intervention strategy. *Clinical Psychology Review, 29,* 695–706. https://doi.org/10.1016/j.cpr.2009.07.003

Liu, J. (2021). Spouse and adult-child dementia caregivers in Chinese American families: Who are more stressed out? *Journal of the American Medical Directors Association, 22*(7), 1512–1517. https://doi.org/10.1016/j.jamda.2020.12.012

Liu, H., Zhou, Z., Fan, X., Wang, J., Sun, H., Shen, C., & Zhai, X. (2020). The influence of left-behind experience on college students' mental health: A cross-sectional comparative study. *International Journal of Environmental Research and Public Health, 17*(5), Article 1511. https://doi.org/10.3390/ijerph17051511

Liu, L., Liu, C., Wang, Y., Wang, P., Li, Y., & Li, B. (2015). Herbal medicine for anxiety, depression and insomnia. *Current Neuropharmacology, 13*(4), 481–493. https://doi.org/10.2174/1570159X1304150831122734

Liu, L.-Y., Zhang, H.-J., Luo, L.-Y., Pu, J.-B., Liang, W.-Q., Zhu, C.-Q., Li, Y.-P., Wang, P.-R., Zhang, Y.-Y., Yang, C.-Y., & Zhang, Z.-J. (2018). Blood and urine metabolomic evidence validating traditional Chinese medicine diagnostic classification of major depressive disorder. *Chinese Medicine, 13,* Article 53. https://doi.org/10.1186/s13020-018-0211-z

Liu, M. (2016). Verbal communication styles and culture. *Oxford Research Encyclopedias: Communication.* Retrieved September 27, 2019, from https://oxfordre.com/communication/view/10.1093/acrefore/9780190228613.001.0001/acrefore-9780190228613-e-162#

Liu, S., Sheng, J., Li, B., & Zhang, X. (2017). Recent advances in non-invasive brain stimulation for major depressive disorder. *Human Neuroscience, 11,* Article 526. https://doi.org/10.3389/fnhum.2017.00526

Liu, W., & Zhang, X. (2000). [*Harvard Girl Liu Yiting*]; 哈佛女孩刘亦婷; Hafo nühai Liu Yiting. Writers Publishing House.

Liu, Z., Qiao, D., Xu, Y., Zhao, W., Yang, Y., Wen, D., Li, X., Nie, X., Dong, Y., Tang, S., Jiang, Y., Wang, Y., Zhao, J., & Xu, Y. (2021). The efficacy of computerized cognitive behavioral therapy for depressive and anxiety symptoms in patients with COVID-19: Randomized controlled trial. *Journal of Medical Internet Research, 23*(5), Article e26883. https://doi.org/10.2196/26883

Liu, Z. M., Ho, S. C., Xie, Y. J., Chen, Y. J., Chen, Y. M., Chen, B., Wong, S. Y.-s., Chan, D., Wong, C. K. M., He, Q., Tse, L. A., & Woo, J. (2016). Associations between dietary patterns and psychological factors: A cross-sectional study among Chinese postmenopausal women. *Menopause, 23*(12), 1294–1302. https://doi.org/10.1097/GME.0000000000000701

Liu, Z. W., Yu, Y., Hu, M., Liu, H. M., Zhou, L., & Xiao, S. Y. (2016). PHQ-9 and PHQ-2 for screening depression in Chinese rural elderly. *PLOS ONE, 11*(3), Article e0151042. https://doi.org/10.1371/journal.pone.0151042

Lloyd's Register Foundation. (2023). Violence and harassment at work. *World Risk Poll 2021*. Retrieved October 20, 2023, from https://wrp.lrfoundation.org.uk/country-results-2021-violence-harassment/world_risk_poll_results_2021_violence_harassment_denmark.pdf, and similar URLs for Finland, Iceland, Norway, Sweden, and Switzerland.

Locke, T. (2019). Global physicians' burnout and lifestyle comparisons. *Medscape*. https://www.medscape.com/slideshow/2019-global-burnout-comparison-6011180#1

Lombardo, G., Mondelli, V., Dazzan, P., & Pariante, C. M. (2021). Sex hormones and immune system: A possible interplay in affective disorders? A systematic review. *Journal of Affective Disorders, 290*, 1–14. https://doi.org/10.1016/j.jad.2021.04.035

Longman, D. P., Shaw, C. N., Varela-Mato, V., Sherry, A. P., Ruettger, K., Sayyah, M., Guest, A., Chen, Y. L., Paine, N. J., King, J. A., & Clemes, S. A. (2021). Time in nature associated with decreased fatigue in UK truck drivers. *International Journal of Environmental Research and Public Health, 18*(6), Article 3158. https://doi.org/10.3390/ijerph18063158

Lopez, A. O., Martinez, M. N., Garcia, J. M., Kunik, M. E., & Medina, L. D. (2021). Self-report depression screening measures for older Hispanic/Latin American adults: A PRISMA systematic review. *Journal of Affective Disorders, 294*, 1–9. https://doi.org/10.1016/j.jad.2021.06.049

Lopez, V., Sanchez, K., Killian, M. O., & Eghaneyan, B. H. (2018). Depression screening and education: An examination of mental health literacy and stigma in a sample of Hispanic women. *BMC Public Health, 18*(1), Article 646. https://doi.org/10.1186/s12889-018-5516-4

Lu, C., & Ng, E. (2019). Healthy immigrant effect by immigrant category in Canada. *Health Reports, 30*(4), 3–11. https://doi.org/10.25318/82-003-x201900400001-eng

Lu, J. G. (2019). Air pollution: A systematic review of its psychological, economic, and social effects. *Current Opinion in Psychology, 32*, 52–65. https://doi.org/10.1016/j.copsyc.2019.06.024

Lu, L., Hu, X., & Jin, X. (2023). IL-4 as a potential biomarker for differentiating major depressive disorder from bipolar depression. *Medicine, 102*(15), e33439. https://doi.org/10.1097/MD.0000000000033439

Lu, Y. R., Rao, Y. B., Mou, Y. J., Chen, Y., Lou, H. F., Zhang, Y., Zhang, D.-X., Xie, H.-Y., Hu, L.-W., & Fang, P. (2019). High concentrations of serum interleukin-6 and interleukin-8 in patients with bipolar disorder. *Medicine, 98*(7), Article e14419. https://doi.org/10.1097/MD.0000000000014419

Lucas, M., Chocano-Bedoya, P., Schulze, M. B., Mirzaei, F., O'Reilly, É. J., Okereke, O. I., Hu, F. B., Willett, W. C., & Ascherio, A. (2014). Inflammatory dietary pattern and risk of depression among women. *Brain, Behavior, and Immunity, 36*, 46–53. https://doi.org/10.1016/j.bbi.2013.09.014

Lucidi, L., Pettorruso, M., Vellante, F., Di Carlo, F., Ceci, F., Santovito, M. C., Di Muzio, I., Fornaro, M., Ventriglio, A., Tomasetti, C., Valchera, A., Gentile, A., Kim, Y.-K., Martinotti, G., Lüdtke, S., Hermann, W., Kirste, T., Beneš, H., & Teipel, S.

(2021). An algorithm for actigraphy-based sleep/wake scoring: Comparison with polysomnography. *Clinical Neurophysiology, 132*(1), 137–145. https://doi.org/10.1016/j.clinph.2020.10.019

Lüdtke, S., Hermann, W., Kirste, T., Beneš, H., & Teipel, S. (2021). An algorithm for actigraphy-based sleep/wake scoring: Comparison with polysomnography. Clinical neurophysiology : official journal of the International Federation of Clinical Neurophysiology, 132(1), 137–145. https://doi.org/10.1016/j.clinph.2020.10.019

Lullau, A. P. M., Haga, E. M. W., Ronold, E. H., & Dwyer, G. E. (2023). Antidepressant mechanisms of ketamine: a review of actions with relevance to treatment-resistance and neuroprogression. *Frontiers in Neuroscience, 17*, 1223145. https://doi.org/10.3389/fnins.2023.1223145

Lumen Learning (2019). *Wealth and Culture in the South*. Retrieved September 28, 2019, from https://courses.lumenlearning.com/ushistory1os2xmaster/chapter/wealth-and-culture-in-the-south/

Lund, J. I., Toombs, E., Radford, A., Boles, K., & Mushquash, C. (2020). Adverse childhood experiences and executive function difficulties in children: A systematic review. *Child Abuse & Neglect, 106*, Article 104485. https://doi.org/10.1016/j.chiabu.2020.104485

Lundeteg, A., Nord, C., Hemberg, C., Ajmal, O., & Dahlgren, T. (2017). *Women CEOs Choose Gender Equality*. AllBright Foundation.

Luppino, F. S., de Wit, L. M., Bouvy, P. F., Stijnen, T., Cuijpers, P., Penninx, B. W., & Zitman, F. G. (2010). Overweight, obesity, and depression: a systematic review and meta-analysis of longitudinal studies. Archives of General Psychiatry, 67(3), 220–229. https://doi.org/10.1001/archgenpsychiatry.2010.2

Lurie, D. I. (2018). An integrative approach to neuroinflammation in psychiatric disorders and neuropathic pain. *Journal of Experimental Neuroscience, 12*. https://doi.org/10.1177/1179069518793639

Lustig, R. H. (2013). Fructose, it's "alcohol without the buzz." *Advances in Nutrition, 4*(2), 226–235. https://doi.org/10.3945/an.112.002998

Luthar, S. S., Small, P. J., & Cicolla, L. (2018). Adolescents from upper middle class communities: Substance misuse and addiction across early adulthood. *Developmental Psychopathology, 30*(1), 315–335. https://doi.org/10.1017/S0954579417000645

Lyall, S. (2007, November 4). In Stetson or wig, he's hard to pin down. *New York Times*. https://www.nytimes.com/2007/11/04/movies/moviesspecial/04lyal.html

Lyoo, Y. C., Ju, S., Kim, E., Kim, J. E., & Lee, J. H. (2014). The Patient Health Questionnaire-15 and its abbreviated version as screening tools for depression in Korean college and graduate students. *Comprehensive Psychiatry, 55*(3), 743–748. https://doi.org/10.1016/j.comppsych.2013.11.011

Lyu, C. P., Pei, J. R., Beseler, L. C., Li, Y. L., Li, J. H., Ren, M., Stallones, L., & Ren, S. P. (2018). Case control study of impulsivity, aggression, pesticide exposure and suicide attempts using pesticides among farmers. *Biomedical and Environmental Science, 31*(3), 242–246. https://doi.org/10.3967/bes2018.031

Ma, J., Li, C., Kwan, M. P., & Chai, Y. (2018). A multilevel analysis of perceived noise pollution, geographic contexts and mental health in Beijing. *International Journal of Environmental Research and Public Health, 15*(7), Article 1479. https://doi.org/10.3390/ijerph15071479

Ma, S., Zhu, Y., & Bresnahan, M. (2021). Chinese international students' face concerns, self-stigma, linguistic factors, and help-seeking intentions for mental health. *Health Communication*, *37*(13), 1631–1639. https://doi.org/10.1080/10410236.2021.1910167

Mackintosh, M., & Kovalev, S. (2006). Commercialization, inequality and transition in health care: The policy challenges in developing and transitional countries. *Journal of International Development*, *18*, 387–391. https://doi.org/10.1002/jid.1289

MacMillan, C. (2020). *The only old-school cabover truck guide you'll ever need*. Smart Trucking. Retrieved September 1, 2021, from https://www.smart-trucking.com/cabover-truck/

Maeda, F., & Nathan, J. H. (1999). Understanding *taijin kyofusho* through its treatment, Morita therapy. *Journal of Psychosomatic Research*, *46*(6), 525–530. https://doi.org/10.1016/s0022-3999(98)00113-5

Maffoni, M. (2021). The cry into the darkness of a burned out physician. *Families, Systems & Health*, *39*(2), 394. https://doi.org/10.1037/fsh0000616

Magnusson, A., Axelsson, J., Karlsson, M. M., & Osakarsson, H. (2000). Lack of seasonal mood change in the Icelandic population: Results of a cross-sectional study. *American Journal of Psychiatry*, *157*(2), 234–238. https://doi.org/10.1176/appi.ajp.157.2.234

Magnusson, N. (2018). The number of female executives in Sweden is rising. *Bloomberg News*, October 16. https://www.bloomberg.com/news/articles/2018-10-16/the-number-of-female-executives-rises-in-sweden-in-new-report

Magovcevic M., Addis M. E. (2008). The Masculine Depression Scale: Development and psychometric evaluation. *Psychology of Men & Masculinity* 9: 117–132. https://doi.org/10.1037/1524-9220.9.3.117

Mahood, S. C. (2011). Medical education: Beware the hidden curriculum. *Canadian Family Physician*, *57*(9), 983–985.

Mair, C., Cunradi, C. B., & Todd, M. (2012). Adverse childhood experiences and intimate partner violence: Testing psychosocial mediational pathways among couples. *Annals of Epidemiology*, *22*(12), 832–839. https://doi.org/10.1016/j.annepidem.2012.09.008

Mäkelä, P., Raitasalo, K., & Wahlbeck, K. (2015). Mental health and alcohol use: A cross-sectional study of the Finnish general population. *European Journal of Public Health*, *25*(2), 225–231. https://doi.org/10.1093/eurpub/cku133

Malfitano, N. (2022, March 3). Parents of UPenn student who committed suicide in 2016 settle wrongful death litigation with school. *Pennsylvania Record*. Retrieved July 24, 2023, from https://pennrecord.com/stories/621208800-parents-of-upenn-student-who-committed-suicide-in-2016-settle-wrongful-death-litigation-with-school

Manago, B., Pescosolido, B. A., & Olafsdottir, S. (2019). Icelandic inclusion, German hesitation and American fear: A cross cultural comparison of mental health stigma and the media. *Scandinavian Journal of Public Health*, *47*(2), 90–98. https://doi.org/10.1177/1403494817750337

Mandell, H., & Spiro, H. (1987). *When Doctors Get Sick*. Plenum Medical Book Company.

Mangory, K. Y., Ali, L. Y., Rø, K. I., & Tyssen, R. (2021). Effect of burnout among physicians on observed adverse patient outcomes: A literature review. *BMC Health Services Research*, *21*(1), Article 369. https://doi.org/10.1186/s12913-021-06371-x

Mannikko, R., Komulainen, P., Schwab, U., Heikkila, H.M., Savonen, K., Hassinen, M., Hanninen, T., Kivipelto, M., & Rauramaa, R. (2015). The Nordic diet and cognition—The DR's EXTRA Study. *British Journal of Nutrition, 114*(2), 231–239. https://doi.org/10.1017/S0007114515001890

Mantani, A., Kato, T., Furukawa, T. A., Horikoshi, M., Imai, H., Hiroe, T., Chino, B., Funayama, T., Yonemoto, N., Zhou, Q., & Kawanishi, N. (2017). Smartphone cognitive behavioral therapy as an adjunct to pharmacotherapy for refractory depression: Randomized controlled trial. *Journal of Medical Internet Research, 19*(11), Article e373. https://doi.org/10.2196/jmir.8602

Mantri, S., Lawson, J. M., Wang, Z., & Koenig, H. G. (2020). Identifying moral injury in healthcare professionals: The moral injury symptom scale-HP. *Journal of Religion and Health, 59*(5), 2323–2340.

Marks, M. (2019). Artificial intelligence-based suicide prediction. *Yale Journal of Health Policy, Law, and Ethics, 21*, 98–121. https://ssrn.com/abstract=3324874

Marsillach, J., Costa, L. G., & Furlong, C. E. (2016). Paraoxonase-1 and early-life environmental exposures. *Annals of Global Health 82*(1): 100–110. https://doi.org/10.1016/j.aogh.2016.01.009

Martin, L. A., Neighbors, H. W., & Griffith, D. M. (2013). The experience of symptoms of depression in men vs. women: Analysis of the National Comorbidity Survey Replication. *JAMA Psychiatry, 70*(10), 1100–1106. https://doi.org/10.1001/jamapsychiatry.2013.1985

Martinez, L. M., Estrada, D., & Prada, S. I. (2019). Mental health, interpersonal trust and subjective well-being in a high violence context. *SSM—Population Health, 8*, Article 100423. https://doi.org/10.1016/j.ssmph.2019.100423

Martins, J., & Brijeshsuku, S. (2018). Phytochemistry and pharmacology of anti-depressant medicinal plants: A review. *Biomedicine Pharmacotherapy, 104*, 343–365. https://doi.org/10.1016/j.biopha.2018.05.044

Maselko, J., Bates, L., Bhalotra, S., Gallis, J. A., O'Donnell, K., Sikander, S., & Turner, E. L. (2017). Socioeconomic status indicators and common mental disorders: Evidence from a study of prenatal depression in Pakistan. *SSM –Population Health, 4*, 1–9. https://doi.org/10.1016/j.ssmph.2017.10.004

Maslach, C., & Jackson, S. E. (1981). The measurement of experienced burnout. *Journal of Occupational Behavior, 2*, 99–113. https://doi.org/10.1002/job.4030020205

Mata, D. A., Ramos, M. A., Bansal, N., Khan, R., Guille, C., Di Angelantonio, E., & Sen, S. (2015). Prevalence of depression and depressive symptoms among resident physicians: A systematic review and meta-analysis. *JAMA, 314*(22), 2373–2383. https://doi.org/10.1001/jama.2015.15845

Matei, R., & Ginsborg, J. (2017). Music performance anxiety in classical musicians—What we know about what works. *British Journal of Psychiatry International, 14*(2), 33–35.

Mathews, B., & Bismark, M. B. (2015). Sexual harassment in the medical profession: Legal and ethical responsibilities. *Medical Journal of Australia, 203*(4), 189–192. https://doi.org/10.5694/mja15.00336

Matsuyama, K. (2015, February 24). Tokyo's elderly turned away amid labor crunch, funding cuts. *Japan Times.* https://www.japantimes.co.jp/news/2015/02/24/national/social-issues/tokyos-elderly-turned-away-amid-labor-crunch-funding-cuts/#.W3y_-s5Kj9Q

Matthews, T. A., Robbins, W., Preisig, M., von Känel, R., & Li, J. (2021). Associations of job strain and family strain with risk of major depressive episode: A prospective cohort study in U.S. working men and women. *Journal of Psychosomatic Research, 147*, Article 110541. https://doi.org/10.1016/j.jpsychores.2021.110541

Mayo Clinic (2021a). *U.S. COVID-19 vaccine rates over time*. Retrieved September 18, 2021, from https://www.mayoclinic.org/coronavirus-covid-19/vaccine-tracker

Mayo Clinic (2021b). *U.S. COVID-19 vaccine tracker: See your state's progress*. https://www.mayoclinic.org/coronavirus-covid-19/vaccine-tracker/

McCrae, R. R., & Costa, P. T. (1987). Validation of the five-factor model of personality across instruments and observers. *Journal of Personality and Social Psychology, 52*(1), 81–90. https://doi.org/10.1037/0022-3514.52.1.81

McCraw, S., Parker, G., Fletcher, K., & Friend, P. (2013). Self-reported creativity in bipolar disorder: Prevalence, types and associated outcomes in mania versus hypomania. *Journal of Affective Disorders, 151*(3), 831–836. https://doi.org/10.1016/j.jad.2013.07.016

McCullough, H. (1985). *Kokin Wakashū: The First Imperial Anthology of Japanese Poetry*. Stanford University Press.

McGregor, G. (2021, August 16). US universities face another school year of too few Chinese students. *Fortune*. https://fortune.com/2021/08/16/us-universities-international-students-china-covid/

McGuire, J. (2010). *Wealth, Health, and Democracy in East Asia and Latin America*. Cambridge University Press.

McHugh, R. K., & Weiss, R. D. (2019). Alcohol use disorder and depressive disorders. *Alcohol Research, 40*, e1–e8. https://doi.org/10.35946/arcr.v40.1.01

McIntyre, R. S., Berk, M., Brietzke, E., Goldstein, B. I., López-Jaramillo, C., Kessing, L. V., Malhi, G. S., Nierenberg, A. A., Rosenblat, J. D., Majeed, A., Vieta, E., Vinberg, M., Young, A. H., & Mansur, R. B. (2020). Bipolar disorders. *Lancet, 396*(10265), 1841–1856. https://doi.org/10.1016/S0140-6736(20)31544-0

McIntyre, R. S., & Calabrese, J. R. (2019). Bipolar depression: The clinical characteristics and unmet needs of a complex disorder. *Current Medical Research and Opinion, 5*, 1–13. https://doi.org/10.1080/03007995.2019.1636017

McIntyre, R. S., Cha, D. S., Kim, R. D., & Mansur, R. B. (2013). A review of FDA-approved treatment options in bipolar depression. *CNS Spectrums, 18*(S1), 4–20. https://doi.org/10.1017/S1092852913000746

McIntyre, R. S., Daniel, D. G., Vieta, E., Laszlovszky, I., Goetghebeur, P. J., Earley, W. R., & Patel, M. D. (2022). The efficacy of cariprazine on cognition: a post hoc analysis from phase II/III clinical trials in bipolar mania, bipolar depression, and schizophrenia. CNS spectrums, 28(3), 319–330. https://doi.org/10.1017/S109285292200013X

McIntyre, R. S., Durgam, S., Kozauer, S. G., Chen, R., Huo, J., Davis, R. E., & Cutler, A. J. (2023). The efficacy of lumateperone on symptoms of depression in bipolar I and bipolar II disorder: Secondary and post hoc analyses. *European Neuropsychopharmacology: The Journal of the European College of Neuropsychopharmacology, 68*, 78–88. https://doi.org/10.1016/j.euroneuro.2022.12.012

McKay, M. P., & Groff, L. (2016). 23 years of toxicology testing fatally injured pilots: Implications for aviation and other modes of transportation. *Accident Analysis and Prevention, 90*, 108–117.

McKinnon, M. (2017, December 7). This website tackles the silent epidemic of men's depression. *HuffPost*. Retrieved July 17, 2021, from https://www.huffpost.com/entry/this-website-tackles-the_b_7936670

McLellan, A. T., Skipper, G. S., Campbell, M., & DuPont, R. L. (2008). Five year outcomes in a cohort study of physicians treated for substance use disorders in the U.S. *BMJ*, 337, Article a2038. https://doi.org/10.1136/bmj.a2038

McNicholas, F., Sharma, S., Oconnor, C., & Barrett, E. (2020). Burnout in consultants in child and adolescent mental health services (CAMHS) in Ireland: A cross-sectional study. *BMJ Open*, *10*(1), Article e030354. https://doi.org/10.1136/bmjopen-2019-030354

Meek, C. B. (2004). The dark side of Japanese management in the 1990s: Karoshi and Ijime in Japanese workplace. *Journal of Managerial Psychology*, *19*, 312–331. doi:10.1108/02683940410527775

Mental Health America (2023). *The State of Mental Health in America*. Retrieved October 10, 2023, from https://mhanational.org/issues/state-mental-health-america

Merriam-Webster (2019). Acculturation. In Merriam-Webster.com dictionary. Retrieved October 9, 2019, from https://www.merriam-webster.com/dictionary/acculturation

Merritt, A. (2000). Culture in the cockpit: Do Hofstede's dimensions replicate? *Journal of Cross-Cultural Psychology*, *31*(3), 283–301. https://doi.org/10.1177/0022022100031003001

Mesoudi, A. (2009). The cultural dynamics of copycat suicide. *PLOS ONE*, *4*(9), Article e7252. https://doi.org/10.1371/journal.pone.0007252

Messias, E., & Flynn, V. (2018). The tired, retired, and recovered physicians: Professional burnout versus major depressive disorder. *American Journal of Psychiatry*, *175*(8), 716–719. https://doi.org/10.1176/appi.ajp.2018.17121325

Messina, M. (2016). Soy and health update: Evaluation of the clinical and epidemiologic literature. *Nutrients*, *8*(12), Article 754. https://doi.org/10.3390/nu8120754

Messina, M., & Gleason, C. (2016). Evaluation of the potential antidepressant effects of soybean isoflavones. *Menopause*, *23*(12), 1348–1360. https://doi.org/10.1097/GME.0000000000000709

Meyers, J. (1999). *Hemingway: A biography*. Da Capo.

Midlarsky, E., Pirutinsky, S., & Cohen, F. (2012). Religion, ethnicity, and attitudes toward psychotherapy. Journal of Religion and Health 51(2): 498–506. https://doi.org/10.1007/s10943-012-9599-4

Miki, T., Eguchi, M., Akter, S., Kochi, T., Kuwahara, K., Kashino, I., Hu, H., Kabe, I., Kawakami, N., Nanri, A., & Mizoue, T. (2018). Longitudinal adherence to a dietary pattern and risk of depressive symptoms: The Furukawa Nutrition and Health Study. *Nutrition*, *48*, 48–54. https://doi.org/10.1016/j.nut.2017.10.023

Miller, A. (2008). *The Drama of the Gifted Child: The Search for the True Self*. Basic Books.

Miller, D. (2017). Physician health programs: "Diagnosing for dollars"? *MDEdge/Psychiatry*, December 5. https://www.mdedge.com/psychiatry/article/153573/depression/physician-health-programs-diagnosing-dollars

Miller, J. (2008). The paradox of popular culture & democracy in America. *Salmagundi*, *157*, 138–152.

Miller, L. (2021). The professional struggles of contemporary Korean women: Origins and consequences of the glass ceiling [Master's thesis, University of San Francisco]. *USF Scholarship*. Retrieved July 27, 2021, from https://repository.usfca.edu/cgi/viewcontent.cgi?article=2186&context=capstone

Milloy, C. (2011, July 24). Amy Winehouse's troubles inspired songs—And then killed the songwriter. *Washington Post.* https://www.washingtonpost.com/local/amy-wineho use-another-tragic-victim-of-manic-depression/2011/07/24/gIQAW3FJXI_story. html?utm_term=.b52cde0988f1

Min, K. B., Kim, H. J., Kim, H. J., & Min, J. Y. (2017). Parks and green areas and the risk for depression and suicidal indicators. *International Journal of Public Health, 62*(6), 647–656. https://doi.org/10.1007/s00038-017-0958-5

Min, S. K. (2004). Treatment and prognosis of *hwabyung*. *Psychiatry Investigation, 1,* 29–36.

Min, S. K., & Suh, S. Y. (2010). The anger syndrome *hwa-byung* and its comorbidity. *Journal of Affective Disorders, 124*(1–2), 211–214. https://doi.org/10.1016/j.jad.2009.10.011

Mindful Aviator (n.d.). https://www.mindfulaviator.com/

Mishima, Y. (1958). *Confessions of a Mask* (M. Weatherby, Trans.). New Directions. (Original work published 1949.)

Mishima, Y. (1959). *The Temple of the Golden Pavilion* (I. Morris, Trans.). Alfred A. Knopf. (Original work published 1956.)

Mishima, Y. (1966). *Death in Midsummer and Other Stories* (E. G. Seidensticker, I. Morris, D. Keene, & G. W. Sargent, Trans.). New Directions. (Original work published 1953.)

Mishima, Y. (1968). *Forbidden Colors* (A. H. Marks, Trans.). Knopf (Original work published 1951 [part 1] and 1953 [part 2].)

Mishima, Y., Ito, S., & Takeda, T. (1956). 中央公論新人賞選評 *Chuokoron shinjinsho senpyo* [Chuokoron's new star—Selection and comments]. Chuokoron Publishing.

Mitchell, A. J., Rao, S., & Vaze, A. (2011). Can general practitioners identify people with distress and mild depression? A meta-analysis of clinical accuracy. *Journal of Affective Disorders, 130*(1–2), 26–36. https://doi.org/10.1016/j.jad.2010.07.028

Miura, K., Olsen, C. M., Rea, S., Marsden, J., & Green, A. C. (2019). Do airline pilots and cabin crew have raised risks of melanoma and other skin cancers? Systematic review and meta-analysis. *British Journal of Dermatology, 181*(1), 55–64. https://doi.org/10.1111/bjd.17586

Miyake, Y., Tanaka, K., Okubo, H., Sasaki, S., & Arakawa, M. (2014). Seaweed consumption and prevalence of depressive symptoms during pregnancy in Japan: Baseline data from the Kyushu Okinawa Maternal and Child Health Study. *BMC Pregnancy and Childbirth, 14,* Article 301. https://doi.org/10.1186/1471-2393-14-301

Miyake, Y., Tanaka, K., Okubo, H., Sasaki, S., Furukawa, S., & Arakawa, M. (2018). Soy isoflavone intake and prevalence of depressive symptoms during pregnancy in Japan: Baseline data from the Kyushu Okinawa Maternal and Child Health Study. *European Journal of Nutrition, 57*(2), 441–450. https://doi.org/10.1007/s00 394-016-1327-5

Mo, P., Cheng, Y., & Lau, J. (2020). Work-related factors on mental health among migrant factory workers in China: Application of the Demand–control and effort–reward imbalance model. *Health & Social Care in the Community, 30*(2), 656–667. https://doi.org/10.1111/hsc.13176

Moeini, R., Memariani, Z., Pasalar, P., & Gorji, N. (2017). Historical root of precision medicine: An ancient concept concordant with the modern pharmacotherapy. *Daru: Journal of Faculty of Pharmacy, Tehran University of Medical Sciences, 25*(1), Article 7. https://doi.org/10.1186/s40199-017-0173-1

Moffa, A. H., Brunoni, A. R., Fregni, F., Palm, U., Padberg, F., Blumberger, D. M., Daskalakis, Z. J., Bennabi, D., Haffen, E., Alonzo, A., & Loo, C. K. (2017). Safety and acceptability of transcranial direct current stimulation for the acute treatment of major depressive episodes: Analysis of individual patient data. *Journal of Affective Disorders, 221*, 1–5. https://doi.org/10.1016/j.jad.2017.06.021

Moksony, F., & Hegedűs, R. (2019). Religion and suicide: How culture modifies the effect of social integration. *Archives of Suicide Research, 23*(1), 151–162. https://doi.org/10.1080/13811118.2017.1406830

Möller-Leimkühler, A. M., & Yücel, M. (2010). Male depression in females? Journal of Affective Disorders, 121(1–2), 22–29. https://doi.org/10.1016/j.jad.2009.05.007

Montana Office of Public Instruction (2020). *Montana Indians: Their History and Location*. https://opi.mt.gov/Educators/Teaching-Learning/Indian-Education-for-All/Indian-Education-Curriculum/montana-indian-their-history-location

Montgomery, S. A., & Åsberg, M. (1979). A new depression scale designed to be sensitive to change. *British Journal of Psychiatry, 134*(4), 382–389. https://doi.org/10.1192/bjp.134.4.382

Moon, D. S. (2014). *Acculturation and the Symptoms of hwa-byung among First- and Second-Generation Korean Americans*. [Doctoral dissertation, Wright Institute]. ProQuest Information & Learning.

Moon, S. J., Hwang, J. S., Kim, J. Y., Shin, A. L., Bae, S. M., & Kim, J. W. (2018). Psychometric properties of the Internet Addiction Test: A systematic review and meta-analysis. *Cyberpsychology, Behavior and Social Networking, 21(8)*, 473–484. https://doi.org/10.1089/cyber.2018.0154

Moreno, O., & Cardemil, E. (2018). The role of religious attendance on mental health among Mexican populations: A contribution toward the discussion of the immigrant health paradox. *The American Journal of Orthopsychiatry, 88*(1), 10–15. https://doi.org/10.1037/ort0000214

Morgan, S., Hanley, G., Cunningham, C., & Quan, H. (2011). Ethnic differences in the use of prescription drugs: A cross-sectional analysis of linked survey and administrative data. *Open Medicine, 5*(2), e87–e93.

Mortier, P. Cuijpers, P., Kiekens, G., Auerbach, R. P., Demyttenaere, K., Green, J. G., Kessler, R. C., Nock, M. K., & Bruffaerts, R. (2018). The prevalence of suicidal thoughts and behaviours among college students: A meta-analysis. *Psychological Medicine, 48*(4), 554–565. https://doi.org/10.1017/S0033291717002215

Mosiołek, A., Pięta, A., Jakima, S., Zborowska, N., Mosiołek, J., & Szulc, A. (2021). Effects of antidepressant treatment on peripheral biomarkers in patients with major depressive disorder (MDD). *Journal of Clinical Medicine, 10*(8), Article 1706. https://doi.org/10.3390/jcm10081706

Mosolov, S. N., Ushkalova, A. V., Kostukova, E. G., Shafarenko, A. A., Alfimov, P. V., Kostyukova, A. B., & Angst, J. (2014). Validation of the Russian version of the Hypomania Checklist (HCL-32) for the detection of bipolar II disorder in patients with a current diagnosis of recurrent depression. *Journal of Affective Disorders, 155*, 90–95. https://doi.org/10.1016/j.jad.2013.10.029

Mossakowski, K. N. (2021). Does Japanese identity buffer stress or intensify symptoms of depression associated with discrimination in Hawai'i? *Hawai'i Journal of Health & Social Welfare, 80*(11), 270–275.

Moutier, C. Y., Myers, M. F., Feist, J. B., Feist, J. C., & Zisook, S. (2021). Preventing clinician suicide: A call to action during the COVID-19 pandemic and beyond. *Academic Medicine, 96*(5), 624–628. https://doi.org/10.1097/ACM.0000000000003972

Mrozek, W., Socha, J., Sidorowicz, K., Skrok, A., Syrytczyk, A., Piątkowska-Chmiel, I., & Herbet, M. (2023). Pathogenesis and treatment of depression: Role of diet in prevention and therapy. *Nutrition, 115*, 112143. https://doi.org/10.1016/j.nut.2023.112143

Mueller, M. A. E., Flouri, E., & Kokosi, T. (2019). The role of the physical environment in adolescent mental health. *Health and Place, 58*, Article 102153. https://doi.org/10.1016/j.healthplace.2019.102153

Mulder, S., & de Rooy, D. (2018). Pilot mental health, negative life events, and improving safety with peer support and a just culture. *Aerospace Medicine and Human Performance, 89*(1), 41–51. https://doi.org/10.3357/AMHP.4903.2018

Müller, R., & Schneider, J. (2017). Noise exposure and auditory thresholds of German airline pilots: A cross-sectional study. *BMJ Open, 7*(5), Article e012913. https://doi.org/10.1136/bmjopen-2016-012913

Muntaner, C., Ng, E., Prins, S. J., Bones-Rocha, K., Espelt, A., & Chung, H. (2015). Social class and mental health: Testing exploitation as a relational determinant of depression. *International Journal of Health Services: Planning, Administration, Evaluation, 45*(2), 265–284. https://doi.org/10.1177/0020731414568508

Murakami, M., & Nakai, Y. (2017). Current state and future prospects for psychosomatic medicine in Japan. BioPsychoSocial Medicine 11: 1. https://doi.org/10.1186/s13030-017-0088-6

Muramatsu, K., Miyaoka, H., Kamijima, K., Muramatsu, Y., Tanaka, Y., Hosaka, M., Miwa, Y., Fuse, K., Yoshimine, F., Mashima, I., Shimizu, N., Ito, H., & Shimizu, E. (2018). Performance of the Japanese version of the Patient Health Questionnaire-9 (J-PHQ-9) for depression in primary care. *General Hospital Psychiatry, 52*, 64–69. https://doi.org/10.1016/j.genhosppsych.2018.03.007

Murayama, H., Nishi, M., Matsuo, E., Nofuji, Y., Shimizu, Y., Taniguchi, Y., Fujiwara, Y., & Shinkai, S. (2013). Do bonding and bridging social capital affect self-rated health, depressive mood and cognitive decline in older Japanese? A prospective cohort study. *Social Science & Medicine, 98*, 247–252. https://doi.org/10.1016/j.socscimed.2013.09.026

Murphy, B. (2018). *Specialty Profiles: These medical specialties have the biggest gender imbalances*. American Medical Association. Retrieved November 1, 2021, from https://www.ama-assn.org/residents-students/specialty-profiles/these-medical-specialties-have-biggest-gender-imbalances

Muse (2023). Discover Muse. http://choosemuse.com

Musu-Gillette, L., de Brey, C., McFarland, J., Hussar, W., Sonnenberg, W., & Wilkinson-Flicker, S. (2017). *Status and Trends in the Education of Racial and Ethnic Groups 2017* (NCES 2017-051). US Department of Education, National Center for Education Statistics. Retrieved September 30, 2019, from https://nces.ed.gov/pubs2017/2017051.pdf

Mutz, J., Edgcumbe, D. R., Brunoni, A. R., & Fu, C. H. Y. (2018). Efficacy and acceptability of non-invasive brain stimulation for the treatment of adult unipolar and bipolar depression: A systematic review and meta-analysis of randomised sham-controlled trials. *Neuroscience and Biobehavioral Reviews, 92*, 291–303. https://doi.org/10.1016/j.neubiorev.2018.05.015

Myers, I., & McCaulley, M. (1985). *Manual: A Guide to the Development and Use of the Myers-Briggs Type Indicator*. Consulting Psychologists.

Na, P. J., Kim, K. B., Lee-Tauler, S. Y., Han, H. R., Kim, M. T., & Lee, H. B. (2017). Predictors of suicidal ideation in Korean American older adults: analysis of the Memory and Aging

Study of Koreans (MASK). *International Journal of Geriatric Psychiatry*, *32*(12), 1272–1279. https://doi.org/10.1002/gps.4608

Nagata, D. K., Kim, J., & Wu, K. (2019). The Japanese American wartime incarceration: Examining the scope of racial trauma. *The American Psychologist*, *74*(1), 36–48. https://doi.org/10.1037/amp0000303

Naito, S. (2013). *Workplace Bullying in Japan*. Japan Institute for Labor Policy and Training. https://www.jil.go.jp/english/reports/documents/jilpt-reports/no.12.pdf#page=119. Retrieved January 7, 2021.

Nakamine, S., Tachikawa, H., Aiba, M., Takahashi, S., Noguchi, H., Takahashi, H., & Tamiya, N. (2017). Changes in social capital and depressive states of middle-aged adults in Japan. *PLOS ONE*, *12*(12), e0189112.

Nam, S. I., & Lincoln, K. D. (2017). Lifetime family violence and depression: The case of older women in Korea. *Journal of Family Violence*, *32*(3), 269–278. https://doi.org/10.1007/s10896-016-9844-9

Nanau, R. M., & Neuman, M. G. (2015). Biomolecules and biomarkers used in diagnosis of alcohol drinking and in monitoring therapeutic interventions. *Biomolecules*, *5*(3), 1339–1385. https://doi.org/10.3390/biom5031339

Nanri, A., Kimury, Y., Matsushita, Y., Ohta, M., Sato, M., Mishima, N., Sasaki, S., & Mizoue, T. (2010). Dietary patterns and depressive symptoms among Japanese men and women. *European Journal of Clinical Nutrition*, *64*(8), 832–839. https://doi.org/10.1038/ejcn.2010.86

Nassauer, S. (2022). Walmart dangles $110,000 starting pay to lure truck drivers. *Wall Street Journal* April 7, 2022. https://www.wsj.com/articles/walmart-raises-pay-to-attract-truck-drivers-11649336400

Nasseri, K., & Moulton, L. (2009). Patterns of death in the first and second generation immigrants from selected Middle Eastern countries in California. *Journal of Immigrant and Minority Health*, *13*, 361–370. https://doi.org/10.1007/s10903-009-9270-7

National Cancer Institute (2021). *Alcohol and Cancer Risk*. Retrieved August 16, 2021, from https://www.cancer.gov/about-cancer/causes-prevention/risk/alcohol/alcohol-fact-sheet

National Center for Education Statistics (2021). *Program for the International Assessment of Adult Competencies. U.S. State and County Estimates*. Retrieved July 4, 2021, from https://nces.ed.gov/surveys/piaac/state-county-estimates.asp

National Center for Health Statistics (2023). Depressive disorder. *The International Classification of Diseases, Tenth Revision, Clinical Modification (ICD-10-CM)*. https://www.cdc.gov/nchs/icd/icd-10-cm.htm. March 31, 2023.

National Committee on Aging, National Committee for Emotional Care Programs, & China Women's Federation Aging Coordination Office (2012). The New 24 Exemplars. https://baike.baidu.hk/item/%E6%96%B0%E4%BA%8C%E5%8D%81%E5%9B%9B%E5%AD%9D/920299

National Institute for Occupational Safety and Health (2019a). *Epworth Sleepiness Scale*. Retrieved July 17, 2021, from https://www.cdc.gov/niosh/work-hour-training-for-nurses/02/epworth.pdf

National Institute for Occupational Safety and Health (2019b). *National Occupational Mortality Surveillance (NOMS)*. Retrieved September 1, 2019, from https://wwwn.cdc.gov/niosh-noms/occupation2.aspx

National Institute of Mental Health (2021). *Research Domain Criteria (RDoC)*. Retrieved November 1, 2021, from https://www.nimh.nih.gov/research/research-funded-by-nimh/rdoc

National Library of Medicine (2019). *Shakespeare and the Four Humors*. https://www.nlm.nih.gov/exhibition/shakespeare/fourhumors.html

National Occupational Mortality Surveillance (2019). *PMR Query System*. https://www.cdc.gov/niosh/topics/noms/query.html

National Vital Statistics System (2019). *National Marriage and Divorce Rate Trends for 2000-2017*. Retrieved October 1, 2019, from https://www.cdc.gov/nchs/nvss/marriage-divorce.htm

Nazerian, R., Korhan, O., & Shakeri, E. (2020). Work-related musculoskeletal discomfort among heavy truck drivers. *International Journal of Occupational Safety and Ergonomics, 26*(2), 233-244. https://doi.org/10.1080/10803548.2018.1433107

Ndjaboué, R., Brisson, C., & Vézina, M. (2012). Organisational justice and mental health: A systematic review of prospective studies. *Occupational and Environmental Medicine, 69*(10), 694-700. https://doi.org/10.1136/oemed-2011-100595

Neill, U. S. (2005). Tom Cruise is dangerous and irresponsible. *The Journal of Clinical Investigation, 115*(8), 1964-1965. https://doi.org/10.1172/JCI26200

Nelson, C. A., Scott, R. D., Bhutta, Z. A., Harris, N. B., Danese, A., & Samara, M. (2020). Adversity in childhood is linked to mental and physical health throughout life. *BMJ (Clinical Research Ed.), 371*, Article m3048. https://doi.org/10.1136/bmj.m3048

Neroien, A., & Chei, B. (2008). Partner violence and health: Results from the first national study on violence against women in Norway. *Scandinavian Journal of Public Health, 36*(2), 161-168. https://doi.org/10.1177/1403494807085188

Newman, R. (1972). Lonely at the top. On *Sail Away*. Warner Bros.

Ng, Q. X., Venkatanarayanan, N., & Ho, C. Y. X. (2017). Clinical use of *Hypericum perforatum* (St John's wort) in depression: A meta-analysis. *Journal of Affective Disorders, 210*, 211-221.

Ng, X., Koh, S. S., Chan, H. W., & Ho, C. Y. X. (2017). Clinical use of curcumin in depression: A meta-analysis. *JAMDA, 18*, 503-508. https://doi.org/10.1016/j.jamda.2016.12.071

Ngomsi, V. (2018, September 14). Mariah Carey has a reported net worth of $520 million—Here's how the pop singer earned it all. *Business Insider*. https://www.businessinsider.com/mariah-careys-net-worth-2018-9?r=UK

Nie, J. B., Li, L., Gillett, G., Tucker, J. D., & Kleinman, A. (2018). The crisis of patient-physician trust and bioethics: lessons and inspirations from China. *Developing World Bioethics* 18(1): 56–64. https://doi.org/10.1111/dewb.12169

Niederkrotenthaler, T., Till, B., Kapusta, N. D., Voracek, M., Dervic, K., & Sonneck, G. (2009). Copycat effects after media reports on suicide: A population-based ecologic study. *Social Science & Medicine, 69*(7), 1085-1090. https://doi.org/10.1016/j.socscimed.2009.07.041

Niedhammer, I., Bertrais, S., & Witt, K. (2021a). Psychosocial work exposures and health outcomes: a meta-review of 72 literature reviews with meta-analysis. *Scandinavian Journal of Work, Environment & Health, 47*(7), 489-508. https://doi.org/10.5271/sjweh.3968

Niedhammer, I., Sultan-Taïeb, H., Parent-Thirion, A., & Chastang, J. F. (2021b). Update of the fractions of cardiovascular diseases and mental disorders attributable to psychosocial work factors in Europe. *International Archives of Occupational and Environmental Health*, *95*, 233–247. https://doi.org/10.1007/s00420-021-01737-4

Nippon Hōsō Kyōkai. (2010). "Muen Shakai: 32,000 'Muenshi' no Shougeki" [The No-relationship Society: The Shock of 32,000 Solitary Deaths]. *Television Documentary Aired* January 31, 2010.

Nippon.com (2022, June 17). Survey finds 40% of Japanese men in their twenties have never dated. *Nippon.com*. https://www.nippon.com/en/japan-data/h01361/

Nippon.com (2023, October 11). No vacation: Less than 20% of Japanese workers take full paid leave. *Nippon.com*. https://www.nippon.com/en/japan-data/h01798/?cx_recs_click=true

Nishitani, N., Kawasaki, Y., & Sakakibara, H. (2019). Insomnia affects future development of depression in workers: A 6-year cohort study. *Nagoya Journal of Medical Science*, *81*(4), 637–645. https://doi.org/10.18999/nagjms.81.4.637

Nishitani, N., & Sakakibara, H. (2010). Job stress factors, stress response, and social support in association with insomnia of Japanese male workers. *Industrial Health, 48(2)*, 178–184. https://doi.org/10.2486/indhealth.48.178

Nissly, T., & Levy, R. (2018). Buprenorphine to treat opioid use disorder: A practical guide. *The Journal of Family Practice*, *67*(9), 544–548.

Nitobe, I. (1900). *Bushido: the soul of Japan: an exposition of Japanese thought*. Philadelphia: Leeds & Biddle.

Niu, L., He, J., Cheng, C., Yi, J., Wang, X., & Yao, S. (2021). Factor structure and measurement invariance of the Chinese version of the Center for Epidemiological Studies Depression (CES-D) scale among undergraduates and clinical patients. *BMC Psychiatry*, *21*(1), Article 463. https://doi.org/10.1186/s12888-021-03474-x

Niu, L., Hoyt, L. T., Shane, J., & Storch, E. A. (2023). Associations between subjective social status and psychological well-being among college students. Journal of American College Health 71(7): 2044–2051. https://doi.org/10.1080/07448481.2021.1954010

Nolan, C. (Director). (2008). *The Dark* [Film]. Warner Bros.

Nomura, K., Yamazaki, Y., Gruppen, L. D., Horie, S., Takeuchi, M., & Illing, J. (2015). The difficulty of professional continuation among female doctors in Japan: A qualitative study of alumnae of 13 medical schools in Japan. *BMJ Open*, *5*(3), Article e005845. https://doi.org/10.1136/bmjopen-2014-005845

Nordberg, J. (2017, December 15). Yes, it happens in Sweden, #Too. *New York Times*. https://www.nytimes.com/2017/12/15/opinion/sunday/sweden-sexual-harassment-assault.html.

Nordic Council of Ministers (2004). *Nordic Nutrition Recommendations 2004 Integrating Nutrition and Physical Activity, 4th edition*. Nordic Council of Ministers.

North, A. C., & Sheridan, L. P. (2009). Death, attractiveness, moral conduct, and attitudes to public figures. *Omega*, *60*(4), 351–363. https://doi.org/10.2190/om.60.4.c

Norton, M. C., Singh, A., Skoog, I., Corcoran, C., Tschanz, J. T., Zandi, P. P., Breitner, J. C. S., Welsh-Bohmer, K. A., & Steffens, D. C.; for the Cache County Investigators. (2008). Church attendance and new episodes of major depression in a community study of older adults: The Cache County Study. *The Journals of Gerontology. Series B, Psychological Sciences and Social Sciences*, *63*(3), 129–137. https://doi.org/10.1093/geronb/63.3.p129

Nowakowski, S., Choi, H., Meers, J., & Temple, J. R. (2016). Inadequate sleep as a mediating variable between exposure to interparental violence and depression severity in adolescents. *Journal of Child & Adolescent Trauma, 9*(2), 109–114. https://doi.org/10.1007/s40653-016-0091-2

Nuñez, A., González, P., Talavera, G. A., Sanchez-Johnsen, L., Roesch, S. C., Davis, S. M., Arguelles, W., Womack, V. Y., Ostrovsky, N. W., Ojeda, L., Penedo, F. J., & Gallo, L. C. (2016). Machismo, marianismo, and negative cognitive-emotional factors: Findings from the Hispanic Community Health Study/Study of Latinos Sociocultural Ancillary Study. *Journal of Latina/o Psychology, 4*(4), 202–217. https://doi.org//10.1037/lat0000050

Nussbaumer-Streit, B., Forneris, C. A., Morgan, L. C., Van Noord, M. G., Gaynes, B. N., Greenblatt, A., Wipplinger, J., Lux, L. J., Winkler, D., & Gartlehner, G. (2019). Light therapy for preventing seasonal affective disorder. *The Cochrane Database of Systematic Reviews, 3*(3), CD011269. https://doi.org/10.1002/14651858.CD011269.pub3

O'Brien, B., Shrestha, S., Stanley, M. A., Pargament, K. I., Cummings, J., Kunik, M. E., Fletcher, T. L., Cortes, J., Ramsey, D., & Amspoker, A. B. (2019). Positive and negative religious coping as predictors of distress among minority older adults. *International Journal of Geriatric Psychiatry, 34*(1), 54–59. https://doi.org/10.1002/gps.4983

O'Dea, B., Larsen, M. E., Batterham, P. J., Calear, A. L., & Christensen, H. (2017). A linguistic analysis of suicide-related Twitter posts. *Crisis, 38*(5), 319–329. https://doi.org/10.1027/0227-5910/a000443

OECD (2023). *Data Explorer*. https://data-explorer.oecd.org [Details of queries provided in footnotes to tables.]

OECD (2023a). Share of births outside of marriage, and childlessness. *OECD Family Database*. Retrieved October 1, 2023, from https://www.oecd.org/els/family/SF_2_4_Share_births_outside_marriage.pdf. and https://www.oecd.org/els/family/SF_2-5-Childlessness.pdf

OECD (2023b). Age-standardized prevalence of diabetes in adults aged over 18. *Health at a Glance 2021: OECD Indicators*, p. 95. OECD iLibrary. Retrieved October 3, 2023, from https://www.oecdilibrary.org

OECD (2023c). Pharmaceutical consumption. *Health at a Glance 2021: OECD Indicators*, p. 240. *OECD iLibrary*. Retrieved October 3, 2023, from https://www.oecd-ilibrary.org.

Oh, K. M., Baird, B., Alqahtani, N., Peppard, L., & Kitsantas, P. (2022). Exploring levels and correlates of depression literacy among older Korean immigrants. *Journal of Cross-cultural Gerontology, 37*(3), 295–313. https://doi.org/10.1007/s10823-022-09461-3

Okuda, M., Olfson, M., Hasin, D., Grant, B. F., Lin, K.-H., & Blanco, C. 2011). Mental health of victims of intimate partner violence: Results from a national epidemiologic survey. *Psychiatric Services, 62*(8), 959–962. https://doi.org/10.1176/ps.62.8.pss6208_0959

Oliff, H. (2017). Graduation rates & American Indian education. *Partnership with Native Americans*. Retrieved September 30, 2019, from http://blog.nativepartnership.org/graduation-rates-american-indian-education/

Oliffe, J. L., Ogrodniczuk, J. S., Gordon, S. J., Creighton, G., Kelly, M. T., Black, N., & Mackenzie, C. (2016). Stigma in male depression and suicide: A Canadian sex comparison study. *Community Mental Health Journal, 52*(3), 302–310. https://doi.org/10.1007/s10597-015-9986-x

Oliffe, J. L., Rossnagel, E., Seidler, Z. E., Kealy, D., Ogrodniczuk, J. S., & Rice, S. M. (2019). Men's depression and suicide. *Current Psychiatry Reports, 21*(10), Article 103. https://doi.org/10.1007/s11920-019-1088-y

Oliveira, D. F. M., Ma, Y., Woodruff, T. K., & Uzzi, B. (2019). Comparison of National Institutes of Health grant amounts to first-time male and female principal investigators. *JAMA, 321*(9), 898–900. https://doi.org/10.1001/jama.2018.21944

Ollove, M. (2018, December 20). Medicaid expansion defeat offers lessons for other states. *Governing*. Retrieved September 28, 2019, from https://www.governing.com/topics/health-human-services/sl-montana-medicaid-expansion-defeat.html

Olson, K. D. (2017). Physician burnout—A leading indicator of health system performance. *Mayo Clinic Proceedings, 92*(11), 1608–1611. https://doi.org/10.1016/j.mayocp.2017.09.008

Omrani, A., Holtzman, N. S., Akiskal, H. S., & Ghaemi, S. N. (2012). Ibn Imran's 10th century Treatise on Melancholy. *Journal of Affective Disorders, 141*(2-3), 116–119. https://doi.org/10.1016/j.jad.2012.02.004

Opie, R. S., Itsiopoulos, C., Parletta, N., Sanchez-Villegas, A., Akbaraly, T. N., Ruusunen, A., & Jacka, F. N. (2016). Dietary recommendations for the prevention of depression. *Nutritional Neuroscience, 20*(3), 161–171. https://doi.org/10.1179/1476830515Y.0000000043

Oquendo, M. A., Bernstein, C. A., & Mayer, L. E. S. (2019). A key differential diagnosis for physicians—Major depression or burnout. *JAMA Psychiatry, 76*(11), 1111–1112. https://doi.org/10.1001/jamapsychiatry.2019.1332

Orban, E., McDonald, K., Sutcliffe, R., Hoffmann, B., Fuks, K. B., Dragano, N., Viehmann, A., Erbel, R., Jockel, K.-H., Pundt, N., & Moebus, S. (2016). Residential road traffic noise and high depressive symptoms after five years of follow-up: Results from the Heinz Nixdorf Recall Study. *Environmental Health Perspectives, 124*(5), 578–585. https://doi.org/10.1289/ehp.1409400

Oreskovich, M. R., Shanafelt, T., Dyrbye, L. N., Tan, L., Sotile, W., Satele, D., West, C. P., Sloan, J., & Boone, S. (2015). The prevalence of substance use disorders in American physicians. *American Journal of Addictions, 24*(1), 30–38. https://doi.org/10.1111/ajad.12173

Organisation for Economic Co-operation and Development (2023). *Income Distribution Database by Country*. https://stats.oecd.org

Osuka, Y., Nishimura, T., Wakuta, M., Takei, N., & Tsuchiya, K. J. (2019). Reliability and validity of the Japan Ijime Scale and estimated prevalence of bullying among fourth through ninth graders: A large-scale school-based survey. *Psychiatry and Clinical Neurosciences, 73*(9), 551–559. https://doi.org/10.1111/pcn.1286

Owens, J. A., & Weiss, M. R. (2017). Insufficient sleep in adolescents: Causes and consequences. *Minerva Pediatrics, 69*(4), 326–336. https://doi.org/10.23736/S0026-4946.17.04914-3

Oxford University Press (n.d.). Acculturation. *Oxford English Dictionary online*. Retrieved June 30, 2023, from www.oed.com.

Oxford University Press (n.d.). Culture. *Oxford English Dictionary*. www.oed.com. Retrieved September 30, 2018.

Ozawa-de Silva, C. (2008). Too lonely to die alone: Internet suicide pacts and existential suffering in Japan. *Culture, Medicine and Psychiatry, 32*(4), 516–551. https://doi.org/10.1007/s11013-008-9108-0

Page, A., Liu, S., Gunnell, D., Astell-Burt, T., Feng, X., Wang, L., & Zhou, M. (2017). Suicide by pesticide poisoning remains a priority for suicide prevention in China: Analysis of national mortality trends 2006–2013. *Journal of Affective Disorders, 208,* 418–423. https://doi.org/10.1016/j.jad.2016.10.047

Pagliai, G., Sofi, F., Vannetti, F., Caiani, S., Pasquini, G., Molino Lova, R., Cecchi, F., Sorbi, S., Macchi, C., & Mugello Study Working Group. (2018). Mediterranean diet, food consumption and risk of late-life depression: The Mugello study. *Journal of Nutrition, Health and Aging, 22*(5), 569–574. https://doi.org/10.1007/s12603-018-1019-3

Paik, J. S., Lee, J. H., Uppal, S., & Choi, W. C. (2020). Intricacies of upper blepharoplasty in Asian burden lids. *Facial Plastic Surgery, 36*(5), 563–574. https://doi.org/10.1055/s-0040-1718391

Pan, X.,-F., Wen, Y., Zhao, Y., Hu, J,-M., Li, S,-Q., Zhang, S.-K., Li, X.-Y., Chang, H., Xue, Q.-P., Zhao, Z.-M., Gu, Y., Li, C.-C., Zhang, Y.-Q., Sun, X.-W., Yang, C.-X., & Fu, C. (2016). Prevalence of depressive symptoms and its correlates among medical students in China: A national survey in 33 universities. *Psychology, Health and Medicine, 21*(7), 882–889.

Pang, K. Y. C. (2000). Symptom expression and somatization among elderly Korean immigrants. *Journal of Clinical Geropsychology, 6*(3), 199–212. https://doi.org/10.1023/A:1009541200013

Pargament, K., Feuille, M., & Burdzy, D. (2011). The Brief RCOPE: Current psychometric status of a short measure of religious coping. *Religions, 2,* 51–76.

Pargament, K. I., Koenig, H. G., & Perez, L. M. (2000). The many methods of religious coping: development and initial validation of the RCOPE. *Journal of Clinical Psychology, 56*(4), 519–543. https://doi.org/10.1002/(sici)1097-4679(200004)56:4<519::aid-jclp6>3.0.co;2-1

ParityTrack.org. (2021). *State parity implementation survey.* Retrieved July 10, 2021, from www.paritytrack.org/reports

Park, B., Cho, H. N., Choi, E., Seo, D. H., Kim, S., Park, Y.-R., Choi, K. S., & Rhee, Y. (2019). Self-perceptions of body weight status according to age-groups among Korean women: A nationwide population-based survey. *PLOS ONE 14*(1), Article e0210486. https://doi.org/10.1371/journal.pone.0210486

Park, C. L., Holt, C. L., Le, D., Christie, J., & Williams, B. R. (2018). Positive and negative religious coping styles as prospective predictors of well-being in African Americans. *Psychology of Religion and Spirituality, 10*(4), 318–326. https://doi.org/10.1037/rel0000124

Park, G. R., Park, E. J., Jun, J., & Kim, N. S. (2017). Association between intimate partner violence and mental health among Korean married women. *Public Health, 152,* 86–94. https://doi.org/10.1016/j.puhe.2017.07.023

Park, H., & Kang, M. Y. (2016). Effects of voluntary/involuntary retirement on their own and spouses' depressive symptoms. *Comprehensive Psychiatry, 66,* 1–8. https://doi.org/10.1016/j.comppsych.2015.11.009

Park, M. (2017, December 7). 8 ways the LDS church addresses mental illnesses. *The Daily Universe.* Retrieved September 28, 2019, from https://universe.byu.edu/2017/12/07/8-ways-the-lds-church-addresses-mental-illnesses/

Park, M., Choi, J., & Lee, H. J. (2020). Flavonoid-rich orange juice intake and altered gut microbiome in young adults with depressive symptom: A randomized controlled study. *Nutrients, 12*(6), Article 1815. https://doi.org/10.3390/nu12061815

Park, N. S., Jang, Y., & Chiriboga, D. A. (2018). Willingness to use mental health counseling and antidepressants in older Korean Americans: The role of beliefs and stigma about depression. *Ethnicity & Health*, *23*(1), 97–110. https://doi.org/10.1080/13557 858.2016.1246429

Park, S., Kim, M. J., Cho, M. J., & Lee, J. Y. (2015). Factors affecting stigma toward suicide and depression: A Korean nationwide study. *The International Journal of Social Psychiatry*, *61*(8), 811–817. https://doi.org/10.1177/0020764015597015

Park, S. I., Cho, Y. G., Kang, J. H., Park, H. A., Kim, K. W., Hur, Y. I., & Kang, H. J. (2013). Sociodemographic characteristics of underweight Korean adults: Korea Nnational Health and Nutrition Examination Survey, 2007-2010. *Korean Journal of Family Medicine*, *34*(6), 385–392. https://doi.org/10.4082/kjfm.2013.34.6.385

Park, Y. J., Kim, H. S., Schwartz-Barcott, D., & Kim, J. W. (2002). The conceptual structure of hwa-byung in middle-aged Korean women. *Health Care for Women International*, *23*(4), 389–397. https://doi.org/10.1080/0739933029008955

Park, K., & Hsieh, N. (2023). A National study on religiosity and suicide risk by sexual orientation. *American Journal of Preventive Medicine*, *64*(2), 235–243. https://doi.org/10.1016/j.amepre.2022.08.020

Parker, G. (2018). The benefits of antidepressants: News or fake news? *British Journal of Psychiatry*, *213*(2), 454–455.

Parker, G., Chan, B., Tully, L., & Eisenbruch, M. (2005). Depression in the Chinese: The impact of acculturation. *Psychological Medicine*, *35*(10), 1475–1483. https://doi.org/10.1017/S0033291705005623

Parker, G. B., Brotchie, H., & Graham, R. K. (2017). Vitamin D and depression. *Journal of Affective Disorders*, *208*, 56–61. https://doi.org/10.1016/j.jad.2016.08.082

Parker, S. (2011). *Balancing act: Regulation of civilian firearms*. In Small Arms Survey 2011. Graduate Institute of International and Development Studies.

Parletta, N., Zarowiecki, D., Cho, J., Wilson, A., Bogomolova, S., Vilani, A., Itsiopoulos, C., Niyonsenga, T., Blunden, S., Meyer, B., Segal, L., Baune, B. T., & O'Dea, K. (2017). A Mediterranean-style dietary intervention supplemented with fish oil improves diet quality and mental health in people with depression: A randomized controlled trial (HELFIMED). *Nutritional Neuroscience*, *22*(7), 474–487. https://doi.org/10.1080/10284 15X.2017.1411320

Paruthi, S., Brooks, L. J., D'Ambrosio, C., Hall, W. A., Kotagal, S., Lloyd, R. M., Malow, B. A., Maski, K., Nichols, C., Quan, S. F., Rosen, C. L., Troester, M. M., & Wise, M. S. (2016). Recommended amount of sleep for pediatric populations: A consensus statement of the American Academy of Sleep Medicine. *Journal of Clinical Sleep Medicine*, *12*(6), 785–786. https://doi.org/10.5664/jcsm.5866

Parvez, M. K., & Richi, V. (2019). Herb–drug interactions and hepatotoxicity. *Current Drug Metabolism*, *20*(4), 275–282. https://doi.org/10.2174/1389200220666190325141422

Pasha, T., & Stokes, P. (2018). Reflecting on the Germanwings disaster: A systematic review of depression and suicide in commercial airline pilots. *Frontiers in Psychiatry*, *9*, Article 86. https://doi.org/10.3389/fpsyt.2018.00086

Patel, R. S., Virani, S., Saeed, H., Nimmagadda, S., Talukdar, J., & Youssef, N. A. (2018). Gender differences and comorbidities in U.S. adults with bipolar disorder. *Brain Sciences*, *8*(9), Article 168. https://doi.org/10.3390/brainsci8090168

Patel, V., Burns, J. K., Dhingra, M., Tarver, L., Kohrt, B. A., & Lund, C. (2018). Income inequality and depression: A systematic review and meta-analysis of the association and a scoping review of mechanisms. *World Psychiatry, 17*(1), 76–89. https://doi.org/10.1002/wps.20492

Payne, K. K. (2019). Median age at first marriage: Geographic variation, 2017. *National Center for Family & Marriage Research*, family profile number 7. https://www.bgsu.edu/ncfmr/resources/data/family-profiles/payne-median-age-first-marriage-geo-fp-19-07.html

Pearce, M. J., Koenig, H. G., Robins, C. J., Nelson, B., Shaw, S. F., Cohen, H. J., & King, M. B. (2015). Religiously integrated cognitive behavioral therapy: A new method of treatment for major depression in patients with chronic medical illness. *Psychotherapy, 52*(1), 56–66. https://doi.org/10.1037/a0036448

Pearce, N., & Davey Smith, G. (2003). Is social capital the key to inequalities in health? *American Journal of Public Health, 93*(1), 122–129. https://doi.org/10.2105/ajph.93.1.122

Peckham, C. (2018). *Medscape national physician burnout & depression report 2018*. https://www.medscape.com/slideshow/2018-lifestyle-burnout-depression-6009235. Retrieved August 31, 2019.

Pedersen, E. R., & Paves, A. P. (2014). Comparing perceived public stigma and personal stigma of mental health treatment seeking in a young adult sample. *Psychiatry Research, 219*(1), 143–150. https://doi.org/10.1016/j.psychres.2014.05.017

Peen, J., Schoevers, R. A., Beekman, A. T., & Dekker, J. (2010). The current status of urban–rural differences in psychiatric disorders. *Acta Psychiatrica Scandinavica, 121*, 84–93. https://doi.org/10.1111/j.1600-0447.2009.01438.x

Peer, S. O., & McGraw, J. S. (2017). Mixed-method study of perfectionism and religiosity among Mormons: Implications for cultural competence and clinical practice. *Issues in Religion and Psychotherapy, 38*(1), Article 12. https://scholarsarchive.byu.edu/irp/vol38/iss1/12

Pelacchi, F., Dell'Osso, L., Bondi, E., Amore, M., Fagiolini, A., Iazzetta, P., Pierucci, D., Gorini, M., Quarchioni, E., Comandini, A., Salvatori, E., Cattaneo, A., Pompili, M., & SALT Study Group. (2022). Clinical evaluation of switching from immediate-release to prolonged-release lithium in bipolar patients, poorly tolerant to lithium immediate-release treatment: A randomized clinical trial. *Brain and Behavior, 12*(3), e2485. https://doi.org/10.1002/brb3.2485

Peña, J., B., Wyman, P. A., Brown, C. H., Matthieu, M. M., Olivares, T. E., Harte, D., & Zayas, L. H. (2008). Immigration generation status and its association with suicide attempts, substance use, and depressive symptoms among Latino adolescents in the USA. *Prevention Science, 9*(4), 299–310. https://doi.org/10.1007/s11121-008-0105-x

Penders, T. M., Stanciu, C. N., Schoemann, A. M., Ninan, P. T., Bloch, R., & Saeed, S. A. (2016). Bright light therapy as augmentation of pharmacotherapy for treatment of depression: A systematic review and meta-analysis. *The Primary Care Companion for CNS Disorders, 18*(5). https://doi.org/10.4088/PCC.15r01906

Perera, S., Eisen, R., Bhatt, M., Bhatnagar, N., de Souza, R., Thabane, L., & Samaan, Z. (2016). Light therapy for non-seasonal depression: Systematic review and meta-analysis. *BJPsych Open, 2*(2), 116–126. https://doi.org/10.1192/bjpo.bp.115.001610

Perreira, K. M., Marchante, A. N., Schwartz, S. J., Isasi, C. R., Carnethon, M. R., Corliss, H. L., Kaplan, R. C., Santisteban, D. A., Vidot, D. C., Van Horn, L., & Delamater, A. M.

(2019). Stress and resilience: Key correlates of mental health and substance use in the Hispanic Community Health Study of Latino Youth. *Journal of Immigrant and Minority Health, 21*(1), 4–13. https://doi.org/10.1007/s10903-018-0724-7

Petersen, M. R., & Burnett, C. A. (2008). The suicide mortality of working physicians and dentists. *Occupational Medicine, 58*(1), 25–29. https://doi.org/10.1093/occmed/kqm117

Peterson, C., Stone, D. M., Marsh, S. M., Schumacher, P. K., Tiesman, H. M., McIntosh, W. L., Lokey, C. N., Trudeau, A.-R. T., Bartholow, B., & Luo, F. (2018). Suicide rates by major occupational group—17 states, 2012 and 2015. *MMWR Morbidity and Mortality Weekly Report, 67*, 1253–1260. https://doi.org/10.15585/mmwr.mm6745a1

Petkus, A. J., Resnick, S. M., Wang, X., Beavers, D. P., Espeland, M. A., Gatz, M., Gruenewald, T., Millstein, J., Chui, H. C., Kaufman, J. D., Manson, J. E., Wellenius, G. A., Whitsel, E. A., Widaman, K., Younan, D., & Chen, J. C. (2022). Ambient air pollution exposure and increasing depressive symptoms in older women: The mediating role of the prefrontal cortex and insula. *The Science of the Total Environment, 823*, 153642. https://doi.org/10.1016/j.scitotenv.2022.153642

Pew Research Center (2018). *Religious Landscape Study*. Retrieved August 5, 2018, from http://www.pewforum.org/religious-landscape-study/

Phelps, J. R., & Ghaemi, S. N. (2006). Improving the diagnosis of bipolar disorder: Predictive value of screening tests. *Journal of Affective Disorders, 92*(2–3), 141–148. https://doi.org/10.1016/j.jad.2006.01.029

Phelps, J. R., & James, J. (2017). Psychiatric consultation in the collaborative care model: The "bipolar sieve" effect. *Medical Hypotheses, 105*, 10–16. https://doi.org/10.1016/j.mehy.2017.06.017

Phillips, J. P. (2016). Workplace violence against health care workers in the U.S. *New England Journal of Medicine, 374*(17), 1661–1669. https://doi.org/10.1056/NEJMra1501998

Phillips, M. R., Yang, G., Zhang, Y., Wang, L., Ji, H., & Zhou, M. (2002). Risk factors for suicide in China: A national case–control psychological autopsy study. *Lancet, 360*, 1728–1736.

Pies, R. (1997). Maimonides and the origins of cognitive-behavioral therapy. *Journal of Cognitive Psychotherapy, 11*, 21–36.

Pies, R. (2007). The historical roots of the "bipolar spectrum": Did Aristotle anticipate Kraeplin's broad concept of manic-depression? *Journal of Affective Disorders, 100*, 7–11.

Pilger, A., Haslacher, H., Meyer, B. M., Lackner, A., Nassan-Agha, S., Nistler, S., Stangelmaier, C., Endler, G., Mikulits, A., Priemer, I., Ratzinger, F., Ponocny-Seliger, E., Wohlschlager-Krenn, E., Teufelhart, M., Tauber, H., Scherzer, T. M., Perkmann, T., Jordakieva, G., Pezawas, L., & Winker, R. (2018). Midday and nadir salivary cortisol appear superior to cortisol awakening response in burnout assessment and monitoring. *Scientific Reports, 8*(1), Article 9151. https://doi.org/10.1038/s41598-018-27386-1

Piven, J. (2004). *The Madness and Perversion of Yukio Mishima*. Praeger.

Poletti, S., Vai, B., Mazza, M. G., Zanardi, R., Lorenzi, C., Calesella, F., Cazzetta, S., Branchi, I., Colombo, C., Furlan, R., & Benedetti, F. (2021). A peripheral inflammatory signature discriminates bipolar from unipolar depression: A machine learning approach. *Progress* in *Neuro-Psychopharmacology & Biological Psychiatry, 105*, Article 110136. https://doi.org/10.1016/j.pnpbp.2020.110136

Pompeii, L. A., Schoenfisch, A. L., Lipscomb, H. J., Dement, J. M., Smith, C. D., & Upadhyaya, M. (2015). Physical assault, physical threat, and verbal abuse perpetrated against hospital workers by patients or visitors in six U. S. hospitals. *American Journal of Industrial Medicine, 58*(11), 1194–1204. https://doi.org/10.1002/ajim.22489

Pompili, M., Innamorati, M., Lamis, D. A., Erbuto, D., Venturini, P., Ricci, F., Serafini, G., Amore, M., & Girardi, P. (2014). The associations among childhood maltreatment, "male depression" and suicide risk in psychiatric patients. *Psychiatry Research, 220*(1–2), 571–578. https://doi.org/10.1016/j.psychres.2014.07.056

Posner, B. (2017, July 14). Chopra: Michael Jackson could have been saved. *Daily Beast.* https://www.thedailybeast.com/chopra-michael-jackson-could-have-been-saved

Post, F. (1996). Verbal creativity, depression and alcoholism. *British Journal of Psychiatry, 168*, 545–555.

Powers, A., Woods-Jaeger, B., Stevens, J. S., Bradley, B., Patel, M. B., Joyner, A., Smith, A. K., Jamieson, D. J., Kaslow, N., & Michopoulos, V. (2020). Trauma, psychiatric disorders, and treatment history among pregnant African American women. Psychological Trauma : Theory, Research, Practice and Policy, 12(2), 138–146. https://doi.org/10.1037/tra0000507

Prasad, F., De, R., Korann, V., Chintoh, A. F., Remington, G., Ebdrup, B. H., Siskind, D., Knop, F. K., Vilsbøll, T., Fink-Jensen, A., Hahn, M. K., & Agarwal, S. M. (2023). Semaglutide for the treatment of antipsychotic-associated weight gain in patients not responding to metformin—A case series. *Therapeutic Advances in Psychopharmacology, 13*, 20451253231165169. https://doi.org/10.1177/20451253231165169

Price, J., Cole, V., Doll, H., & Goodwin, G. M. (2012). The Oxford Questionnaire on Emotional Side-Effects of Antidepressants (OQuESA): Development, validity, reliability and sensitivity to change. *Journal of Affective Disorders, 140*(1), 66–74. https://doi.org/10.1016/j.jad.2012.01.030

Price, E. C., Gregg, J. J., Smith, M. D., & Fiske, A. (2018). Masculine traits and depressive symptoms in older and younger men and women. American Journal of Men's Health 12(1): 19–29. https://doi.org/10.1177/1557988315619676

Pridmore, S., Skerritt, P., & Ahmadi, J. (2004). Why do doctors dislike treating people with somatoform disorder? *Australasian Psychiatry, 12*(2), 134–138. https://doi.org/10.1080/j.1039-8562.2004.02085.x

Puthran, R., Zhang, M. W., Tam, W. W., & Ho, R. C. (2016). Prevalence of depression amongst medical students: A meta-analysis. *Medical Education, 50*(4), 456–468. https://doi.org/10.1111/medu.12962

Putnam, R. (2000). *Bowling alone: The collapse and revival of American community.* Simon and Schuster.

Puzo, Q., Mehlum, L., & Qin, P. (2018). Rates and characteristics of suicide by immigration background in Norway. *PLOS ONE, 13*(9), Article e0205035. https://doi.org/10.1371/journal.pone.0205035

Qiu, P., Caine, E. D., Hou, F., Cerulli, C., Wittink, M. N., & Li, J. (2016). The prevalence of distress and depression among women in rural Sichuan Province. PloS One 11(8): e0161097. https://doi.org/10.1371/journal.pone.0161097

Qiu, X., Shi, L., Kubzansky, L. D., Wei, Y., Castro, E., Li, H., Weisskopf, M. G., & Schwartz, J. D. (2023). Association of long-term exposure to air pollution with late-life depression in older adults in the US. JAMA Network Open, 6(2), e2253668. https://doi.org/10.1001/jamanetworkopen.2022.53668

Quan, Y., Wang, Z.-Y., Xiong, M., Xiao, Z.-T., & Zhang, H.-Y. (2014). Dissecting traditional Chinese medicines by omics and bioinformatics. *Natural Product Communications*, 9(9), 1391–1396. https://doi.org/10.1177/1934578X1400900942

Quirk, S. E., Williams, L. J., O'Neil, A., Pasco, J. A., Jacka, F. N., Housden, S., Berk, M., & Brennan, S. L. (2013). The association between diet quality, dietary patterns and depression in adults: A systematic review. *BMC Psychiatry*, 13, Article 175. https://doi.org/10.1186/1471-244X-13-175

Racz, S. J., McMahon, R. J., & Luthar, S. S. (2011). Risky behavior in affluent youth: Examining the co-occurrence and consequences of multiple problem behaviors. *Journal of Child and Family Studies*, 20(1), 120–128. https://doi.org/10.1007/s10826-010-9385-4

Radloff, L. S. (1977). The CES-D Scale: A self-report depression scale for research in the general population. *Applied Psychological Measurement*, 1(3), 385–401. https://doi.org/10.1177/014662167700100306

Raffler, N., Rissler, J., Ellegast, R., Schikowsky, C., Kraus, T., & Ochsmann, E. (2017). Combined exposures of whole-body vibration and awkward posture: A cross sectional investigation among occupational drivers by means of simultaneous field measurements. *Ergonomics*, 60(11), 1564–1575. https://doi.org/10.1080/00140139.2017.1314554

Rainie, L., Keeter, S., & Perrin, A. (2019, July 22). *Trust and Distrust in America*. Pew Research Center. Retrieved July 5, 2021, from https://www.pewresearch.org/politics/2019/07/22/trust-and-distrust-in-america/

Rajbhandary, S., & Basu, K. (2010). Working conditions of nurses and absenteeism: Is there a relationship? An empirical analysis using National Survey of the Work and Health of Nurses. *Health Policy*, 97(2–3), 152–159. https://doi.org/10.1016/j.healthpol.2010.04.010

Ramakrishnan, A., Sambuco, D., & Jagsi, R. (2014). Women's participation in the medical profession: Insights from experiences in Japan, Scandinavia, Russia, and eastern Europe. *Journal of Women's Health*, 23(11), 927–934. https://doi.org/10.1089/jwh.2014.4736

Randhawa, P. J. (2019, May 23). Doctor left destitute after seeking help from physician health program. *5 on Your Side: Investigations*. https://www.ksdk.com/article/news/local/doctor-left-destitute-after-seeking-help-from-physician-health-program/63-99720f38-5c5c-43c6-9c4c-c0f522ddc8c4

Rankin, A. (2018). *Mishima, Aesthetic Terrorist*. University of Hawaii Press.

Rasmus, P., & Kozłowska, E. (2023). Antioxidant and anti-inflammatory effects of carotenoids in mood disorders: An overview. *Antioxidants*, 12(3), 676. https://doi.org/10.3390/antiox12030676

Rassy, J., Bardon, C., Dargis, L., Côté, L. P., Corthésy-Blondin, L., Mörch, C. M., & Labelle, R. (2021). Information and communication technology use in suicide prevention: Scoping review. *Journal of Medical Internet Research*, 23(5), Article e25288. https://doi.org/10.2196/25288

Rathert, C., Williams, E. S., & Linhart, H. (2018). Evidence for the quadruple aim: A systematic review of the literature on physician burnout and patient outcomes. *Medical Care, 56*(12), 976–984. https://doi.org/10.1097/MLR.0000000000000999

Ravindran, A. V., Balneaves, L. G., Faulkner, G., Ortiz, A., McIntosh, D., Morehouse, R. L., Ravindran, L., Yatham, L. N., Kennedy, S. H., Lam, R. W., MacQueen, G. M., Milev, R. V., Parikh, S. V., & CANMAT Depression Work Group (2016). Canadian Network for Mood and Anxiety Treatments (CANMAT) 2016 clinical guidelines for the Management of Adults with Major Depressive Disorder: Section 5. Complementary and alternative medicine treatments. *Canadian Journal of Psychiatry, 61*(9), 576–587. https://doi.org/10.1177/0706743716660290

Recupero, P., Pinals, D. A., Candilis, P., Hoge, S. K., Buchanan, A., Swartz, M., Fisher, C. E., Janofsky, J., Anfang, S., Devido, J., Datta, V., Benedek, E., & Sidor, M. (2017). *Resource Document on Recommended Best Practices for Physician Health Programs*. American Psychiatric Association.

Redden, E. (2019, May 30). International student well-being. *Inside Higher Ed*. Retrieved September 29, 2019, from https://www.insidehighered.com/news/2019/05/31/panel-focuses-mental-health-needs-international-students

Reed, D. B., & Cronin, J. S. (2003). Health on the road: issues faced by female truck drivers. *AAOHN Journal: Official Journal of the American Association of Occupational Health Nurses, 51*(3), 120–125.

Reeves, G. M., Tonelli, L. H., Anthony, B. J., & Postolache, T. T. (2007). Precipitants of adolescent suicide: Possible interaction between allergic inflammation and alcohol intake. *International Journal of Adolescent Medicine and Health, 19*(1), 37–43. https://doi.org/10.1515/ijamh.2007.19.1.37

Reher, D., & Requena, M. (2018). Living alone in later life: A global perspective. *Population and Development Review, 44*(3), 427–454. https://doi.org/10.1111/padr.12149

Reifels, L, Mishara, B. L., Dargis, L., Vijayakumar, L., Philips, M. R., & Pirkis, J. (2019). Outcomes of community-based suicide prevention approaches that involve reducing access to pesticides: A systematic literature review. *Suicide and Life-Threatening Behavior, 49*(4), 1019–1031. https://doi.org/10.1111/sltb.12503

Reinert, M., Fritze, D. & Nguyen, T. (2022). *The State of Mental Health in America 2023*. Mental Health America, Alexandria VA.

Reis, C., Mestre, C., Canhão, H., Gradwell, D., & Paiva, T. (2016a). Sleep complaints and fatigue of airline pilots. *Sleep Science, 9*(2), 73–77. https://doi.org/10.1016/j.slsci.2016.05.003

Reis, C., Mestre, C., Canhao, H., Gradwell, D., & Paiva, T. (2016b). Sleep and fatigue differences in the two most common types of commercial flight operations. *Aerospace Medicine and Human Performance, 87*(9), 811–815. https://doi.org/10.3357/AMHP.4629.2016

Reisch, T., Steffen, T., Habenstein, A., & Tschacher, W. (2013). Change in suicide rates in Switzerland before and after firearm restriction resulting from the 2003 "Army XXI" reform. *American Journal of Psychiatry, 170*(9), 977–984. https://doi.org/10.1176/appi.ajp.2013.12091256

Remembering Heath Ledger (2017, May 4). [Interview]. *Interview*. https://www.interviewmagazine.com/film/new-again-heath-ledger-1

Ren, L., & Chen, G. (2017). Rapid antidepressant effects of Yueju: A new look at the function and mechanism of an old herbal medicine. *Journal of Ethnopharmacology, 203*, 226–232. https://doi.org/10.1016/j.jep.2017.03.042

Reno, E., Brown, T. L., Betz, M. E., Allen, M. H., Hoffecker, L., Reitinger, J., Roach, R., & Honigman, B. (2018). Suicide and high altitude: An integrative review. *High Altitude Medicine & Biology, 19*(2), 99–108. https://doi.org/10.1089/ham.2016.0131

Rentfrow, P. J., Gosling, S. D., Jokela, M., Stillwell, D. J., Kosinski, M., & Potter, J. (2013). Divided we stand: three psychological regions of the United States and their political, economic, social, and health correlates. Journal of Personality and Social Psychology, 105(6), 996–1012. https://doi.org/10.1037/a0034434

Resnik, P., De Choudhury, M., Musacchio Schafer, K., & Coppersmith, G. (2021). Bibliometric studies and the discipline of social media mental health research. Comment on "Machine learning for mental health in social media: Bibliometric study." *Journal of Medical Internet Research*, 23(6), Article e28990. https://doi.org/10.2196/28990

Riano, N. S., Linos, E., Accurso, E. C., Sung, D., Linos, E., Simard, J. F., & Mangurian, C. (2018). Paid family and childbearing leave policies at top US medical schools. *JAMA*, 319(6), 611–614. https://doi.org/10.1001/jama.2017.19519

Ricciuti, M. D. (2019). Memorandum and Order on Defendants' Motions to Dismiss in Civil Action No. 18-2603. (W. Tang vs. President and Fellows of Harvard College). https://masslawyersweekly.com/wp-content/blogs.dir/1/files/2019/09/Tang-v.-Harvard.pdf. Accessed August 1, 2024.

Rice, S. M., Aucote, H. M., Eleftheriadis, D., & Möller-Leimkühler, A. M. (2018). Prevalence and co-occurrence of internalizing and externalizing depression symptoms in a community sample of Australian male truck drivers. *American Journal of Men's Health*, 12(1), 74–77. https://doi.org/10.1177/1557988315626262

Rice, S. M., Fallon, B. J., Aucote, H. M., & Möller-Leimkühler, A. M. (2013). Development and preliminary validation of the Male Depression Risk Scale: Furthering the assessment of depression in men. *Journal of Affective Disorders*, 151(3), 950–958. https://doi.org/10.1016/j.jad.2013.08.013

Rice, S. M., Kealy, D., Seidler, Z. E., Oliffe, J. L., Levant, R. F., & Ogrodniczuk, J. S. (2020). Male-type and prototypal depression trajectories in men experiencing mental health problems. *International Journal of Environmental Research and Public Health*, 17(19), Article 7322. https://doi.org/10.3390/ijerph17197322

Rice, S. M., Oliffe, J. L., Kealy, D., & Ogrodniczuk, J. S. (2018). Male depression subtypes and suicidality: Latent profile analysis of internalizing and externalizing symptoms in a representative Canadian sample. *The Journal of Nervous and Mental Disease*, 206(3), 169–172. https://doi.org/10.1097/NMD.0000000000000739

Riddell, C. A., Harper, S., Cerdá, M., & Kaufman, J. S. (2018). Comparison of rates of firearm and nonfirearm homicide and suicide in black and white non-Hispanic men, by U.S. State. *Annals of Internal Medicine*, 168(10), 712–720. https://doi.org/10.7326/M17-2976

Right to work law. (2021). In *Wikipedia*. https://en.wikipedia.org/wiki/Right-to-work_law#U.S._states_with_right-to-work_laws

Rizvi, S. J., Pizzagalli, D. A., Sproule, B. A., & Kennedy, S. H. (2016). Assessing anhedonia in depression: Potentials and pitfalls. *Neuroscience and Biobehavioral Reviews*, 65, 21–35. https://doi.org/10.1016/j.neubiorev.2016.03.004

Ro, A. (2014). Occupational mobility and depression among the foreign-born in the United States. *Journal of Immigrant and Minority Health*, 16(6), 1149–1156. https://doi.org/10.1007/s10903-013-9945-y

Roberts, M. E., Han, K., & Weed, N. C. (2006). Development of a scale to assess *hwa-byung*, a Korean culture-bound syndrome, using the Korean MMPI-2. *Transcultural Psychiatry*, 43(3), 383–400. https://doi.org/10.1177/1363461506067715

Roberts, S., Arseneault, L., Barratt, B., Beevers, S., Danese, A., Odgers, C. L., Moffitt, T. E., Reuben, A., Kelly, F. J., & Fisher, H. L. (2019). Exploration of NO2 and PM2.5 air pollution and mental health problems using high-resolution data in London-based children from a UK longitudinal cohort study. Psychiatry Research, 272, 8–17. https://doi.org/10.1016/j.psychres.2018.12.050

Robinson, N., & Bergen, S. E. (2021). Environmental risk factors for schizophrenia and bipolar disorder and their relationship to genetic risk. Current knowledge and future directions. *Frontiers in Genetics, 12*, Article 686666. https://doi.org/10.3389/fgene.2021.686666

Rockett, R., & Smith, G. S. (1993). Covert suicide among elderly Japanese females: Questioning unintentional drownings. *Social Science & Medicine, 36*(11), 1467–1472.

Roh, S., Lee, S. U., Soh, M., Ryu, V., Kim, H., Jang, J. W., Lim, H. Y., Jeon, M., Park, J. I., Choi, S., & Ha, K. (2016). Mental health services and R&D in South Korea. *International Journal of Mental Health Systems, 10*, 45. https://doi.org/10.1186/s13033-016-0077-3

Rohlman, D. S., Ismail, A. A., Rasoul, G. A., Bonner, M. R., Hendy, O., Mara, K., Wang, K., & Olson, J.R. (2016). A 10-month prospective study of organophosphorus pesticide exposure and neurobehavioral performance among adolescents in Egypt. *Cortex; A Journal Devoted to the Study of the Nervous System and Behavior 74*: 383–395. https://doi.org/10.1016/j.cortex.2015.09.011

Rolin, D., Whelan, J., & Montano, C. B. (2020). Is it depression or is it bipolar depression? *Journal of the American Association of Nurse Practitioners, 32*(10), 703–713. https://doi.org/10.1097/JXX.0000000000000499

Romo, M. L., George, G., Mantell, J. E., Mwai, E., Nyaga, E., Strauss, M., Odhiambo, J. O., Govender, K., & Kelvin, E. A. (2019). Depression and sexual risk behavior among long-distance truck drivers at roadside wellness clinics in Kenya. *Peer Journal, 7*, Article e7253. https://doi.org/10.7717/peerj.7253

Rosenbloom, R., & Batalova, J. (2022). *Mexican immigrants in the United States*. Migration Policy Institute. Retrieved August 15, 2023 from https://www.migrationpolicy.org/article/mexican-immigrants-united-states

Ross, J., Hua, S., Perreira, K. M., Hanna, D. B., Castañeda, S. F., Gallo, L. C., Penedo, F. J., Tarraf, W., Hernandez, R., Vega Potler, N., Talavera, G. A., Daviglus, M. L., Gonzalez, F., 2nd, Kaplan, R. C., & Smoller-Wassertheil, S. (2019). Association between immigration status and anxiety, depression, and use of anxiolytic and antidepressant medications in the Hispanic Community Health Study/Study of Latinos. Annals of Epidemiology, 37, 17–23.e3. https://doi.org/10.1016/j.annepidem.2019.07.007

Rosta, J., & Aasland, O. G. (2016). Doctors' working hours and time spent on patient care in the period 1994–2014. *Tidsskriftet den Norske Legeforening, 136*, 1355–1359. https://doi.org/10.4045/tidsskr.16.0011

Rotenstein, L. S., Ramos, M. A., Torre, M., Segal, J. B., Peluso, M. J., Guille, C., Sen, S., & Mata, D. A. (2016). Prevalence of depression, depressive symptoms and suicidal ideation among medical students: A systematic review and meta-analysis. *JAMA, 316*(21), 2214–2236. https://doi.org/10.1001/jama.2016.17324

Roy, A. L., Godfrey, E. B., & Rarick, J. R. (2016). Do we know where we stand? Neighborhood relative income, subjective social status, and health. *American Journal of Community Psychology, 57*(3–4), 448–458. https://doi.org/10.1002/ajcp.12049

Rugel, E. J., Carpiano, R. M., Henderson, S. B., & Brauer, M. (2019). Exposure to natural space, sense of community belonging, and adverse mental health outcomes across an urban region. *Environmental Research, 171*, 365–377. https://doi.org/10.1016/j.env res.2019.01.034

Rugulies, R., Aust, B., & Madsen, I. E. (2017). Effort–reward imbalance at work and risk of depressive disorders. A systematic review and meta-analysis of prospective cohort studies. *Scandinavian Journal of Work, Environment, and Health, 43*(4), 294–306. https://doi.org/10.5271/sjweh.3632

Ruiz, R. J., Newman, M., Records, K., Wommack, J. C., Stowe, R. P., & Pasillas, R. M. (2019). Pilot study of the mastery lifestyle intervention. *Nursing Research, 68*(6), 494–500. https://doi.org/10.1097/NNR.0000000000000384

Russell, R., Metraux, D., & Tohen, M. (2017). Cultural influences on suicide in Japan. *Psychiatry and Clinical Neurosciences, 71(1)*, 2–5. https://doi.org/10.1111/pcn.12428

Ryu, S. Y., Crespi, C. M., & Maxwell, A. E. (2013). Drinking patterns among Korean adults: Results of the 2009 Korean Community Health Survey. *Journal of Preventive Medicine and Public Health, 46*(4), 183–191. https://doi.org/10.3961/jpmph.2013.46.4.183

Saadat, N., Lydic, T. A., Misra, D. P., Dailey, R., Walker, D. S., & Giurgescu, C. (2020). Lipidome profiles are related to depressive symptoms and preterm birth among African American women. *Biological Research for Nursing, 22*(3), 354–361. https://doi.org/10.1177/1099800420923032

Saavedra, K., & Salazar, L. A. (2021). Epigenetics: A missing link between early life stress and depression. *Advances in Experimental Medicine and Biology, 1305*, 117–128. https://doi.org/10.1007/978-981-33-6044-0_8

Sabry, W. M., & Vohra, A. (2013). Role of Islam in the management of psychiatric disorders. *Indian Journal of Psychiatry, 55*(S2), S205–S214. https://doi.org/10.4103/0019-5545.105534

Saeki, U. (Ed.). (1981). *Kokin Wakashu 古今和歌集* [Anthology of ancient and modern poetry]. Iwanami Bunko.

Sahle, B. W., Reavley, N. J., Li, W., Morgan, A. J., Yap, M., Reupert, A., & Jorm, A. F. (2021). The association between adverse childhood experiences and common mental disorders and suicidality: An umbrella review of systematic reviews and meta-analyses. *European Child & Adolescent Psychiatry, 31*, 1489–1499. https://doi.org/10.1007/s00 787-021-01745-2

Saijo, Y., Chiba, S., Yoshioka, E., Kawanishi, Y., Nakagi, Y., Itoh, T., Sugioka, Y., Kitaoka-Higashiguchi, K., & Yoshida, T. (2014). Effects of work burden, job strain and support on depressive symptoms and burnout among Japanese physicians. *International Journal of Occupational Medicine and Environmental Health, 27*(6), 980–992. https://doi.org/10.2478/s13382-014-0324-2

Saito, M., Kondo, N., Aida, J., Kawachi, I., Koyama, S., Ojima, T., & Kondo, K. (2017). Development of an instrument for community-level health related social capital among Japanese older people: The JAGES Project. *Journal of Epidemiology, 27*(5), 221–227. https://doi.org/10.1016/j.je.2016.06.005

Saito, M., Kondo, N., Oshio, T., Tabuchi, T., & Kondo, K. (2019). Relative deprivation, poverty, and mortality in Japanese older adults: A six-year follow-up of the JAGES Cohort Survey. *International Journal of Environmental Research and Public Health, 16*(2), 182. https://doi.org/10.3390/ijerph16020182

Saitō, T. (2013). *Hikikomori: Adolescence Without End* (J. Angles, Trans.). University of Minnesota Press. (Original work published 1998.)

Salazar, J. W., Meisel, K., Smith, E. R., Quiggle, A., McCoy, D. B., & Amans, M. R. (2019). Depression in patients with tinnitus: A systematic review. *Otolaryngology—Head and Neck Surgery* 161(1): 28–35. https://doi.org/10.1177/0194599819835178

Salas-Wright, C. P., Kagotho, N., & Vaughn, M. G. (2014). Mood, anxiety, and personality disorders among first and second-generation immigrants to the United States. *Psychiatry Research*, *220*(3), 1028–1036. https://doi.org/10.1016/j.psychres.2014.08.045

Salas-Wright, C. P., Vaughn, M. G., Goings, T. C., Miller, D. P., & Schwartz, S. J. (2018). Immigrants and mental disorders in the United States: New evidence on the healthy migrant hypothesis. *Psychiatry Research*, *267*, 438–445. https://doi.org/10.1016/j.psychres.2018.06.039

Sánchez-Vidaña, D. I., Ngai, S. P., He, W., Chow, J. K., Lau, B. W., & Tsang, H. W. (2017). The effectiveness of aromatherapy for depressive symptoms: A systematic review. *Evidence-Based Complementary and Alternative Medicine*, *2017*, Article 5869315. https://doi.org/10.1155/2017/5869315

Sanchez-Villegas, A., Zazpe, I., Santiago, S., Perez-Cornago, A., Martinez-Gonzalez, M. A., & Lahortiga-Ramos, F. (2018). Added sugars and sugar-sweetened beverage consumption, dietary carbohydrate index and depression risk in the Seguimiento Universidad de Navarra (SUN) project. *British Journal of Nutrition*, *119*(2), 211–221. https://doi.org/10.1017/S0007114517003361

Sanhueza, C., Ryan, L., & Foxcroft, D. R. (2013). Diet and the risk of unipolar depression in adults: Systematic review of cohort studies. *Journal of Human Nutrition and Dietetics*, *26*(1), 56–70. https://doi.org/10.1111/j.1365-277X.2012.01283.x

Sanlorenzo, M., Wehner, M. R., Linos, E., Kornak, J., Kainz, W., Posch, C., Vujic, I., Johnston, K., Gho, D., Monico, G., McGrath, J. T., Osella-Abate, S., Quaglino, P., Cleaver, J. E., & Ortiz-Urda, S. (2015). The risk of melanoma in airline pilots and cabin crew: A meta-analysis. *JAMA Dermatology*, *151*(1), 51–58. https://doi.org/10.1001/jamadermatol.2014.1077

Sarchiapone, M., Mandelli, L., Carli, V., Iosue, M., Wasserman, C., Hadlaczky, G., Hoven, C. W., Apter, A., Balazs, J., Bobes, J., Brunner, R., Corcoran, P., Cosman, D., Haring, C., Kaess, M., Keeley, H., Kereszteny, A., Kahn, J.-P., Postuvan, V., ... Wasserman, D. (2014). Hours of sleep in adolescents and its association with anxiety, emotional concerns, and suicidal ideation. *Sleep Medicine*, *15*(2), 248–254. https://doi.org/10.1016/j.sleep.2013.11.780

Sarno, E., Moeser, A. J., & Robison, A. J. (2021). Neuroimmunology of depression. *Advances in Pharmacology*, *91*, 259–292. https://doi.org/10.1016/bs.apha.2021.03.004

Sarris, J., Murphy, J., Mischoulon, D., Papakostas G. I., Fava, M., Berk, M., & Ng, C. H. (2016). Adjunctive nutraceuticals for depression: A systematic review and meta-analyses. *American Journal of Psychiatry*, *173*(6), 575–587. https://doi.org/10.1176/appi.ajp.2016.15091228

Sarris, J., O'Neil, A., Coulson, C. E., Schweitzer, I., & Berk, M. (2014). Lifestyle medicine for depression. *BMC Psychiatry*, *14*, Article 107. https://doi.org/10.1186/1471-244X-14-107

Sartorius, N., Chiu, H., Heok, K. E., Lee, M.-S., Ouyang, W. C., Sato, M., Yang, Y. K., & Yu, X. (2014). Name change for schizophrenia. *Schizophrenia Bulletin*, *40*(2), 255–258. https://doi.org/10.1093/schbul/sbt231

Sasaki, N., Carrozzino, D., & Nishi, D. (2021). Sensitivity and concurrent validity of the Japanese version of the Euthymia scale: a clinimetric analysis. *BMC Psychiatry, 21*(1), 482. https://doi.org/10.1186/s12888-021-03494-7

Sasaki, N., & Nishi, D. (2023). Euthymia scale as a protective factor for depressive symptoms: a one-year follow-up longitudinal study. *BMC Research Notes, 16*(1), 230. https://doi.org/10.1186/s13104-023-06512-x

Sasdelli, A., Lia, L., Luciano, C. C., Nespeca, C., Berardi, D., & Menchetti, M. (2013). Screening for bipolar disorder symptoms in depressed primary care attenders: Comparison between Mood Disorder Questionnaire and Hypomania Checklist (HCL-32). *Psychiatry Journal*, 548349. https://doi.org/10.1155/2013/548349

Sathappan, A. V., Luber, B. M., & Liansby, S. H. (2019). The dynamic duo: Combining noninvasive brain stimulation with cognitive interventions. *Progress in Neuropsychopharmacology and Biological Psychiatry, 89*, 347–360. https://doi.org/10.1016/j.pnpbp.2018.10.006

Sathyanarayanan, G., Vengadavaradan, A., & Bharadwaj, B. (2019). Role of yoga and mindfulness in severe mental illnesses: A narrative review. *International Journal of Yoga, 12*(1), 3–28. https://doi.org/10.4103/ijoy.IJOY_65_17

Satia, J. A. (2010). Dietary acculturation and the nutrition transition: An overview. *Applied Physiology Nutrition and Metabolism, 35*(2), 219–223. https://doi.org/10.1139/H10-007

Sato, M. (2006). Renaming schizophrenia: A Japanese perspective. *World Psychiatry, 5*(1), 53–55.

Sato, R., Kawanishi, C., Yamada, Tl, Hasegawa, H., Ikeda, H., Kato, D., Furuno, T., Kishida, I., & Hirayasu, Y. (2006). Knowledge and attitude towards suicide among medical students in Japan: Preliminary study. *Psychiatry and Clinical Neurosciences, 60*(5), 558–562.

Savage, M., Devine, F., Cunningham, N., Taylor, M., Li, Y., Hjelbrekke, J., Le Roux, B., Friedman, S., & Miles, A. (2013). A new model of social class? Findings from the BBC's Great British Class Survey Experiment. *Sociology, 47*(2), 219–250. https://doi.org/10.1177/0038038513481128

Sawada, N., Uchida, H., Suzuki, T., Watanabe, K., Kikuchi, T., Handa, T., & Kashima, H. (2009). Persistence and compliance to antidepressant treatment in patients with depression: A chart review. *BMC Psychiatry, 9*, Article 38. https://doi.org/10.1186/1471-244X-9-38

Scheepers, R., Silkens, M., van den Berg, J., & Lombarts, K. (2020). Associations between job demands, job resources and patient-related burnout among physicians: Results from a multicentre observational study. *BMJ Open, 10*(9), Article e038466. https://doi.org/10.1136/bmjopen-2020-038466

Schein, E., & Van Maanen, J. (2013). *Career Anchors* (4th ed.). Wiley.

Schell, T. L., Cefalu, M., Griffin, B. A., Smart, R., & Morral, A. R. (2020). Changes in firearm mortality following the implementation of state laws regulating firearm access and use. *Proceedings of the National Academy of Sciences, 117*(26), 14906–14910. https://doi.org/10.1073/pnas.1921965117

Schernhammer, E. S., & Colditz, G. A. (2004). Suicide rates among physicians: A quantitative and gender assessment (meta-analysis). *American Journal of Psychiatry, 161*, 2295–2302. https://doi.org/10.1176/appi.ajp.161.12.2295

Schmechel, D. E. (2007). Art, alpha-1-antitrypsin polymorphisms and intense creative energy: Blessing or curse. *Neurotoxicology, 28*, 899–914. https://doi.org/10.1016/j.neuro.2007.05.011

Schmechel, D. E., & Edwards, C. L. (2012). Fibromyalgia, mood disorders, and intense creative energy: A1AT polymorphisms are not always silent. *Neurotoxicology, 33*(6), 1454–1472. https://doi.org/10.1016/j.neuro.2012.03.001

Schneiderjobs.com (2023). How much does it cost to get a CDL? *Schneiderjobs.com*. Retrieved July 4, 2023, from https://schneiderjobs.com/blog/cost-to-get-cdl.

Schnyder, N., Panczak, R., Groth, N., & Schultze-Lutter, F. (2017). Association between mental health–related stigma and active help-seeking: Systematic review and meta-analysis. *British Journal of Psychiatry, 210*(4), 261–268. https://doi.org/10.1192/bjp.bp.116.189464

Schwenk, T. L., Davis, L., & Wimsatt, L. A. (2010). Depression, stigma and suicidal ideation in medical students. *JAMA, 304*(11), 1181–1190. https://doi.org/10.1001/jama.2010.1300

Schwenk, T. L., Gorenflo, D. W., & Leja, L. M. (2008). A survey of the impact of being depressed on the professional status and mental health care of physicians. *Journal of Clinical Psychiatry, 69*(4), 619–620. https://doi.org/10.4088/jcp.v69n0414

Scott, A. J., Webb, T. L., Martyn-St James, M., Rowse, G., & Weich, S. (2021). Improving sleep quality leads to better mental health: A meta-analysis of randomised controlled trials. *Sleep Medicine Reviews, 60*, 101556. https://doi.org/10.1016/j.smrv.2021.101556

Seabrook, E. M., Kern, M. L., Fulcher, B. D., & Rickard, N. S. (2018). Predicting depression from language-based emotion dynamics: Longitudinal analysis of Facebook and Twitter status updates. *Journal of Medical Internet Research, 20*(5), Article e168. https://doi.org/10.2196/jmir.9267

Sege, R., Nykiel-Bub, L., & Selk, S. (2015). Sex differences in institutional support for junior biomedical researchers. *JAMA, 314*(11), 1175–1177. https://doi.org/10.1001/jama.2015.8517

Seidler, M. (1983). Kant and the Stoics on suicide. *Journal of the History of Ideas, 44*(3), 429–453. https://doi.org/10.2307/2709175

Selhub, E. M., Logan, A. C., & Bested, A. C. (2014). Fermented foods, microbiota, and mental health: Ancient practice meets nutritional psychiatry. *Journal of Physiological Anthropology, 15*(33), Article 2. https://doi.org/10.1186/1880-6805-33-2

Sellström, E., Bremberg, S., & O'campo, P. (2011). Yearly incidence of mental disorders in economically inactive young adults. *European Journal of Public Health, 21*(6), 812–814. https://doi.org/10.1093/eurpub/ckq190

Semmer, N. K., Jacobshagen, N., Meier, L. L., Elfering, A., Beehr, T. A., Kälin, W., & Tschan, F. (2015). Illegitimate tasks as a source of work stress. *Work and Stress, 29*(1), 32–56. https://doi.org/10.1080/02678373.2014.1003996

Sen, S., Kranzler, H. R., Krystal, J. H., Speller, H., Chan, G., Gelernter, J., & Guille, C. (2010). A prospective cohort study investigating factors associated with depression during medical internship. *Archives of General Psychiatry, 67*(6), 557–565. https://doi.org/10.1001/archgenpsychiatry.2010.41

Seo, Y. A., Chung, H. C., & Kim, Y. A. (2019). Experience and acceptance of cosmetic procedures among Korean women in their 20s. *Aesthetic Plastic Surgery, 43*(2), 531–538. https://doi.org/10.1007/s00266-018-1257-0

Seo, Y. A., & Kim, Y. A. (2020). Factors affecting acceptance of cosmetic surgery in adults in their 20s–30s. *Aesthetic Plastic Surgery*, *44*(5), 1881–1888. https://doi.org/10.1007/s00 266-020-01761-8

Serrano-Medina, A., Ugalde-Lizárraga, A., Bojorquez-Cuevas, M. S., Garnica-Ruiz, J., González-Corral, M. A., García-Ledezma, A., Pineda-García, G., & Cornejo-Bravo, J. M. (2019). Neuropsychiatric disorders in farmers associated with organophosphorus pesticide exposure in a rural village of northwest méxico. International Journal of Environmental Research and Public Health, 16(5), 689. https://doi.org/10.3390/ijerph16050689

Seshagiri, B. (1998). Occupational noise exposure of operators of heavy trucks. *American Industrial Hygiene Association Journal*, *59*(3), 205–213. https://doi.org/10.1080/154281 19891010479

Settanni, M., & Marengo, D. (2015). Sharing feelings online: Studying emotional well-being via automated text analysis of Facebook posts. *Frontiers in Psychology*, *6*, Article 1045. https://doi.org/10.3389/fpsyg.2015.01045

Sha, F., Chang, Q., Law, Y. W., & Yip, P. S. F. (2018). Suicide rates in China, 2004–2014: Comparing data from two sample-based mortality surveillance systems. *BMC Public Health*, *18*, Article 239. https://doi.org/10.1186/s12889-018-5161-y

Shafiee, A., Jafarabady, K., Seighali, N., Mohammadi, I., Rajai Firouz Abadi, S., Abhari, F. S., & Bakhtiyari, M. (2024). Effect of saffron versus selective serotonin reuptake inhibitors (SSRIs) in treatment of depression and anxiety: A Meta-analysis of randomized controlled trials. Nutrition Reviews, nuae076. Advance online publication. https://doi.org/10.1093/nutrit/nuae076

Shanafelt, T., Goh, J., & Sinsky, C. (2017). The business case for investing in physician well-being. *JAMA Internal Medicine*, *177*(12), 1826–1832. https://doi.org/10.1001/jamain ternmed.2017.4340

Shanafelt, T. D., & Noseworthy, J. H. (2017). Executive leadership and physician well-being. *Mayo Clinic Proceedings*, *92*(1), 129–146. https://doi.org/10.1016/j.may ocp.2016.10.004

Shapiro, D., Dundar, A., Huie, F., Wakhungu, P., Yuan, X., Nathan, A., & Hwang, Y. A. (2017). *Completing College: A National View of Student Attainment Rates by Race and Ethnicity. Fall 2010 Cohort* (Signature Report No. 12b). National Student Clearinghouse Research Center.

Sharma, A., Sharp, D. M., Walker, L. G., & Monson, J. R. (2008). Stress and burnout in colorectal and vascular surgical consultants working in the UK National Health Service. *Psychooncology*, *17*, 570–576. https://doi.org/10.1002/pon.1269

Shattell, M., Apostolopoulos, Y., Collins, C., Sonmez, S., & Fehrenbacher, C. (2012). Trucking organization and mental health disorders of truck drivers. *Issues in Mental Health Nursing*, *33*, 436–444. https://doi.org/10.3109/01612840.2012.665156

Shay, J. (2014). Moral injury. *Psychoanalytic Psychology*, *31*, 182–191. https://doi.org/10.1037/a0036090

Sheehan, D. V. (2015). *Mini International Neuropsychiatric Interview 7.0*. Medical Outcomes Systems.

Sheikh, A. (2005). Jinn and cross-cultural care. *Journal of the Royal Society of Medicine*, *98*(8), 339–340. https://doi.org/10.1258/jrsm.98.8.339

Shen, H., Zhang, L., Xu, C., Zhu, J., Chen, M., & Fang, Y. (2018). Analysis of misdiagnosis of bipolar disorder in an outpatient setting. *Shanghai Archives of Psychiatry, 30*(2), 93–101. https://doi.org/10.11919/j.issn.1002-0829.217080

Shen, S., Li, Y., Zhou, M., Zhang, C., Jiang, Y., & Kang, Y. (2013). Depression status and associated factors in Chinese occupational truck drivers. *Cell Biochemistry and Biophysics, 67*(3), 1497–1500. https://doi.org/10.1007/s12013-013-9651-3

Shields, M., Dimov, S., Kavanagh, A., Milner, A., Spittal, M. J., & King, T. L. (2021). How do employment conditions and psychosocial workplace exposures impact the mental health of young workers? A systematic review. *Social Psychiatry and Psychiatric Epidemiology, 56*(7), 1147–1160. https://doi.org/10.1007/s00127-021-02077-x

Shiffman, S., Stone, A. A., & Hufford, M. R. (2008). Ecological momentary assessment. *Annual Review of Clinical Psychology, 4*, 1–32. https://doi.org/10.1146/annurev.clinpsy.3.022806.091415

Shigemura, J., Ogawa, T., Yoshino, A., Sato, Y., & Nomura, S. (2010). Predictors of antidepressant adherence: Results of a Japanese internet-based survey. *Psychiatry and Clinical Neurosciences, 64*(2), 179–186. https://doi.org/10.1111/j.1440-1819.2009.02058.x

Shin, C., Ko, Y. H., An, H., Yoon, H. K., & Han, C. (2020). Normative data and psychometric properties of the Patient Health Questionnaire-9 in a nationally representative Korean population. *BMC Psychiatry, 20*(1), Article 194. https://doi.org/10.1186/s12888-020-02613-0

Shin, S., Saito, E., Inoue, M., Sawada, N., Ishihara, J., Takachi, R., Nanri, A., Shimazu, T., Yamaji, T., Iwasaki, M., Sasazuki, S., & Tsugane, S. (2016). Dietary pattern and breast cancer risk in Japanese women: the Japan Public Health Center-based Prospective Study (JPHC Study). The British Journal of Nutrition, 115(10), 1769–1779. https://doi.org/10.1017/S0007114516000684

Shoman, Y., Marca, S. C., Bianchi, R., Godderis, L., van der Molen, H. F., & Guseva Canu, I. (2021). Psychometric properties of burnout measures: A systematic review. *Epidemiology and Psychiatric Sciences, 30*, Article e8. https://doi.org/10.1017/S2045796020001134

Shorrocks, A., Davies, J., & Lluberas, R (2022). *Credit Suisse Global Wealth Databook 2022*, pp. 14–17 and 119–122. Zürich, Credit Suisse.

Siegel, M. B., & Boine, C. C. (2020). The Meaning of Guns to Gun Owners in the U.S.: The 2019 National Lawful Use of Guns Survey. *American Journal of Preventive Medicine, 59*(5), 678–685. https://doi.org/10.1016/j.amepre.2020.05.010

Siegrist, J. (1996). Adverse health effects of high-effort/low-reward conditions. *Journal of Occupational Health Psychology, 1*(1), 27–41. https://doi.org//1076-8998.1.1.27

Siegrist, J. (2021). Psychosoziale arbeitsbelastungen und erkrankungsrisiken: Wissenschaftliche evidenz und praktische konsequenzen [Psychosocial stress at work and disease risks: Scientific evidence and implications for practice]. *Der Internist, 62*, 893–898. https://doi.org/10.1007/s00108-021-01105-x

Siegrist, J., & Li, J. (2016). Associations of extrinsic and intrinsic components of work stress with health: A systematic review of evidence on the effort-reward imbalance model. *International Journal of Environmental Research and Public Health, 13*(4), 432. https://doi.org/10.3390/ijerph13040432

Siegrist, J., Shackelton, R., Link, C., Marceau, L., von dem Knesebeck, O., & McKinlay, J. (2010). Work stress of primary care physicians in the US, UK and German health care systems. *Social Science & Medicine, 71*(2), 298–304. https://doi.org/10.1016/j.socscimed.2010.03.043

Siegrist, J., & Wege, N. (2020). Adverse psychosocial work environments and depression: A narrative review of selected theoretical models. *Frontiers in Psychiatry, 11*, Article 66. https://doi.org/10.3389/fpsyt.2020.00066

Sigurdsson, B., Palsson, S. P., Aevarsson, O., Olafsdottir, M., & Johannsson, M. (2014). Saliva testosterone and cortisol in male depressive syndrome, a community study. The Sudurnesjamenn study. *Nordic Journal of Psychiatry, 68(8)I*, 579–587. https://doi.org/10.3109/08039488.2014.898791

Sigurdsson, B., Palsson, S. P., Aevarsson, O., Olafsdottir, M., & Johannsson, M. (2015). Validity of Gotland Male Depression Scale for male depression in a community study: The Sudurnesjamenn study. *Journal of Affective Disorders, 173*, 81–89. https://doi.org/10.1016/j.jad.2014.10.065

Silverman, E. K. (2016). Risk of lung disease in PI MZ heterozygotes. Current status and future research directions. *Annals of the American Thoracic Society, 13*(S4). https://doi.org/10.1513/AnnalsATS.201507-437KV

Silverman, S. (2010). *The Bedwetter: Stories of Courage, Redemption, and Pee*. HarperCollins.

Simon, M., Chang, E. S., Zeng, P., & Dong, X. (2013). Prevalence of suicidal ideation, attempts, and completed suicide rate in Chinese aging populations: A systematic review. *Archives of Gerontology and Geriatrics, 57*(3), 250–256. https://doi.org/10.1016/j.archger.2013.05.006

Singh, A. (2017). The "scourge of Korea": Stress and suicide in Korean society. *Berkeley Political Review*, October 31. Retrieved May 4, 2019, from https://bpr.berkeley.edu/2017/10/31/the-scourge-of-south-korea-stress-and-suicide-in-korean-society/

Sinha, A., Shariq, A., Said, K., Sharma, A., Jeffrey Newport, D., & Salloum, I. M. (2018). Medical comorbidities in bipolar disorder. *Current Psychiatry Reports, 20*(5), Article 36. https://doi.org/10.1007/s11920-018-0897-8

Siripala, T. (2018). Japan's births and marriages spiral to record low. *The Diplomat*, January 4. https://thediplomat.com/2018/01/japans-births-and-marriages-spiral-to-record-low/

Sit, D., & Haigh, S. (2019). Use of "Lights" for bipolar depression. *Current Psychiatry Reports, 21*(6), 45. https://doi.org/10.1007/s11920-019-1025-0

Skarupski, K. A., Tangney, C. C., Li, H., Evans, D. A., & Morris, M. C. (2013). Mediterranean diet and depressive symptoms among older adults over time. *The Journal of Nutrition, Health & Aging, 17*(5), 441–445. https://doi.org/10.1007/s12603-012-0437-x

Skodo, A. (2018, December 6). Sweden: By turns welcoming and restrictive in its immigration policy. *Migration Information Source*. https://www.migrationpolicy.org/article/sweden-turns-welcoming-and-restrictive-its-immigration-policy

Slater, P. (1990). *The Pursuit of Loneliness*. Beacon Press. (Original work published 1970)

Slingsby, B. T., Plotnikoff, G. A., Mizuno, T., & Akabayashi, A. (2007). Physician strategies for addressing patient adherence to prescribed psychotropic medications in Japan: A qualitative study. *Journal of Clinical Pharmacy and Therapeutics, 32*(3), 241–245. https://doi.org/10.1111/j.1365-2710.2007.00816.x

Sluggett, L., Wagner, S. L., & Harris R. L. (2019). Sleep duration and obesity in children and adolescents. *American Journal of Diabetes, 43*(2), 146–152. https://doi.org/10.1016/j.jcjd.2018.06.006

Smith, C. A., Armour, M., Lee, M., Wang, L., & Hay, P. J. (2018). Acupuncture for depression. *Cochrane Database of Systematic Reviews*. https://doi.org/10.1002/14651858.CD004046.pub4

Smith, N. D., & Kawachi, I. (2014). State-level social capital and suicide mortality in the 50 U.S. states. *Social Science and Medicine, 120*, 269–277. https://doi.org/10.1016/j.socsci med.2014.09.007

Smith, P. N., & Cukrowicz, K. C. (2010). Capable of suicide: A functional model of the acquired capability component of the interpersonal-psychological theory of suicide. *Suicide & Life-Threatening Behavior, 40*(3), 266–275. https://doi.org/10.1521/suli.2010.40.3.266

Smith, S. (2020). These beautiful truck drivers are changing the stereotype. *CDL Life*, August 14. https://cdllife.com/2020/these-beautiful-truck-drivers-are-changing-the-stereotype/

Smith, S. G., Chen, J., Basile, K. C., Gilbert, L. K., Merrick, M. T., Patel, N., Walling, N., & Jain, A. (2017). *National Intimate Partner and Sexual Violence Survey (NISVS): 2010–2012 State Report*. Retrieved October 15, 2019, from https://www.cdc.gov/violencepre vention/pdf/NISVS-StateReportBook.pdf

Snaith, R. P., Hamilton, M., Morley, S., Humayan, A., Hargreaves, D., & Trigwell, P. (1995). A scale for the assessment of hedonic tone: The Snaith-Hamilton Pleasure Scale. *British Journal of Psychiatry, 167*, 99–103. https://doi.org/10.1192/bjp.167.1.99

Snarr, J. D., Heyman, R. E., & Slep, A. M. (2010). Recent suicidal ideation and suicide attempts in a large-scale survey of the U.S. Air Force: Prevalences and demographic risk factors. *Suicide & Life-threatening Behavior, 40*(6), 544–552. https://doi.org/10.1521/suli.2010.40.6.544

Sobowale, K., Zhou, N., Fan, J., Liu, N., & Sherer, R. (2014). Depression and suicidal ideation in medical students in China: A call for wellness curricula. *International Journal of Edical Education, 5*, 31–36. https://doi.org/10.5116/ijme.52e3.a465

Social Capital Project (2018). *The Geography of Social Capital in America*. SCP Report 1–18. page 20.

Social Security Administration (2020, October). *Annual Statistical Report on the Social Security Disability Insurance Program, 2019*. Retrieved July 10, 2021, from https://www.ssa.gov/policy/docs/statcomps/di_asr/2019/index.html

Soler, J. K., Yaman, H., Esteva, M., Dobbs, F., Asenova, R. S., Katic, M., Ozvacic, Z., Desgranges, J. P., Moreau, A., Lionis, C., Kotanyi, P., Carelli, F., Nowak, P. R., Azeredo, Z. A. S., Marklund, E., Churchill, D., & Ungan, M. (2008). Burnout in European family doctors: The EGPRN study. *Family Practice, 25*(4), 245–265. https://doi.org/10.1093/fampra/cmn038

Sommeiller, E., & Price, M. (2018). *The New Gilded Age*. Economic Policy Institute. https://www.epi.org/publication/the-new-gilded-age-income-inequality-in-the-u-s-by-state-metropolitan-area-and-county/

Son, J., & Feng, Q. (2019). In social capital we trust? *Social Indicators Research, 144*(1), 167–189. https://doi.org/10.1007/s11205-018-2026-9

Song, J., Jiang, R., Chen, N., Qu, W., Liu, D., Zhang, M., Fan, H., Zhao, Y., & Tan, S. (2021). Self-help cognitive behavioral therapy application for COVID-19-related mental health problems: A longitudinal trial. *Asian Journal of Psychiatry, 60*, 102656. https://doi.org/10.1016/j.ajp.2021.102656

Song, T., Han, X., Du, L., Che, J., Shi, S., Fu, C., Gao, W., Lu, J., & Ma, G. (2018). The role of neuroimaging in the diagnosis and treatment of depressive disorder: A recent review. *Current Pharmaceutical Design, 24*(22), 2515–2523. https://doi.org/10.2174/138161 2824666180727111142

Song, Y. N., Zhang, G. B., Zhang, Y. Y., & Su, S. B. (2013). Clinical applications of omics technologies on ZHENG differentiation research in Traditional Chinese Medicine. *Evidence-based Complementary and Alternative Medicine, 2013*:989618. https://doi.org/10.1155/2013/989618

Spoerri, A., Zwahlen, M., Bopp, M., Gutzwiller, F., & Egger, M.; for the Swiss National Cohort Study (2010). Religion and assisted and non-assisted suicide in Switzerland: National Cohort Study. *International Journal of Epidemiology*, *39*(6), 1486–1494. https://doi.org/10.1093/ije/dyq141

Sriharan, A., Ratnapalan, S., Tricco, A. C., Lupea, D., Ayala, A. P., Pang, H., & Lee, D. D. (2020). Occupational stress, burnout, and depression in women in healthcare during COVID-19 pandemic: Rapid scoping review. *Frontiers in Global Women's Health*, *1*, Article 596690. https://doi.org/10.3389/fgwh.2020.596690

Srivastava, S., Childers, M. E., Baek, J. H., Strong, C. M., Hill, S. J., Warsett, K. S., Wang, P. W., Akiskal, H. S., Akiskal, K. K., & Ketter, T. A. (2010). Toward interaction of affective and cognitive contributors to creativity in bipolar disorders: A controlled study. *Journal of Affective Disorders*, *125*(1–3), 27–34. https://doi.org/10.1016/j.jad.2009.12.018

Srivastava, S., & Ketter, T. (2010). The link between bipolar disorders and creativity: Evidence from personality and temperament studies. *Current Psychiatry Reports*, *12*, 522–530. https://doi.org/10.1007/s11920-010-0159-x

Statista Research (2024). Population distribution South Korea 2023, by religion. https://www.statista.com/statistics/996013/south-korea-population-distribution-by-religion/. Accessed August 1, 2024.

Statistics Bureau of Japan (2023a). *Statistical Handbook of Japan 2023*, p. 17,18.

Statistics Bureau of Japan (2023b). *Statistical Handbook of Japan 2023*, p. 12,13.

Statistics Bureau of Japan (2023c). *Statistical Handbook of Japan 2023*, p. 131.

Statistics Denmark (2019). Fertility. https://dst.dk/en/Statistik/emner/borgere/befolkning/fertilitet. Accessed August 1, 2024.

Statistics Norway (2018). *Women and Men in Norway*. https://www.ssb.no/en/befolkning/artikler-og-publikasjoner/_attachment/347081?_ts=1632b8bcba0

Statistics Sweden (2024). Number of persons with foreign or Swedish background (detailed division) by region, age, and sex. Year 2002–2023. https://www.statistikdatabasen.scb.se/pxweb/en/ssd/START__BE__BE0101__BE0101Q/UtlSvBakgFin/. Accessed October 1, 2024.

Steidel, A. G., & Contreras, J. M. (2003). A new familism scale for use with Latino populations. *Hispanic Journal of Behavioral Sciences*, *25*(3), 312–330. https://doi.org/10.1177/0739986303256912

Stein, E. M., Gennuso, K. P., Ugboaja, D. C., & Remington, P. L. (2017). The epidemic of despair among White Americans: Trends in the leading causes of premature death, 1999–2015. *American Journal of Public Health*, *107*(10), 1541–1547. https://doi.org/10.2105/AJPH.2017.303941

Stene-Larsen, K., & Reneflot, A. (2019). Contact with primary and mental health care prior to suicide: A systematic review of the literature from 2000 to 2017. *Scandinavian Journal of Public Health*, *47*(1), 9–17. https://doi.org/10.1177/1403494817746274

Stewart, S., & Thompson, D. R. (2015). Does comedy kill? A retrospective, longitudinal cohort, nested case–control study of humour and longevity in 53 British comedians. *International Journal of Cardiology*, *180*, 258–261. https://doi.org/10.1016/j.ijcard.2014.11.152

Stiles, B. M., Fish, A. F., Vandermause, R., & Malik, A. M. (2018). The compelling and persistent problem of bipolar disorder disguised as major depression disorder: An integrative review. *Journal of the American Psychiatric Nurses Association*, *24*(5), 415–425. https://doi.org/10.1177/1078390318784360

Stogios, N., Humber, B., Agarwal, S. M., & Hahn, M. (2023). Antipsychotic-induced weight gain in severe mental illness: Risk factors and special Considerations. *Current Psychiatry Reports*, 10.1007/s11920-023-01458-0. https://doi.org/10.1007/s11920-023-01458-0

Stoker, G. C. (2019). Impressions of a Pilot. *Live Journal*. Retrieved September 1, 2019, from https://war-poetry.livejournal.com/787393.html

Stoor, J. P. A., Berntsen, G., Hjelmeland, H., & Silviken, A. (2019). "If you do not *birget* [manage] then you don't belong here": A qualitative focus group study on the cultural meanings of suicide among Indigenous Sámi in Arctic Norway. *International Journal of Circumpolar Health, 78(1)*, Article 1565861. https://doi.org/10.1080/22423 982.2019.1565861

Størmer, C. C. L., Laukli, E., Høydal, E. H., & Stenklev, N. C. (2015). Hearing loss and tinnitus in rock musicians: A Norwegian survey. *Noise & Health, 17*(79), 411–421. https://doi.org/10.4103/1463-1741.169708

Størmer, C. C. L., Sorlie, T., & Stenklev, N. C. (2017). Tinnitus, anxiety, depression and substance abuse in rock musicians a Norwegian survey. *The International Tinnitus Journal, 21*(1), 50–57.

Strawbridge, R., Young, A. H., & Cleare, A. J. (2017). Biomarkers for depression: Recent insights, current challenges and future prospects. *Neuropsychiatric Disease and Treatment, 13*, 1245–1262. https://doi.org/10.2147/NDT.S114542

Strub, S., & Moser, M. S. (2010). Risiko und Verbreitung sexueller Belästigung am Arbeitsplatz – Zahlen zur Situation in der Schweiz [Risk and extent of sexual harassment in the workplace-figures documenting the situation in Switzerland]. *Arbeit, 19*(1), 21–36. https://doi.org/10.1515/arbeit-2010-0104.

Stulz, N., Pichler, E.-M., Kawohl, W., & Hepp, U. (2018). The gravitational force of mental health services: Distance decay effects in a rural Swiss service area. *BMC Health Services Research, 18*, Article 81. https://doi.org/10.1186/s12913-018-2888-1

Su, S., Li, X., Lin, D., Xu, X., & Zhu, M. (2013). Psychological adjustment among left-behind children in rural China: the role of parental migration and parent-child communication. Child: Care, Health and Development 39(2): 162–170. https://doi.org/10.1111/j.1365-2214.2012.01400.x

Su, Q., Yu, B., He, H., Zhang, Q., Meng, G., Wu, H., Du, H., Liu, L., Shi, H., Xià, Y., Guo, X., Liu, X., Li, C., Bao, X., Gu, Y., Fang, L., Yu, F., Yang, H., Sun, S., Wang, X., ... Niu, K. (2016). Nut consumption is associated with depressive symptoms among Chinese adults. *Depression and Anxiety, 33*(11), 1065–1072. https://doi.org/ 10.1002/da.22516

Subramaniam, M., Abdin, E., Picco, L., Pang, S., Shafie, S., Vaingankar, J. A., Kwok, K. W., Verma, K., & Chong, S. A. (2017). Stigma towards people with mental disorders and its components—A perspective from multi-ethnic Singapore. *Epidemiology and Psychiatric Sciences, 26*(4), 371–382. https://doi.org/10.1017/S2045796016000159

Suchy-Dicey, A., Verney, S. P., Nelson, L. A., Barbosa-Leiker, C., Howard, B. A., Crane, P. K., & Buchwald, D. S. (2020). Depression symptoms and cognitive test performance in older American Indians: The Strong Heart Study. *Journal of the American Geriatrics Society, 68*(8), 1739–1747. https://doi.org/10.1111/jgs.16434

Sugg N. (2015). Intimate partner violence: prevalence, health consequences, and intervention. The Medical Clinics of North America, 99(3), 629–649. https://doi.org/10.1016/j.mcna.2015.01.012

Suh, S. (2013). Stories to be told: Korean doctors between *hwa-byung* (fire-illness) and depression, 1970–2011. *Culture, Medicine and Psychiatry, 37*(1), 81–104. https://doi.org//10.1007/s11013-012-9291-x

Sūn Sīmiǎo (2019). *Essential Prescriptions for Emergencies* (S. Wilms, Translator.). Happy Goat Publications.

Sun, A., & Wu, X. (2023). Efficacy of non-pharmacological interventions on improving sleep quality in depressed patients: A systematic review and network meta-analysis. *Journal of Psychosomatic Research, 172*, 111435. https://doi.org/10.1016/j.jpsychores.2023.111435

Sun, L., & Zhang, J. (2016). Medically serious suicide attempters with or without plan in rural China. *Journal of Nervous and Mental Disease, 204*(11), 851–854.

Sun, T., Gao, L., Li, F., Shi, Y., Xie, F., Wang, J., Wang, S., Zhang, S., Liu, W., Duan, X., Liu, X., Zhang, Z., Li, L., & Fan, L. (2017). Workplace violence, psychological stress, sleep quality and subjective health in Chinese doctors: A large cross-sectional study. *BMJ Open, 7*(12), Article e017182. https://doi.org/10.1136/bmjopen-2017-017182

Sun, X., Qin, X., Zhang, M., Yang, A., Ren, X., & Dai, Q. (2021). Prediction of parental alienation on depression in left-behind children: A 12-month follow-up investigation. *Epidemiology and Psychiatric Sciences, 30*, Article e44. https://doi.org/10.1017/S2045796021000329

Suzuki, K. (2018). 死んだ後もひとりぼっち…孤独死を防ぐには？ [Even after death, remaining alone. How can lonely deaths be prevented?] *Yomiuri Online*, January 29. Retrieved August 21, 2018, from https://www.yomiuri.co.jp/fukayomi/ichiran/20180123-OYT8T50069.html?page_no=1

Suzuki, K., Takei, N., Kawai, M., Minabe, Y., & Mori, N. (2003). Is *taijin kyofusho* a culture-bound syndrome? *The American Journal of Psychiatry, 160*(7), Article 1358. https://doi.org/10.1176/appi.ajp.160.7.1358

Suzuki, T., Miyaki, K., Tsutsumi, A., Hashimoto, H., Kawakami, N., Takahashi, M., Shimazu, A., Inoue, A., Kurioka, S., Kakehashi, M., Sasaki, Y., & Shimbo, T. (2013). Japanese dietary pattern consistently relates to low depressive symptoms and it is modified by job strain and worksite supports. *Journal of Affective Disorders, 150*(2), 490–498. https://doi.org/10.1016/j.jad.2013.04.044

Svrluga, S., & Wan, W. (2023, August 25). Yale to update policies after lawsuit over student mental health. *The Washington Post*. https://www.washingtonpost.com/education/2023/08/25/yale-settlement-mental-health-lawsuit/

Swiss Federal Statistical Office (2015). *Swiss Agriculture: Pocket Statistics*, 2015. https://www.bfs.admin.ch/asset/en/349914

Swiss Federal Statistical Office (2019). *Population: Current Situation and Change*. https://www.bfs.admin.ch/bfs/en/home/statistics/population/effectif-change.html

Swissinfo.ch (2017). Report highlights depression gulf between Swiss language regions. Swissinfo.ch, October 29. 2017. https://www.swissinfo.ch/eng/society/report-highlights-depression-gulf-between-swiss-language-regions/43633960#.

Swissinfo.ch (2017, October 29). Report highlights depression gulf between Swiss language regions. *Swiss Broadcasting Corporation*. https://www.swissinfo.ch/eng/report-highlights-depression-gulf-between-swiss-language-regions/43633960

Swissinfo.ch (2018). Almost 40% of Swiss residents have a migration background. *Swiss Broadcasting Corporation*. https://www.swissinfo.ch/eng/demography_almost-40--of-swiss-residents-have-a-migration-background/44468978

Szewczyk, B., Szopa, A., Serefko, A., Poleszak, E., & Nowak, G. (2018). The role of magnesium and zinc in depression: Similarities and differences. *Magnesium Research*, *31*(3), 78–89. https://doi.org/10.1684/mrh.2018.0442

Tafur, M. M., Crowe, T. K., & Torres, E. (2009). A review of *curanderismo* and healing practices among Mexicans and Mexican Americans. *Occupational Therapy International*, *16*(1), 82–88. https://doi.org/10.1002/oti.265

Tahara, M. (Trans.). (1980). *Tales of Yamato: A Tenth-century Poem-tale*. University Press of Hawaii.

Tai, C. (2018, October 14). Being ugly hurts in Korea: Why it's so hard to say no to K-beauty. *South China Morning Post*. Retrieved May 4, 2019, from https://www.scmp.com/week-asia/society/article/2167875/being-ugly-hurts-south-korea-why-its-so-hard-say-no-k-beauty

Takagi, M. (2016). Japan's oldest-old population in the Edo period (2): An attempt to use historical materials of the Naoshima Island, Uwajima and Sendai Domain, 1720–1872. *Ritsumeikan Sangyo Shakai Ronshu*, *52*(1), 109–130.

Takaki, J., Taniguchi, T., Fukuoka, E., Fujii, Y., Tsutsumi, A., Nakajima, K., & Hirokawa, K. (2010). Workplace bullying could play important roles in the relationships between job strain and symptoms of depression and sleep disturbance. *Journal of Occupational Health*, *52*(6), 367–374. https://doi.org/10.1539/joh.l10081

Takaki, J., Taniguchi, T., & Hirokawa, K. (2013). Associations of workplace bullying and harassment with pain. *International Journal of Environmental Research and Public Health*, *10*(10), 4560–4570. https://doi.org/10.3390/ijerph10104560

Tamblyn, R., Bates, D. W., Buckeridge, D. L., Dixon, W., Forster, A. J., Girard, N., Haas, J., Habib, B., Kurteva, S., Li, J., & Sheppard, T. (2019). Multinational comparison of new antidepressant use in older adults: A cohort study. *BMJ Open*, *9*(5), Article e027663. https://doi.org/10.1136/bmjopen-2018-027663

Tamir, M., Schwartz, S. H., Oishi, S., & Kim, M. Y. (2017). The secret to happiness: Feeling good or feeling right? *Journal of Experimental Psychology: General*, *146*(10), 1448–1459. https://doi.org/10.1037/xge0000303

Tan, T. X. (2014). Major depression in China-to-US immigrants and US-born Chinese Americans: Testing a hypothesis from culture-gene co-evolutionary theory of mental disorders. *Journal of Affective Disorders*, *167*, 30–36. https://doi.org/10.1016/j.jad.2014.05.046

Tang v. President and Fellows of Harvard College, et al. (2018, September 11). Plaintiff's complaint and request for jury trial (Mass. Sup. Ct.).

Tani, Y., Fujiwara, T., Kondo, N., Noma, H., Sasaki, Y., & Kondo, K. (2016). Childhood socioeconomic status and onset of depression among Japanese older adults: The JAGES prospective cohort study. *American Journal of Geriatric Psychiatry*, *24*(9), 717–726. https://doi.org/10.1016/j.jagp.2016.06.001

Taniguchi, T., Takaki, J., Hirokawa, K., Fujii, Y., & Harano, K. (2016). Associations of workplace bullying and harassment with stress reactions: A two-year follow-up study. *Industrial Health*, *54*(2), 131–138. https://doi.org/10.2486/indhealth.2014-0206

Tarasov, V. V., Ivanets, N. N., Svistunov, A. A., Chubarev, V. N., Kinkulkina, M. A., Tikhonova, Y. G., Syzrantsev, N. S., Chubarev, I. V., Muresanu, C., Somasundaram, S. G., Kirkland, C. E., & Aliev, G. (2021). Biological mechanisms of atypical and melancholic major depressive disorder. *Current Pharmaceutical Design*, *27*(31), 3399–3412. https://doi.org/10.2174/1381612827666210603145441

Tarumi, S. (2005). New dysthymic type of depression fostered by modern society. *Clinical Medicine, 34,* 687–694.

Taylor, C. L. (2017). Creativity and mood disorder: A systematic review and meta-analysis. *Perspectives on Psychological Science, 12,* 1040–1076. https://doi.org/10.1177/1745691617699653

Taylor, M. (2012). Not with a bang but a whimper. *Anthropoetics, 18*(1), Article 1801. http://anthropoetics.ucla.edu/category/ap1801

Taylor, P. (ed.) (2013). *The Rise of Asian Americans* (pp. 53–36). Pew Research Center. https://www.pewresearch.org/social-trends/2012/06/19/the-rise-of-asian-americans/.

Teo, A. R. (n.d.). *Dr. Alan Teo.* www.dralanteo.com

Teo, A. R., Chen, C. I., Kubo, H., Katsuki, R., Sato-Kasai, M., Shimokawa, N., Hayakawa, K., Umene-Nakano, W., Aikens, J. E., Kanba, S., & Kato, T. A. (2018). Development and validation of the 25-item Hikikomori Questionnaire (HQ-25). *Psychiatry and Clinical Neurosciences, 72*(10), 780–788. https://doi.org/10.1111/pcn.12691

Teo, A. R., & Gaw, A. C. (2010). Hikikomori, a Japanese culture-bound syndrome of social withdrawal? A proposal for DSM-5. *The Journal of Nervous and Mental Disease, 198*(6), 444–449. https://doi.org/10.1097/NMD.0b013e3181e086b1

TheLocal.se. (2015, April 13). Sweden the "least religious" nation in the Western world. *The Local.* https://www.thelocal.se/20150413/swedes-least-religious-in-western-world

Theorell, T., Perski, A., Akerstedt, T., Sigala, F., Ahlberg-Hulten, G., Svensson, J., & Peneroth, P. (1988). Changes in job strain in relation to changes in physiological state. A longitudinal study. *Scandinavian Journal of Work and Environmental Health, 14,* 189–196.

Theroux, P. (2015). *Deep South: Four Seasons on Back Roads.* Boston: Houghton Mifflin Harcourt.

Thiese, M. S., Moffitt, G., Hanowski, R. J., Kales, S. N., Porter, R. J., & Hegmann, K. T. (2015). Commercial driver medical examinations: Prevalence of obesity, comorbidities, and certification outcomes. *Journal of Occupational and Environmental Medicine, 57,* 659–665. https://doi.org/10.1097/JOM.0000000000000422

Thomas, J. L., Jones, G. N., Scarinci, I. C., Mehan, D. J., & Brantley, P. J. (2001). The utility of the CES-D as a depression screening measure among low-income women attending primary care clinics. *International Journal of Psychiatry in Medicine, 31*(1), 25–40. https://doi.org/10.2190/FUFR-PK9F-6U10-JXRK

Thomas, K. J. A. (2012). *A Demographic Profile of Black Caribbean immigrants in the United States.* Migration Policy Institute.

Thomason, M. E., Hendrix, C. L., Werchan, D., & Brito, N. H. (2021). Social determinants of health exacerbate disparities in COVID-19 illness severity and lasting symptom complaints. *MedRxiv: The Preprint Server for Health Sciences.* https://doi.org/10.1101/2021.07.16.21260638

Thommasen, H. V., Lavanchy, M., Connelly, I., Berkowitz, J., & Grzybowski, S. (2001). Mental health, job satisfaction, and intention to relocate. Opinions of physicians in rural British Columbia. *Canadian Family Physician, 47,* 737–744.

Thompson, R., Lawrance, E. L., Roberts, L. F., Grailey, K., Ashrafian, H., Maheswaran, H., Toledano, M. B., & Darzi, A. (2023). Ambient temperature and mental health: A systematic review and meta-analysis. *The Lancet Planetary Health, 7*(7), e580–e589. https://doi.org/10.1016/S2542-5196(23)00104-3

Thomson, I. (2004). *Primo Levi: A Life.* Picador.

Thonney, J., Kanachi, M., Sasaki, H., & Hatayama, T. (2006). Guilt and shame in Japan: Data provided by the thematic apperception test in experimental settings. *North American Journal of Psychology, 8*, 85–98.

Thorpe, A., Fagerlin, A., Drews, F. A., Shoemaker, H., Brecha, F. S., & Scherer, L. D. (2024). Predictors of COVID-19 vaccine uptake: an online three-wave survey study of US adults. BMC Infectious Diseases, 24(1), 304. https://doi.org/10.1186/s12879-024-09148-9

Thun, S., Halsteinli, V., & Løvseth, L. (2018). A study of unreasonable illegitimate tasks, administrative tasks, and sickness presenteeism amongst Norwegian physicians: An everyday struggle? *BMC Health Services Research, 18*(1), Article 407. https://doi.org/10.1186/s12913-018-3229-0

Times Higher Education (2021). Keio University. *World University Rankings*. Retrieved May 15, 2021, from https://www.timeshighereducation.com/world-university-rankings/keio-university

Ting, J. Y., & Hwang, W.-C. (2009). Cultural influences on help-seeking attitudes in Asian American students. *American Journal of Orthopsychiatry, 79*(1), 125–132.

Toivonen, T., Norasakkunkit, V., & Uchida, Y. (2011). Unable to conform, unwilling to rebel? Youth, culture, and motivation in globalizing Japan. *Frontiers in Psychology, 2*, Article 207. https://doi.org/10.3389/fpsyg.2011.00207

Toma, S., MacIntosh, B. J., Swardfager, W., & Goldstein, B. I. (2018). Cerebral blood flow in bipolar disorder: A systematic review. *Journal of Affective Disorders, 241*, 505–513.

Torok, M., Han, J., Baker, S., Werner-Seidler, A., Wong, I., Larsen, M. E., & Christensen, H. (2020). Suicide prevention using self-guided digital interventions: A systematic review and meta-analysis of randomised controlled trials. *The Lancet Digital Health, 2*(1), e25–e36. https://doi.org/10.1016/S2589-7500(19)30199-2

Tóth, B., Hegyi, P., Lantos, T., Szakács, Z., Kerémi, B., Varga, G., Tenk, J., Pétervári, E., Balaskó, M., Rumbus, Z., Rakonczay, Z., Bálint, E. R., Kiss, T., & Csupor, D. (2019). The efficacy of saffron in the treatment of mild to moderate depression: A meta-analysis. *Planta Medica, 85*(1), 24–31. https://doi.org/10.1055/a-0660-9565

Transport Canada (2023). Psychiatry (SSRIs). *Handbook for Civil Aviation Medical Examiners*. Retrieved October 1, 2023 from https://tc.canada.ca/en/aviation/publications/handbook-civil-aviation-medical-examiners-tp-13312#psychiatry-ssris

Trimble, M. (2012). *Why People Like to Cry*. Oxford University Press.

Troxel, W. M., Helmus, T. C., Tsang, F., & Price, C. C. (2016). Evaluating the impact of whole-body vibration (WBV) on fatigue and the implications for driver safety. *Rand Health Quarterly, 5*(4), Article 6.

Truck Drivers Jobs (2023). Is it safe to be a female truck driver? *Truck Drivers Jobs*. Retrieved August 15, 2023, from https://truckdriversjobs.net/cdl-jobs-for-women/.

Tsai, F. J., Huang, Y. H., Liu, H. C., Huang, K. Y., Huang, Y. H., & Liu, S. I. (2014). Patient health questionnaire for school-based depression screening among adolescents. *Pediatrics, 133*(2), e402–e409. https://doi.org/10.1542/peds.2013-0204

Tsai, M.-Y., Chen, S.-Y., & Lin, C.-C. (2017). Theoretical basis, application, reliability, and sample size estimates of a meridian energy analysis device for traditional Chinese medicine research. *Clinics, 72*(4), 254–257. https://doi.org/10.6061/clinics/2017(04)10

Tsitsika, A., Janikian, M., Schoenmakers, T. M., Tzavela, E. C., Olafsson, K., Wójcik, S., Macarie, G, F., Tzavara, C., The EU NET ADB Consortium, & Richardson, C. (2014). Internet addictive behavior in adolescence: A cross-sectional study in seven European countries. *Cyberpsychology, Behavior and Social Networks*, *17*(8), 528–535. https://doi.org/10.1089/cyber.2013.0382

Tsuno, K., Kawakami, N., Tsutsumi, A., Shimazu, A., Inoue A., Odagiri, Y., Yoshikawa, T., Haratani, T., Shimomitsu, T., & Kawachi, I. (2015). Socioeconomic determinants of bullying in the workplace: A national representative sample in Japan. *PLOS ONE*, *10*(3), Article e0119435. https://doi.org/10.1371/journal.pone.0119435

Tucker, J. S., Pollard, M. S., & Green, H. D., Jr. (2021). Associations of social capital with binge drinking in a national sample of adults: The importance of neighborhoods and networks. *Health & Place*, *69*, Article 102545. https://doi.org/10.1016/j.healthplace.2021.102545

Tummala-Narra, P., Li, Z., Yang, E. J., Xiu, Z., Cui, E., & Song, Y. (2021). Intergenerational family conflict and ethnic identity among Chinese American college students. *The American Journal of Orthopsychiatry*, *91*(1), 36–49. https://doi.org/10.1037/ort0000515

Ueno, Y. (Ed.) (2008). Matsuo Bashō: *Oinokobuki/sarashinakiko/saganikki*. Izumi Shoin.

UK Civil Aviation Authority (2013, March 10). *Class 1–2 certification—Depression*. Retrieved September 1, 2019, from http://www.caa.co.uk/Aeromedical-Examiners/Medical-standards/Pilots-(EASA)/Conditions/Mental-health/Mental-health-GM/

UK Civil Aviation Authority (2023). *Mental Health Guidance Material*. Retrieved September 1, 2023 from https://www.caa.co.uk/aeromedical-examiners/medical-standards/pilots/conditions/mental-health/mental-health-guidance-material-gm/

Umegaki, Y., & Todo, N. (2017). Psychometric properties of the Japanese CES-D, SDS, and PHQ-9 depression scales in university students. *Psychological Assessment*, *29*(3), 354–359. https://doi.org/10.1037/pas0000351

United Health Foundation (2020). *America's Health Rankings*. Retrieved July 7, 2021, from https://www.americashealthrankings.org/explore/annual

United Health Foundation (2023). *America's Health Rankings*. Self-rated mental health status incuding suicidal ideation. Retrieved August 10, 2023, from www.americashealthrankings.org

U.S. Census Bureau (2015). *Asian/Pacific American Heritage Month: May 2015*. Retrieved September 27, 2019, from https://www.census.gov/newsroom/facts-for-features/2015/cb15-ff07.html

U. S. Census Bureau (2021). American Community Survey 2020: ACS 5-Year Estimates. Table B04006: People Reporting Ancestry. https://data.census.gov/table/ACSDT5Y2020.B04006. Accessed August 20, 2024.

U.S. Census Bureau (2022). *Wealth and asset ownership for households, by type of asset and selected characteristics: 2020*. Retrieved March 29, 2023, from https://www.census.gov/data/tables/2020/demo/wealth/wealth-asset-ownership.html

U.S. Census Bureau (2023a). *America's Families and Living Arrangements*: 2023. https://www.census.gov/data/tables/2023/demo/families/cps-2023.html. Accessed August 1, 2024.

U.S. Census Bureau (2023b). *American Community Survey 2021*. Selected Population Profile in the United States. Table S0201. Retrieved October 5, 2023, from https://data.census.gov/table?t=-09&g=010XX00US.

U.S. Census Bureau (2023c). *Explore Census Data*. https://data.census.gov. Details of specific queries appear in footnotes to the tables that cite their data.

U.S. Census Bureau (2023d). *Household Pulse Survey: Measuring Social and Economic Impacts during the Coronavirus Pandemic*. https://www.census.gov/programs-surveys/household-pulse-survey.html. Accessed September 1, 2023.

U.S. Census Bureau (2023e). *American Community Survey 2020*. Table B02015 Asian Alone by Selected Groups. https://data.census.gov/table?q==ACSDT5Y2020.B02015

U.S. Census Bureau (2024a). *Profile of Los Angeles County by race and ethnicity*. https://data.census.gov/profile/Los_Angeles_County,_California?g=050XX00US06037#race-and-ethnicity. Accessed August 1, 2024.

U.S. Census Bureau (2024b). Poverty Status in the Past 12 Months. *American Community Survey*, Table S1701. https://data.census.gov/table/ACSST5Y2022.S1701?g=010XX00US$0400000. Accessed August 1, 2024.

U.S. Environmental Protection Agency (2023). *Toxics Release Inventory (TRI) Program*. https://www.epa.gov/toxics-release-inventory-tri-program

U.S. Federal Reserve (2023). *Economic Well-Being of U.S. Households in 2020*. https://www.federalreserve.gov/publications/2021-supplemental-appendixes-report-economic-well-being-us-households-2020-appendix-B.html. Accessed September 1, 2023.

USA Facts (2021). *COVID Vaccine Tracker*. Retrieved July 1, 2021, from https://usafacts.org/visualizations/covid-vaccine-tracker-states/

USA Facts (2023). US Coronavirus Vaccine Tracker. https://usafacts.org/visualizations/covid-vaccine-tracker-states/. Accessed October 1, 2024.

Usuda, K., Nishi, D., Okazaki, E., Makino, M., & Sano, Y. (2017). Optimal cut-off score of the Edinburgh Postnatal Depression Scale for major depressive episode during pregnancy in Japan. *Psychiatry and Clinical Neurosciences*, 71(12), 836–842. https://doi.org/10.1111/pcn.12562

Vaa Stelling, B. E., & West, C. P. (2021). Faculty disclosure of personal mental health history and resident physician perceptions of stigma surrounding mental illness. *Academic Medicine: Journal of the Association of American Medical Colleges*, 96(5), 682–685. https://doi.org/10.1097/ACM.0000000000003941

Valdivieso-Mora, E., Peet, C. L., Garnier-Villarreal, M., Salazar-Villanea, M., & Johnson, D. K. (2016). A systematic review of the relationship between familism and mental health outcomes in Latino Population. *Frontiers in Psychology*, 7, Article 1632. https://doi.org/10.3389/fpsyg.2016.01632

Vance, J. D. (2016). *Hillbilly Elegy: A memoir of a family and culture in crisis*. New York: Harper.

van Dalfsen, J. H., & Markus, C. R. (2018). The influence of sleep on human hypothalamic–pituitary–adrenal (HPA) axis reactivity: A systematic review. *Sleep Medicine Reviews*, 39, 187–194. https://doi.org/10.1016/j.smrv.2017.10.002

VanderWeele, T. J., Li, S., Tsai, A. C., & Kawachi, I. (2016). Association between religious service attendance and lower suicide rates among US women. *JAMA Psychiatry*, 73(8), 845–851. https://doi.org/10.1001/jamapsychiatry.2016.1243

Van Orden, K. A., Witte, T. K., Cukrowicz, K. C., Braithwaite, S. R., Selby, E. A., & Joiner, T. E., Jr. (2010). The interpersonal theory of suicide. *Psychological Review*, 117(2), 575–600. https://doi.org/10.1037/a0018697

van Wendel de Joode, B., Mora, A. M., Lindh, C. H., Hernández-Bonilla, D., Córdoba, L., Wesseling, C., Hoppin, J.A., & Mergler, D. (2016). Pesticide exposure and neurodevelopment in children aged 6–9 years from Talamanca, Costa Rica. *Cortex; A Journal Devoted to the Study of the Nervous System and Behavior* 85: 137–150. https://doi.org/10.1016/j.cortex.2016.09.003

Varda, B. K., & Glover, M., 4th (2018). Specialty board leave policies for resident physicians requesting parental leave. *JAMA*, 320(22), 2374–2377. https://doi.org/10.1001/jama.2018.15889

Vasiliu O. (2023a). Impact of SGLT2 inhibitors on metabolic status in patients with psychiatric disorders undergoing treatment with second-generation antipsychotics. *Experimental and Therapeutic Medicine, 25*(3), 125. https://doi.org/10.3892/etm.2023.11824

Vasiliu O. (2023b). Therapeutic management of atypical antipsychotic-related metabolic dysfunctions using GLP-1 receptor agonists: A systematic review. *Experimental and Therapeutic Medicine, 26*(1), 355. https://doi.org/10.3892/etm.2023.12054

Vellante, M., Zucca, G., Preti, A., Sisti, D., Rocchi, M. B., Akiskal, K. K., & Akiskal, H. S. (2011). Creativity and affective temperaments in non-clinical professional artists: An empirical psychometric investigation. *Journal of Affective Disorders, 135*(1–3), 28–36. https://doi.org/10.1016/j.jad.2011.06.062

Verhaak, A. M. S., Williamson, A., Johnson, A., Murphy, A., Saidel, M., Chua, A. L., Minen, M., & Grosberg, B. M. (2021). Migraine diagnosis and treatment: A knowledge and needs assessment of women's healthcare providers. Headache 61(1): 69–79. https://doi.org/10.1111/head.14027

Vermeulen, E., Stronks, K., Visser, M., Brouwer, I. A., Schene, A. H., Mocking, R. J., Colpo, M., Bandinelli, S., Ferrucci, L., & Nicolaou, M. (2016). The association between dietary patterns derived by reduced rank regression and depressive symptoms over time: The Invecchiare in Chianti (InCHIANTI) study. *The British Journal of Nutrition, 115*(12), 2145–2153. https://doi.org/10.1017/S0007114516001318

Vilagut, G., Forero, C. G., Barbaglia, G., & Alonso, J. (2016). Screening for depression in the general ICD with meta-analysis. *PLOS ONE, 11*(5), Article e0155431. https://doi.org/10.1371/journal.pone.0155431

Violence against doctors: Why China? Why now? What next? (2014). *Lancet, 383*(9922), 1013. https://doi.org/10.1016/S0140-6736(14)60501-8

Virta, J. J., Heikkilä, K., Perola, M., Koskenvuo, M., Räihä, I., Rinne, J. O., & Kaprio, J. (2013). Midlife sleep characteristics associated with late life cognitive function. Sleep 36(10): 1533 -1541A. https://doi.org/10.5665/sleep.3052

Viscelli, S. (2016, May). Truck stop: How one of America's steadiest jobs turned into one of its most grueling. *The Atlantic*. Retrieved July 11, 2019, from https://www.theatlantic.com/business/archive/2016/05/truck-stop/481926/

Vogel, L. (2016). Bullying still rife in medical training. *CMAJ, 188*(5), 321–322. https://doi.org/10.1503/cmaj.109-5237

Vorderwülbecke, F., Feistle, M., Mehring, M., Schneider, A., & Linde, K. (2015). Aggression and violence against primary care physicians—A nationwide questionnaire survey. *Deutsches Arzteblatt International, 112*(10), 159–165. https://doi.org/10.3238/arztebl.2015.0159

Wade, R., Jr, Cronholm, P. F., Fein, J. A., Forke, C. M., Davis, M. B., Harkins-Schwarz, M., Pachter, L. M., & Bair-Merritt, M. H. (2016). Household and community-level Adverse Childhood Experiences and adult health outcomes in a diverse urban population. *Child Abuse & Neglect, 52*, 135–145. https://doi.org/10.1016/j.chiabu.2015.11.021

Wadley, A. L., Iacovides, S., Roche, J., Scheuermaier, K., Venter, W., Vos, A. G., & Lalla-Edward, S. T. (2020). Working nights and lower leisure-time physical activity associate with chronic pain in southern African long-distance truck drivers: A cross-sectional study. *PLOS ONE, 15*(12), Article e0243366. https://doi.org/10.1371/journal.pone.0243366

Wagstaff, A. S., & Arva, P. (2009). Hearing loss in civilian airline and helicopter pilots compared to air traffic control personnel. *Aviation, Space, and Environmental Medicine, 80*(10), 857–861. https://doi.org/10.3357/asem.1991.2009

Wakefield, J. D., & Schmitz, M. F. (2017). Symptom quality versus quantity in judging prognosis: Using NESARC predictive validators to locate uncomplicated major depression on the number-of-symptoms severity continuum. *Journal of Affective Disorders*, *208*, 325–329. https://doi.org/10.1016/j.jad.2016.09.015

Wålinder, J., & Rutzt, W. (2001). Male depression and suicide. *International Clinical Psychopharmacology*, *16*, S21–S24. https://doi.org/10.1097/00004850-200103002-00004

Walker, C. (2008). *Depression and civilization: The politics of mental health in the twenty-first century*. Springer.

Wall, M., Schenck-Gustafsson, K., Minucci, D., Sendén, M. G., Løvseth, L. T., & Fridner, A. (2014). Suicidal ideation among surgeons in Italy and Sweden—a cross-sectional study. *BMC Psychology*, *2*(1), 53. https://doi.org/10.1186/s40359-014-0053-0

Walton, E. C. (2018). Asian Americans in small-town America. *Contexts* 17(4), 18–23. https://journals.sagepub.com/doi/10.1177/1536504218812864

Wan, W. (2023, January 19). Yale changes mental health policies for students in crisis. *The Washington Post*. https://www.washingtonpost.com/education/2023/01/18/yale-mental-health-policies-change/

Wang, W., Zhang, H., Washburn, D. J., Shi, H., Chen, Y., Lee, S., Du, Y., & Maddock, J. E. (2018). Factors influencing trust towards physicians among patients from 12 hospitals in China. *American Journal of Health Behavior* 42(6): 19–30. https://doi.org/10.5993/AJHB.42.6.3

Wang, B., Han, L., Wen, J., Zhang, J., & Zhu, B. (2020). Self-poisoning with pesticides in Jiangsu Province, China: A cross-sectional study on 24,602 subjects. *BMC Psychiatry*, *20*(1), Article 545. https://doi.org/10.1186/s12888-020-02882-9

Wang, C., Tian, Z., & Luo, Q. (2023). The impact of exercise on mental health during the COVID-19 pandemic: a systematic review and meta-analysis. *Frontiers in Public Health*, *11*, 1279599. https://doi.org/10.3389/fpubh.2023.1279599

Wang, C. J., Yang, T. F., Wang, G. S., Zhao, Y. Y., Yang, L. J., & Bi, B. N. (2018). Association between dietary patterns and depressive symptoms among middle-aged adults in China in 2016–2017. *Psychiatry Research*, *260*, 123–129. https://doi.org/10.1016/j.psychres.2017.11.052

Wang, F., Kessels, H. W., & Hu, H. (2014). The mouse that roared: Neural mechanisms of social hierarchy. *Trends in Neurosciences*, *37*(11), 674–682. https://doi.org/10.1016/j.tins.2014.07.005

Wang, J., Zhao, Q., Liu, T., An, M., & Pan, Z. (2019). Career orientation and its impact factors of general practitioners in Shanghai, China: A cross-sectional study. *BMJ Open*, *9*(3), Article e021980. https://doi.org/10.1136/bmjopen-2018-021980

Wang, M., Armour, C., Wu, Y., Ren, F., Zhu, X., & Yao, S. (2013). Factor structure of the CES-D and measurement invariance across gender in mainland Chinese adolescents. *Journal of Clinical Psychology*, *69*(9), 966–979. https://doi.org/10.1002/jclp.21978

Wang, M., & Liu, L. (2014). Parental harsh discipline in mainland China: Prevalence, frequency and coexistence. *Child Abuse and Neglect*, *38*, 1128–1137. https://doi.org/10.1016/j.chiabu.2014.02.016

Wang, P., & Chen, Z. (2013). Traditional Chinese medicine ZHENG and OMICS convergence: A systems approach to post-genomics medicine in a global world. *OMICS*, *17*(9), 451–459. https://doi.org/10.1089/omi.2012.0057

Wang, R., Liu, Y., Xue, D., & Helbich, M. (2019). Depressive symptoms among Chinese residents: How are the natural, built, and social environments correlated? *BMC Public Health*, *19*(1), Article 887. https://doi.org/10.1186/s12889-019-7171-9

Wang, W., Bian, Q., Zhao, Y., Li, X., Wang, W., Du, J., Zhang, G., Zhou, Q., & Zhao, M. (2014). Reliability and validity of the Chinese version of the Patient Health Questionnaire (PHQ-9) in the general population. *General Hospital Psychiatry*, *36*(5), 539–544. https://doi.org/10.1016/j.genhosppsych.2014.05.021

Wang, Y. (2008). 围炉夜话 Wéi Lú Yè Huà [*Fireside chat*]. Zhonghua Book Company. (Original work published 1854)

Wang, Y. (2017, June 7). 40 Years of "gaokao" after Mao. *Sixth Tone*. Retrieved May 24, 2019, from http://www.sixthtone.com/news/1000306/40-years-of-gaokao-after-mao

Wang, Y., Chen, Z., Guo, F., Huang, Z., Jiang, L., Duan, Q., & Zhang, J. (2017). Sleep patterns and their association with depression and behavior problems among Chinese adolescents in different grades. *PsyCh Journal*, *6*, 253–262. https://doi.org/10.1002/pchj.189

Wang, Y.-Y., Xu, D. D., Liu, R., Yang, Y., Grover, S., Ungvari, G. S., Hall, B. J., Wang, G., & Xiàng, Y.-T. (2019). Comparison of the screening ability between the 32-item Hypomania Checklist (HCL-32) and the Mood Disorder Questionnaire (MDQ) for bipolar disorder: A meta-analysis and systematic review. *Psychiatry Research*, *273*, 461–466. https://doi.org/10.1016/j.psychres.2019.01.061

Wang, Y.-Y., Xiao, L., Rao, W.-W., Chai, J.-X., & Zhang, S.-F. (2019). The prevalence of depressive symptoms in "left-behind children" in China: A meta-analysis of comparative studies and epidemiological surveys. *Journal of Affective Disorders*, *244*, 209–216. https://doi.org/10.1016/j.jad.2018.09.066

Wasserman, D., Hoven, C. W., Wasserman, C., Wall, M., Eisenberg, R., Hadlaczky, G., Kelleher, I., Sarchiapone, M., Apter, A., Balas, J., Bobes, J., Brunner, R., Corcoran, P., Cosman, D., Guillemin, F., Haring, C., Iosue, M., Kaess, M., Kahn, J.-P., . . . Carli, V. (2015). School-based suicide prevention programmes: The SEYLE cluster-randomised, controlled trial. *Lancet*, *385*(9977), 1536–1544. https://doi.org/10.1016/S0140-6736(14)61213-7

Weaver, A., Taylor, R. J., & Himle, J. (2015). Depression and mood disorder among African American and White women—Reply. *JAMA Psychiatry*, *72*(12), 1257. https://doi.org/10.1001/jamapsychiatry.2015.2202

Weaver, A., Himle, J. A., Taylor, R. J., Matusko, N. N., & Abelson, J. M. (2015). Urban vs rural residence and the prevalence of depression and mood disorder among African American women and Non-Hispanic White women. *JAMA Psychiatry*, *72*(6), 576–583. https://doi.org/10.1001/jamapsychiatry.2015.10

Weenink, J. W., Kool, R. B., Bartels, R. H., & Westert, G. P. (2017). Getting back on track: A systematic review of the outcomes of remediation and rehabilitation programmes for healthcare professionals with performance concerns. *BMJ Quality and Safety*, *26*(12), 1004–1014. https://doi.org/10.1136/bmjqs-2017-006710

Wei, L., Champman, S., Li, X., Li, X., Li, S., Chen, R., Bo, N., Chater, A., & Horne, R. (2017). Beliefs about medicines and non-adherence in patients with stroke, diabetes mellitus and rheumatoid arthritis: A cross-sectional study in China. *BMJ Open*, *7*(10), Article e017293. https://doi.org/10.1136/bmjopen-2017-017293

Weigl, M., Schneider, A., Hoffmann, F., & Angerer, P. (2015). Work stress, burnout, and perceived quality of care: A cross-sectional study among hospital pediatricians. *European Journal of Pediatrics, 174*(9), 1237–1246. https://doi.org/10.1007/s00431-015-2529-1

Wekenborg, M. K., Hill, L. K., Thayer, J. F., Penz, M., Wittling, R. A., & Kirschbaum, C. (2019). The longitudinal association of reduced vagal tone with burnout. *Psychosomatic Medicine, 81*(9), 791–798. https://doi.org/10.1097/PSY.0000000000000750

Wenger, J. (2008). Freedom isn't free: Voices from the truck driving industry. *New Solutions, 18*(4), 481–491. https://doi.org/10.2190/ns.18.4.e

Wernette, M. J., & Emory, J. (2017). Student bedtimes, academic performance, and health in a residential high school. *Journal of School Nursing, 33*(4), 264–268. https://doi.org/10.1177/1059840516677323

West, C. P., Dyrbye, L. N., Sloan, J. A., & Shanafelt, T. D. (2009). Single item measures of emotional exhaustion and depersonalization are useful for assessing burnout in medical professionals. *Journal of General Internal Medicine, 24*(12), 1318–1321. https://doi.org/10.1007/s11606-009-1129-z

Wible, P. (2015). Commentary: Do physician health programs increase physician suicides? *Medscape*, August 28. https://www.medscape.com/viewarticle/850023

Wikipedia (2023a). List of U.S. states and territories by elevation.

Wikipedia (2023b) List of ethnic groups in the United States by household income. https://en.wikipedia.org/wiki/List_of_ethnic_groups_in_the_United_States_by_household_income#cite_note-byancestry2-6. Accessed September 1, 2023.

Wilcox, W. B., & DeRose, L. (2017). *World Family Map 2017: Mapping Family change and Child Well-Being Outcomes*. Social Trends Institute. Retrieved October 14, 2019, from http://socialtrendsinstitute.org/upload/worldfamilymap-2019-051819final.pdf

Willie, T. C., & Kershaw, T. S. (2019). An ecological analysis of gender inequality and intimate partner violence in the United States. *Preventive Medicine, 118*, 257–263. https://doi.org/10.1016/j.ypmed.2018.10.019

Willie, T. C., Kershaw, T., & Sullivan, T. P. (2018). The impact of adverse childhood events on the sexual and mental health of women experiencing intimate partner violence. *Journal of Interpersonal Violence, 36*(11–12), 5145–5166. https://doi.org/10.1177/0886260518802852

Willoughby, A. R., Alikhani, I., Karsikas, M., Chua, X. Y., & Chee, M. W. L. (2023). Country differences in nocturnal sleep variability: Observations from a large-scale, long-term sleep wearable study. *Sleep Medicine, 110*, 155–165. https://doi.org/10.1016/j.sleep.2023.08.010

Wilson, D., Driller, M., Johnston, B., & Gill, N. (2021). The effectiveness of a 17-week lifestyle intervention on health behaviors among airline pilots during COVID-19. *Journal of Sport and Health Science, 10*(3), 333–340. https://doi.org/10.1016/j.jshs.2020.11.007

Winehouse, A. (2006). Rehab [Song]. On *Back to Black*. Island Records.

Wing, T. (2017). Climate change, green development and the Indigenous struggle for cultural preservation in Arctic Norway. *Climate Institute*, November 28. http://climate.org/climate-change-green-development-and-the-indigenous-struggle-for-cultural-preservation-in-arctic-norway/

Winter, G., Hart, R. A., Charlesworth, R. P. G., & Sharpley, C. F. (2018). Gut microbiome and depression: What we know and what we need to know. *Review of Neuroscience, 29*(6), 629–643. https://doi.org/10.1515/revneuro-2017-0072

Wirz-Justice, A., & Terman, A. M. (2022). CME: Light therapy: Why, what, for whom, how, and when (and a postscript about darkness). *Praxis, 110*(2), 56–62. https://doi.org/10.1024/1661-8157/a003821

Wisti, E. (2017, July 21). We have nothing worse than death to fear. *The Awl*. https://www.theawl.com/2017/07/we-have-nothing-worse-than-death-to-fear/

Wong, R., Wu, R., Guo, C., Lam, J. K., & Snowden, L. R. (2012). Culturally sensitive depression assessment for Chinese American immigrants: Development of a comprehensive measure and a screening scale using an item response approach. *Asian American Journal of Psychology*, *3*(4), 230–253. https://doi.org/10.1037/a0025628

Wong, W. C., Tam, S. M., & Leung, P. W. (2007). Cross-border truck drivers in Hong Kong: Their psychological health, sexual dysfunctions and sexual risk behaviors. *Journal of Travel Medicine*, *14*(1), 20–30. https://doi.org/10.1111/j.1708-8305.2006.00085.x

Woo, J., Chang, S. M., Hong, J. P., Lee, D. W., Hahm, B. J., Cho, S. J., Park, J. I., Jeon, H. J., Seong, S. J., Park, J. E., & Kim, B. S. (2019). The association of childhood experience of peer bullying with DSM-IV psychiatric disorders and suicidality in adults: Results from a nationwide survey in Korea. Journal of Korean Medical Science, 34(46), e295. https://doi.org/10.3346/jkms.2019.34.e295

Woodard, C. (2011). *American Nations*. Viking Penguin.

Woodward, A., Lipari, R., & Eaton, W. (2017). Occupations and the prevalence of major depressive episode in the National Survey on Drug Use and Health. *Psychiatric Rehabilitation Journal*, *40*(2), 172–178. https://doi.org/10.1037/prj0000251

Woodyard, C. (2019). Women are increasingly joining the deadly world of truck driving, confronting sexism and long days. *USA TODAY*, March 9. https://www.usatoday.com/story/news/nation/2019/03/09/women-truck-drivers-shortage-opportunities-pay-big-rigs/2845083002/

World Bank (2019). World development indicators: Rural population (% of total population). https://databank.worldbank.org/data/reports.aspx?source=world-development-indicators

World Bank (2021). GDP per capita (constant 2010 US$), Republic of Korea. Retrieved May 18, 2021, https://data.worldbank.org/indicator/NY.GDP.PCAP.CD?locations=KR

World Bank (2023a). GDP per capita (current US$). Retrieved October 1, 2023 from https://data.worldbank.org/indicator/NY.GDP.PCAP.CD?locations=JP&view=chart

World Bank (2023b).Life expectancy at birth, total (years) -Japan. Retrieved October 1, 2023 from https://data.worldbank.org/indicator/SP.DYN.LE00.IN?locations=JP.

World Economic Forum (2020). *The Global Social Mobility Report 2020: Equality, Opportunity and a New Economic Imperative*. https://www3.weforum.org/docs/Global_Social_Mobility_Report.pdf

World Economic Forum (2023). *Global Gender Gap Report 2023*. Retrieved October 1, 2023, from https://www3.weforum.org/docs/WEF_GGGR_2023.pdf

World Health Organization (1992). *The ICD-10 Classification of Mental and Behavioral Disorders: Clinical Descriptions and Diagnostic Guidelines*.

World Health Organization (2018). *Global Status Report on Alcohol and Health 2018*. Geneva: World Health Organization; pp. 221, 316, 319, 322.

World Health Organization (2023). Global status report on physical activity 2022: Country profiles. https://www.who.int/publications/i/item/9789240064119. Accessed October 1, 2024.

World Population Review (2021). *Prison Population by State*. Retrieved July 4, 2021, from https://worldpopulationreview.com/state-rankings/prison-population-by-state

World Population Review (2024a). *Age at First Marriage by Country*. Retrieved October, 1, 2024, from https://worldpopulationreview.com/country-rankings/age-at-first-marriage-by-country

World Population Review (2024b). *Average Age of Having First Child by Country*. Retrieved October 1, 2024, from https://worldpopulationreview.com/country-rankings/average-age-of-having-first-child-by-country

World Values Survey Association (2023). *The Inglehart-Welzel World Cultural Map*. https://www.worldvaluessurvey.org/WVSNewsShow.jsp?ID=467. Accessed August 1, 2024.

Worley S. L. (2018). The extraordinary importance of sleep: The detrimental effects of inadequate sleep on health and public safety drive an explosion of sleep research. *Pharmacy and Therapeutics, 43*(12), 758–763.

Wu, A. C., Donnelly-McLay, D., Weisskopf, M. G., McNeely, E., Betancourt, T. S., & Allen, J. G. (2016). Airplane pilot mental health and suicidal thoughts: A cross-sectional descriptive study via anonymous web-based survey. *Environmental Health, 15*(1), Article 121. https://doi.org/10.1186/s12940-016-0200-6

Wu, C., Chiang, M., Harrington, A., Kim, S., Ziedonis, D., & Fan, X. (2018). Racial disparity in mental disorder diagnosis and treatment between non-Hispanic White and Asian American patients in a general hospital. *Asian Journal of Psychiatry, 34*, 78–83. https://doi.org/10.1016/j.ajp.2018.04.019

Wu, H., Cai, Z., Yan, Q., Yu, Y., & Yu, N. N. (2021). The impact of childhood left-behind experience on the mental health of late adolescents: Evidence from Chinese college freshmen. *International Journal of Environmental Research and Public Health, 18*(5), Article 2778. https://doi.org/10.3390/ijerph18052778

Wu, J. (2008). *The scholars* (G. Yang, Trans.). Silk Pagoda.

Wu, J., Yeung, A. S., Schnyer, R., Wang, Y., & Mischoulon, D. (2012). Acupuncture for depression: A review of clinical applications. *Canadian Journal of Psychiatry, 57*(7), 397–405. https://doi.org/10.1177/070674371205700702

Wu, R., Zhu, H., Wang, Z. J., & Jiang, C. L. (2021). A large sample survey of suicide risk among university students in China. *BMC Psychiatry, 21*(1), Article 474. https://doi.org/10.1186/s12888-021-03480-z

Wu, S., Wang, X., Wu, Q., Zhai, F., & Gao, Q. (2017). Acculturation-based family conflict: A validation of Asian American Family Conflict Scale among Chinese Americans. *PsyCh Journal, 6*(4), 294–302. https://doi.org/10.1002/pchj.183

Wu, Y., Levis, B., Riehm, K. E., Saadat, N., Levis, A. W., Azar, M., Rice, D. B., Boruff, J., Cuijpers, P., Gilbody, S., Ioannidis, J. P. A., Kloda, L. A., McMillan, D., Patten, S. B., Shrier, I., Ziegelstein, R. C., Akena, D. H., Arroll, B., Ayalon, L., ... Thombs, B. D. (2019). Equivalency of the diagnostic accuracy of the PHQ-8 and PHQ-9: A systematic review and individual participant data meta-analysis. *Psychological Medicine, 50*(8), 1368–1380. https://doi.org/10.1017/S0033291719001314

Wu, Y., Levis, B., Sun, Y., He, C., Krishnan, A., Neupane, D., Bhandari, P. M., Negeri, Z., Benedetti, A., & Thombs, B. D. (2021). Accuracy of the Hospital Anxiety and Depression Scale Depression subscale (HADS-D) to screen for major depression: Systematic review and individual participant data meta-analysis. *BMJ, 373*, Article n972. https://doi.org/10.1136/bmj.n972

Wu, Y.-C. (2016). A disorder of *qi*: Breathing exercise as a cure for neurasthenia in Japan, 1900–1945. *Journal of the History of Medicine and Allied Sciences, 71*(3), 322–344. https://doi.org/10.1093/jhmas/jrv029

Wu, Y. T., Prina, A. M., Jones, A., Matthews, F. E., & Brayne, C. (2015). Older people, the natural environment and common mental disorders: Cross-sectional results from the Cognitive Function and Ageing Study. BMJ Open, 5(9), Article e007936. https://doi.org/10.1136/bmjopen-2015-007936

Wurm, W., Vogel, K., Holl, A., Ebner, C., Bayer, D., Mörkl, S., Szilagyi, I.-S., Hotter, E., Kapfhammer, H.-P., & Hoffmann, P. (2016). Depression–burnout overlap in physicians. *PLOS ONE, 11*(3), Article e0149913. https://doi.org/10.1371/journal.pone.0149913

Xia, N.-G., Lin, J.-H., Ding, S.-Q., Dong, F.-R., Shen, J.-Z., Du, Y.-R., Wang, X.-S., Chen, Y.-Y., Zhu, Z.-G., Zheng, R.-Y., & Xu, H.-Q. (2019). Reliability and validity of the Chinese version of the Patient Health Questionnaire 9 (C-PHQ-9) in patients with epilepsy. *Epilepsy & Behavior, 95*(5), 65–69. https://doi.org/10.1016/j.yebeh.2019.03.049

Xianguo Kong v. Trustees of the University of Pennsylvania (2018). https://info.feldmanshepherd.com/hubfs/Complaint%20-%20FILED%20-%20Redacted.pdf?t=1523387373569&utm_campaign=Kong_%20Press%20Release&utm_source=hs_email&utm_medium=email&_hsenc=p2ANqtz-_uqDtYNYn0F4__lcJSY-UC6n4g7_BuBant07NZOy6tKbuGpjTEoXjU-luFVNotDoEQVojx

Xiao, Y. (1992). [*The History of Zhuangyuan*]; 狀元史話; Zhuangyuan shihua. Chongqing Publishing House.

Xiong, M., Li, Y., Tang, P., Zhang, Y., Cao, M., Ni, J., & Xing, M. (2018). Effectiveness of aromatherapy massage and inhalation on symptoms of depression in Chinese community-dwelling older adults. *Journal of Alternative and Complementary Medicine, 24*(7), 717–724. https://doi.org/10.1089/acm.2017.0320

Xu, K. (2019). Holistic disease of the times—The catastrophe of exam-oriented education. *Zhiru*. https://zhuanlan.zhihu.com/p/21651116

Xu, Z., Zhang, S., Huang, L., Zhu, X., Zhao, Q., Zeng, Y., Zhou, D., Wang, D., Kuga, H., Kamiya, A., & Qu, M. (2018). Altered resting-state brain activities in drug-naïve major depressive disorder assessed by fMRI: Associations with somatic symptoms defied by yin-yang theory of traditional Chinese medicine. *Frontiers in Psychiatry, 9*, Article 195. https://doi.org/10.3389/fpsyt.2018.00195

Yaghmour, N. A., Brigham, T. P., Richter, T., Miller, R. S., Philibert, I., Baldwin, D. C., Jr., & Nasca, T. J. (2017). Causes of death of residents in ACGME-accredited programs 2000 through 2014: Implications for the learning environment. *Academic Medicine, 92*(7), 976–983. https://doi.org/10.1097/ACM.0000000000001736

Yale College Programs of Study. (2023). Academic regulations: J. Time away and return: Postponement, leave of absence, medical leave of absence, and withdrawal. *Bulletin of Yale University*, updated January 2023. https://catalog.yale.edu/ycps/academic-regulations/leave-of-absence-withdrawal-reinstatement/

Yalin, N., & Young, A. H. (2020). Pharmacological treatment of bipolar depression: What are the current and emerging options? *Neuropsychiatric Disease and Treatment, 16*, 1459–1472. https://doi.org/10.2147/NDT.S245166

Yamaguchi, A., Kim, M.-S., Oshio, A., & Akutsu, S. (2016). Relationship between bicultural identity and psychological well-being among American and Japanese older adults. *Health Psychology Open, 3*(1). https://doi.org/10.1177/2055102916650093

Yamaguchi, M. (2018, March 9). Japan Finance Ministry confirms death of official in scandal. *AP News*. https://www.apnews.com/7ff8022d80334935871776a22364f8f2

Yamashita, T., Bardo, A. R., Millar, R. J., & Liu, D. (2020). Numeracy and preventive health care service utilization among middle-aged and older adults in the U.S. *Clinical Gerontologist, 43*(2), 221–232. https://doi.org/10.1080/07317115.2018.1468378

Yamazaki, Y., Kozono, Y., Mori, R., & Marui, E. (2011). Difficulties facing physician mothers in Japan. *Tohoku Journal of Experimental Medicine, 225*(3), 203–209.

Yan, Y. (2018). The ethics and politics of patient-physician mistrust in contemporary China. *Developing World Bioethics*, *18*(1), 7–15. https://doi.org/10.1111/dewb.12155

Yang, A. C., Tsai, S. J., Yang, C. H., Shia, B. C., Fuh, J. L., Wang, S. J., Peng, C. K., & Huang, N. E. (2013). Suicide and media reporting: a longitudinal and spatial analysis. *Social Psychiatry and Psychiatric Epidemiology*, *48*(3), 427–435. https://doi.org/10.1007/s00127-012-0562-1

Yang, H. C., Xiang, Y. T., Liu, T. B., Han, R., Wang, G., Hu, C., Li, L.-J., Wang, X.-P., Peng, H.-J., Si, T.-M., Fang, Y.-R., Yuan, C.-M., Lu, Z., Hu, J., Chen, Z.-Y., Huang, Y., Sun, J., Li, H.-C., Zhang, J.-B., & Angst, J. (2012). Hypomanic symptoms assessed by the Hypomania Checklist (HCL- 32) in patients with major depressive disorder: A multicenter trial across China. *Journal of Affective Disorders*, *143*(1–3), 203–207. https://doi.org/10.1016/j.jad.2012.06.002

Yang, S. J., Kim, J. M., Kim, S. W., Shin, I. S., & Yoon, J. S. (2006). Bullying and victimization behaviors in boys and girls at South Korean primary schools. *Journal of the American Academy of Child and Adolescent Psychiatry*, *45*(1), 69–77. https://doi.org/10.1097/01.chi.0000186401.05465.2c

Yang, Y. (2003). Demon and confinement: The disposal of psychiatric patients by the Song people. *Journal of History of Taiwan Normal University*, *31*, 37–90.

Yang, T., Wang, J., Huang, J., Kelly, F. J., & Li, G. (2023). Long-term exposure to multiple ambient air pollutants and association with incident depression and anxiety. *JAMA Psychiatry*, *80*(4), 305–313. https://doi.org/10.1001/jamapsychiatry.2022.4812

Yao, H., Wang, P., Tang, Y. L., Liu, Y., Liu, T., Liu, H., Chen, Y., Jiang, F., & Zhu, J. (2021). Burnout and job satisfaction of psychiatrists in China: a nationwide survey. *BMC Psychiatry* 21(1): 593. https://doi.org/10.1186/s12888-021-03568-6

Yatham, L. N., Kennedy, S. H., Parikh, S. V., Schaffer, A., Bond, D. J., Frey, B. N., Sharma, V., Goldstein, B. I., Rej, S., Beaulieu, S., Alda, M., MacQueen, G., Milev, R. V., Ravindran, A., O'Donovan, C., McIntosh, D., Lam, R. W., Vazquez, G., Kapczinski, F., . . . Berk, M. (2018). Canadian Network for Mood and Anxiety Treatments (CANMAT) and International Society for Bipolar Disorders (ISBD) 2018 guidelines for the management of patients with bipolar disorder. *Bipolar Disorders*, *20*(2), 97–170. https://doi.org/10.1111/bdi.12609

Yau, W. Y., Chan, M. C., Wing, Y. K., Lam, H. B., Lin, W., Lam, S. P., & Lee, C. P. (2014). Noncontinuous use of antidepressant in adults with major depressive disorders—A retrospective cohort study. *Brain and Behavior*, *4*(3), 390–397. https://doi.org/10.1002/brb3.224

Ye, G. F., Thatipamala, P., & Siegel, M. (2022). Assessment of reasons for ownership and attitudes about policies among firearm owners with and without children. *JAMA Network Open*, *5*(1), e2142995. https://doi.org/10.1001/jamanetworkopen.2021.42995

Ye, G. Y., Davidson, J. E., Kim, K., & Zisook, S. (2021). Physician death by suicide in the U.S.: 2012–2016. *Journal of Psychiatric Research*, *134*, 158–165. https://doi.org/10.1016/j.jpsychires.2020.12.064

Ye, X., Shu, H. L., Feng, X., Xia, D. M., Wang, Z. Q., Mi, W. Y., Yu, B., Zhang, X. L., & Li, C. (2020). Reliability and validity of the Chinese version of the Patient Health Questionnaire-9 (C-PHQ-9) in patients with psoriasis: A cross-sectional study. *BMJ Open*, *10*(7), Article e033211. https://doi.org/10.1136/bmjopen-2019-033211

Yen, S., Robins, C. J., & Lin, N. (2000). A cross-cultural comparison of depressive symptom manifestation: China and the United States. *Journal of Consulting and Clinical Psychology*, *68*(6), 993–999. https://doi.org/10.1037//0022-006x.68.6.993

Yeung, A., Chan, R., Mischoulon, D., Sonawalla, S., Wong, E., Nierenberg, A. A., & Fava, M. (2004). Prevalence of major depressive disorder among Chinese-Americans in primary care. *General Hospital Psychiatry, 26*(1), 24–30. https://doi.org/10.1016/j.genhospps ych.2003.08.006

Yeung, A., Chang, D., Gresham, R., Nierenberg, A., & Fava, M. (2004). Illness beliefs of depressed Chinese American patients in primary care. *The Journal of Nervous and Mental Disease, 192*(4), 324–327. https://doi.org/10.1097/01.nmd.0000120892.96624.00

Yeung, A., Martinson, M. A., Baer, L., Chen, J., Clain, A., Williams, A., Chang, T. E., Trinh, N.-H. T., Alpert, J. E., & Fava, M. (2016). The effectiveness of telepsychiatry-based culturally sensitive collaborative treatment for depressed Chinese American immigrants: A randomized controlled trial. *The Journal of Clinical Psychiatry, 77*(8), e996–e1002. https://doi.org/10.4088/JCP.15m09952

Yeung, A., Trinh, N. H., Chang, T. E., & Fava, M. (2011). The Engagement Interview Protocol (EIP): Improving the acceptance of mental health treatment among Chinese immigrants. *International Journal of Culture and Mental Health, 4*(2), 91–105. https://doi.org/10.1080/17542863.2010.507933

Yeung, A., Wang, F., Feng, F., Zhang, J., Cooper, A., Hong, L., Wang, W., Griffiths, K., Bennett, K., Bennett, A., Alpert, J., & Fava, M. (2018). Outcomes of an online computerized cognitive behavioral treatment program for treating Chinese patients with depression: A pilot study. *Asian Journal of Psychiatry, 38*, 102–107. https://doi.org/10.1016/j.ajp.2017.11.007

Yeung, K. S., Hernandez, M., Mao, J. J., Haviland, I., & Gubili, J. (2018). Herbal medicine for depression and anxiety: A systematic review with assessment of potential psycho-oncologic relevance. *Phytotherapy Research, 32*(5), 865–891. https://doi.org/10.1002/ptr.6033

Yeung, W.-F., Chung, K.-F., Ng, K.-Y., Yu, Y.-M., Zhang, S.-P., Ng, B. F.-L., & Ziea, E. T.-C. (2015). Prescription of Chinese herbal medicine in pattern-based traditional Chinese medicine treatment for depression: A systematic review. *Evidence-Based Complementary and Alternative Medicine, 2015*, Article 160189. https://doi.org/10.1155/2015/160189

Yim, I. S., & Kofman, Y. B. (2018). The psychobiology of stress and intimate partner violence. *Psychoneuroendocrinology, 105*, 9–24. https://doi.org/10.1016/j.psyneuen.2018.08.017

Ying, Y., Lee, P. A., Tsai, J. L., Lee, Y. J., & Tsang, M. (2001). Relationship of young adult Chinese Americans with their parents: Variation by migratory status and cultural orientation. *American Journal of Orthopsychiatry, 71*, 342–349. https://doi.org/10.1037/0002-9432.71.3.342

Ying, Y. W. (1988). Depressive symptomatology among Chinese-Americans as measured by the CES-D. *Journal of Clinical Psychology, 44*(5), 739–746. https://doi.org/10.1002/1097-4679(198809)44:5<739::aid-jclp2270440512>3.0.co;2-0

Yoon, B. H., Angst, J., Bahk, W. M., Wang, H. R., Bae, S. O., Kim, M. D., Jung, Y.-E., Min, K. J., Lee, H.-B., Won, S., Hong, J., Choi, M. S., Jon, D.-I., & Woo, Y. S. (2017). Psychometric properties of the Hypomania Checklist-32 in Korean patients with mood disorders. *Clinical Psychopharmacology and Neuroscience, 15*(4), 352–360. https://doi.org/10.9758/cpn.2017.15.4.352

Yoshikawa, E., Nishi, D., and Matsuoka, Y. J. (2016). Association between frequency of fried food consumption and resilience to depression in Japanese company workers: A cross-sectional study. *Lipids in Health and Disease, 15*(1), Article 156. https://doi.org/10.1186/s12944-016-0331-3

Young, J., Savoy, C., Schmidt, L. A., Saigal, S., & Van Lieshout, R. J. (2019). Child sleep problems and adult mental health in those born at term or extremely low birth weight. *Sleep Medicine, 53*, 28–34. https://doi.org/10.1016/j.sleep.2018.09.007

Young, R., Sweeting, H., & Ellaway, A. (2011). Do schools differ in suicide risk? The influence of school and neighbourhood on attempted suicide, suicidal ideation and self-harm among secondary school pupils. *BMC Public Health, 11*, Article 874. https://doi.org/10.1186/1471-2458-11-874

Youngclaus, J., & Fresne, J. A. (2020). *Physician Education Debt and the Cost to Attend Medical School: 2020 Update*. Association of American Medical Colleges. Published online: https://store.aamc.org/downloadable/download/sample/sample_id/368.

Youssef, J., & Deane, F. P. (2013). Arabic-speaking religious leaders' perceptions of the causes of mental illness and the use of medication for treatment. *Australia and New Zealand Journal of Psychiatry, 47*(11), 1041–1050. https://doi.org/10.1177/0004867413499076

Yu, J., Cheah, C. S., & Calvin, G. (2016). Acculturation, psychological adjustment, and parenting styles of Chinese immigrant mothers in the United States. *Cultural Diversity & Ethnic Minority Psychology, 22*(4), 504–516. https://doi.org/10.1037/cdp0000091

Yu, L., Cao, Y., Wang, Y., Liu, T., MacDonald, A., Bian, F., Li, X., Wang, X., Zhang, Z., Wang, P. P., & Yang, L. (2023). Mental health conditions of Chinese international students and associated predictors amidst the pandemic. Journal of Migration and Health, 7, 100185. https://doi.org/10.1016/j.jmh.2023.100185

Yu, S., Guo, X., Yang, H., Zheng, L., & Sun, Y. (2015). Soybeans or soybean products consumption and depressive symptoms in older residents in rural northeast China: A cross-sectional study. *Journal of Nutrition, Health and Aging, 19*(9), 884–893. https://doi.org/10.1007/s12603-015-0517-9

Yu, Y., & Yu, H. (Eds.). (2012). *Èrshísì Xiào* 二十四孝 [*Twenty-four exemplars of filial piety*]. Yuelu Publisher.

Yue, A., Gao, J., Yang, M., Swinnen, L., Medina, A., & Rozelle, S. (2018). Caregiver depression and early child development: A mixed-methods study from rural China. Frontiers in Psychology 9: 2500. https://doi.org/10.3389/fpsyg.2018.02500

Zalsman, G., Hawton, K., Wasserman, D., van Heeringen, K., Arensman, E., Sarchiapone, M., Carli, V., Höschl, C., Barzilay, R., Balazs, J., Purebl, G., Kahn, J. P., Sáiz, P. A., Lipsicas, C. B., Bobes, J., Cozman, D., Hegerl, U., & Zohar, J. (2016). Suicide prevention strategies revisited: 10-year systematic review. *The Lancet Psychiatry, 3*(7), 646–659. https://doi.org/10.1016/S2215-0366(16)30030-X

Zeng, Y., Lin, R., Liu, L., Liu, Y., & Li, Y. (2019). Ambient air pollution exposure and risk of depression: A systematic review and meta-analysis of observational studies. *Psychiatry Research, 276*, 69–78. https://doi.org/10.1016/j.psychres.2019.04.019

Zeng, Z. (2008). *Xiao Jing—The Classic of Xiao: With English Translation* (X. Feng, Trans.). Tsoi Dug.org. Retrieved May 24, 2019, from http://www.tsoidug.org/Xiao/Xiao_Jing_Transltn.pdf

Zhang, H., Chi, P., Long, H., & Ren, X. (2019). Bullying victimization and depression among left-behind children in rural China: Roles of self-compassion and hope. *Child Abuse & Neglect, 96*, Article 104072. https://doi.org/10.1016/j.chiabu.2019.104072

Zhang, H., Zhou, H., & Cao, R. (2021). Bullying victimization among left-behind children in rural China: Prevalence and associated risk factors. *Journal of Interpersonal Violence, 36*(15–16), NP8414–NP8430. https://doi.org/10.1177/0886260519843287

Zhang, J. (2010). Marriage and suicide among Chinese rural young women. *Social Forces, 89*(1), 311–326.

Zhang, J., Conwell, Y., Zhou, L., & Jiang, C. (2004). Culture, risk factors and suicide in rural China: A psychological autopsy case control study. *Acta Psychiatrica Scandinavica, 110*(6), 430–437. https://doi.org/10.1111/j.1600-0447.2004.00388.x

Zhang, J., Fang, L., Wu, Y. W., & Wieczorek, W. F. (2013). Depression, anxiety, and suicidal ideation among Chinese Americans: A study of immigration-related factors. *The Journal of Nervous and Mental Disease, 201*(1), 17–22. https://doi.org/10.1097/NMD.0b013e31827ab2e2

Zhang, J., & Lv, J. (2014). Psychological strains and depression in Chinese rural populations. *Psychology, Health & Medicine, 19*(3), 365–373. https://doi.org/10.1080/13548506.2013.808752

Zhang, J., Sun, W., Kong, Y., & Wang, C. (2012). Reliability and validity of the Center for Epidemiological Studies Depression Scale in 2 special adult samples from rural China. *Comprehensive Psychiatry, 53*(8), 1243–1251. https://doi.org/10.1016/j.comppsych.2012.03.015

Zhang, J., & Zhou, L. (2009). A case control study of suicides in China with and without mental disorder. *Crisis, 30*(2), 68–72. https://doi.org/10.1027/0227-5910.30.2.68

Zhang, Y., Folarin, A. A., Sun, S., Cummins, N., Bendayan, R., Ranjan, Y., Rashid, Z., Conde, P., Stewart, C., Laiou, P., Matcham, F., White, K. M., Lamers, F., Siddi, S., Simblett, S., Myin-Germeys, I., Rintala, A., Wykes, T., Haro, J. M., Penninx, B. W., ... RADAR-CNS Consortium. (2021). Relationship between major depression symptom severity and sleep collected using a wristband wearable device: Multicenter longitudinal observational study. *JMIR mHealth and uHealth, 9*(4), e24604. https://doi.org/10.2196/24604

Zhang, Y., Ting, R., Lam, M., Lam, J., Nan, H., Yeung, R., Yang, W., Ji, L., Weng, J., Wing, Y.-K., Sartorius, N., & Chan, J. C. N. (2013). Measuring depressive symptoms using the Patient Health Questionnaire-9 in Hong Kong Chinese subjects with type 2 diabetes. *Journal of Affective Disorders, 151*(2), 660–666. https://doi.org/10.1016/j.jad.2013.07.014

Zhang, Y., Wang, J., Ye, Y., Zou, Y., Chen, W., Wang, Z., & Zou, Z. (2023). Peripheral cytokine levels across psychiatric disorders: A systematic review and network meta-analysis. Progress in neuro-psychopharmacology & biological psychiatry, 125, 110740. https://doi.org/10.1016/j.pnpbp.2023.110740

Zhang, Y. L., Liang, W., Chen, Z. M., Zhang, H. M., Zhang, J. H., Weng, X. Q., Yang, S.-C., Zhang, L., Shen, L.-J., & Zhang, Y.-L. (2013). Validity and reliability of Patient Health Questionnaire-9 and Patient Health Questionnaire-2 to screen for depression among college students in China. *Asia-Pacific Psychiatry, 5*(4), 268–275. https://doi.org/10.1111/appy.12103

Zhang, Z. (1999). *Shang Han Lun: On Cold Damage, Translation and Commentaries* (Edited and translated by Mitchell, C., Ye, F., & Wiseman, N.). Paradigm Publications.

Zhang, Z. (2012). *Jin gui yao lue: Essential prescriptions of the golden cabinet, translations and commentaries* (N. Wiseman & S. Wilms, Trans.). Paradigm Publications.

Zhao, D., & Zhang, Z. (2019). Changes in public trust in physicians: empirical evidence from China. Frontiers of Medicine 13(4): 504–510. https://doi.org/10.1007/s11684-018-0666-4

Zhao, Q., Guo, R., Fan, Z., Hu, L., Hu, Z., & Liu, Y. (2023). Medical conditions and preference of Traditional Chinese Medicine: Results from the China Healthcare Improvement Evaluation Survey. Patient Preference and Adherence 17: 227–237. https://doi.org/10.2147/PPA.S398644

Zheng, K., & West-Olatunji, C. A. (2016). Mental health concerns of mainland Chinese international students in the United States: A literature review. *Vistas Online*. Article 20. https://www.counseling.org/docs/default-source/vistas/article_20fcbf24f16116603abcacff0000bee5e7.pdf?sfvrsn=4

Zheng, L., Sun, Z., Liu, C., Zhang, J., Jin, Y., & Jin, H. (2023). Acupuncture-adjuvant therapies for treating perimenopausal depression: A network meta-analysis. *Medicine*, *102*(33), e34694. https://doi.org/10.1097/MD.0000000000034694

Zhichao, H., Ching, L. W., Huijuan, L., Liang, Y., Zhiyu, W., Weiyang, H., Zhaoxiang, B., & Linda, Z. L. D. (2021). A network meta-analysis on the effectiveness and safety of acupuncture in treating patients with major depressive disorder. *Scientific Reports*, *11*(1), 10384. https://doi.org/10.1038/s41598-021-88263-y

Zhou, S., & Cheung, M. (2017). *Hukou* system effects on migrant children's education in China: Learning from past disparities. *International Social Work*, *60*(6), 1327–1342. https://doi.org/10.1177/0020872817725134

Zhou, Y., Xu, J., & Rief, W. (2020). Are comparisons of mental disorders between Chinese and German students possible? An examination of measurement invariance for the PHQ-15, PHQ-9 and GAD-7. *BMC Psychiatry*, *20*(1), Article 480. https://doi.org/10.1186/s12888-020-02859-8

Zhu, W., Wang, L., & Yang, C. (2018). Corruption or professional dignity: An ethical examination of the phenomenon of "red envelopes" (monetary gifts) in medical practice in China. *Developing World Bioethics*, *18*(1), 37–44. https://doi.org/10.1111/dewb.12152

Zhu, X., Shek, D., & Dou, D. (2021). Factor structure of the Chinese CES-D and invariance analyses across gender and over time among Chinese adolescents. *Journal of Affective Disorders*, *295*, 639–646. https://doi.org/10.1016/j.jad.2021.08.122

Zhu, Y., Wu, Z., Sie, O., Cai, Y., Huang, J., Liu, H., Yao, Y., Niu, Z., Wu, X., Shi, Y., Zhang, C., Liu, T., Rong, H., Yang, H., Peng, D., & Fang, Y. (2020). Causes of drug discontinuation in patients with major depressive disorder in China. *Progress in Neuro-psychopharmacology & Biological Psychiatry*, *96*, 109755. https://doi.org/10.1016/j.pnpbp.2019.109755

Zhuang, W., Liu, S. L., Xi, S. Y., Feng, Y. N., Wang, K., Abduwali, T., Liu, P., Zhou, X. J., Zhang, L., & Dong, X. Z. (2023). Traditional Chinese medicine decoctions and Chinese patent medicines for the treatment of depression: Efficacies and mechanisms. Journal of Ethnopharmacology, 307, 116272. https://doi.org/10.1016/j.jep.2023.116272

Zhuo, L. B., Yao, W., Yan, Z., Giron, M., Pei, J. J., & Wang, H. X. (2020). Impact of effort reward imbalance at work on suicidal ideation in ten European countries: The role of depressive symptoms. *Journal of Affective Disorders*, *260*, 214–221. https://doi.org/10.1016/j.jad.2019.09.007

Zierau, F., Bille, A., Rutz, W., & Bech, P. (2002). The Gotland Male Depression Scale: A validity study in patients with alcohol use disorder. *Nordic Journal of Psychiatry*, *56*(4), 265–271. https://doi.org/10.1080/08039480260242750

Zigmond, A. S., & Snaith, R. P. (1983). The Hospital Anxiety and Depression Scale. *Acta Psychiatrica Scandinavica*, *67*(6), 361–370. https://doi.org/10.1111/j.1600-0447.1983.tb09716.x

Zimmerman, M., Chelminski, I., Young, D., Dalrymple, K., & Martinez, J. H. (2014). A clinically useful self-report measure of the DSM-5 mixed features specifier of major depressive disorder. *Journal of Affective Disorders*, *168*, 357–362. https://doi.org/10.1016/j.jad.2014.07.021

Zimmerman, M., & Holst, C. G. (2018). Screening for psychiatric disorders with self-administered questionnaires. *Psychiatry Research, 270,* 1068–1073. https://doi.org/10.1016/j.psychres.2018.05.022

Zimmermann, M., & Papa, A. (2019). Causal explanations of depression and treatment credibility in adults with untreated depression: Examining attribution theory. *Psychology and Psychotherapy, 93*(3), 537–554. https://doi.org/10.1111/papt.12247

Zock, J. P., Verheij, R., Helbich, M., Volker, B., Spreeuwenberg, P., Strak, M., Janssen, N. A. H., Dijst, M., & Groenewegen, P. (2018). The impact of social capital, land use, air pollution and noise on individual morbidity in Dutch neighbourhoods. *Environment International, 121*(Pt. 1), 453–460. https://doi.org/10.1016/j.envint.2018.09.008

Zou, L., Yeung, A., Li, C., Wei, G. X., Chen, K. W., Kinser, P. A., Chan, J. S. M., & Ren, Z. (2018). Effects of meditative movements on major depressive disorder: A systematic review and meta-analysis of randomized controlled trials. *Journal of Clinical Medicine, 7*(8), Article 195. https://doi.org/10.3390/jcm7080195

Zou, X., Cheng, Y., & Nie, J. B. (2018). The social practice of medical guanxi (personal connections) and patient–physician trust in China: An anthropological and ethical study. *Developing World Bioethics, 18*(1), 45–55. https://doi.org/10.1111/dewb.12164

Zou, P., Siu, A., Wang, X., Shao, J., Hallowell, S. G., Yang, L. L., & Zhang, H. (2021). Influencing factors of depression among adolescent Asians in North America: A systematic review. Healthcare 9(5): 537. https://doi.org/10.3390/healthcare9050537

Index

For the benefit of digital users, indexed terms that span two pages (e.g., 52–53) may, on occasion, appear on only one of those pages.

Tables and figures are indicated by *t* and *f* following the page number.

A1AT (alpha-1 antitrypsin) deficiency, 562–63
Aaliyah, 548*t*
ABCs. *See* American-born Chinese
abuse, 203–6. *See also* adverse childhood events (ACEs); maltreatment
accidental deaths. *See* unnatural deaths
acculturation
    and communication styles, 80–81
    and intergenerational cultural conflict, 232–38
    overview, 93–95
    to patient role, 158
    and therapeutic strategy for Chinese patients, 281–85
acculturative family distancing (AFD), 93–94, 233, 234–35, 237
acculturative stress
    in Chinese international students, 229–30
    and depression, 95
    in Korean American families, 373–76, 375*t*
    overview, 93–94
ACEs. *See* adverse childhood events (ACEs); maltreatment
acquired capacity for suicide (ACS), 101, 102–3, 102*t*, 368, 369–70
active noise reduction, 643–44, 664
acupuncture, 148, 168, 173
adolescence
    and achievement pressure in upper-middle-class families, 133
    among Korean Americans, 373–74
    Chinese CES-D use during, 276–77
    culture-related issues interfering with sleep in, 143
    environmental hazards, exposure to during, 144
    hikikomori in, 328
    hypomanic behavior in, 57
    in Nordic nations and Switzerland, 396–97, 396*t*
    substance use in, 146
    in upper class, 135
adult traumatic events, culturally-related, 96–98
adverse childhood events (ACEs). *See also* maltreatment
    in American regional cultures, 443–44, 476, 481–83, 482*t*
    among creative professionals, 544
    and normalization of trauma, 95–96
    in South Korean culture, 356–57, 376
aesthetics, Japanese, 301–4
AFD (acculturative family distancing), 93–94, 233, 234–35, 237
African American Protestant churches, 466–67. *See also* Black Americans
age. *See also* adolescence; children; older people; young adults
    and alcohol use in Nordic countries and Switzerland, 390–92
    and American suicide rates by level of urbanization, 453*t*
    and China's suicide mortality trend, 258–59, 259*f*
    at death of pop superstars, 548*t*
    and depression across American regions, 11–17, 12*t*, 13*t*
    and depression and suicide in older Chinese Americans, 262–63
    and depression during COVID-19 pandemic, 514*t*, 516
    and depression in Nordic countries and Switzerland, 383
    discrimination based on, in occupational cultures, 92–93, 640–41
    and effect of social capital on depression in China, 76
    and expressions of hypomania, 54–55
    and female-to-male suicide rate ratio in China, 261–62
    and financial aspects of airline pilots' careers, 640–41
    and harmful drinking in Korean culture, 358
    and household net worth by race/ethnicity, 116, 116*t*
    and income inequality in Nordic countries and Switzerland, 386*t*, 390–92
    intersection with cultural identity, 88–93
    and interstate variations in suicide mortality, 444–45
    and MDD, suicide, and unnatural deaths in Japan, 297, 298*t*

age (*cont.*)
  and peak interval for MDD in Nordic nations and Switzerland, 381, 382*t*, 383, 428
  and regional differences in epidemiology of MDD, BPD, and suicide, 499, 500*t*, 501*t*, 504*t*
  and relationship between religious affiliation and suicide, 103
  and socioeconomic status, 116, 116*t*
  state poverty rates by, 474*t*
  and suicide among Korean Americans, 374–76, 375*t*
  and suicide in American regions, 508–10, 508*t*, 509*t*, 511, 512
  and suicide in Korea, 342–43, 367–69, 367*t*, 375*t*
  and suicide mortality among Asian Americans, 374–76, 375*t*
  and suicide mortality in retired pilots, 637–38
  and suicide mortality rate in Nordic nations and Switzerland, 382*t*, 383, 427*t*, 428
  and truck driving, 658–59
  and unnatural deaths in Chinese culture, 259–60, 260*t*, 261*t*
  and use of depression symptom questionnaires with Japanese patients, 340–41
AI (artificial intelligence), 59, 83
aimai (ambiguity), in Japanese culture, 309
airline pilots
  anticipated stigma of depression among, 153–54
  concealment of depression among, 632–35
  culture of, 638–39
  demographics and financial aspects among, 640–43
  and depression screening questionnaires, 46
  female, special issues of, 639–40
  health conditions, impact on, 635–36
  occupational hazards for, 643–46
  overview, 627–30
  regulations and institutional stigma affecting, 630–32
  stigma and choice of treatment by, 636–37
  suicide by active and retired, 637–38
  working around stigma and denial, 646–51
airplane crashes, 628–30
air pollution, 494*t*, 495, 664–65
Akutagawa, Ryūnosuke, 542
Alabama. *See* Deep South region (United States)
Alaskan Natives. *See* American Indians
alcohol use/alcohol use disorders. *See also* binge drinking
  and American regional cultures, 12*t*
  among airline pilots, 628, 646
  among creative professionals, 521–22, 527, 533–34, 544–45, 552, 557–58
  among physicians, 618–19
  among truck drivers, 666–67, 680–81
  in Finland, 397–401
  in Nordic nations and Switzerland, 394–96, 395*t*
  relation to culture and depression, 145–46
  in South Korean culture, 358–59
Alcohol Use Disorders Identification Test–Concise, 400
Allman, Duane, 548*t*
Almost Nearly Perfect People, An (Booth), 384
alpha-1 antitrypsin (A1AT) deficiency, 562–63
al-Razi, Abi Bakr Muhammad ibn Zakariyya (Rhazes), 176
alternative diagnostic criteria for clinical depression, 32–33
alternative medicine. *See* complementary, alternative, and integrative medicine (CAIM)
alternative treatment for depression, 156–57
altitude, and depression risk, 17, 493, 494*t*
amae (dependence), in Japanese culture, 309
AMAS (Aviation Medicine Advisory Service), 651
ambiguity (*aimai*), in Japanese culture, 309
American baby boom generation, 89
American-born Chinese (ABCs). *See also* Chinese students at American universities
  depression risk in, 202
  intergenerational cultural conflicts affecting, 232–38
  Luchang Wang's story, 210–12
  Luke Tang's story, 208–10
  representative suicides of, 214*t*
  suicidality in, 202
American Indians
  in Montana, 441
  overview, 431–32
  population of in specific states, 451*t*
  in Southwest, 471
  and state poverty rates, 474*t*
  and urban-rural differences in suicide rates, 453*t*
American Psychiatric Association (APA), 23–24, 25–32
American regional cultures
  behavioral and environmental risk factors across, 480–87, 482*t*, 484*t*, 486*t*
  depression during COVID-19 pandemic in, 512–17, 514*t*
  describing, 435–40
  educational differences among, 467–72, 467*t*
  environmental influences on depression risk in, 493–98, 494*t*
  and epidemiology of MDD, bipolar disorder, and suicide, 499–505, 500*t*, 501*t*, 502*t*, 504*t*

firearm culture differences among, 490–93, 491*t*
general discussion, 518
income inequality and poverty in, 472–80, 473*t*, 474*t*, 479*t*
individualism/collectivism in, 63–64
lessons from cultural comparison of pairs of states, 447–48
lifestyle risk factors for depression in, 487–90, 488*t*
mental health variations across, 444–46
overview, 430–33
personality and mental health in, 443–44
power distance in, 65
race and ethnicity in, 450–53, 451*t*
regional personality in, 459–63, 460*t*, 464*t*
regions with hybrid cultures, 440–43
religion, depression, and suicide in, 465–67
rural–urban population distribution in, 446, 448–50, 449*t*, 452–53, 453*t*, 454*t*, 477
and salient categories of immigrants to the United States, 433–35
seeing through cultural lens, 11–17, 12*t*, 13*t*
social capital, variation among, 455–59, 457*t*
and socioeconomic status, 115
suicide rate variability among, 453*t*, 505–12, 507*t*, 508*t*, 509*t*
Anatomy of Dependence, The (Doi), 309
Anatomy of Melancholy (Burton), 181–82
ancestry of Americans, 453–54, 454*t*
ancient medical systems. *See* traditional medicine
anger illness (*hwa-byung*), South Korea, 147, 343, 347–53, 351*t*
anhedonia
among airline pilots, 634–35
in diagnosis of MDD, 26–27, 28
in interpersonal-neuropsychiatric model (IPNP) of suicide, 107–8
anime, psychologically oriented, 313–14
anticipated stigma, 151, 153–54
antidepressant foods, 177–78, 189–90, 191*t*, 192–93
antidepressant treatment
for airline pilots, 630–32, 637
for bipolar patients, 49, 51–52
Chinese patient adherence to, 241–42, 287–91
for creative professionals, 530–33
culture and choice of treatment, 155–56
electroacupuncture as adjunct to, 168
for highly educated people, 471–72
in Iceland, 423
individualizing with biomarkers, 35–36
for Japanese patients, 338–41
for *kokoro no kaze* in Japan, 319–20
and mistrust in the United States, 498
for physician-patients, 623–24

for South Korean patients, 377–79
stigmatization of, 152
targeting biomarkers as indicator of progress, 150
antifeminism, in Norway, 415–16
antipsychotic drugs, 51, 538–39
APA (American Psychiatric Association), 23–24, 25–32
Appalachia
behavioral and environmental risk factors in, 480–87, 482*t*, 484*t*, 486*t*
educational attainment in, 467–72, 467*t*
environmental influences on depression risk in, 493–98, 494*t*
epidemiology of MDD, bipolar disorder, and suicide in, 499–505, 500*t*, 501*t*, 502*t*, 504*t*
firearm culture in, 490–93, 491*t*
income inequality and poverty in, 472–80, 473*t*, 474*t*, 479*t*
and lessons from cultural comparison of pairs of states, 447–48
lifestyle risk factors for depression in, 487–90, 488*t*
overview, 436–37
primary ancestries in, 453–54, 454*t*
race and ethnicity of population of, 450–53, 451*t*
regional personality in, 459–63, 460*t*, 464*t*
religious identity in, 464*t*, 465–67
rural–urban population distribution in, 449*t*, 452–53, 453*t*
social capital in, 456–59, 457*t*
suicide rates in, 452–53, 453*t*, 505–12, 507*t*, 508*t*, 509*t*
and truck crash risk, 655
Arabic and Islamic medicine, traditional, 162, 175–80, 185–87
Aretaeus of Cappadocia, 165
Aristotle, 164–65
Arizona. *See* Southwest region (United States)
aromatherapy, 683
artificial intelligence (AI), 59, 83
artists, 523. *See also* creative talent
Ashkenazic Jewish Americans, 241
Asian American Family Conflict Scale (FCS), 235
Asian Americans. *See also* Chinese Americans; Japanese Americans; Korean Americans
in Connecticut, Utah, and the United States, 13*t*
depression among during COVID-19 pandemic, 515–16, 517
difficulty of categorizing, 432
and educational debt among physicians, 609–10
gender and depression prevalence among, 517

Asian Americans (*cont.*)
  income inequality and poverty among, 472-73, 474*t*
  and median household income by race and ancestry, 117*t*
  population of in specific states, 451*t*
  in rural areas, 452-53
  and state poverty rates, 472-73, 474*t*
  stigma of depression among, 154-55
  suicide among, 375-76, 375*t*
  underutilization of mental health services by, 263-64
  urban-rural differences in suicide rates for, 452, 453*t*
assimilation, 94
asylum seekers, in Sweden, 410
atypical depression, 317
audience, importance to creative professionals, 534-35
auscultation (*wén*), in TCM, 168-69
Australian Civil Aviation Safety Authority, 631-32
authoritarian parenting, 237
authoritative parenting, 237
authority, and power distance, 64-65
autonomy, and intergenerational cultural conflict, 236-37
availability of highly lethal means of self-harm, 102*t*, 109-10, 256, 258
Aviation Medicine Advisory Service (AMAS), 651
Avicenna (Abu Ali Al-Hussein Ibn Abdulla Ibn Sina), 177-78
awareness, cultural. *See* cultural awareness
Ayurvedic medicine, 149, 162. *See also* traditional medicine

baby boom generation, 89
background, cultural, 61. *See also* cultural identity
baihe bing (lily disease), in TCM, 170, 171*t*
ba no kuuki wo yomu (reading the air), Japan, 309-10
Bashō, Matsuo, 6
Basic Questions (*Suwen*), *Huangdi Neijing*, 169
BBC (British Broadcasting Corporation), 114-15
beauty of imperfection/beauty of serene melancholy (*wabi-sabi*), Japan, 302-3
Beck Depression Inventory (BDI)
  assessing patients from other cultures with, 273
  Chinese version of, 266-67, 268-69
  Korean version of, 370, 372
  screening for depression with, 38-39, 41-42, 43-44, 45-47
  subthreshold conditions, sensitivity to, 274
behavioral activation, 102*t*, 104-5, 368

behavioral activation therapy, 107-8, 177-78
behavioral inhibition, 102*t*, 105-6, 368
behavioral risk factors, in American regional cultures, 480-90, 482*t*, 484*t*, 486*t*, 488*t*
Behavioral Risk Factor Surveillance Survey, 490, 491-92, 491*t*
belly (*hara*), Japan, 320
benchmarking of care processes, 586
"Benefits of Antidepressants, The" (Parker), 498
Bennington, Chester, 548*t*
Bern Illegitimate Tasks Scale, 606
biànzhèng lùnzhì (pattern recognition and treatment determination), in TCM, 170-72, 171*t*
bicultural individuals, 80-81, 93-94, 338
Big Five personality traits, in regional cultures, 459, 460*t*
binge drinking
  in American regional cultures, 487-89, 488*t*
  cultural normalization of, 145-46
  in Finland, 145-46, 397-401
  in Nordic nations and Switzerland, 394-96, 395*t*
  in South Korea, 145-46, 347, 358
biofeedback, 649
biomarkers
  of bipolar spectrum disorders, 57-59
  of burnout, 597-98
  of depression, and cross-cultural dialogue, 149-51
  in diagnosis of clinical depression, 34-36
  and stigmatization of depression, 149-50
bipolar spectrum. *See also* clinical depression; stigmatization of depression; treatment
  in American regional cultures, 444, 499, 500-1, 500*t*, 501*t*
  among airline pilots, 153-54, 630, 632, 636
  among creative professionals, 522, 523-26, 527-29, 530, 534-35, 538-42, 543-44, 545, 546-47, 557, 560-62, 563-66
  among physicians, 619-24
  among truck drivers, 675
  biomarkers for, 57-59
  bipolar depression, defined, 50
  bipolar disorder, defined, 50
  in Chinese students at American universities, 202, 205-6, 208-10, 241
  in classical Greco-Roman medicine, 164-65
  comorbidities of, 48-49
  culturally aware assessment of, 36
  diagnosis of, 50-51, 52
  historical context of stigma related to, 180-82, 194
  in Japanese culture, 333-34
  linking American regional cultures to epidemiology of, 499-505, 500*t*, 501*t*, 502*t*, 504*t*
  middle zone of, 36-38

in Norwegian culture, 416–17
overview, 48
in scope of clinical depression, 25
screening depressed patients for, 49, 59
screening questionnaires for, 52–57, 54t, 56t
in South Korea, 342–43
in Switzerland, 426
in traditional Arabic and Islamic medicine, 176–77, 185
in traditional Chinese medicine, 169, 170, 173–74, 175
traditional medicine as complementary treatment for, 196–97
treatment overview, 49, 51–52
in the upper class, 137–38
birth rates, in Nordic countries and Switzerland, 388–89
bisphenol-A (BPA)–containing plastics, 190–92
Black Americans, 451t
 African American Protestant churches, 466–67
 and American regional cultures, 431
 in Connecticut, Utah, and the United States, 13t
 in the Deep South, 437
 depression among during COVID-19 pandemic, 514t, 515–16
 and educational debt among physicians, 609–10
 median household income among, 116–18, 117t
 pregnant low-income women among, 483
 state poverty rates for, 474t
 and urban-rural differences in depression, 124, 452, 453t
Blake, K. R., 418–19
bloodletting, 163–64, 169
blood relations (chi-en), Japan, 308
Boeing 737 Max airplane, 642–43
Bolan, Marc, 548t
Bondevik, Kjell Magne, 414
bonding social capital, 74–75, 76, 124, 308
Bonham, John, 548t
Boomers, 89
Booth, Michael, 384
BPA (bisphenol-A)–containing plastics, 190–92
brain, in classical Greco-Roman medicine, 163–64
breath (ki), Japan, 320–21
Breen, Lorna, 571
bridging social capital, 74–75, 76
Brief Religious Coping Scale (Brief RCOPE), 84–85, 85t, 465–66
British Broadcasting Corporation (BBC), 114–15
British immigration to the United States, 436–37
Brooks, E. M., 465

Brooks, R. C., 418–19
Buddhism, 298–99, 354, 369
built in front (tatemae), Japan, 312
bullying
 ijime in Japan, 321–23
 of physicians in training, 588–89
 in South Korean culture, 365–66
burnout
 among physicians, overview of, xv, 591–97
 biomarkers of, 597–98
 distinguishing from moral injury in physicians, 609
 and middle zone of depression, 38
 overview, 572
 treatment of in physicians, 598–600
Burton, Robert, 181–82
Bushidō (Inazō Nitobe), 325

cabover truck design, 663
CADS-9 (Chinese American Depression Scale), 271–73
CAIM (complementary, alternative, and integrative medicine), 162, 169, 194–97
canned foods, 190–92
Canon of Medicine (Avicenna), 177
capital, and social class, 114–15. See also social capital
career anchors, of physicians, 579–81
Carey, Mariah, 527, 529
Carpenter, Karen, 548t
Catholicism, 103, 104, 466
CBI (Copenhagen Burnout Inventory), 595–97
CBT (cognitive-behavioral therapy), 186–87, 282–83, 339–40, 649
CCHR (Citizens Commission on Human Rights), 529–30
CDL (commercial driver's license), 659, 677
celebrities. See also creative talent
 defined, 523
 influence of on broader culture, 529–30
 lonely at the top phenomenon among, 130, 553–54
 and parasocial relationships and culture of fandom, 554–55
 personalized treatment for, 566–67, 570
 suicide among, 365, 369–70, 554–55
 and toxicity of pop music stardom, 547–53, 548t
Celsus, Aulus Cornelius, 165–66
Center for Epidemiologic Studies Depression Scale (CES-D)
 assessing patients from other cultures with, 273
 Chinese version, 266–67, 268–69, 274–81
 Japanese patients, using with, 340–41
 Korean version, 370, 372
 screening for depression with, 38–39, 40–41, 42, 43–47

Central Midwest. *See* Midwest region (United States)
certification, for truck drivers, 676
Chang, Wendy, 214*t*
chemical exposures, 144, 494*t*, 495–97
chest (*mune*), Japan, 320
chi-en (blood relations or community/neighborhood ties), Japan, 308
children. *See also* adverse childhood events (ACEs)
  abandonment of parents by, in Japanese culture, 4–8
  bullying of, in Japan, 321–23
  bullying of, in South Korea, 365–66
  cultural expectations regarding, 90
  culture-related issues interfering with sleep among, 143
  deprivation of, and depression in old age, 332
  and exposure to environmental hazards, 144
  and face, in South Korea, 360
  and filial piety in Chinese culture, 9–11, 222–25
  gun safety in homes with, 490–91
  left-behind, in China, 252–54
  maltreatment of, in South Korea, 357, 376
  poverty among, in American regions, 476
  traumatic events experienced by, 95–96
  upper class, 134, 135, 136
Chinese American Depression Scale (CADS-9), 271–73
Chinese Americans. *See also* American-born Chinese; Chinese students at American universities
  depression among during COVID-19 pandemic, 517
  depression and suicide in older, 262–64
  depression in other Asian Americans versus, 375–76
  expression of depression among, 264–66
  intergenerational cultural conflicts affecting, 232–38
  shift in typical views of depression by, 280–81
  suicide among, 375–76, 375*t*
  therapeutic strategy for, 281–85
Chinese Australians, 283, 284–85
Chinese BDI, 266–67, 268–69
Chinese CES-D, 266–67, 268–69, 274–81
Chinese culture. *See also* Chinese Americans; Chinese students at American universities; traditional Chinese medicine (TCM)
  and acculturation, stigma, and therapeutic strategy, 281–85
  adherence to antidepressant medication in, 285–91
  and choice of treatment, 156
  communication style in, 79
  concealment of negative emotion in, 228–29
  and contemporary relationship of mainstream and traditional medicine, 183–85, 188–89
  cultural customization of PHQ-9 for, 271–73
  culturally aware depression screening and rating for, 266–71
  and depression and suicide in rural China, 254–62, 259*f*, 260*t*, 261*t*
  education, role in, 216–22
  expression of negative emotions in, 246, 247*t*
  face, upward comparison, and climbing the ivy in, 225–28
  family culture of Japan versus, 300
  filial piety in, 222–25
  left-behind persons in, 249–62, 259*f*, 260*t*, 261*t*
  overview, 201
  seeing through cultural lens, 9–11
  shift in typical views of depression in, 276–81
  social capital in, 76, 77–78
  stigmatization of mental illness in, 183–84, 188–89, 239–40, 254, 265, 281–85
  trust in, 73–74, 285–91
  varied faces of depression in, 274–81
Chinese PHQ-9, 266–67, 268–71
Chinese students at American universities
  cases of depression ending in suicide among, 201–16, 214*t*
  Chinese CES-D use with, 276
  concealment of negative emotion by, 228–29
  and education in Chinese history and culture, 216–22
  encounters with student health and counseling services by, 238–43
  expression of negative emotions by, 246, 247*t*
  face, upward comparison, and climbing the ivy among, 225–28
  and filial piety, 222–25
  general suggestions for universities regarding, 244–46
  intergenerational cultural conflicts affecting, 232–38
  international students, issues of, 229–32
  overview, xvi, 201–2
  potential for social media analysis among, 243–44
  university responses to mental health issues among, 291–92
Choi, Jin-sil, 365, 369–70
Chopra, Deepak, 545
Christianity. *See also* Catholicism; Protestantism
  LDS Christians (aka Mormons), 441–42, 465

in South Korea, 354, 369
and suicide, 103, 104
chronic obstructive pulmonary disease (COPD), 413
chronobiological disruption. *See also* sleep
 among airline pilots, 643
 among truck drivers, 659–60
 culture-related issues with, 29
 and susceptibility to depression, 143
Church of Jesus Christ of Latter-day Saints (LDS Church), 441–42, 465
cigarette smoking
 in American regional cultures, 488*t*, 489–90
 in Denmark, 413
cinnamon, 177–78
Citizens Commission on Human Rights (CCHR), 529–30
civilian flight training, 641
class, social. *See* socioeconomic status
classical Greco-Roman medicine, 162, 163–67
classical musicians, 556–57
Classic of Filial Piety, The (*Xiàojīng*), 223
"cleaning one's name", e.g., by suicide (*haji wo susugu*), Japan, 324–25
climbing the ivy (*páténg*), in Chinese culture, 227–28
Cline, Patsy, 548*t*
clinical depression. *See also* bipolar spectrum; cultural identity; cultural lens, depression through; occupational cultures; suicide and suicidality; traditional medicine
 alternative diagnostic criteria for, 32–33
 in American regional cultures, 499, 501–5
 during COVID-19 pandemic, 512–17, 514*t*
 and culture-related issues with diagnosis of MDD, 25–32
 defined, 24–25
 depression screening questionnaires for, 38–47
 evolving Western concept of, 187–88
 and middle zone of depression and bipolar illness, 36–38
 overview, 23–25, 161
 suggested criteria for, 33–36
Clinically Useful Depression Outcome Scale supplemented with questions for DSM-5 mixed features (CUDOS-M), 55–56, 56*t*
Cobain, Kurt, 548*t*
cognition, in diagnosis of depression, 30–31, 34
cognitive-behavioral therapy (CBT), 186–87, 282–83, 339–40, 649
cognitive social capital, 74–76, 77–78
collaborative care for Chinese patients, 282, 285
Collective Efficacy indicator (Social Capital Project), 456
collectivism, 42, 63–64, 63*t*

college students, Chinese. *See* Chinese students at American universities
comedians, 560–62
commercial driver's license (CDL), 659, 677
commodification (commercialization) of healthcare, 584–88
common cold of the spirit (*kokoro no kaze*), Japan, 319–20
communication issues, in intergenerational cultural conflicts, 233–35
communication style
 as dimension of culture, 79–81
 in Finland, 403
 in Japanese culture, 309–12
 seeing through cultural lens, 17–21
Community Health sub-index (Social Capital Project), 456
community ties (*chi-en*), Japan, 308
comorbidities, 48–49, 562–63
competition between Chinese parents, 226–27
complaints, against physicians, 588
complementary, alternative, and integrative medicine (CAIM), 162, 169, 194–97
composers, 557. *See also* creative talent
comprehensive approaches to health. *See* traditional medicine
conditions, use of term in book, 24
Confucianism
 in Chinese culture, 216–19, 222–28
 and filial piety, 9–11, 222–25
 in Japanese culture, 298–301
 in South Korean culture, 354–57, 362, 369
 suicide in, 100
Connecticut, 11–17
connection (*en*) concept, Japan, 7–8, 308
controlling behavior of men toward female partners, 418–20
Cooke, Sam, 548*t*
COPD (chronic obstructive pulmonary disease), 413
Copenhagen Burnout Inventory (CBI), 595–97
co-pilots, 638–39. *See also* airline pilots
coping, religious, 84–86, 85*t*
copycat suicides, 369–70, 554–55
Cornell, Chris, 548*t*
corporal punishment, in South Korea, 357, 376
cosmetic surgery, in South Korean culture, 360–65
cosmic rays, airline pilot exposure to, 643
counseling
 for airline pilots, 650–51
 Chinese student encounters with, 238–43
 for physician burnout, 598–99
country musicians, 558, 559. *See also* creative talent
county-level *kējǔ*, China, 217–18
"Covert Suicide Among Elderly Japanese Females" (Rockett and Smith), 303–4

COVID-19 pandemic
  depression across American regional cultures during, 512–17, 514t
  and depression in physicians, 571–72
  job strain during, 120
  mental health consequences of, xvii, 685
  and mistrust in the United States, 430–31
  moral injury to physicians during, 121, 607
  and prevalence of clinical depression, 91
  and short-term versus long-term orientation, 69
  sickness presenteeism among physicians during, 590
  and socioeconomic status, 113, 118
  and subjective social status as determinant of health, 130–31
  and tightness-looseness of American regions, 462
crashes
  airplane, 628–30
  of large trucks, 654–55
creative talent
  audience, importance of to, 534–35
  avoidance of treatment among, 539–40
  clinical assessment of, 526–29, 567–69
  comedians, 560–62
  culture of creative professions, 529–33
  and issues of specific musical genres, 555–60
  life narratives and courses of illness among, 563–66
  lonely at the top phenomenon among, 553–54
  misdiagnosis of depression among, 542–43
  normalization or mischaracterization of mood disorders among, 137, 540–42
  overview, xv–xvi, 521–26
  parasocial relationships and culture of fandom among, 554–55
  personalized treatment for, 566–70
  productivity, relationship to illness among, 543–45
  remissions among, effect on work, 535–39, 536f, 537f
  stigmatization of depression among, 527, 529, 539–40
  suicide and premature death among, 533–34
  and toxicity of pop music stardom, 547–53, 548t
  undiagnosed medical problems in, 562–63
  working conditions of, 546–47
cross-cultural dialogue, and biomarkers of depression, 149–51
Cruise, Tom, 529–30
"Cry Into the Darkness of a Burned Out Physician, The" (Maffoni), 591
CUDOS-M (Clinically Useful Depression Outcome Scale supplemented with questions for DSM-5 mixed features), 55–56, 56t

cultural antidepressants, 123–24
cultural awareness
  in clinical context, 159–60
  defined, 149
  when prescribing antidepressants to Chinese patients, 288–91
  when screening and rating depression in Chinese people, 266–71
cultural background, 61. See also cultural identity
cultural capital, 114–15
cultural dimensions of interpersonal-neuropsychiatric model of suicide. See interpersonal-neuropsychiatric model of suicide
cultural homelessness, 94–95, 237–38, 515–16
cultural humility, 149
cultural identity. See also American regional cultures; Chinese culture; Japanese culture; Nordic nations; occupational cultures; socioeconomic status; South Korean culture; Switzerland; traditional medicine
  and acculturation, 93–95
  of airline pilots, 638–39
  and biomarkers of depression and cross-cultural dialogue, 149–51
  and choice of treatment for depression, 155–57
  and communication styles, 79–81
  and cultural awareness in clinical context, 159–60
  and diet, 140–42
  and dimensional characterization of cultures, 62–63
  and environmental hazards, 143–44
  and individualism/collectivism, 63–64, 63t
  and indulgence/restraint, 70–71, 70t
  and inference from metaphor and word choice, 81–83
  intersection of age and gender with, 88–93
  and lifestyle and environmental factors, 140
  and masculinity/femininity, 67–68, 67t
  and normalization of trauma, 95–98
  overview, 60–62
  "patient" role as, 157–58, 277–78
  and perspective of traditional medical systems, 147–49
  and phenomenology of depression, 146–47
  of physicians, 577–78, 587
  and power distance, 64–66, 65t
  and psychoactive substance use, 145–46
  and religious identity, 83–87, 85t
  and short-term orientation/long-term orientation, 68–70, 69t
  and sleep, 142–43
  and social capital, 74–78
  and stigma of depression, 151–55

and subjective social status, 132–33
and suicidality, 110–12
and trust, 72–74
and uncertainty avoidance, 66–67, 66t
cultural lens, depression through. *See also* clinical depression; cultural identity
  bipolar spectrum, 52–57
  culturally aware criteria for clinical depression, 32–36
  depression screening questionnaires, 38–47
  issues with diagnosis of MDD, 25–32
  middle zone depression, 36–38
  overview, xv–xix, 3, 21–22
  suicidality, 110–12
cultural map, Inglehart-Welzel, 385–88, 391f
Cultural Revolution (China), 184, 219–21
culture, defined, 60
curanderismo, 148–49
cured meats, 190–92
Curtis, Ian, 548t
cyclothymia, 50, 52, 523–24. *See also* bipolar spectrum
cytokines, 58

daimyō (local lords), Japan, 299–300
Daoism, 167–68, 298–99
death-life-view (*shisei-kan*), Japan, 325
death(s). *See also* premature death; suicide and suicidality; unnatural deaths
  of despair, in the United States, 435–36, 458–59, 505–8, 507t
  disconnected (*muenshi*), Japan, 6, 331
  in Japanese culture, 325
  lonely (*kodokushi*), in Japan, 6–8, 298, 331–33
  of older people in Japan, 4–8
  from overwork (*karōshi*), in Japan, 298, 305–7
  recurrent thoughts of, in diagnosis of MDD, 31
debt, educational, among physicians, 580–81, 609–11
debtor-operators, in trucking, 657
Deep South region (United States)
  behavioral and environmental risk factors in, 480–87, 482t, 484t, 486t
  culture of, 437–38
  educational attainment in, 467–72, 467t
  environmental influences on depression risk in, 493–98, 494t
  epidemiology of MDD, bipolar disorder, and suicide in, 499–505, 500t, 501t, 502t, 504t
  firearm culture in, 490–93, 491t
  income inequality and poverty in, 472–80, 473t, 474t, 479t
  and lessons from cultural comparison of pairs of states, 447–48
  lifestyle risk factors for depression in, 487–90, 488t
  primary ancestries in, 453–54, 454t
  race and ethnicity of population of, 450–53, 451t
  regional personality in, 459–63, 460t, 464t
  religious identity in, 464t, 465–67
  rural–urban population distribution in, 449t, 452–53, 453t
  social capital in, 456–59, 457t
  suicide rates in, 452–53, 453t, 505–12, 507t, 508t, 509t
Delaware Bay region (United States), 436
Delaware River region (United States), 436
demand–control imbalance
  among physicians, 600–2, 604
  among truck drivers, 653, 659–60
  in middle-class and upper-middle-class jobs, 120
Demand–Control–Support Questionnaire, 604
De Medicina (Celsus), 165–66
Democratic People's Republic of Korea (North Korea), 345
demographics
  of airline pilots, 640–43
  and American regional cultures, 13t, 450–52, 451t
  in Nordic countries and Switzerland, 384, 388–93
Denmark. *See also* Nordic nations
  demographic and cultural differences with other Nordic nations, 384
  diet and depression in, 393–94, 394t
  historical context of, 411–12
  hygge culture in, 412–13
  intimate partner violence (IPV) in, 412
  MDD prevalence in, 381–83, 382t
  overview of culture, 380–81
  pleasure-seeking culture in, 413–14
  sexual harassment in, 406–7, 407t
  suicide in, 381, 382t, 383, 427t
denormalization of trauma, 97–98
dependence (*amae*), in Japanese culture, 309
depersonalization (DP), in MBI, 593, 594
depressed phase of bipolar I disorder, 25
depressing foods, 190–92, 192t
depression screening questionnaires. *See also* Beck Depression Inventory (BDI); Center for Epidemiologic Studies Depression Scale (CES-D); Patient Health Questionnaire 9-item (PHQ-9)
  for Chinese American patients, 265
  culturally aware, for Chinese patients, 266–71
  for detection of bipolar spectrum disorders, 52–57, 54t, 56t
  for externalized depression, 388
  Hypomania Checklist (HCL-32), 52–55, 54t, 57, 620

depression screening questionnaires (*cont.*)
   for Japanese patients, 312, 329, 340–41
   for masculine depression, 388, 668–69, 671*t*
   Mood Disorder Questionnaire (MDQ), 52–53
   overview, 38–47
   Oxford Depression Questionnaire (ODQ), 532
   Patient Health Questionnaire 15-item (PHQ-15), 371
   Patient Health Questionnaire 2-item (PHQ-2), 513–15
   Patient Health Questionnaire 8-item (PHQ-8), 33, 39, 40
   positive predictive value of, 43
   for South Korean patients, 370–73
   translations of, 47
despair, deaths of, 435–36, 458–59, 505–8, 507*t*
diagnosis of depression
   alternative diagnostic criteria for clinical depression, 32–33
   among creative professionals, 526–29
   in bipolar spectrum, 50–51, 52
   in classical Greco-Roman medicine, 163
   culture-related issues with, 25–32
   failure of, 17–21
   suggested criteria for, 33–36
   in traditional Chinese medicine, 168–69
   versus undiagnosed cases, xvii
   in upper-class patients, 137
Diagnostic and Statistical Manual, Fifth Edition, Text Revision (DSM-5-TR), APA, 23–24, 25–32
diagnostic interviews, 45–46
diān (epilepsy), in TCM, 169
diān kuáng (bipolar disorder), in TCM, 169–70
diet
   of airline pilots, suggestions for improving, 647–48
   in Nordic nations and Switzerland, 393–97, 394*t*, 395*t*, 396*t*
   relation to culture and depression, 140–42
   in traditional medicine, 189–94, 191*t*, 192*t*
   traditional versus modern diets, 190, 192–93
differential item functioning (DIF), 46–47
digital biomarkers, of bipolar spectrum disorders, 57–58
dimensional characterization of cultures, 387
   communication styles in, 79–81
   individualism/collectivism in, 63–64, 63*t*
   indulgence/restraint in, 70–71, 70*t*
   masculinity/femininity in, 67–68, 67*t*
   overview, 62–63
   power distance in, 64–66, 65*t*
   short-term orientation/long-term orientation in, 68–70, 69*t*
   social capital in, 74–78
   trust in, 72–74
   uncertainty avoidance in, 66–67, 66*t*

direct communication, 79–80
disability benefits, 501–5, 504*t*
discipline, harsh. *See also* adverse childhood events (ACEs)
   in Chinese culture, 203, 205, 224
   in South Korean culture, 357, 376
disconnected deaths (*muenshi*), Japan, 6, 331
discrimination. *See also* stigmatization of depression
   and acculturation, 94
   among upper-class people, 136
   among upper-middle-class people, 132–33
   based on age, 92–93
   based on gender, 390, 581–83, 639–40
   based on perceived cultural identities, 61
   based on religious identity, 86–87, 466
   racial, in the Deep South, 437
   and social capital, 77–78
   toward Chinese Americans, 237–38
   toward Japanese Americans, 337–38
   toward people with depression, 151–55
disease, use of term in book, 24
"Disenchanted Self, The" (Brooks), 465
disengagement scale, in OBI, 595
disorders, use of term in book, 24
distress. *See also* financial distress
   in diagnosis of MDD, 32
   idioms of, 149
   suicide as involving, 101
divorce
   in American regional cultures, 482*t*, 484–85
   in Finland, 403
doctors. *See* physicians
dogs, as companions for truck drivers, 667–68, 683–84
Doi, Takeo, 309
Doll's House, A (Ibsen), 415
domestic violence, 481, 482*t*, *See also* intimate partner violence (IPV)
downward comparison, 131
DP (depersonalization), in MBI, 593, 594
Drake, Nick, 548*t*
drinking culture. *See also* alcohol use/alcohol use disorders; binge drinking
   among Korean Americans, 373–74
   in Finland, 397–401
   in South Korea, 347, 358–60
driven dysphoria, 104–5, 543–44
dropping out of college, 119
drowning deaths, in Japan, 297, 298*t*, 303–4
drug use. *See* substance use/substance use disorders
DSM-5-TR (*Diagnostic and Statistical Manual, Fifth Edition, Text Revision*), APA, 23–24, 25–32
dysfunction, in diagnosis of MDD, 32
dysthymia. *See* clinical depression

eating habits. *See* diet
economic capital, 114–15
economic issues, in Nordic countries and Switzerland, 386t, 388–93, *See also* financial distress; poverty
economics of airline industry, 640–43
education
  and American regional cultures, 467–72, 467t
  and depression during COVID-19 pandemic, 514t, 516
  as determinant of socioeconomic status, 121–24, 126
  and performance on cognitive screening tests, 31
  role in Chinese history and culture, 216–22
educational debt, among physicians, 580–81, 609–11
EE (emotional exhaustion), in MBI, 593, 594
effort–reward imbalance (ERI)
  among physicians, 600–1, 602, 604–5
  among truck drivers, 653
  in middle-class and upper-middle-class jobs, 120
EIP (Engagement Interview Protocol), 265–66
Eisen, Carl, 648–49
elaborate speech, 80
electroacupuncture, 168
electronic medical records (EMRs), 585–86
elite, classification of, 115
elite universities, Chinese students at. *See* Chinese students at American universities
emergent service workers, 115
eminent creators. *See also* creative talent
  decline in function, effect on, 564
  defined, 523
  influence on broader culture, 526, 529–30
  treatment of, 539–40, 566–67, 570
emotional blunting, 531–33, 623–24
emotional distancing, cultural conflict expressed as, 233
emotional exhaustion (EE), in MBI, 593, 594
emotional states, Japanese metaphors for, 319–21
empathy, informed, 159–60
emphysema, 562–63
employment. *See* job strain/stress; occupational cultures; work
EMRs (electronic medical records), 585–86
en (connection or tie) concept, Japan, 7–8, 308
energy (*ki* or spirit), Japan, 320–21
energy, in diagnosis of clinical depression, 34
engagement, facilitating in Chinese American patients, 265–66
Engagement Interview Protocol (EIP), 265–66
English immigration to the United States, 436–37

enhancement of function, treatment focusing on, 678–79
environment
  and American regional cultures, 13t, 17, 480–87, 482t, 484t, 486t, 493–98, 494t
  and cultural identity, overview, 140
  hazardous, risk to physicians, 588
  hazards in, in relation to culture and depression, 143–44
  influence on suicide rates, 111
  in interpersonal-neuropsychiatric (IPNP) model of suicide, 102t
  quality of, and social capital, 76–77
epilepsy, 164, 169, 562
ERI. *See* effort–reward imbalance
esketamine, 569
Essential Prescriptions from the Golden Cabinet (Jīn Guì Yào Lüè), Zhang, 170
established middle class, 115
ethnicity. *See also* cultural identity
  and American regional cultures, 431–33, 450–53, 451t
  and contrasting mortality trends in the United States, 435–36
  and cultural antidepressants, 124
  and depression during COVID-19 pandemic, 512–13, 514t, 515–17
  and income inequality and poverty in the United States, 472–73, 474t
  and relationship between social capital and depression, 77–78
  and socioeconomic status, 116–18, 116t, 117t
  state poverty rates by, 474t
  and upper-class status, 136
European ancestries of Americans, 453–54, 454t
European medicine. *See* Western medicine
Euthymia Scale, 312, 340–41
Evangelical Protestantism, 463, 485
evidence-based practice guidelines, 586–87
examinations, focus on in Chinese culture, 216–22
exhaustion scale, in OBI, 595
experience of pain, in IPNP model of suicide, 102t, 106–7
experience of pleasure, in IPNP model of suicide, 102t, 107–8
externalizing behavior. *See also* male depression
  in American regional cultures, 501–3
  among truck drivers, 668, 669–70, 674
  and childhood poverty, 476
  in men in Nordic countries and Switzerland, 388, 400–1
  in middle zone depression, 37–38
  screening for, 39–40
  and social class, 124–25
  in truck drivers, 656

FAA (Federal Aviation Administration), 630–31, 632, 651
face
　in Chinese culture, 225–28, 231–32
　in South Korean culture, 360–65
facial cosmetic procedures, in South Korean culture, 360–65
fame and fortune, sudden, 552–53
families
　and face, in South Korea, 360
　in Japanese culture, 299, 300
　Korean American, acculturative stress in, 373–76, 375t
　lonely, 129–30
　South Korean, generational differences in, 346
familismo (familism), in American Southwest, 438–39
family. *See also* children; parents
family distancing, acculturative, 93–94, 233, 234–35, 237
Family Interaction sub-index (Social Capital Project), 455
Family Unity sub-index (Social Capital Project), 455
fans
　and culture of fandom, 554–55
　importance of to creative professionals, 534–35
Far West. *See* Mountain States, United States
fatal airplane crashes, 628–30
fatal truck crashes, 654, 655
fatigue
　among airline pilots, 634–35, 639, 645–46
　in diagnosis of MDD, 30
FCS (Asian American Family Conflict Scale), 235
fear of personal relations disorder (*taijin kyofusho*), Japan, 307–8
Federal Aviation Administration (FAA), 630–31, 632, 651
Federal Motor Carrier Safety Administration (FMCSA), 676
federal regulations for truck drivers, 661–62
femininity/masculinity (gender role differentiation), 67–68, 67t
feminism, in Norway, 415–16
filial piety
　in Chinese culture, 9–11, 222–25
　in Japanese culture, 7, 300
　in South Korean culture, 360, 368
financial distress. *See also* poverty; socioeconomic status
　and ability to treat depression, 118–19
　among airline pilots, 635–36, 640–43
　among Chinese international students, 231
　among physicians, 580–81, 609–11
　and depression during COVID-19 pandemic, 513–15, 514t

and short-term versus long-term orientation, 69–70
and suicide in South Korea, 366, 368
Finland. *See also* Nordic nations
　binge drinking in, 145–46, 397–401
　communication style of, 403
　demographic and cultural differences with other Nordic nations, 384
　immigrants in, 411
　MDD prevalence in, 381–83, 382t
　overview of culture, 380–81
　sauna use in, 401
　sexual harassment in, 407, 407t
　sisu concept and historical trauma in, 402–4
　suicide in, 381, 382t, 383, 404, 427t, 428
　weapons ownership in, 404
firearm, suicide by, 12t, 15–16, 508–11, 508t, *See also* gun ownership
fire illness (*hwa-byung*), South Korea, 147, 343, 347–53, 351t
first-class medical certificates for airline pilots, 630–32
five elements (*wǔ xíng*), in TCM, 167–68
flight engineers, 639
FMCSA (Federal Motor Carrier Safety Administration), 676
food deserts, 141–42
foods. *See also* diet
　antidepressant, 177–78, 189–90, 191t, 192–93
　depressing, 190–92, 192t
fùèrdài (rich second generation), in China, 225–26
Fukazawa, Shichirō, 4–5, 6
function, treatment focusing on enhancement of, 678–79

Galen, 166
gaman (patience), Japan, 323
Gao, Yanding, 203–4
gaokao (national examination), China, 219–21
Gaye, Marvin, 548t
GBD (Global Burden of Disease) database, 380–81
GDS (Geriatric Depression Scale), Korean version, 372–73
Gelfand, M. J., 461
gender
　and acceptance of hypomanic behavior, 57
　and adolescent mental health in Nordic nations and Switzerland, 396t, 397
　in American Southwest culture, 438, 439–40
　and Chinese CES-D, 277
　and depression and suicide in Chinese Americans, 263
　and depression during COVID-19 pandemic, 514t, 515–17
　and depression in Switzerland, 428–29

and HCL-32 scores, 53–55
inequality in medical field, 581–84
intersection with cultural identity, 88–93
and physician burnout, 596
and psychometrics of depression questionnaires, 43–44
and regional differences in epidemiology of MDD, BPD, and suicide, 499, 500t, 501t, 502t
and somatic expression of depression, 278
state poverty rates by, 474t, 477
and suicide in rural China, 254–62, 259f, 260t, 261t
suicide mortality for Asian Americans based on, 374–75, 375t
and suicide rates for creative professionals, 533
gender equality
in American regional cultures, 441–42
in Connecticut, Utah, and the United States, 13t
and controlling behavior by men, 418–20
and intimate partner violence (IPV), 485–87
in Nordic countries and Switzerland, 387–88
in Norway, 414, 415–16
in South Korean culture, 354–57
in Sweden, 406
in the United States, 430
gender role differentiation, 67–68, 67t
Generation 1.5. See also Chinese students at American universities
Chinese American, 202, 212–13, 214t
and intergenerational cultural conflicts, 232–38
Korean American, 373, 378
genetic risk factors, and stigma of depression, 154
geniuses of the arts and sciences. See creative talent
Geriatric Depression Scale (GDS), Korean version, 372–73
German language, metaphor and word choice in, 82
Germanwings Flight 9525, 629
Geschwind syndrome, 562
ginger, 177–78
Global Burden of Disease (GBD) database, 380–81
global financial crisis of 2008, 420
globalization, xvi
Gotland Male Depression Scale (GMDS), 388, 668–69, 671t
Great British Class Survey (BBC), 114–15
Greater Appalachia, 436–37. See also Appalachian culture
Greco-Roman medicine, 162, 163–67
grit (sisu), Finland, 402–4
grounded pilots, 635–36

group consciousness (shūdan ishiki), Japan, 307–8
guilt
in diagnosis of MDD, 30
in Japanese culture, 323–24
survival, 565
gun ownership
in the Deep South, 437–38
in Finland, 404
interstate differences in, 490–93, 491t
in Switzerland, 427–28
Guo, Heng "Nikita", 203–6
Guo Jujing, 9

HADS (Hospital Anxiety and Depression Scale), 633
Haggard, Merle, 652
haji (internalized shame), Japan, 299, 323–25
haji wo susugu ("cleaning one's name", e.g., by suicide), Japan, 324–25
han (South Korean national emotion), 346–47
happiest countries. See Nordic nations; Switzerland
hara (belly), Japan, 320
harassment. See also bullying; sexual harassment
of physicians in training, 588–89
power, in Japanese culture, 321–23
harmful drinking, 358–59, 373–74. See also alcohol use/alcohol use disorders; binge drinking
Harrington, J. R., 461, 463
harsh discipline. See also adverse childhood events (ACEs)
in Chinese culture, 203, 205, 224
in South Korean culture, 357, 376
Hashimoto, R., 316–17
HCL-32 (Hypomania Checklist), 52–55, 54t, 57, 620
health
change in, as criteria for clinical depression, 33
hazards for airline pilots, 643–46
hazards for truck drivers, 660–66
risk factors in American regional cultures, 487–90, 488t
healthcare
commodification of, 584–88
depression risks in, 120, 121
truck driver access to, 660
health conditions. See medical conditions
health insurance, for truck drivers, 653, 666
healthy immigrant effect, 435
hearing loss
among airline pilots, 643–44
among musicians, 556, 560
among truck drivers, 663–64
heart (kokoro), Japan, 319, 320–21

heart metaphors, in Chinese language, 246, 247t
heart qi deficiency, in TCM, 170, 171t
heavy drinking. *See* binge drinking
Hedda Gabler (Ibsen), 415
Hemingway, Ernest, 540, 541–42
Hendrix, Jimi, 548t
herbal remedies for depression
    in classical Greco-Roman medicine, 163–64
    risks of self-treatment with, 196–97
    similarity between prescription antidepressants and, 148
    in traditional Chinese medicine, 170–73, 171t
hierarchical relationships
    in Japanese culture, 299–300
    in medical settings, 588–89
    in South Korean culture, 354–57
high-context communication style, 17–21, 79, 309–12
higher education. *See also* Chinese students at American universities
    in American regional cultures, 467–72, 467t
    socioeconomic status and, 119, 126
highly educated immigrants to the United States, 434
highly lethal means of self-harm, availability of, 102t, 109–10, 256, 258
hikikomori (prolonged and severe social withdrawal), Japan, 298, 327–30
Hikikomori Questionnaire (HQ-25), 329
Hillbilly Elegy (Vance), 95
Hinduism, 100
hip-hop musicians, 558, 559. *See also* creative talent
Hippocrates, 163–64
Hispanic Americans
    in the American Southwest, 450–51, 471
    in Connecticut, Utah, and the United States, 13t
    depression among during COVID-19 pandemic, 514t, 515–17
    and income inequality and poverty, 474t
    and median household income by race and ancestry, 117t
    population of in specific states, 451t
    in rural areas, 452–53
    in the Southwest, 438–40
    and state poverty rates, 474t
Hispanos, in the American Southwest, 438, 450–51
Hofstede, Geert, 60, 62–63, 387
holistic views of health. *See* traditional medicine
hollow disease, 205
home safety, and gun ownership, 490
homicidal ideation in airline pilots, 628–30
hon'ne (true sound), Japan, 312
hope, in IPNP model of suicide, 102t, 108
hopeless and despairing feeling (*zetsubō-kan*), Japan, 311

Hospital Anxiety and Depression Scale (HADS), 633
hospitalization, psychiatric, in South Korea, 376–77
hours of service (HOS) rules, for truck drivers, 661–62
Household Pulse Survey Wave 39 (U.S. Census Bureau), 512–13
Houston, Whitney, 548t
HQ-25 (Hikikomori Questionnaire), 329
Huangdi Neijing (*The Yellow Emperor's Inner Canon*), China, 167–68, 169–70
hùkǒu (resident registration) system, China, 249–50, 251–52
humiliating treatment, of physicians in training, 588–89. *See also* bullying
humility, cultural, 149
humors
    in classical Greco-Roman medicine, 163, 164, 165, 166
    in traditional Arabic and Islamic medicine (TAIM), 176–77
hwa-byung (fire illness/anger illness), South Korea, 147, 343, 347–53, 351t
Hwa-Byung Rating Scale, 350, 351t
hygge culture, in Denmark, 412–13
hypersomnia, in diagnosis of MDD, 29
hypnotic drugs, 542–43
hypomania. *See also* bipolar spectrum
    in bipolar spectrum, 50–51, 52
    in classical Greco-Roman medicine, 165
    screening with CUDOS-M, 55–57, 56t
    in upper-class people, 137
Hypomania Checklist (HCL-32), 52–55, 54t, 57, 620
hypoxia, airline pilot exposure to, 643

Ibn Imran, Ishaq, 176–77
Ibn Sina, Abu Ali Al-Hussein Ibn Abdulla (Avicenna), 177–78
Ibsen, Henrik, 415
ICD-10-CM (*International Classification of Diseases, 10th Revision, Clinical Modification*), National Center for Health Statistics, 23–24
Iceland. *See also* Nordic nations
    cultural antidepressants in, 421–22
    demographic and cultural differences with other Nordic nations, 384
    general discussion, 420–23
    MDD prevalence in, 381–83, 382t
    overview of culture, 380–81
    stigmatization of depression in, 422–23
    suicide in, 381, 382t, 383, 427t
ichigo ichie (one opportunity, one encounter), Japan, 302
ICI (Intercultural Conflict Inventory), 235–36
idioms of distress, 149

ijime (bullying), Japan, 321–23
ikigai (reason to live) concept, Japan, 82, 108–9, 384–85
"illegal immigrants," in the United States, 433–34
illegitimate tasks, and job stress, 600–1, 603, 606
illness. *See also* medical conditions
  in classical Greco-Roman medicine, 163
  in traditional Chinese medicine, 168
  use of term in book, 24
  words chosen to name, and stigmatization, 180
immigrants. *See also* Chinese Americans; cultural identity; Japanese Americans; Korean Americans
  acculturation of, 93–94
  in ancestries of American regions, 432–33
  British, 436–37
  and cultural antidepressants, 123–24
  diet and depression among, 141–42
  dietary acculturation among, 193
  exposure to environmental hazards among, 144
  Japanese, 301, 336–37
  mortality trends among, 435–36
  in Nordic nations, 408–9, 410–11, 419–20
  population of in specific states, 451*t*
  sleep and depression among, 142–43
  social class and mood disorder epidemiology among, 127
  in Switzerland, 392
  to the United States, salient categories of, 433–35
immune-inflammatory signature, 58
imperfection, beauty of (*wabi-sabi*), Japan, 302–3
Imperial Examination (*kējǔ*), China, 216–19
impermanence (*mujō*), Japan, 301–2
"Impressions of a Pilot" (Stoker), 627
improvisational musicians, 559. *See also* creative talent
impulsive suicide, 490, 491–92
incarceration rates, in American regions, 476–77
income
  and depression during COVID-19 pandemic, 514*t*, 516
  insecurity of, socioeconomic status and, 118–19
  stratification of social classes based on, 113–16, 121–24, 126
income inequality. *See also* socioeconomic status
  in American regional cultures, 472–80, 473*t*, 474*t*, 479*t*
  in Nordic countries and Switzerland, 386*t*, 390–92

  and power distance, 65
  and social capital, 78
  in the United States, 431
India, suicide in, 100
Indian Ayurvedic medicine, 149, 162. *See also* traditional medicine
indirect communication, 79–80
individualism, 63–64, 63*t*
indulgence/restraint, 70–71, 70*t*
inference from metaphor and word choice, 81–83
informed empathy, 159–60
Inglehart-Welzel World Cultural Map, 385–87, 391*f*
injuries, among truck drivers, 662
inquiry (*wèn*), in TCM, 168–69
insanity, in classical Greco-Roman medicine, 165–66
insecticides, organophosphate, 495
insomnia, 29, 142, 307, 542–43
inspection (*wàng*), in TCM, 168–69
Institutional Health sub-index (Social Capital Project), 456, 458–59
institutionalized stigma of depression
  in airline industry, 153–54, 630–32, 636–37
  overview, 153–54
  in trucking industry, 676–78
instrumental social capital, 74–75
integrative medicine. *See* complementary, alternative, and integrative medicine (CAIM)
Intercultural Conflict Inventory (ICI), 235–36
interdependent self-construal, in Japanese culture, 307–8, 340–41
intergenerational cultural conflicts in Chinese families, 232–38
interleukins, 58
internalized shame (*haji*), Japan, 299, 323–25
International Classification of Diseases, 10th Revision, Clinical Modification (ICD-10-CM), National Center for Health Statistics, 23–24
international students, depression among, 470–71. *See also* Chinese students at American universities
internet
  access to in American rural areas, 446
  internet-based psychotherapy, 282–83
  use in Iceland, 423
internment of Japanese Americans during World War II, 335, 336, 337–38
interns, medical, 575–76, 588–90
interpersonal aspects of depression, 42
interpersonal-neuropsychiatric (IPNP) model of suicide
  acquired capacity for suicide (ACS) in, 101, 102–3, 102*t*, 368, 369–70

interpersonal-neuropsychiatric (IPNP) model of suicide (*cont.*)
  availability of highly lethal means of self-harm in, 102*t*, 109–10, 256, 258
  behavioral activation in, 102*t*, 104–5, 368
  behavioral inhibition in, 102*t*, 105–6, 368
  experience of pain in, 102*t*, 106–7
  experience of pleasure in, 102*t*, 107–8
  hope in, 102*t*, 108
  and interstate variability in suicide, 505
  and issues of Korean women, 368
  and Japanese culture, 325
  overview, 101, 102*t*
  perceived burdensomeness (PB) in, 101–4, 102*t*, 325, 368
  and physician-patients, 624
  reason to live in, 108–9
  thwarted belongingness (TB) in, 101–4, 102*t*, 325, 368
interpersonal-psychological theory of suicide (IPTS), 101
interview-based standards of diagnosis, 45–46
intimate partner violence (IPV)
  in American regional cultures, 443–44, 485–87, 486*t*
  among Korean Americans, 374
  in Denmark, 412
  in Finland, 403–4
  in Norway, 418–20
  in South Korea, 355–57
involuntary hospitalization, in South Korea, 376–77
Iowa. *See* Midwest region (United States)
IPNP. *See* interpersonal-neuropsychiatric model of suicide
IPTS (interpersonal-psychological theory of suicide), 101
IPV. *See* intimate partner violence (IPV)
Islam
  depression and suicide in, 87, 102–3
  traditional medicine in, 162, 175–80, 185–87
Ivy League education, importance in Chinese culture, 227–28

Jackson, Michael, 545, 562–63
Jamison, Kay, 523
Jang Ja-Yeon, 365
Japanese Americans
  communication style of, 80–81
  and connections with Japanese culture, 308
  depression in, 334–38, 375–76
  suicide among, 375–76, 375*t*
Japanese culture
  aesthetics and depression in, 301–4
  alternative to psychiatry in, 313–14
  and changing economic situation in Japan, 295–97, 300–1, 317
  communication style in, 79, 309–12
  and cultural concerns in antidepressant treatment, 338–41
  disconnected deaths (*muenshi*) in, 6, 331
  family relationships in, 299, 300
  filial piety in, 222
  and gender-related challenges in medicine, 583
  indulgence versus restraint in, 70–71
  inference from metaphor and word choice in, 82
  interdependent self-construal in, 307–8
  and intersection of age and gender with ethnic identity, 88–89
  lonely death (*kodokushi*) in, 6–8, 298, 331–33
  metaphors for emotional states in, 319–21
  modern type depression in, 314–19
  normalization of bullying in, 321–23
  overview, 10–11, 293–98
  presentations of depression in, 298, 303, 327
  problems in recognition of bipolarity in, 333–34
  prolonged and severe social withdrawal (*hikikomori*) in, 298, 327–30
  psychometric studies of depression rating scales in, 44
  reason to live (*ikigai*) in, 108–9
  samurai culture in, modern consequences of, 304–7
  seeing through cultural lens, 4–8
  shame and suicide in, 323–27
  shin-gata utsu-byo (new type depression) in, 152
  social capital in, 77
  stigmatization of depression in, 180, 313
  suicide rates in, 297–98, 298*t*
  syncretism and Yamato spirit in, 298–301
  woman physicians in, parental leave for, 590
Japanese rule in Korea, 345
jazz musicians, 558, 559. *See also* creative talent
jeong (South Korean national emotion), 347
Jin, Shengyu, 214*t*
jīngluò (meridians), in TCM, 167–68
Jīn Guì Yào Lüè (*Essential Prescriptions from the Golden Cabinet*), Zhang, 170
jinn possession, in Islamic culture, 185–86
job satisfaction, and physician career anchors, 580
job strain
  among physicians, 573–74, 578, 600–7, 620–21
  among truck drivers, 653, 659–60
  in Japanese culture, 305–7
  in middle-class or upper-middle-class jobs, 120
John Henryism, 124

Joint Economic Committee of the U.S. Senate, 455–59, 457*t*
joint suicide, 100
Jones, Brian, 548*t*
Joplin, Janis, 548*t*
jōshi (lovers' suicide), 324–25

Kalaichandran, Amitha, 589
Kampo (traditional Japanese medicine), 162, 175
karojisatsu (overwork suicide), Japan, 305
karōshi (death from overwork), Japan, 298, 305–7
karyu rojin (low-class older people), Japan, 332–33
Kato, T. A., 316–17
Kawabata, Yasunari, 542–43
kējŭ (*Imperial Examination*), China, 216–19
Kenny, Dianna, 547–52
Kentucky. *See* Appalachian culture
ketamine, 569
K-GDS (Korean Geriatric Depression Scale), 372–73
ki (spirit or energy), Japan, 320–21
Kitanaka, Junko, 326–27
Kobayashi, Makoto, 314–16
kodokushi (lonely death), Japan, 6–8, 298, 331–33
kokoro (heart), Japan, 319, 320–21
Kokoro-App, 339–40
kokoro no kaze (common cold of the spirit), Japan, 319–20
Kong, Ao "Olivia", 212–13
Korean Americans. *See also* South Korean culture
  binge drinking among, 145–46
  family acculturative stress in, 373–76, 375*t*
  overview, 343
  rating and screening for depression, 370–73
  similarities between South Koreans and, 344
  stigmatization of depression and barriers to treatment among, 377–79
  suicide among, 374–76, 375*t*
Korean Geriatric Depression Scale (K-GDS), 372–73
Korean PHQ-9, 370–71
Korean War, 345
kuáng, in TCM, 169

lagom culture, Sweden, 409
Lakoff, Daniel, 589
lamotrigine, 51
Lapps (Sámi people), in Norway, 417–18
Latino Americans. *See* Hispanic Americans
latitude, and depression risk, 493–95, 494*t*
LDS Church (Church of Jesus Christ of Latter-day Saints), 441–42, 465
leaves of absence policies at universities, 210–12, 240, 245, 291–92

Ledger, Heath, 526–27, 528–29
Lee, Mike, 455
left-behind people, in China
  children, 252–54
  depression and suicide rates in rural areas, 254–62, 259*f*, 260*t*, 261*t*
  migration within China due to economic growth, 251–53
  older adults, 252–53, 254
  wives, 249–51, 252–53, 254, 256
  Xiaojuan Wang's story, 249–51
lethal means of self-harm, availability of, 102*t*, 109–10, 256, 258
Levi, Primo, 565
Li, Yangkai, 214*t*
liǎn (face), in Chinese culture, 225
licensed practical nurses (LPNs), demand-control imbalance for, 120
life expectancy, and socioeconomic status, 92
life force (*qi*), in TCM, 167–68, 170–72, 171*t*
lifestyle
  across American regional cultures, 487–90, 488*t*
  of airline pilots, adjusting, 644–49
  of creative professionals, modifying, 569
  and cultural identity, 140
  and diet, 140–42
  of physicians, adjusting, 621
  and psychoactive substance use, 145–46
  and sleep, 142–43
  of truck drivers, modifying, 683
LiftAffect, 650–51
light therapy, 51, 493–95
lily disease (*bǎihé bìng*), in TCM, 170, 171*t*
Língshū (*Spiritual Pivot*), *Huangdi Neijing*, 169–70
linking social capital, 74–75
literacy, in American regional cultures, 469, 470
lithium, 51, 538–39
Liu, Andrea, 214*t*
Liu, Kaifeng, 214*t*
Liu, Weiwei "Linka", 206–7
liver qì stagnation, in TCM, 170, 171*t*
local lords (daimyō), Japan, 299–300
loneliness
  among truck drivers, 666–68
  Japanese appreciation for, 301–4
  and socioeconomic status, 129–30
  and upper-class status, 136
lonely at the top phenomenon, 130, 553–54
lonely death (*kodokushi*) in Japan, 6–8, 298, 331–33
lonely families, 129–30
long COVID, 130–31
long-haul truck drivers. *See* truck drivers
long-term orientation, 68–70, 69*t*
looseness-tightness, in American regional cultures, 459–63, 460*t*, 475–76

Los Angeles metropolitan area, 516
loss of license insurance for airline pilots, 635–36
lovers' suicide (*jōshi* or *shinjū*), 324–25
low-class older people (*karyu rojin*), Japan, 332–33
low-context communication style, 17–21, 79
lower class, 114, 143
lower-middle class, 127–28
lower-upper class, 114, 134–35, 136
loyalty, in Japanese culture, 300
LPNs (licensed practical nurses), demand-control imbalance for, 120
Lu, Xiao, 214*t*
Lubitz, Andreas, 629

machismo gender role, in American Southwest, 438, 439–40
MADRS (Montgomery-Åsberg depression rating scale), 81–82
Maffoni, M., 591
Maimonides (Moses ben Maimon), 178
mainstream medicine. *See* Western medicine
major airlines, 641–42
major depressive disorder (MDD). *See also* clinical depression
  in adult immigrants from poorer countries, 127
  in American regional cultures, 444–45, 499–503, 500*t*, 501*t*
  biochemical markers of, 58
  in Chinese patients, 280
  Chinese PHQ-9 use to screen for, 269–71
  during COVID-19 pandemic, 513
  in creative professionals, 525–26
  and culture-related issues with diagnosis, 25–32
  defined, 23
  depression screening questionnaires for, 38–47
  diagnosis of, 25, 50
  in Japan, 297–98, 317–18, 327, 340, 341
  linking American regional cultures to epidemiology of, 499–505, 500*t*, 501*t*, 502*t*, 504*t*
  in Nordic countries, 381–83, 382*t*, 414
  in old age, 91
  and post-traumatic embitterment disorder, 352–53
  in South Korea, 342–43, 371, 372–73
  in Switzerland, 381–83, 382*t*, 428
major depressive episodes (MDEs), 50, 51, 525
Malaysia Airlines Flight 370, 630
male depression
  in American regional cultures, 501–3
  among physicians, 622
  among truck drivers, 668–70, 670*t*, 671*t*, 674
  in Finland, 400–1

measurement with Gotland Male Depression Scale (GMDS), 388, 668–69, 671*t*
  and middle zone depression, 37–38
  in Nordic countries and Switzerland, 388
  in truck drivers, 656
male superiority, in South Korean culture, 354–57
male white-collar workers, depression in Japanese, 293–95, 317
maltreatment. *See also* adverse childhood events (ACEs)
  of children in South Korea, 357, 376
  as risk factor for suicidal ideation, 262–63
  and suicide of Chinese students, 203–6
manga, psychologically oriented, 313–14
mania. *See also* bipolar spectrum
  in classical Greco-Roman medicine, 165
  in diagnosis of MDD versus bipolar depression, 50–51, 52
  in medieval European medicine, 181
  in traditional Arabic and Islamic medicine (TAIM), 176–77
marianismo gender role, in American Southwest, 438, 440
marneros, in classical Greco-Roman medicine, 165
marriage. *See also* intimate partner violence (IPV)
  in American regional cultures, 484–85
  and changing economic situation in Japan, 296–97
  conflict in as common cause for *hwa-byung*, 349
  cultural expectations regarding, 89–90
  in Finland, 403
  and mental health in rural China, 254–56
  in Nordic countries and Switzerland, 388–89
  and stigma of depression, 154
masculine culture
  of airline industry, and underdiagnosis of depression, 634–35
  in Finland, 400–1
  of truck drivers, 654, 668–70, 670*t*, 671*t*
  in the United States, 501–3
Masculine Depression Risk Scale (MDRS-22), 668–69, 670*t*
Masculine Depression Scale (MDS), 668–69
masculinity/femininity (gender role differentiation), 67–68, 67*t*
Maslach Burnout Inventory (MBI), 593, 594
Massachusetts. *See* New England region (United States)
MAT (medication-assisted treatment), 570
maternity leave, 306, 589–90
Mayo Clinic, 599–600
MBI (Maslach Burnout Inventory), 593, 594
MBTI (Myers-Briggs Type Indicator), 523–24

MDD (major depressive disorder). *See also* clinical depression
  in adult immigrants from poorer countries, 127
  in American regional cultures, 444–45, 499–503, 500*t*, 501*t*
  biochemical markers of, 58
  in Chinese patients, 280
  Chinese PHQ-9 use to screen for, 269–71
  during COVID-19 pandemic, 513
  in creative professionals, 525–26
  and culture-related issues with diagnosis, 25–32
  defined, 23
  depression screening questionnaires for, 38–47
  diagnosis of, 25, 50
  in Japan, 297–98, 317–18, 327, 340, 341
  linking American regional cultures to epidemiology of, 499–505, 500*t*, 501*t*, 502*t*, 504*t*
  in Nordic countries, 381–83, 382*t*, 414
  in old age, 91
  and post-traumatic embitterment disorder, 352–53
  in South Korea, 342–43, 371, 372–73
  in Switzerland, 381–83, 382*t*, 428
MDEs (major depressive episodes), 50, 51, 525
MDQ (Mood Disorder Questionnaire), 52–53
MDRS-22 (Masculine Depression Risk Scale), 668–69, 670*t*
MDS (Masculine Depression Scale), 668–69
meats, cured, 190–92
media
  coverage of celebrity suicides by, 554–55
  trust in, 458–59
medical certificates, for airline pilots, 630–32
medical conditions
  in airline pilots, 635–36
  associated with depression, 489–90
  comorbidities of bipolar disorder, 48–49
  creative professional deaths from, 534
  musculoskeletal, 501–3, 504*t*, 662
  in physicians, review of by treating clinician, 621–22
  and sickness presenteeism among physicians, 590
  in truck drivers, 654, 678, 681
  undiagnosed, in creative professionals, 562–63
medical examination, for truck drivers, 676–77
medical interns, 575–76, 588–90
medical leaves of absence from universities, 210–12, 240, 245, 291–92
medical licensing boards (MLBs), 614–18
medical profession, depression risks in, 120, 121. *See also* physicians
medical research, gender-related challenges in, 582

medical school
  depression during, 575–76
  mental health education in, 243
  stigma of depression in, 612–14
medical systems, ancient. *See* traditional medicine
medication-assisted treatment (MAT), 570
medications. *See also* antidepressant treatment
  abuse by creative professionals, 545
  antipsychotic, 51, 538–39
  Asian Americans, rate of psychotropic use by, 263–64
  assessing use in truck drivers, 680–81
  Chinese attitude toward, 241–42, 287–91
  and clinical assessment of creative professionals, 526–27
  for creative professionals, 538–39, 559, 569
  culture and choice of, 155–56
  hypnotic, 542–43
  for medical disorders, affecting mood state, 563
  for physician-patients, 623–24
  rate of use by Asian Americans, 263–64
  suicidal patients seeking, 112
  targeting biomarkers as indicator of progress, 150
  as treatment during COVID-19 pandemic, 514*t*
  trust issues related to, 73–74
medieval European medicine, 181
meditation, 648–49
Meiji period, Japan, 300–1
melancholia, 25, 163, 176–78, 181–82
Melancholy III (Munch), 536*f*, 536
men. *See also* gender; intimate partner violence (IPV); male depression
  culture and phenomenology of depression in, 147
  externalizing behavior in, 124–25
  facial cosmetic procedures for in South Korea, 362
  and *hikikomori* in Japanese culture, 327–30
  IPV victimization of, 485–87, 486*t*
  in Japan, and changes in economic situation, 293–95, 296–97
  machismo gender role for, in American Southwest, 438, 439–40
  with modern type depression in Japan, 314–19
  psychologically controlling behavior toward female partner, 418–20
  suicide among in Switzerland and Nordic countries, 427–28, 427*t*, 429
  suicide by in the United States, 508–10, 509*t*, 511–12
mental distress, suicide as involving, 101
mental health
  across American regional cultures, 443–46
  of refugees in the United States, 434

mental health services
  in American regional cultures, 15–16, 444, 446, 448–50
  Chinese student encounters with, 238–43
  income inequality and poverty and access to, 477–80, 479t
  scarcity of in rural China, 254
  underutilization by Asian Americans, 263–64
  underutilization by Chinese Americans, 264
mental illness. *See also* bipolar spectrum; clinical depression
  changing views of in China, 183–84
  versus clinical depression, 25
  in contemporary Islamic societies, 185–86
  use of term in book, 24
  words chosen to name, link to stigmatization, 180
Mercury, Freddie, 548t
meridians (*jīngluò*), in TCM, 167–68
metal musicians, 556, 558. *See also* creative talent
metaphors
  for emotional states, Japanese, 319–21
  in German language, 82
  for heart, in Chinese language, 246, 247t
  inference from, 81–83
  in Spanish language, 82
methaqualone, 542–43
metropolitan areas as American regional cultures, 442–43, 475
Mexican Americans, 438–40, 450–51, 516
Miami metropolitan area, 442–43, 516–17
mianzi (face), in Chinese culture, 225–26
Michael, George, 548t
middle-aged men
  depression in Japanese white-collar workers, 293–95, 317
  suicide by in Japan, 325–26
middle class, 114, 115, 120–21, 127–29
middle zone depression, 25, 36–38, 149–52
Midlands culture
  behavioral and environmental risk factors in, 480–87, 482t, 484t, 486t
  educational attainment in, 467–72, 467t
  environmental influences on depression risk in, 493–98, 494t
  epidemiology of MDD, bipolar disorder, and suicide in, 499–505, 500t, 501t, 502t, 504t
  firearm culture in, 490–93, 491t
  income inequality and poverty in, 472–80, 473t, 474t, 479t
  and lessons from cultural comparison of pairs of states, 447–48
  lifestyle risk factors for depression in, 487–90, 488t
  overview, 436, 440–41
  primary ancestries in, 453–54, 454t
  race and ethnicity of population of, 450–53, 451t
  regional personality in, 459–63, 460t, 464t
  religious identity in, 464t, 465–67
  rural–urban population distribution in, 449t, 452–53, 453t
  social capital in, 456–59, 457t
  suicide rates in, 452–53, 453t, 505–12, 507t, 508t, 509t
Midwest region (United States)
  ancestry of population, 432–33
  behavioral and environmental risk factors in, 480–87, 482t, 484t, 486t
  educational attainment in, 467–72, 467t
  environmental influences on depression risk in, 493–98, 494t
  epidemiology of MDD, bipolar disorder, and suicide in, 499–505, 500t, 501t, 502t, 504t
  firearm culture in, 490–93, 491t
  income inequality and poverty in, 472–80, 473t, 474t, 479t
  and lessons from cultural comparison of pairs of states, 447–48
  lifestyle risk factors for depression in, 487–90, 488t
  overview, 440–41
  primary ancestries in, 453–54, 454t
  race and ethnicity of population of, 450–53, 451t
  regional personality in, 459–63, 460t, 464t
  religious identity in, 464t, 465–67
  rural–urban population distribution in, 449t, 452–53, 453t
  social capital in, 456–59, 457t
  suicide rates in, 452–53, 453t, 505–12, 507t, 508t, 509t
migraine, 675–76
migration within China, 251–53. *See also* left-behind people, in China
mileage, compensation for truck drivers based on, 657–58
military service, in South Korea, 372
mindfulness, 302, 648–49
Mini International Neuropsychiatric Interview (MINI), 45, 312
Minnesota. *See* Midwest region (United States)
minority populations, concentrations in American regions, 451–52
Mishima, Yukio, 540–41
MISS-HP (Moral Injury Symptoms Scale of Health Professionals), 608–9
Mississippi. *See* Deep South region (United States)
mistreatment, of physicians in training, 588–89. *See also* maltreatment

mistrust
  in American regional cultures, 517
  of physicians, in Chinese patients, 285–91
  in the United States, 430–31, 458–59, 497–98
mixed features, depression with, 50–51, 52. *See also* bipolar spectrum
mixed race persons, 94–95, 450, 451*t*, 514*t*, 515–16
MLBs (medical licensing boards), 614–18
modern type depression (MTD), Japan, 152, 298, 314–19, 334, 594
money, worries about. *See* financial distress
mono no aware (pathos of things), Japan, 301–2
Montana. *See* Mountain States, United States
Montgomery-Åsberg depression rating scale (MADRS), 81–82
mood, in diagnosis of MDD, 27–28
Mood Disorder Questionnaire (MDQ), 52–53
MoodGYM program, 283
Moon, Keith, 548*t*
moral injury, 121, 573–74, 587, 607–9, 655
Moral Injury Symptoms Scale of Health Professionals (MISS-HP), 608–9
Mormons (LDS Christians), 441–42, 465
Morrison, Jim, 548*t*
motives for entering medical profession, 578–81
Mountain States (Far West), United States
  behavioral and environmental risk factors in, 480–87, 482*t*, 484*t*, 486*t*
  educational attainment in, 467–72, 467*t*
  environmental influences on depression risk in, 493–98, 494*t*
  epidemiology of MDD, bipolar disorder, and suicide in, 499–505, 500*t*, 501*t*, 502*t*, 504*t*
  firearm culture in, 490–93, 491*t*
  income inequality and poverty in, 472–80, 473*t*, 474*t*, 479*t*
  and lessons from cultural comparison of pairs of states, 447–48
  lifestyle risk factors for depression in, 487–90, 488*t*
  overview, 441–42
  primary ancestries in, 453–54, 454*t*
  race and ethnicity of population of, 450–53, 451*t*
  regional personality in, 459–63, 460*t*, 464*t*
  religious identity in, 464*t*, 465–67
  rural–urban population distribution in, 449*t*, 452–53, 453*t*
  social capital in, 456–59, 457*t*
  suicide rates in, 452–53, 453*t*, 505–12, 507*t*, 508*t*, 509*t*
MTD (modern type depression), Japan, 152, 298, 314–19, 334, 594

muenshi (disconnected deaths), Japan, 6, 331
mujō (impermanence), Japan, 301–2
multiracial people. *See* mixed race persons
Munch, Edvard, 535–36, 536*f*, 537*f*
mune (chest), Japan, 320
murder–suicides involving airplane crashes, 628–30
Murray, Conrad, 545
musculoskeletal conditions, 501–3, 504*t*, 662
musicians. *See* creative talent
Muslim culture. *See* Islam
Myers-Briggs Type Indicator (MBTI), 523–24

Naked Woman in a Landscape (Munch), 536, 537*f*
Narayama Bushiko (Fukazawa), 4–5, 6
National Center for Education Statistics, 470
National Center for Health Statistics, 23–24
national cultures. *See* cultural identity
national emotions, South Korea, 346–47
national examination (*gaokao*), China, 219–21
National Institute for Occupational Safety and Health (NIOSH), 637–38
National Institute of Mental Health (NIMH), 26, 187–88
national-level *kējǔ*, China, 217–18
National Occupational Mortality Surveillance (NOMS) system, 637–38
Native Americans. *See* American Indians
natural disasters, and social capital, 78
Nebraska. *See* Midwest region (United States)
negative emotion
  concealment of in Chinese culture, 228–29
  expression of in Chinese language, 246, 247*t*
  Japanese words and phrases describing, 311–12
negative religious coping, 84–86, 85*t*
negative thoughts and/or feelings, as criteria for clinical depression, 33–34
neighborhood social capital, 76–77
neighborhood ties (*chi-en*), Japan, 308
neighboring states, cultural comparison of. *See* American regional cultures
Neomexicanos, in American Southwest, 438, 450–51
neurasthenia, 183–85
neurological diseases, and bipolar disorders, 48–49
Neuroticism-Extraversion-Openness Personality Inventory (NEO-PI), 523–24
neurotoxic pesticides, 144
new affluent workers, 115
New England region (United States)
  behavioral and environmental risk factors in, 480–87, 482*t*, 484*t*, 486*t*
  culture of, 436
  educational attainment in, 467–72, 467*t*
  environmental influences on depression risk in, 493–98, 494*t*

New England region (United States) (*cont.*)
  epidemiology of MDD, bipolar disorder, and suicide in, 499–505, 500*t*, 501*t*, 502*t*, 504*t*
  firearm culture in, 490–93, 491*t*
  income inequality and poverty in, 472–80, 473*t*, 474*t*, 479*t*
  and lessons from cultural comparison of pairs of states, 447–48
  lifestyle risk factors for depression in, 487–90, 488*t*
  primary ancestries in, 453–54, 454*t*
  race and ethnicity of population of, 450–53, 451*t*
  regional personality in, 459–63, 460*t*, 464*t*
  religious identity in, 464*t*, 465–67
  rural–urban population distribution in, 449*t*, 452–53, 453*t*
  social capital in, 456–59, 457*t*
  suicide rates in, 452–53, 453*t*, 505–12, 507*t*, 508*t*, 509*t*
  and truck crash risk, 655
New Hampshire. *See* New England region (United States)
Newman, Randy, 554
New Mexico. *See* Southwest region (United States)
new money, 122, 134–37
New Orleans metropolitan area, 442–43
New Twenty-Four Filial Exemplars, The (Xi), 10
new type depression. *See* modern type depression, Japan
New York metropolitan area, 442–43, 475
NIBS (non-invasive brain stimulation), 649–50
NIMH (National Institute of Mental Health), 26, 187–88
NIOSH (National Institute for Occupational Safety and Health), 637–38
Nitobe, Inazō, 325
nitrate exposure, 190–92
noise exposure
  among airline pilots, 643–44
  among musicians, 556, 560
  among truck drivers, 663–64
NOMS (National Occupational Mortality Surveillance) system, 637–38
non-Hispanic Whites
  in Connecticut, Utah, and the United States, 13*t*
  deaths of despair among, 435–36
  depression among during COVID-19 pandemic, 514*t*, 515–16
  European ancestries of, 453–54, 454*t*
  income inequality and poverty among, 474*t*
  and median household income by race, 117*t*
  population in specific states, 451*t*
  state poverty rates by, 474*t*
  suicide mortality for, 374–75, 375*t*
  and urban–rural differences in suicide rates, 453*t*

non-invasive brain stimulation (NIBS), 649–50
non-pharmacological treatment of depression, 156–57
Nordic diet, 192–93, 394
Nordic nations
  Danish culture, 411–14
  demographic and cultural differences among, 384, 388–93
  diet and depression in, 393–97, 394*t*, 395*t*, 396*t*
  Finnish culture, 397–404
  gender equality in medical specialties in, 583–84
  Icelandic culture, 420–23
  immigrants in, 411
  MDD prevalence in, 381–83, 382*t*
  Norwegian culture, 414–20
  overview, xv, 380–84, 382*t*
  sexual harassment in, 404–8, 407*t*
  social, economic, and demographic issues in, 386*t*, 388–93
  suicide in, 381, 382*t*, 383, 385, 427*t*
  Swedish culture, 404–11, 407*t*
  values and cultural dimensions of, 385–88, 391*f*
  and World Happiness Survey, 384–85
normalization
  of binge drinking, 145–46
  of bullying, in Japanese culture, 321–23
  of depression, 124, 576–77
  of hypomania in the upper class, 137
  of mood disorders in creative professionals, 540–42
  of trauma, cultural, 95–98
North Korea (Democratic People's Republic of Korea), 345
Norway. *See also* Nordic nations
  bipolar spectrum in, 416–17
  cultural antidepressants in, 416
  demographic and cultural differences with other Nordic nations, 384
  gender equality in, 414, 415–16
  immigrants in, 419–20
  intimate partner violence (IPV) in, 418–20
  MDD prevalence in, 381–83, 382*t*
  overview of culture, 380–81
  public investment in mental health services in, 414, 416–17
  Sámi people in, 417–18
  suicide in, 381, 382*t*, 383, 427*t*
Notorious B.I.G., 548*t*
numeracy, in American regional cultures, 469–70
nutritional insufficiencies, 150–51
nutritional supplements, 196–97, 648, 684

obasute (*ubasute*/*oyasute*), Japan, 4–6
obesity
  in American regional cultures, 487–89, 488*t*
  among airline pilots, 644, 647

among truck drivers, 660
and depression risk, 141
OBI (Oldenburg Burnout Inventory), 595
obstetrician/gynecologists (ob-gyns), 483
obstructive sleep apnea (OSA), 489–90, 644–45, 680
occupational burnout. See burnout
occupational cultures. See also airline pilots; creative talent; physicians; truck drivers
    age discrimination in, 92–93
    and depression risks of middle-class and upper-middle-class jobs, 120–21
    normalization of trauma in, 96–98
    and sleep, 142–43
Ochs, Phil, 548t
ODQ (Oxford Depression Questionnaire), 532
Oldenburg Burnout Inventory (OBI), 595
older people
    Chinese American, 262–64
    creative professionals, 564–65, 566
    intersection of age and gender with ethnic identity, 88–89, 90–93
    in Japan, abandonment and death of, 4–8
    Korean American, 374–76, 375t, 377–78
    left-behind, in China, 252–53, 254
    physicians, 588
    poverty among, in Nordic countries and Switzerland, 386t, 390–92
    South Korean, depression in, 346, 372–73
    suicide by in South Korea, 367–69, 367t
    suicide by in the United States, 510, 512
    unnatural deaths among Japanese, 303–4, 331–33
    unnatural deaths and suicide in Chinese culture, 259–60, 260t
old money, 122, 135, 136
olfaction (wén), in TCM, 168–69
omega-3 fatty acid supplementation, 648
omics technologies, 172
one opportunity, one encounter (ichigo ichie), Japan, 302
opioids
    overdose deaths related to, 506–8, 507t
    violent attacks on physicians from patients seeking, 587–88
Oregon. See Pacific Northwest region (United States)
organizational connections (sha-en), Japan, 308
organizational culture affecting physicians, 577–78, 584–88
organizational injustice, 600–1, 602–3, 605–6
organizational programs for reducing burnout, 598–600
organophosphate exposure, 495–96. See also pesticides
OSA (obstructive sleep apnea), 489–90, 644–45, 680
other specified depressive disorder, 24
others' perceptions, as facet of cultural identity, 61–62

outdoor recreation, 683–84
outside mental health services, university support for, 240–41, 246
overdose deaths, 506–8, 507t
overwork suicide (karojisatsu), Japan, 305
owner-operators, in trucking, 657, 658, 674
Oxford Depression Questionnaire (ODQ), 532
oyasute (ubasute/obasute), 4–6

PA (personal accomplishment), in MBI, 593, 594
Pacific Northwest region (United States)
    behavioral and environmental risk factors in, 480–87, 482t, 484t, 486t
    educational attainment in, 467–72, 467t
    environmental influences on depression risk in, 493–98, 494t
    epidemiology of MDD, bipolar disorder, and suicide in, 499–505, 500t, 501t, 502t, 504t
    firearm culture in, 490–93, 491t
    income inequality and poverty in, 472–80, 473t, 474t, 479t
    and lessons from cultural comparison of pairs of states, 447–48
    lifestyle risk factors for depression in, 487–90, 488t
    overview, 442
    primary ancestries in, 453–54, 454t
    race and ethnicity of population of, 450–53, 451t
    regional personality in, 459–63, 460t, 464t
    religious identity in, 464t, 465–67
    rural–urban population distribution in, 449t, 452–53, 453t
    social capital in, 456–59, 457t
    suicide rates in, 452–53, 453t, 505–12, 507t, 508t, 509t
paid leave, Japanese attitude toward, 306
pain, experience of in IPNP model of suicide, 102t, 106–7
panbi (upward comparison), 131, 226–28
parasocial relationships (PSRs), 554–55
parents
    and face, in South Korea, 360
    and filial piety in Chinese culture, 9–11, 222–25
    impact of social class of, 121–22
    older, abandonment of in Japan, 4–8
    parental leave for physicians in training, 589–90
    parenting style and intergenerational cultural conflict, 237
    suicide by older, in South Korea, 368
    upper-middle-class, and subjective social status, 133
Park, Su-jin, 363–65
Parker, G., 284, 498
particulate air pollution, 494t, 495

pàténg (climbing the ivy), in Chinese culture, 227–28
paternity leave, 306, 589–90
pathos of things (*mono no aware*), Japan, 301–2
patience (*gaman*), Japan, 323
Patient Health Questionnaire 15-item (PHQ-15), 371
Patient Health Questionnaire 2-item (PHQ-2), 513–15
Patient Health Questionnaire 8-item (PHQ-8), 33, 39, 40
Patient Health Questionnaire 9-item (PHQ-9)
  airline pilots, assessment with, 633–35
  alternative diagnostic criteria for clinical depression, 33
  assessing patients from other cultures with, 273
  and burnt-out physicians, 594–95
  Chinese version, 266–67, 268–71
  cultural customization for Chinese patients, 271–73
  Japanese version, 312, 341
  Korean version, 370–71
  screening for depression with, 38–40, 42, 43–44, 45–47
  subthreshold conditions, insensitivity to, 274
patient-related burnout scale, in CBI, 595–97
patient role
  acculturating to, 157–58
  in Chinese culture, 277–78
  physician acceptance of, 614
pattern recognition and treatment determination (*biànzhèng lùnzhì*), in TCM, 170–72, 171t
PB (perceived burdensomeness), 101–4, 102t, 325, 368
PCPs. *See* physicians; primary care physicians
peer counseling for airline pilots, 650–51
People's Republic of China. *See* Chinese culture
perceived burdensomeness (PB), 101–4, 102t, 325, 368
perfectionism, in South Korean culture, 362
performance anxiety, 556
performing artists, 523, 539–40, 546, 547, 552, 564. *See also* creative talent
perpetual foreigner stereotype, 237–38
personal accomplishment (PA), in MBI, 593, 594
personal burnout scale, in CBI, 595–96, 597
personality
  in American regional cultures, 443–44
  among creative professionals, 523–24
  regional, 459–63, 460t, 464t
  and social capital, 78
personalized medicine, 352, 566–70, 623–24, 626

pesticides, 144, 256, 258, 495–96
pharmacotherapy. *See* medications
phenomenology of depression, 146–47
phenotypes of clinical depression
  in TCM, 170–72, 171t
  use of screening questionnaires to identify, 267
Philanthropic Health indicator (Social Capital Project), 456
PHPs (physician health programs), 616–19
PHQ-15 (Patient Health Questionnaire 15-item), 371
PHQ-2 (Patient Health Questionnaire 2-item), 513–15
PHQ-8 (Patient Health Questionnaire 8-item), 33, 39, 40
PHQ-9. *See* Patient Health Questionnaire 9-item
physical abuse of children in South Korea, 357, 376. *See also* adverse childhood events (ACEs)
physical environment
  and American regional cultures, 493–98, 494t
  hazardous, physicians working in, 588
  and suicide rates, 111
physical inactivity, in American regional cultures, 487–89, 488t
physical symptoms of depression. *See also* somatic symptoms of depression
  and culture and phenomenology of depression, 146–47
  in diagnosis of clinical depression, 34
  in *hwa-byung*, 348–49
physical violence toward partners. *See* intimate partner violence (IPV)
physician health programs (PHPs), 616–19
physicians
  avoidance of treatment among, 611–12, 614
  biomarkers of burnout in, 597–98
  burnout among, 591–97
  Chinese patient trust in, 285–91
  clinical assessment of creative professionals, 526–27
  clinical care of, 619–24
  and commodification of healthcare, 584–88
  cultural identities of, 577–78
  and depression risks in medical profession, 120, 121
  and environmental influences in American regions, 496–98
  financial distress among, 580–81, 609–11
  gender-related challenges for, 581–84
  job stress among, 573–74, 578, 600–7
  moral injury to, 573–74, 587, 607–9
  motives for entering profession and career anchors, 578–81
  overview, xv

overwork of Japanese, 305–6
psychiatrists as clinician of choice for
 treating, 622–23, 625–26
 relationship with Japanese patients, and
  adherence, 339
 sickness presenteeism, 590
 stigmatization of depression among, 573,
  575–76, 611–18
 substance abuse by, 618–19
 suicide among, 571, 572, 574, 624–25
 in traditional Arabic and Islamic medicine
  (TAIM), 178–79
 in traditional Chinese medicine (TCM), 173
 in training, 575–76, 588–90
 treatment of burnout in, 598–600
 trust in, 72–74
 vulnerability to depression, 571–77
 working conditions for, 584–88
Pike, Roland, 672–73
pilots. See airline pilots
plastic surgery, in South Korean culture,
  360–65
pleasure, experience of in IPNP model of
  suicide, 102t, 107–8
pleasure-seeking
 in Denmark, 413–14
 in Japanese culture, 333–34
PMRs (proportional mortality ratios) for
  suicide in pilots, 637–38
pollution, 494t, 495–97
popular musicians, 547–53, 548t, 556, 557–58,
  See also creative talent
population screening for depression. See
  depression screening questionnaires
positive mental health, education in skills to
  build, 242, 243
positive predictive value, of depression
  screening questionnaires, 43
positive religious coping, 84–86, 85t
positive thoughts and/or feelings, in diagnosis
  of clinical depression, 34
Post, Felix, 523
postpartum depression (PPD), 90, 483–84
post-traumatic embitterment disorder
  (PTED), 352–54, 353t
poverty. See also financial distress;
  socioeconomic status
 in American regional cultures, 472–80, 473t,
  474t, 479t
 in Nordic countries and Switzerland, 386t,
  390–92
 of older people in Japan, 331, 332–33
 of older people in South Korea, 346, 368
power distance, 64–66, 65t
power harassment, in Japanese culture, 321–23
PPD (postpartum depression), 90, 483–84
practice to cultivate qi (qìgōng), in TCM, 169
precariat, classification of, 115

pregnancy, among physicians in training, 590
premature death. See also unnatural deaths
 of creative professionals, 533–39, 536f, 537f,
  547–53, 548t, 558, 561
 of truck drivers, 654
primary care physicians (PCPs). See also
  physicians
 acculturation, stigma, and strategy for
  Chinese patients, 281–82, 285
 consultation by depressed Chinese
  Americans, 264–65
 and environmental influences on
  depression, 498
 failure to recognize depression and
  suicidality, 17–21
 integration of mainstream with traditional
  or complementary medicine, 195–96
 use of depression screening questionnaires
  by, 267
 visits to prior to suicide, 112
primary prevention of suicide, 242–43
primed perception, 159–60
Prince, 548t, 562
processed foods diets, 190
productivity, relationship to illness in creative
  professionals, 543–45
professional burnout. See burnout
professional cultures. See occupational cultures
prolonged and severe social withdrawal
  (hikikomori), Japan, 298, 327–30
propofol, 545
proportional mortality ratios (PMRs) for
  suicide in pilots, 637–38
Protestantism
 African American churches, 466–67
 in American regional cultures, 463
 and divorce, 485
 and suicide, 103, 104
provincial-level kējǔ, China, 217–18
PSRs (parasocial relationships), 554–55
psychiatric hospitalization in South Korea,
  376–77
psychiatry. See also treatment
 acculturation, stigma, and strategy for
  Chinese patients, 282, 284–85
 celebrities allied against, 529–30
 contemporary relationship with traditional
  medicine, 182–89
 disparagement and devaluation of in
  medical schools, 614
 physician-patients, 622–23, 625–26
 shinryonaika as alternative to in Japan,
  313–14
 use of depression screening questionnaires
  in, 267
 view of suicide in Japanese, 326–27
psychoactive substance use. See substance use/
  substance use disorders

psychological impact of medical conditions in pilots, 635–36
psychologically controlling behavior of men toward female partners, 418–20
psychological services, Chinese student encounters with, 238–43
psychology, contemporary relationship with traditional medicine, 182–89
psychomotor agitation or retardation, in diagnosis of MDD, 29–30
psychosomatic internal medicine (*shinryōnaikai*), Japan, 313–14
psychosomatic nature of depression, 146–47. *See also* somatic symptoms of depression
psychosomatic syndromes, 37. *See also hwa-byung*, South Korea
psychotherapy
  acculturation, stigma, and strategy for Chinese patients, 282–83
  for airline pilots, 637, 649, 650
  Ashkenazic Jewish American attitude toward, 241
  Chinese attitude toward, 240–41
  during COVID-19 pandemic, 514*t*
  for creative talent, 536–38
  culture as determinant of attitudes toward, 156
  integrating religious concepts into, 186–87
psychotic depression, 25, 629
psychotropic medications. *See* medications
PTED (post-traumatic embitterment disorder), 352–54, 353*t*
Pursuit of Loneliness, The (Slater), 130

qì (vital energy/life force), in TCM, 167–68, 170–72, 171*t*
qiè (palpation), in TCM, 168–69
qìgōng (practice to cultivate qi), in TCM, 169
Quaker immigrants to the United States, 436
quantitative performance measures in healthcare, 586
questionnaires. *See* depression screening questionnaires

race. *See also* ancestry of Americans; cultural identity; ethnicity
  and American regional cultures, 431–32, 450–53, 451*t*
  and cultural antidepressants, 124
  and depression during COVID-19 pandemic, 512–13, 514*t*, 515–17
  and discrimination toward minorities, 94–95
  and income inequality and poverty in the United States, 472–73, 474*t*
  and socioeconomic status, 116–18, 116*t*, 117*t*
  state poverty rates by, 474*t*
racism, in American Deep South, 437

rap musicians, 558, 559
RDoC (Research Domain Criteria), NIMH, 26, 187–88
reading the air (*ba no kuuki wo yomu*), Japan, 309–10
reason to live
  assessing in creative professionals, 568–69
  assessing in truck drivers, 681
  ikigai concept, Japan, 82, 108–9, 384–85
  in interpersonal-neuropsychiatric (IPNP) model of suicide, 102*t*, 108–9
recurrent thoughts of death, in diagnosis of MDD, 31
Redding, Otis, 548*t*
refugees, 410, 434
regional airlines, 641–42
regional personality, 459–63, 460*t*, 464*t*, *See also* American regional cultures
regulations
  in airline industry, 630–32
  for truck drivers, 661–62, 666, 672
reindeer herding, by Sámi people, 417–18
relational social capital, 74–76
relaxation, systematic, 648–49
religious identity
  in American regional cultures, 438, 441–42, 463, 464*t*, 465–67
  in Chinese culture, 216–19, 222–28
  and cultural antidepressants, 124
  and divorce, 485
  and *hwa-byung*, 350
  in Japanese culture, 298–301
  overview, 83–87, 85*t*
  and reason to live, 109
  religion-based treatment, 186–87
  in South Korean culture, 354–57, 362, 369
  and stigmatization of depression, 181
  and suicide, 102–4
Renaissance, 181–82
Republic of Korea. *See* South Korean culture
Research Domain Criteria (RDoC), NIMH, 26, 187–88
resident physicians, 575–76, 588–90
resident registration (*hùkǒu*) system, China, 249–50, 251–52
resilience, education in skills to build, 242
restraint/indulgence, 70–71, 70*t*
retail, demand–control imbalance in, 120
retirement
  cultural identity and, 88–89
  in Japan, 295–96
  of physicians, 611, 625
  in South Korea, 368–69
  suicide of pilots in, 637–38
Rhazes (Abi Bakr Muhammad ibn Zakariyya al-Razi), 176
rich second generation (*fùèrdài*), in China, 225–26

INDEX 825

right hemisphere lesions, in Japanese people, 310–11
right-to-work laws, 661
Risk Screening Environmental Indicators (RSEI) score, EPA, 493, 494t
Rockett, R., 303–4
rock musicians, 556, 558, 560. See also creative talent
romanticizing of mood disorders, 539
Rong, Xin, 214t
Rúlín Wàishǐ (*The Scholars*), Wu, 219
rural–urban populations. See also left-behind people, in China
  and American regional cultures, 446, 448–50, 449t, 452–53, 453t, 477
  migration within China, 251–53
  in Norway, 417
  in Switzerland, 392–93, 423–27
Russia, in Finnish history, 402

SAD (seasonal affective disorder), 422, 493
sadness, Japanese appreciation for, 301–4
saffron, 177–78
St. John's wort, 163–64, 181
SAMe (S-adenosylmethionine), 648
Sámi people (Lapps), in Norway, 417–18
samurai culture, Japan, 299–300, 304–7
San Francisco Bay Area, United States, 442, 475, 517
sati tradition (India), 100
Saudi Arabia, female resident physicians in, 583
saunas, in Finnish culture, 401
Savage, Mike, 114–15
schizophrenia, 180, 313
school
  bullying at, in South Korea, 365–66
  modern type depression and, in Japan, 314–19
  normalization of bullying in Japanese culture, 321–23
Scream, The (Munch), 535–36
screening questionnaires. See depression screening questionnaires
seasonal affective disorder (SAD), 422, 493
seasonality of mood disorders, 493–95
secular-rational values, 386–87, 391f
selective serotonin reuptake inhibitors (SSRIs), 530–32, 631
Selena, 548t
self-blame, among physicians, 578
self-construal in Japanese culture, 307–8, 340–41
self-critical nature of creative professionals, 564–65
self-definition, 61. See also cultural identity
self-effacing speech, 80
self-enhancing speech, 80

self-expression values, 386–87, 391f
self-harm, availability of highly lethal means of, 102t, 109–10, 256, 258
self-neglect, deaths from, 99–100
self-shaming, in Japanese culture, 323–24
self-stigma, 151, 152–53, 573, 677. See also stigmatization of depression
serene melancholy, beauty of (*wabi-sabi*), Japan, 302–3
serotonin and norepinephrine reuptake inhibitor (SNRI) antidepressants, 531–32
SES. See income inequality; poverty; socioeconomic status
seven-level model of social class, 114
sexual harassment
  in Denmark, 406–7, 407t
  of female truck drivers, 674
  in Finland, 407, 407t
  in Japanese culture, 322–23
  in South Korean culture, 365
  in Sweden, 404–8, 407t
  in Switzerland, 428–29
  of women medical students and physicians, 581–82
sexuality
  in later life, cultural expectations regarding, 90–91
  and pleasure-seeking culture in Denmark, 413
sha-en (organizational connections), Japan, 308
Shah, Zaharie Amad, 630
Shakur, Tupac, 548t
shamans, in TCM, 173–74
shame, and suicide in Japanese culture, 323–27
Shānghán Zábìng Lùn (*Treatise on Cold Damage Disorders*), Zhang, 170
SHAPS (Snaith-Hamilton Pleasure Scale), 107
shin-gata utsu-byo. See modern type depression (MTD), Japan
shinjū (lovers' suicide), 324–25
shinryōnaika (psychosomatic internal medicine), Japan, 313–14
Shintō, in Japanese culture, 298–99
shisei-kan (death-life-view), Japan, 325
shōgun era, Japan, 299–300
short-term orientation, 68–70, 69t
shūdan ishiki (group consciousness), Japan, 307–8
sickness presenteeism, 590
Silicon Valley, United States, 442, 475
Silverman, Sarah, 561–62
Singapore, unnatural deaths and suicide in, 259–62, 260t, 261t
single motherhood, in American regional cultures, 483–84, 484t
single-person households, in Nordic countries and Switzerland, 389, 392

sisu (grit), Finland, 402–4
Slater, Philip, 130
slavery, in the Deep South, 437, 456–58, 461
sleep
    among airline pilots, 634–35, 639, 643, 644–46, 647–48
    among Chinese students, 218–19
    among truck drivers, 659–60
    and biomarkers of depression, 35
    in diagnosis of clinical depression, 34
    in Japanese culture, 307, 333
    relation to culture and depression, 142–43
smartphone apps, 339–40
Smith, G. S., 303–4
smoking
    in American regional cultures, 488*t*, 489–90
    in Denmark, 413
Snaith-Hamilton Pleasure Scale (SHAPS), 107
SNRI (serotonin and norepinephrine reuptake inhibitor) antidepressants, 531–32
social capital
    in American regional cultures, 435–36, 455–59, 457*t*
    dimensions of, 74–78
    of Japanese people outside of Japan, 308
    overview, 62
    and problematic drinking in South Korea, 359–60
    and social class, 114–15, 127–30
Social Capital Project (Joint Economic Committee of the U.S. Senate), 455–59, 457*t*
social class. *See* socioeconomic status
social environment
    in Nordic countries and Switzerland, 388–93
    and suicide rates, 111–12
social media analysis, 243–44
Social Mobility Index, 389–90
Social Security Disability Insurance (SSDI), 501–5, 504*t*
Social Support sub-index (Social Capital Project), 456
social withdrawal, prolonged and severe (*hikikomori*), Japan, 298, 327–30
socioeconomic status (SES). *See also* income inequality; poverty
    acculturative stress when improving, 95
    and age, 116, 116*t*
    and American regional cultures, 13*t*, 16–17
    conflicting determinants of, 121–24
    depression risks of middle-class and upper-middle-class jobs, 120–21
    and environmental hazards, 143
    and higher education, 119
    and income-based stratification, 113–16
    and income insecurity, 118–19
    and judgments about hypomanic symptoms, 55–56
    and life expectancy, 92
    and mood disorder epidemiology, 126–30
    and mood disorder phenomenology, 124–26
    in Nordic countries and Switzerland, 389–90, 392
    overview, 113
    and race/ethnicity, 116–18, 116*t*, 117*t*
    subgroups, awareness of differences between, 116–18
    and subjective social status, 130–33
    in the United States, 431
    upper class, troubles of, 133–39
sodium nitrate, 190–92
somatic symptoms of depression
    and acculturation of Chinese patients, 281–84, 285
    in American regional cultures, 501–4
    among Chinese Americans, 264–65
    among truck drivers, 677
    and Chinese CES-D, 276–81
    in Chinese culture, 270, 271
    in diagnosis of clinical depression, 34
    in diagnosis of MDD, 31–32
    in *hwa-byung*, 348–49
    and socioeconomic status, 125–26
    in South Korean patients, 371
somatoform syndromes, 37
somatopsychic nature of depression, 146–47
Song Dynasty, China, 173–74
Southern California, 442, 516
Southern culture. *See* Deep South region (United States)
South Korean culture. *See also* Korean Americans
    binge drinking, 145–46, 347, 358
    communication style of, 79
    Confucianism in, 354–57
    cosmetic surgery and face, 360–65
    culture and choice of treatment, 156
    depression-related syndromes reflecting, 347–54, 351*t*, 353*t*
    drinking culture, 358–60
    filial piety, 222
    han national emotion, 346–47
    historical context, 345–46
    jeong national emotion, 347
    overview, 11, 342–45
    phenomenology of depression, 147
    rating and screening for depression, 370–73
    sexual harassment and bullying, 365–66
    social capital, 76
    stigma of depression and barriers to treatment, 376–79
    suicide in, 342–43, 359, 365, 366–70, 367*t*, 374–75, 377
Southwest region (United States)
    behavioral and environmental risk factors in, 480–87, 482*t*, 484*t*, 486*t*

culture of, 438–40
educational attainment in, 467–72, 467t
environmental influences on depression risk in, 493–98, 494t
epidemiology of MDD, bipolar disorder, and suicide in, 499–505, 500t, 501t, 502t, 504t
firearm culture in, 490–93, 491t
income inequality and poverty in, 472–80, 473t, 474t, 479t
and lessons from cultural comparison of pairs of states, 447–48
lifestyle risk factors for depression in, 487–90, 488t
primary ancestries in, 453–54, 454t
race and ethnicity of population of, 450–53, 451t
regional personality in, 459–63, 460t, 464t
religious identity in, 464t, 465–67
rural–urban population distribution in, 449t, 452–53, 453t
social capital in, 456–59, 457t
suicide rates in, 452–53, 453t, 505–12, 507t, 508t, 509t
Spanish language, metaphor and word choice in, 82
special issuance of medical certificates for airline pilots, 630–31
specificity, of depression screening questionnaires, 43
spirit (*ki* or energy), Japan, 320–21
Spiritual Pivot (Língshū), Huangdi Nejing, 169–70
spleen qì deficiency, in TCM, 170, 171t
SSDI (Social Security Disability Insurance), 501–5, 504t
SSRIs (selective serotonin reuptake inhibitors), 530–32, 631
SSS (subjective social status), 130–33, 226–27, 318–19
stars. *See also* creative talent
defined, 523
lonely at the top phenomenon among, 553–54
and parasocial relationships and culture of fandom, 554–55
toxicity of pop music stardom, 547–53, 548t
states, cultures in different. *See* American regional cultures
status seeking within upper class, 134–35
stereotyping, 61, 237–38
stigmatization of depression
in airline industry, 630–32, 636–37, 646–51
among creative professionals, 527, 529, 539–40
among physicians, 573, 575–76, 611–18
among truck drivers, 676–78
based on biomarkers, 149–50

in Chinese culture, 183–84, 188–89, 239–40, 254, 265, 281–85
concerns about in persons with new money, 137
in contemporary Islamic societies, 185–86
culture-dependent nature of, 151–55
in Iceland, 422–23
in interpersonal-neuropsychiatric (IPNP) model of suicide, 101
in Japanese culture, 180, 313
and middle zone of depression, 38
in South Korean culture, 376–79
and tightness–looseness of American regions, 462
and traditional medicine, 180–82, 194
stoicism, in Japanese culture, 305, 306, 325
Stoker, G. C., 627
STOP-BANG questionnaire for OSA, 680
stress. *See* acculturative stress; job strain/stress
structural competency, 149
structural social capital, 74–75
Structured Clinical Interview for DSM-5, 45
structured clinical interviews, 45–46
student health services, Chinese student encounters with, 238–43
students, depression among. *See also* Chinese students at American universities
in medical school, 575–76, 612–14
overview, 470–71
subgroups, among racial/ethnic groups, 116–18
subjective social status (SSS), 130–33, 226–27, 318–19
substance use/substance use disorders
and American regional cultures, 12t, 16–17
among creative professionals, 521–22, 527, 533–34, 544–45, 552, 557–58, 570
among physicians, 618–19
among truck drivers, 680–81
and bipolar spectrum, 48
opioid overdose deaths, 506–8, 507t
relation to culture and depression, 145–46
subsyndromal hypomania, 50–51, 52. *See also* bipolar spectrum
subsyndromal MDD. *See* clinical depression
successful creators, 523. *See also* creative talent
suicide and suicidality. *See also* interpersonal-neuropsychiatric model of suicide; unnatural deaths
across American regional cultures, 11–17, 12t, 444–45, 452–53, 453t, 458–59, 463, 499, 505–12, 507t, 508t, 509t
and alcohol consumption, 359
among airline pilots, 637–38
among Chinese Americans, 262–64, 375–76, 375t
among Chinese students at American universities, 201–16, 214t

suicide and suicidality (*cont.*)
  among creative professionals, 533–39, 536*f*, 537*f*, 541–42, 543, 545, 554–55, 564, 568–69
  among Japanese Americans, 375–76, 375*t*
  among Korean Americans, 374–76, 375*t*
  among physicians, 571, 572, 574, 624–25
  and CES-D use, 42
  in China, 9–11, 249, 251, 254–62, 259*f*, 260*t*, 261*t*
  and communication styles, 17–21
  depression questionnaires sensitive to, 274
  in diagnosis of MDD, 31
  educational interventions for prevention of, 242–43
  exclusion from culturally aware criteria for clinical depression, 33
  in Finland, 404, 428
  and gun ownership and storage, 490, 491–92
  inference from metaphor and word choice, 82
  interpersonal-psychological theory of, 101
  Islamic view of, 179
  in Japan, 8, 297–98, 303–4, 323–27
  linking regional cultures to epidemiology of, 499–505, 500*t*, 501*t*, 502*t*, 504*t*
  in Nordic nations, 381, 382*t*, 383, 385, 427*t*
  overview, xv–xvii, 99–101
  in PHQ-9, 40
  relationship between religion and, 466
  and religious coping, 84–85
  in South Korea, 342–43, 359, 365, 374–75, 377
  in Switzerland, 381, 382*t*, 383, 385, 393, 426, 427–28, 427*t*, 429
  through cultural lens, 110–12
  truck drivers, assessing risk for, 681
  and university responses to student mental health issues, 291–92
suicide-homicides involving airplane crashes, 628–30
Sun, Andrew, 214*t*
Sun, Jing, 218–19
Sūn, Sīmiǎo, 173
supernatural model of illness, 173–74, 178–79, 185–86
supplements, 196–97, 648, 684
Su, Qin, 218–19
survival guilt, 565
survival values, 386–87, 391*f*
Sùwèn (*Basic Questions*), *Huangdi Neijing*, 169
Sweden. *See also* Nordic nations
  cultural paradoxes in, 409–10
  demographic and cultural differences with other Nordic nations, 384
  in Finnish history, 402
  gender equality in medical specialties in, 583–84
  historical context of, 406
  immigrants in, 408–9, 410–11
  lagom culture in, 409
  MDD prevalence in, 381–83, 382*t*
  overview of culture, 380–81, 408–9
  sexual harassment in, 404–8, 407*t*
  suicide in, 381, 382*t*, 383, 427*t*
Switzerland
  bipolar spectrum in, 426
  demographic and cultural differences within, 383–84
  diet and depression in, 393–97, 394*t*, 395*t*, 396*t*
  general discussion, 423–29
  MDD prevalence in, 381–83, 382*t*
  overview of culture, 380–81
  rural–urban divide in, 392–93, 423–27
  social, economic, and demographic issues in, 388–93, 386*t*
  suicide in, 381, 382*t*, 383, 385, 393, 426, 427–28, 427*t*, 429
  values and cultural dimensions in, 385–88, 391*f*
  women's mental health in, 428–29
syncretism, in Japanese culture, 298–301
systematic relaxation, 648–49

taijin kyofusho (TKS or fear of personal relations disorder), Japan, 307–8
TAIM (traditional Arabic and Islamic medicine), 162, 175–80, 185–87
Taiwan, unnatural deaths and suicide in, 259–61, 260*t*, 261*t*
talking about depression, cultural differences in, 79–81
Tang, Luke, 208–10
Tang, Xiaolin, 214*t*
tatemae (built in front), Japan, 312
TB (thwarted belongingness), 101–4, 102*t*, 325, 368
TCM. *See* traditional Chinese medicine
technical middle class, 115
Temperament Evaluation of Memphis, Pisa, and San Diego Autoquestionnaire (TEMPS-A), 523–24
temperature, and depression risk, 493, 494*t*
temporal lobe epilepsy (TLE), 562
tests, focus on in Chinese culture, 216–22
Tezuka, Osamu, 314
thwarted belongingness (TB), 101–4, 102*t*, 325, 368
Tian, Miaoxiu, 214*t*
Tidewater culture, United States, 436
tie (*en*) concept, Japan, 7–8, 308
tightness–looseness, in American regional cultures, 459–63, 460*t*, 475–76
tinnitus
  among airline pilots, 643–44
  among musicians, 556, 560
  among truck drivers, 663–64
TKM (traditional Korean medicine). *See* traditional Chinese medicine

TKS (*taijin kyofusho*), Japan, 307–8
TLE (temporal lobe epilepsy), 562
Tokugawa shogunate, 299–300
torture, in classical Greco-Roman medicine, 166
tortured genius myth, 539. *See also* creative talent
toxic exposure, 494t, 495–97
traditional Arabic and Islamic medicine (TAIM), 162, 175–80, 185–87
traditional Chinese medicine (TCM)
   contemporary relationship with mainstream medicine, 183–85, 188–89
   diagnostic process in, 168–69
   general discussion, 174–75
   herbal remedies for depression in, 148
   Huangdi Neijing, 167–68, 169–70
   mood disorders in *Língshū*, 169–70
   overview, 162, 167–68
   personalized, holistic approach to treatment in, 288
   phenotypes of clinical depression in, 170–72, 171t
   during Song Dynasty, 173–74
   Sūn Sīmiǎo, 173
   treatment of depression in, 169, 170–73, 171t, 174–75
   Zhang Zhòngjǐng, 170
   zhèng concept in, 168, 170–72, 171t
traditional diets, 140–42, 190, 192–93
traditional Korean medicine (TKM). *See* traditional Chinese medicine (TCM)
traditional medicine. *See also* traditional Chinese medicine (TCM)
   Arabic and Islamic (TAIM), 162, 175–80, 185–87
   contemporary relationship of mainstream approaches and, 182–89
   diet and depression in, 189–94, 191t, 192t
   European, 181–82
   Greco-Roman, 163–67
   integrative medicine, 194–97
   overview, 147–49, 161–62
   stigma of depression in, 180–82
traditional values, 386–87, 391f, 392
traditional working class, 115
training
   aviation, 641
   physicians in, 575–76, 588–90
translations of depression questionnaires, 47
Transport Canada, 631
trauma
   cultural normalization of, 95–98
   in South Korean culture, 346
Treatise on Cold Damage Disorders (*Shānghán Zábìng Lùn*), Zhang, 170
Treatise on Melancholy (Ibn Imran), 176–77
treatment
   of airline pilots, 630–32, 636–37, 646–51
   barriers to, in South Korean culture, 376–79

   of bipolar spectrum patients, 49, 51–52
   of burnout, 598–600
   of Chinese patients, 281–85, 287–91
   in classical Greco-Roman medicine, 163–64, 165–66
   in complementary, alternative, and integrative medicine, 194–97
   during COVID-19 pandemic, 514t
   of creative professionals, 529–33, 536–40, 559, 565–70
   culture and choice of, 155–57
   electroacupuncture as adjunct to antidepressants, 168
   and environmental influences on depression, 496–98
   of *hwa-byung*, 349–50
   in Iceland, 423
   importance of numeracy to, 469–70
   and income inequality and poverty, 477–78
   individualizing with biomarkers, 35–36
   integrating religious concepts into, 186–87
   of Japanese patients, 338–41
   of *kokoro no kaze* in Japan, 319–20
   of medical conditions associated with depression, 489–90
   in medieval European medicine, 181
   of modern type depression (MTD), 318
   and moral injury to physicians, 587, 607
   overview, xvii
   of physicians, 611–12, 614, 622–24
   targeting biomarkers as indicator of progress, 150–51
   in traditional Arabic and Islamic medicine (TAIM), 176–78
   in traditional Chinese medicine (TCM), 169, 170–73, 171t, 174–75
   in traditional medical systems, 147–49
   of truck drivers, 677, 678–79, 680, 682–84
   of upper-class patients, 137–39, 475
trephination, 181
tristitia (sadness), in classical Greco-Roman medicine, 165–66
truck drivers
   clinical evaluation of, 679–82
   and effort–reward imbalance, 120
   female, 672–76
   institutional and personal stigma of depression among, 676–78
   loneliness among, 666–68
   occupational culture of, 654–55, 668–70, 670t, 671t, 683–84
   occupational hazards for, 660–66
   overview, 652–57
   relationships with jobs, 671–72
   treatment for, 678–79, 680, 682–84
   working conditions of, 657–60
"Truck Driver's Blues" (Haggard), 652
"Truck Driving Woman" (Wilson & Pike), 672–73
true sound (*hon'ne*), Japan, 312

trust
   in American regional cultures, 437, 458–59, 497–98, 517
   of Chinese patients in physicians, 285–91
   and cultural identity, 72–74
   in dimensional characterization of cultures, 62
   in physicians, and commodification of healthcare, 585
   and social capital, 74, 75, 76
   in the United States, 430–31
Trust in Physician Scale, 286
turmeric, 177–78
Twenty-Four Filial Exemplars, The (Guo Jujing), 9

ubasute (*obasute/oyasute*), Japan, 4–6
ultraviolet-A radiation, airline pilot exposure to, 643
uncertainty avoidance, 66–67, 66t
underclass, 114, 122, 123–24
understated speech, 80
underweight women, in South Korean culture, 362
undocumented immigrants in the United States, 433–34
unemployment, of youth in Sweden, 409–10. *See also* financial distress
United Kingdom
   Civil Aviation Authority, 631
   social class in, 114–15
university students, Chinese. *See* Chinese students at American universities
unmarried mothers, in American regional cultures, 483–84
unnatural deaths. *See also* suicide and suicidality
   in American regional cultures, 505–8, 507t
   among creative professionals, 521–22, 533–39, 536f, 537f, 547–53, 548t, 558
   among truck drivers, 654
   in Chinese culture, 259–60, 260t
   in Japanese culture, 297, 298t, 303–4
   overview, 99–100
unspecified depressive disorder, 24
unspecified mood disorder, 24
upper class, 114, 122, 133–39
upper-middle class
   depression risks of jobs for, 120–21
   and mood disorder epidemiology, 129–30
   in seven-level model of social class, 114
   subjective social status, 131–33
   upper class persons identifying as, 134
Upper Midwest. *See* Midwest region (United States)
upper-upper class, 114
upward comparison (*panbi*), 131, 226–28

urban populations. *See* rural–urban populations
U.S. Census Bureau Household Pulse Survey Wave 39, 512–13
U.S. Environmental Protection Agency Risk Screening Environmental Indicators (RSEI) score, 493, 494t
Utah, 11–17, 441–42

vacation days, Japanese attitude toward, 306
values
   in Inglehart-Welzel World Cultural Map, 386–87, 391f
   in intergenerational cultural conflicts, 233, 234, 235
   in Nordic countries and Switzerland, 385–88, 391f
Vance, J. D., 95
van Zandt, Ronnie, 548t
vibration, as health risk for truck drivers, 662–63
violence against physicians, 587–88
visual artists, major depressive episodes among, 525. *See also* creative talent
vital energy (*qi*), in TCM, 167–68, 170–72, 171t
vitamin D insufficiency/deficiency, 192–93
vortioxetine, 532

wabi-sabi (beauty of imperfection/beauty of serene melancholy), Japan, 302–3
wàng (inspection), in TCM, 168–69
Wang, Annie, 214t
Wang, Luchang, 210–12
Wang, Xiaojuan, 249–51
Wang, Ziwen, 214t
Washington (state). *See* Pacific Northwest region (United States)
Washington, DC metropolitan area, 442, 475
WBV (whole-body vibration), 662–63
wealth. *See also* income inequality; socioeconomic status
   as determinant of socioeconomic class, 121–24
   versus face, in Chinese culture, 225–26
   and power distance, 64–65
weapons ownership. *See* gun ownership
wearable devices to track sleep and activity, 29–30, 35, 57–58, 546–47, 598, 649, 682
weight
   changes in, and diagnosis of MDD, 29
   of women in South Korean culture, 362
wén (auscultation/olfaction), in TCM, 168–69
wèn (inquiry), in TCM, 168–69
Wenger, Julia, 671–72
Western diets, 140–41, 190

Western Europe
  MDD prevalence and suicide in, 381, 382*t*
  suicide mortality rate in, 367–68, 367*t*
Western medicine. *See also* physicians
  contemporary relationship with traditional medicine, 182–89
  integration with traditional or complementary medicine, 194–97
  stigmatization of depression in history of Europe, 181–82
West Virginia. *See* Appalachian culture
white-collar workers, depression in Japanese, 293–95, 314–19
whole-body vibration (WBV), 662–63
whole foods diets, 190
Williams, Robin, 555
Wilson, Johnny, 672–73
Winehouse, Amy, 521–22, 526–27, 530, 562–63
Wisconsin. *See* Midwest region (United States)
withdrawal, among creative professionals, 534–35
women's mental health. *See also* gender; intimate partner violence (IPV); sexual harassment
  airline pilots, 639–40
  and American regional cultures, 16, 438, 440, 441–42
  among Korean Americans, 373–74
  and Chinese CES-D, 277
  creative professionals, 552
  in Denmark, 412–13
  and economic situation in Japan, 296
  externalizing behavior, 388
  and facial cosmetic procedures in South Korea, 360–65
  and gender inequality in South Korea, 354–57
  hwa-byung, 347–52
  intersection of age and gender with ethnic identity, 89–91
  left-behind wives in China, 249–51, 252–53, 254, 256, 257–58
  in Nordic countries and Switzerland, 383
  older Chinese Americans, 263
  physicians, 581–84, 589–90
  in rural China, 254–57, 261–62
  somatic expression of depression, 278
  suicide in American regions, 508–9, 508*t*, 510, 511
  suicide in South Korea, 367–68, 367*t*
  in Switzerland, 428–29
  truck drivers, 672–76
  work–family conflict for physicians, 603
  working-class women with children, 128
word choice, inference from, 81–83
work. *See also* airline pilots; creative talent; occupational cultures; physicians; truck drivers
  Chinese international student worries about, 231
  and gender inequality in South Korea, 354–55
  Japanese attitude toward, 305–7
  modern type depression and, 314–19
  normalization of bullying at in Japan, 321–23
  sexual harassment at, in South Korea, 365
working class, 114, 127–28, 434
working poor, 114, 121–24
work-related burnout scale, in CBI, 595–97
World Cultural Map, Inglehart-Welzel, 385–87, 391*f*
World Happiness Report, xv, 380
World Happiness Survey, 384–85
World Values Survey (WVS), 385
World War II, 335, 336, 337–38
worthlessness, feelings of, 30
writers, 525–26, 565. *See also* creative talent
Wu Jingzi, 219
wǔ xíng (five elements), in TCM, 167–68
Wyoming. *See* Mountain States (Far West), United States

Xiàojīng (*The Classic of Filial Piety*), 223
xiùcái title (China), 217–18

Yale University, 210–12, 291–92
Yamato Monogatari anthology (Japan), 5–6
Yamato spirit (Japan), 298–301
Yankee culture
  behavioral and environmental risk factors in, 480–87, 482*t*, 484*t*, 486*t*
  educational attainment in, 467–72, 467*t*
  environmental influences on depression risk in, 493–98, 494*t*
  epidemiology of MDD, bipolar disorder, and suicide in, 499–505, 500*t*, 501*t*, 502*t*, 504*t*
  firearm culture in, 490–93, 491*t*
  income inequality and poverty in, 472–80, 473*t*, 474*t*, 479*t*
  and lessons from cultural comparison of pairs of states, 447–48
  lifestyle risk factors for depression in, 487–90, 488*t*
  in Midwest, 440–41
  overview, 436
  primary ancestries in, 453–54, 454*t*
  race and ethnicity of population of, 450–53, 451*t*
  regional personality in, 459–63, 460*t*, 464*t*
  religious identity in, 464*t*, 465–67
  rural–urban population distribution in, 449*t*, 452–53, 453*t*
  social capital in, 456–59, 457*t*
  suicide rates in, 452–53, 453*t*, 505–12, 507*t*, 508*t*, 509*t*

Yan Zhitui, 219
Yellow Emperor's Inner Canon, The (*Huangdi Neijing*), China, 167–68, 169–70
Yeung, Albert, 265–66
yin and yang, 167–68
Yoshida, Jane, 334–36
Young, Neil, 562
young adults
 creative professionals, 565–66
 hikikomori in, 328
 male, depression in South Korean, 372
 with modern type depression in Japan, 314–19
 unemployed, in Sweden, 409–10
young-old, 92

youth. *See* adolescence
yueju herbal remedy, 148
yūgen principle, Japan, 303
Yuichiro, Yasuda, 314

Zen Buddhism, 299
Zeng, Shen (Zengzi), 223
zetsubō-kan (hopeless and despairing feeling), Japan, 311
Zhang, J., 258
Zhang, Shuqin, 214*t*
 Zhāng Zhòngjīng, 170
zhèng, in TCM, 168, 170–72, 171*t*
zhuàngyuán title, in China, 217–18